CURRAN'S ATLAS *of* HISTOPATHOLOGY

REVISED BY

R.C.CURRAN

MD · FRCP(Lond.) · FRCPath · FRS (Edin.) · FFPathRCPI

AND

J. CROCKER

MA · MD (Cantab) · FRCPath · Hon MRCP (Lond.)

4TH REVISED EDITION

WITH 810 PHOTOMICROGRAPHS

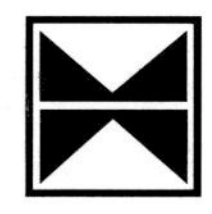

HARVEY MILLER PUBLISHERS
OXFORD UNIVERSITY PRESS

Originating Publisher HARVEY MILLER LTD 17/19 Elsworthy Road · London NW3 3DS · England

Published in conjunction with OXFORD UNIVERSITY PRESS
Great Clarendon Street · Oxford OX2 6DP

Oxford University Press is a department of the University of Oxford.
It furthers the University's objective of excellence in research, scholarship,
and education by publishing worldwide in
Oxford · New York
Athens · Auckland · Bangkok · Bogotá · Buenos Aires · Calcutta · Cape Town
Chennai · Dar es Salaam · Delhi · Florence · Hong Kong · Istanbul · Karachi · Kuala Lumpur
Nairobi · Paris · São Paulo · Singapore · Taipeh · Tokyo · Toronto · Warsaw
with associated companies in Berlin · Ibadan

Oxford is a registered trade mark of Oxford University Press in the UK and in certain other countries.

Distributed in the United States by OXFORD UNIVERSITY PRESS, INC. · New York

First edition published 1966
Reprinted with minor revisions 1967, 1968,1969,1970
Second edition published 1972
Reprinted 1973, 1975(twice), 1976, 1977, 1978, 1979, 1981, 1982, 1983
Third edition published 1985
Reprinted 1988, 1990, 1993, 1995
Fourth edition published 2000

ISBN 0192632205

British Library Cataloguing in Publication Data
Data available

Illustrations originated by Schwitter AG · Basel · Switzerland
Printed and bound in Italy by Grafiche Milani S.p.A. · Milano · Italy

Contents

Preface to 4th edition

THIS NEW EDITION of the Colour Atlas of Histopathology contains many significant changes and additions. It includes a considerable number of new illustrations and accompanying texts that reflect the ever-widening range and amount of extremely sensitive and highly specific techniques. These techniques are now so highly developed that alterations in tissue structure are almost always detectable, frequently down to the molecular level, including alterations in DNA. These methods have an even greater portential for diagnosing illness both rapidly and, generally, accurately. The techniques, developed partly by Professor Crocker, are based largely on Immunohistochemistry and In-situ hybridisation (see METHODS, below).

With the exception of Chapter 10, which has been revised by Professor D.B. Brewer, all other chapters in the Atlas have been written by us. Our illustrations are largely based on the hematoxylin and eosin (HE) technique, and a great deal of study has been devoted to a re-interpretation of many variations in tissue morphology and function. One or more of three types of arrows have been placed on most of the illustrations, which makes recognition of 'targets' in most lesions and illnesses much swifter. The effect is an impressive aid to diagnosis.

Since the Preface to the Third Edition of this Atlas contained much invaluable information about the nature of disease, we have decided to reprint it here, in this new adition, without any alteration.

R.C.Curran & J.Crocker

Preface to 3rd edition (1985)

THROUGHOUT its long history, pathology has been concerned with the study of the derangements of tissue structure and function that occur in disease, and the correlation of these changes with clinical signs and symptoms. This clinico-pathological approach, which made pathology the foundation of clinical practice, remains as valid as ever. In recent years the rate of advance of the subject has accelerated greatly with the introduction of a steadily widening range of techniques of great sensitivity, many applicable to paraffin sections, which allow the histopathologist to identify, with a high degree of specificity, cells and their products. At the same time new clinical methods (endoscopy, needle biopsy, etc.) have provided the pathologist with samples of fresh tissues and cells, sometimes repeatedly, from virtually every part of the body. The contribution that the pathologist can make to clinical practice and the understanding of disease has been enormously enhanced by these twin developments, There can be no doubt that for the foreseeable future pathology will retain its place as a basic part of the undergraduate curriculum.

Histopathology has the unique advantage of making visible the body's many complex systems and their interactions and malfunctions in disease; and the first edition of this Atlas was produced with the intention of providing the student, in a vivid and readily assimilable form, a means of acquiring a clear understanding of the basis of the many diseases that he or she will encounter in clinical practice, whether in hospital or in general practice. The Atlas was first published in 1966 and it was well received throughout the world. It was translated into six languages and it has been reprinted each year. On each occasion the question of revision was considered and in 1972 about one-twentieth of the contents were changed. However, histopathology is (or was until recently) a slowly-evolving science and it was decided to wait until a thorough revision could be justified. The time for this has arrived and this third edition is virtually a new book in both format and content.

An important feature of previous editions was the large size of the page, which enabled the student to compare 18 illustrations at one time. The format of the new edition, howver, allows for larger illustrations which provide increased information; and at the same time the student has the greater convenience in using, carrying and storing a smaller-sized volume. The number of pictures has been increased from 765 to 804 and two-thirds (545) are new. The area of each picture has now been almost doubled and the advantages of this will, it is hoped, be immediately obvious.

The great majority of the illustrations are based on paraffin sections stained with hematoxylin and eosin, the method in routine use. Other techniques, in more or less common use (some using cryostat sections), have been included, where they make a specific contribution; and the potential of the newer immunohistochemical methods will be apparent from the examples included.

The general arrangement of the contents has been retained, with a chapter on each of the main systems of the organs of the body. There is also an introductory chapter of a general nature which aims to demonstrate the more important reactions of the tissues in disease and at the same time teach the student the basic language of histopathology, thereby enabling him or her to read and assess the significance of changes in tissue as revealed by microscopy. This proved to be a popular feature of previous editions and it has been extended. The text has been re-written, and along with a description of the contents of each picture a limited amount of clinical information about the lesion and its pathogenesis is given. Most of the conditions are common or fairly common diseases, but occasional examples of rare lesions have been included when they illustrate a pathological process with particular clarity. It must be emphasised, however, that the book remains an Atlas, the primary purpose of which is to convey information in a visual form. It is meant to complement existing textbooks, and prior study of the Atlas will, it is hoped, make the better textbooks both more intelligible and more pleasurable to read.

A comprehensive index has been provided, and a limited number of cross-references have been inserted in the text, mainly in Chapter 1, to augment it and to integrate its contents with the rest of the book.

The book is intended primarily for undergraduate students but experience with its predecessors suggests that it is likely to prove useful to postgraduate students training in pathology or another clinical discipline.

Acknowledgements

Most of the illustrations in the Atlas are based on cases dealt with in the course of the routine hospital service provided for the Hospitals of the Birmingham Central Health District, and I wish to pay tribute to Mr. K. J. Reid, Senior Chief Medical Laboratory Scientific Officer and his colleagues for the consistently high quality of the preparations which they have produced. Mr. Sidney Whitfield, Chief MLSO, was directly responsible for much of the work and he also supplied the section of schistosomiasis of liver (11.18) from his personal collection. Two other individuals merit special mention: first, Mrs Mary Guibarra, who prepared many of the sections of tumours; and Mr. John Gregory who performed the immunohistochemical techniques.

Some of the illustrations in Chapter 5 are from sections kindly loaned by Professor R. S. Patrick (Glasgow), and some in Chapter 12 are from slides provided by the late Dr. C. W. Taylor, pathologist to Birmingham Women's Hospital for many years. The section of the Stein-Leventhal ovary was provided by Professor J. R. Tighe (St. Thomas's Hospital, London).

A number of illustrations are based on cases referred to the Department of Pathology and I am grateful to the following for access to the cases: Dr. T. G. Ashworth, Walsgrave Hospital, Coventry; Dr. B. W. Codling; Gloucestershire Royal Hospital, Gloucester; Dr. N. D. Gower, Hallam Hospital, Sandwell, Birmingham; Dr. P. S. Hasleton, Wythenshawe Hospital, Manchester; Dr. F. Kurrein, Royal Infirmary, Worcester; Dr. A. M. Light, Good Hope District General Hospital, Sutton Coldfield; Dr. J. Martin, Taiwan Hospital, Abu Dhabi, U.A.E.; Dr. J. Rokos, Staffordshire General Infirmary, Stafford; Dr. T. P. Rollason, Maelor General Hospital, Wrexham; Dr. D. I. Rushton, Maternity Hospital, Birmingham; Dr. W. Shortland-Webb, Dudley Road Hospital, Birmingham; and Dr. Carol M. Starkie, Selly Oak Hospital, Birmingham.

The pathologist to whom the cases were referred was usually my colleague, Professor E. L. Jones. Professor Jones also gave generously of his time and advice in many other ways during the preparation of the Atlas, and without his help it is doubtful whether this new edition would have appeared.

The manuscript was typed by Mrs. Valerie Adkins and Miss G. L. Parkinson, and I thank them for their hard work and patience.

Finally, I must pay a special tribute to Harvey and Elly Miller. As on previous occasions their advice and professional skills were invaluable at all stages of preparation of the volume and I am pleased to have this opportunity to acknowledge my indebtedness to them.

We wish to acknowledge the help given by Mrs Jane Starzinsky, Miss Keely Jenner, Dr Simon Trotter and Professor Simon Herrington; and Professor Roy Weller supplied photomicrographs. Dr Catherine Crocker assisted with organisation of figure legends. John Crocker's photographs were taken by means of a Leitz Orthomat E photomicroscope. Photographic assistance was provided by The Medical Illustration Department, Birmingham Heartlands Hospital.

Methods

Brooke's stain: stains growth hormone-containing (acidophil) cells in the pituitary orange and prolactin-containing cells red.
Dialyzed iron method: stains acid mucins, and particularly those of the connective tissue, blue
Gough-Wentworth technique: thin (300 μm) unstained slices of whole lung (inflated and fixed).
Grimelius's silver method: stains argyrophil materials (such as 5-hydroxytryptamine) black.
Grocott's methenamine silver method: stains fungi black.
Hematoxylin and eosin (HE): combination of basophil (purple) nuclear stain and acidophil (pink) cytoplasmic stains in routine use.
Indirect antibody immunoperoxidase method: for detecting antigens in cryostat or paraffin sections by means of polyclonal or monoclonal antibodies. Examples shown are based on the peroxidase-antiperoxidase (PAP) sequence; a brown reaction product indicates the site of the antigen in the tissues.
Loyez (iron hematoxylin) method: stains myelin blue-black.
Periodic acid-Schiff (PAS) sequence: stains carbohydrates, and particularly epithelial mucin and glycogen, purplish-red (magenta).
Periodic acid-silver (PAsilver) method: stains basement membrane (particularly in kidney) and fungi, black.
Perls' method (Prussian Blue reaction): stains ferric iron, particularly haemosiderin, blue.
Thin resin-embedded (½–1 μm) sections: facilitates study of the finer details of cell and tissue structure.
Gordon and Sweet's method: silver deposition method staining fine connective tissue fibres (including basement membranes and newly-formed collagen), black.
Solochrome cyanin: stains myelin blue.
Sudan IV: stains lipid orange-red.
Toluidine blue: reveals periodic striations in muscle cells (e.g. To confirm that a tumour is a rhabdomyosarcoma).
Van Gieson: stains collagenous fibrous tissue purplish-red. Sometimes combined with Weigert's method for elastic fibres (Weigert-Van Gieson).
Von Kossa: stains bone salts black (in sections of undecalcified tissue).
Weigert's method (Miller's modification): stains elastic fibres blue-black.
Ziehl-Neelson (ZN) technique: stains myobacteria, (e.g. *M. Tuberculosis*) purplish-red.
Immunohistochemistry: An antibody is applied to the section. The antibody reacts with the antigen in question and is raised in, for example, mice or sheep. A second and/or third antibody to mouse or sheep is applied. These second or tertiary antibodies are labelled with a chemical which is then demonstrated tinctorially. Thus, a specific colour (usually brown) localises the antigen, indirectly. Two different antigens may be demonstrated by the sequential application of antibodies linked to agents which give contrasting colours (such as brown and purple).
In-situ hybridisation: An oligonucleotide probe is applied to the section after appropriate treatment. The probe is complementary to the DNA sequence of interest. Binding is then demonstrated by the sequential application of antibodies linked to agents which give contrasting colours (such as brown and purple).

Atlas of Histopathology

1.1 Acute inflammation

Acute inflammation is the early response of a tissue to injury, generally developing quickly and tending to subside within a few days. It does not invariably do so however. The mucous membrane of this patient's colon was acutely inflamed (ulcerative colitis). Acute inflammation is typically of short duration, but in this case the acute inflammation of the mucosa persisted for some months and eventually spread to the anal canal. The anal canal (left) is lined with stratified squamous epithelium, within which there are many polymorph leukocytes, mainly neutrophils, most of them close to the surface of the mucosal epithelium (arrow). The submucosa, is markedly hyperemic, containing several small thin-walled vessels, dilated and full of blood (thick arrow). Many polymorphs (double arrow) are visible within these vessels, arranged alongside the elongated endothelial cells. The connective tissue between the vessels is pale and edematous, from the presence of inflammatory exudate (e.g. centre). In addition to the many neutrophil polymorph leukocytes, there are also lymphocytes and plasma cells, evidence which shows that this acute inflammatory reaction is superimposed on a subacute or chronic lesion. HE ×230

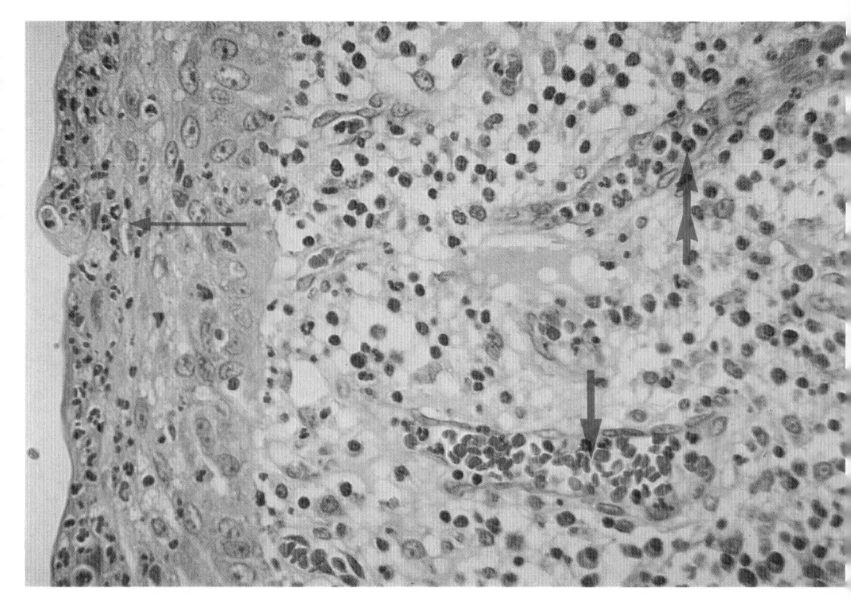

1.2 Acute inflammation

In acute inflammation, the flow of blood to the inflamed area is greatly increased. The flow eventually slows, and the polymorphs move towards the periphery of the stream, where they come into contact with the endothelial cells which line the blood vessels and to which they have a strong tendency to adhere. The small vessel shown here, a capillary or post-capillary venule in the mesentery of an acutely inflamed appendix, is enormously dilated, and an almost continuous layer of polymorphs is adhering to the endothelial surface (arrow). This is 'pavementing' of the endothelium. In the inflamed tissues, the permeability of the blood vessels increases and the polymorphs migrate actively between the endothelial cells, through the vessel wall and then into the surrounding tissues, towards the cause of the inflammation (chemotaxis). Plasma proteins also travel by the same route, but passively, from the blood into the tissues, as may occasional red cells and platelets. This vessel is so dilated that the blood flow has probably stopped. That is, stasis has developed. HE ×335

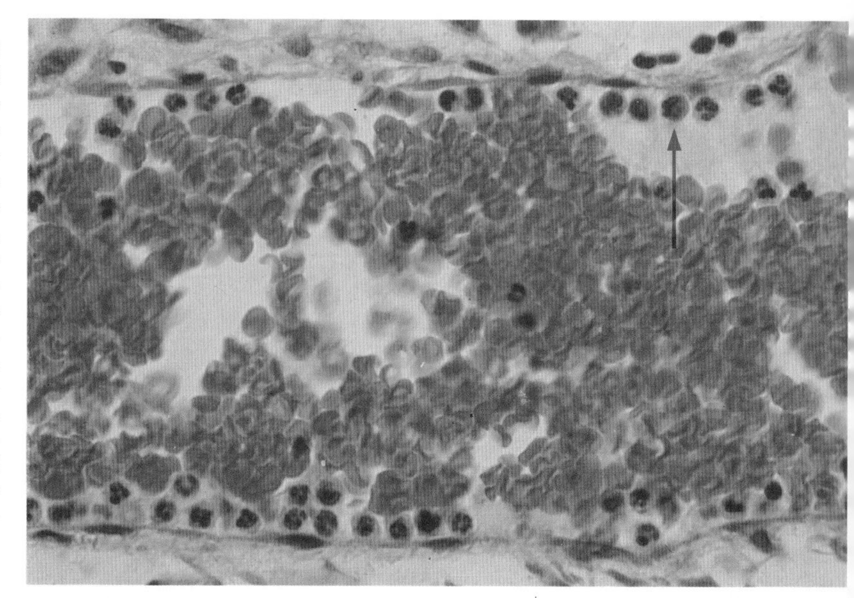

1.3 Acute inflammation: abscess

When the agent causing an acute inflammatory reaction is persistent (e.g. pyogenic staphylococci), emigration of polymorphs to the site of the inflammatory stimulus (often bacterial) may continue until they form a mass in the tissues. Some surrounding tissue is invariably killed (necrosis) by the inflammatory agent and enzymes released by polymorphs. An abscess thus forms, as a thick exudate, containing polymorphs, necrotic tissue elements and serous fluid. The colour of the pus tends to vary with the type of infective agent, staphylococcus aureus for example typically producing creamy yellow pus, whereas streptococcal pus is usually "thin". When a thick exudate collects in the skin, it constitutes a pustule (pus-filled vesicle). This lesion is a pustule at an early stage in its formation. Large numbers of polymorph leukocytes have migrated from the small blood vessels in the dermis (bottom) into the stratified squamous epithelium of the skin, and they are starting to collect together within the epithelium (arrow). HE ×335

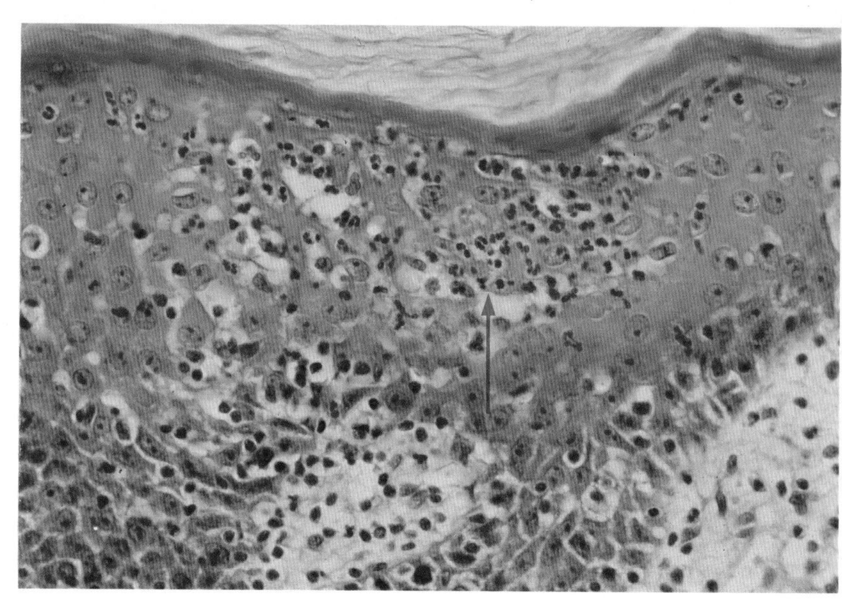

1.4 Acute inflammation: pustule

A pustule is a visible collection pus in or beneath the epidermis. It is generally located in a hair follicle or in the pore of a sweat gland. Pustule of this type are unilocular as rule, whereas multilocular pustules with several compartments usually originate from a spongiotic vesicle within the epidermis. This is a fully-formed pustule, a small ovoid abscess (thin arrow) within the upper epidermis which is causing the epithelial surface to bulge upwards. The surface of the skin over the pustule is covered with a fairly thick layer of strongly eosinophil keratin but it is starting to break down over the centre of the pustule. Neutrophil polymorphs are the main constituent of the contents of the pustule, but many eosinophilic keratinous 'squames' also mingle with the polymorphs. At higher magnification, necrotic (non-keratinized) epithelial cells were also visible within the abscess. The connective tissues of the dermis are also inflamed and fairly heavily infiltrated with inflammatory cells (thick arrow).

HE ×150

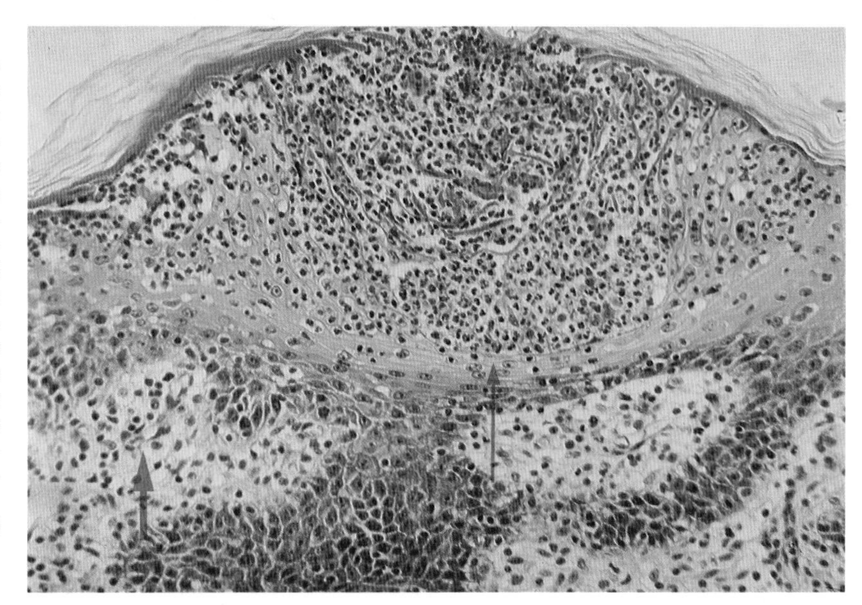

1.5 Pyemic abscess: myocardium

In addition to the primary focus, pyemia is a general septicemia, with pyogenic organisms in significant numbers in the bloodstream, which forms multiple pus-filled abscesses (secondary foci of suppuration) in various parts of the body. An abscess is always accompanied by destruction of tissue, and in acute inflammation it takes the form of a localized area of liquefactive necrosis in an organ or tissue. This abscess is in the wall of the left ventricle. It is an ovoid mass (centre), destroying and displacing the muscle fibres of the myocardium. The fibres nearest the abscess are necrotic (double arrow) and lack viable nuclei, having been killed by the toxins from the deeply basophilic colonies of *Staphylococcus pyogenes* in the centre of the abscess. The abscess contains also degenerate polymorphs and macrophages, fibrin (thin arrows) and red cells. There is also an infiltrate of acute inflammatory cells and red cells in the interstitial tissues of the myocardium (top). The small thin-walled blood vessel (thick arrow) is greatly dilated.

HE ×150

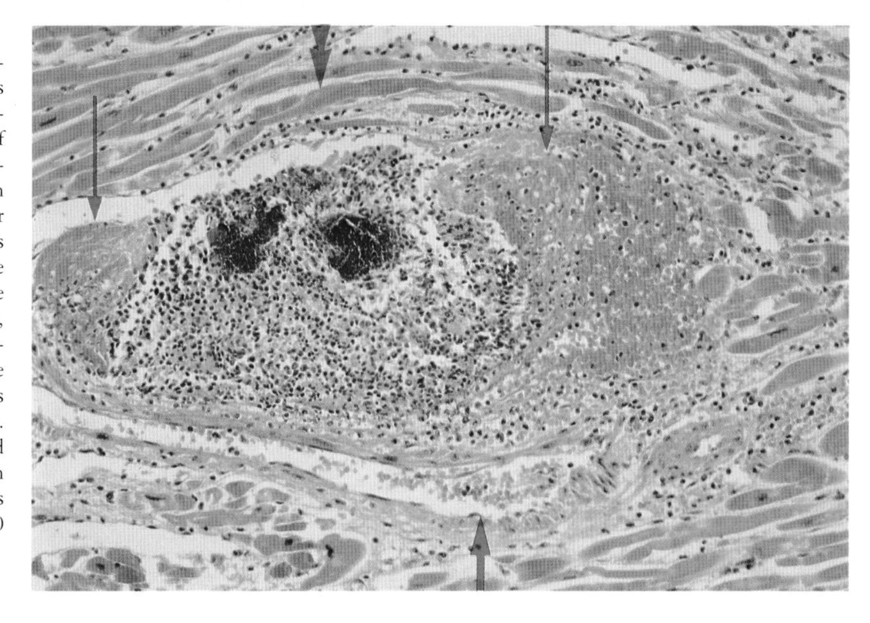

1.6 Pyemic abscess: myocardium

Pyemia is usually a very serious illness. There is no evidence of encapsulation of the abscess by granulation tissue or fibrous tissue, and the patient survives for only a few days. This is another of the many small abscesses which were present in the wall of the ventricle of the heart. The pus consists of large numbers of polymorph leukocytes (most of which are necrotic and disintegrating) and fewer macrophages, as well as two prominent deeply stained colonies of *Staphylococcus pyogenes* (thin arrow). Fragments of necrotic heart muscle fibres (thick arrows), killed by the toxins from the bacteria and the polymorph enzymes, are also present. The serous fluid component of the pus is unstained and not visible. Although deeply stained nuclei are still visible in the myocardial fibres at the periphery of the abscess, the fibres are probably necrotic. The small blood vessels (right side) adjacent to the abscess are dilated.

HE ×235

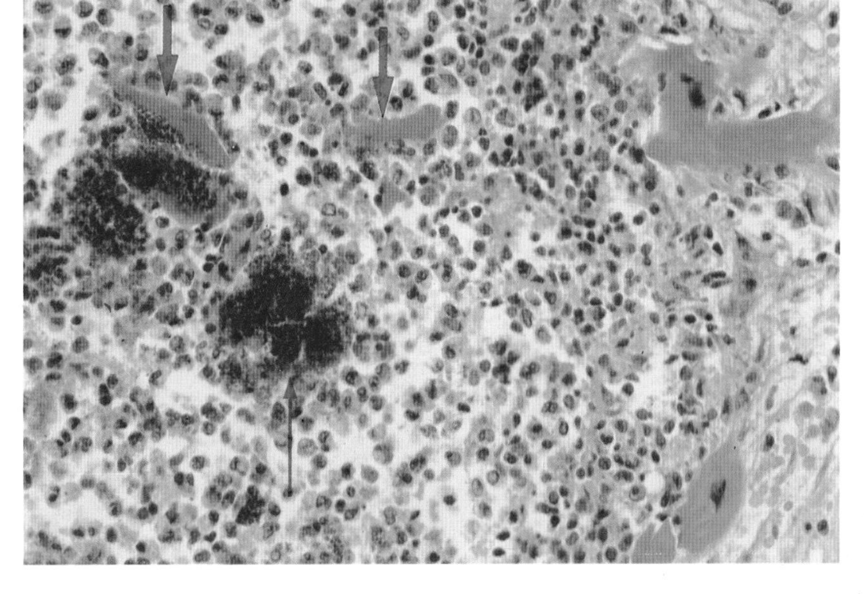

1.7 Acute inflammation: abscess

Sometimes pyogenic (pus-forming) microorganisms get into a wound and cause acute inflammation which may advance to suppuration and abscess formation. This is particularly liable to happen if there is foreign material (including fibrin and blood clot) in the wound. This is a surgical wound, 3 weeks old. The stratified squamous epithelium (left) has healed, but in the dermis there is a collection of pus which consists mainly of polymorph leukocytes, macrophages and necrotic tissue cells. The strongly eosinophilic material (thin arrow) consists of fibrin and keratin squames. The microorganisms responsible for the formation of pus are not visible (unstained), and the clear (empty) clefts contained foreign material which dissolved during processing of the tissue for histology. Infection of a surgical wound, causing inflammation and more notably suppuration, delays or arrests healing and leads to the formation of increased amounts of fibrous tissue. HE ×215

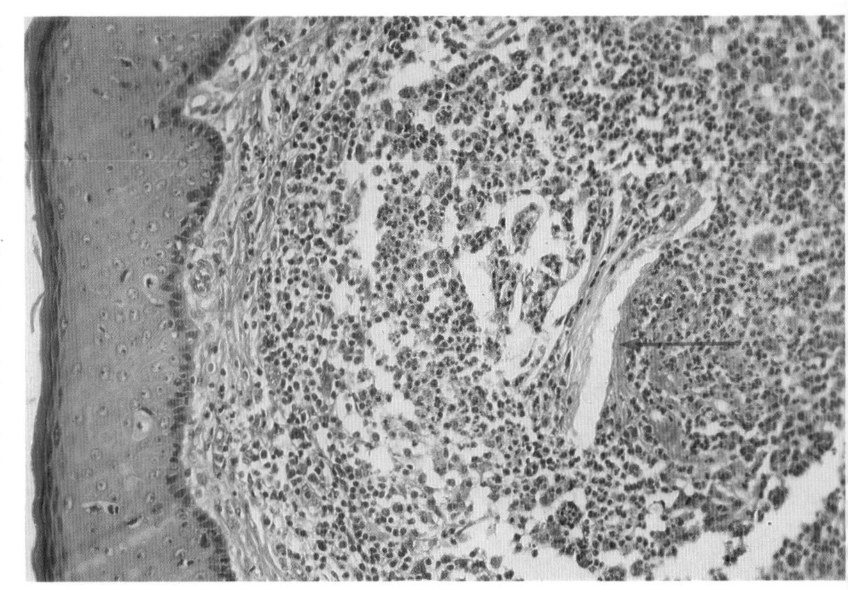

1.8 Fungal abscess: hand

Infection of the tissues with Madurella species gives rise to a chronic disease (Maduramycosis) which is caused by a variety of fungi. The organism is found in the soil or on plants, and lesions are accordingly located more often in the foot than in the hand. They usually take the form of multiple abscesses which discharge pus and cause considerable destruction of tissue (including bone). A man of 40 developed a lump in the subcutaneous tissues of his right hand. After it had persisted for several months, it was resected. The excised specimen (5 × 3 × 2cm) was composed of firm, white fibrofatty tissue in which there were several hard irregular yellow areas. This is one of the yellow areas. It is an abscess, containing several colonies (thin arrow) of the fungus *Madurella grisea*. The colonies lie in pus consisting of deeply stained polymorphs (thick arrow) and an outer zone of larger paler-staining macrophages (double arrow).

HE ×150

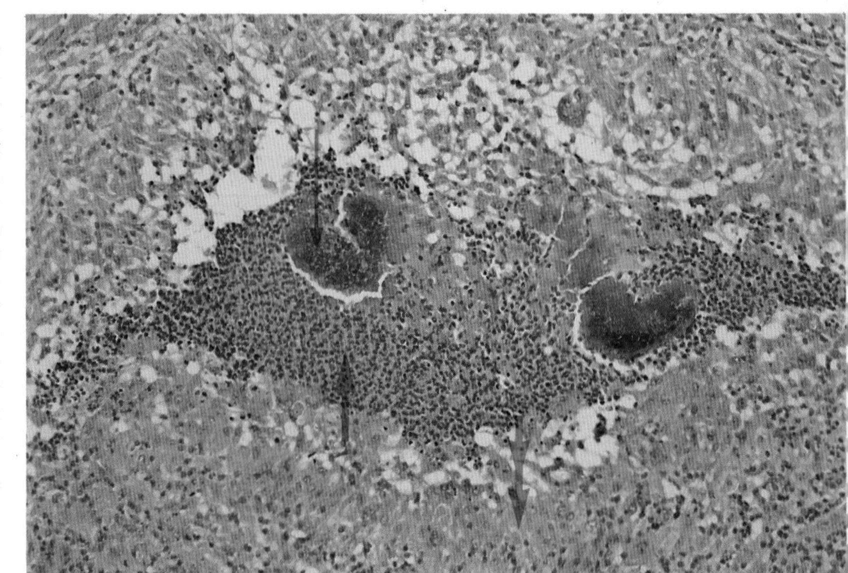

1.9 Infective (mycotic) aneurysm: cerebral artery

An infective (mycotic) aneurysm is produced by growth of microorganisms in the arterial wall. It is usually a complication of bacterial endocarditis, the bacteria setting up a destructive inflammatory lesion which may weaken the vessel wall and allow it to bulge. This patient had infective endocarditis in which vegetations, consisting of platelets and fibrin and containing microorganisms, form on the valve cusps of the heart. Material tends to break away from the vegetations and impact in small blood vessels, including the vasa vasorum of the arteries. The wall of the artery has been destroyed, only a thin layer of degenerate muscle remaining (thin arrow). The thick muscle of the wall has been largely replaced by a pus-like exudate of polymorph leukocytes, fibrin strands and macrophages; and a mass of deep red thrombus (thick arrow) in which there are colonies (dark blue) of bacteria (double arrow), projects into the lumen.

HE ×135

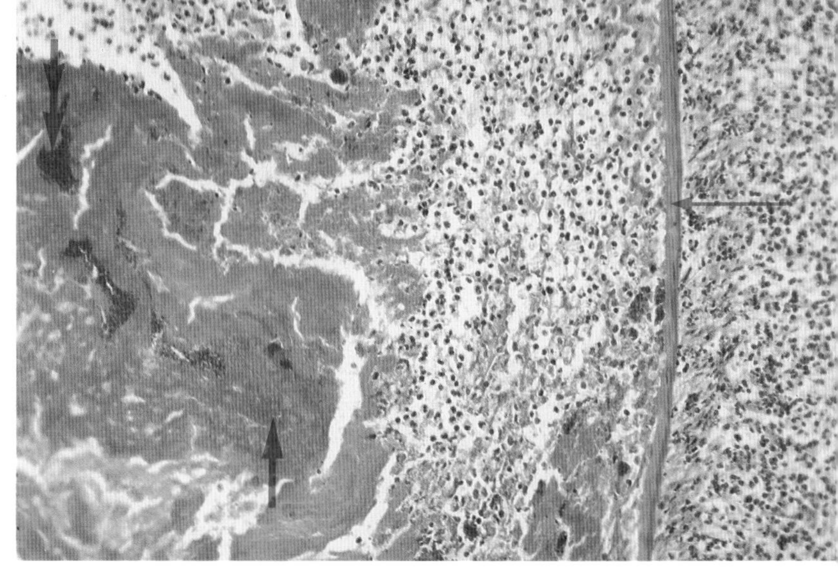

1.10 Eosinophil leukocytes

The role of eosinophil leukocytes is linked to the body's immune response, perhaps through the ingestion of antigen-antibody complexes. Unlike neutrophil polymorphs, eosinophil leukocytes do not release enzymes which destroy the tissues and cause an abscess to form. They are characteristically associated with the response of the tissues to parasites. This lesion is from the chronic disease Onchocerciasis, caused by the filarial worm *Onchocerca volvulus*. This field illustrates tissues that contain a necrotic worm, but the worm is deeper in the tissues and not visible. There is a small blood vessel (thin arrow), along with moderate numbers of lymphocytes and plasma cells. The vessel and cells however are surrounded by a very large number of eosinophil polymorphs (thick arrow). There is also some loose connective tissue. The eosinophil polymorphs are binucleated and have with deep red granular cytoplasm.

HE ×200

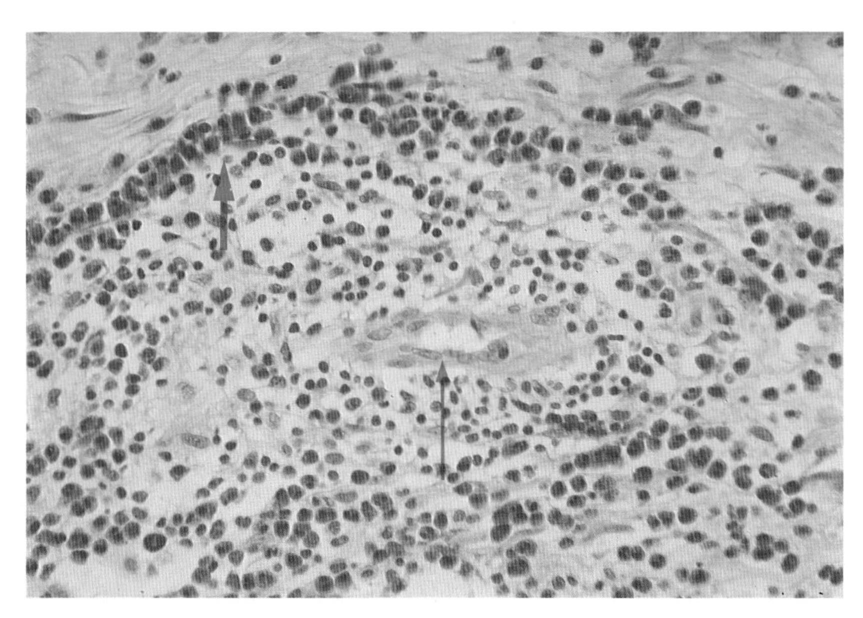

1.11 Macrophages: gall bladder

Macrophages circulate in the blood as monocytes and leave the bloodstream via post-capillary venules. They take part in the resolution of acute inflammatory responses. They are very efficient scavengers, with lysosomal enzymes which can destroy not only neutrophil leukocytes but also a very wide range of substances. After an acute inflammatory reaction subsides, they readily remove necrotic debris. This is the gall bladder of a woman of 71 who had suffered from cholecystitis for many years. The wall of the gall bladder was much thicker than normal and there were many chronic abscesses in the wall. With the exception of a few degenerate polymorphs (thin arrows), the cells are very large macrophages (activated, with an increased content of lysosomes), each cell having a single vesicular (sac-like) nucleus (containing a prominent nucleolus) and abundant granular and vacuolated cytoplasm. Whole cells (polymorphs and red cells) and cell fragments are present in many of the macrophages (thick arrows).

HE ×575

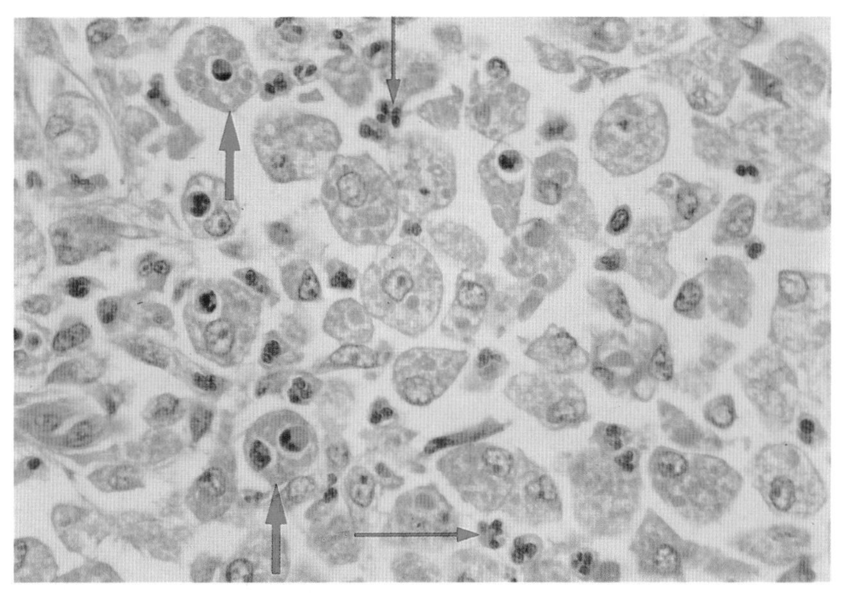

1.12 Xanthogranulomatous reaction: gallbladder

Xanthogranulomatous reaction in a gallbladder immunostained for the antigen CD68, which is a marker of histiocytes. This demonstrates numerous 68-positive foamy (vacuolated lipid-containing) histiocytes with their brown reaction product.

In the cytoplasm of histiocytes in the mucosa lining the gall bladder, there is patchy deposition of (doubly refractile) lipids (cholesterol esters), producing a characteristic distinct macroscopic yellowish flecking pattern (cholesterosis), described as a "strawberry" gall bladder. The lipids may form larger deposits which may develop into eventually polypoidal nodules. The nodules are often associated with cholesterol stones within the gall bladder.

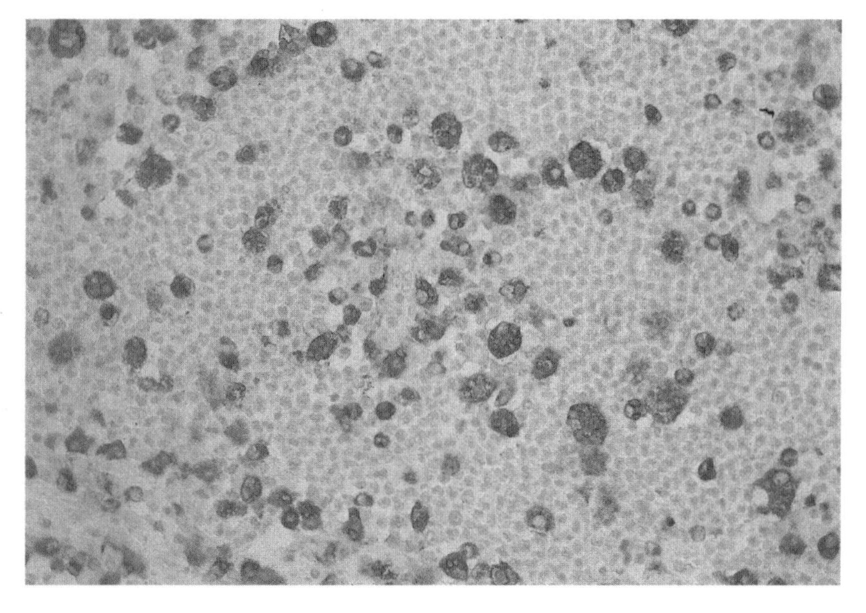

1.13 Programmed cell death ("apoptosis")

Apoptotic body with crescentic degenerate areas. Apoptosis or 'programmed cell death' occurs on an individual cell basis; that is, single cells surrounded by viable neighbours and dying one by one. The apoptotic cell has unique characteristic morphological features, best seen at the electron microscope level but also detectable with the light microscope. The changes include condensation of the nucleus, shrivelling of the cell and accumulation of the chromatin round the inner parts of the nuclear membrane to form crescentic structures (thick arrow), as shown. Apoptotic cells shrink and break into fragments which are rapidly removed by phagocytosis. The process thereby differs from necrosis and is not associated with an inflammatory response.

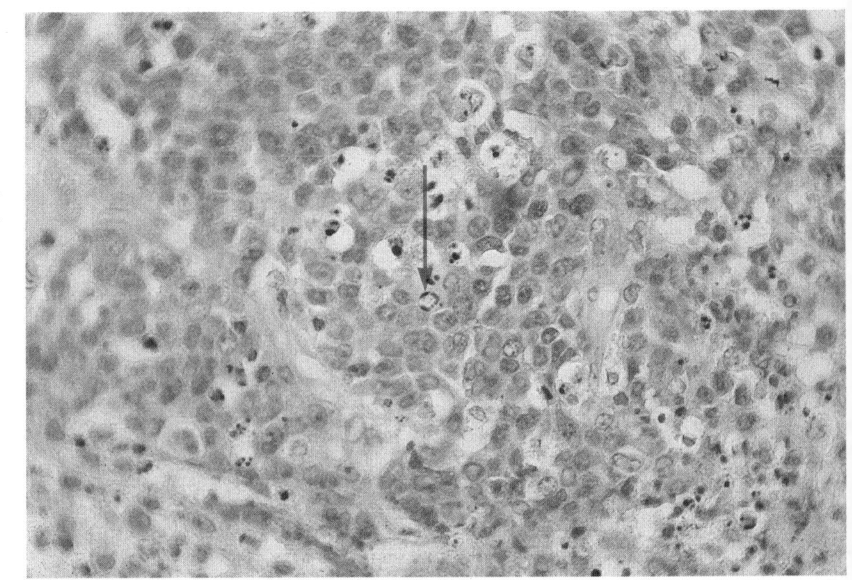

1.14 Chronic abscess: cholesterol granuloma

When an abscess persists for a long time, there is continued destruction of cells, the number of neutrophil polymorphs falling and the macrophage and lymphocyte population steadily increasing. Lipid, derived from the degenerated (necrotic) cells and possibly from the blood, collects. Cholesterol crystals and sometimes also globules of neutral fat may increase in number sufficiently to produce a yellow colour. The lesion is termed a cholesterol granuloma, a granulomatous lesion in which cholesterol ester crystals are surrounded by foreign body giant cells, in a mass of fibrotic granulation tissue. The material in this field is from a chronic abscess in the mastoid process. In addition to many closely packed macrophages, lymphocytes and extravasated red cells, it contains numerous multinucleated giant cells (thick arrows) which line the elongated clear (empty) spaces previously occupied by large cholesterol crystals (dissolved in preparation for histology). HE ×235

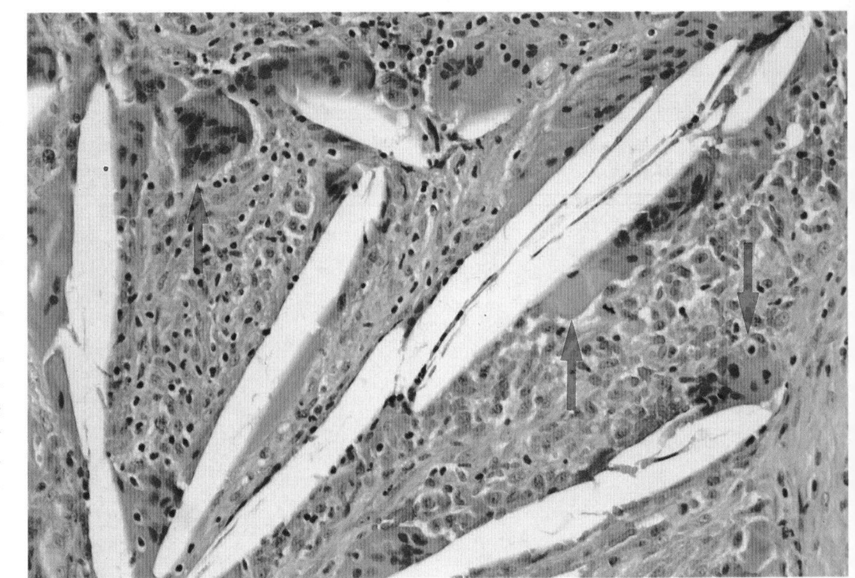

1.15 Hypersensitivity reaction to penicillin: skin

In the skin, the pattern of reaction to drugs varies widely, but is generally a non-specific dermatitis. In more acute lesions, vesicles and bullae may form. In this case a woman of 52 developed a skin rash after treatment with penicillin, which acts as a hapten (incomplete antigen) that combines with serum or tissue proteins. The epidermis (left) is edematous, with separation of the epithelial cells (spongiosis) and formation of a vesicle (thin arrow) beneath the keratinous surface. There are numerous polymorph leukocytes within the epithelium; and eosinophil leukocytes and detached epithelial cells within the vesicle. The upper dermis is edematous, from the presence of pinkish exudate. There is a fairly intense infiltrate of inflammatory cells, mainly around the dilated small blood vessels (thick arrow). The inflammatory cells are a mixture of eosinophil leukocytes, lymphocytes and macrophages. HE ×235

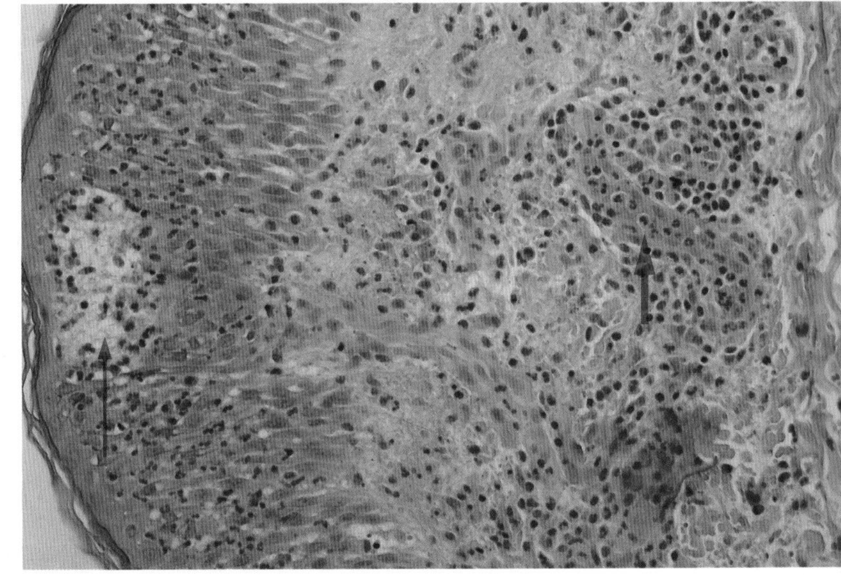

1.16 Hypersensitivity reaction to penicillin: skin

This is a more advanced lesion than that shown in 1.15. A large vesicle (bulla) has formed (left) within the epidermis. It is roughly spherical and contains weakly stained eosinophilic fluid and small numbers of polymorphs (mostly eosinophil leukocytes). The bulla is surrounded by a wall of epithelial cells, both superficial and deep to it (arrows). For a bulla of this size to form within the epidermis, there must be loss of cohesion and separation of the keratinocytes (acanthocytes), that is, acantholysis. There is a considerable number of detached epithelial cells within the bulla, many of them necrotic and lacking a nucleus. The dermis (right) is fairly heavily infiltrated with inflammatory cells (eosinophils, lymphocytes and macrophages) but does not appear to be hyperemic.

HE ×150

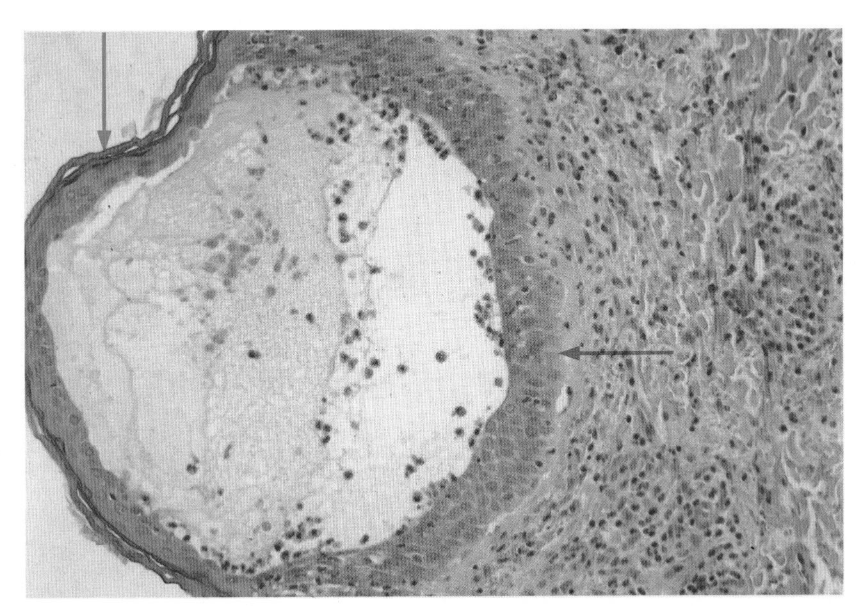

1.17 Herpes zoster: skin

Herpes zoster is an acute inflammatory disease of the cerebral ganglia and ganglia of the posterior nerve roots outside the central nervous system, generally in the lower cervical or dorsal region. The disease is a recrudescence of a latent Varicella (chickenpox virus) infection and occurs as immunity to the virus falls and affects adults, particularly the elderly. The ganglia (groups of gangliocytes) are infiltrated by lymphocytes, and many gangliocytes are destroyed. In the skin supplied by the sensory nerve related to the ganglion, there is pain and hyperalgesia, followed by erythema and formation of vesicles which are full of a serous or even hemorrhagic fluid. This shows a cutaneous vesicle, typically intraepidermal and multilocular, traversed by strands of necrotic cells and cell walls. Swollen and necrotic cells (balloon cells) (thick arrows) lie free within the vesicle. Beneath the vesicle the upper dermis is edematous and hyperemic, and heavily infiltrated by lymphocytes in one area (thin arrow). HE ×150

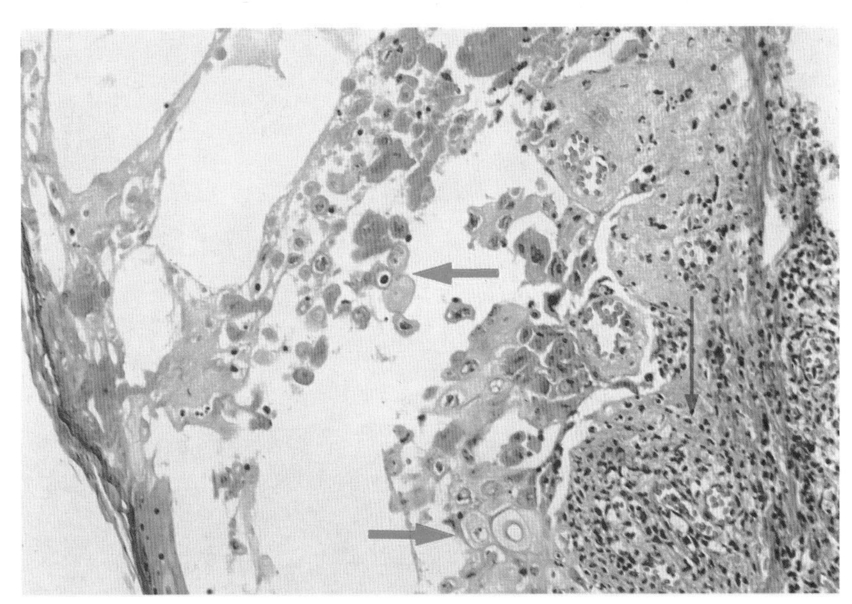

1.18 Acute anterior poliomyelitis: spinal cord

Anterior poliomyelitis is an inflammation of the anterior horns of the grey substance of the spinal cord. The poliomyelitis virus is neurotropic, destroying the large motor neurons in the anterior horns of the spinal cord and brainstem. Paralysis of the muscles results. Although there may be an initial polymorph response, viruses characteristically evoke a lymphocytic response in the tissues. This shows a small blood vessel (cut in two places) in the lumbar cord, close to an acutely inflamed anterior horn. The vessel is dilated (thin arrow), reflecting the hyperemia of the inflamed tissue; and it is surrounded by a 'cuff' of deeply stained small lymphocytes (thick arrow). The adjacent white matter (bottom) is degenerate, showing extreme edema and vacuolation (double arrow). The lymphocytic infiltration of the tissues may persist for some months after the acute phase of the illness.

HE ×135

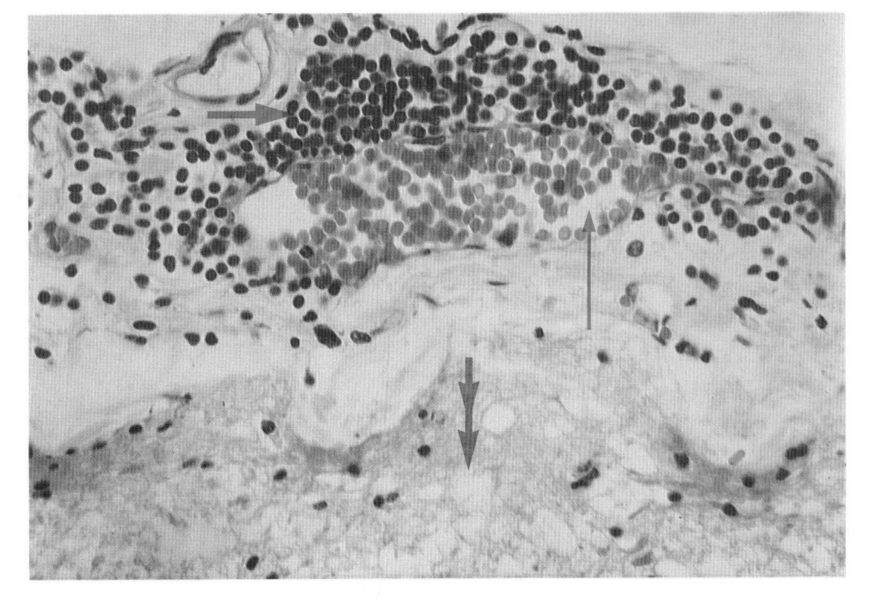

1.19 Rheumatoid nodule: skin

Rheumatoid arthritis is one of the range of overlapping diseases which share some form of disorder of the autoimmune system. In a minority of patients with rheumatoid arthritis, one or more subcutaneous nodules develop in the subcutaneous tissues and produce dome-shaped elevations of the skin, usually adjacent to a joint or bursa. Most nodules cause no symptoms or disability and generally persist for years. Necrosis of collagenous tissue in the nodules is a common manifestation. This is part of a small cutaneous nodule. There are numerous thick-walled small blood vessels (thin arrow) in the nodule, a feature of the early stages of its formation. On the left, the collagenous fibres are necrotic and deeply eosinophilic like fibrin (thick arrow). The change is therefore described as fibrinoid necrosis. Although fibrinoid material is formed from disintegrating collagen, fibrin can be demonstrated in it. The tissues are infiltrated by small numbers of lymphocytes and macrophages. HE ×235

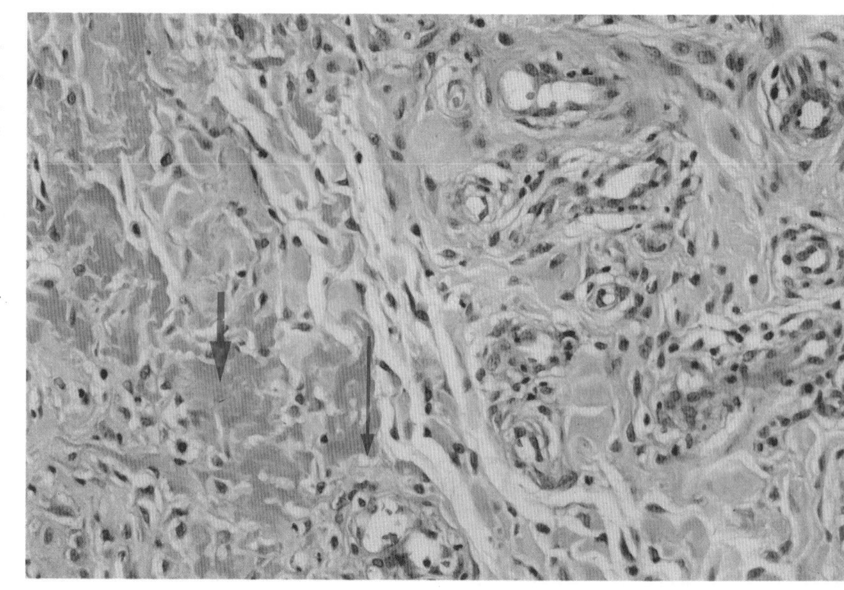

1.20 Gumma: brain

Gummas consist of tissue resembling granulation tissue. They occur in the tertiary stage of syphilis. Although there are only a few spirochetes (*Treponema pallidum*) in the gumma, there is generally extensive necrosis of the tissue, and the cells are mostly lymphocytes and plasma cells, the latter often in considerable numbers. Healing tends to lead to extensive fibrous tissue formation. This shows part of a gumma of brain. There are mature plasma cells (thick arrows), lying in collagenous fibrous tissue. Small lymphocytes and macrophages are also present. The numerous plasma cells have well-defined densely eosinophilic cytoplasm in which there a single moderately-sized nucleus, usually located at one pole of the cell. The chromatin frequently takes the form of dense clumps, distributed around the periphery of the nucleus in a 'clock-face' or 'cart-wheel' pattern. Plasma cells synthesize immunoglobulin, and the bluish-pink colour of the cytoplasm is caused by the abundant rough endoplasmic reticulum in the cytoplasm. HE ×375

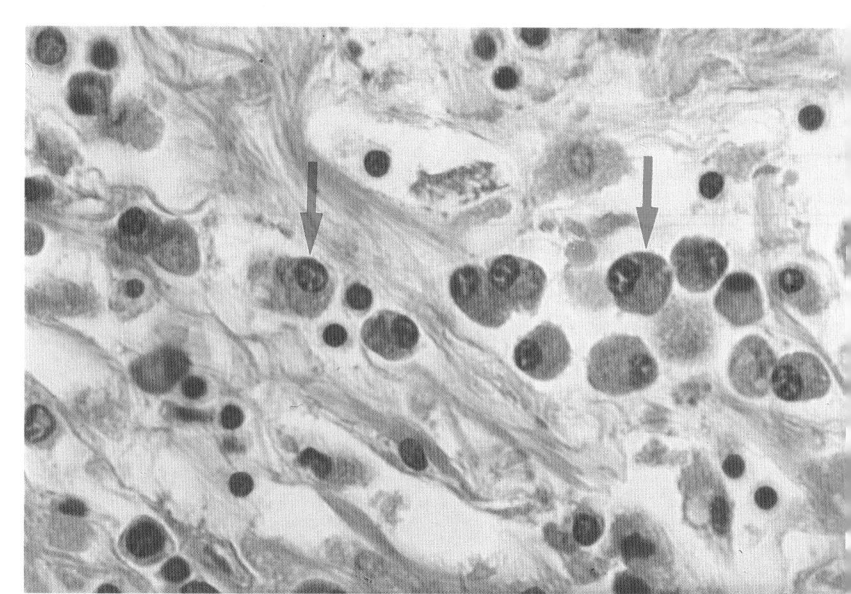

1.21 Plasma cell with immunoglobulin inclusions

Chronic inflammatory tissue, including a plasma cell which is so stimulated that it is accumulating immunoglobulin crystals (thick arrow) in large refractile vesicles (Russell bodies) containing IgM. Consequently the plasma cell resembles a distorted raspberry (morular cell of Mott or "Mott body"). One example is chronic meningitis and focal encephalitis, in which haracteristic morular cells of Mott can be seen in perivascular cuffs of lymphocytes and plasma cells.

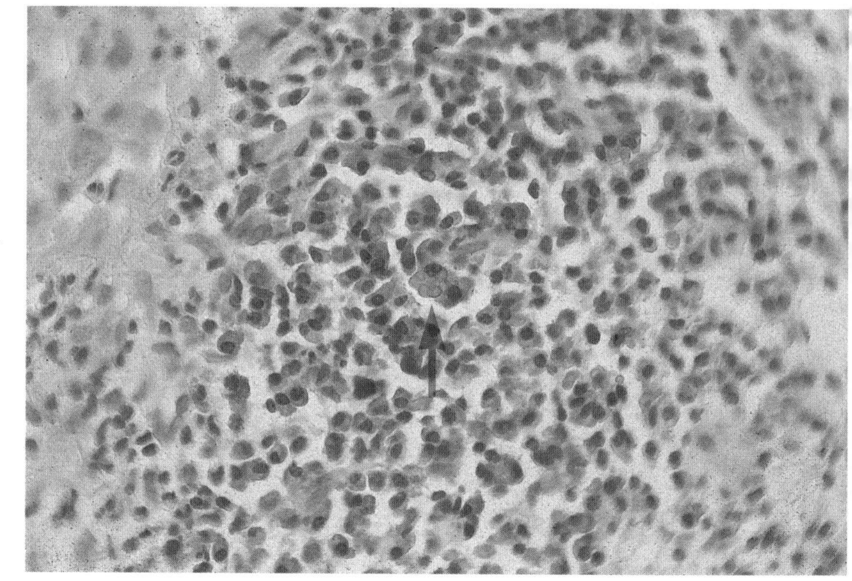

1.22 Fat necrosis: skin

When the fat cells of adipose tissue die (fat necrosis), the neutral fat in their cytoplasm is released extracellularly. The fat is then ingested by macrophages, which split the fat into fatty acids and glycerol. Release of the fat can excite a marked inflammatory reaction, with the eventual production of much fibrous tissue. In this fatty tissue, all the fat cells (adipocytes) have died and released their fat which appears as large clear round spaces. These are droplets of 'free' (i.e. extracellular) neutral fat (dissolved during tissue processing), and each space which contained a droplet is surrounded by a ring of macrophages which are ingesting the fat. Each macrophage has a compact basophilic nucleus and abundant cytoplasm with a pale pinkish colour. The cytoplasm has a granular or 'frosted-glass' texture (thin arrow), caused by the presence in it of many small droplets of fat which are undergoing digestion by lysosomal enzymes. One macrophage appears to be in mitosis (thick arrow). HE ×135

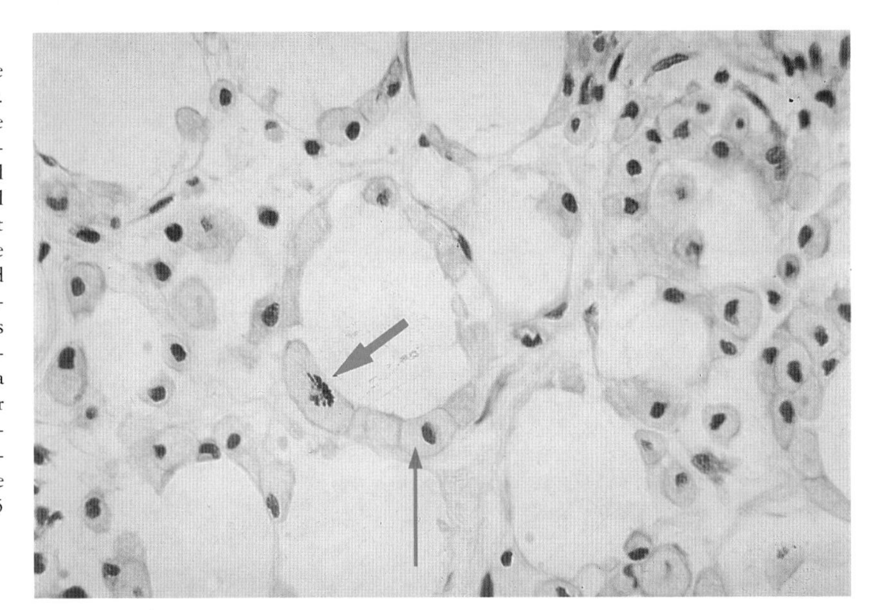

1.23 Fat necrosis: skin

To allow lipids to be demonstrated in histological sections, it is necessary to avoid reagents which dissolve fat. 'Frozen' (cryostat) sections are therefore used. This is a cryostat section of the same lesion as that shown in 1.22, stained with a solution of Sudan IV in alcohol (the dye does not dissolve in water). The round droplets of extracellular ('free') fat, which initially occupied the large central spaces, were readily dissolved by the alcohol of the staining solution and lost from the tissue section. In contrast, macrophages surround the circular spaces, and their abundant cytoplasm is occupied by large numbers of small droplets of fat which have taken up the dye from the Sudan IV solution and been thereby stained a bright orange-red colour (arrow). Sudan IV ×135

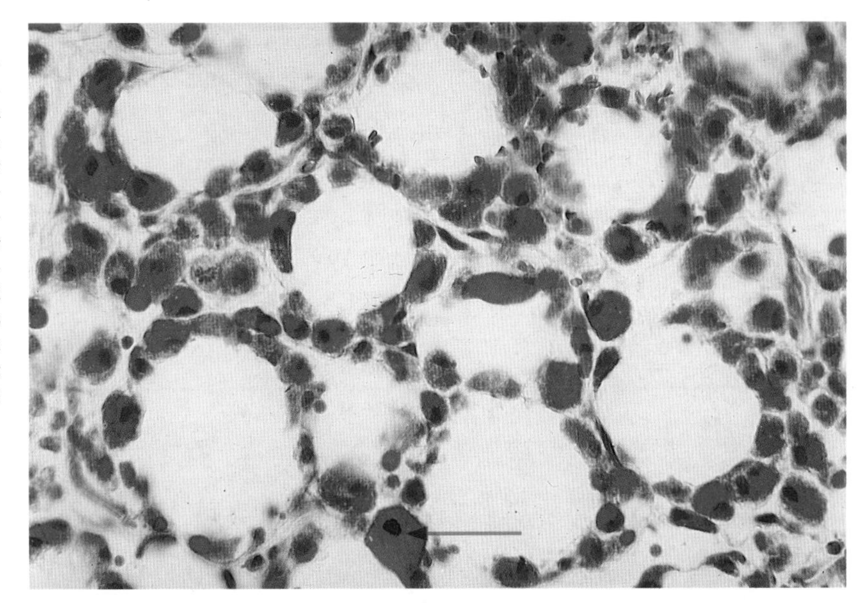

1.24 Melanosis coli

In melanosis coli, the mucous membrane of the colon is black or dark brown. A woman of 63 had the proximal half of the colon resected for carcinoma. The mucosa of the ascending colon was dark brown, almost black, in colour. The lumen of the colon is on the left but not visible. The deeper parts of several colonic glands are shown, with the muscularis mucosae on the right (thick arrow). Each gland is lined by a single layer of mucus-secreting columnar cells (thin arrow), and between the glands in the lamina propria there is a collection of mononuclear macrophages, each with a large amount of light brown cytoplasm (double arrow). The brown colour of the cytoplasm is produced by the presence of a dark pigment (not true melanin) which is thought to be synthesized by enzymic action in the wall of the colon, from amino acids absorbed from the lumen of the colon. Chronic constipation is believed to predispose to melanosis coli. The condition is symptomless and of no pathological significance.

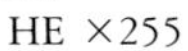

HE ×255

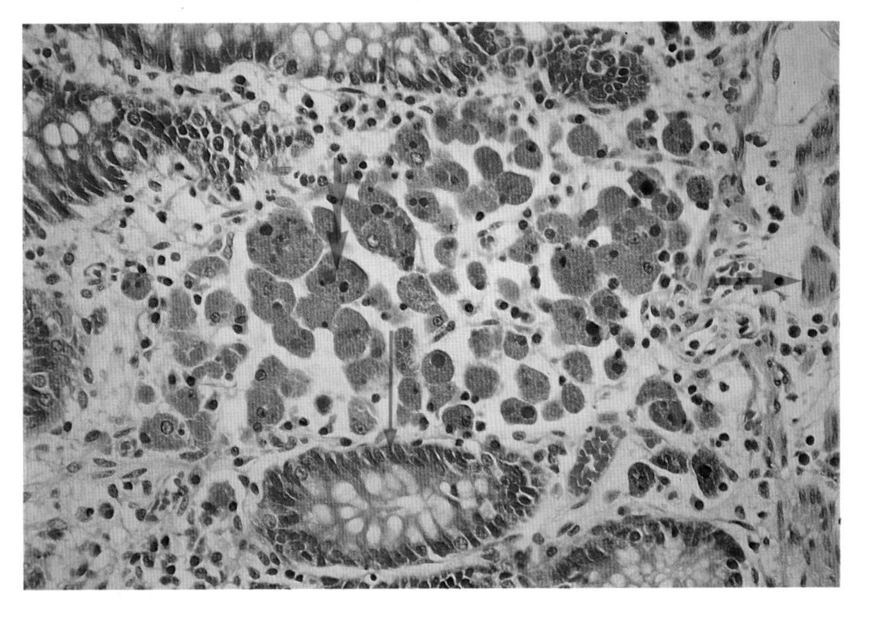

1.25 Macrophages: lung

Macrophages are large highly phagocytic cells with a small oval, sometimes indented, nucleus. Small particles (1μm or less) of carbon-containing dust (smoke) are often present in the atmosphere of cities and are consequently inhaled by the inhabitants. The particles readily reach the alveoli, where they are ingested by the pulmonary macrophages and carried by the lymphatics to the lymph nodes. Many carbon-laden phagocytes remain within the lung and pleura however, and if the load of dust is heavy, anthracosis results. In this case the amount of dust present was moderate. The pleura is thicker and more fibrous than normal (thin arrow), and within it there are elongated collections of macrophages laden with black (carbon) particles (thick arrow), as well as a population of small lymphocyte-like cells. Adjoining the pleura there are several dilated pulmonary alveoli, lined by a single layer of cuboidal cells which have replaced the normal flat lining cells. Within the alveoli there are numerous round phagocytes (double arrow) with brown-coloured cytoplasm and a small dark nucleus. HE ×310

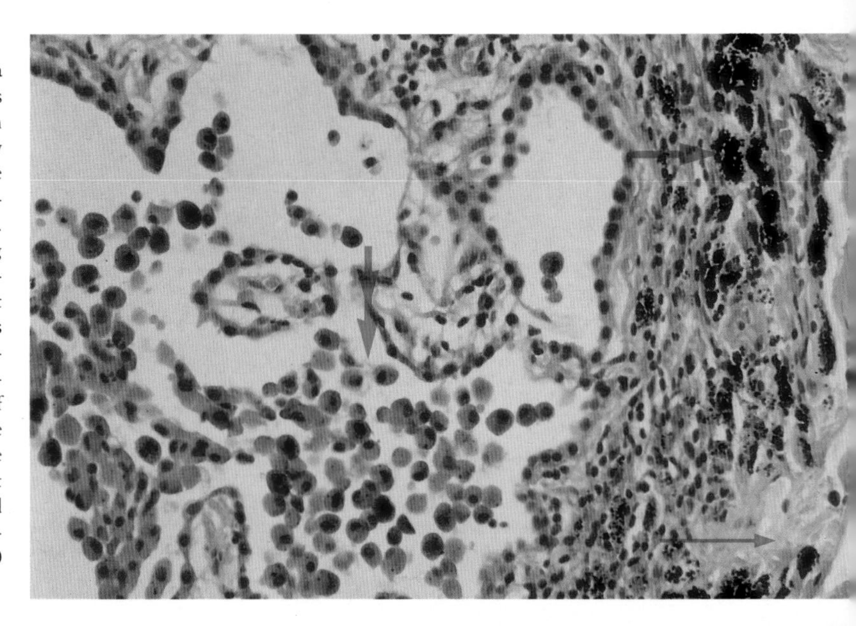

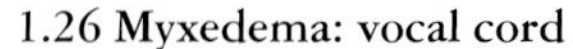

1.26 Myxedema: vocal cord

In myxedema there is increase in the connective tissue mucins throughout the body, and this accounts, for example, for the thickening of the skin. The larynx is also involved, the vocal cords swelling and the voice becoming coarse and low-pitched. This shows part of a swollen vocal cord. The surface of the cord is just out of the picture on the left, and some striated muscle fibres (in cross-section) of the larynx are visible on the right (thin arrow). Between these two tissues there is a broad sheet of stromal connective tissue with a large amount of solid-looking matrix but no visible small blood vessels. The matrix has a greatly increased content of basophilic connective tissue mucin, which has stained a fairly uniform purplish-blue colour (thick arrow), and in which there is moderate population of evenly distributed connective tissue cells. Each of these cells has a deeply basophilic nucleus (most of the nuclei are round), in clear cleft-like space. The space however is probably just the greatly swollen (vacuolated) cytoplasm of each connective tissue cell. HE ×120

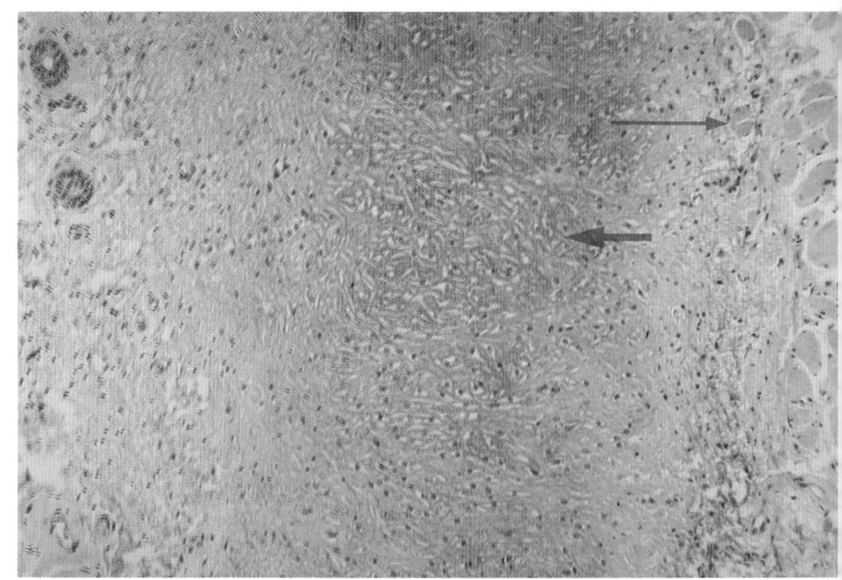

1.27 Sarcoidosis: larynx

Sarcoidosis is a granulomatous disease of unknown etiology, and it is characterized by the presence of follicles composed of epithelioid cells. The lesions may originate in almost any tissue, but the intrathoracic tissues are most often involved. This is the anterior commissure of the larynx of a 48-year-old woman. The stratified squamous epithelium, with a surface layer of eosinophilic keratin, is greatly attenuated but intact. There is an infiltrate of small lymphocytes within the basal layers of the epithelium, but in the underlying connective tissue there is a much heavier infiltrate of small basophilic lymphocytes and of larger epithelioid cells. The epithelioid cells, each which has a considerable amount of strongly eosinophilic cytoplasm, are arranged in several round follicles (thin arrows); and there is a multinucleated giant cell of Langhans type in one of the follicles (thick arrow). Langhans-type giant cells are often present in considerable numbers and may contain asteroid bodies in their cytoplasm. Healing of sarcoid lesions tends to produce much fibrous tissue which can interfere with the functions of a tissue. HE ×190

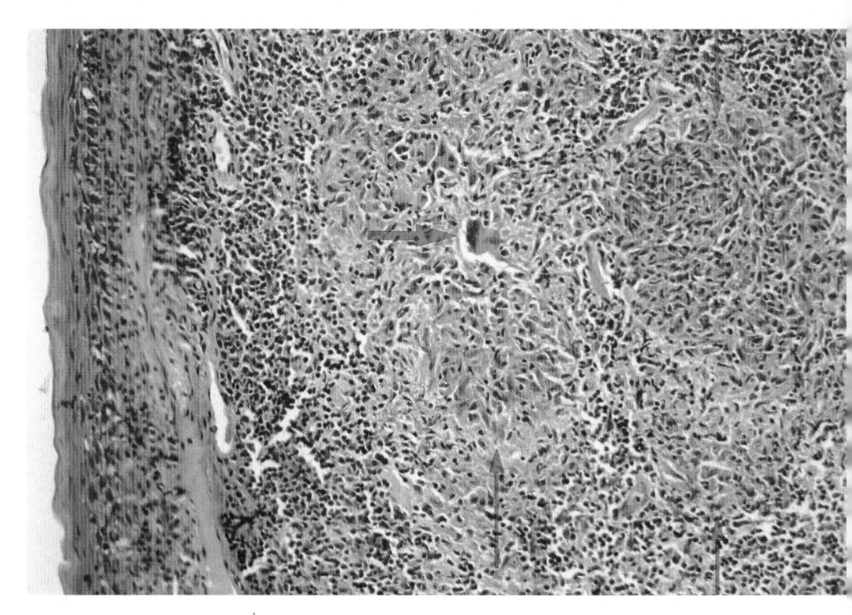

1.28 Sarcoidosis: lymph node

Sarcoidosis is a chronic progressive granulomatous condition of unknown etiology, involving almost any organ or tissue typified by the presence of rounded collections (follicles) of epithelioid cells. Sarcoid follicles do not undergo necrosis (caseation). Healing may however lead to considerable fibrosis. The clinical manifestations of the disease reflect the sites of greatest involvement by the lesions. Lymph nodes, particularly in the mediastinum and cervical region, are often affected. The lymphoid tissue of this node has been largely replaced by two follicles composed of large epithelioid cells (thin arrow) with eosinophilic cytoplasm and vesicular nuclei. Several multinucleated giant cells (thick arrow) of the Langhans type are also present. A large laminated shell-like nodular mass (double arrow), stained blue-black because of its content of calcium, is present in the larger follicle. This is a Schaumann body. Fibrous tissue has formed at the periphery of the follicles.

HE ×235

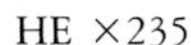

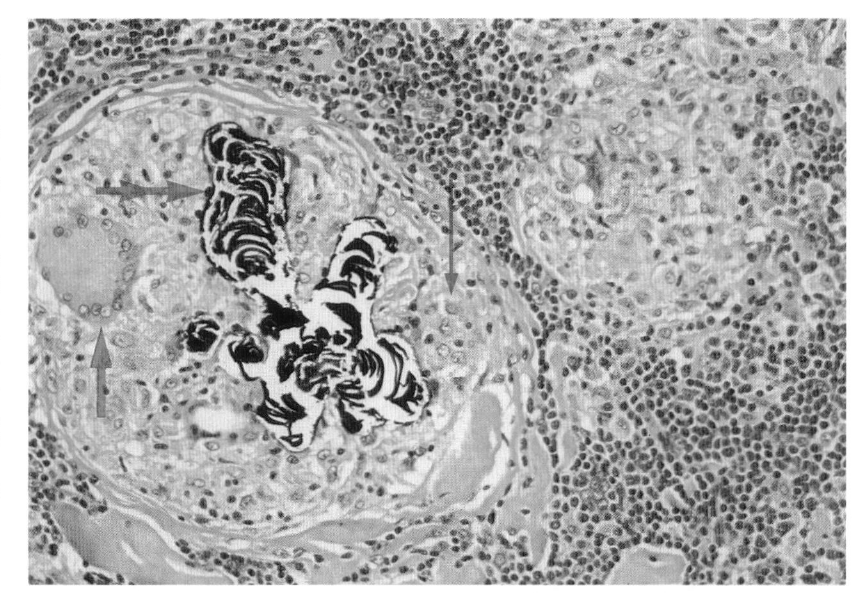

1.29 Infarct: lung

An infarct of lung is usually a dark red hemorrhagic wedge-shaped mass, with its 'base' on the pleural surface. Blood enters the dead tissue from neighbouring arteries and veins and distends the infarct. Occlusion of a branch of the pulmonary artery is not sufficient by itself to cause infarction, and increased pulmonary venous pressure is usually also present. Presumably it acts by impairing pulmonary blood flow, but other factors may also play a part. In this case, the patient had severe mitral stenosis. Histologically the walls of the pulmonary alveoli are necrotic and thickened by the greatly distended tortuous capillaries (full of fused red cells) (thin arrows). The alveolar air spaces contain large numbers of desquamated and (presumably) necrotic cells with pyknotic nuclei, red cells and cell debris (much of it derived from red cells). However the identities of the various cells, mostly endothelial and alveolar epithelial cells shed from the capillaries and the alveolar walls, cannot be determined. There is also abundant fibrin in the air spaces. The connective tissue of the pleura (thick arrow) is infiltrated by extravasated red cells and fibrin.

HE ×150

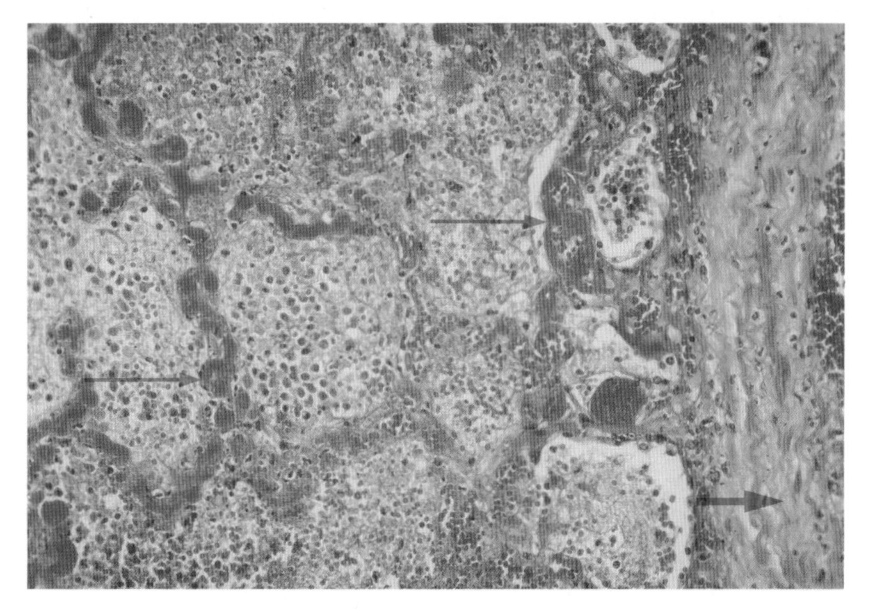

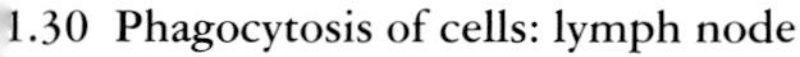

1.30 Phagocytosis of cells: lymph node

Removal of effete or damaged cells of all types is one of the functions of macrophages, and they do so very effectively by means of the wide range of hydrolytic enzymes in their lysosomes. In this case there was a deposit of metastatic tumour, from an unknown primary tumour, in a lymph node in the axilla of the patient. This is a widely dilated lymphatic sinus in the node and within it there are numerous very large phagocytic cells (thin arrow). The nuclei of the large phagocytes are very large pale and vesicular (thick arrow), and in the very abundant well-defined cytoplasm of each cell there are many ingested cells. Some of the ingested cells have round deeply basophilic nuclei of moderate size, whereas the nuclei in other ingested cells are frankly pyknotic or fragmented and necrotic (double arrow). The precise nature of the phagocytosed cells uncertain. Some may be lymphoid cells but some are almost certainly neoplastic.

HE ×860

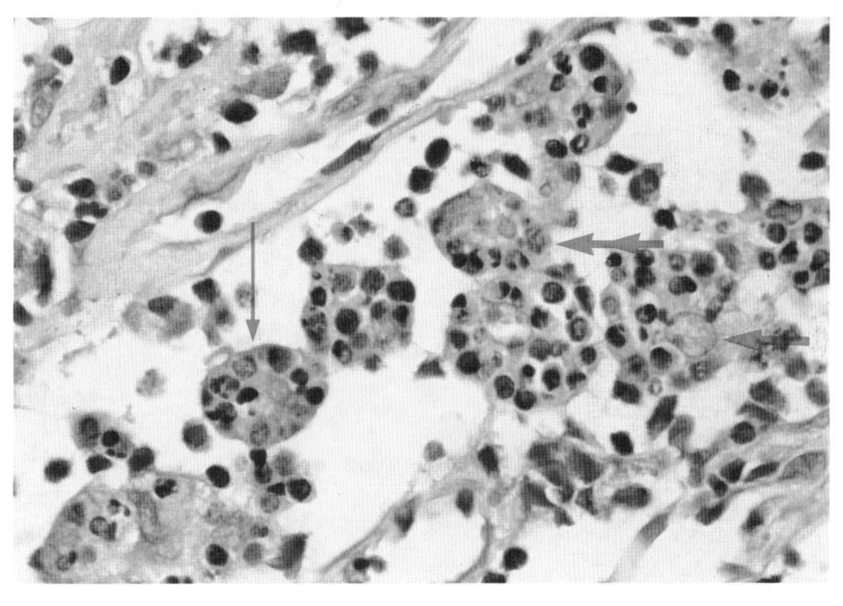

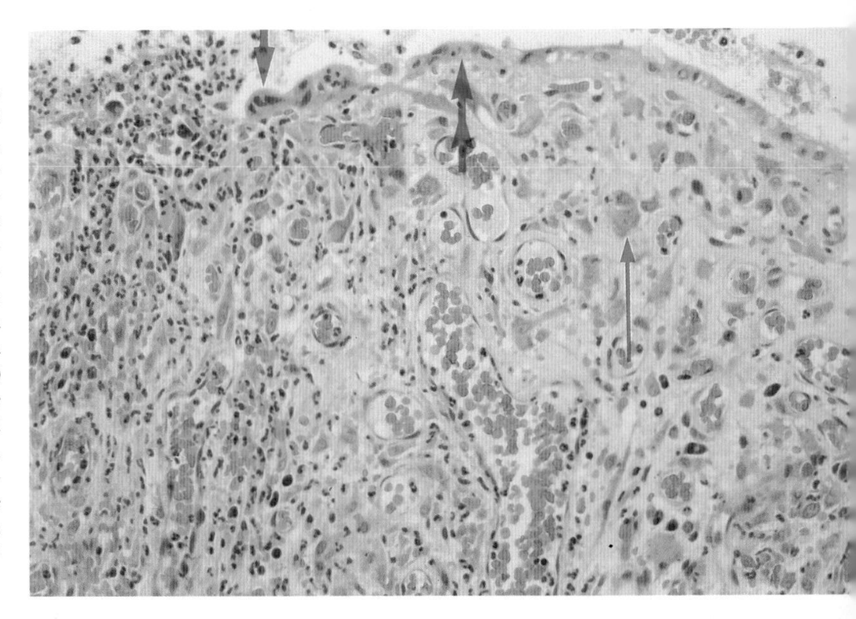

1.31 Healing ulcer (resected juvenile polyp): rectum

Juvenile polyps are benign globoid lesions and sometimes multiple (juvenile polyposis coli). A man of 20 suffered from rectal bleeding, and a small ovoid mass (2 × 1cm), attached by a short stalk to the rectal mucosa, was resected. It proved to be juvenile polyp, It consists of expanded and inflamed lamina propria, associated with crypt dilatation. In this field it resembles vascular granulation tissue and contains large numbers of dilated thin-walled blood vessels, large mononuclear phagocytes (thin arrow), and small numbers of lymphocytes and plasma cells. Most of the surface of the polyp is covered with a single layer of pleomorphic epithelial cells (double arrow) but at one point there is an area of ulceration where these cells are lacking (top left). At the edge of the ulcerated area the epithelial cells are proliferating and heaped up, and their nuclei are basophilic and pleomorphic (thick arrow). In the tissue beneath the ulcerated area, the number of inflammatory cells is markedly increased, with polymorph leukocytes predominating. HE ×235

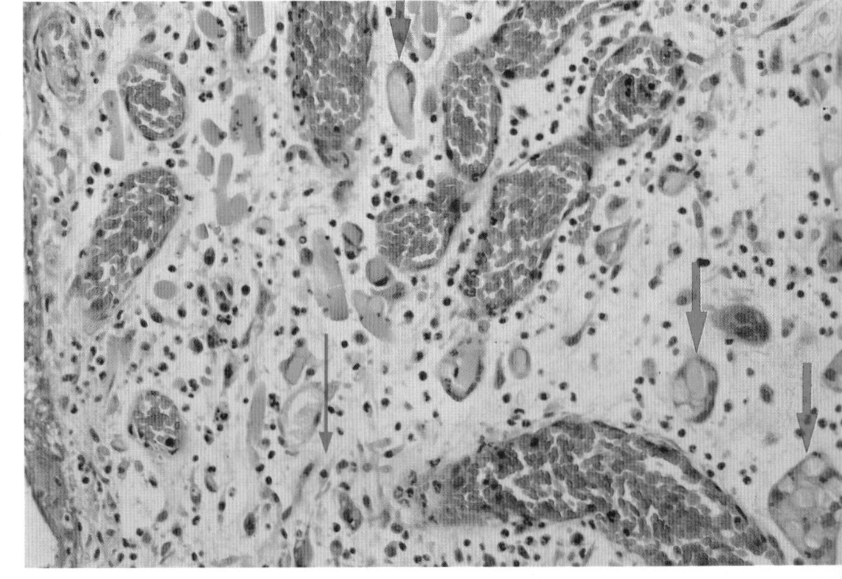

1.32 Foreign-body granuloma: healed wound of skin

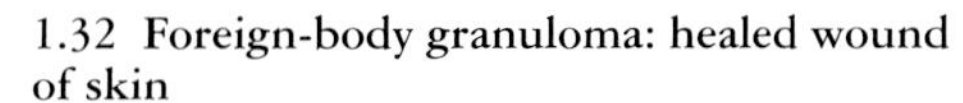

A foreign-body granuloma is a localized histiocytic skin reaction to a foreign body in the tissues. A woman of 40 developed small soft irregular elevated nodules in the scar of a healed surgical incision of the skin, and this is one of the nodules. It is granulation tissue, consisting of many large and greatly dilated thin-walled blood vessels, moderate numbers of lymphocytes and plasma cells, and a small population of elongated plump active-looking fibroblasts (thin arrow). The most notable component however is the presence of many large or very large (giant) phagocytes. In most of the largest cells there are multiple nuclei, and their cytoplasm contains pale-staining fragments of foreign material (thick arrows). When examined by polarized light, the material proved to be birefringent and identified as nylon suture material from the original surgical incision. The nodules therefore were 'stitch granulomas'. HE ×235

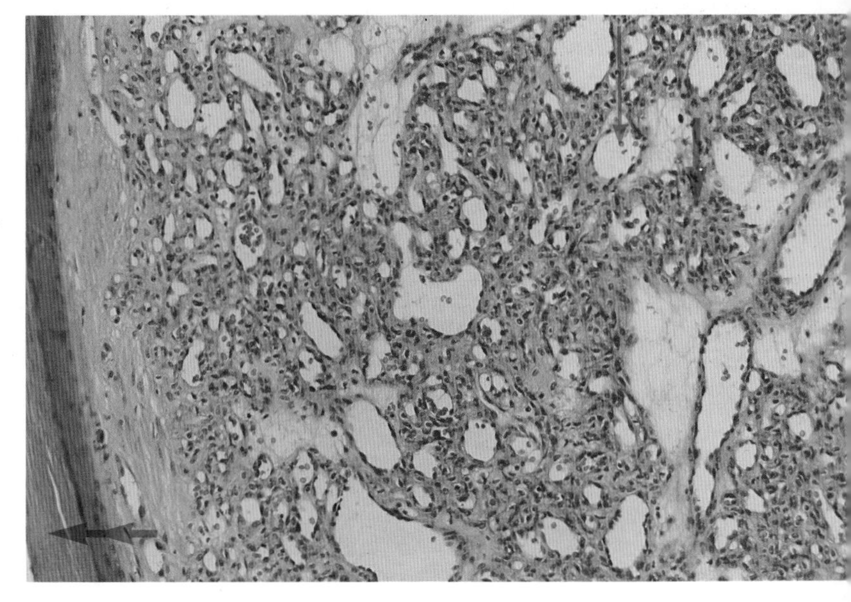

1.33 Pyogenic granuloma: skin

A pyogenic granuloma is a soft red pedunculated nodule, the surface of which is sometimes ulcerated. The nodule grows rapidly and tends to recur on removal, but it is thought by some to be reactive rather truly neoplastic. Occasionally it originates in a capillary hemangioma which has been traumatized, but in other instances it is probably derived from exuberantly-growing granulation tissue. This lesion is in the skin and it consists mainly of large numerous closely packed thin-walled blood vessels (thin arrow), some very dilated but many small and with little or no lumen (thick arrow). The predominant cells are endothelial cells and the resemblance to capillary hemangioma is close. There are relatively few lymphocytes and plasma cells in the edematous connective tissue between the vessels. The epidermis is flattened and stretched over the lesion, but the surface, covered with a thick layer of keratin (double arrow), is intact. The end-result of healing is a fibrous scar. HE ×150

1.34 Organization of thrombus: vein

Organization is the replacement of blood clots (thrombi) by fibrous tissue. Thrombus in the lumen of a blood vessel is 'foreign' material, and the body removes it by the process of organization. Small thin-walled blood vessels penetrate the thrombus, accompanied by fibroblasts and macrophages. The macrophages ingest the fibrin, red cells and platelets, and eventually fibroblasts convert the thrombus into a fibrous cord. The organizing tissue is sterile and few polymorphs are present, in contrast to the large numbers in the granulation tissue of a healing wound. This shows a small vein in which organization of the thrombus is well advanced. The wall of the vein is on the right (thin arrow). Deeply eosinophilic thrombus (thick arrow) adheres to the wall and fills the lumen. The thrombus has been widely penetrated by numerous thin-walled channels (double arrow) which have converted the thrombus into a spongy mass. Within the channels, which are lined by endothelium and widely patent, there is a sparse population red cells and leukocytes. HE ×215

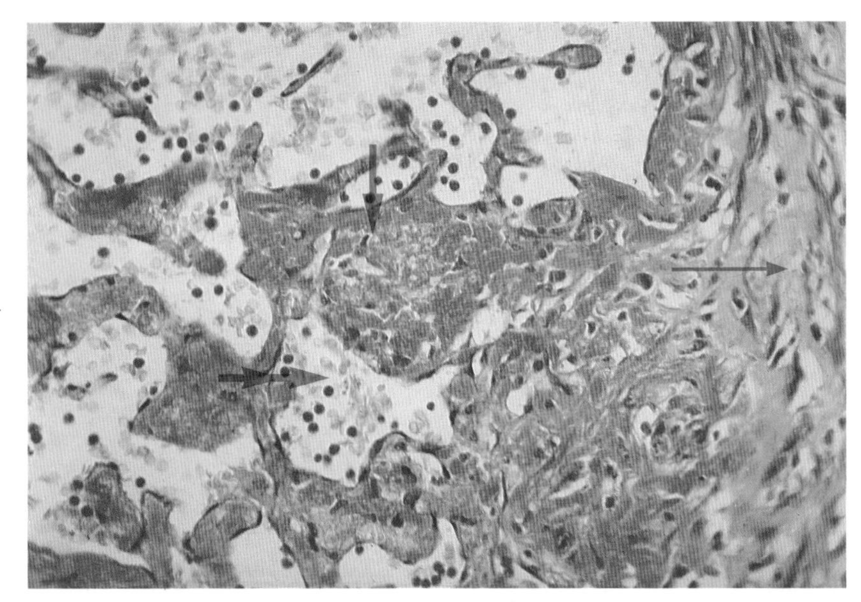

1.35 Healing ulcer: ileum

This field shows part of an extensively ulcerated area of the ileal mucosa which is now healing. The lesion has been caused by Crohn's disease (regional ileitis), and it can involve any part of the intestinal tract, from oral cavity to anus. It is most common site however in the terminal ileum. It may affect individuals of any age, but most are young adults. The lumen of the intestine is at the top, and the hypertrophied muscularis mucosae of the intestinal wall is just visible (thin arrow). The normal villous structure of the mucosa has been destroyed, and replaced by a thin layer of granulation tissue consisting of large numbers of dilated blood vessels and a sparse population of inflammatory cells, including large macrophages (thick arrow), lymphocytes and plasma cells. Covering the surface of the granulation tissue there is a layer of closely packed tall columnar epithelial cells (double arrow). Some restoration of the normal architecture of the ileum may take place in time, but villi are unlikely to form in an area as severely damaged as this. HE ×360

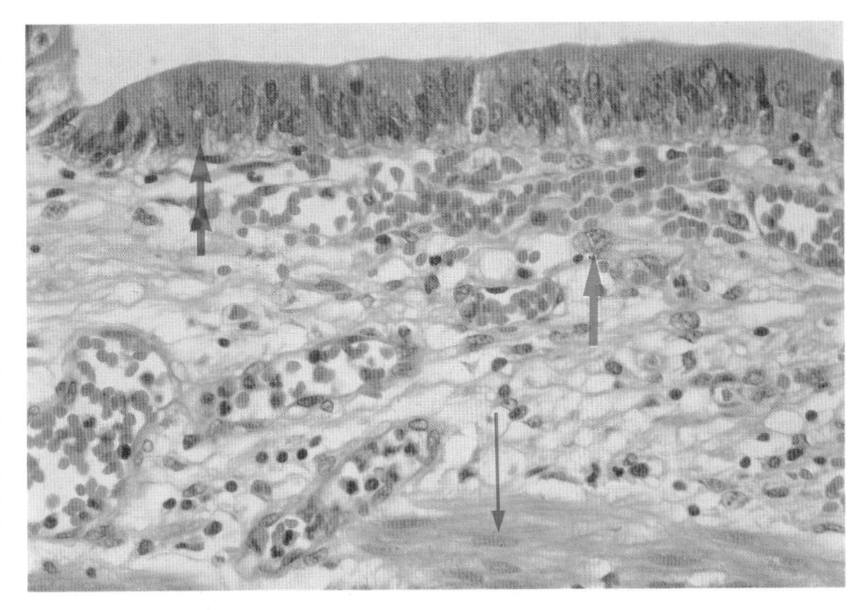

1.36 Healing ulcer: skin

A melanoma developed on the calf of a woman aged 55. It was removed surgically, but a small part of the incision failed to heal and left an area of persistent ulceration which was resected some weeks later. This shows the margin of the ulcer. A sheet of stratified squamous epithelium (thin arrows) is growing over and largely covering a layer of granulation tissue, leaving part of the ulcerated area still visible (top right). The sheet of epithelium is stratified and covered with necrotic cells and keratinous debris. Rete ridges however are lacking. The granulation tissue (centre and bottom) which previously formed the floor of the ulcer is mature, consisting mainly of abundant collagen fibres and thick-walled small blood vessels (thick arrow). Small groups of inflammatory cells are also present (double arrow). HE ×235

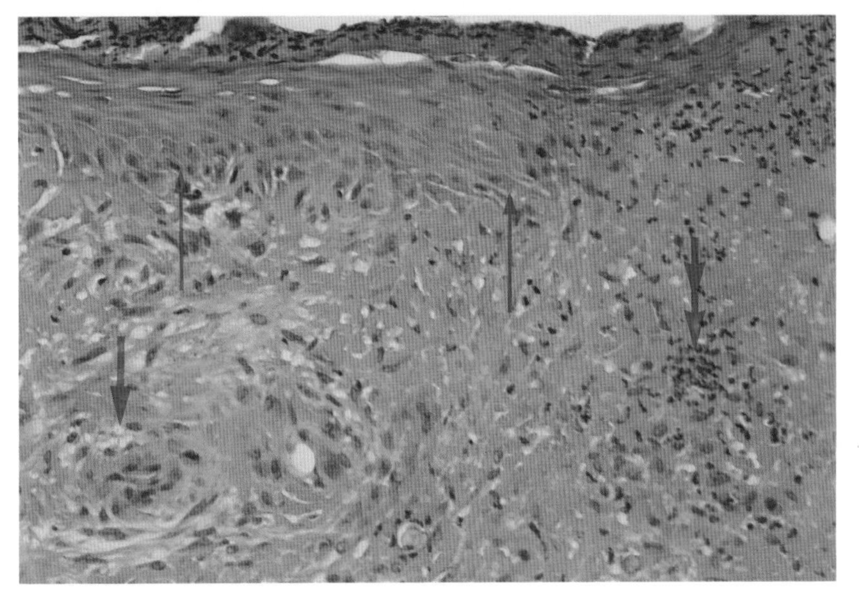

1.37 Healed wound: cornea

The cornea (top), a transparent structure, rests on a thick pink hyaline basement membrane (Bowman's membrane, or anterior limiting layer) (thick arrow) and its external surface is covered with stratified squamous epithelium. Beneath Bowman's membrane there is a thick layer of avascular collagenous fibrous tissue of the cornea. The cornea had been incised surgically two months prior to removal of the eye, and the healed wound is visible as a 'gap' in the stroma, filled with connective tissue and many fibrocytes (double arrow). However the collagen fibres in it lack the regular orientation of the large collagenous fibres of the stroma, and there are no small blood vessels, the new tissue therefore being avascular. Bowman's membrane has also been breached in the wound, and the epithelium covering the gap in it (thin arrow) is much thinner than the normal epithelium on each side of the wound. HE ×134

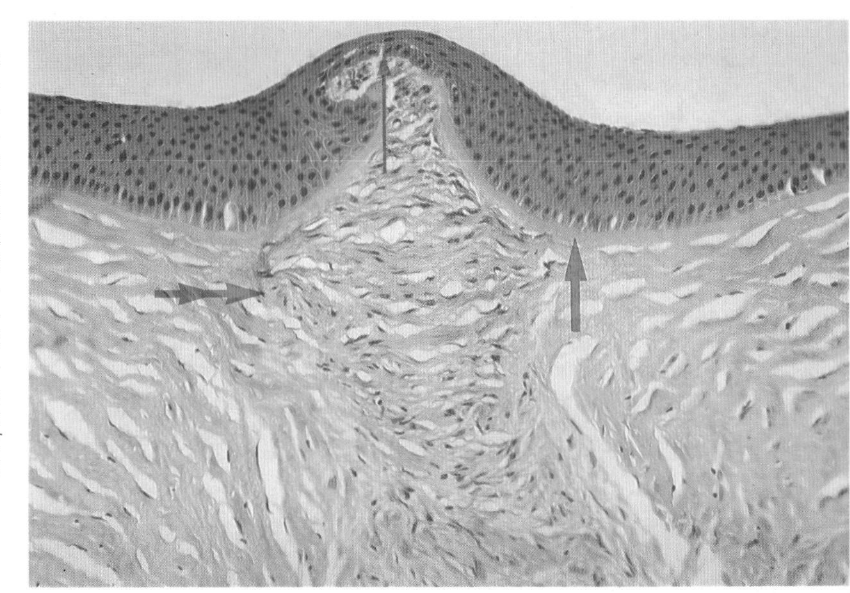

1.38 Healed wound: skin

A wound of skin that heals quickly and completely eventually becomes relatively inconspicuous, and even histologically restoration of the epithelium and collagenous tissues of the dermis may be so complete as to make the site difficult to identify. However the dermal elastic fibres fail to regenerate as a rule, and stains for elastic tissue generally reveal a gap in the connective tissues of the dermis, even when the wound is old and apparently completely healed. This is a surgical wound which had been healed for some months. The surface epithelium (thin arrow) is intact and fairly normal-looking, apart from the fact that it is relatively flat and lacks well-formed rete ridges. The normal dermis (thick arrow) adjacent to the wound is rich in very dark-staining elastic fibres, whereas in the scar tissue of the healed wound there are no elastic fibres (double arrow). Elastic stain ×55

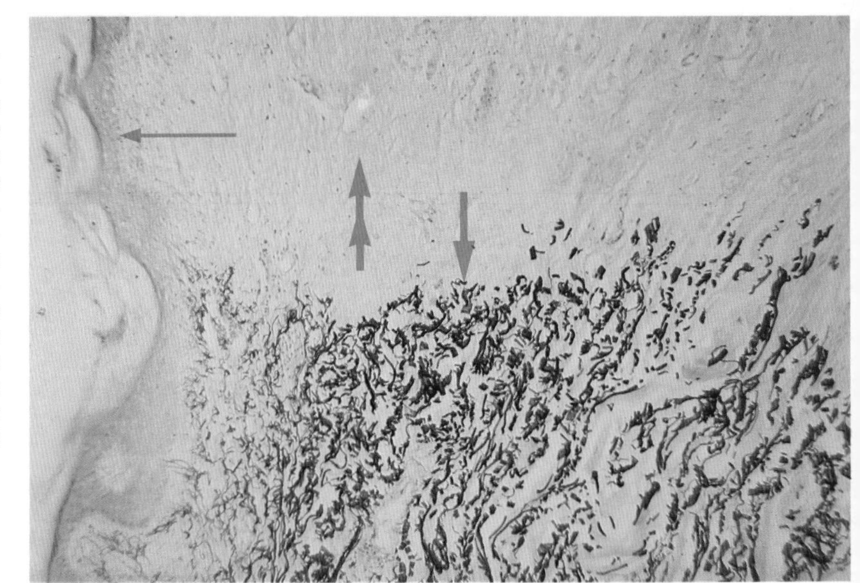

1.39 Keloid in healed wound: skin

The main structural component in a healed wound of skin is collagen, but keloid sometimes develops in a healing wound. An abnormally large amount of collagen is laid down in the wound, and forms a sharply elevated irregularly-shaped scar which grows to such an extent that it bulges above the surface of the adjacent skin. The epidermis and dermis (thin arrow) appear normal, but the deeper dermis and subcutaneous tissues are replaced by very broad bands of hyaline eosinophilic collagen (thick arrow), much larger and thicker than e.g. the collagen fibres in the dermis immediately adjacent to the epidermis. Even at this magnification it is obvious that the fibroblasts associated with the keloid fibres are much larger and active-looking (double arrow) when compared with normal fibroblasts. Black people are more liable to develop keloid than white individuals, and in this case there is a high concentration of dark pigment (melanin) in the basal layer of epithelial cells in the skin.

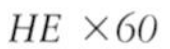

HE ×60

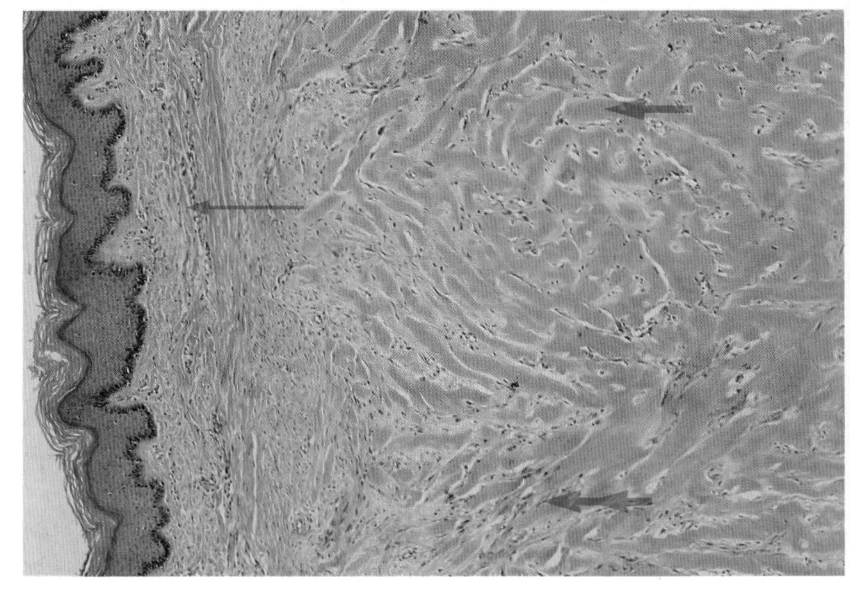

1.40 Healing fracture: rib

When a bone fractures, a fibrin clot forms and is generally replaced by a meshwork of woven bone. Osteoblasts are the counterpart of the fibroblasts of collagenous tissue and are derived from the 'resting' osteocytes of the periosteum and endosteum of the bone. They play the major role in restoring the structure of the bone, responding rapidly to lay down woven bone in somewhat haphazard fashion and occasionally cartilage. This tissue is callus and it effects temporary repair. The normal cortical bone is on the right (thin arrow), and the other tissue (centre and left) is the 'external' callus, i.e. the callus on the external aspect of the bone. It consists of thick trabeculae of woven bone (thick arrow) and vascular connective tissue. The surfaces of the bone trabeculae are covered with large active-looking osteoblasts (double arrows) which will lay down dense lamellar bone. There is also some cartilage (left margin) superficial to the woven bone. HE ×95

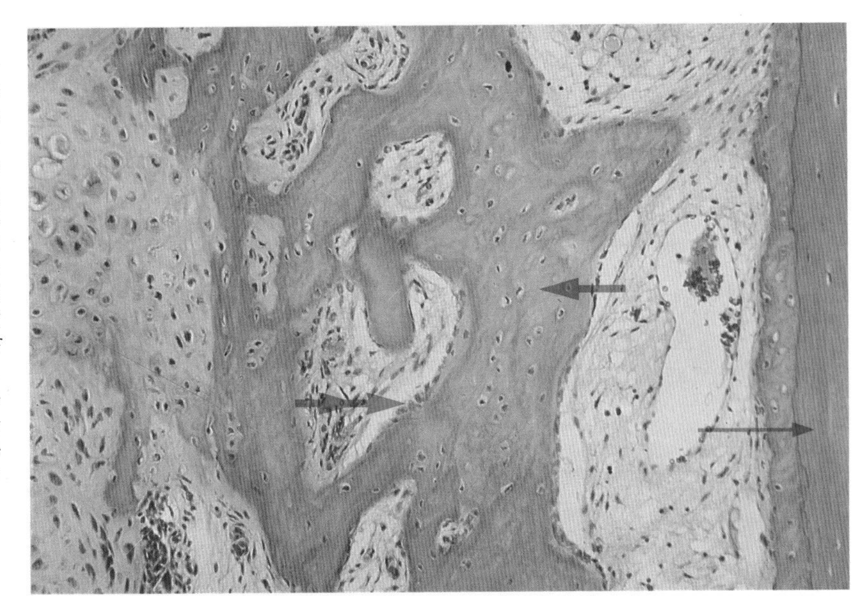

1.41 Healing fracture: rib

A collar of callus, formed by the periosteum of a long bone and called external callus, is shown here in some detail. It consists of trabeculae of new bone and cartilage (centre and left). The new bone is coarse-fibred ('woven') bone (thin arrows), with osteocytes distributed throughout the basophilic matrix and elongated prominent osteoblasts (thick arrow) covering most of the surface of the trabeculae. The chondrocytes in the solid matrix of the cartilage vary considerably in size, from very large (double arrow) to small spindle-shaped forms, and their arrangement is somewhat disorderly. During the process of remodelling the callus (internal and external), trabeculae of dense lamellar bone are laid down in orderly fashion and the cartilage is removed, thereby reforming the cortex of the bone. In this way, if the ends of the broken bone have been correctly apposed, the normal bone structure can be restored completely. HE ×200

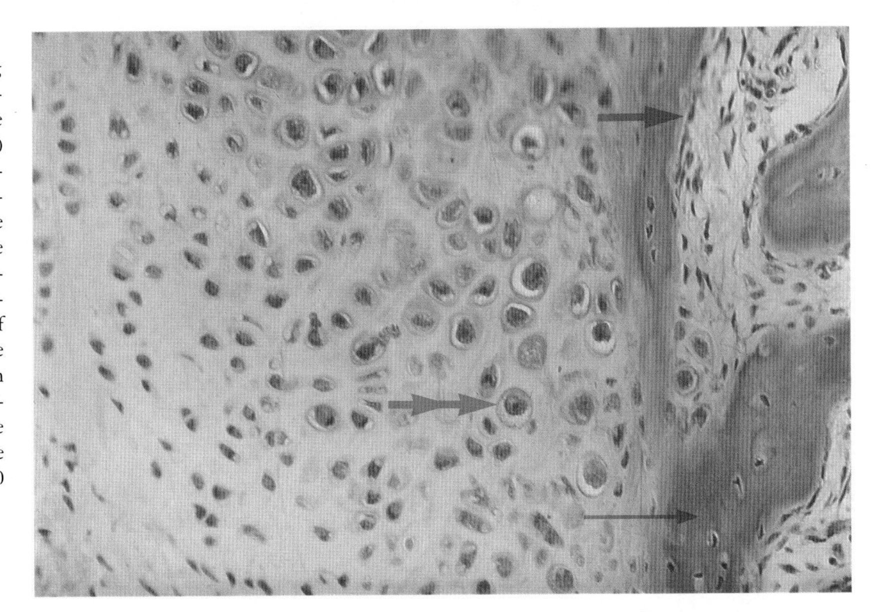

1.42 Hyperostosis: Ewing's tumour in femur

Hyperostosis means hypertrophy of bone (reactive bone formation). The bone-forming cells of the periosteum and/or endosteum may be stimulated in various ways other than by a fracture, e.g. by the presence of a low-grade inflammatory lesion or by a slowly growing neoplasm, most commonly a meningioma (rapidly growing tumours destroy the bone rather than stimulate it). In this case the patient had a Ewing's tumour of the femur which was invading and disrupting the cortical bone of the shaft. The periosteum has reacted and its external surface is covered with a layer of very cellular fibrous tissue (thin arrow) which has grown outwards (down, in this field) and formed a much thicker layer of osteogenic connective tissue. There are numerous trabeculae of woven bone (double arrow) in this osteogenic connective tissue and they are aligned at right angles to the femoral cortex. The osteocytes in the woven bone are typically large and round or ovoid in shape. In places there are many osteoblasts (thick arrow) on the surfaces of the trabeculae. HE ×150

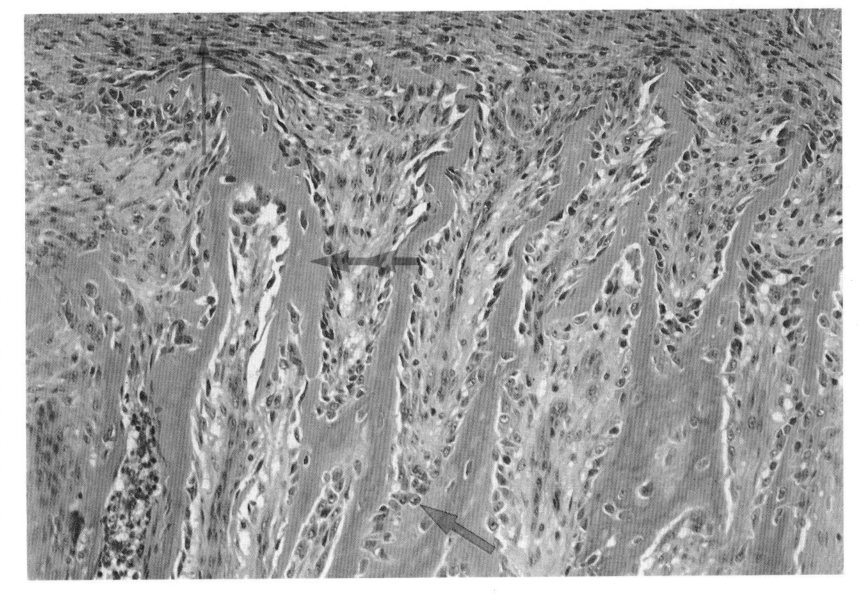

1.43 Pilomatricoma of skin: foreign-body giant cells

Pilomatricoma is a benign sharply-circumscribed calcifying epithelial neoplasm (calcified epithelioma), derived from hair matrix cells. It is usually firm spheroidal intracutaneous mass, 1-3 cm dia, The neoplastic cells mature and die, becoming eosinophilic keratinized 'shadow' or 'ghost' cells without nuclei. The necrotic cells are foreign to the tissues and phagocytes attempt to remove them. This tumour was in the skin of the upper arm of a man of 31, and this small part of it consists of a weakly eosinophilic sheet (upper two-thirds of field) in which there are many small pale ovoid foci, each of which lacks a nucleus. These are (necrotic) 'ghost' cells (thin arrow). The sheet of necrotic cells is being attacked by a layer of very active-looking closely-apposed phagocytes, most of them very large multinucleated cells (foreign-body giant cells) (thick arrow). The ghost cells frequently calcify and this makes them even more resistant to phagocytosis.

HE ×440

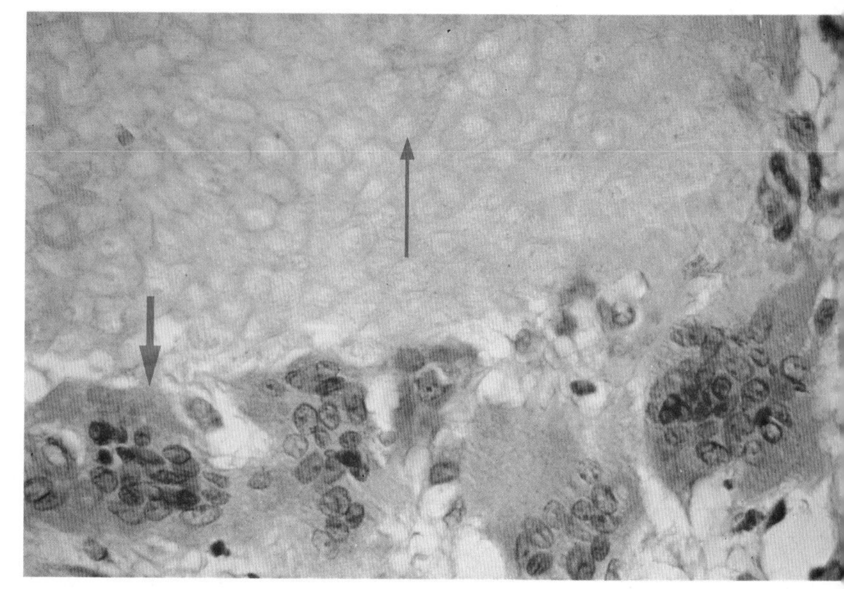

1.44 Plasmacytoma: chest wall

A plasmacytoma is a focal neoplasm (solitary myeloma) of plasma cells. Outside the bone marrow is termed an extramedullary plasmacytoma. A man of 58 developed a swelling on his chest wall, and the mass (15x12x10cm), which appeared to be encapsulated, was removed surgically, along with part of a rib. Histologically it consists of neoplastic plasma cells of varying degrees of differentiation, but many look mature (thin arrows). Phagocytes mingle with the neoplastic cells and most are giant multinucleated cells (thick arrow) which ingest large quantities of amorphous material. The material is amyloid, staining positively with Congo Red and then showing green (anomalous) birefringence when examined with polarized light. Some of the amyloid material is extracellular. The amyloid is derived from immunoglobulin, and since neoplastic plasma cells secrete an abnormal immunoglobulin, amyloid is frequently present in plasmacytomas and multiple myelomas.

HE ×360

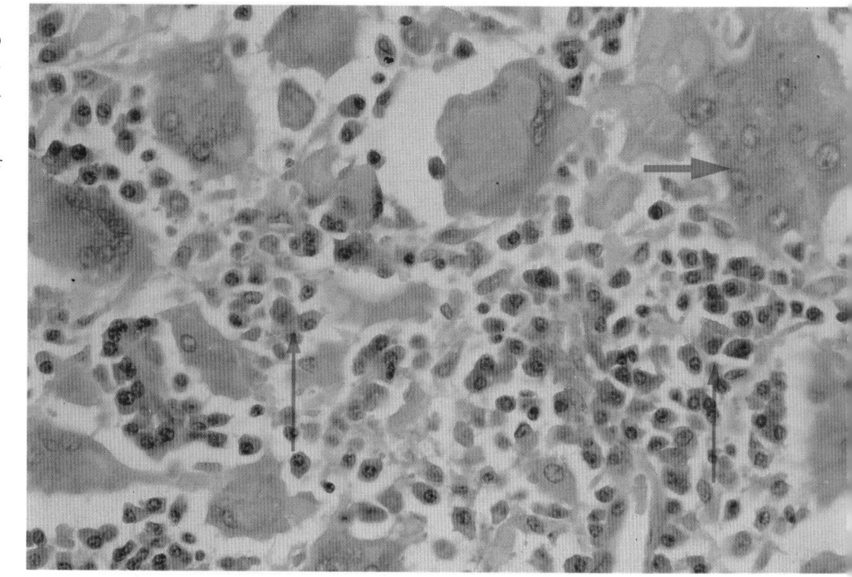

1.45 Schistosomiasis: rectum

Schistosomiasis (sometimes called bilharziasis) of the intestine is caused by trematode parasites (flukes). Flukes of *Schistosomiasis mansoni* live mainly in the inferior and superior mesenteric veins but migrate to deposit their eggs in venules, generally of the colon. Most of the ova laid by the female worm pass through the rectal mucosa and are excreted, but some remain in the tissues. This shows the granulomatous reaction to the ova in a specimen of rectal mucosa. Between the bases of three mucosal glands there is a dense infiltrate of inflammatory cells, consisting (centre and right of centre) of numerous large macrophages with abundant pale-staining cytoplasm (thin arrow), and collections of eosinophil leukocytes (thick arrow). Lymphocytes are also present. No ova are visible. The granulomatous reaction tends to produce fibrous thickening, occasionally very marked, of the wall of the intestine. Eggs lodging in the liver may give rise to peripheral fibrosis, hepatosplenomegaly and ascites.

HE ×150

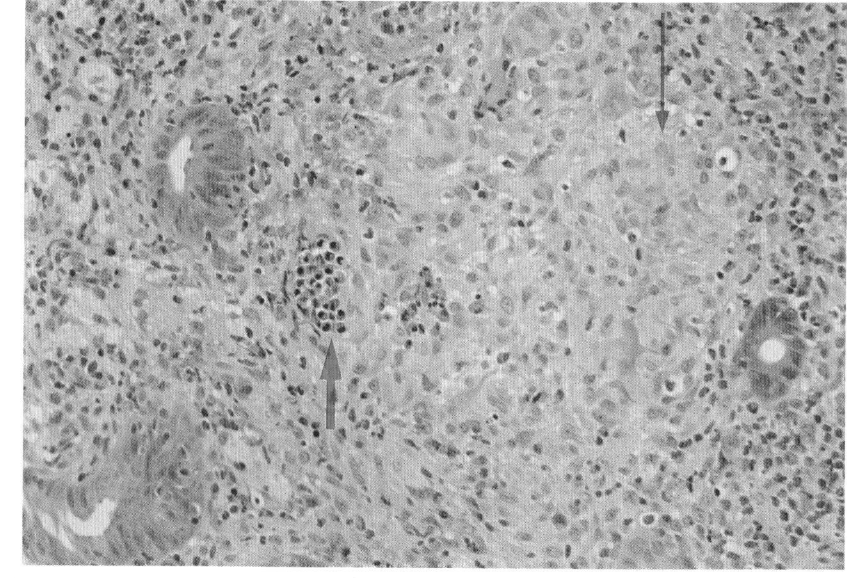

1.46 Phagocytosis of lipid: skin

The patient was a man with a considerably raised level of plasma lipids (hyperlipidemia). Deposits of lipid in his skin led to the formation of yellow nodules (xanthomas). One of the nodules had been traumatized and the lipid was dispersed in the dermis, where it was phagocytosed by macrophages. Many of the macrophages are very large (giant foreign-body) cells with a large amount of eosinophilic cytoplasm and multiple pale vesicular nuclei (thick arrows) in many of which there is a central nucleolus. The cytoplasm of the giant cells is vacuolated in places but the most prominent features are the large empty (clear) clefts in the cytoplasm which had contained cholesterol crystals (the cholesterol dissolved in reagents). There are also prominent eosinophilic asteroid (star-shaped) bodies (thin arrow) in three of the giant cells. The smaller macrophages, for example, have finely granular (frosted-glass) cytoplasm. The significance of asteroid bodies is not known. HE ×360

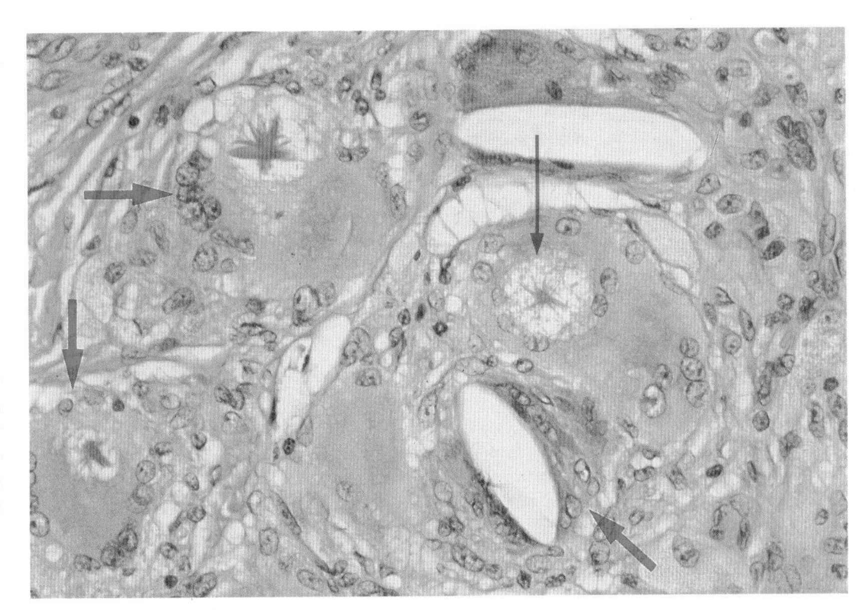

1.47 Malakoplakia

In malakoplakia, soft patches develop on the mucous membrane of a hollow organ and occasionally, in chronic cystitis, they take the form rounded plaques (1-2cm dia) in the bladder wall. Although malakoplakia usually affects the bladder, this lesion was in perinephric (retroperitoneal) fat. It is a very cellular granulation tissue, consisting largely of closely packed plasma cells, lymphocytes and large macrophages, but accompanied also by small plump endothelium-lined blood vessels (double arrow). The smaller cells are mature plasma cells and lymphocytes in roughly equal numbers. The many macrophages (thin arrows) have abundant eosinophilic well-defined cytoplasm and in some of them there are various distinctive 'inclusions'. One of these inclusions is basophilic and spherical (thick arrow), the deep blue-black colour being caused by its rich content of calcium and iron. Inclusions of this type were numerous throughout the tissue and are termed Michaelis-Gutmann bodies. HE ×360

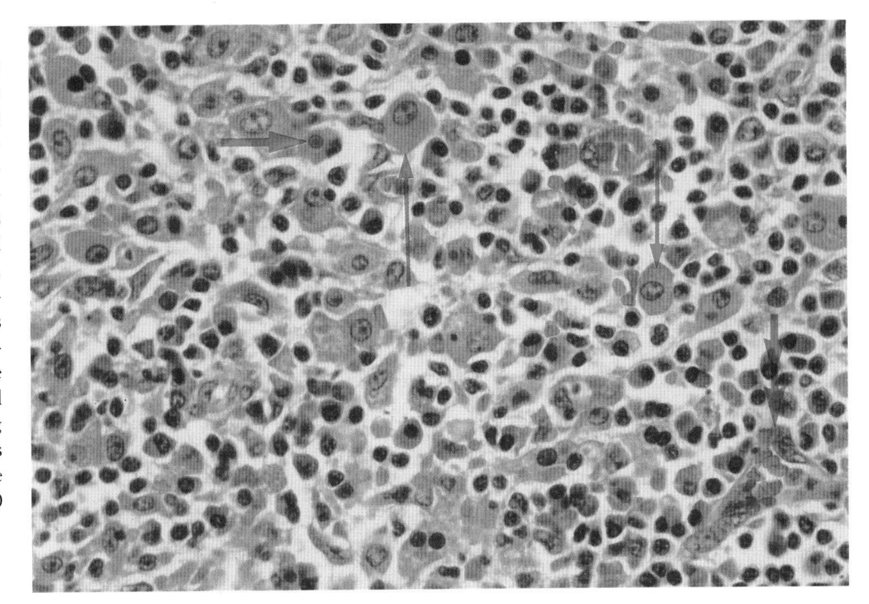

1.48 Orbital pseudotumour

Orbital pseudotumour is a distinctive chronic inflammatory reaction in the orbital tissues of the eye, which may closely resemble a neoplasm and often becomes bilateral. Its etiology is unknown but the process may be of the same type as that which occurs in retroperitoneal fibrosis. An autoimmune basis has been postulated but without clear evidence. This is a fairly early lesion and it is therefore very cellular with minimal fibrosis. The cells are mainly eosinophil polymorphs (thick arrow), leukocytes and lymphocytes but a few macrophages and plasma cells are also present. A lesion of this structure may be mistaken for Hodgkin's disease. The 'onion-skin' thickening of the adventitia of the small artery (thin arrow) is a non-specific inflammatory response but reminiscent of the changes that affect small arteries in the spleen in systemic lupus erythematosus. Sometimes there is also considerable fibroblastic activity, and older lesions tend to become progressively more fibrous. HE ×135

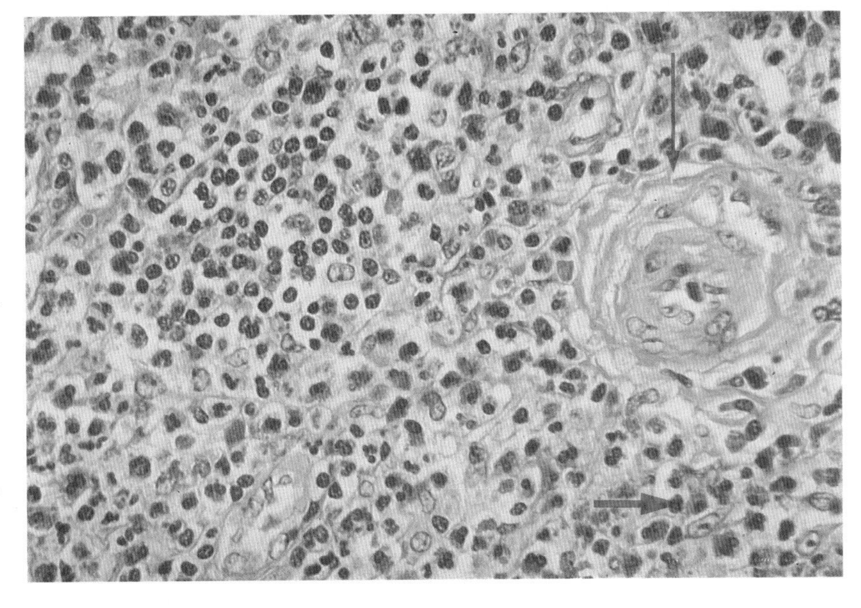

1.49 Hyaline (Mallory) bodies: liver

Mallory bodies are deeply eosinophilic and consist of hyaline reticulum (effete cytoplasmic organelles), within hepatocytes in nutritional cirrhosis. Mallory bodies are characteristically found in livers damaged by chronic alcohol abuse, but similar bodies are occasionally seen in non-alcoholic cirrhosis. They can also be produced in livers of animals experimentally by toxins. This is a cirrhotic liver. Almost all the hepatocytes are swollen, with edematous vacuolated cytoplasm (ballooning degeneration) (thin arrows). Some hepatocytes, however, have large round 'clear' (empty) spaces in their cytoplasm which were occupied by droplets of neutral fat (which dissolved in reagents); and several of the very swollen hepatocytes contain a deeply eosinophilic round Mallory body (thick arrows). Liver cells are prone to accumulate droplets of fat in their cytoplasm from various causes, including abuse of alcohol, chronic malnutrition and obesity. HE ×135

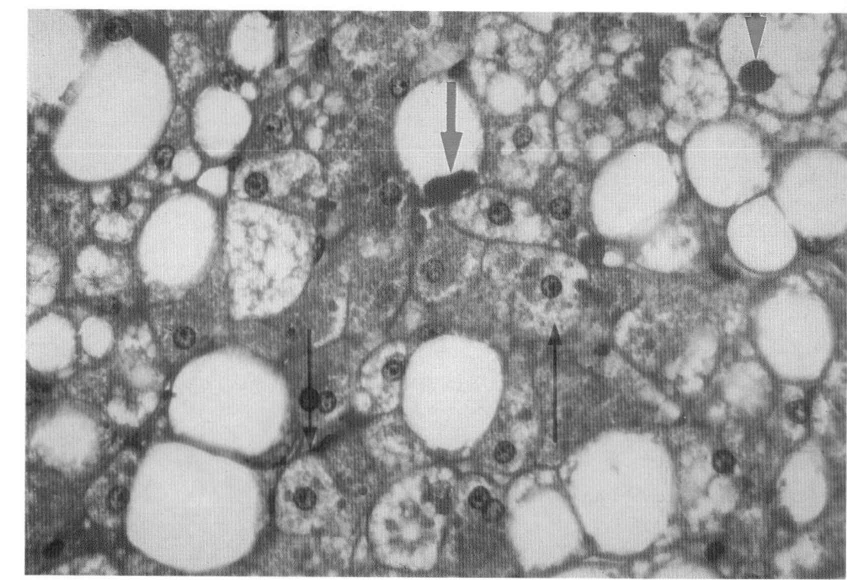

1.50 Actinic elastosis: skin

Actinic (solar or senile) elastosis is the term applied to degeneration of the connective tissues of the dermis. This form of degeneration is commonly seen in skin repeatedly exposed to sunlight, particularly the face of elderly individuals and especially those who are fair-skinned. A man of 62 had a basal cell carcinoma removed surgically from the skin of his forehead. This field illustrates the changes in the dermis, some distance from the tumour. Most of the long thick eosinophilic collagenous fibres have lost most of their nuclei and are fragmenting into slender basophilic fibres (thick arrows). The slender basophilic fibres are tortuous and resemble elastic fibres. They also stain with special stains for true elastic fibres, and the change in the collagenous fibres is therefore generally termed 'elastotic' degeneration. The change is probably caused by the ultraviolet component of sunlight, and the same factors are also involved in the development of basal cell carcinoma. HE ×360

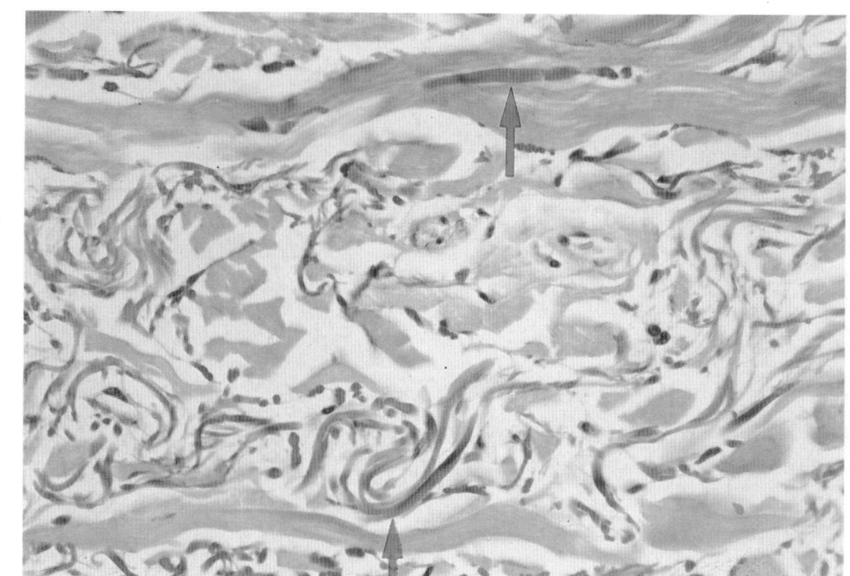

1.51 Radiodermatitis: skin

When skin is exposed to biologically effective levels of ionizing radiation (X-rays) an inflammatory reaction occurs. In this case a tumour was excised from the skin, three months after the skin had been exposed to comparatively large (therapeutic) doses of ionizing radiation. The tumour is not in the field, and the epidermis is thickened and markedly edematous, with wide separation of the epithelial cells (thin arrow). There is also no keratin on the surface of the epidermis, keratinization having failed. Numerous red cells (thick arrow) have leaked into the epidermis from the extremely dilated blood vessels in the dermis. The vessels are also surrounded by a densely eosinophilic cuff of fibrinous exudate (double arrow). The dermal connective tissues are diffusely and heavily infiltrated by inflammatory cells. There is no clear separation of the dermis into upper and deeper dermis. Skin as severely damaged as this, and lacking a protective layer of keratin, is very prone to ulceration. HE ×55

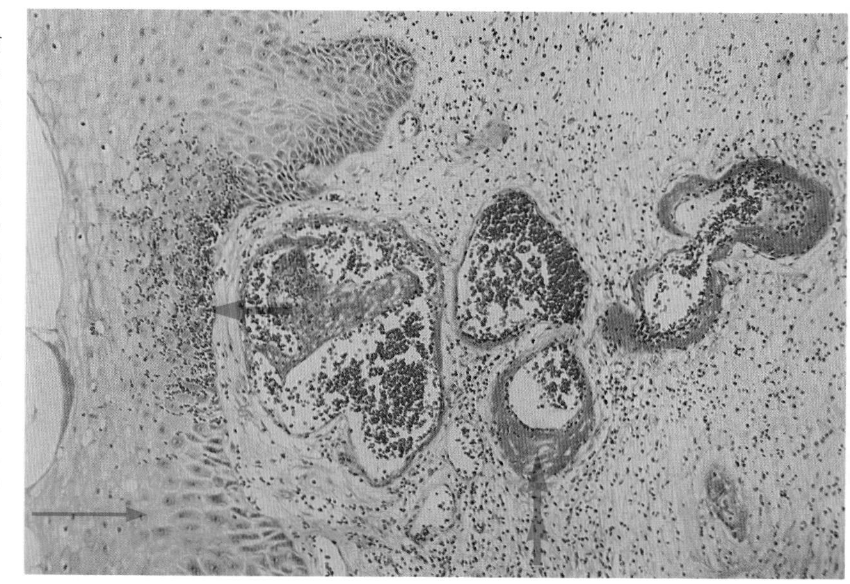

1.52 Myelofibrosis: bone marrow

In myelofibrosis there is progressive fibrosis of the hemopoietic bone marrow which appears to be reactive to an associated myeloproliferative disorder. This is a specimen of bone marrow from the iliac crest of a person with myelofibrosis. The disease is at an early stage, with large numbers of the various types of hemopoietic cells: erythrocytes (thin arrow), granulocytes and multinucleated megakaryocytes (thick arrow). These cells are closely packed and surround fat cells (large clear ovoid spaces, the fat having dissolved in reagents). Elsewhere it is even more noticeable that the amount of fat in the marrow is less than normal, the fat cells having been almost completely replaced by hemopoietic cells. The megakaryocytes in particular have increased greatly in number, and some of them are morphologically abnormal. As the disease progresses, the cellularity of the marrow decreases and fibrous tissue increases; and even at this stage an increase in reticulin fibres is readily detectable by special stains. HE ×360

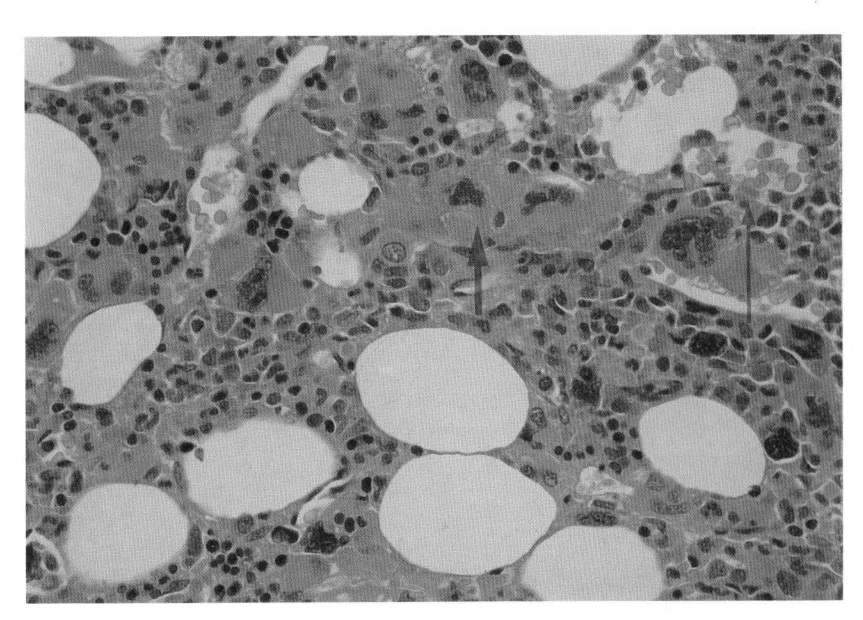

1.53 Squamous metaplasia and dysplasia: bronchus

Metaplasia is the transformation of one type of differentiated tissue into another. Thus in a gall bladder containing a calculus, the mucus-secreting columnar epithelium tends to undergo metaplasia to the reputedly more resistant stratified squamous epithelium; and when the mucosa lining the bronchi is 'irritated' by e.g. carcinogenic substances (benzpyrene, etc.), it too tends to develop foci of squamous metaplasia and dysplasia. The mucosal tissue in this field was resected from the bronchus of a man who was a heavy cigarette smoker. The normal mucin-secreting pseudostratified ciliated columnar epithelium of the bronchial mucosa has disappeared and been replaced by thick stratified squamous epithelium, the surface cells of which are tending to keratinize (thin arrow). The epithelial cells in the basal layers are large, closely packed and very pleomorphic (double arrows). They also have large vesicular nuclei which are extremely pleomorphic. There is also increased mitotic activity (thick arrow). HE ×135

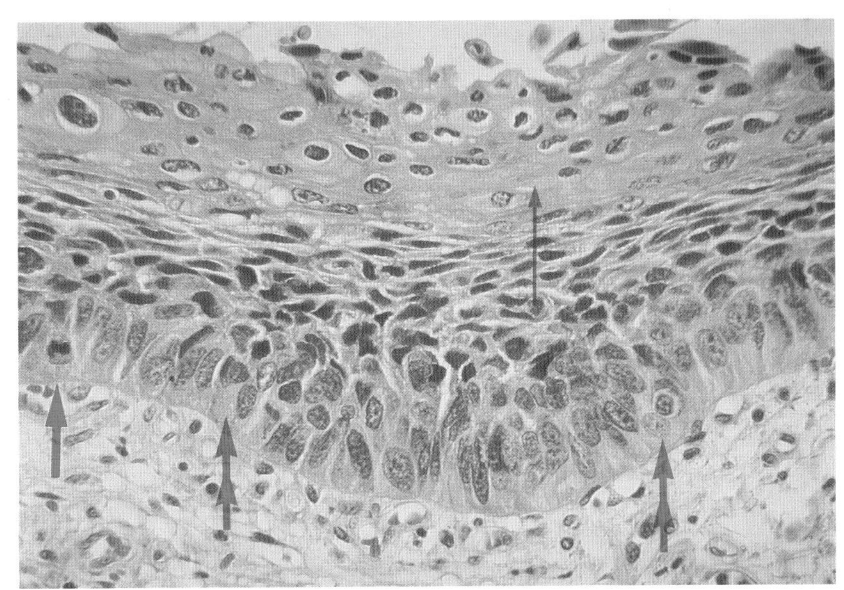

1.54 Dysplasia: bladder

In dysplasia, cell and tissue structure is disorganized, sometimes so markedly as to obscure the identity of the tissue and be termed anaplastic. A man of 67 who had worked for many years in the rubber industry developed severe recurrent cystitis, for which he underwent total cystectomy. The mucosa (thin arrows) lining the bladder is very dysplastic. The epithelial cells are large and show only a slight tendency to stratification. They have eosinophilic cytoplasm and large nuclei, each of which contains a prominent central nucleolus (thick arrow). The submucosa (lower half of field) is very vascular (double arrow), and in it there is an inflammatory infiltrate of lymphocytes and plasma cells, as well as some eosinophilic exudate. The dysplastic changes in the epithelium were almost certainly produced by carcinogenic substances such as beta-naphthylamine previously used in the rubber industry. Careful search however revealed no evidence of carcinoma in the bladder. HE ×360

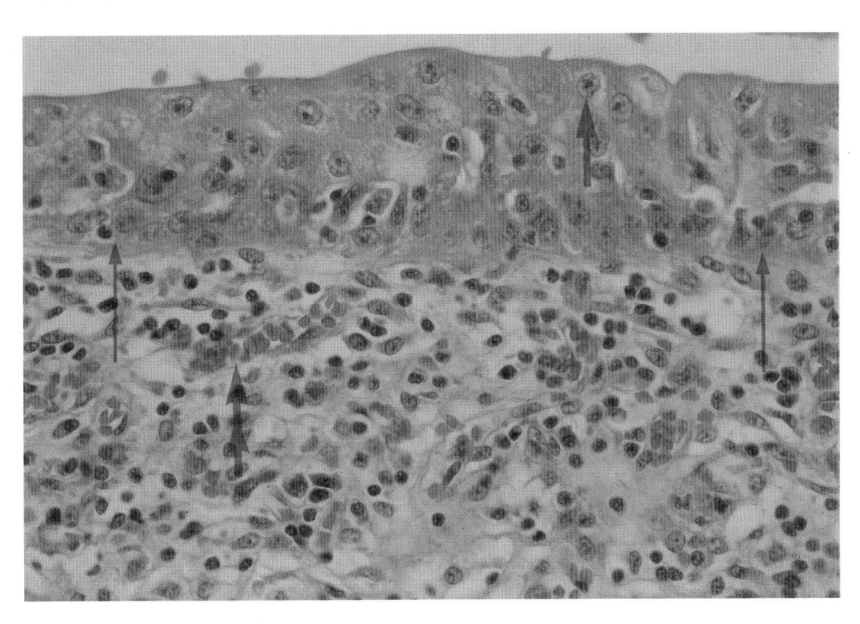

1.55 Hemangioma: skin

A hemangioma is a benign tumour composed of newly-formed blood vessels. This was a small red-blue lesion in the skin of the eyelid. Histologically it is sponge-like, consisting of relatively large dilated blood-filled sinus-like spaces, with thin walls of fibromuscular tissue (arrow), lined by flat endothelial cells. The sinus-like vascular spaces interconnect with one another. This type of structure is characteristic of the cavernous type of hemangioma. However cavernous hemangiomas are not true tumours but hamartomas, i.e. benign tumour-like nodules (malformations) in which there is localized over-production of a tissue. Hamartomas are present at birth, grow in step with the other tissues of the individual, show little tendency to spontaneous involution but stop growing when body growth is complete. HE ×150

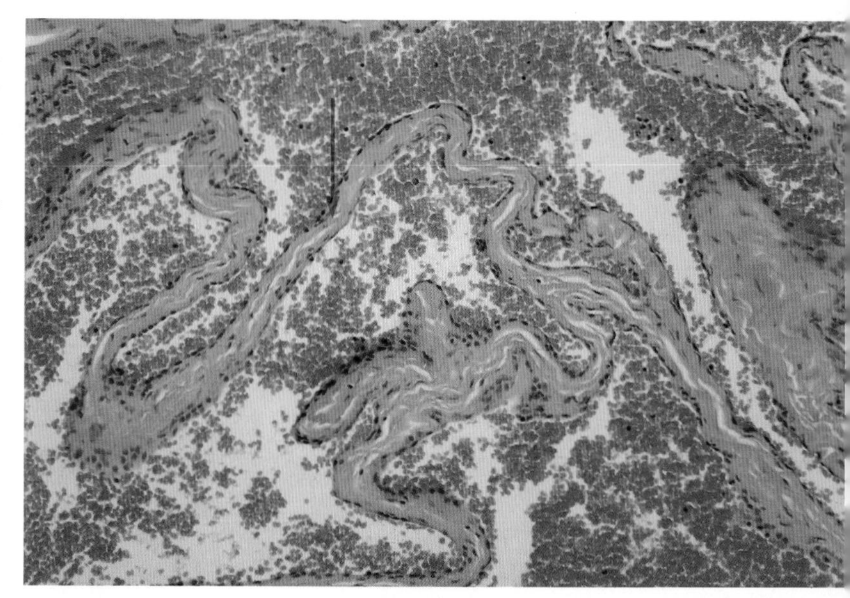

1.56 Epidermal cyst: skin

A cyst is a fluid-filled cavity which arises from dilatation of a pre-existing structure and is generally lined by epithelium. This is a trichilemmal (pilar or keratin) type of cyst which is almost always located on the scalp and is never found on hairless skin. The cyst is lined by stratified squamous epithelium , and the cyst cavity is full of desquamated densely eosinophilic keratinized cells (double arrow). The epithelial cells adjacent to the contents of the cyst are large pale cells with abundant weakly eosinophilic cytoplasm (thick arrow). Underlying these (left margin of field) are much smaller eosinophilic cells with deeply basophilic nuclei (thin arrow). The basal layer is a single row of small cuboidal epithelial cells (left margin). There is no layer of granular cells (keratinocytes), the pale cells undergoing very rapid keratinization without that stage of maturation. HE ×135

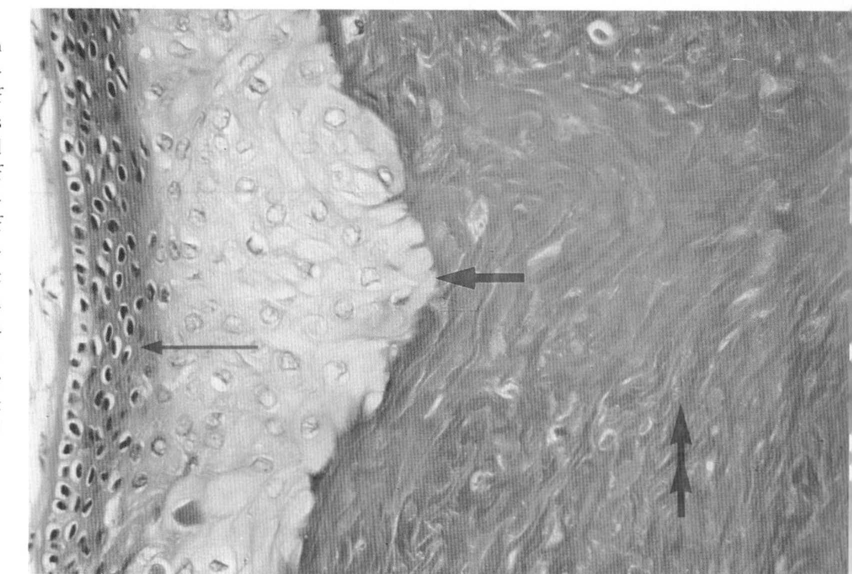

1.57 Squamous papilloma: tonsil

This is the right tonsil of a man of 35. The tonsil is out of sight on the right, and this shows part of a warty arborescent mass 4cm in height which was growing from its surface. Its structure, shown here, is that of a papilloma arising from stratified squamous epithelium. It consists of finger-like papilliform processes with well-vascularized connective tissue core, covered with a thick layer of stratified squamous epithelium, seen here in longitudinal section and also in cross-section (thin arrows). There is a fairly intense infiltrate of chronic inflammatory cells in the connective tissue of the cores of the papilliform processes and in the underlying tissues. Between the finger-like processes there are deep clefts, some containing cell debris (thick arrow). Other types of epithelium also give rise to papillomas in the oropharynx and larynx. HE ×60

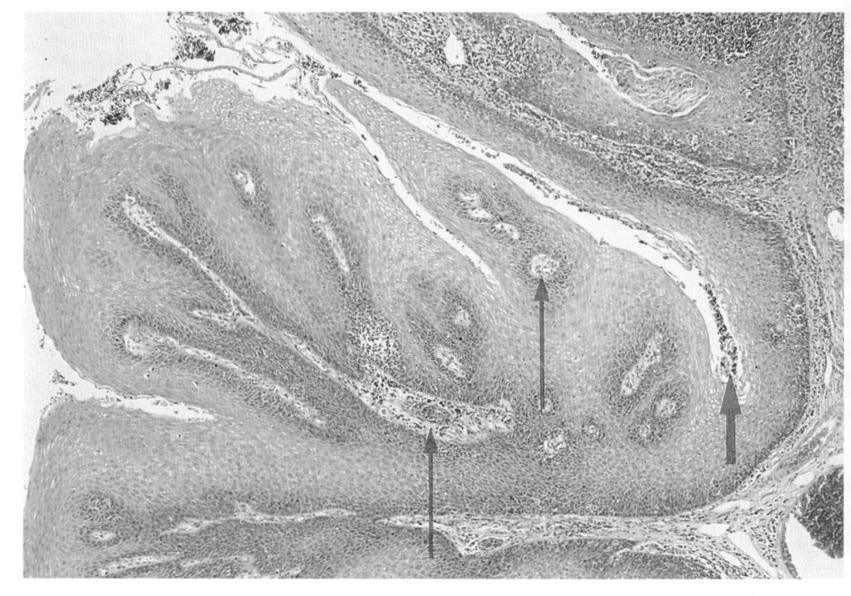

1.58 Tubular adenoma: rectum

This lesion is a tubular adenoma from the rectum of a man of 79. Papillary adenoma of the colon are generally polypoid and they often have a central slender stalk. They show a small but definite tendency to undergo malignant change. However, the tendency to become malignant is even greater in villous papillomas, large soft papillary polyps in the colon. Beneath the tubular adenoma (centre and left), the normal mucosal glands of the colonic mucosa, lined by mucus-secreting epithelium, are seen in cross-section (thin arrow). Each of the papilliform processes of the adenoma consists of a slender core of vascular connective tissue (thick arrows), covered with a thick layer of closely packed tall columnar epithelial cells (double arrow) which show considerable dedifferentiation and dysplasia. Their nuclei are large and basophilic, and apparently form several layers. Mucus secretion is greatly reduced; and at higher magnification occasional mitotic figures were evident. No invasion of the connective tissue of the stalks however had occurred. HE ×100

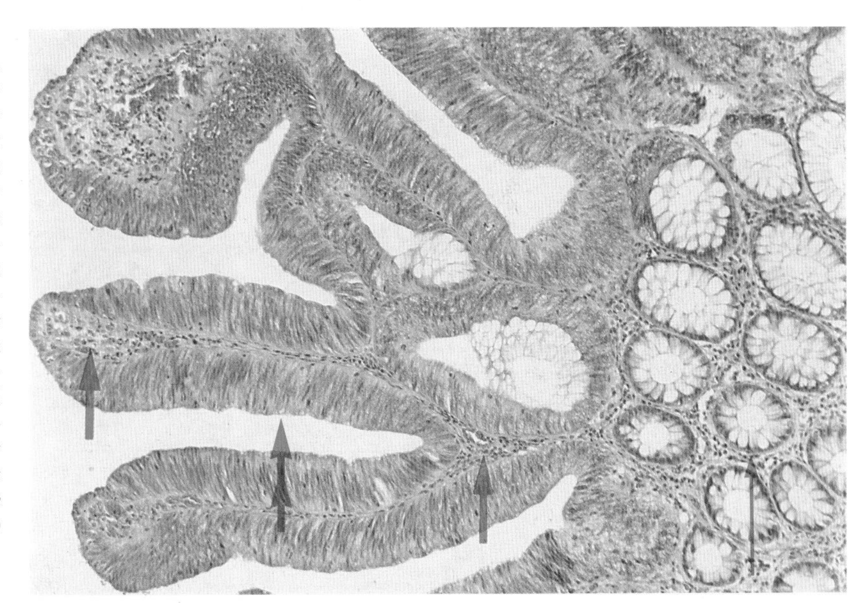

1.59 Leiomyosarcoma

A sarcoma is a tumour composed of tissue resembling embryonic connective tissue, and it is often highly malignant. A leiomyosarcoma is a malignant neoplasm consisting of large spindle-shaped cells of smooth muscle. A leiomyosarcoma is a comparatively rare tumour, which tends to spread by the bloodstream to distant sites to form metastases. This tumour was in the scrotum. Histologically it is a highly cellular tissue, consisting of interlacing bundles (thin arrow) of large elongated cells, some very elongated, with ovoid vesicular nuclei and abundant eosinophilic cytoplasm. The nuclei of the tumour cells are pleomorphic, some being very large and basophilic (thick arrow). All have prominent nucleoli. There are occasional mitoses. The cells are poorly-differentiated smooth muscle cells, and they are arranged in a somewhat haphazard pattern which does not occur in normal tissues. With special techniques myofibrils can be demonstrated in their cytoplasm. HE ×135

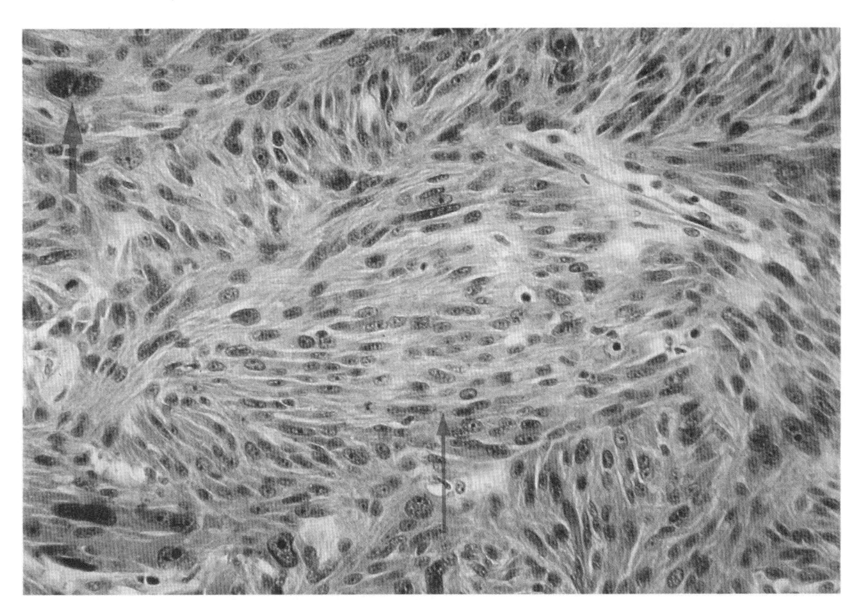

1.60 Carcinoma in lymphatics: caecum

This is a section of caecal mucosa and submucosa. The mucosa was macroscopically normal, and its glands (left half), seen in cross-section, are microscopically normal. The muscularis mucosae (double arrow) is intact. A primary carcinoma of caecum (not illustrated) was located several cm from the mucosa, and it was removed surgically along with part of the colon. In the submucosa (right half) there are collections, varying widely in size, of basophilic malignant (carcinoma) cells. Some of the tumour cells lie close to the muscularis mucosae and others form gland-like spaces (thick arrows). However the collections that lie within the distended lymphatic channels (thin arrows) are much larger, and are probably finger-like cords of tumour cells which have spread from the primary growth and infiltrated adjacent lymphatic channels. Lymphatic permeation is one reason for excising a considerable portion of normal-looking bowel around a carcinoma. HE ×80

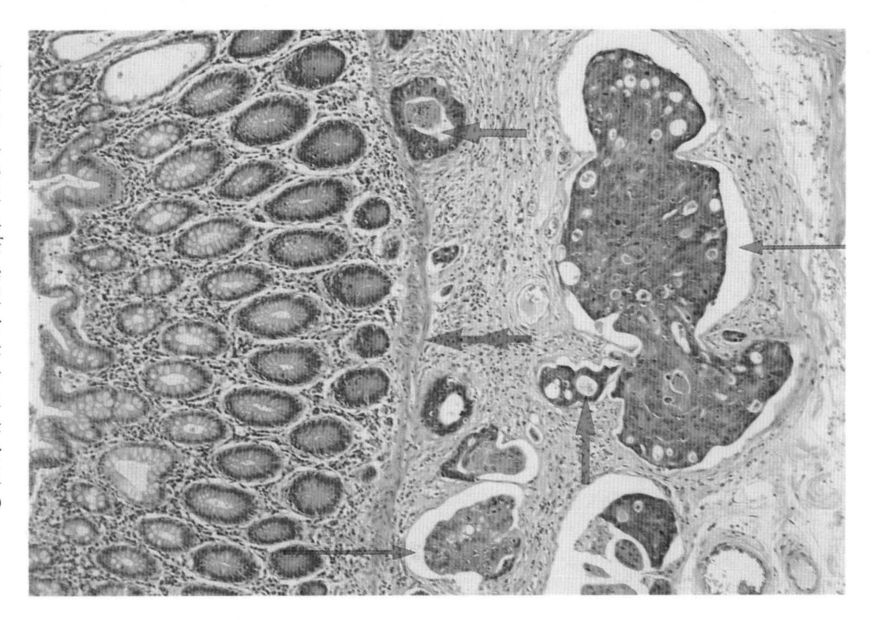

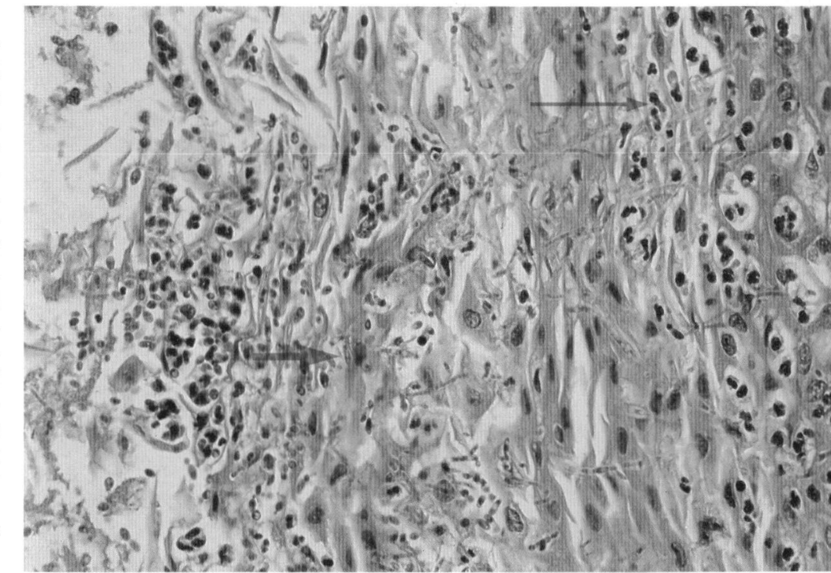

2.1 Candidiasis: esophagus

Candidiasis is caused by the yeast-like fungus *Candida (Monilia) albicans*. It is an organism of low virulence, and lesions are confined as a rule to the surface of mucous membranes as white patches on the mucosa, of cheeks, tongue and pharynx. Proliferating Candida may also form a thrush-like membrane on the surface of the epithelium lining the esophagus of individuals with a terminal illness. The organism invades deeper tissues only when the body's defences are lowered. This is a section of a plaque on the surface of the esophageal mucosa. The lumen of the esophagus is at the left margin. The epithelial lining is mildly inflamed, and the more-superficial squamous epithelial cells (thick arrow) are separated by inflammatory edema and forming clefts. A layer of desquamating squamous cells and inflammatory cells has formed on the mucosal surface. Inflammatory cells (mostly polymorph leukocytes) (thin arrow) are present in all layers of the epithelium, including the deeper layer of large polygonal eosinophilic squamous epithelial cells. HE ×360

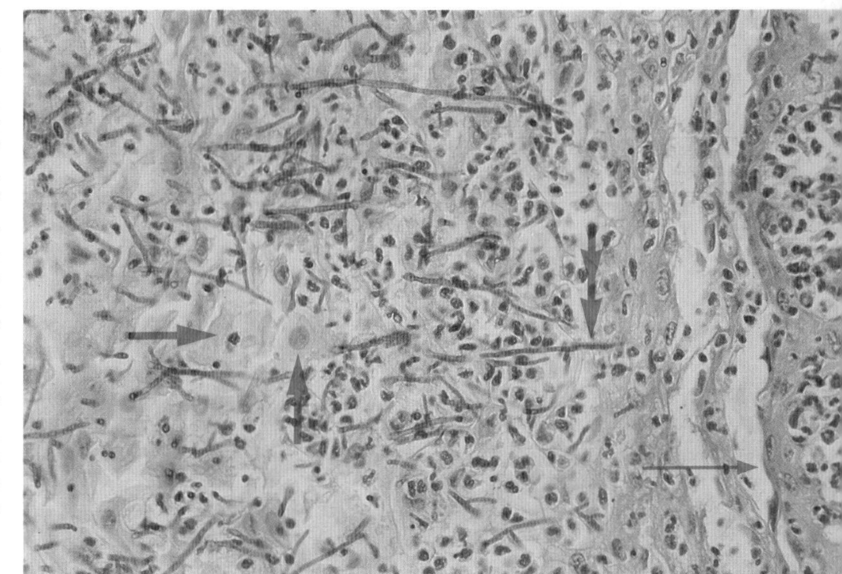

2.2 Candidiasis: esophagus

This is the same lesion as that in 2.1, and faintly basophilic hyphae are just detectable in it. However *Candida albicans* hyphae do not stain well in HE preparations, and this section has therefore been treated with the periodic acid-Schiff (PAS) method, which stains the hyphae of *Candida albicans* an intense purple-red colour. This esophageal lesion consists of a thick layer (centre and left of field) of stratified squamous epithelial cells, the more superficial part is a sheet of large desquamating squamous epithelial cells (thick arrows) which is tending to separate from the still-intact layer of basal epithelial cells (thin arrow) resting on the submucosa. Moderate numbers of polymorph leukocytes and lymphocytes are scattered throughout the layer of epithelial cells and the submucosa. The most prominent feature however is the web of very long purple-red branching hyphae (approx. 1μm thick) (double arrow) which have penetrated the plaque (of desquamated squamous epithelial cells) down to the basal layer of epithelial cells on the right. HE ×360

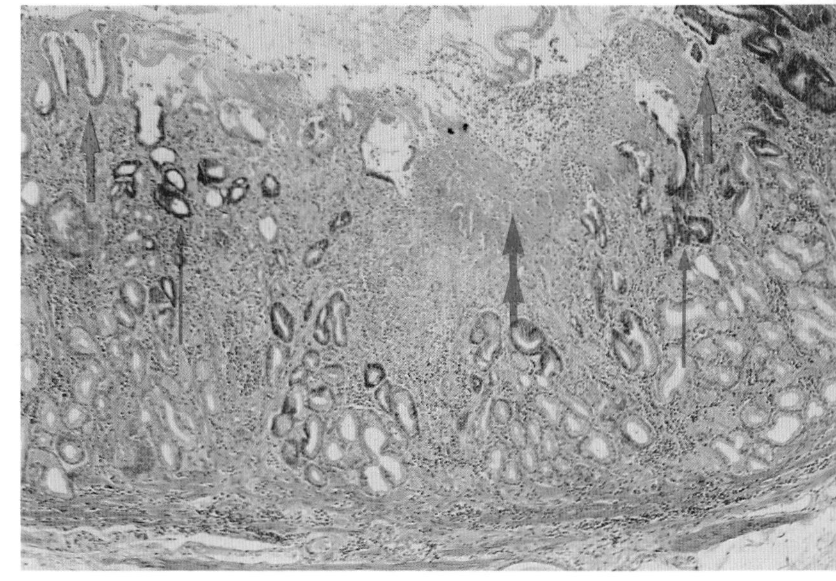

2.3 Erosion (acute peptic ulcer): stomach

Most erosions of the gastric mucosa measure from 1 to 5mm across, and are rarely more than 1cm dia. Erosions are often multiple and may be the source of considerable hemorrhage. An erosion does not extend beyond the muscularis mucosae, but an acute ulcer does so, although it does not usually breach the muscle coats. In this field, the lumen of the stomach is at the top and the muscularis mucosae is visible at the bottom. In the more superficial part of the mucosa, there is a saucer-shaped erosion, an area of ulceration, produced by necrosis and destruction of the superficial glandular tissue (thick arrow)s). The erosion is very shallow, and its floor consists largely of necrotic tissue and cells (double arrow). The viable mucosa, beneath the necrotic tissue and at both sides of it, is infiltrated with inflammatory cells; and along its margin (at the bottom of the necrotic mucosal tissue but particularly on each side of the erosion), the most superficial glands in the underlying (viable) mucosa are distorted, deeply basophilic and partly necrotic (thin arrows). HE ×60

:.4 Chronic peptic ulcer: stomach

:hronic peptic ulcers are generally round or ovoid. They :end to penetrate deeply into or through the stomach /all, and complete disruption of the muscle coats is gen- rally accepted as the criterion for classifying a peptic ul- er as chronic. The most common complications of hronic peptic ulceration are hemorrhage, perforation nd penetration (extension through the whole thickness f the gastric wall into an adjacent organ). In this exam- le, the ulcer (centre) is well-defined and looks 'punched- out', having penetrated through both the basophilic gas- ric mucosa (thin arrows) and the eosinophilic muscle oats (thick arrow). The mucosa is slightly redundant on he right, overhanging the edge of the crater to a certain xtent, but the mucosa looks fairly normal in general and s not heaped up in the same way as in a malignant lesion. The walls of the crater are steep, and remnants of the nuscle coat are visible in the left and right sides of the rater walls. The floor of the crater is flat, consisting of a hick layer of collagenous fibrous tissue and, on its sur- ace, a densely-eosinophilic band of necrotic tissue (dou- ble arrow). HE ×7

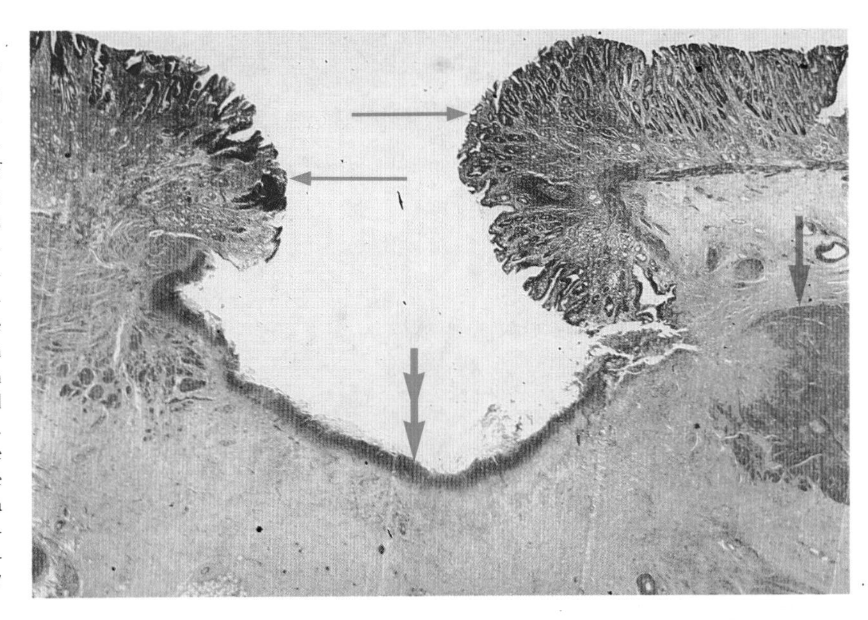

:.5 Chronic peptic ulcer: stomach

:hronic peptic ulcers of the stomach are most common n the lesser curvature, whereas chronic peptic ulcers in he duodenum (much more common than gastric ulcers) occur within 2cm of the pylorus. This is the same chronic gastric peptic ulcer as in 2.4, at higher magnification. The crater of the ulcer is just visible at the top and the tis- ue which forms the floor of the ulcer crater fills the rest of he field. The most superficial layer consists of a thin layer of deeply eosinophilic fibrinous exudate and fragments of necrotic cells (thin arrows). Beneath this layer there is a much thicker layer of mature well-formed granulation issue. The granulation tissue is very vascular, consisting of numerous widely dilated thin-walled blood vessels thick arrows) and a fairly large population of macro- phages and other chronic inflammatory cells. Polymorph eukocytes are seemingly absent. When the ulcer heals, epithelial cells grow across the surface of the granulation issue, and when continuity of the epithelium has been restored, the granulation tissue matures into fibrous tis- sue. As time passes, the fibrosis increases and eventually becomes the dominant feature of the ulcer. HE ×135

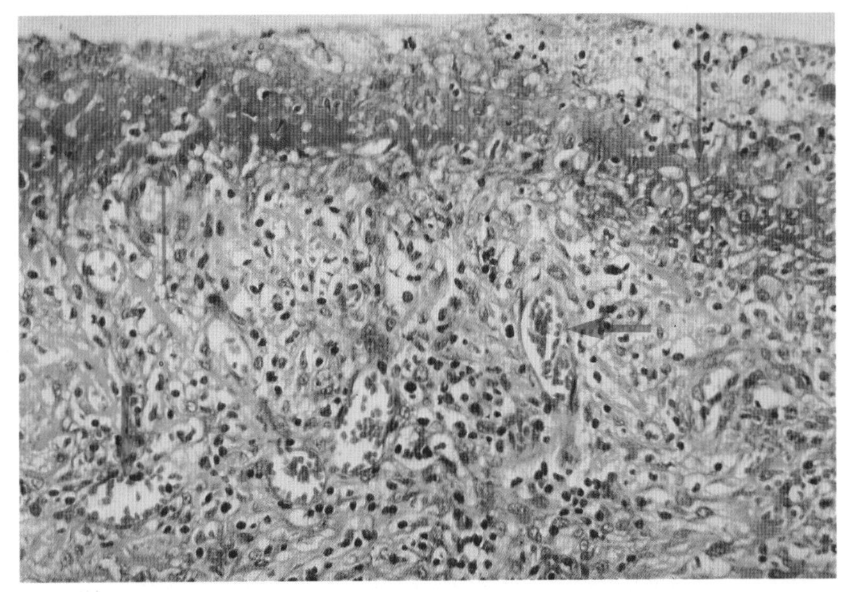

2.6 Atrophic gastritis: stomach

In the common forms of chronic gastritis, the mucosa is usually atrophic and thinner than normal, and the gastric glands are shortened and widely separated. A man of 61 had a partial gastrectomy for chronic peptic ulcer, and this is a section of mucosa several cm from the ulcer crater. There is complete loss of the parietal and chief cells, and the mucosa consists of irregular glands lined by large numbers of cuboidal or columnar epithelial cells, many of them containing large droplets of mucin (goblet cells) (thick arrows). The surface of the epithelium had a villous structure, similar to that of the small intestine: 'intestinal metaplasia' of the mucosa. There are numerous lymphocytes in the submucosa, and a large lymphoid follicle (thin arrow). The eosinophilic muscularis mucosae (double arrow) is markedly thickened. When the submucosal lymphoid tissue is markedly increased and lymphoid follicles with germinal centres are present, the term chronic follicular gastritis is applied. Follicular gastritis is commonly seen in stomachs in which a chronic peptic ulcer is present. In peptic ulceration of the duodenum, chronic gastritis when present is usually confined to the antral region of the stomach. HE ×60

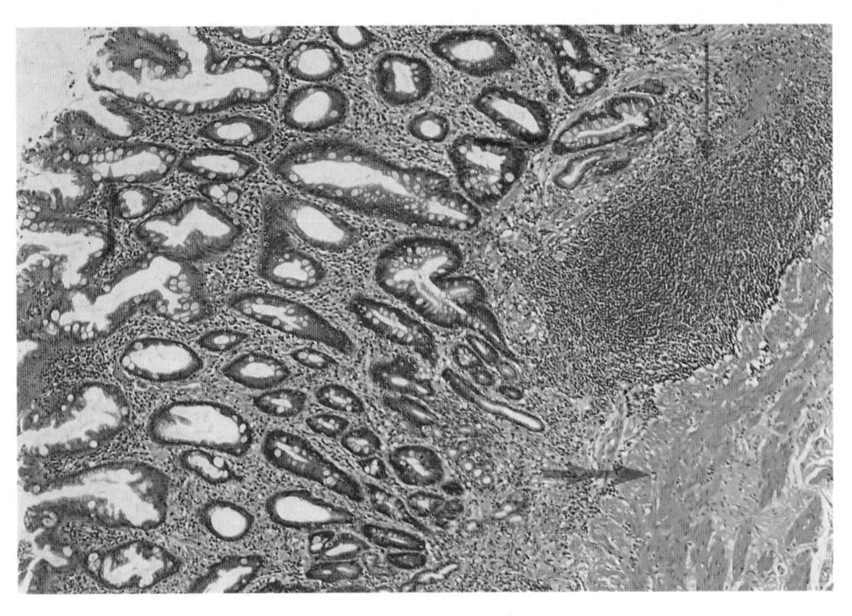

2.7 Atrophic gastritis: stomach

Chronic gastritis is often associated with gastric carcinoma, and it has been suggested that the larger the tumour the more extensive the lesion. Polypoid carcinomas and adenomatous polyps are regularly associated with severe gastric atrophy, but there is still some doubt about there being such a firm predisposition. This is a portion of mucosa from the pyloric canal of the stomach of a man of 78 with a gastric carcinoma. It is a superficial part of the mucosa, with the lumen of the stomach at the top. The mucosa is atrophic and composed entirely of small irregular and rather tortuous glands (arrows), lined by distended mucin-filled goblet cells of 'intestinal' type. No oxyntic or chief (peptic) cells remain. There are no villi of small-intestine type, and the mucosa resembles more closely that of the colon. The number of inflammatory cells in the stroma is fairly small. HE ×150

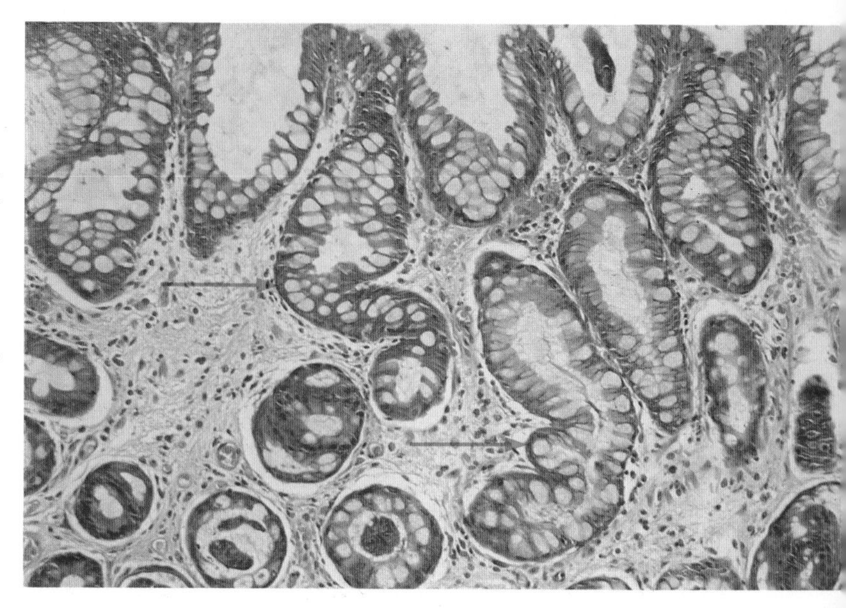

2.8 Superficial gastritis: stomach

Superficial gastritis is most common in the antral region of the stomach. It may persist for years, or it may become more severe and change to atrophic gastritis. A man of 37 had a partial gastrectomy for recurrent duodenal ulcer. Macroscopically, the mucosa of the antral region appeared flatter than normal, but histologically there is little evidence of atrophy. This shows only the superficial mucosa, with the lumen of the stomach just visible on the left. The glands are tortuous (many in cross-section) and most are lined by plump cuboidal or columnar epithelial cells with vesicular ovoid nuclei and eosinophilic cytoplasm which secretes little or no mucin (thin arrow). The epithelial cells show considerable mitotic activity. Between the glands there is a dense infiltrate of inflammatory cells (double arrows), consisting mainly of lymphocytes and plasma cells, and a smaller population of leukocytes (eosinophil and neutrophil. These changes are reactive and commonly seen in glands associated with an inflammatory lesion. Some pyloric glands, lined by a single layer of tall pink mucin-filled cells (thick arrows) with small basophilic flattened nuclei, are also visible.
HE ×150

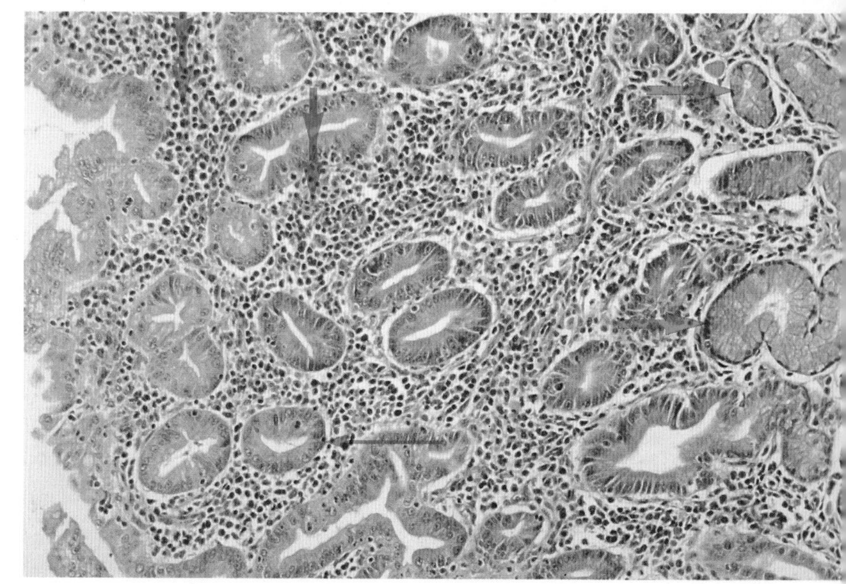

2.9 Chronic (follicular) gastritis (Type B) - *Helicobacter pylori organism*

Section of gastric mucosa from a patient with gastritis, showing in most cases numerous minute curved bacillary organisms (spirilliform *Helicobacter pylori*) (arrow), closely apposed to the layer of mucus covering the surface epithelium and glandular lumina. These organisms are known to be associated with active gastritis and particularly with its progression to malignant lymphoma or adenocarcinoma.

Helicobacter-induced gastritis is possibly the commonest type, and it can affect any part of the stomach. It may lead to the development of gastric and duodenal ulcers, and the age variation is wide, including children. There is an intense infiltrate of plasma cells in the foveolar zone of the mucosa, with variable involvement of the glandular zone, and a mixed acute and chronic inflammatory cell reaction in the underlying lamina propria. There are often signs also of depletion or degradation of mucin.

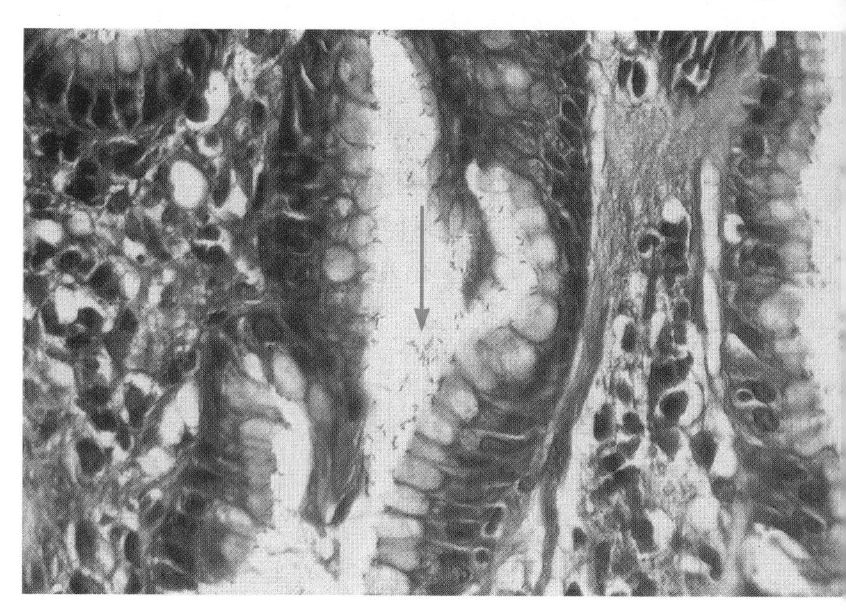

2.10 Hypertrophic gastritis: stomach

In hypertrophic gastritis (also called gastric rugal hypertrophy), the gastric mucosal folds (rugae) are enlarged in both breadth and length, and simulate the convolutions of the brain. The lesion can also be confused with carcinoma or malignant lymphoma. In some lesions, the macroscopic appearance is not caused by thickening of the mucosa but by an increased amount of connective tissue in the submucosa. In this case, the patient was a 67-year-old woman suspected of having gastric carcinoma. This is the mucosa from the fundus of the stomach, showing parts of several greatly enlarged rugae. The broad cores of the rugae consist of much edematous and fibrous connective tissue (thick arrow). The surface of the rugae and the greatly elongated associated glands are covered (mostly) by a single layer of very large columnar cells (thin arrow) with their cytoplasm distended by a large quantity of eosinophilic mucin. Small numbers of chronic inflammatory cells are present in the connective tissue of the rugae. HE ×60

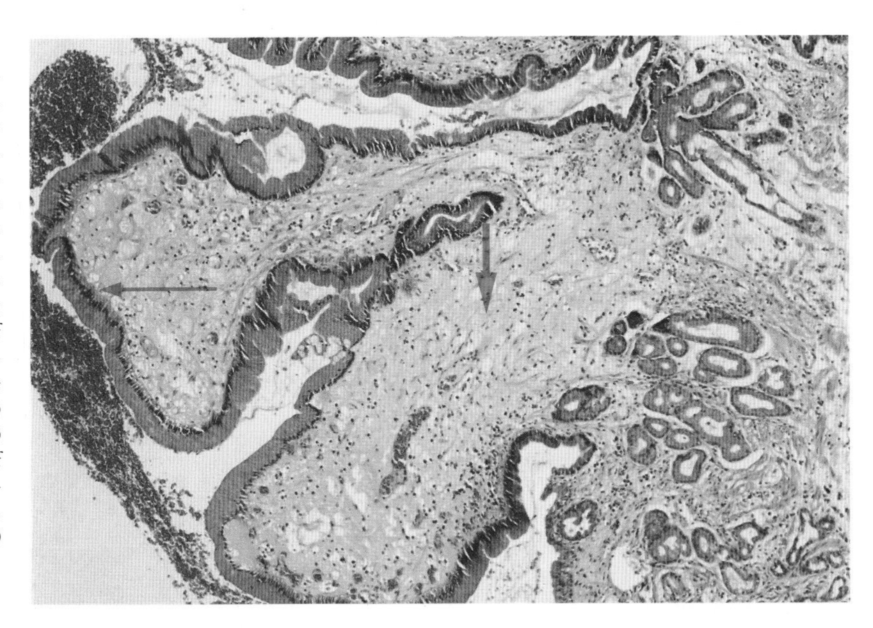

2.11 Epithelial dysplasia: stomach

Dysplasia means abnormal (atypical) cellular proliferation; or, in other words, alteration of the size, shape and organization of adult cells (usually epithelial). Mitotic activity is increased but the mitotic figures are normal. In the stomach, dysplasia of the glandular epithelium is seen occasionally in chronic gastritis with intestinal metaplasia, and the difficulty is to distinguish it from intramucosal carcinoma. This is the antral mucosa, highly magnified, of a woman of 62. The glands, noticeably distorted, are lined by closely packed cuboidal or tall columnar epithelial cells, with large ovoid hyperchromatic (darkly stained) nuclei which show considerable pleomorphism (thin arrow). The polarity of the glandular epithelial cells is severely disturbed, and the mucin-secreting activity of the cells is greatly reduced, with only a relatively small droplet of pale mucin at the apex of each cell (thick arrow). Among the epithelial cells there are fairly numerous mitoses. Between the glands there is a fairly intense infiltrate of inflammatory cells, including polymorph leukocytes, lymphocytes and plasma cells. HE ×460

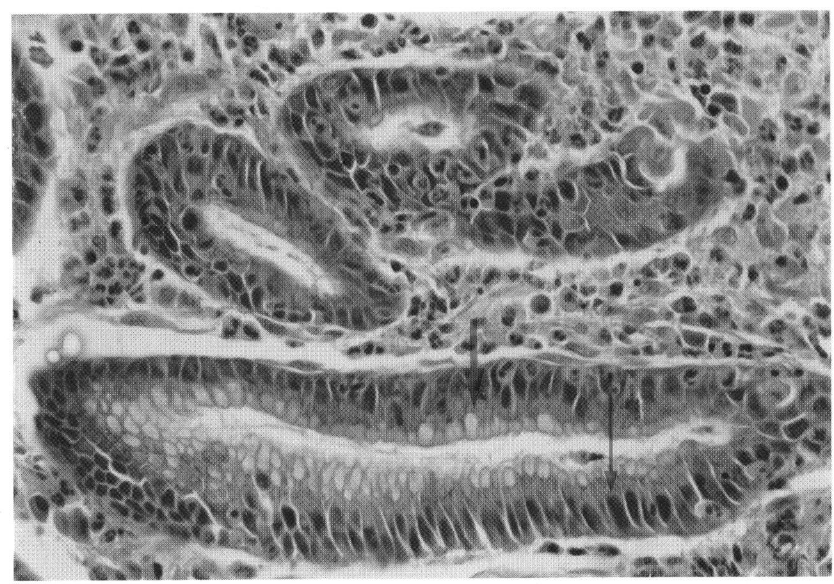

2.12 Adenocarcinoma: stomach

Carcinoma of stomach may arise in any part of the stomach. There has been some increase in number in the cardiac region, but most are located in the antrum. Incomplete forms of intestinal metaplasia, in which goblet cells are associated with atypical mucin-secreting epithelium, may be associated with development of carcinoma. Gastric carcinomas can assume a wide range of forms, but they almost always have the features of mucin-secreting adenocarcinoma. This is the mucosa from the lesser curvature of the stomach of a man of 70 who had a partial gastrectomy for carcinoma of stomach. The lumen of the stomach is on the left and the muscularis mucosae (thin arrow) on the right. The mucosa is thickened, with numerous papillary projections on the surface, and the normal glandular pattern of the gastric mucosa has been replaced by an extensive irregular network of extremely pleomorphic malignant glands (thick arrows). The glands are 'intestinal-type' glands, lined by deeply basophilic epithelial cells and surrounded by an intense infiltrate of chronic inflammatory cells. There is probably also early penetration of the eosinophilic fibres of the muscularis mucosae. HE ×30

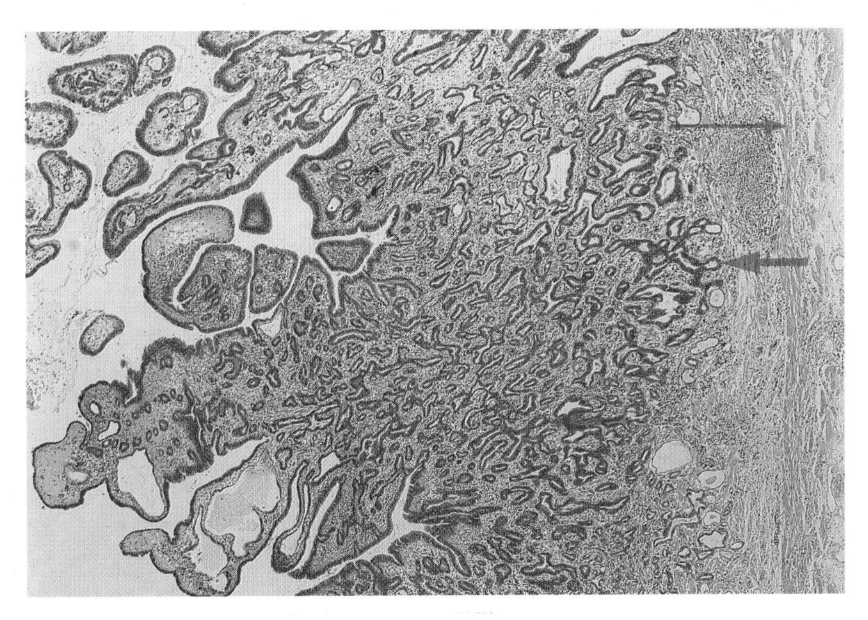

2.13 Adenocarcinoma: stomach

This is the same tumour as in **2.11**. This field shows, at high magnification, the malignant epithelial cells which cover the surface of the (only partly visible) very distorted papilliform projections and line the glands. The malignant cells are very crowded tall columnar epithelial cells which form several layers of large basophilic nuclei (thin arrows). The nuclei are pleomorphic and vesicular and many of them contain prominent nucleoli. They also show considerable mitotic activity (thick arrows). There are small quantities of pale mucin in their cytoplasm (readily demonstrable by special stains). The connective tissue of the mucosa is infiltrated with a moderate number of chronic inflammatory cells. Although the carcinomatous change is confined to the mucosa in this part of the stomach and the appearances are those of a superficial polypoid lesion, elsewhere the tumour had invaded the stomach wall deeply. It had not, however, metastasized to the regional nodes. HE ×360

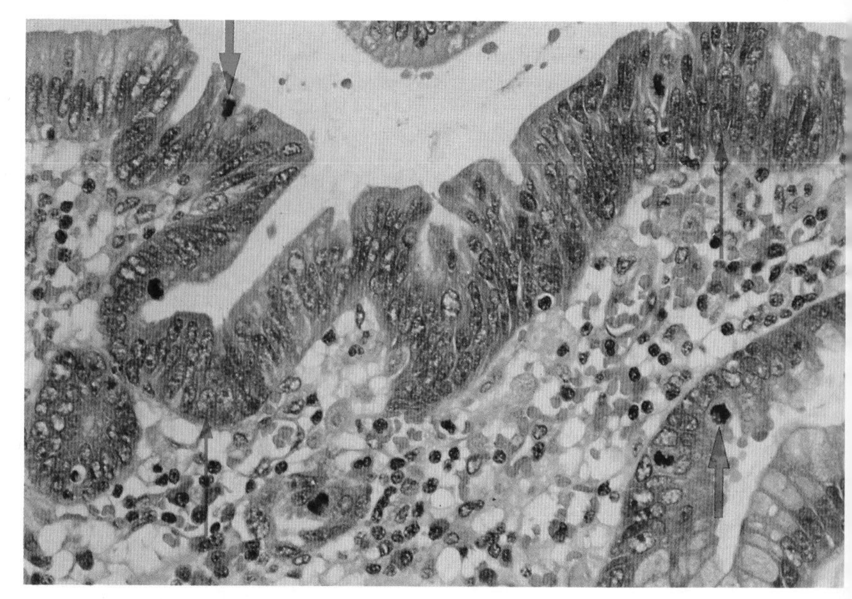

2.14 Adenocarcinoma: stomach

Carcinomas of stomach can be classified (roughly) into two groups: intestinal-type carcinomas, which form large glands lined by a single layer of tall columnar cells (as in carcinoma of colon), and diffuse carcinomas, in which the malignant cells are smaller and form few or no acini. A man of 75 had a partial gastrectomy for carcinoma of stomach. Macroscopically the mucosa was flat, but irregularly thickened and superficially ulcerated in places. Histologically, it is a superficial spreading form of carcinoma, in which the malignant cells are confined to the mucosa. The lumen of the stomach is hardly visible on the left and there is a thick eosinophilic muscularis mucosae (thin arrow) on the right. In the superficial mucosa the glands, greatly reduced in number, are elongated, very slender and lined by atrophic epithelium (thick arrows). Between the glands there are large numbers of closely packed eosinophilic tumour cells. In the basal layers of the mucosa however there are relatively normal pyloric-type glands (double arrow), lined by a single layer of cells with a much strongly eosinophilic cytoplasm. There is a dense infiltrate of chronic inflammatory cells around these glands and also in the muscularis mucosae. HE ×60

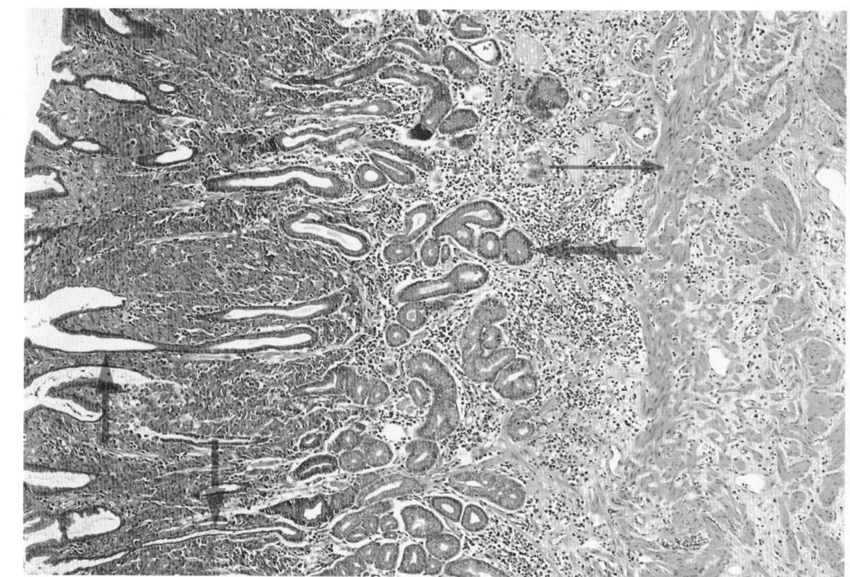

2.15 Adenocarcinoma: stomach

This is the same tumour as in **2.14**, at higher magnification. The lumen of the stomach is at the top. The surviving glands, only partly visible, are widely separated and lined by epithelial cells of widely varying size. The basal parts of two glands are lined by very flat atrophic cells (thin arrows), whereas the cells lining more superficial parts of the glands are cuboidal or large mucin-secreting columnar (non-neoplastic) cells (double arrow). Between and beneath these glands there is a sheet of closely packed large cells, each with a pale vesicular nucleus (often containing a nucleolus) and a considerable amount of eosinophilic cytoplasm. In the cytoplasm of many of the cells there is a very large weakly eosinophilic droplet of mucin (thick arrows). Special stains showed that the mucin filled the cytoplasm and pushed the nucleus of the cell to one side, thereby giving it a signet-ring appearance. All these large cells are malignant epithelial cells which have spread widely through the upper gastric mucosa but have not yet penetrated deeply, even to the muscularis mucosae. Examination of the lymph nodes revealed no metastases.

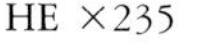
HE ×235

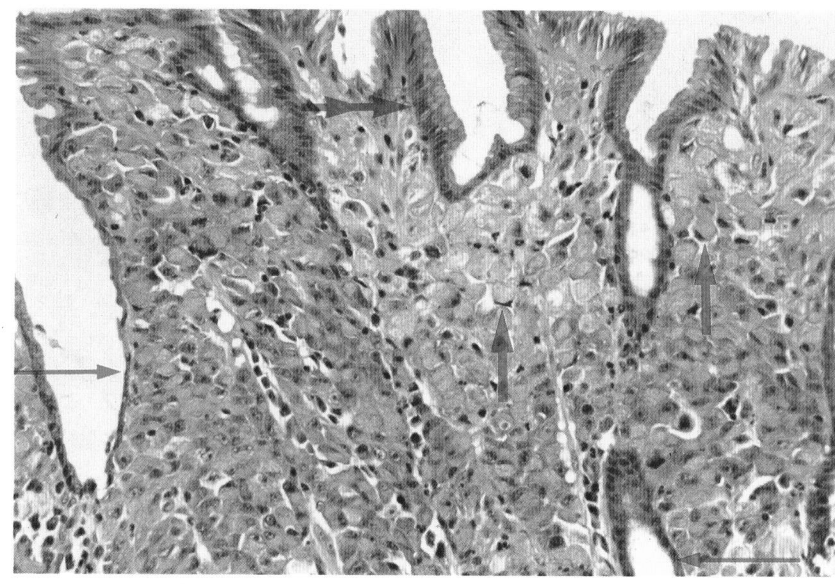

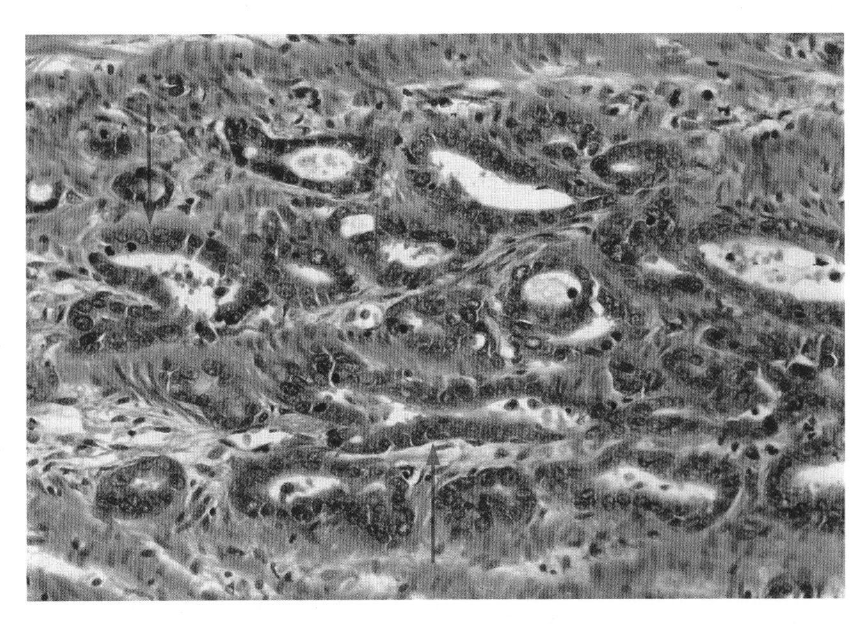

2.16 Adenocarcinoma: stomach

There are two main types of carcinoma of stomach. The first type is associated with the presence of metaplastic intestinal epithelium and generally forms glandular structures (as in 2.11 and 2.13) characterized by a more diffuse infiltrative pattern, the malignant cells forming sheets consisting of single cells or small groups of cells but very few glands (as in 2.14 and 2.15). A phase of intraepithelial or intramucosal neoplasia, characterized by distortion of the normal mucosal gland pattern and varying degrees of epithelial dysplasia, may precede either type of tumour. This field is from the muscle coat underlying a malignant (carcinomatous) ulcer which was present on the lesser curvature of the stomach. This part of the tumour consists of unusually well-formed glands, which are invading the eosinophilic muscle fibres (top and bottom). The glands are malignant and lined by a single layer of cuboidal epithelial cells (arrows) with round or ovoid strongly basophilic nuclei but only a relatively small amount of cytoplasm which is apparently not secreting mucin. The tumour cells show considerable mitotic activity however. HE ×235

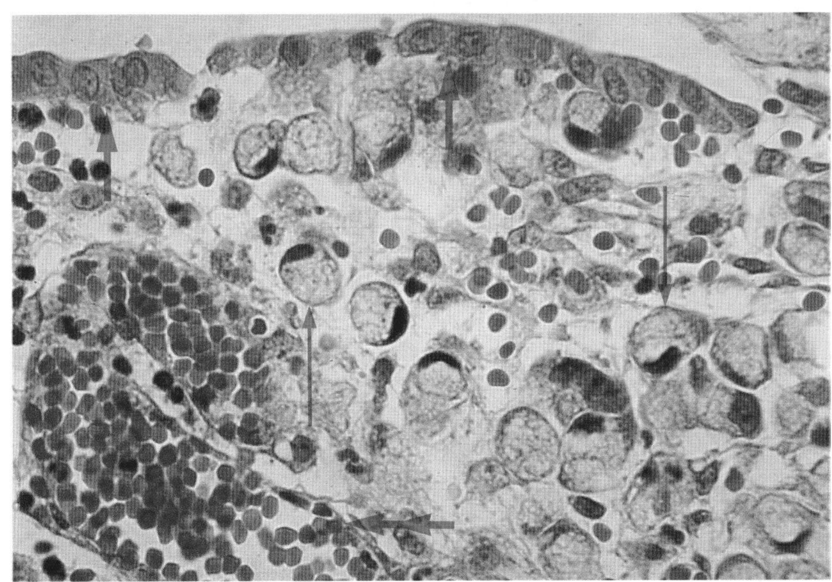

2.17 Adenocarcinoma: stomach

This is a diffuse infiltrating type of carcinoma. At the top of this field, the peritoneal (serosal) surface of the stomach is visible and it consists of a single layer of plump cuboidal cells (thick arrows) with a large round or ovoid nucleus. It is apparently intact, but large malignant epithelial cells (thin arrows) have penetrated the stomach wall to reach the serosa, where they form a cluster of these cells in the subserosa, alongside a very dilated thin-walled blood vessel (double arrow). They are round signet-ring cells, the cytoplasm of which is distended by a large droplet of pale-staining granular mucin. The mucin has pushed the dark-staining kidney- or bean-shaped nucleus against the cell membrane on one side of the cell and so caused the cells to look like signet rings. Nevertheless tumour cells of this type readily penetrate the gastric serosa, to reach the peritoneal cavity where they may grow (peritoneal carcinomatosis) or spread to other organs such as the ovaries (transcelomic spread). Gastric carcinoma can also spread to the liver in the portal bloodstream. HE ×400

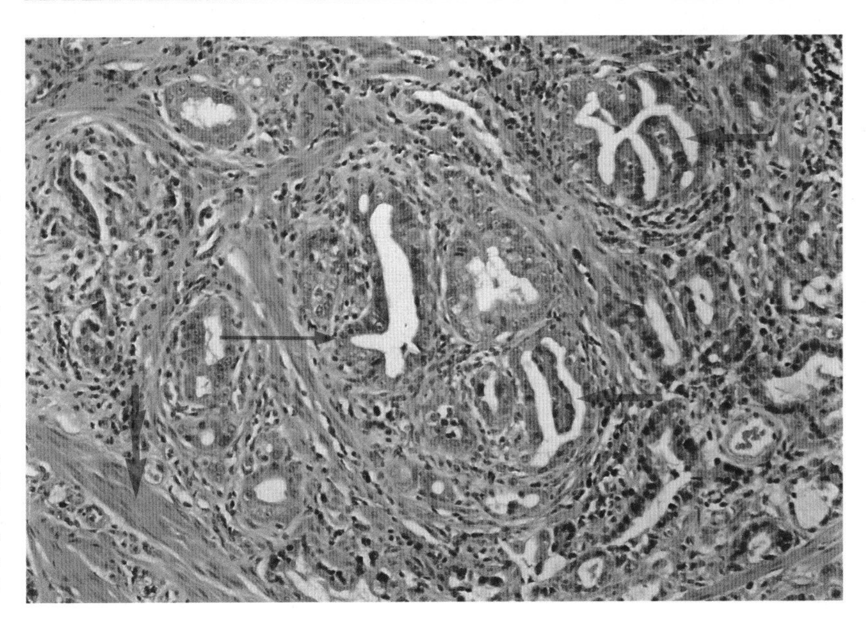

2.18 Adenocarcinoma: ampulla of Vater

Carcinomas of the ampulla of Vater are often small and they can arise in various parts of the ampulla of Vater, such as the terminal part of the common bile duct or the ampulla itself or the duodenal mucosa. They are usually well differentiated, and they tend to form papillary outgrowths into the lumen of the duodenum. Like carcinomas of the bile duct, they may produce clinical signs by obstructing the flow of biliary and pancreatic secretions. This tumour consists of glandular acini which are very irregular in size and shape. The glands are lined (mostly) by a single layer of very pleomorphic epithelial cells which have varying amounts of cytoplasm but tend to be cuboidal (thin arrow). Some of the epithelial cells have relatively large round vesicular nuclei which contain a prominent nucleolus. The lining epithelial cells also form small papillary projections (thick arrows) into the lumen of the glands. The epithelial cells are mitotically active in this field, and the glands appear to be infiltrating the abundant stroma, which consists of fibrous tissue and haphazardly arranged eosinophilic smooth muscle fibres (double arrow). The latter may be part of the wall of the duodenum. There is also a sparse infiltrate of chronic inflammatory cells. HE ×150

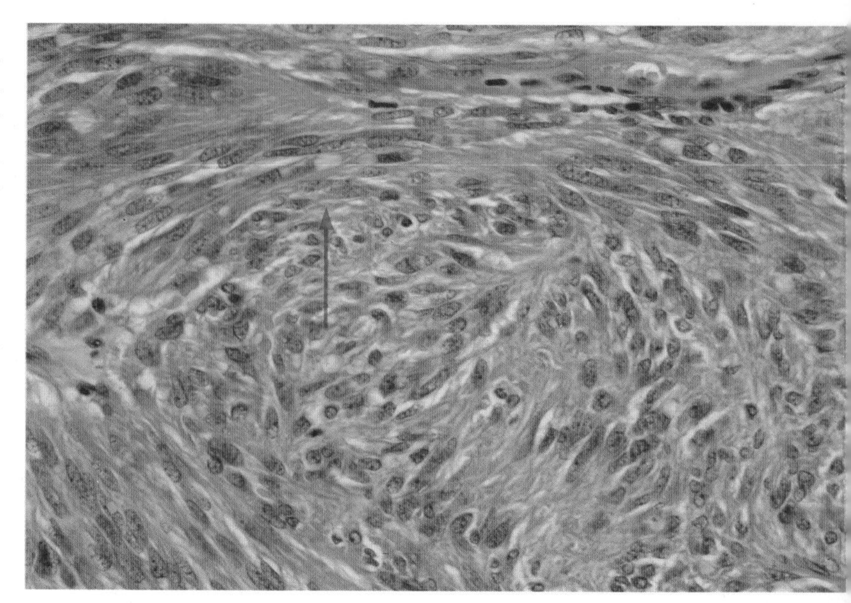

2.19 Leiomyoma: stomach

The majority of benign mesenchymal tumours of stomach are leiomyomas. Most are small, less than 1cm dia and sometimes multiple, but a few may be large and bulge into the lumen of the stomach or intraperitoneally. The tumour is usually located beneath the mucosa, where it forms a round or ovoid mass. Ulceration may give rise to serious hemorrhage. This lesion was an ovoid mass (5 × 4 × 4cm) in the anterior wall of the stomach of a man of 75. It was well demarcated and apparently encapsulated but there was an area (2 × 1cm) of ulceration of the gastric mucosa (stretched over the tumour), and there had been clinical evidence of recurring hemorrhage over a long period. The tumour consists of interlacing bundles of large elongated cells (arrow) with much eosinophilic cytoplasm and large elongated (blunt-ended) vesicular nuclei which tend to form palisades. They are smooth muscle cells, and special stains confirms that little collagen is present. There are no mitotic figures but a small number was found in other parts of the tumour. Despite the mitotic activity and cellularity of the tumour, it was regarded as benign. HE ×360

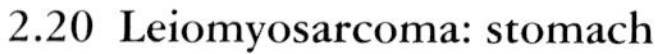

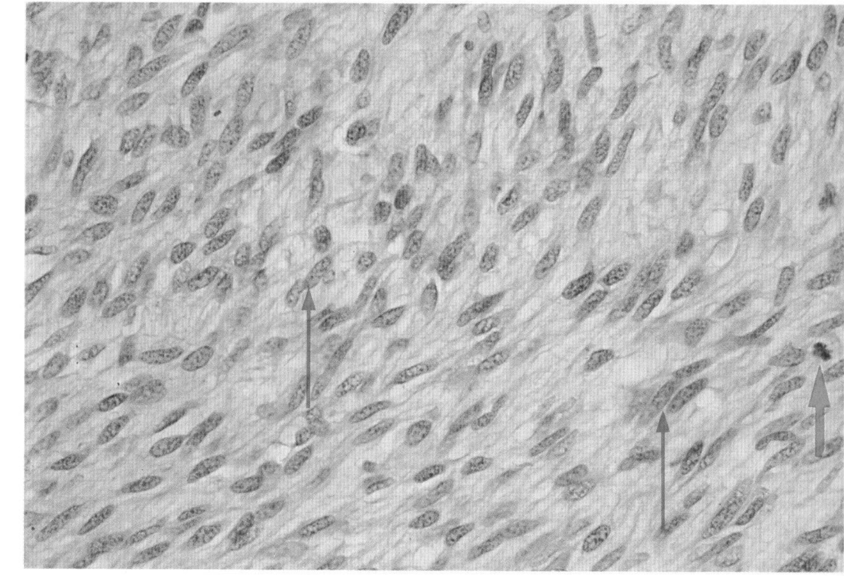

2.20 Leiomyosarcoma: stomach

Most smooth muscle tumours of the stomach are well-differentiated, but a small minority of lesions are usually several cm dia, consisting of very numerous closely packed cells with bizarre hyperchromatic nuclei, are malignant. This field is from a leoimyosarcoma, and it consists of elongated cells, fairly uniformly orientated, with pale elongated round-ended vesicular nuclei (thin arrows) in which there are several small nucleoli. The cells also have a considerable amount of eosinophilic cytoplasm which has a decidely fibrillary texture, and special stains confirmed the presence of myofibrils. Only one mitosis is visible (thick arrow) but elsewhere in the tumour there are, on average, 3-6 mitoses per high-power field. Since the most important criterion for malignancy is the mitotic activity of the tumour cells, the tumour is regarded as a leiomyosarcoma. Malignancy was also confirmed by the presence of secondary deposits in the peritoneal cavity. Leiomyosarcoma of stomach does not metastasize to lymph nodes but secondary deposits may occur in the liver and lungs. HE ×360

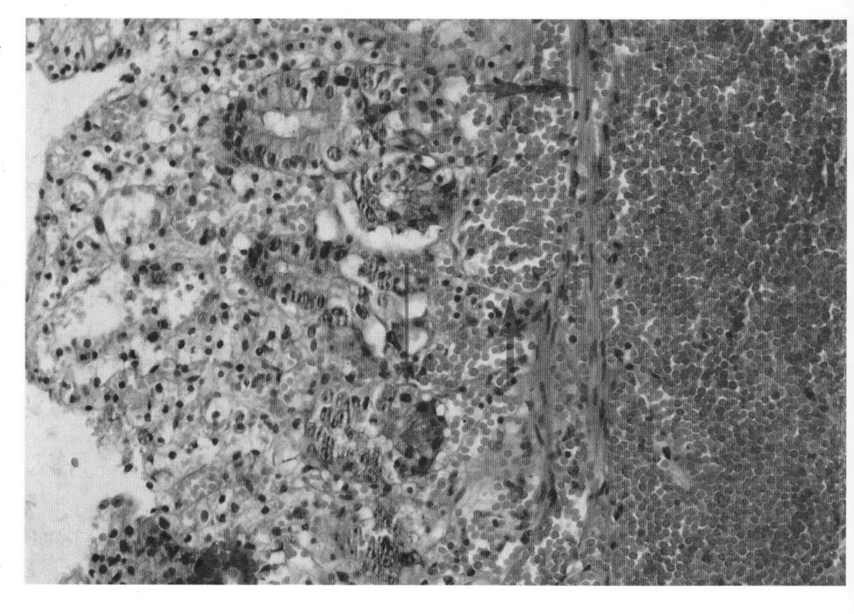

2.21 Infarct: ileum

Infarction is tissue necrosis, caused by reduction or loss of blood supply. In the small intestine, infarction can result from either venous or arterial obstruction. usually a major artery (usually the superior mesenteric) is occluded. However venous infarction may occur, following mechanical occlusion of mesenteric veins (in a twisted a loop of intestine). In this infarct of the small intestine, there is extensive necrosis of the mucosa, and the intestinal villi (left) have lost their surface layer of tall epithelial cells and collapsed. The crypts of the glands (thin arrow), although they appear somewhat degenerate, are still lined by epithelial cells with deeply stained round nuclei. The small blood vessels (thick arrow) underlying the crypts are greatly dilated. The muscularis mucosae itself seems to be viable, consisting of elongated smooth muscle cells (double arrow) which retain their well-stained elongated nuclei. Characteristically there is also, beneath the muscularis mucosae, extensive hemorrhage into the infarcted tissue, in the form of a large collection of extravasated deeply red blood on the right. HE ×235

2.22 Celiac disease (gluten enteropathy): jejunum

Celiac disease is intestinal malabsorption caused by hypersensitivity to gluten, and it reduces the absorptive surface of the intestine to a remarkable extent. The patient in this case was hypersensitive to wheat gluten and examination with the dissecting microscope showed great reduction in the height of the villi (partial villus atrophy), mostly in the duodenum and upper part of the jejunum but not in the ileum. In a normal intestine, the villi are covered by single layer of tall columnar epithelial cells, but in this field the villus that is demonstrated is markedly atrophic. Instead of being slender and finger-shaped, the villus is very short and broad (leaf- or spade-shaped) and covered with a layer of small cuboidal or low-columnar epithelial cells, irregular in size and shape. The epithelial cells rest on a greatly thickened and hyaline basement membrane. Beneath (and within) the basement membrane there are dilated small blood vessels (thin arrows), a small number of lymphocytes and a much larger number of round plasma cells, each with an eccentric nucleus (located at one pole of the cell) (thick arrows). There are also a few lymphocytes between the epithelial cells. HE ×200

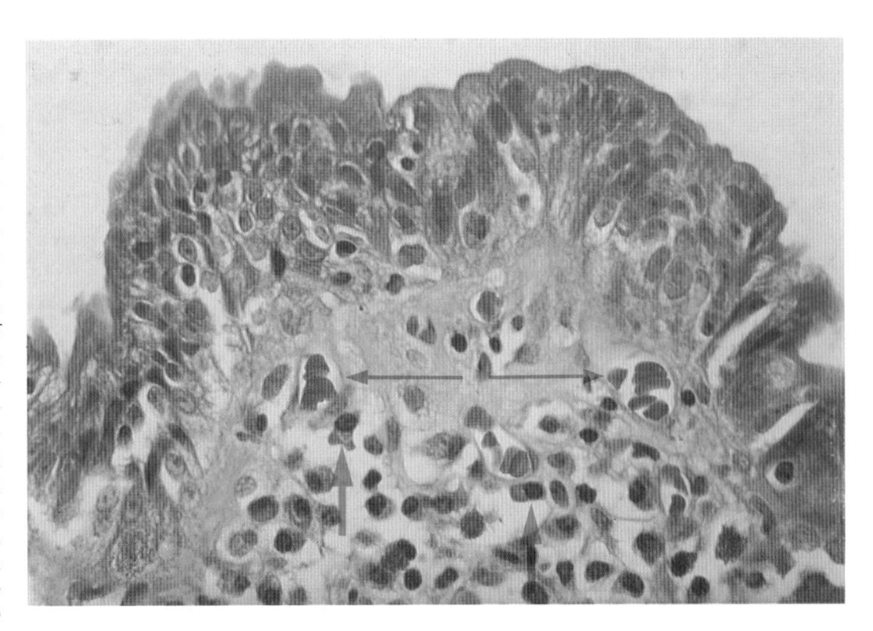

2.23 Intestinal lymphangiectasis: ileum

In intestinal lymphangiectasis, an uncommon condition, the villi containing the dilated lymphatics are shortened and distorted. Consequently the flow of lymph from the small intestine is obstructed, which leads to malabsorption of fat and fat-related vitamins. Fat is lost in congenital forms of lymphangiectasis, associated with malformation of lymphatics, and lymphocytes which may cause immunodeficiency are also lost, as may protein-rich fluid into the lamina propria and then into the lumen of the gut (protein-losing enteropathy). In this field, there is a single villus, projecting (leftwards) into the lumen of the small intestine. The villus is markedly swollen, from the presence in its core of a greatly-dilated lymphatic vessel (thin arrow), around which there are dilated small blood vessels. The surface of the villus is covered with a single layer of tall columnar epithelial cells (thick arrow), with much eosinophilic cytoplasm and ovoid basal nuclei. The epithelial cells appear normal. All the other villi in the biopsy specimen showed similar features. HE ×360

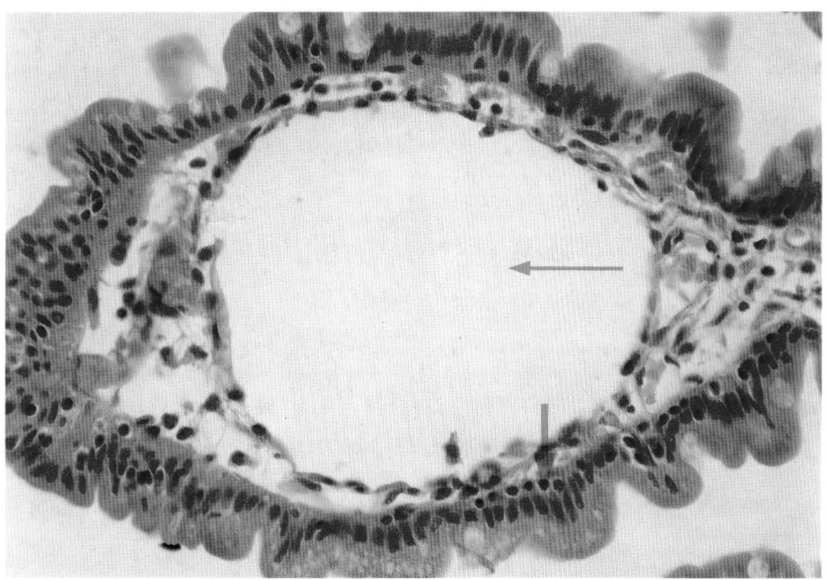

2.24 Typhoid (enteric) fever: ileum

Typhoid fever is a systemic infection caused by *Salmonella typhi*. The bacilli attach themselves to the epithelium lining the small intestine and penetrate it to reach the submucosa, where they are ingested by neutrophils and macrophages. The bacilli are not killed by the phagocytes but proliferate within them. Peyer's patches and the lymphoid follicles swell and many become necrotic, with ulceration of the overlying mucosa. Hemorrhage and perforation of the wall of the intestine are liable to occur. The patient in this case had been ill for about 10 days, and the lymphoid tissue in this Peyer's patch has been replaced by large macrophages (thick arrows) with a considerable amount of eosinophilic cytoplasm and round vesicular nuclei. Mingling with them are similar cells containing a smaller deeply basophilic nucleus, lymphocytes and plasma cells, but no polymorph leukocytes. Necrosis is occurring, the tissue consisting only of cytoplasmic and nuclear debris (thin arrow), but a Gram's stain would reveal large numbers of typhoid bacilli. During recovery, the necrotic cells are phagocytosed and the epithelium quickly spreads over the ulcerated area, producing very little scarring. The thin-walled blood vessel at the right margin is greatly dilated (double arrow). HE ×135

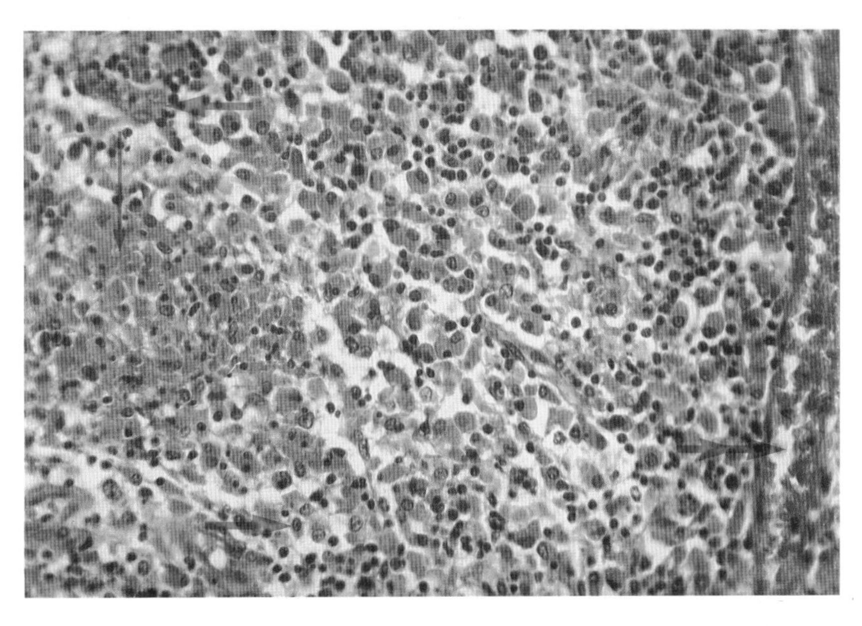

2.25 Crohn's disease

Although the cause of Crohn's disease is still unknown, the disease closely resembles tuberculosis, and an atypical mycobacterium has been (and still is) regarded as the most likely etiological agent. The lesions in the intestine are patchy, and although the intervening mucosa may appear normal, it tends to be become edematous and produce a cobblestone pattern. A woman of 51 had 42cm of terminal ileum and 10cm of caecum removed for Crohn's disease. The mucosa of the ileum was inflamed, with extensive patchy ulceration (which tends to be linear) and loss of the normal mucosal pattern. The mucosa of the caecum showed an irregular 'mosaic' pattern. The mesentery of the small intestine was greatly thickened. This is the caecum, with the lumen of the bowel on the left. There is intense edema of the mucosa and submucosa, with diffuse infiltration with weakly eosinophilic fluid. The lymphatics in the submucosa (thin arrows) and the mucosa (thick arrows) are dilated. Chronic inflammatory cells are present in moderate numbers, mostly beneath the surface epithelium (left). Red-staining Paneth cells can be detected in the crypts of the colonic glands. HE ×60

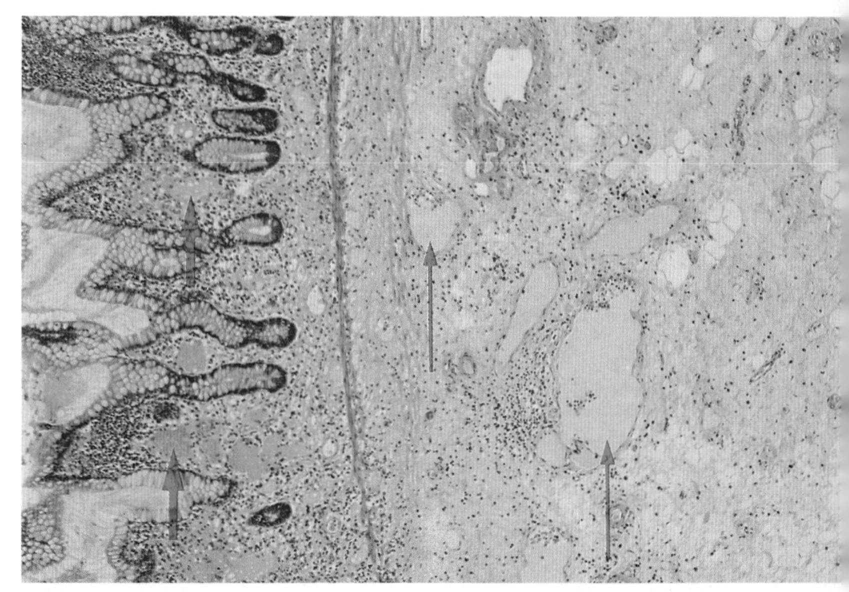

2.26 Crohn's disease: ileum

In Crohn's disease, the process is inflammatory. Whereas in ulcerative colitis the lesions are essentially mucosal, Crohn's disease usually involves all layers of the bowel wall (transmural inflammation). Healing produces fibrous tissue which, along with the inflammatory edema, is liable to thicken and obstruct the intestine, thereby producing a common complication of Crohn's disease. In this case, the disease was confined to the ileum, and this field shows part of the affected mucosa and submucosa. On both sides of the intact muscularis mucosae (thin arrow) the tissues are heavily infiltrated by extremely large numbers of inflammatory cells. Most of them are lymphocytes and plasma cells, but there is also a large crypt abscess (double arrow). The abscess has developed in a greatly distended crypt, in one intestinal gland, and it consists (almost exclusively) of polymorph leukocytes. Epithelial cells line only part of the crypt, the bottom of which is disrupted, and most of the cells are flattened (thick arrow). Crypt abscesses are associated more with ulcerative colitis than with Crohn's disease. HE ×135

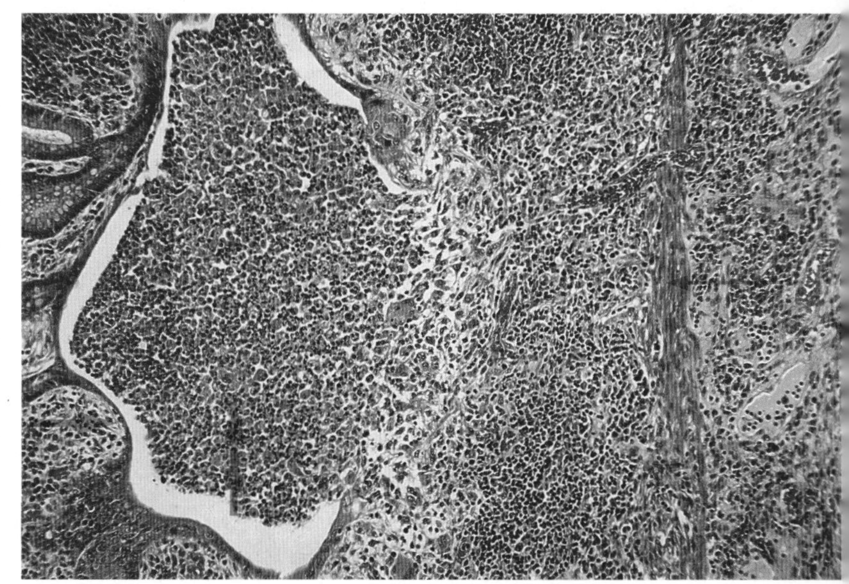

2.27 Crohn's disease: anal canal

In Crohn's disease, all layers of the intestinal wall are inflamed; that is, transmural inflammation. The most constant (and diagnostic) features of the inflammatory process are focal infiltrates of lymphocytes and non-caseating epithelioid cell granulomas which resemble a sarcoid granuloma. Epithelioid granulomas may be present not only in the bowel wall and mesentery but also in the associated lymph nodes. Their presence helps to distinguish the Crohn' disease from ulcerative colitis but they may be difficult to detect. This lesion is in the anal canal. The canal is lined with a fairly thick layer of stratified squamous epithelial cells (thick arrows) with round or ovoid pale vesicular nuclei, in some of which there is a prominent nucleolus. Occasional polymorph leukocytes and lymphocytes infiltrate the squamous epithelial cells, and in the submucosa there is a follicular collection (thin arrow) of large epithelioid cells, surrounded by a small number of lymphocytes and other chronic inflammatory cells. The epithelioid cells have pleomorphic vesicular nuclei and much eosinophilic cytoplasm, and some of them are degenerate. Multinucleated giant cells are often present along with the epithelioid cells within the follicle. HE ×200

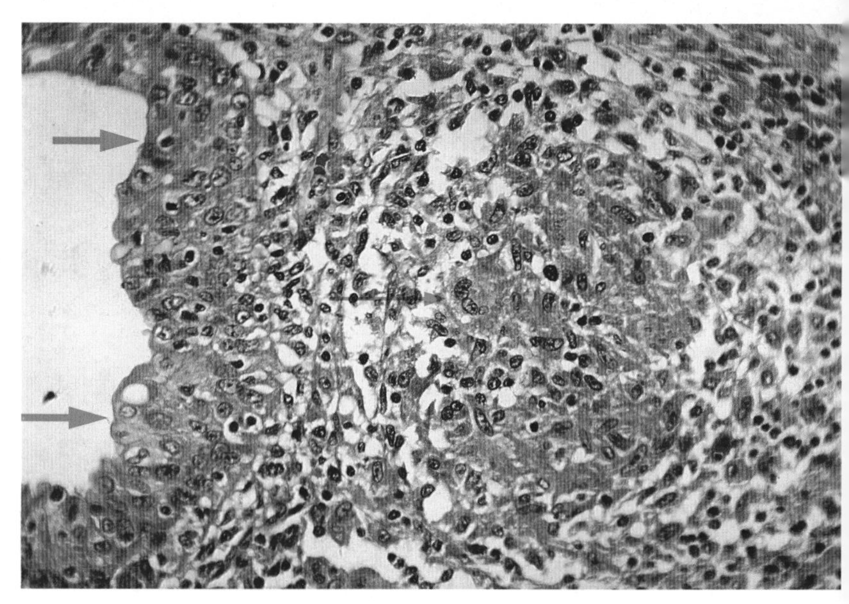

2.28 Ulcerative colitis: colon

In ulcerative colitis the inflammatory process is relatively superficial compared with Crohn's disease, but the mucosa may be extensively ulcerated and hemorrhage may be severe. The mucosa between the ulcerated areas tends to project as pseudopolyps. This shows the mucosa of the colon, with the lumen at the top of the field. The mucosa is acutely inflamed and intensely hyperemic, and its surface is covered with a single layer of epithelial cells which vary greatly in size and shape (thin arrows). In the mucosa there is also a fairly dense infiltrate of inflammatory cells and it is particularly intense (double arrow) in the region of the muscularis mucosae. The majority of the glands are irregular in shape, apparently having been compressed by the swollen interglandular tissue. The epithelial cells lining the glands vary in form from atrophic and almost completely flattened to low cuboidal). However several other glands are distended with mucus and inflammatory cells (thick arrows), and one of them (top centre arrow) resembles a crypt abscess, the contents appearing pus-like. HE ×60

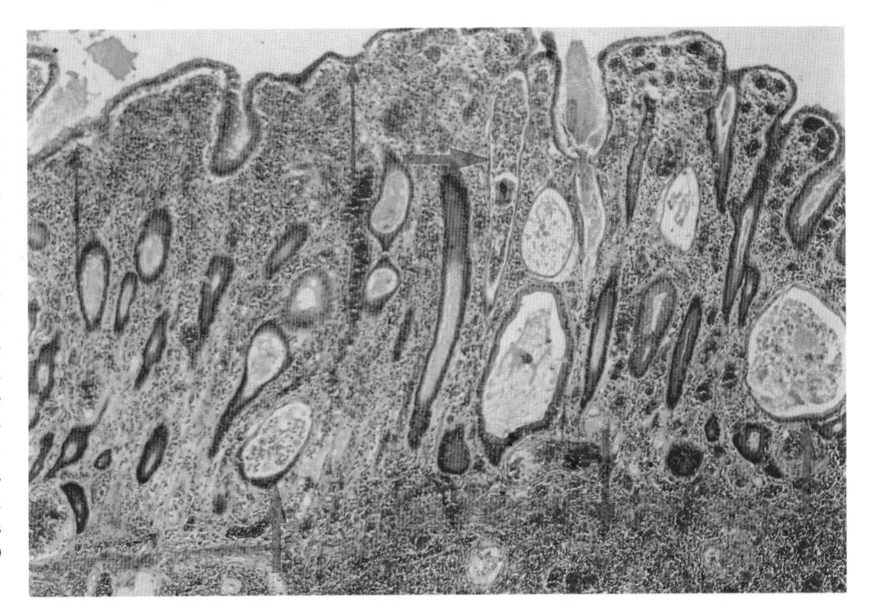

2.29 Ulcerative colitis: colon

Ulcerative colitis is a disease of colonic epithelium, which undergoes recurrent damage and attempts at regeneration. Characteristic features of the condition are depletion of goblet cells, abnormal crypts and crypt abscesses. This is part of the colonic mucosa is from **2.28**, at higher magnification. Only a small part of the mucosal surface (lower left) is visible and it is covered with single layer of cuboidal or low columnar epithelial cells (thin arrow), with eosinophilic cytoplasm which appears to secrete very little mucin. The glands are lined by a single layer of flat elongated and severely attenuated cells (thick arrow); and several of the glands (top half of field) are filled with strongly eosinophilic secretion and some cell fragments. One gland (along bottom of field) is packed pus-like material (crypt abscess) which consists of closely packed cell debris, mainly from degenerate polymorph leukocytes but also necrotic macrophages. A giant multinucleated cell is also present in the gland (double arrow). Between all the glands the mucosa is intensely hyperemic, with large numbers of considerably dilated small blood vessels. HE ×235

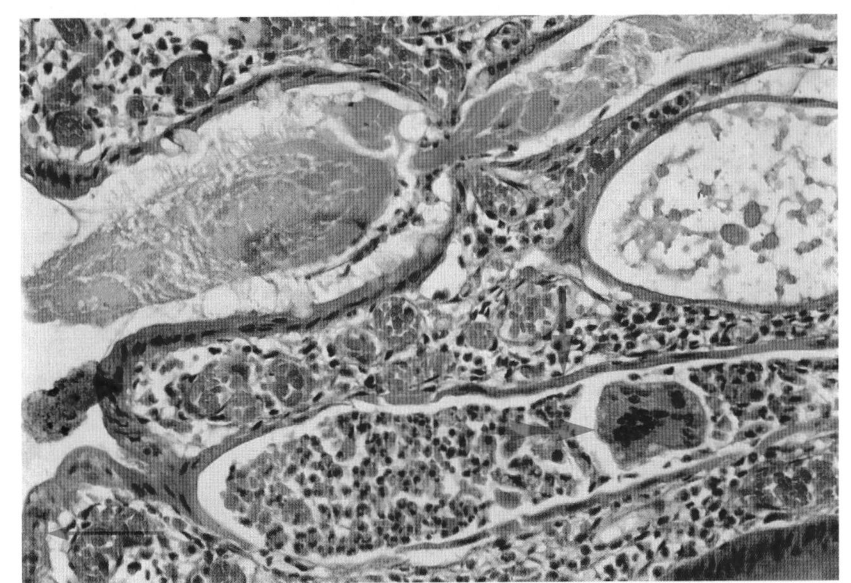

2.30 Ulcerative colitis: colon

The behaviour of ulcerative colitis (mainly as diarrhea) can vary widely, from mild and self-limiting to acute and fulminating, with numerous exacerbations and remissions over many years. Although the disease is primarily a disease of the colon and generally confined to it, the terminal ileum is also affected ('back-wash' ileitis) in a significant number of cases. In long-standing ulcerative colitis, there is an increased risk of carcinoma and it may arise at several sites. This a section of the colon from a long-standing case of ulcerative colitis. The lumen of the colon is just visible on the left (double arrow). The wall of the colon is thinner than normal. The mucosa and submucosa have been replaced by vascular granulation tissue (left half of picture) in which there are many dilated small blood vessels (thick arrow), as well as numerous plasma cells and lymphocytes. Small numbers of similar cells are present in the connective tissue beneath the serosal surface of the peritoneum (extreme right) and throughout the very atrophic eosinophilic muscle fibres (thin arrow) which form the wall of the colon. HE ×60

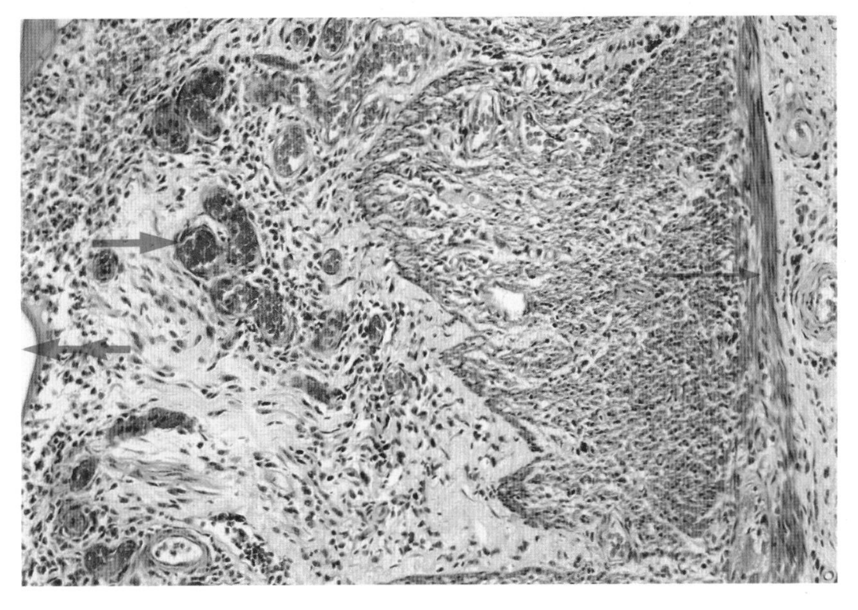

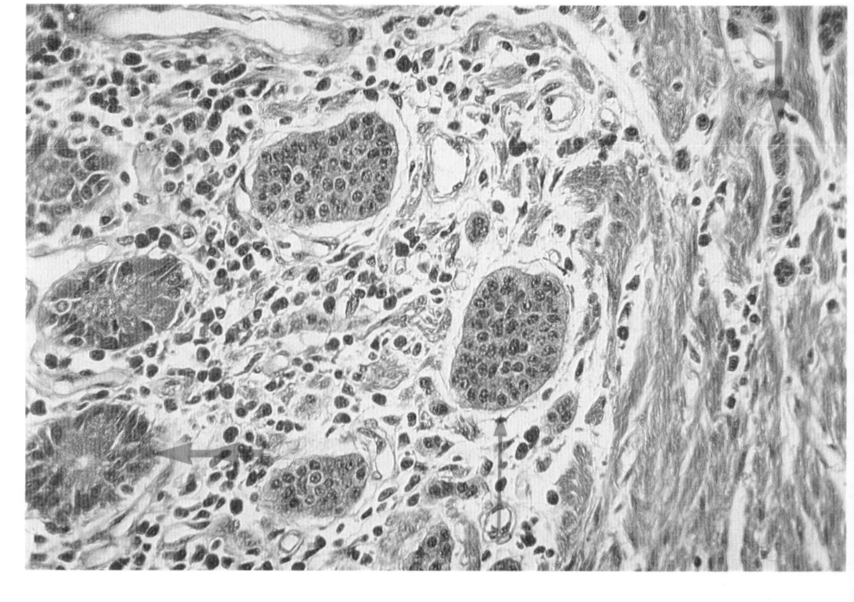

2.31 Carcinoid tumour: caecum

Carcinoid tumours generally take the form of small submucosal (generally) nodules, sometimes yellow but often grey. They arise from Kulchitsky cells (of the diffuse endocrine system) which secrete 5-hydroxytryptamine (serotonin). Carcinoid tumours of the alimentary tract are usually located in the ileum but may metastasize to the lymph nodes and liver. Extensive secondary deposits may give rise to the carcinoid syndrome. This field is from a small nodule in the wall of the caecum. The crypts of the intestinal glands are just visible (in cross-section) on the left (double arrow), and in the submucosa between the glands and the muscle coats on the right, there are several compact solid groups (surrounded by a thin basement membrane) of uniform polyhedral cells (thin arrow) with a moderate amount of cytoplasm and round or ovoid vesicular nuclei. Smaller groups of cells (thick arrow) are invading the eosinophilic muscle fibres. There is no mitotic activity among the tumour cells. In the tissues between the groups of tumour cells there are many eosinophil leukocytes. HE ×135

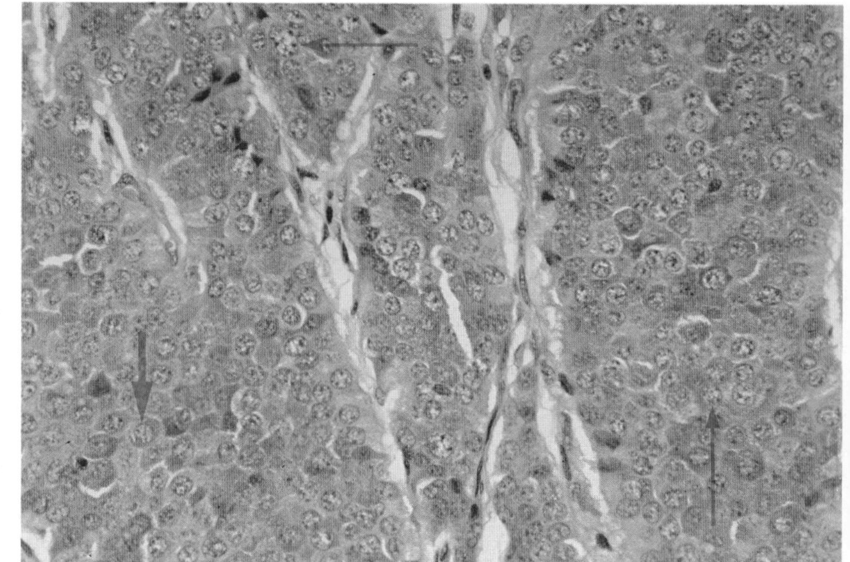

2.32 Secondary carcinoid tumour: lymph node

Carcinoid tumours are slow-growing lesions which invade locally but do not metastasize readily. Occasionally however very small tumours may be associated with distant metastases. Carcinoid tumours are usually asymptomatic, but sometimes endocrine secretion produces systemic effects. This is a metastatic deposit in a lymph node in the neck, from a primary tumour of unknown origin. It consists of groups of closely packed cells of uniform type. The cells have large round vesicular nuclei (thin arrows) in which the chromatin forms small clumps, a characteristic feature of cells of this type; and in some cells, particularly those situated towards the centre of the cords of cells, the cytoplasm is well-defined and intensely eosinophilic (thick arrow). No mitoses are evident. Membrane-bound dense core granules may be demonstrated in the cytoplasm, and special stains can detect argentaffin granules at the periphery of cytoplasm (2.33). Delicate bands of stromal connective tissue run between the groups of tumour cells. Macroscopically, bands of fibrous tissue may cause kinking & partial obstruction of the intestine. HE ×360

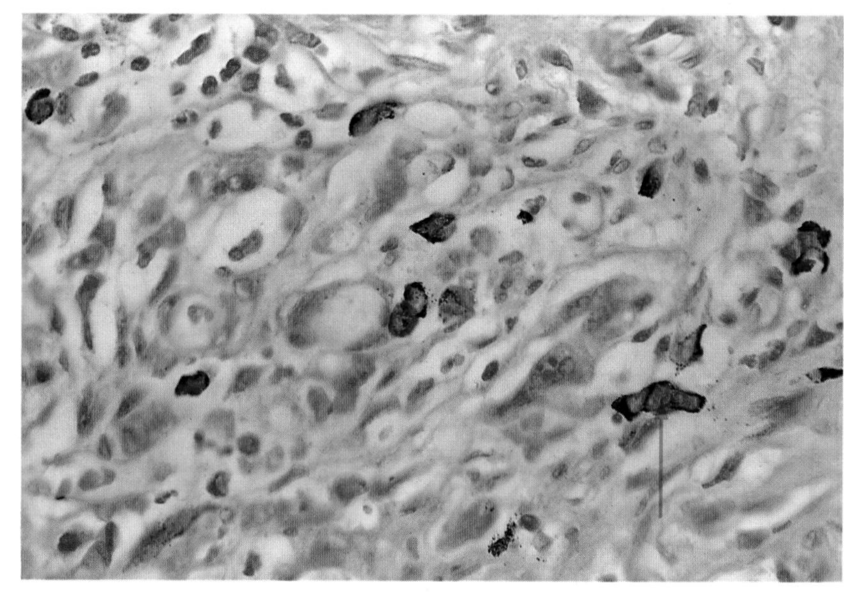

2.33 Carcinoid tumour: appendix

Carcinoid tumours may be found in various sites in the gastrointestinal tract, and most often in appendix & rectum. They may also be located in the gallbladder & (rarely) in teratomatous ovarian tumours. The neoplastic cells may be arranged in solid nests, trabeculae, anastomosing bands or (uncommonly) ribbons & rosette-like formations. This tumour was found in the wall of an acutely inflamed appendix from a woman of 62. Its colour was yellow, following fixation in formalin, and it has penetrated the muscle coats to the serosa. This is a histological section which has been stained by the Grimelius technique (an argyrophil method), using a silver-containing reagent; and another solution has been used to 'develop' the sites of deposition of the silver in the section. The cytoplasm of the carcinoid cells is a dense black colour, and the nuclei are orange-red (from the counterstain) (arrow). Carcinoid tumours of the proximal parts of the alimentary tract (duodenum and stomach) and of the lung tend to be argentaffin-negative; that is, they do not react directly with silver nitrate solutions but are usually positive with argyrophil methods such as the Grimelius technique. Grimelius method ×575

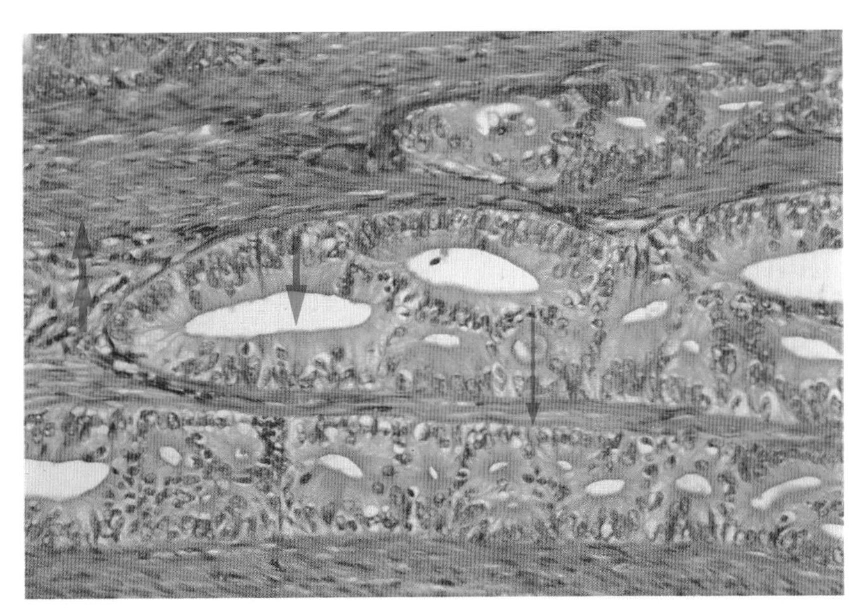

2.34 Adenocarcinoma: small intestine

Primary adenocarcinomas of the small intestine are uncommon and exhibit a wide range of growth patterns. Most tumours of this type arise in the duodenum, in the region of the ampulla of Vater (2.18) and form papillary growths, but elsewhere carcinoma of the small intestine tends (like colonic carcinoma) to encircle the bowel wall and form ulcerating or annular stenosing growths which produce stenosis and obstruction of the intestine. This tumour consists of greatly elongated malignant glands and acini of widely varying size, lined by tall columnar cells with eosinophilic cytoplasm and a 'brush' border at their apex (thick arrow), and closely resembling the normal columnar epithelium of the glands of the small intestine. The nuclei of the tumour cells are closely packed, ovoid or round and vesicular, with some tendency to layering. They are however fairly regular in size and shape. Arranged in parallel columns, the malignant glands (thin arrow) are invading the eosinophilic muscle fibres (double arrow) of the intestinal wall. Mitotic activity is low elsewhere in the tumour.

HE ×235

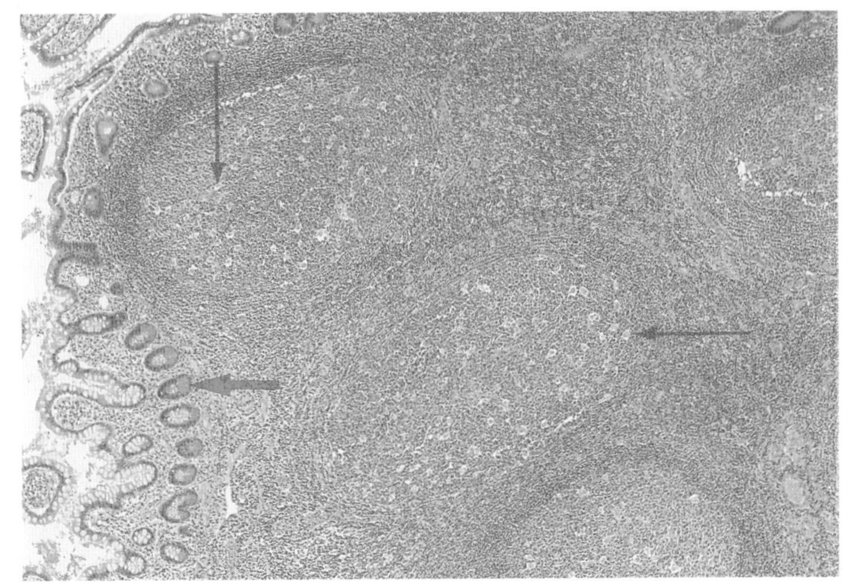

2.35 Lymphoid hyperplasia: ileum

Lymphoid hyperplasia (pseudolymphoma) in the small intestine is rare and, macroscopically, it is generally indistinguishable from lymphoma or carcinoma. The condition may be focal and take the form of a single mass, which may lead to intussusception; or it may be more diffuse, appearing as small nodules of lymphoid tissue scattered throughout the intestine (this latter is often associated with infection by *Giardia lamblia*). In this case, the lesion is a single large mass of extremely hyperplastic lymphoid tissue which projects into the lumen of the ileum on the left. The mucosa (left margin) is stretched over the lymphoid tissue, in which there are very large reactive germinal centres. In the germinal centres there are many macrophages with much pale or clear cytoplasm which, against the background of a large population of deeply basophilic small lymphocytes, produces a 'starry--sky' pattern (thin arrows). The villi of the mucosa overlying the lymphoid tissue are reduced in height, and the epithelial cells on the mucosal surface and lining the glands are mostly mucin-secreting goblet cells. The cores of the villi are distended with lymphocytes, and in one part of the mucosa (double arrow) there are no villi. Deeply eosinophilic Paneth cells (thick arrow) are prominent in the crypts of Lieberkühn. HE ×60

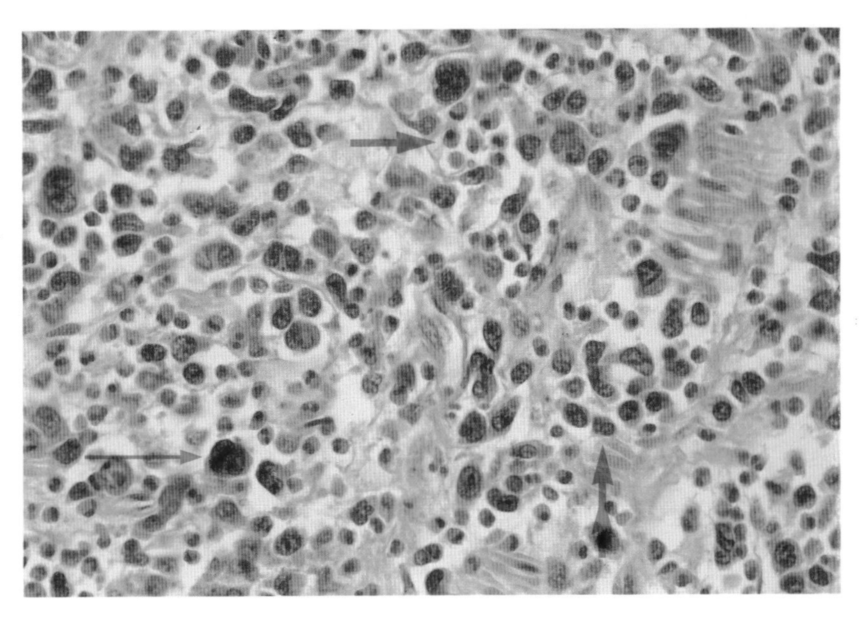

2.36 Immunoblastic lymphoma: small intestine

Lymphomas arising outside the alimentary tract may involve it secondarily but lymphomas sometimes arise in the gut itself (usually the ileum), often in association with celiac disease or related malabsorption syndromes. They generally form a large polypoid mass but there are sometimes multiple masses. This lesion, in the small intestine, is a high grade immunoblastic lymphoma, consisting of large immunoblasts (B- or T-type). The immunoblasts sometimes show varying degrees of plasmablastic or plasmacytic differentiation. In this field, the immunoblasts are large or very large round cells (thin arrow) with a moderate amount of cytoplasm and large very pleomorphic and deeply basophilic nuclei which vary widely in size and shape. In many of the nuclei the chromatin pattern is coarse and the larger nuclei are clearly vesicular. Some of the immunoblasts are binucleated. The immunoblasts (double arrow) are invading the smooth muscle fibres in the wall of the intestine and are accompanied by a large number of much smaller eosinophil leukocytes (thick arrow). HE ×360

2.37 *Enterobius vermicularis* (Oxyuriasis): appendix

Infestation with *Enterobius vermicularis* is common in some countries and it particularly affects children. It is a small worm (threadworm or pinworm), 10-12mm long, and it is acquired by ingesting eggs which hatch in the ileum as larvae. The larvae then emigrate to the appendix and large intestine, and may congregate in the appendix in numbers large enough to fill its lumen. The worms are occasionally found in appendices resected surgically, but they are not the cause of appendicitis. In this appendix, the lumen is dilated and contains several worms which have been cut in various planes. The outer coat of the worm consists of eosinophilic amorphous chitin (thin arrow), and the viscera are clearly visible inside the worms. The mucosa (thick arrow) lining the appendix is thick, with numerous elongated glands surrounded by a dense population of small basophilic lymphocytes and lymphoid follicles. There is pus-like material (double arrow) in the lumen of the appendix, but the mucosal surface is intact. HE 75

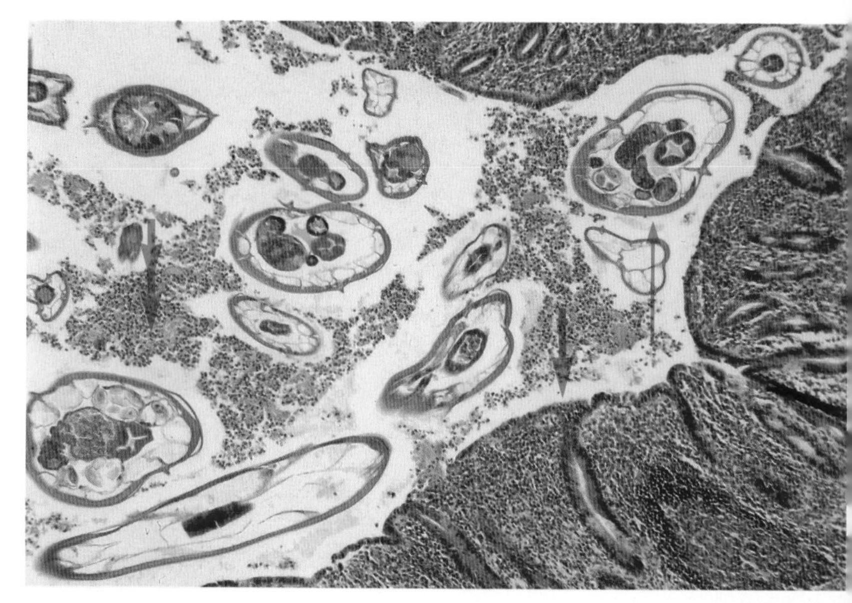

2.38 *Enterobius vermicularis* (Oxyuriasis): appendix

Enterobius vermicularis is an active parasite, and can migrate considerable distances in the individual; for example, it may cause pruritus ani, or (uncommonly) a gravid female worm may migrate up the female genital tract and reach the peritoneal cavity via the uterus and Fallopian tubes. An appendix 9cm long was removed at operation from a woman of 21. It was not macroscopically inflamed but the lumen contained several threadworms. This lesion is in the submucosa of the appendix. It takes the form of an oval sheet of cells, consisting of large numbers of eosinophilic epithelioid macrophages (thin arrow), a smaller population of small lymphocytes and occasional elongated fibroblasts, surrounded by a dense population of the small lymphocytes of the appendiceal lymphoid tissue. In the centre of the sheet the cells are necrotic and consist of bluish-red necrotic debris (double arrow). In the debris there is a fragment of a threadworm (thick arrow), which confirms that the lesion is a granuloma, produced by a threadworm which has invaded the wall of the appendix, presumably from the lumen. The lumen of the appendix did contain several worms. HE ×150

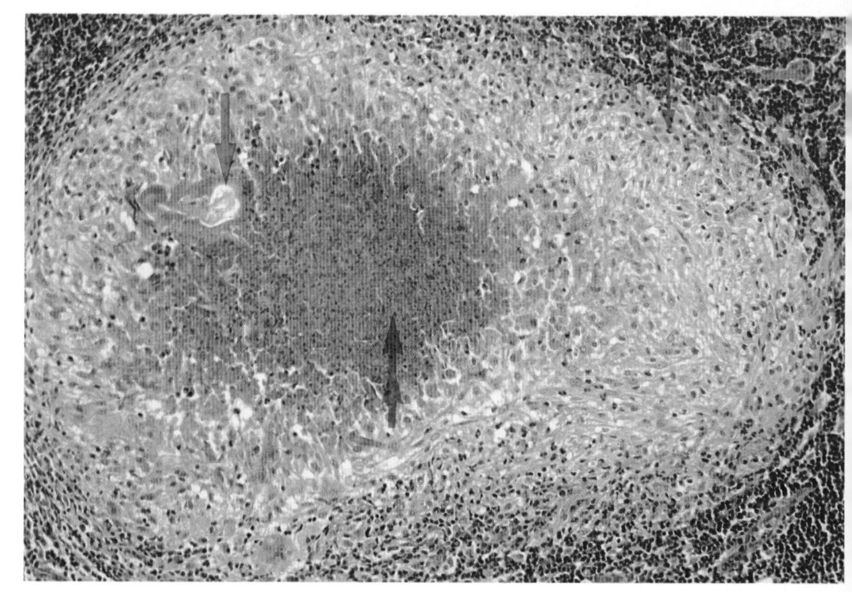

2.39 Acute appendicitis

Acute appendicitis is still common in Europe and the USA but uncommon in many other parts of the world, including Asia and Africa, probably for reasons of diet. The acute inflammatory process tends to spread along the muscular and serous coats, particularly if the lumen is obstructed. It may also spread to the peritoneal surface, and form fibrinous adhesions which enclose the appendix in a cavity, along with bacteria and many polymorph leukocytes. The number of leukocytes may be sufficient to form an abscess containing pus; that is, periappendiceal abscess formation. Gangrene may develop distal to the obstruction in the appendix, and perforation and peritonitis may follow. This field shows the wall of the appendix, with the lumen at the top. The mucosa has been largely destroyed and only a few remnants of the glands remain (double arrow). The blood vessels in the submucosa are greatly dilated (thick arrow). Large numbers of polymorph leukocytes have infiltrated the submucosa and the wall of smooth muscle fibres. The infiltrate is greatest in the submucosa, where it amounts to pus formation (suppuration) (thin arrow). There is also an exudate of fibrin and polymorphs on the peritoneal surface (bottom margin). HE ×60

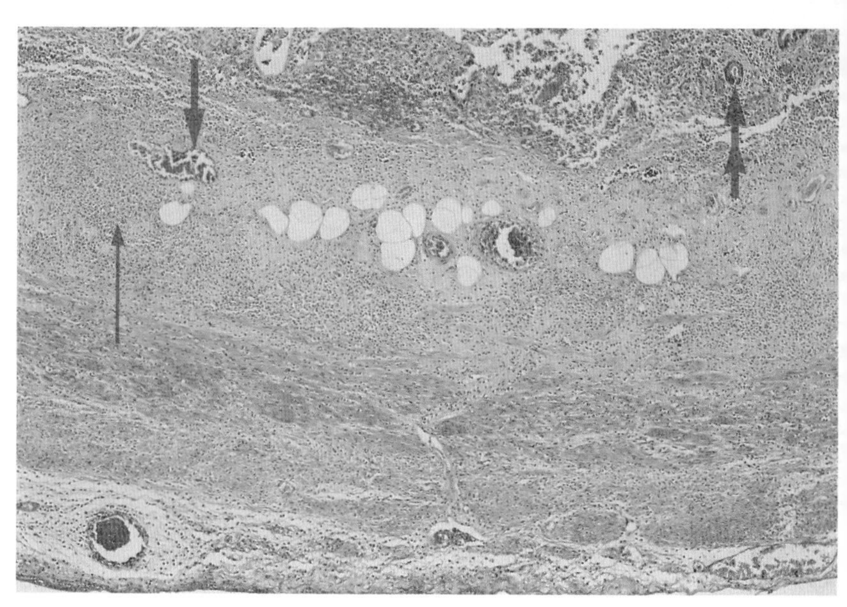

2.40 Acute appendicitis

Acutely inflamed appendices are swollen and the blood vessels appear intensely congested. Yellowish plaques of fibrin form on the peritoneal surface of the appendix, which makes the surface look rough. The mucosa lining the lumen is usually ulcerated, and large numbers of neutrophil leukocytes infiltrate the wall of the appendix deeply, and often as far as the serosa (transmural inflammation). Serosal inflammation usually also indicates peritoneal inflammation. This shows the same muscle coats of the appendix as in 2.39, at higher magnification. The smooth muscle fibres, cut in cross-section (thin arrow), are slightly vacuolated but still viable, and their nuclei are pale oval and vesicular. There is also a sparse infiltrate of macrophages and lymphocytes in the muscle coats. However, the adjacent bundles of slender smooth muscle fibres (thick arrow), cut longitudinally, are separated by a pus-like inflammatory exudate (double arrows) which consists mostly of large numbers of polymorph leukocytes and a small number of chronic inflammatory cells.

HE ×150

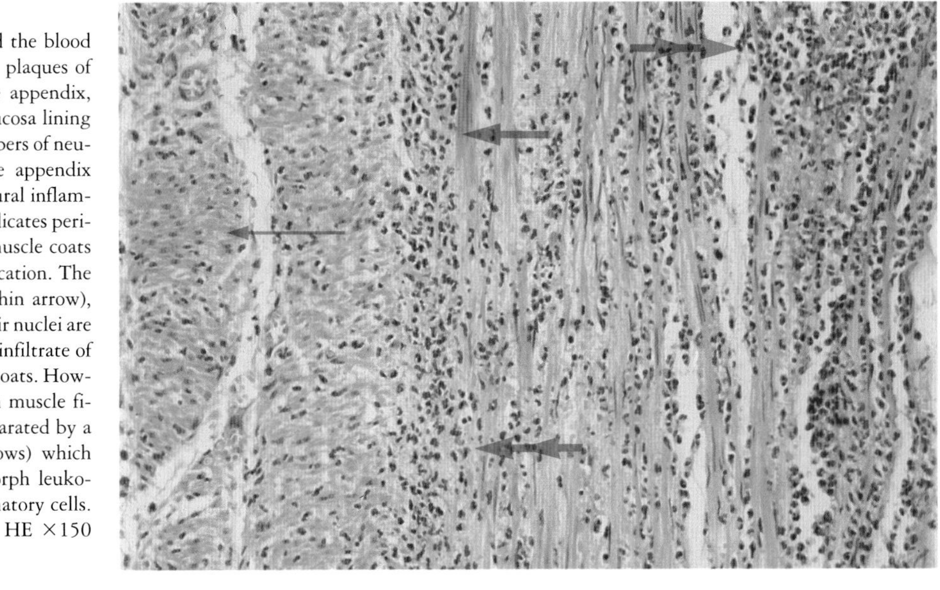

2.41 Acute appendicitis

This is an acutely inflamed appendix, infiltrated by an intense eosinophilic inflammatory exudate. There is also a fibrinous exudate on the peritoneal surface of the organ. Histologically, near the tip of the appendix, there is a focal lesion of the mucosa, with infiltration of the mucosa by large numbers of polymorph leukocytes. A large elongated gland, lined by a single layer of cuboidal epithelial cells, extends down into the mucosa. The base of the gland is ulcerated (thick arrow) and it is surrounded by a cuff of pus-like exudate (an abscess) (thin arrows). There is also a small amount of pus in the lumen of the affected gland (centre). The more superficial part of the gland is also encircled by pus-like exudate, and adjoining it part of the normal lymphoid tissue of the appendix is visible (double arrow). Acute appendicitis probably starts in this way, with a suppurative lesion (abscess) at the bottom of a crypt; but spread of the lesion to involve the whole appendix is greatly enhanced when the appendiceal lumen is obstructed, e.g. by a fecalith.

HE ×150

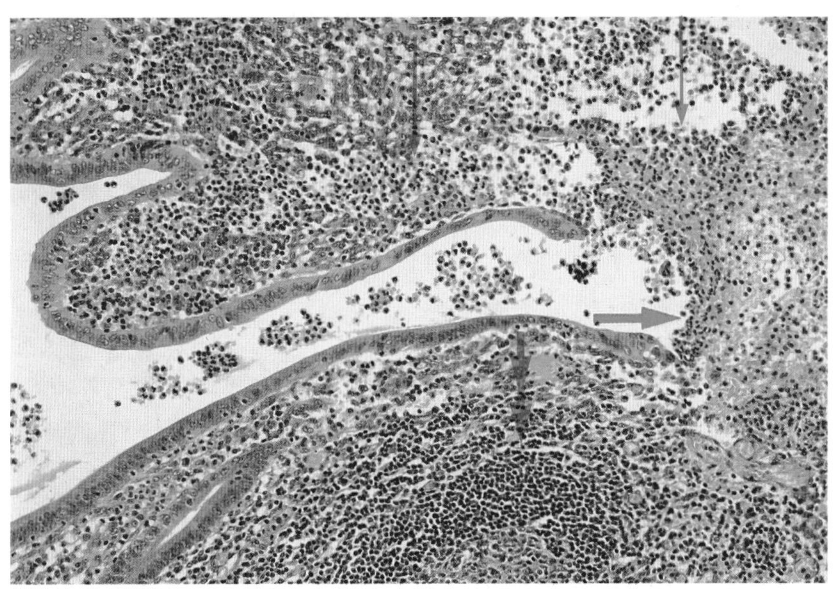

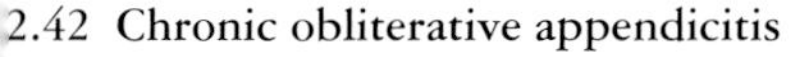

2.42 Chronic obliterative appendicitis

Previously, a patient with vague abdominal symptoms was liable to be diagnosed as chronic appendicitis, but chronic appendicitis is now generally regarded as a non-existent diagnosis. In older subjects, the lumen of the appendix is often obliterated by fibrosis, partly or completely, from the tip of the organ downwards. These changes may have been produced by previous episodes of acute inflammation, but they are much more likely to be the result of an ageing process in which the mucosal lymphoid tissue atrophies and is replaced by fibrous tissue. This field is from an appendix removed surgically for 'chronic appendicitis'. Both mucosa and submucosa of the appendix have disappeared, and the lumen is completely blocked (centre and left of field) by fat (thick arrow), fibrous tissue and thick-walled blood vessels (double arrow). The muscle coats of the wall of the appendix (thin arrow) appear to be relatively normal, and there is no cellular or vascular evidence for 'inflammation'.

HE ×60

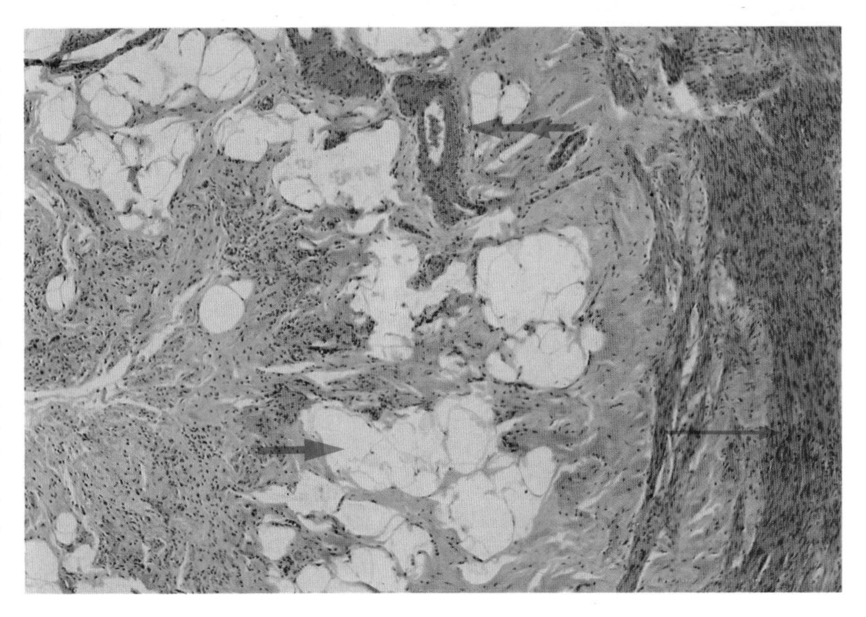

2.43 Hirschsprung's disease: colon

Hirschsprung's disease (idiopathic megacolon) is a congenital disorder which usually becomes evident soon after birth. The defect is one of innervation, the parasympathetic ganglion cells being absent (aganglionosis) from the intramural and submucosal plexuses (Meissner's and Auerbach's) of the distal part of the colon. Accordingly, coordinated propulsive movement does not occur in the abnormal (distal) colon, although the sigmoid colon and rectum usually appear normal. Consequently, it is the proximal (normal) part of the colon that is distended and may become acutely obstructed. The muscle coats of this (proximal) part of the colon undergo hypertrophy, if the patient survives. Unusually, the whole colon may show the abnormality, the aganglionic segment extending to the anus. Characteristically, in this field there are no ganglion cells, most of the field being occupied by a branch of the myenteric plexus. The nerve fibres appear hypertrophied (arrow), and elsewhere there are prominent bundles of nerve fibres in the muscularis mucosae. HE ×360

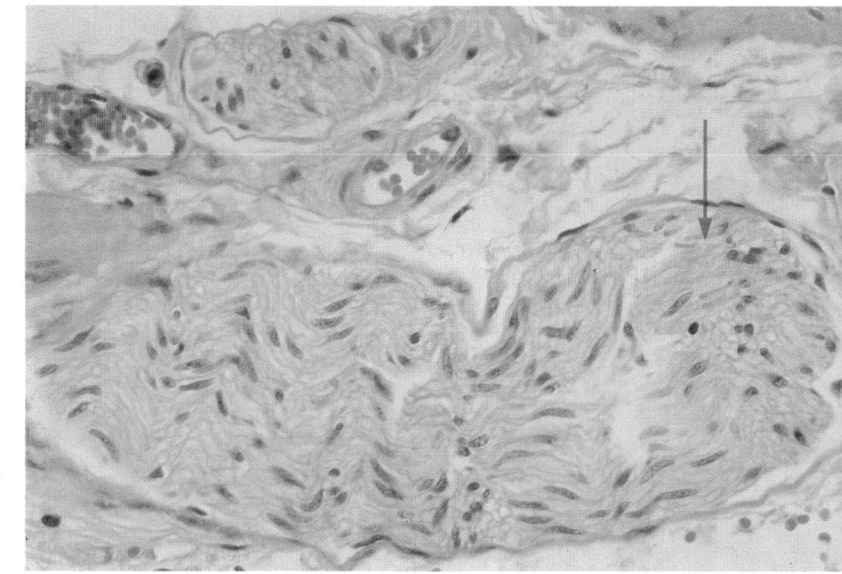

2.44 Pneumatosis intestinalis: colon

In pneumatosis intestinalis, soft polypoid (grape-like) swellings project into the lumen of the colon may cause intestinal obstruction. The swellings are gas-filled cysts and are located in the submucosa. The condition, which may affect the colon or small intestine, is sometimes associated with chronic lung disease or secondary to some other disease of the gastrointestinal tract. The swellings, which give the mucosa a 'cobble-stone' or 'pebbled' appearance, may be misdiagnosed as neoplastic lesions. The mucosa of the colon is at the top and left side of this field. It appears normal, as does the muscularis mucosae (thin arrow). In the submucosa, there is a large round cystic space which is completely empty (double arrow). The wall of the cystic space varies greatly in thickness, from very this to a thick layer of fibrous tissue (beneath the muscularis mucosae). The cystic space is lined, only in parts, by large and very large cells (thick arrows) with deeply eosinophilic cytoplasm, the other parts being lined only by fibrous tissue. There are scattered lymphocytes in the vicinity of the cystic cavity. The gas in the cystic cavity is not air but the product of bacterial action. HE ×60

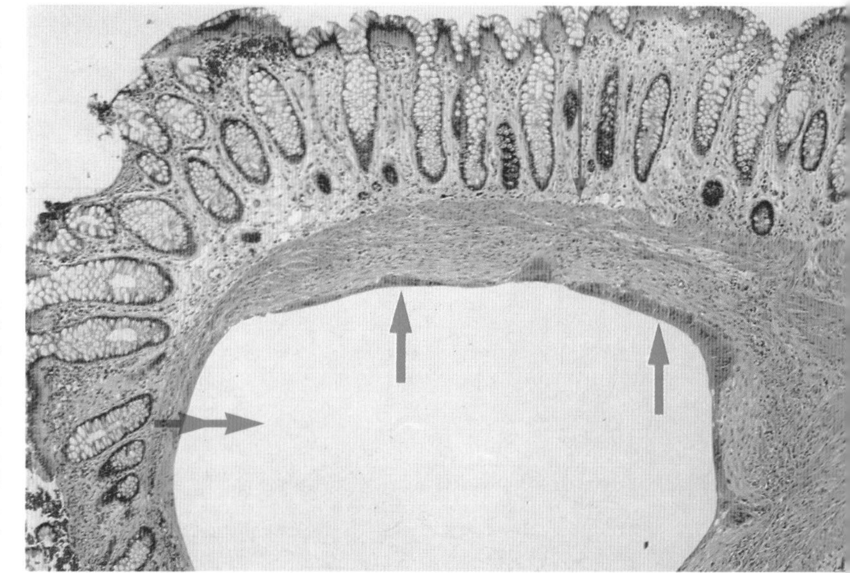

2.45 Pneumatosis intestinalis: colon

This is the same cyst and its wall as in 2.44, at higher magnification. Only a small segment of the cystic cavity is visible (double arrow), and it is lined by a single layer of closely apposed giant multinucleated cells (macrophages) with large amount of deeply eosinophilic cytoplasm (thin arrow). Presumably these giant cells should be regarded as a granulomatous reaction to the gas in the cystic cavity. The surfaces of the giant cells facing the lumen are flat, giving the lining of the cystic cavity a 'smooth' surface. The very basophilic parts of the crypts of the colonic glands are just visible at the top margin. The muscularis mucosae beneath the crypts is intact, and the elongated smooth muscle fibres of which it consists appear normal and fully viable. Between the muscularis mucosae and the giant cells lining the cystic cavity, there is a fairly thick layer band of eosinophilic collagenous fibrous tissue (thick arrow). Small numbers of lymphocytes and plasma cells are present in the connective tissues on both sides of the muscularis mucosae. HE ×235

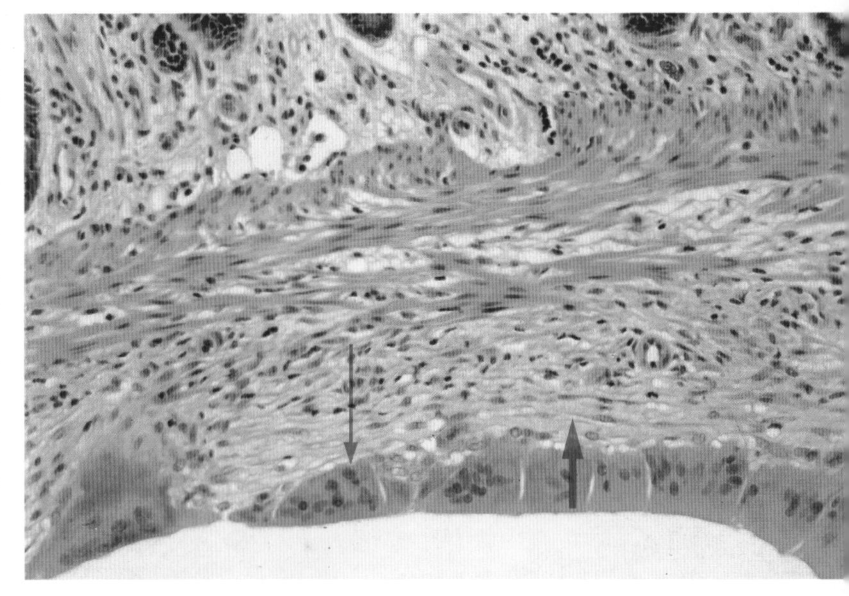

2.46 Pseudomembranous colitis

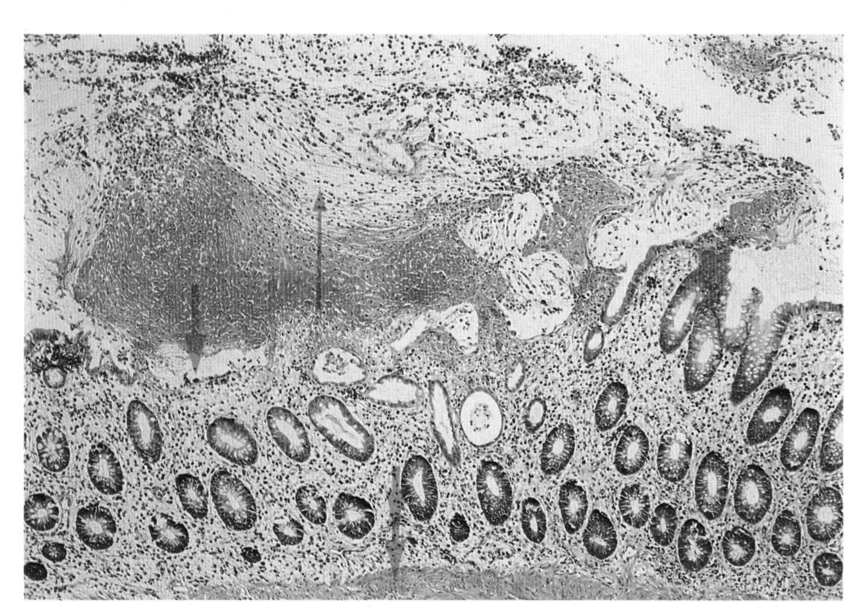

Some patients develop colitis after treatment with broad-spectrum antibiotics, such as lincomycin and clindamycin, which depress the normal flora. The watery diarrhea produced in this way may last for weeks. The pseudomembranous form of antibiotic-induced colitis however is probably caused by the anaerobic organism, *Clostridium difficile*, the toxin from which damages the wall of the bowel sufficiently to cause superficial necrosis of the mucous nmembrane. A biopsy of the mucosa may be required to establish the diagnosis. This is a specimen of rectal mucosa from a woman of 43 who developed post-operative diarrhea. The surface of the mucosa is covered with a fairly thick pseudomembrane which tends to assume a mushroom shape, the so-called 'summit' lesion. The membrane is a mixture of mucus (unstained) (thin arrow), large numbers of inflammatory cells (mainly polymorphs) and eosinophilic material (mainly fibrin and red cells). The mucosa underlying the pseudomembrane is ulcerated (thick arrow), the result of necrosis of the most superficial layer of the mucosa, but the deeper parts of the colonic glands are fully viable and remain. The muscularis mucosae (double arrow) appears normal.

HE ×60

2.47 Pseudomembranous colitis

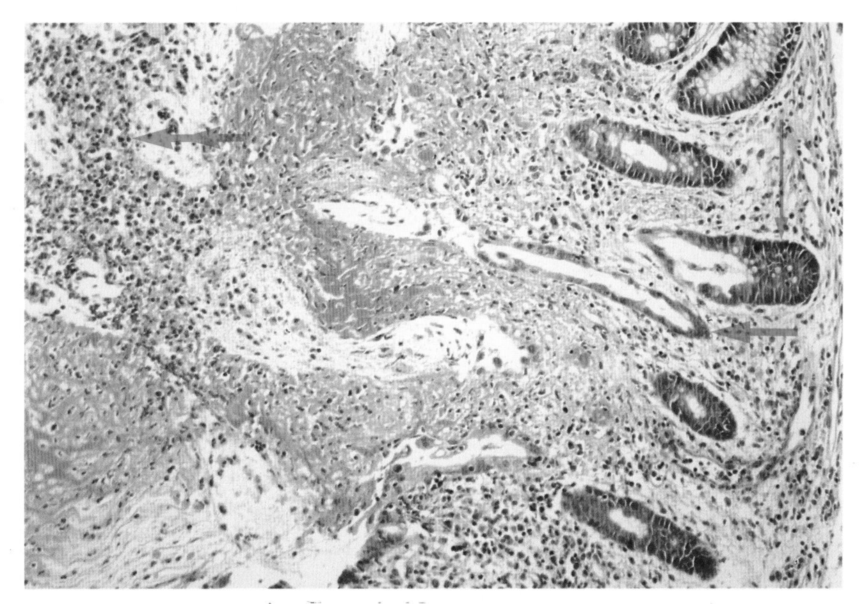

This is the same lesion as in 2.46, at higher magnification. Intestinal pseudomembranes are the products of bacteria of low invasive capacity (including *Clostridium difficile*) but producing potent exotoxins. In this field, the pseudomembrane is composed of deeply eosinophilic fibrin, very pale or colourless epithelial mucus and large numbers of small basophilic inflammatory cells of various types (double arrow), trapped in the weakly stained mucus. The pseudomembrane is firmly adherent to the surface of the colonic mucosa, and underlying it the most superficial parts of the mucus-secreting glands in the mucosa are necrotic. As a result, the mucosal surface is superficially ulcerated, but the damaged slightly distorted glands (thick arrow) are attempting to regenerate. In contrast however, the deeper parts of the partly-necrotic mucosal glands have survived (thin arrow). There is also an infiltrate of various types of inflammatory cells between the glands.

HE ×150

2.48 Epithelial dysplasia: colon

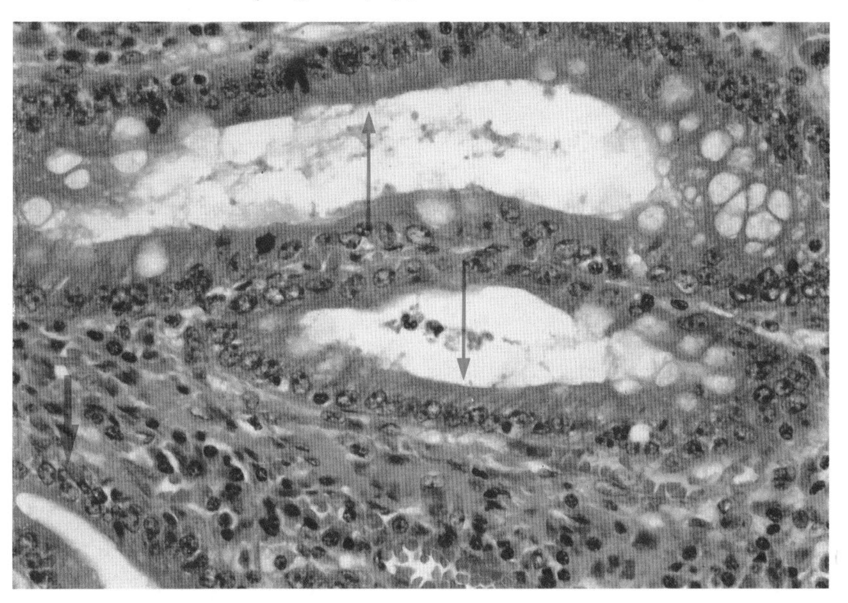

When dysplastic changes are being assessed, it is important to avoid areas that are actively inflamed, to prevent confusion with reactive changes. In patients with ulcerative colitis, there frequently are dysplastic changes in the colonic epithelium which may precede the development of malignancy and therefore a significantly increased risk of developing carcinoma of colon. In this tissue, resected from a woman of 62 with long-standing ulcerative colitis, there are two longitudinally-sectioned glands and a small part of another gland (thick arrow). The two larger glands are dysplastic, and lined by pleomorphic cuboidal or low-columnar epithelial cells (thin arrows). In both glands only a minority of the epithelial cells show active secretion of mucin, the others having uniform eosinophilic cytoplasm. The nuclei in the smaller of the two glands are round vesicular and fairly regular, but the nuclei in many of the closely packed cells lining the larger gland are significantly more pleomorphic and hyperchromatic. There are one or more prominent nucleoli in the epithelial cells in both glands. There is also mitotic activity in the cells lining the larger gland. There is a moderate infiltrate of small lymphocytes in the tissues adjacent to the glands.

HE ×150

2.49 Tubulovillous adenoma: colon

Adenomatous polyps are common lesions in the colon and occasionally undergo malignant change to adenocarcinoma. Tubular adenomas begin as flat lesions, 1-2mm dia, but tend to enlarge and become spheroidal (up to 3cm dia). They consist of elongated branching crypts which ramify and lack a stalk. However this tumour, cut longitudinally, is a tubulovillous adenoma, a combination of tubular and villous adenomas which takes the form of a polyp, a pedunculated mass of hyperchromatic epithelial cells attached to the wall of the colon by a slender stalk. The stalk of connective tissue (double arrow) is covered for most of its length with a mucosa consisting of normal-looking glands lined by a single layer of mature pale mucus-secreting epithelial cells (thin arrow). These pale epithelial cells gradually merge into the mass (the head of the polyp) which consists of large numbers of closely packed glands and tubules (thick arrows), irregular in size and shape, lined by deeply basophilic epithelial cells. The epithelium covering the surface of the polyp is not invading the stalk. HE x12

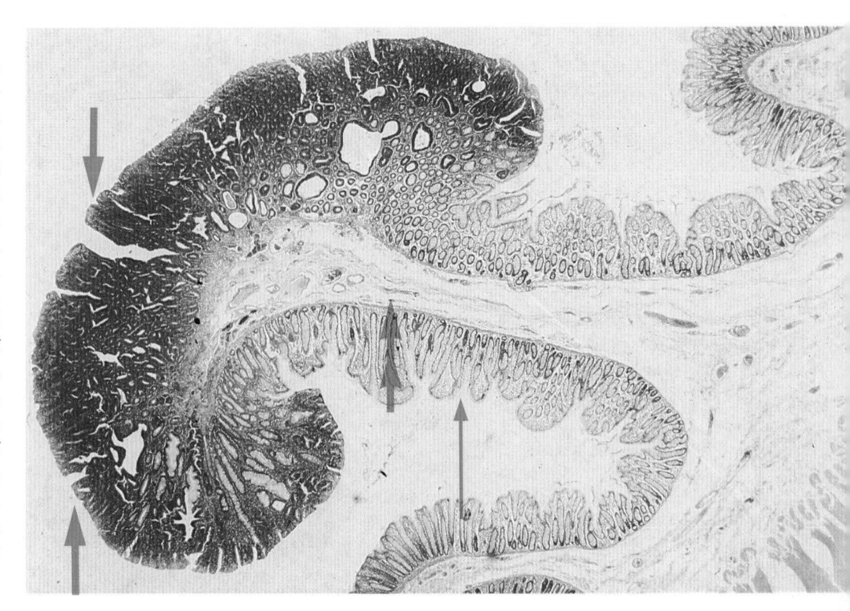

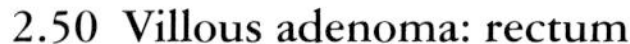

2.50 Villous adenoma: rectum

Villous adenomas (villous papillomas), less common than tubular adenomas, arise anywhere in the colon, but mostly in the rectum. They are generally more than 4cm dia, ovoid soft and flat and often without a stalk. The surface is covered with fine villous processes. A man of 68 had a large (10 × 6cm) villous adenoma of the rectum which was removed surgically. The tissue resected consists of papilliform processes, of varying lengths, growing more or less directly from the surface of the rectal mucosa. The tip of one villus is visible in this field, and covered with closely packed tall columnar epithelial cells with basophilic (round-ended) nuclei, elongated and heavily stratified (arrow). The epithelial cells on the surface of the villus and lining the glands secrete modest amounts of mucus. Mitotic activity was not detected but, at higher magnification, occasional mitotic figures were visible. The stalk of the villus has not been invaded, and the two glands (in cross-section) are enclosed in well-formed basement membrane. The core of the villus is infiltrated with lymphocytes and plasma cells. Villous papillomas of this type tend to become malignant (carcinomatous). HE x235

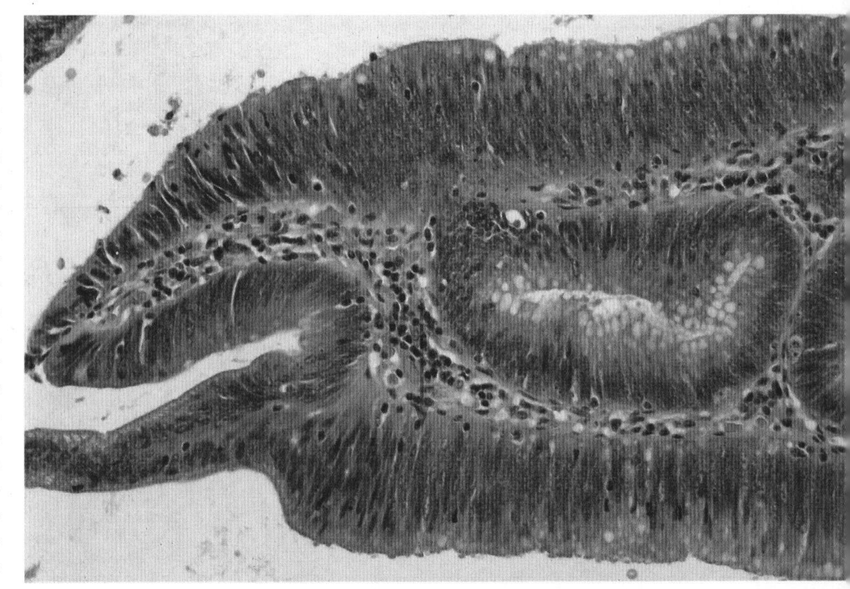

2.51 Villous adenoma: appendix

Villous adenoma, usually a single lesion of older age groups, tends to be located in the sigmoid colon or rectum. It consists of fine fronds, which sometimes branch, and a delicate core of collagenous tissue. Its surface is lined by a single layer of closely apposed tall columnar cells. It usually grows, encircling the lumen of the colon, but occasionally it has a short and thick stalk. Loss of fluid and electrolytes from a large lesion may cause hyponatremia, hypokalemia and dehydration. This villous adenoma in the appendix of a man aged 54, was unusual in that it was a small lesion which blocked the lumen of the appendix and produced a mucocele. It consists of slender papillae, each with a core of delicate connective tissue, heavily infiltrated with small round basophilic lymphocytes (thick arrow) and covered with tall columnar epithelial cells. Most of the epithelial cells have a large amount of deeply eosinophilic cytoplasm (thin arrow), but a minority are goblet cells, containing a large apical droplet of pale mucin (double arrow). The elongated vesicular round-ended nuclei show no pleomorphism. HE x150

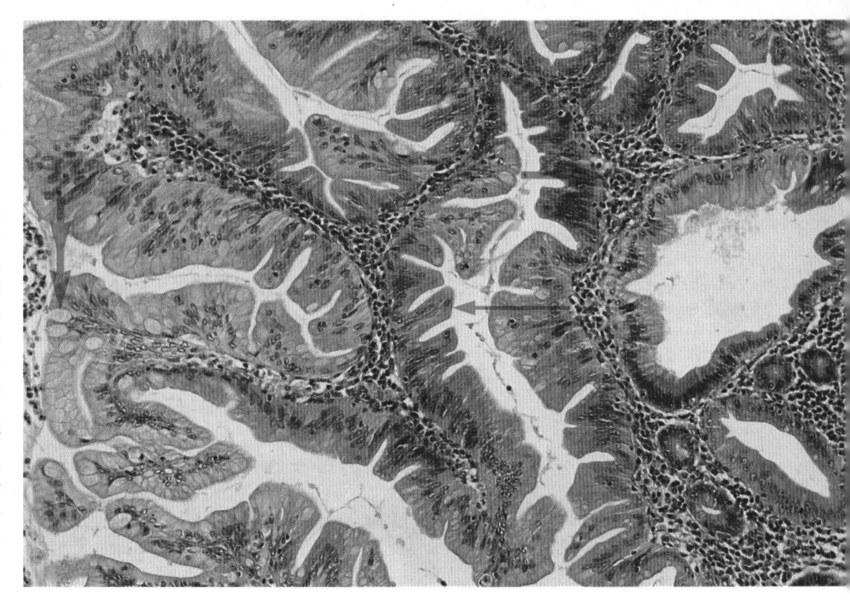

2.52 Villous adenoma: appendix

Sometimes a villous adenoma secretes large amounts of mucin, which cause diarrhea. Foci of dysplasia and carcinoma-in-situ are more common in villous adenomas than in tubular adenomas, and villous adenomas should be resected adequately. This is the same villous adenoma as in 2.51, at higher magnification. This field is occupied by the tip of one villous process. It has a core consisting of delicate connective tissue, a central small blood vessel, small round lymphocytes, plasma cells and a few macrophages. The core of the villous process is covered by a prominent basement membrane (double arrow), on which there is layer of large very tall columnar epithelial cells (thin arrow), very closely apposed to each other. The epithelial cells have a considerable amount of eosinophilic cytoplasm, and in a minority of them there is a large pale apical ovoid droplet of epithelial mucin (goblet-type epithelial cells). The epithelial nuclei are ovoid, vesicular and very regular in size and shape (thick arrow). There is no mitotic activity. There is some crowding of the nuclei, which may have been emphasized by oblique sectioning of the tissue. HE ×360

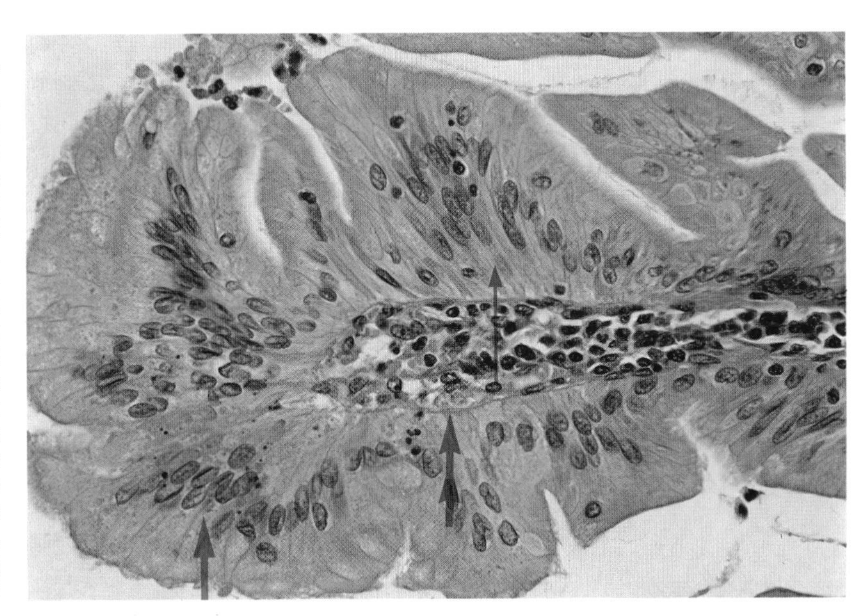

2.53 Adenocarcinoma: colon

Carcinoma of colon takes various forms, such as a fungating mass in the caecum and ascending colon, a hard infiltrating mass in the transverse, descending and sigmoid colon, and a flat ulcer in the rectum. Occasionally a carcinoma of colon has a stalk. Macroscopically this tumour took the form of an ulcer with a heaped-up ('rolled') edge, and it is now visible, histologically, in cross-section in this field. Normal colonic mucosa is just visible at the upper right margin, and it is continuous with a much thicker and more basophilic layer of malignant epithelium at the top right side of the field. This in turn merges with the raised mass of deeply-staining tumour cells (thin arrow) which constitutes the rolled edge of the ulcer. The ulcer crater is on the left of this rolled edge, and the floor of the ulcer (thick arrows) is a layer of carcinomatous tissue, consisting of malignant cells which are invading downwards and laterally, destroying the muscle coats and invading the pericolonic fat. Some eosinophilic muscle fibres survive (double arrow), and there are small basophilic lymphoid follicles in the unstained pericolonic fat. HE ×4

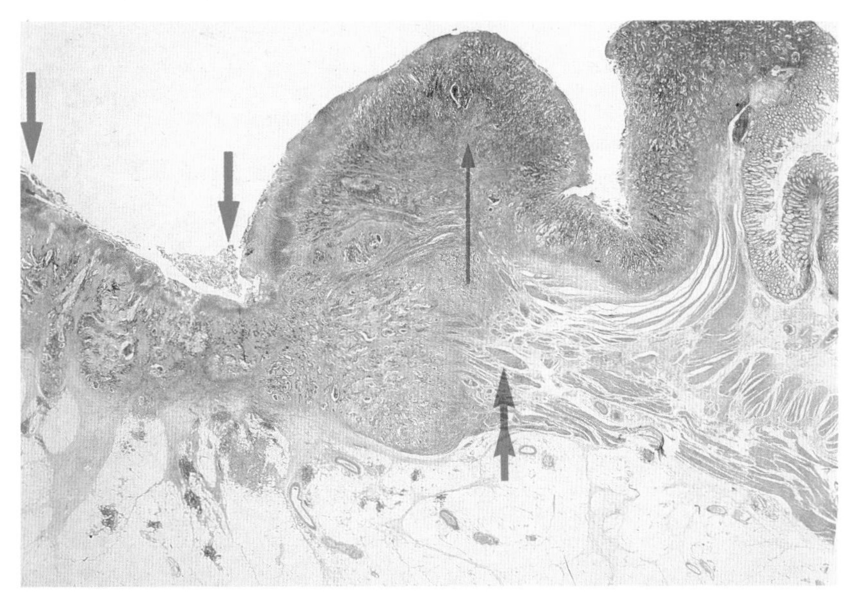

2.54 Adenocarcinoma: colon

Adenocarcinoma of colon tends to spread not only by direct invasion and by the lymphatic channels, but also does so by the portal vein to the liver. Most carcinomas form long tubules, lined by moderately pleomorphic tall columnar epithelial cells, which ramify through bowel wall. This tumour, which invaded the wall of the colon and penetrated to the pericolonic tissues, is poorly-differentiated and in this field it consists of two sheets of large malignant cells with eosinophilic cytoplasm and ovoid or round moderately pleomorphic vesicular nuclei (thin arrow). In both sheets, the tumour cells have formed several small acini containing mucinous material (thick arrows) but the lining cells show little evidence of active mucin secretion. Special stains and electron microscopy however usually reveal many other minor 'micro-acini', even in a fairly anaplastic lesion like this one. The two sheets of tumour cells are also separated by a thick band of fibrous tissue and many lymphocytes and plasma cells; and within the larger mass of cells there is an area of necrosis (double arrow). At higher magnification, considerable mitotic activity is detectable in the tumour cells. HE ×200

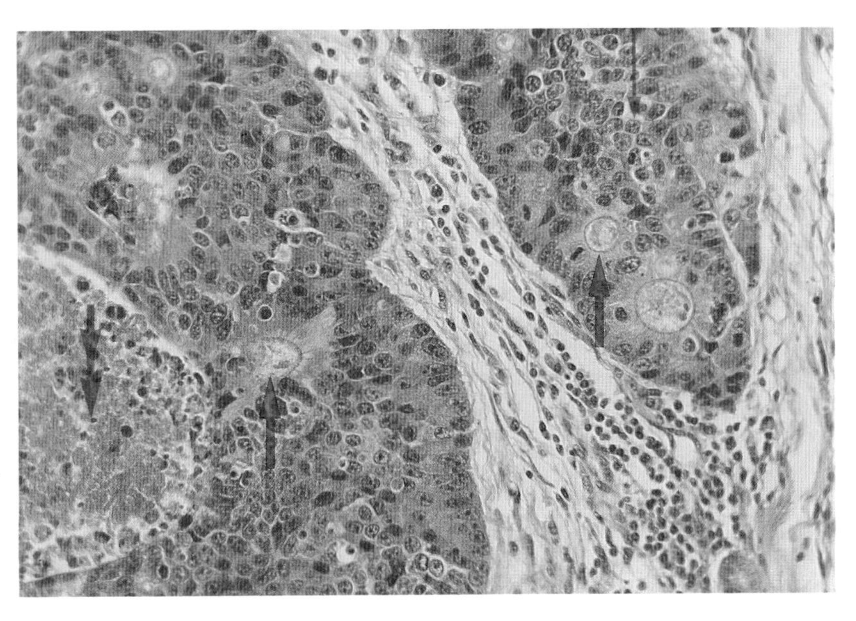

2.55 Benign lymphoid polyp: rectum

A lymphoid polyp (occasionally termed focal lymphoid hyperplasia) is a small soft polypoid mass or nodule of lymphoid tissue It is most often located in the rectal submucosa, and covered with smooth intact mucosa. It projects into the rectum, where it may cause bleeding or prolapse. Its etiology is probably inflammatory, the result of infection or injury. Similar lesions sometimes arise in the colon or small intestine, usually in children. Lymphoid polyps are generally multiple but they rarely cause symptoms or complications. This lesion vaguely resembles a small lymph node, but it has neither a proper capsule nor sinusoids, and consists instead of large sheets or clumps of small lymphocytes (thin arrow), separated by strands of vascular connective (thick arrow). Prominent germinal centres frequently form in the cellular sheets and clumps. Higher-power examination confirmed that the lymphoid tissue is mature and not lymphomatous. The lesion is probably hamartomatous in nature. Accurate diagnosis of this type of lesion is important, since lymphomas sometimes occur as primary lesions of the colon.

HE ×40

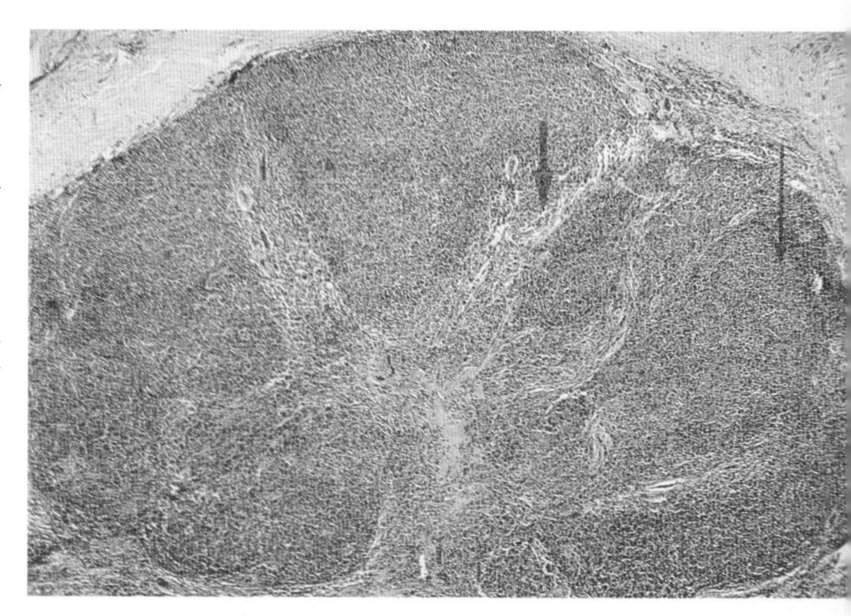

2.56 Lymphoplasmacytic lymphoma: colon

Lymphoplasmacytic lymphomas (also called LP immunocytoma) are of low grade malignancy and consists generally (but not exclusively) of numerous small lymphocyte-like (lymphoplasmacytic) cells, plasma cells and relatively few immunoblasts. In this case, a section of sigmoid colon and rectum 30cm long was removed surgically from woman aged 81 who had diverticulosis. Multiple diverticula were present in the resected segment, and in addition the mucosa of the whole of the resected bowel was heavily infiltrated with neoplastic cells. The infiltrate extended also into the pericolonic fat, where they formed multiple nodules. This field shows a section of colonic mucosa and submucosa, with the pale mucus-secreting glands at the left margin. Beneath the eosinophilic lamina propria there is a dense diffuse infiltrate of closely packed small cells with basophilic nuclei (mostly lymphoplasmacytic cells, at high magnification). The infiltrate extends deeply into the submucosal tissues, and throughout it there are numerous irregular deposits of amorphous strongly eosinophilic amyloid-like material (thick arrows). The lymphoplasmacytic cells also extend upwards into the mucosa, between the glands and up to the mucosal surface (thin arrow). HE ×60

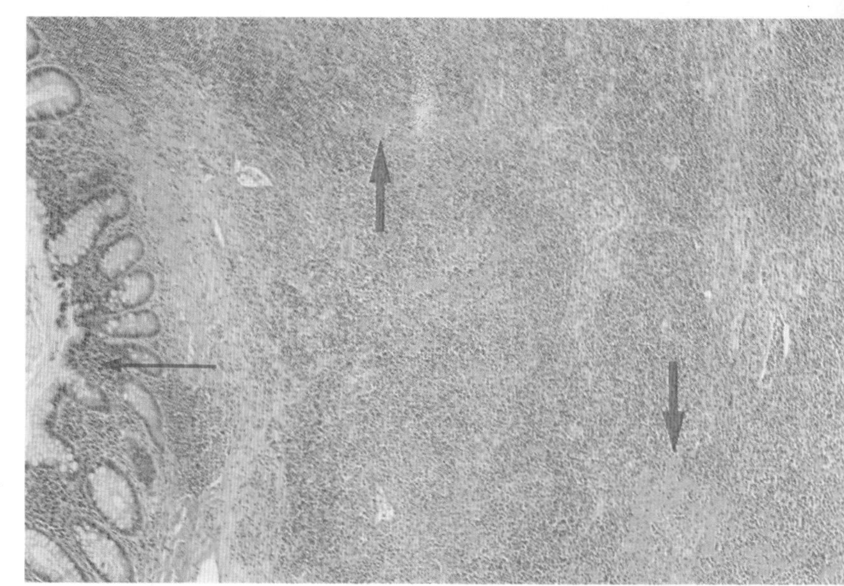

2.57 Lymphoplasmacytic lymphoma: colon

This shows a small part of the lymphoplasmacytic lymphoma in **2.56**, at higher magnification. The neoplastic cells, in general, appear comparatively well-differentiated, with well-defined cytoplasmic borders. Many of the cells are lymphocyte-like, with a small round basophilic nucleus (often with granular chromatin) and only a little cytoplasm (thin arrow). Mingling with the lymphocyte-like cells are numerous lymphoplasmacytic cells, slightly larger than the lymphocyte-like cells and with more cytoplasm. Also present are fairly numerous plasma cells, characteristically with abundant eosinophilic cytoplasm and a compact (eccentric) nucleus, located at one pole of the cell. In the cytoplasm of some of the plasma cells there is a pale (less deeply eosinophilic) juxtanuclear 'halo', and in other plasma cells the chromatin in the nuclei has a 'clock-face pattern. Also present (as a rule) are numerous histiocytes, larger than the other cells, each with a large relatively pale vesicular nucleus (thick arrow). Between the neoplastic cells of various types, there are small masses of amorphous strongly eosinophilic amyloid-like material (double arrow).

HE ×575

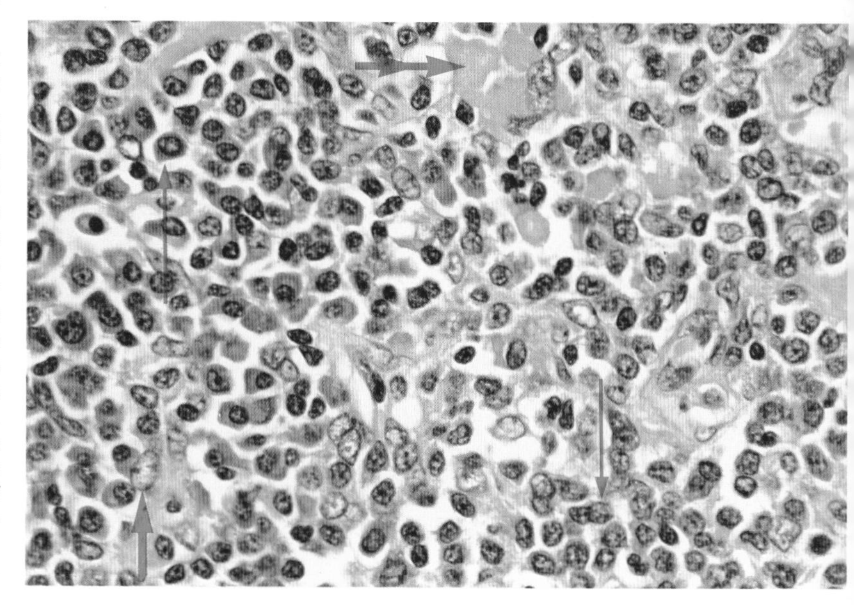

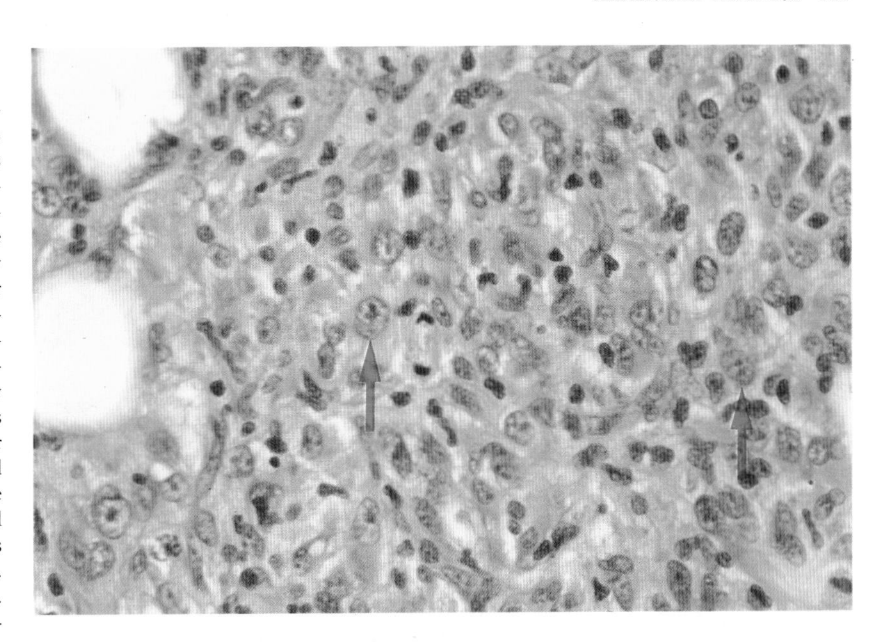

:.58 Malignant fibrous histiocytoma: etroperitoneum

'here are large numbers of histiocytes in some lympho-ytic lymphomas and care should be taken to identify this ype of lesion accurately. Malignant fibrous histiocytomas re thought to arise from primitive mesenchymal or fi-roblastic cells, and tend to be located in deeper struc-ures than the benign form. The macroscopic appearance f the tumour tends to be non-specific, but generally akes the form of well-circumscribed fleshy nodular or nultinodular mass. The cut surface may be slightly yel-ow (high fat content) or myxoid. Histologically, it is diffi-ult to predict the tumour's behaviour, since very pleo-norphic cells and numerous atypical mitoses do not truly ndicate malignancy. This field, at high magnification, is rom a large mass in the retroperitoneum. The tumour ells (thick arrows) have large vesicular round or ovoid uclei and much eosinophilic cytoplasm, in which there re a number of enzymes (detected by histochemical nethods) characteristic of macrophage lysosomes alpha-1- antichymotrypsin, lysozyme and cathepsin B). n each nucleus there is a prominent central nucleolus. The small deeply basophilic nuclei are mainly lympho-ytic, although a few polymorph leukocytes are also pres-nt. HE x470

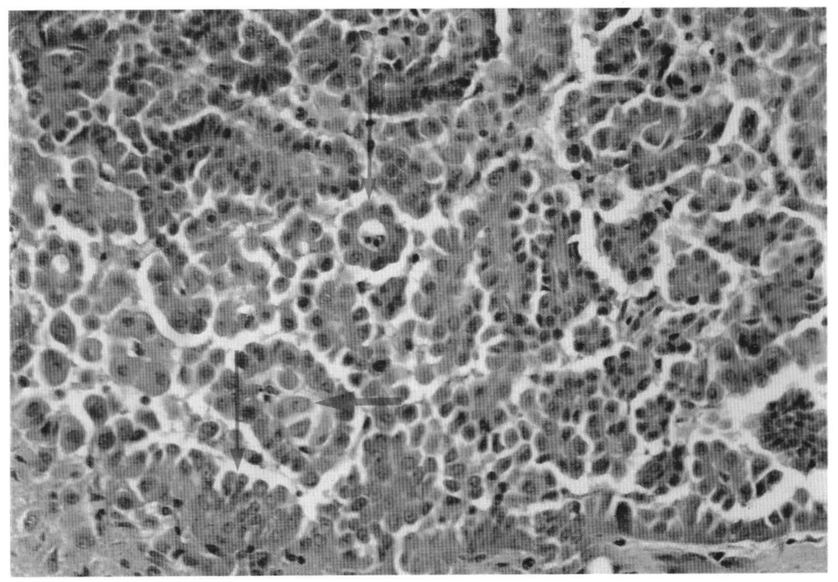

2.59 Mesothelioma: peritoneal cavity

There is a close link between inhalation of asbestos fibres nd mesothelioma, and mesotheliomas in the pleural cav-ty may spread through the diaphragm to the peritoneal avity. Primary mesothelioma of the peritoneal cavity nay occur however, and the diffuse type tends to spread widely over the peritoneal surface and form multiple nod-les or plaques. Distant metastasis is unusual however. This primary peritoneal lesion has spread throughout the eritoneal cavity and is growing on the surface of the mall intestine (just visible at bottom margin). The tu-nour consists of large numbers of closely packed slender apillae of varying length, separated by 'interpapillary lefts' and covered with a single layer of mesenchymal ells (thin arrows). The centre of each papilla is a small ound space or it is occupied by a small amount of deli-ate connective tissue or a few cells (thick arrow). The nesenchymal cells (many peg-shaped) are of a uniform ize, with a moderate amount of well-defined eosinophilic ytoplasm. Their nuclei are mostly round, basophilic and esicular. Many nuclei contain a fairly prominent nucleo-us. HE x235

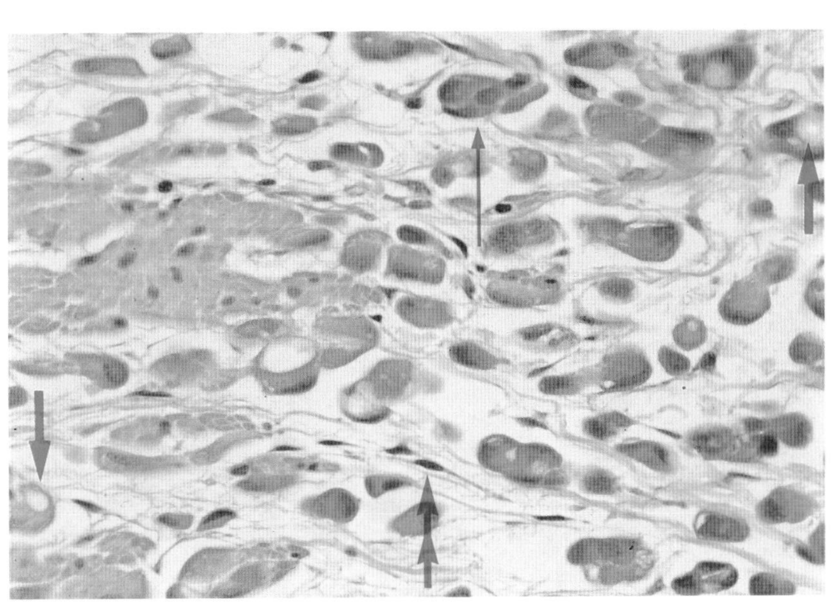

2.60 Mesothelioma: peritoneal cavity

Peritoneal mesotheliomas may be solitary benign lesions or solitary diffuse ones. This is a malignant peritoneal nesothelioma, invading the muscle coat of the small ntestine. The neoplastic mesenchymal cells are enetrating between eosinophilic fragments of smooth nuscle and accompanied by very loose pale-staining nyxoid connective tissue and slender fibrocytes (double rrow). The mesenchymal cells are large (thin arrow) but ariable in size and shape, some elongated and others normous. They all have a large quantity of eosinophilic ytoplasm and a small inconspicuous nucleus. The ytoplasmic boundaries are well-defined, and there are lear (empty) vacuoles (thick arrows) in the cytoplasm of nany cells. Mesotheliomas secrete hyaluronic acid which resumably occupied the cytoplasmic vacuoles initially; nd hyaluronic acid in the stromal tissue confirms the liagnosis. HE x360

3.1 Osteopetrosis: vertebra

Osteopetrosis (marble bone disease) is a group of rare diseases in which the normal resorption of bone by osteoclasts fails. Uniformly thickened dense bones form instead, and their cortical and cancellous regions are often indistinguishable. The infantile type is recessively inherited and causes death early in life. In the milder dominantly-inherited form, the symptoms are often minimal and the disorder is discovered by routine X-ray. In the less severe form, the disease may not be manifest until near adolescence. All bones may be affected but membranous bones (skull etc.) tend to be spared. Resorption of cartilage matrix and of cortical bone is defective. The bulky new bone may encroach on the marrow cavity and interfere with hemopoiesis and, with the exit foramina of nerves, disturbance of function. The bones are thickened and dense, but brittle and fracture readily. This vertebral body.consists of extremely deformed tightly-packed thick trabeculae of eosinophilic bone (thin arrow) and irregular sheets of curved poorly cellular extremely pale cartilaginous matrix (thick arrows). Many lacunae appear to lack a viable osteocyte. Islands of cellular hemopoietic tissue (double arrow) survive. HE ×90

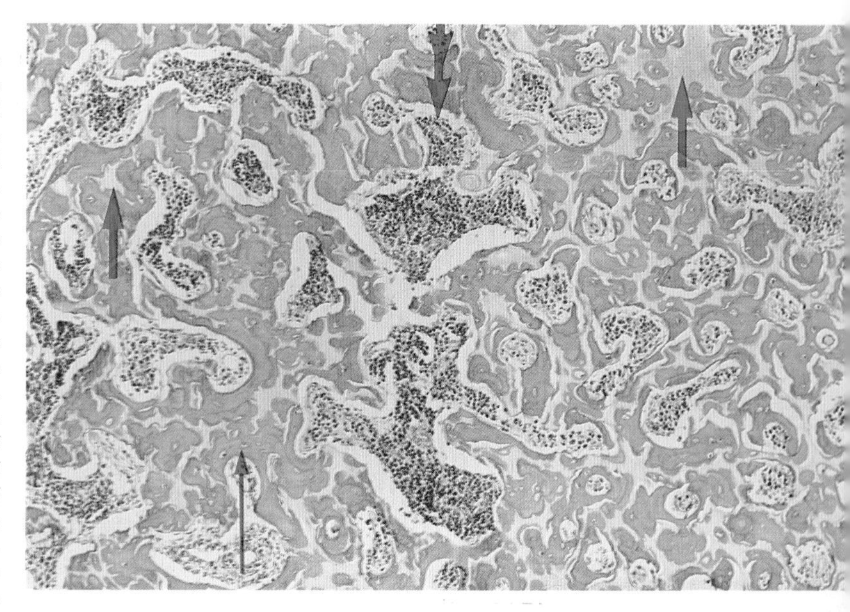

3.2 Osteopetrosis: vertebra

Osteoclasts which function abnormally are responsible for the defect in normal bone resorption which produces osteopetrosis. The changes are an increased tendency to fractures and osteomyelitis, encroachment on marrow space (leading to anaemia and extramedullary hematopoiesis) and compression of cranial nerves. This shows part of the same lesion as in 3.1. The trabeculae of bone are broad and their shape abnormal. The centres of the trabeculae consist of pale-staining homogeneous material (thick arrow) which closely resembles cartilage matrix and in which there are no chondrocytes. The surfaces of the trabeculae consist of layers of eosinophilic bone matrix (thin arrows) but they contain relatively few osteocytes. Between the trabeculae there are small foci of densely packed hemopoietic cells. In osteopetrosis, there seems also to be defective ossification, since the bone in the trabeculae is woven (coarse-fibred) bone and lacks compact trabeculae of lamellar bone. Moreover the number of osteoclasts is small, and resorption of cartilage is defective. HE ×215

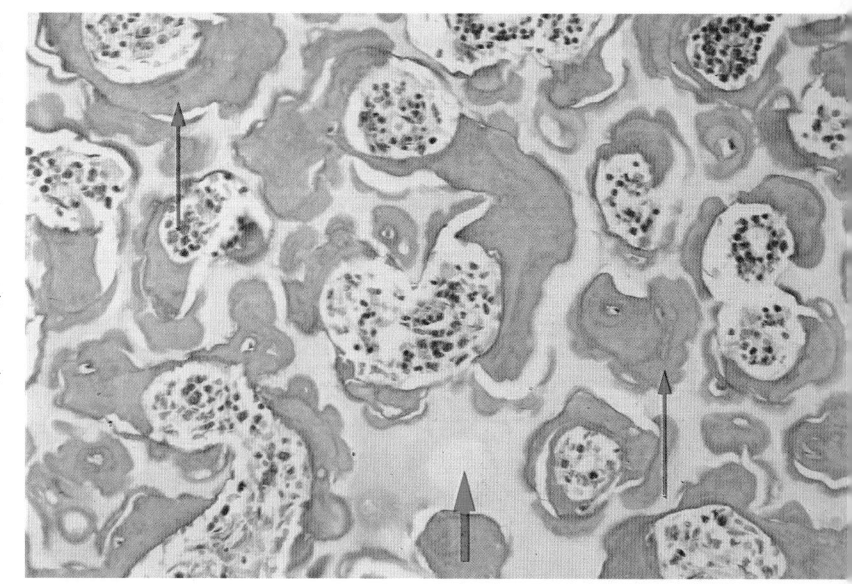

3.3 Fibrous dysplasia: bone

Fibrous dysplasia is a focal slowly expanding lesion in which the bone is replaced by fibroblasts, collagen and irregular trabeculae of bone. There are two distinct forms of fibrous dysplasia: the monostotic, in which only one bone is affected, at any age; and the polyostotic, with lesions in many bones which cause deformities and fractures. In monostotic lesions the affected area is replaced by proliferating fibroblasts in which there are scattered irregularly shaped trabeculae of bone which lack the usual rim of osteoblasts. The lesions in the polyostotic form are on one side of the body and accompanied by endocrine abnormalities (most often precocious puberty in the female), termed Albright's syndrome. There is often also patchy brown pigmentation of the skin on the same side as the bone lesions. In this case, the medullary cavity of an affected rib is expanded by a distinctive type of tissue which consists of highly cellular but loosely-textured vascular connective tissue (thick arrows). In the connective tissue there are trabeculae of deeply eosinophilic woven (coarse-fibred) bone (thin arrows), characteristically curved or sickle-shaped (spicules) with no osteoblasts on the surface. HE ×150

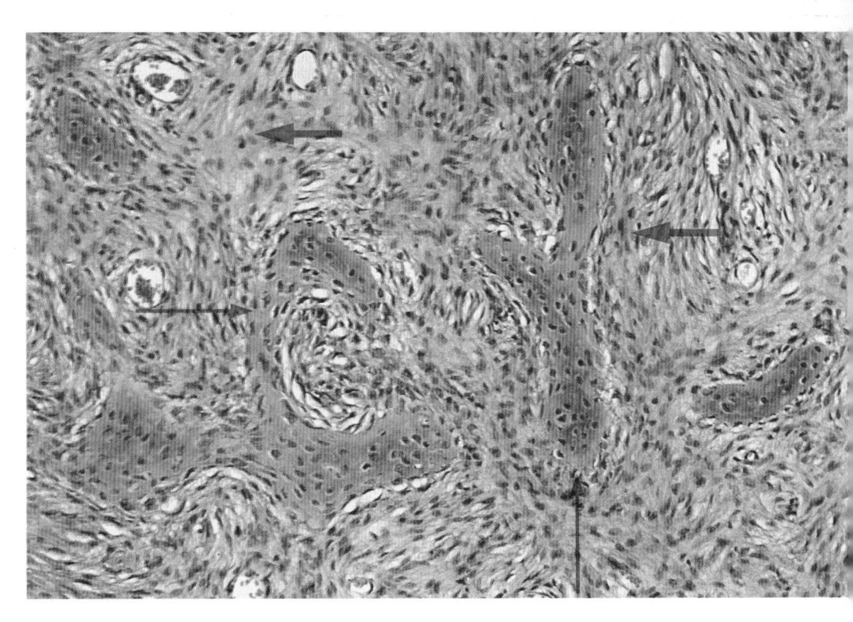

3.4 Osteomyelitis: bone

Most cases of pyogenic osteomyelitis occur in previously healthy active individuals. A wide range of bacteria can cause suppurative lesions of bone but in most cases the organism is *Staphylococcus aureus*. The infection may reach the bone locally, following a compound fracture (with damage to the skin) or via the bloodstream. The latter is the route in young people (less than 20 years of age). The site of entry of the organism is usually not apparent and the bacteremia is subclinical. If treatment is inadequate, pus may spread in the medullary cavity and beneath the periosteum. In this case, the trabeculae of dense cortical bone (thick arrow) are being eroded by the sheet of pus which fills the medullary cavity (thin arrow). The pus consists of large numbers of polymorph leukocytes and large round macrophages, accompanied by thick strands of eosinophilic fibrinous material. Considerable necrosis of bone is liable to occur in osteomyelitis, often through damage to the blood supply, but in this lesion the osteocytes in the bone lacunae retain their nuclear staining.

HE ×150

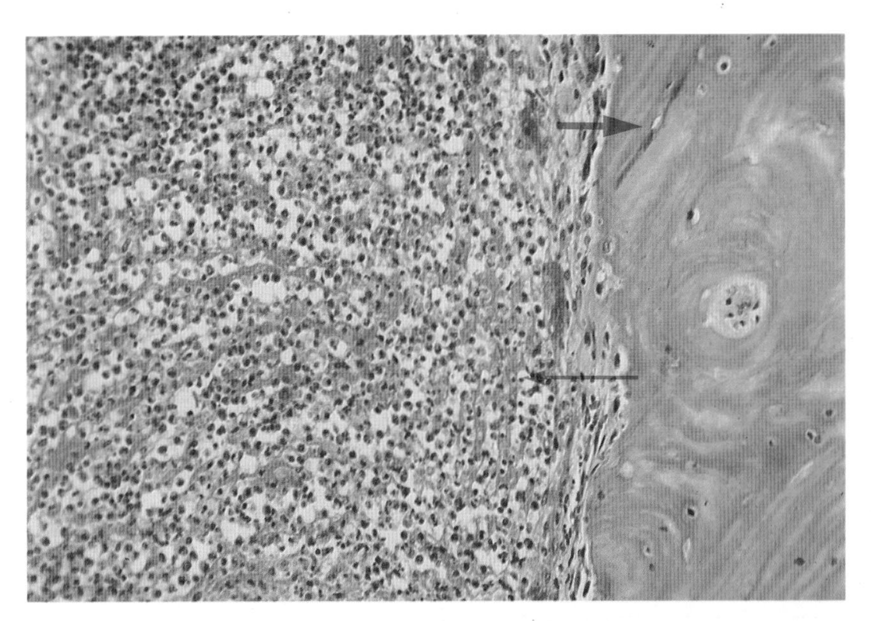

3.5 Osteomyelitis: bone

The long bones of the extremities are most often involved, and the infection tends to begin in the region of the metaphysis, at the most vascular site and most frequently in a lower limb. The probable mechanism for causing osteomyelitis is considered to be mild trauma in association with small hematomas that become infected by blood-borne staphylococci. Osteomyelitic lesions which are treated inadequately tend to become chronic, the outcome being extensive necrosis of existing bone as well as formation of much new reactive bone by the periosteum and endosteum. This lesion is a chronic pyogenic lesion of bone, taking the form of a sheet of reactive (new) woven bone. The new bone consists of an interlacing network of intensely basophilic trabeculae of woven (coarse-fibred) bone (thick arrows). The osteocytes in the woven bone are characteristically large and round and have basophilic ovoid nuclei. Between the trabeculae there is much pale amorphous material (thin arrows), surrounded by slender fibrocytes. Woven bone is usually not a permanent tissue and is normally removed by osteoclasts. It may be replaced by trabeculae of lamellar bone. HE ×135

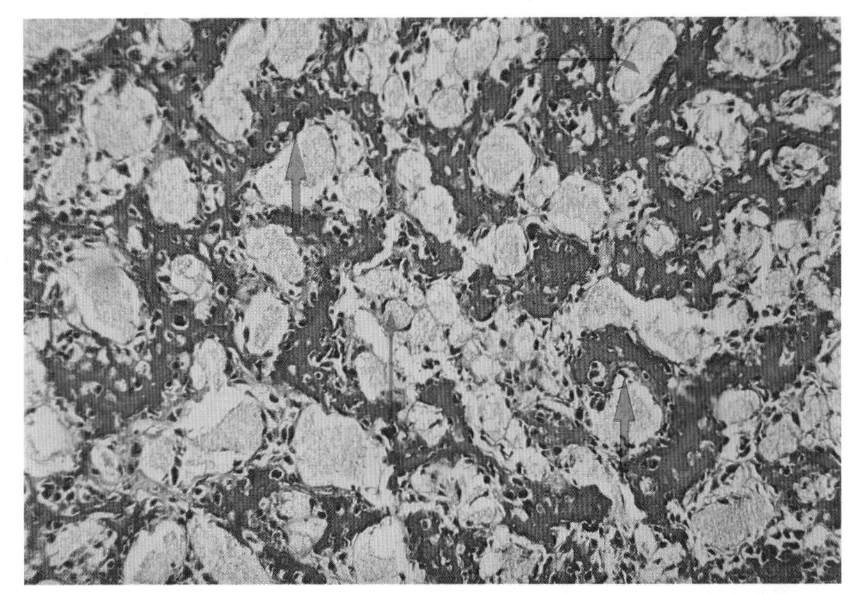

3.6 Tuberculous osteomyelitis: bone

Tuberculous osteomyelitis is a disease of children and young adults, and unpasteurized milk was often the source of infection. The disease has become less and less common in parts of the world however, where infection of lungs and intestine is well controlled, but it is still common in developing countries. The tubercle bacillus (*Mycobacterium tuberculosis*) infects bone via the bloodstream. The lesion tends to start at the metaphysis but synovial membrane is also susceptible. It has an insidious onset, with low-grade fever and loss of weight. Destruction of bone and synovial membranes may be considerable, and the necrotic tissue may liquefy to form a 'cold abscess'. This part of this lesion consists of tuberculous granulation tissue, rich in large macrophages with abundant pale cytoplasm and a relatively small nucleus (thin arrow), small lymphocytes and scant epithelioid macrophages. There are also relatively few capillaries. There is also a deeply eosinophilic necrotic trabecula of bone (thick arrow) which is necrotic and the osteocyte lacunae in it are empty. Between the necrotic bone trabecula and the sheet of viable granulation tissue there is deeply eosinophilic necrotic tissue (double arrow) which would appear caseous on macroscopic examination. HE ×55

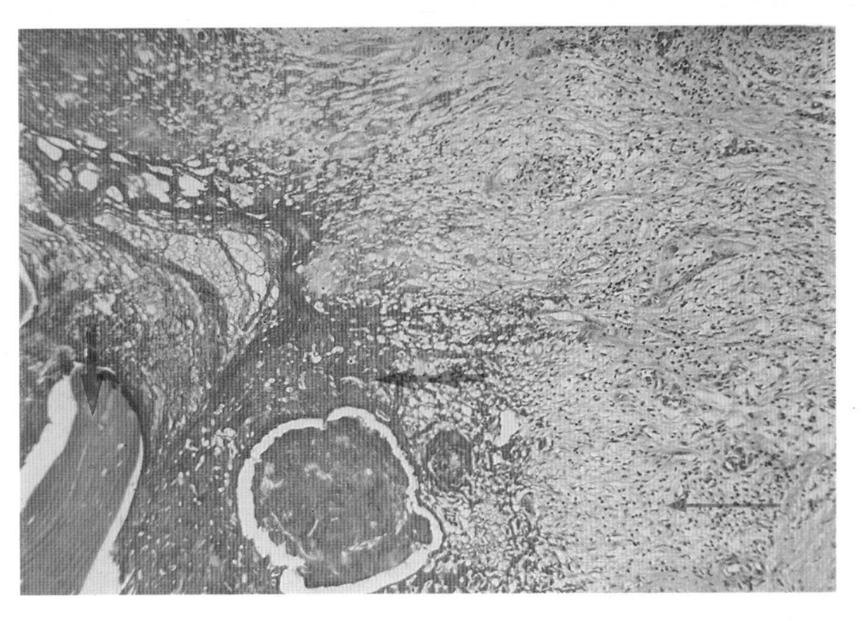

3.7 Necrosis (post-irradiation): cartilage

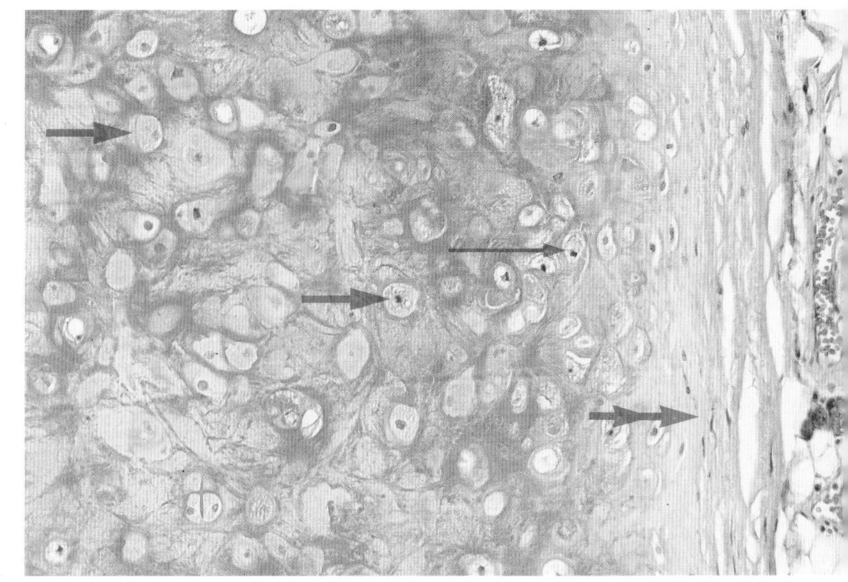

Tissues exposed to ionizing radiation show damage to collagen, which becomes densely hyalinized and the blood vessels may become telangiectatic, with thick hyalinized walls. Fibroblasts and endothelial cells are enlarged and the nuclei are damaged. Necrosis of cartilage is a fairly common and often troublesome complication of X-ray therapy, particularly when high pressure oxygen is used. In this case therapeutic X-irradiation had been given to the skin overlying the cartilage 3 months previously. The perichondrium consists of collagenous fibrous tissue (double arrow) and dilated small blood vessels. Many of the perichondrial fibrocytes are nucleated and probably viable, and in the sheet of hyaline cartilage underlying the perichondrium a few peripheral chondrocytes (thin arrow) still have small but pyknotic nuclei. All the other chondrocytes in the sheet of hyaline cartilage are large but necrotic and unstained (thick arrow). In addition, the matrix between the chondrocytes has lost its characteristic basophilia and stains red (the chondrocyte nuclei which lose their basophilia tend to stain red). The cartilage is therefore almost certainly completely necrotic. Necrotic cartilage can be removed by macrophages, but this generally takes a long time and the result is generally considerable fibrous scarring. HE ×150

3.8 Chondrodermatitis nodularis helicis: ear

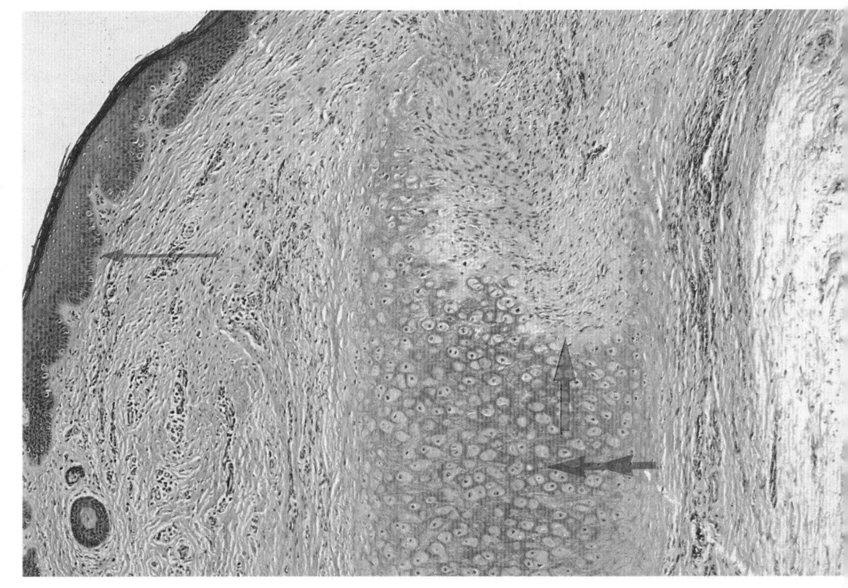

Chondrodermatitis nodularis helicis is characterized by the presence of one or more small very tender nodules on the apex of the helix of the ear. The lesion is present more often in males and is considered to be the effect of trauma. Necrosis of the underlying cartilage of the ear is usually present and was thought to be the prime lesion. Necrosis of dermal collagen may however be the first event. The nodules generally ulcerate, and chronic inflammatory cells infiltrate the perichondrium of the underlying cartilage. This lesion was in the left ear of a woman of 74. The squamous epithelium (thin arrow) is not ulcerated. There is a fairly intense perivascular infiltrate of basophilic chronic inflammatory cells in the dermis and also in the sheet of fibrous tissue beneath the auricular cartilage. The matrix of the cartilage is brightly eosinophilic (double arrow). Many of the chondrocytes in it have no nucleus. and the nuclei in the other chondrocytes are small and pyknotic. Part of the sheet of cartilage has been invaded and destroyed by vascular connective tissue (thick arrow). HE ×60

3.9 Chondrodermatitis nodularis helicis: ear

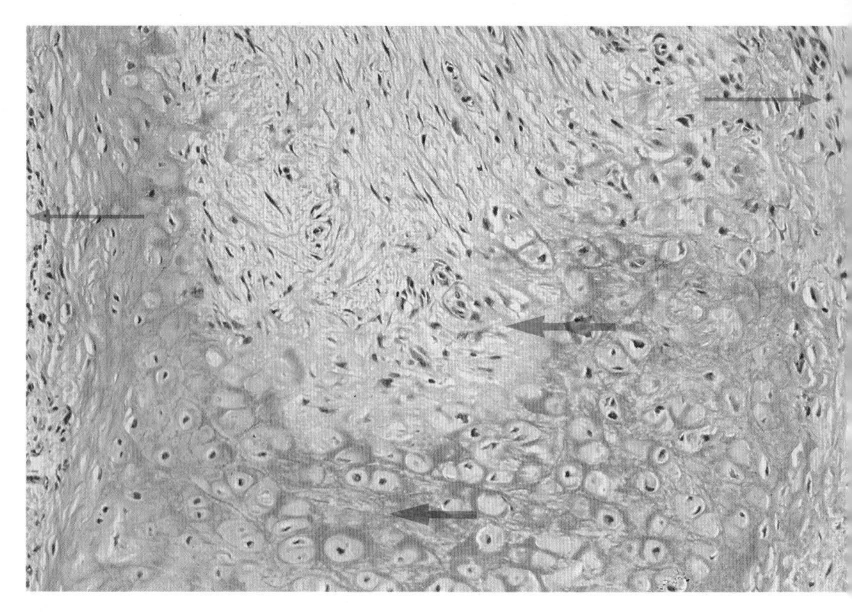

This is part of the lesion in 3.8, at higher magnification. On each side of the sheet of cartilage there is a layer of perichondrial connective tissue (thin arrows). The matrix of the cartilage is a deep bluish-red colour and granular (thick arrow). It has been invaded and eroded by pale delicate connective tissue (double arrow), in which there are numerous spindle-shaped fibroblasts and fibrocytes and also occasional macrophages. Many of the chondrocytes lack nuclei, and in the others the nucleus is small and pyknotic. This sheet of auricular cartilage is almost certainly wholly necrotic, despite the presence of nuclei in some chondrocytes. Living cartilage is very resistant to phagocytic attack, and the dense cartilage matrix of necrotic cartilage also protects the dead chondrocytes from macrophages. HE ×150

3.10 Hyperparathyroidism (osteitis fibrosa cystica): bone

Bone changes are caused by elevated levels of parathyroid hormone (PTH) and they occur in both primary and secondary hyperthyroidism. The effects on bone structure include both bone resorption by osteoclasts and new bone formation by osteoblasts. Severe focal bone resorption and destruction may be sufficient to lead to nodular space-occupying masses, composed of cysts and fibrous tissue and termed 'brown tumours' (the brown colour is produced by the considerable amount of hemosiderin). Sometimes the number of giant cells (osteoclasts) in these 'tumours' may sufficiently great as to confuse this condition with true giant-cell tumours of bone. In this example, one side of the trabeculae of normal mature lamellar bone is under active attack by numerous osteoclasts (thin arrows). As a result, most of the bone has been almost completely eroded and replaced by a large amount of pale cellular connective tissue within which there are dilated thin-walled blood vessels and fairly extensive hemorrhage. Basophilic trabeculae of new (woven) bone (thick arrows) project from other side of the fragments of lamellar bone. HE ×135

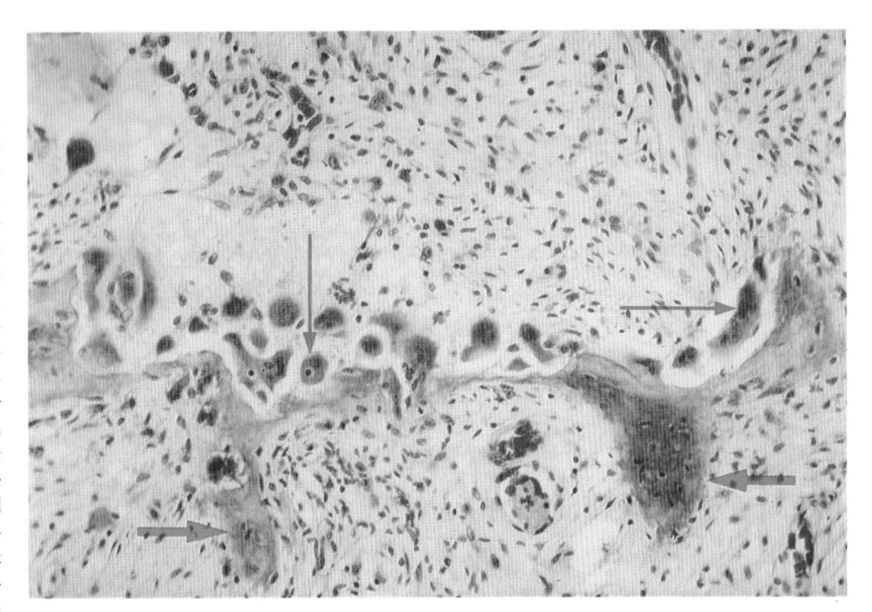

3.11 Rickets: costochondral junction

Rickets is a disease of children, and in developing countries most cases are caused by deficiency of vitamin D. The disease is characterized by failure of mineralization of osteoid in bone with abnormalities of bone growth. Newly formed bone matrix fails to calcify and remains as osteoid. At the epiphyses, the cartilage matrix fails to mineralize. The unmineralized cartilage resists resorption, and its replacement by bone can not take place. The epiphyses enlarge but growth of bone is retarded. In this example of the disease, the eosinophilic collagenous fibrous periosteum is at the top, and beneath it there is broad sheet of bluish hyaline epiphyseal cartilage (left). The intercellular matrix (left) of the cartilage is uncalcified, and the thick disorderly columns of chondrocytes (thin arrows) cause the epiphysis to bulge. The metaphysis consists of small but dilated thin-walled blood vessels (thick arrows) and elongated trabeculae of widely varying size and shape which contain both basophilic cartilage and eosinophilic osteoid. Basophilic hemopoietic cells (double arrow) are visible in the marrow cavity. HE ×60

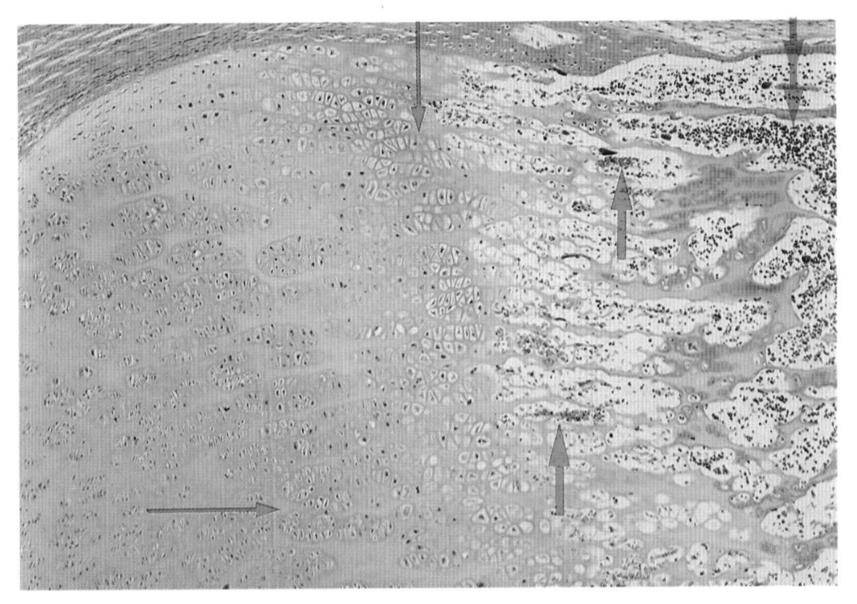

3.12 Rickets: costochondral junction

This is part of the same lesion as in 3.11, higher magnification. It consists of a large sheet of epiphyseal cartilage, composed of bluish matrix and large fully viable proliferating chondrocytes. Some of the chondrocytes are arranged singly and the others in clusters of widely varying sizes (double arrow). The chondrocytes also vary greatly in size and most of them have an ovoid basophilic nucleus. Some however appear to lack a nucleus but absence of a nucleus may be a technical artefact. There is no evidence of calcification of the matrix. At the metaphysis (right margin), the chondrocytes are arranged in elongated columns of closely packed cartilage cells which are becoming increasingly disordered (thin arrows). Correspondingly, as the chondrocytes approach the metaphysis, the intercellular matrix becomes more and more attenuated until there are only thin walls between the columns of cartilage cells. Further right, the small blood vessels are widely dilated and thin-walled (thick arrow), and they appear to penetrate between the columns of cartilage cells with difficulty. Few osteoblasts accompany the blood vessels. HE ×150

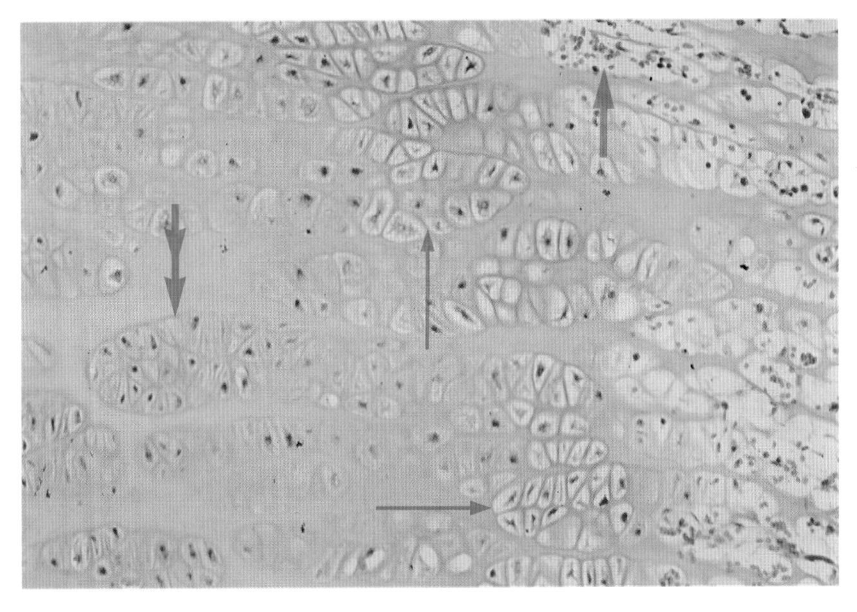

3.13 Paget's disease: skull

Paget's disease (osteitis deformans) is a fairly common condition affecting men and women equally. The etiology is unknown. The disease is focal, and lesions may be found in the vertebrae, pelvis, skull and long bones (other than the ribs). In the early stages the bone is soft and vascular with active resorption of bone, but later bone formation predominates and the bone becomes very thick and dense but brittle. Microscopically the trabeculae are very broad, and running through them there is an irregular pattern (a 'mosaic') of highly irregular cement lines (thin arrows). The pattern confirms that previously there have been numerous repeated patchy and disordered episodes of bone resorption and formation. In the pale myxoid connective tissue between the bone trabeculae there are greatly dilated thin-walled blood vessels, and layers of osteoblasts (thick arrows) on the surface of the trabeculae are forming new bone. Elsewhere on the trabecular surface there is very active resorption of bone by osteoclasts (double arrows), leading to 'notching' of the trabeculae. HE ×150

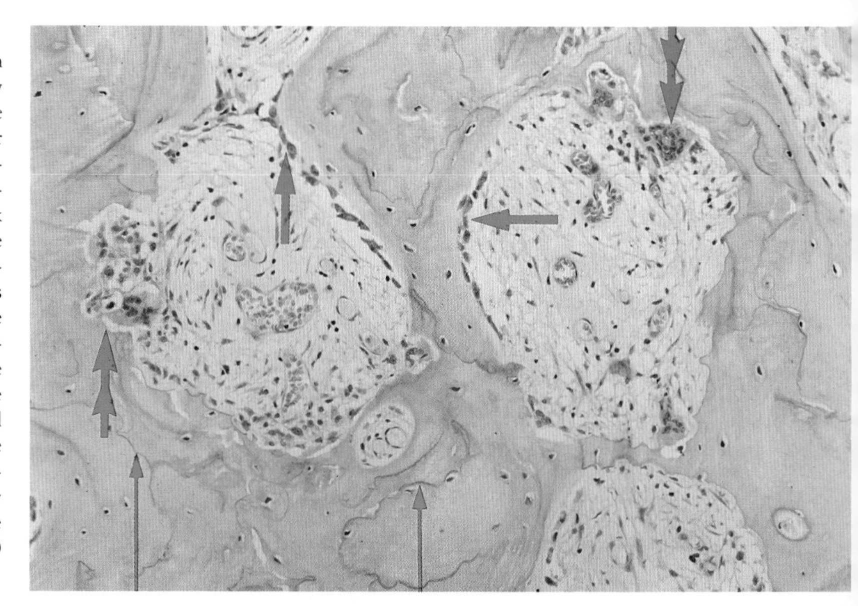

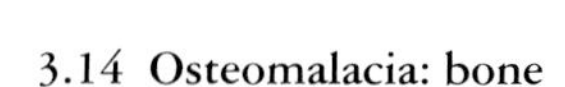

3.14 Osteomalacia: bone

Osteomalacia ('soft bone') is a structural abnormality of bone and it is the counterpart in adults of rickets in children. Where bone is being formed, it is inadequately calcified and 'soft', and non-calcified bone matrix (osteoid) is present in abnormally large amounts. This is a biopsy specimen of bone from the iliac crest of a man of 52 with adult-type Fanconi 'rickets'. The histological section has been cut without prior decalcification of the bone, and the bone salts remain in the bone. Only parts of the several trabeculae of lamellar bone are calcified, and it has been stained black by the von Kossa method. The remaining parts of the trabeculae are a deep orange-red colour (arrows), signifying that they consist of (uncalcified) osteoid. The layer of osteoid on the surfaces of normal bone lamellae is usually thin, but in this specimen the layer of osteoid is many times thicker than normal (up to 200μm thick) and thereby demonstrates very severe osteomalacia.

Von Kossa-neutral red ×80

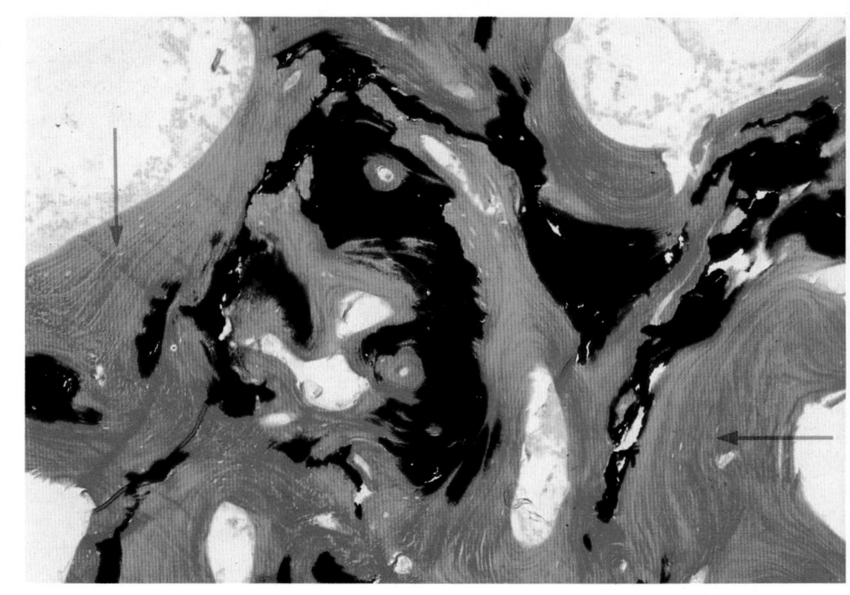

3.15 Osteoporosis: bone

Osteoporosis is a decrease in the total mass of bone without structural abnormalities. There is increased 'porosity' or rarefaction of the bone, and it represents a form of atrophy. The bone present is adequately calcified; that is, the quantity but not the quality of the bone is reduced. The total mass of the affected bones is decreased, and the bony cortex and trabeculae are thinned. Senile osteoporosis is present to some extent in most individuals more than 50 years of age, being generally more severe in women after the menopause. Endocrine diseases and environmental factors (decreased physical activity, inadequate diet etc.) may also play a role. In this example of osteoporosis, the bone trabeculae are remarkably thin and delicate (thin arrow) and widely spaced. They are however fully calcified. There is no osteoclastic activity, and the osteoblasts on the surface of the trabeculae are flat and inconspicuous. Fatty marrow (thick arrow) fills the large spaces between the trabeculae. The cause of osteoporosis in this case is more likely to be increased resorption rather than decreased formation. HE ×55

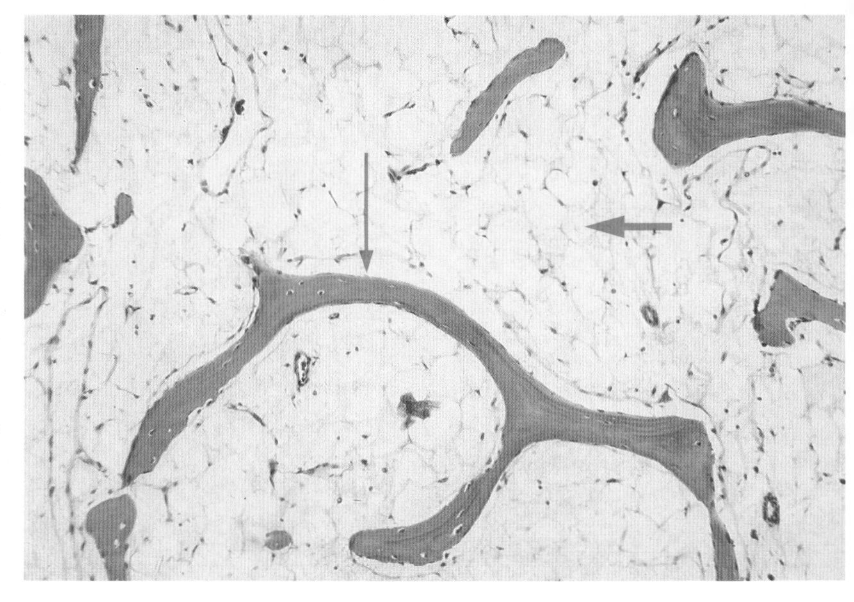

3.16 Aneurysmal bone cyst: vertebra

Aneurysmal bone cyst is a very uncommon benign lesion which affects young people, less than 20 years of age. It is found in a variety of sites, affecting vertebrae and flat bones rather than long bones. It is large destructive lesion, consisting of soft hemorrhagic tissue which is usually multicystic. It erodes the bone eccentrically and expands it, and there is usually a thin layer of normal bone at the outer surface of the lesion. This histological section of tissue is from a lesion in a vertebral body. It consists of large thin-walled endothelium-lined blood vessels (double arrow), cellular fibrous connective tissue, and large numbers of various types of cells, including small lymphocytes, multinucleated giant cells of the osteoclast type (thin arrows) and sheets of plump spindle-shaped fibroblastic cells, most of which have abundant eosinophilic cytoplasm. Also present are ill-formed trabeculae of weakly eosinophilic osteoid (thick arrow). Extensive hemorrhage has occurred from the large blood vessels.

HE ×60

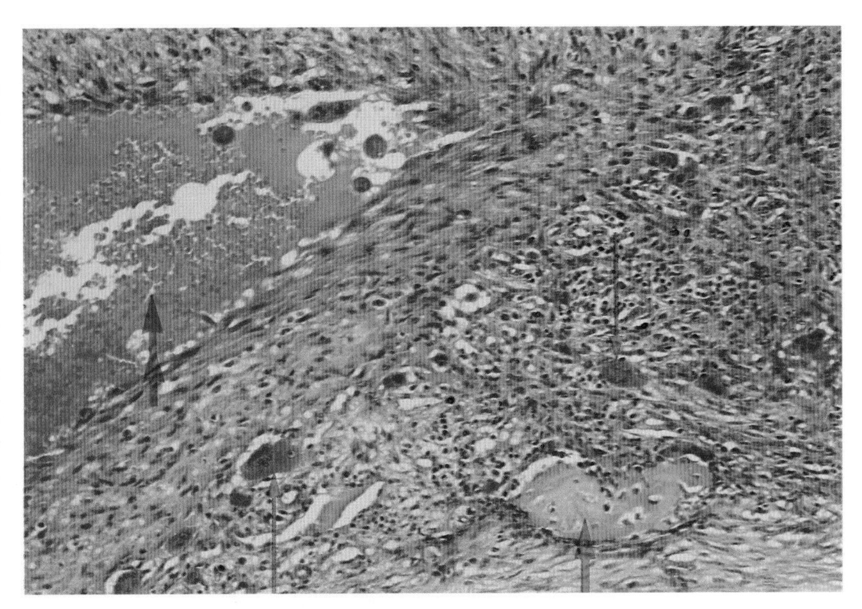

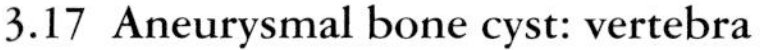

3.17 Aneurysmal bone cyst: vertebra

X-rays show that an aneurysmal bone cyst is a typically well-circumscribed lytic lesion which greatly expands and bulges the involved bone eccentrically. This tissue is part of the same lesion as in 3.16, at higher magnification. In it there is a large very dilated blood vessel (top left), lined with an incomplete layer of flat endothelial cells (and sometimes vascular granulation tissue) and supported by a sheet of eosinophilic cellular connective tissue (double arrow). Alongside this connective tissue there is a larger area of much looser (vacuolated) myxomatous connective tissue, containing multinucleated (osteoclast-type) giant cells (thin arrow), elongated fibroblasts and dilated thin-walled blood vessels. There are also many round cells scattered throughout both types of connective tissue. At the margin of the myxomatous tissue there is a trabecula of eosinophilic osteoid (thick arrow), almost acellular. There is usually also a considerable amount of hemosiderin in this lesion. Aneurysmal bone cyst is curable by adequate surgical excision, and it is therefore important to distinguish it from giant-cell tumour of bone or from vascular osteosarcoma.

HE ×150

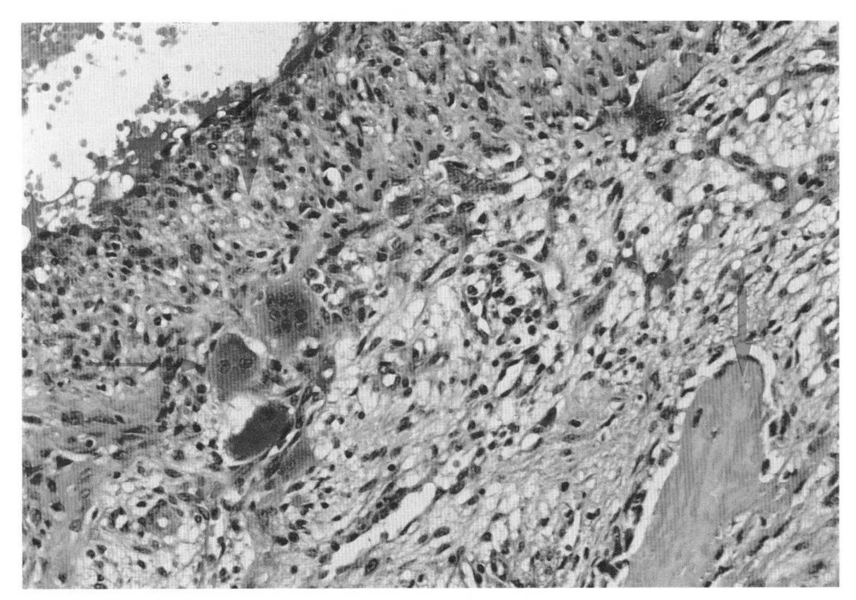

3.18 Hemangiopericytoma: femur

Hemangiopericytomas are uncommon and considered to originate from pericytes. They arise in any part of the body, including bone. Most are well-localized lesions, spheroidal and usually less than 5cm dia, but a minority recur locally and occasionally metastasize. This lesion in the femur is a well-differentiated tumour, reminiscent of a glomus tumour, and composed of cords of cells, separated by a delicate stroma consisting largely of thin-walled blood vessels. Some of the blood vessels contain blood (double arrow) but the other blood vessels are collapsed and inconspicuous (thick arrows). The blood vessels are lined by endothelial cells, and a reticulin (silver) stain revealed a continuous basement membrane between the endothelial cells and the neoplastic cells. The nuclei of the tumour cells are round or ovoid and regular in size and shape. They are also weakly vesicular and contain very finely granular chromatin (thin arrow). The cytoplasm is eosinophilic, moderate in amount and its margins are ill-defined. There are usually also several small vacuoles. There is no mitotic activity in this area and few mitoses could be found elsewhere in the tumour.

HE ×360

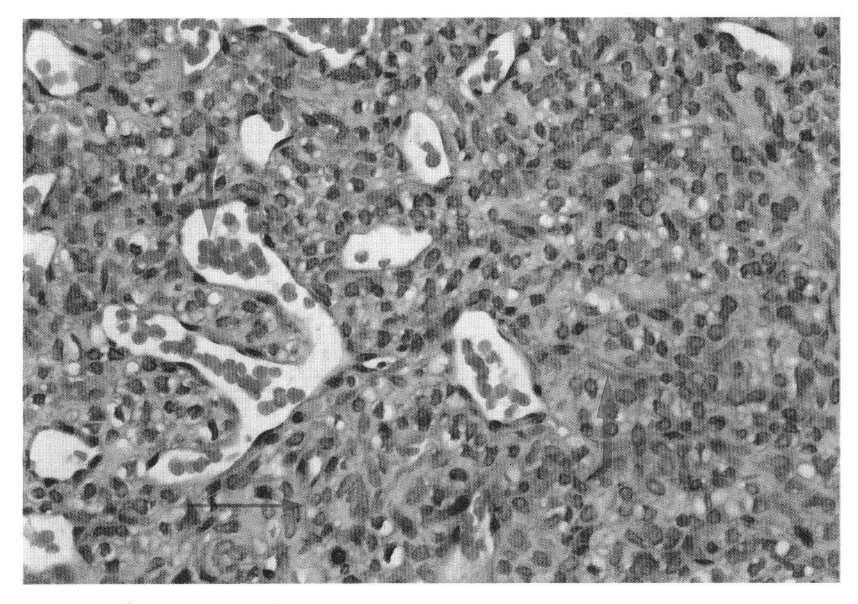

3.19 Eosinophilic granuloma: bone

Eosinophilic granuloma is one of the three related diseases included in the term histiocytosis × and typified by the presence, in the skin, of Langerhans cells which contain tennis racket-shaped Birbeck granules (visible in the EM). It is a relatively benign well-demarcated unilocular disease, consisting of Langerhans cells and a wide range of other cells. This is an osteolytic lesion (2cm dia) (visible with X-rays) in the temporal bone of a man of 33. Histologically it consists of a diffuse infiltrate of histiocytes with foamy (finely vacuolated) cytoplasm (thin arrow), eosinophil leukocytes (left margin), lymphocytes, and multinucleated giant (Touton-type) cells with a large quantity of granular cytoplasm, around the periphery of which there is a long row of nuclei (thick arrow). Strands of fibrous tissue are also present in the lesion. There was also evidence of invasion of the temporal muscle. After adequate surgical excision an eosinophilic granuloma does not usually recur. HE x270

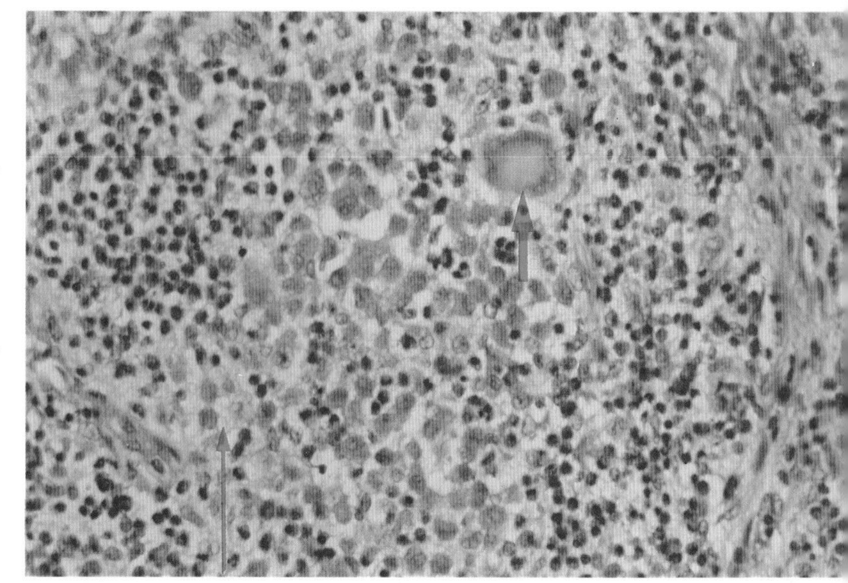

3.20 Osteochondroma: femur

Osteochondroma (osteocartilaginous exostosis) is the most common benign bone neoplasm, generally in subjects less than 20 years of age. Most tumours are solitary, but rarely multiple osteochondromas occur in familial distribution (termed diaphyseal aclasis, multiple exostoses) with an autosomal dominant inheritance. A typical tumour consists of a stalk of mature bone and a cap of hyaline cartilage, and it may grow large enough to press on local structures. Its surface is often lobulated. This small sessile hard mass attached to the shaft of the femur near the knee-jointconsists, histologically, of trabeculae of mature bone (thin arrow) and a broad outer sheet of hyaline cartilage (double arrow). The bluish cartilage matrix is being eroded by numerous dilated thin-walled blood vessels (thick arrow).The surface of the cartilage is smooth and covered with connective tissue (left margin) which is continuous (elsewhere) with the periosteum of the femur. Growth of an osteochondroma is similar to that which occurs at the epiphysis, with the cap of cartilage acting like the epiphyseal plate. Malignant transformation of solitary osteochondromas is very rare, with the cartilage transforming into a chondrosarcoma.

HE x120

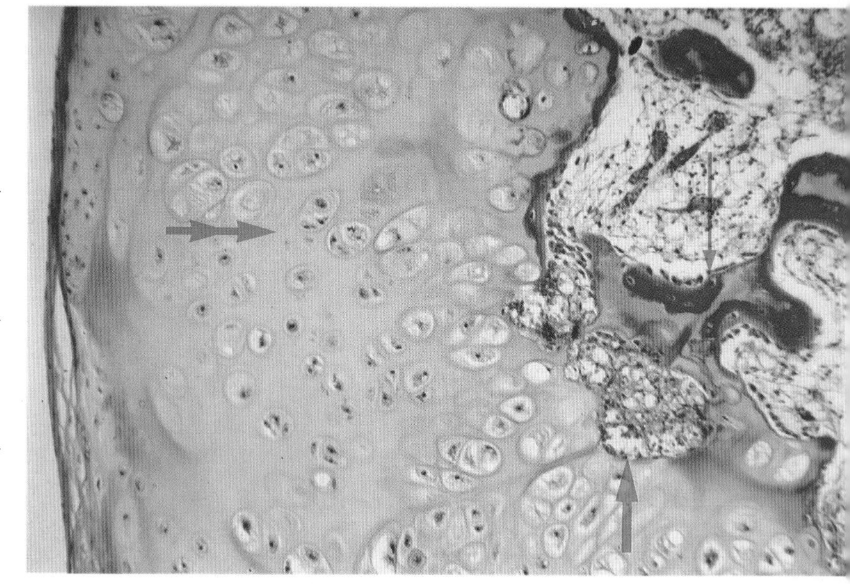

3.21 Giant-cell tumour: bone

Giant-cell tumours of bone (osteoclastomas) are malignant, and inadequately resected lesions recur locally. About 10% metastasize. It is a tumour of adults, usually 20-40 years of age, and tends to be located at the end of long bones, where it forms an expansile locally destructive mass which may invade the knee-joint. The cut surface is usually red and hemorrhagic, with dark brown areas and fibrous-walled cystic spaces filled with blood. This tumour in the head of the fibula is sarcoma-like, consisting of large numbers of highly pleomorphic neoplastic cells of unknown origin, many spindle-shaped, and also many multinucleated giant cells which resemble osteoclasts (arrows). The neoplastic cells vary in size and shape, from elongated fibroblast-like to large round forms. The equally pleomorphic nuclei in the neoplastic cells are pale and vesicular and nearly always contain a prominent nucleolus. The connective tissue in the tumour does not form osteoid or bone, but it is actively growing and determines the degree of malignancy. HE x215

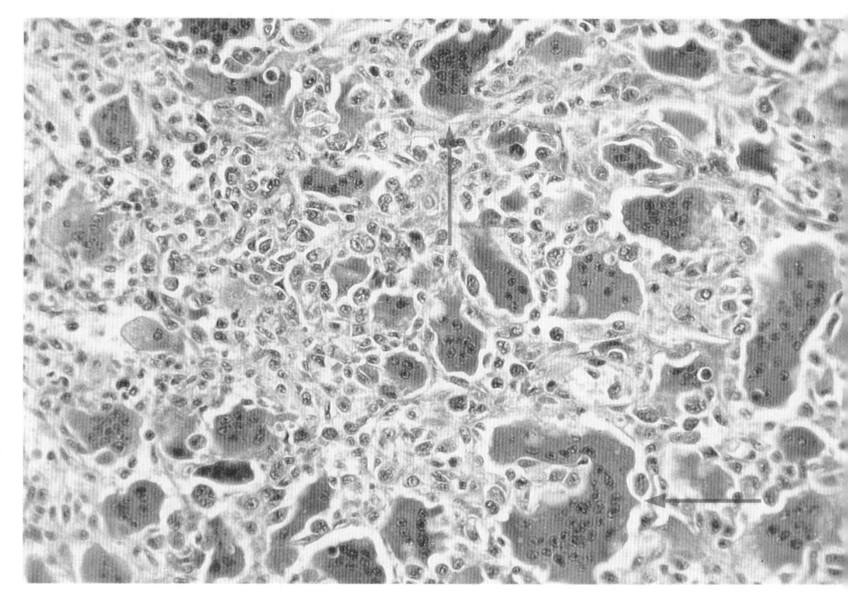

3.22 Osteoid osteoma: bone

Osteoid osteoma is an uncommon small (less than 1.5cm) benign neoplasm which causes intense pain. It occurs mainly in the 10-30 age group and more often in males than females. It is located in the cortex of the metaphysis in bones of the limbs, hands and feet or vertebral column. The sharply demarcated lesion is a central nidus, sharply demarcated and surrounded by a rim of sclerotic bone, and composed of highly vascular osteoblastic connective tissue and osteoid. The tumour also contains much uncalcified (eosinophilic) osteoid and large numbers of proliferating osteoblasts. It also induces an osteosclerotic reaction in the surrounding bone. This example was in the head of the ulna. It consists of very irregular sheets and trabeculae of eosinophilic osteoid (thin arrow) and bluish (basophilic) bone (mineralized osteoid) (thick arrow). In the vascular connective tissue between the sheets and trabeculae of osteoid and bone there is a large population of cells of various types and sizes, including many osteoblasts arranged along the surface of the trabeculae (double arrow). Resection of the lesion is curative.

HE ×120

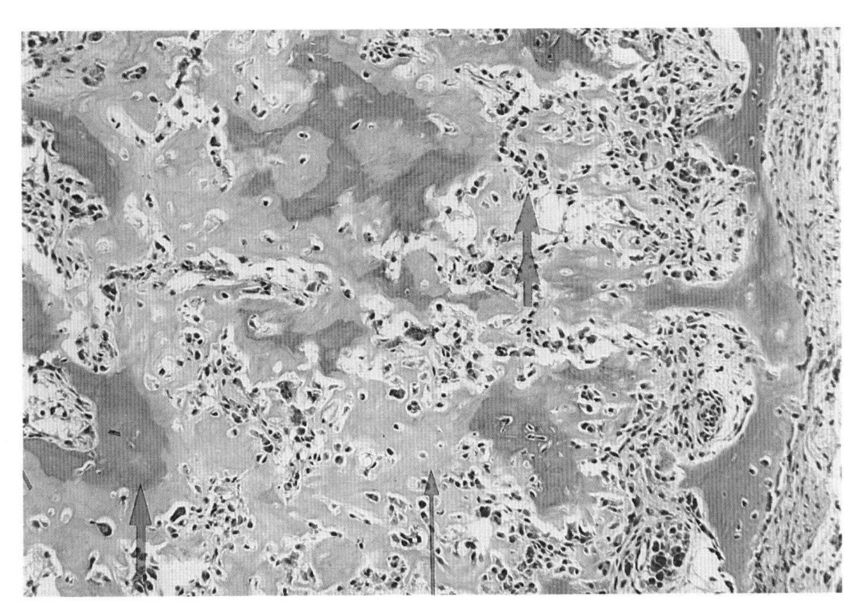

3.23 Osteoblastoma: bone

Osteoblastoma (giant osteoid osteoma) is a benign tumour, in the medulla of the epiphysis. It is rarely aggressive and arises in the 10-30 age group, the same range as that in patients with an osteoid osteoma. The two types of tumour are also located in the same sites but with different frequencies. Histologically also, osteoblastoma is similar to osteoid osteoma, resembling its nidus, but it is usually a bigger lesion (more than 2cm dia), does not cause pain, and does not induce a sclerotic reaction in the surrounding bone. This specimen is composed of closely packed small irregular trabeculae of very eosinophilic osteoid (thick arrow), the surfaces of which are covered with a single layer (more or less) of very many active-looking large pleomorphic osteoblasts (thin arrow) with round or ovoid deeply basophilic nuclei and abundant strongly eosinophilic cytoplasm. Many of the osteoblasts on the surfaces of the trabeculae have a 'tear-drop' shape, whereas the many individual osteoblasts in the connective tissue between the trabeculae are (approximately) round.

HE ×235

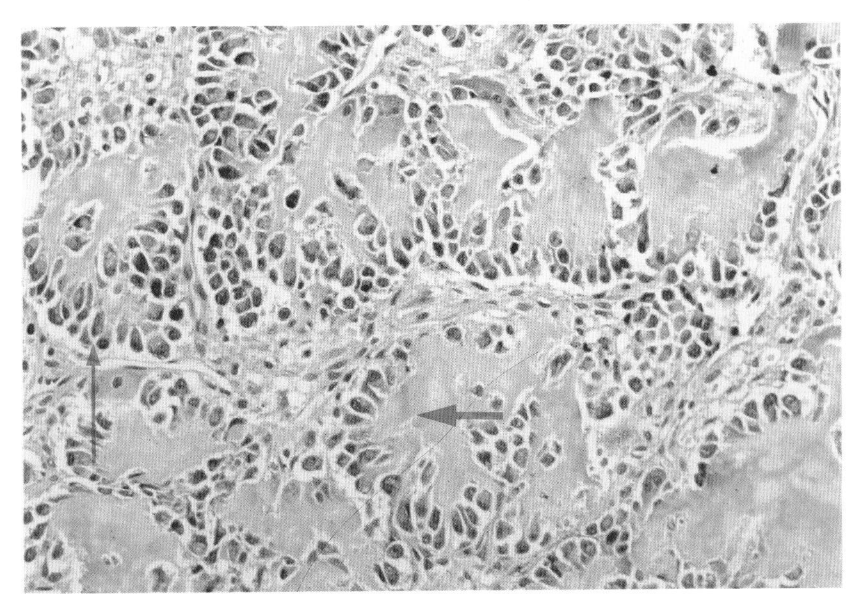

3.24 Osteosarcoma: bone

Apart from the cases developing in older people with Paget's disease of bone, osteosarcoma is a highly malignant tumour of children and young adults under 25 years of age. It tends to develop in the medullary cavity of the metaphysis of a long bone, and many of the tumours are located around the knee. The presence of varying amounts of osteoid establishes the diagnosis. Cartilage also often forms, and the amount may be considerable (chondroblastic osteosarcoma). The tumour invades expands the periosteum, sometimes breaking through it, and it metastasizes readily by the bloodstream to the lungs. The prognosis is poor. This tumour consists of pleomorphic abnormal osteoblasts, often anaplastic, and small irregular trabeculae of eosinophilic osteoid (double arrow). The malignant osteoblasts have large pleomorphic vesicular nuclei, with a large number of mitotic figures, often abnormal (thin arrow). The nuclei contain finely granular chromatin and in many of the nuclei there is a prominent nucleolus. A few multinucleated giant cells are also present (thick arrow). The malignant cells also frequently produce bone and cartilage.

HE ×360

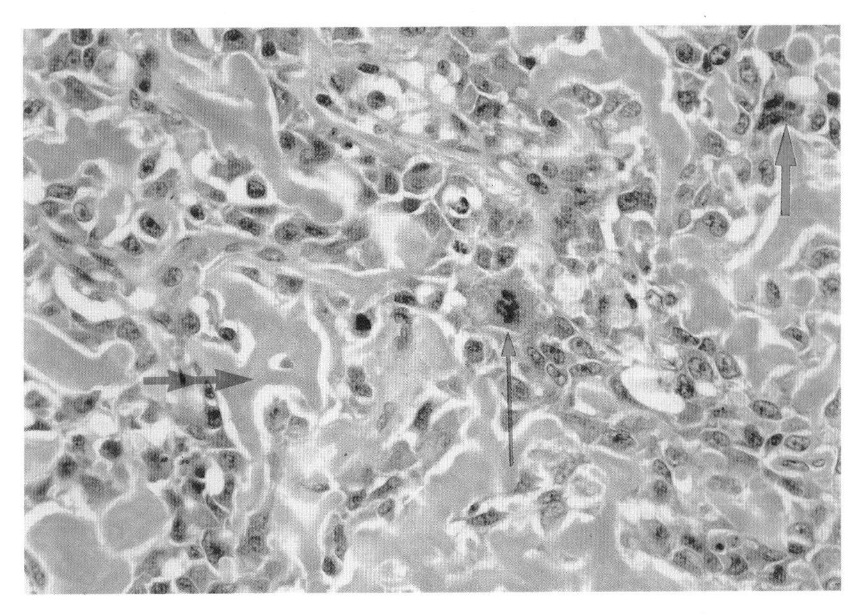

3.25 Chordoma: bone

Chordoma is a slow-growing lobulated nodular mass which arises in remnants of the notochord in the vertebral bodies and intervertebral discs. Chordomas are malignant and grow slowly but inexorably. About half of them are located 1) in the sacrococcygeal region, where it compresses the cauda equina; 2) at the clivus, from which it extends into the posterior fossa, compressing the brainstem; and 3) in the suprasellar region, where it compresses the pituitary stalk and third ventricle. The cut surface of chordomas is soft and gelatinous, and the tumours are very difficult to remove completely by surgery. There is also a very high rate of recurrence and usually a fatal outcome. Microscopically a chordoma consists of sheets of large cells with regular ovoid nuclei and a large amount of cytoplasm, distended by one or more large vacuoles which contain pale grey gelatinous or mucoid material (thin arrows). These cells are sometimes called physaliferous cells. In other parts of this tumour, vacuolation of the cytoplasm is much less pronounced. The sheets of tumour cells are separated by strands of vascular fibrous tissue stroma (thick arrow). There is no mitotic activity. HE ×235

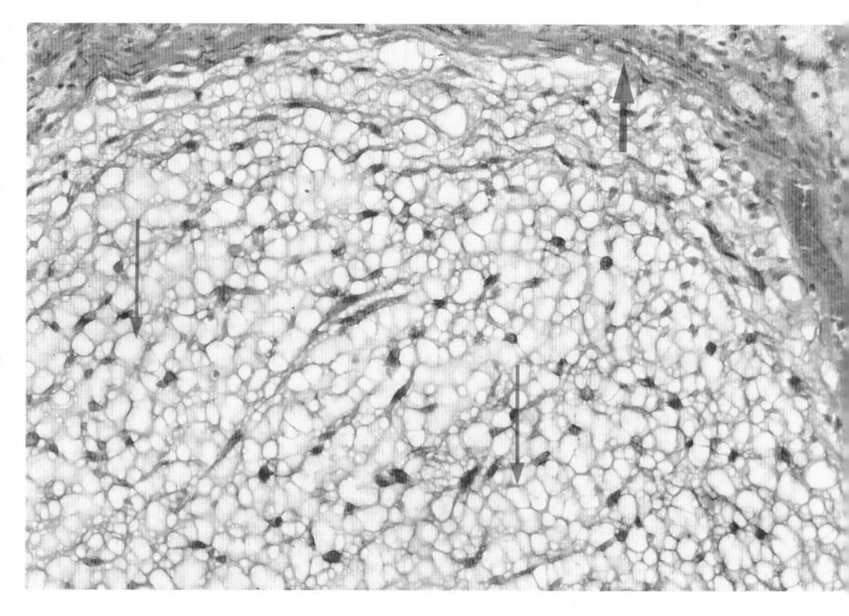

3.26 Fibrous cortical defect (non-ossifying fibroma): bone

Fibrous cortical defect is a benign sharply delineated lesion of the long bones of adolescents, which starts near the epiphysis but moves away from it as the bone grows. A non-ossifying fibroma is similar to a fibrous cortical defect except that it occurs within a bone and is usually larger. Neither it nor fibrous cortical defect is a true neoplasm, but both are associated with a defect in the epiphyseal plate and a fracture sometimes occurs through the lesion. The presenting symptom is usually pain, but most of the lesions are free of symptoms and slowly resolve. Macroscopically fibrous cortical defect is generally brown or dark red in colour, and this one, in the femur of a girl of 13, was brown to the naked eye. Histologically it consists of interlacing bundles of moderately cellular collagenous fibrous tissue (thin arrow), rich in plump spindle-shaped cells with elongated nuclei. Macrophages and small lymphocytes are also present in the fibrous tissue, along with numerous compact (osteoclast-like) multinucleated giant cells (thick arrow). HE ×235

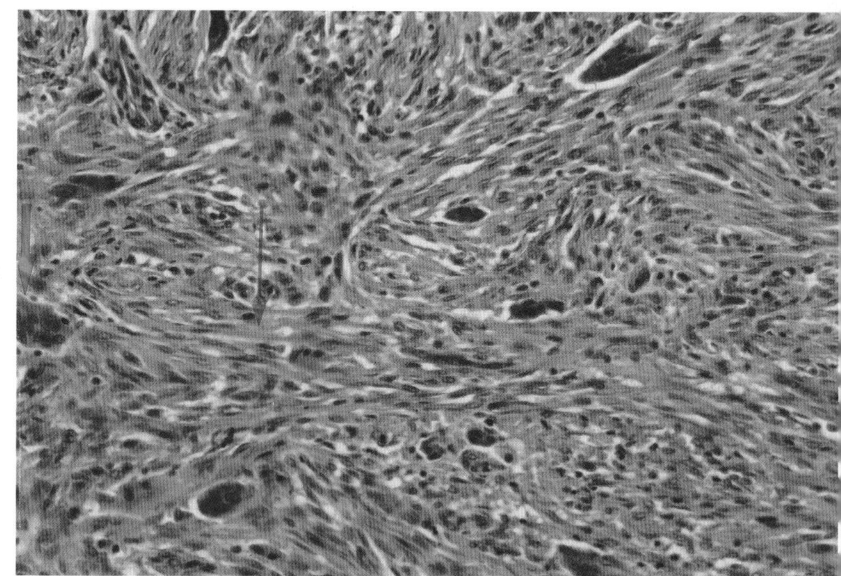

3.27 Fibrous cortical defect (non-ossifying fibroma): bone

Fibrous cortical defect is sharply demarcated by a scalloped plate of sclerotic bone which always abuts on the cortex. Sometimes a storiform pattern is evident in the fibrous tissue of fibrous cortical defects, and clusters of fat-filled macrophages and deposits of hemosiderin are often also present in the lesion. There is no evidence of bone trabecula formation. In this fibrous cortical defect, which had (macroscopically) a characteristic brown colour, consists of fibrous tissue, large numbers of elongated fibroblasts (stained red) with elongated blunt-ended nuclei, and large numbers of macrophages of various shapes, including many elongated fibroblast-like forms. Within the cytoplasm of the round macrophages (and many of the fibroblast-like cells) there are large amounts of hemosiderin which has been stained deeply blue by Perls' method (Perls' method colours hemosiderin blue). There is virtually no hemosiderin however within the many red-stained multinucleated giant cells (thick arrows). Perls' method ×360

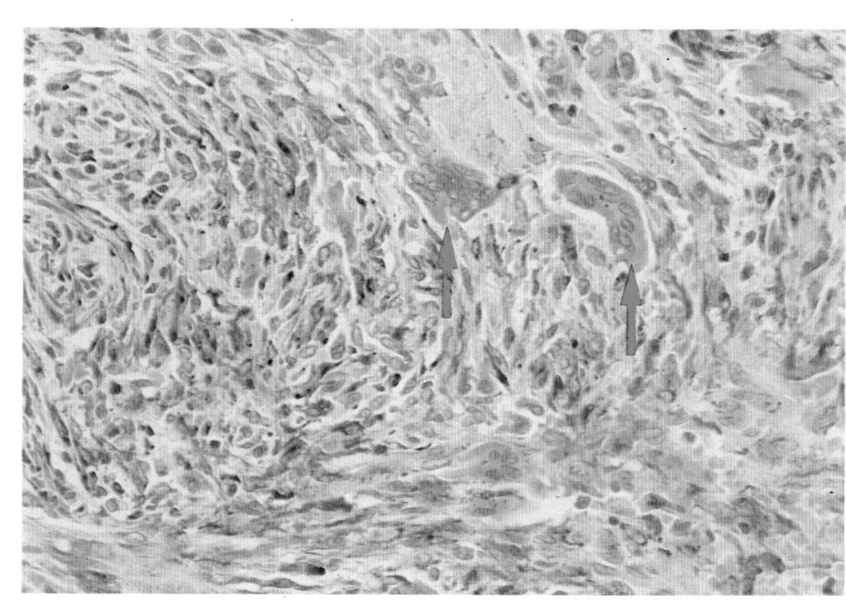

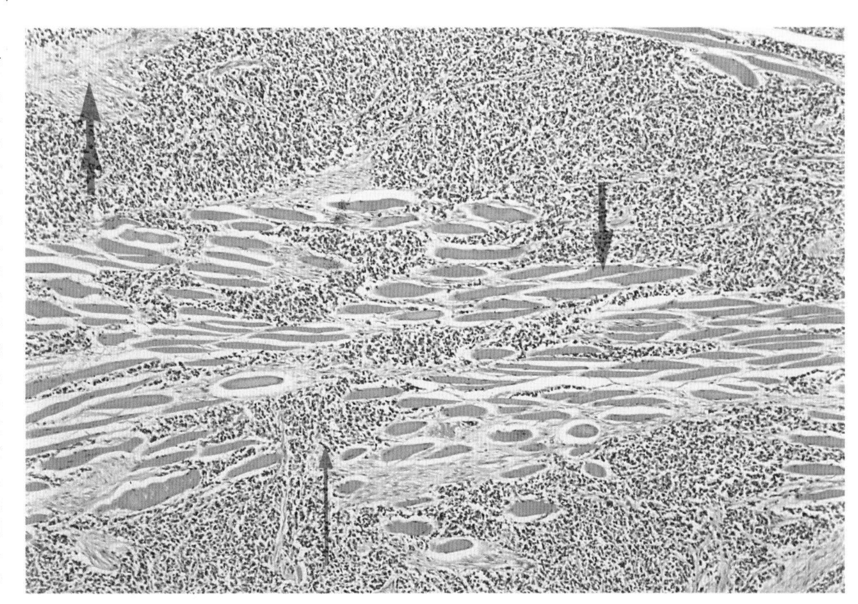

3.28 Ewing's sarcoma: scapula

Ewing's sarcoma is an uncommon malignant neoplasm of children and young adults (5-30 years of age), with a 25% survival rate. Males are affected twice as often as females. Most lesions are located in the diaphysis of the bones of the limbs or pelvis but may be found in other sites. The tumour is of uncertain origin but probably arises from primitive neuroectodermal cells, the presence of the t(11-22) translocation helping to distinguish Ewing's sarcoma from neuroblastoma (which often shows partial monosomy 1). The patient often has pain in the site of the tumour and also pyrexia. Osteomyelitis may be suspected. The tumour metastasizes readily and the prognosis is poor. This lesion originated in the scapula but it grew rapidly and invaded the associated muscles. This shows broad sheets of small anaplastic proliferating small round cells (thin arrow) with compact spheroidal or ovoid hyperchromatic nuclei (with a high mitotic rate), infiltrating between deeply eosinophilic striated muscle fibres (thick arrow), many of which are compressed and atrophic. There are also some bundles of paler collagenous fibrous tissue (double arrow). HE ×60

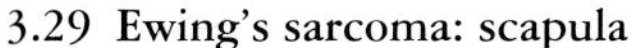

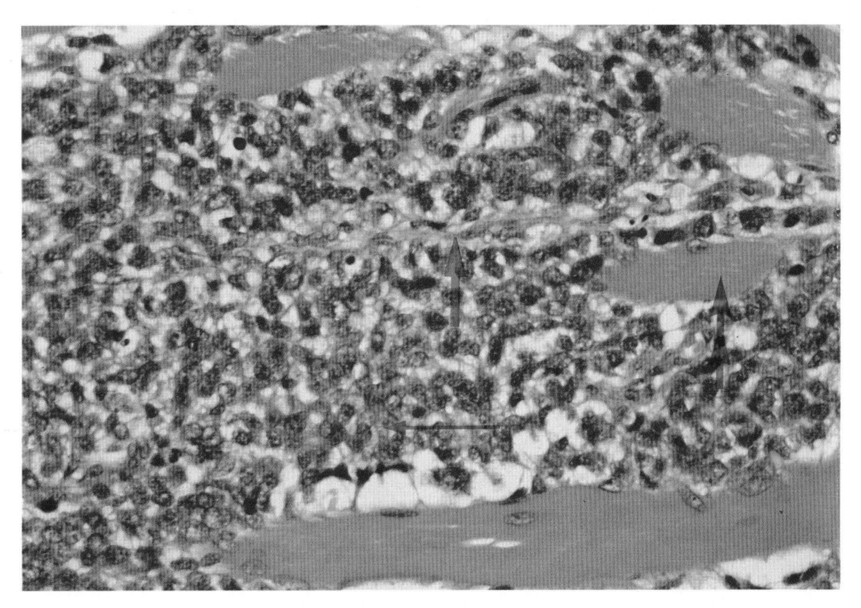

3.29 Ewing's sarcoma: scapula

Ewing's sarcoma is soft and friable, with areas of necrosis and hemorrhage. It grows rapidly, and expands to destroy the medullary cavity, bony cortex and surrounding soft tissues. By means of X-rays, it has the appearance, in the diaphysis, of a radiolucent lesion which infiltrates the cortex and destroys it from within. It also tends to spread by the bloodstream at an early stage. The presence of periodic acid-Schiff (PAS)-positive glycogen in the cytoplasm and of antigen 0-13 (by immunohistochemical techniques), as well as chromosomal translocation abnormality, are helpful diagnostic features. This is part of the same tumour as in **3.28**, at higher magnification. The tumour cells (thin arrow) have round vesicular nuclei (about twice the size of a lymphocyte nucleus) which show only slight pleomorphism. The cytoplasm is scant and heavily vacuolated and the cytoplasmic boundaries indistinct. The stroma consists of small blood vessels (thick arrow). There are a few pyknotic nuclei but no mitoses are present in this field. However they were numerous elsewhere. The striated muscle fibres are atrophic and probably fragmented (double arrow). HE ×360

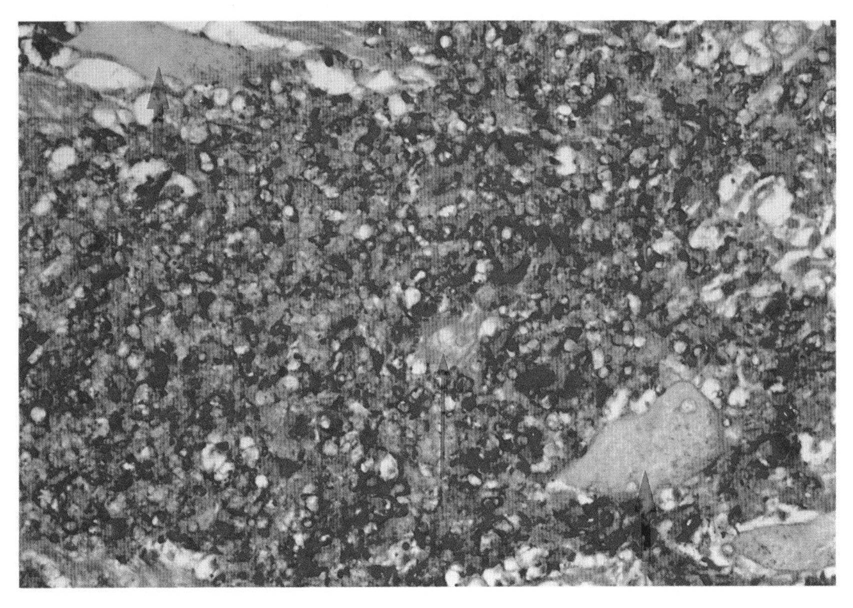

3.30 Ewing's sarcoma: scapula

In the sparse ill-defined cytoplasm of the cells of a Ewing's tumour there are few organelles (including mitochondria) and no neurosecretory granules or neuron-specific esterase (NSE). Nor is there any desmin, vimentin or keratin. In this part of the same lesion as in **3.29** and **3.30**, the vacuolated cytoplasm of the malignant cells contains a considerable amount of glycogen, and its presence is an important diagnostic criterion. The histological section has been reacted by the periodic acid-Schiff (PAS) method which stains the glycogen a deep purplish-red colour. The cytoplasm of all the tumour cells reacts positively. A histological section pretreated with diastase was PAS-negative, confirming that the substance in the cytoplasm was glycogen and readily destroyed by the diastase. The small blood vessels of the stroma (thin arrow) and the striated muscle fibres (thick arrows), without treatment with diastase, do not stain PAS-positively for glycogen. PAS ×360

3.31 Rheumatoid arthritis

Rheumatoid arthritis is a chronic systemic disease of unknown etiology. There is a progressive and potentially deforming inflammatory arthritis, involving many joints and particularly those of the hands and feet. The synovial membrane lining an affected joint is inflamed and hyperplastic, and proliferates to form swollen congested thick villous processes which project into the joint space. The villous processes consist of fleshy granulation tissue (termed pannus) in which there are numerous lymphocytes (mostly T helper cells) and plasma cells. The cartilaginous lining of the joint may be destroyed and fibrous ankylosis of the joint results. This is the capsule and synovial lining of an inflamed joint. The synovial cells have proliferated, and the joint (top) is now lined by a thick multicelled layer of elongated synovial cells with eosinophilic cytoplasm (thin arrows). The fibrous capsule of the joint is hyperemic with dilated blood vessels (thick arrow) and heavily infiltrated with chronic inflammatory cells, mainly lymphocytes which have formed a lymphoid follicle (double arrow). HE ×150

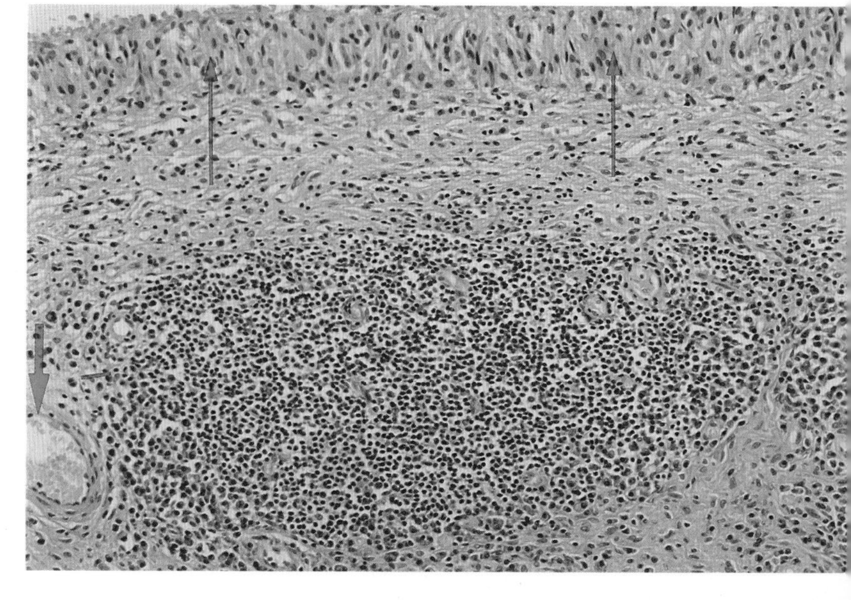

3.32 Rheumatoid arthritis

In rheumatoid arthritis, nodules (1-2 cm dia) often develop in the subcutaneous tissues, often in the skin at the elbows. They are granulomas, consisting of a central sheet of deeply eosinophilic fibrous tissue which has undergone fibrinoid necrosis, surrounded by palisaded histiocytes. In the joints, on the other hand, there are generally large numbers of neutrophil leukocytes in the synovial fluid but they are scarce in synovial tissue. This is a synovial villus, and it is projecting into the same joint as in 3.31. It consists of connective tissue covered with an irregular layer of flat synovial cells with a moderate amount of cytoplasm and a pleomorphic nucleus. The connective tissue is vascular, with numerous dilated small blood vessels (thin arrows), and its stroma is heavily infiltrated with chronic inflammatory cells, many of which are mature plasma cells. Two Russell bodies (thick arrows), effete plasma cells with red-stained cytoplasm, are present. HE ×310

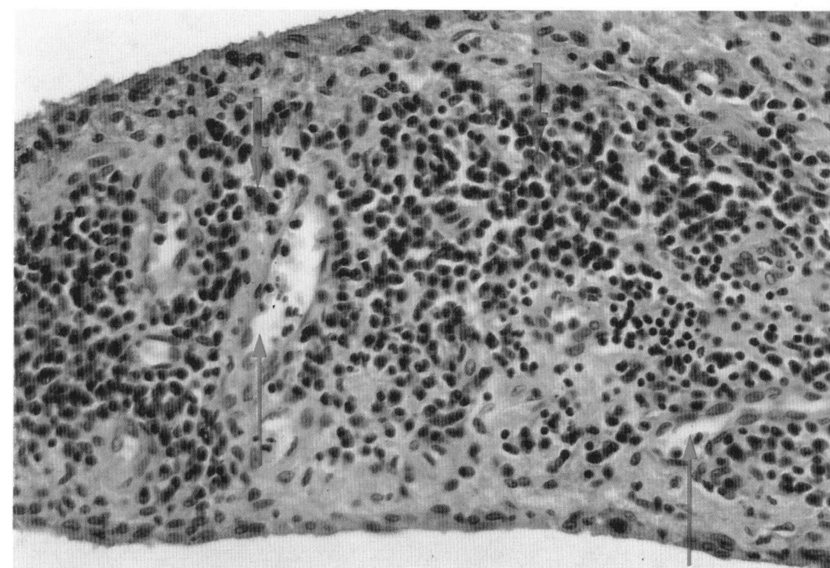

3.33 Rheumatoid arthritis: metacarpophalangeal joint

Pannus, which consists of granulation tissue and many lymphocytes and plasma cells, erodes articular cartilage, subchondral bone, peri-articular ligaments and tendons, leading to progressive destruction of joints. Initially, in this joint, pannus (vascular connective tissue and many chronic inflammatory cells) has grown across the surface of the metacarpal from the capsule of the joint and obliterated the joint space. At the same time it has destroyed the articular cartilage, which would normally have been present on the upper surface, and also the underlying deeply eosinophilic dense lamellar bone of the metacarpal (double arrow). Now, as shown here, the affected joint consists of the eroded head of the metacarpal at the bottom and, above it, covered by a sheet of pale fibrous connective tissue (thin arrow) in which there are several small blood vessels and only a few small lymphocytes. A few small pale-staining fragments of cartilage matrix (thick arrow) remain in the connective tissue. This is clearly a fully ankylosed joint.

HE ×200

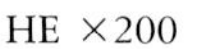

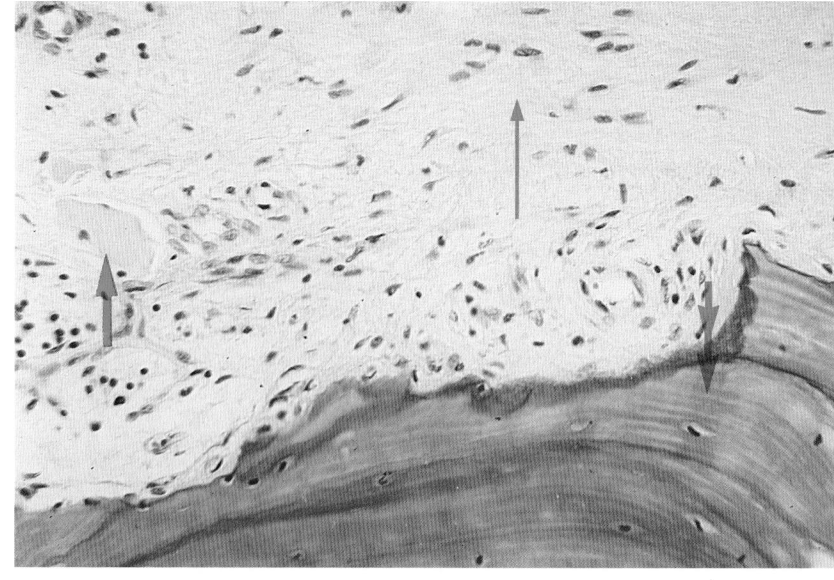

3.34 Synovial chondromatosis

Synovial osteochondromatosis is an uncommon condition of unknown etiology, which sometimes gives rise to pain and swelling. It usually affects the knee but sometimes he hip-joint, and is characterized by the presence of multiple foci of cartilaginous metaplasia in the synovial membrane lining the joint, with the synovial cells proliferating to form nodules of cartilage and bone. Sometimes fragments containing the new tissue break off and become oose bodies within the joint. Movement of the joint is ometimes limited, and may lock intermittently. The outcome may be osteoarthrosis. The condition is reputedly benign but local recurrence occasionally takes place. Most of the new tissue is a type of connective tissue which resembles immature cartilage, with abundant pale bluish ntercellular matrix and large well-spaced ovoid cells thin arrow). In several areas however the tissue is more ikely to be cartilaginous, consisting of more mature-ooking chondrocytic cells in basophilic matrix (double arrow). In other parts of the lesion the proliferating synovial tissue has undergone hyaline degeneration (thick arrows). HE x150

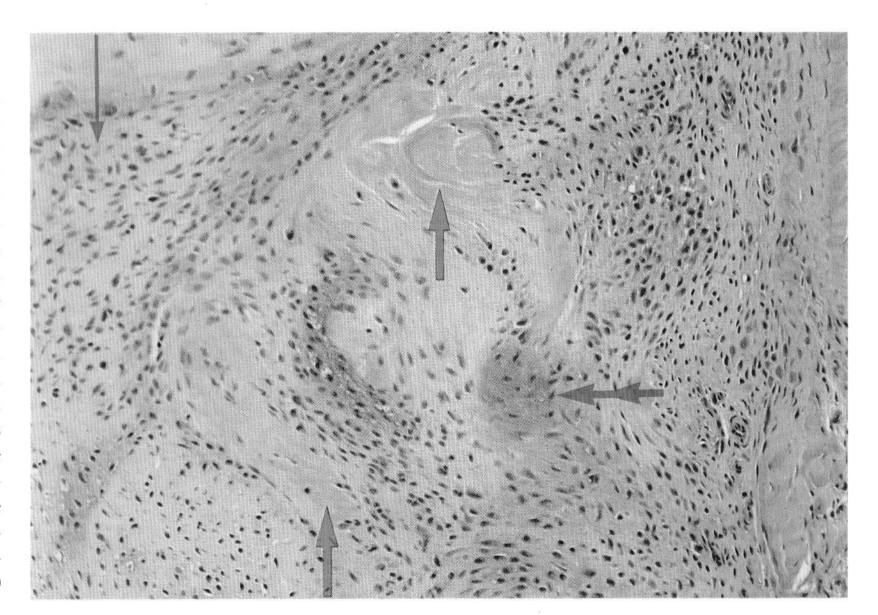

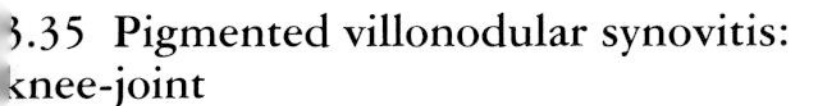

3.35 Pigmented villonodular synovitis: knee-joint

Villonodular synovitis, probably an inflammatory lesion, occurs in young adults and usually involves a large joint knee, ankle, hip, etc.). The synovial lining of the joint proliferates and fills the joint with villous outgrowths papillary processes), dark orange-brown in colour from the presence of large amounts of hemosiderin. It is a benign lesion, but complete excision of all the papillary processes is difficult and recurrence not infrequent. Malignant change does not take place. Large numbers of elongated villi (thick arrows) project into the knee joint from the thick fibrous capsule (thin arrow). The villi, which have a core of vascular connective tissue, consist of proliferating synovial epithelial cells, lymphocytes, plasma cells and histiocytes. At higher magnification, many of histiocytes appear foamy and contain lipid and hemosiderin, and multinucleated giant cells are often present. Generally however, the villi are slender and delicate, and ack the bulky infiltrate of lymphocytes and plasma cells n the synovial villi in rheumatoid arthritis. The histological appearances of this lesion resemble so-called giant-cell tumour of tendon sheath. HE x80

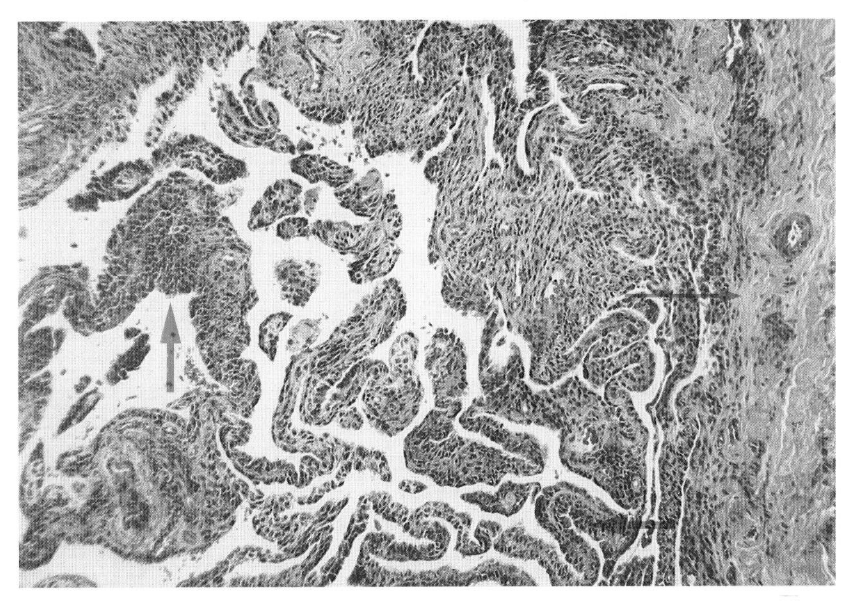

3.36 Giant-cell tumour of tendon sheath

There is uncertainty as to whether giant-cell tumour of tendon sheath (benign fibrous histiocytoma), a common benign lesion involving the synovium, is a true neoplasm or an inflammatory reaction (nodular synovitis). It usually arises within the joint (usually the knee) or in the tendon sheaths in the hands and feet. In a tendon, the lesion is a well-defined firm round rubbery mass (0.3-3 cm dia) with a grey or brown cut surface, whereas in the knee it is similar but often pedunculated and sometimes multiple. The yellowish-brown mass is benign, but pressure may cause atrophy of neighbouring structures. Histologically it consists of cellular fibrous tissue in which there are many histiocytes with ill-defined eosinophilic cytoplasm (thin arrows), some of it vacuolated (foamy), as well as macrophages, multinucleated giant cells (double arrow) and fibroblasts. Many macrophages contain a large amount of golden-brown hemosiderin (thick arrow). The surface of the tumour is covered with the flattened synovial cells lining the tendon sheath.

HE x335

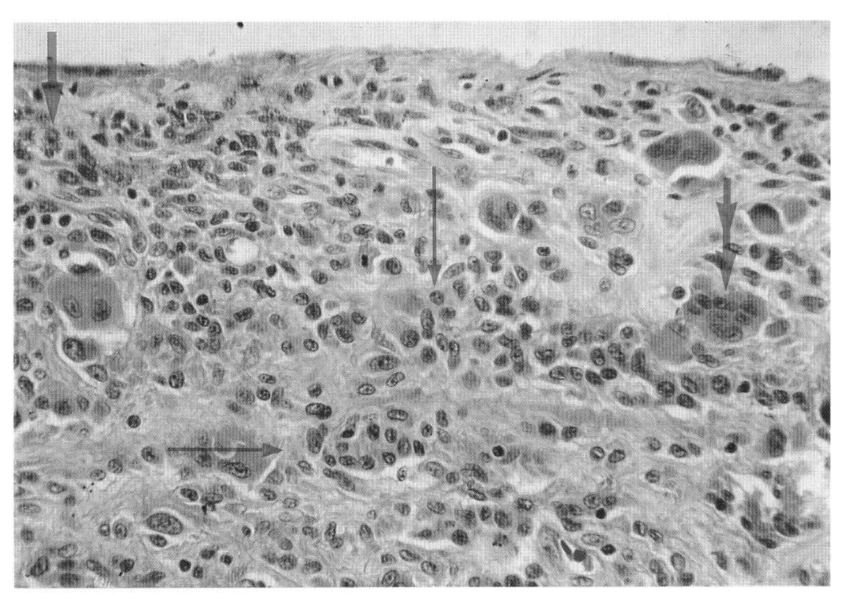

3.37 Bursitis: elbow

When a bursa forms over the olecranon (the proximal bony projection of the ulna at the elbow) and then becomes inflamed, it is termed olecranon bursitis (also called student's elbow). It is caused most often as a result of repeated trauma. The bursa is distended with watery fluid at first, but hemorrhage sometimes occurs, and altered blood and fibrin are often present. Granulation tissue forms and the wall of the bursa becomes thick and vascular and eventually fibrosed, containing only a sparse exudate of lymphocytes and plasma cells. The wall of this bursa consists of a sheet vascular granulation tissue and young connective tissue (thin arrow), in which there are large numbers of dilated capillaries, macrophages, elongated fibroblasts and chronic inflammatory cells. The wall is lined with a single layer of flattened synovial cells (thick arrow), and projecting from it, into the lumen, are long dense strands of fibrin (stained a dense red colour) (double arrow). In chronic bursitis long strands of fibrous tissue may form in the lumen. HE ×135

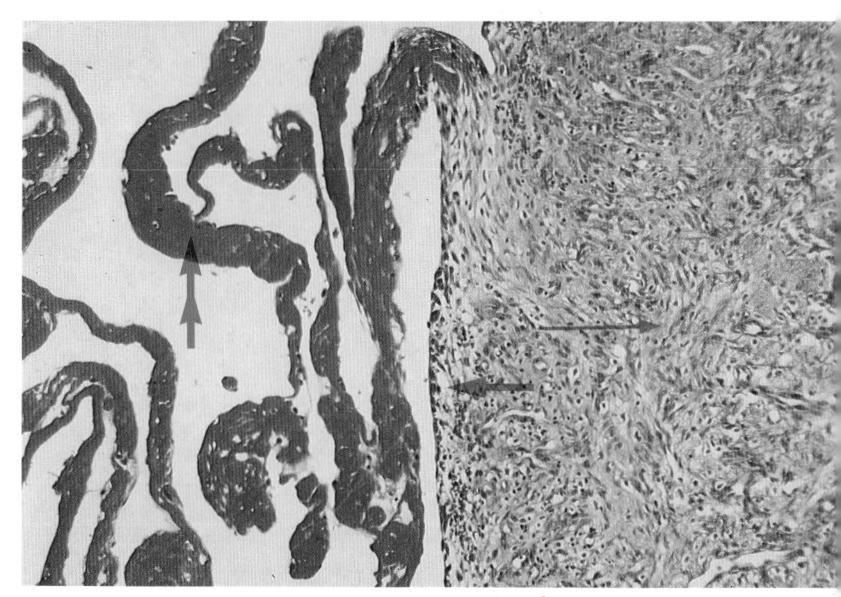

3.38 Osteoarthrosis: hip joint

Osteoarthrosis, sometimes termed (inaccurately) osteoarthritis, is a disease of the elderly. It is not an inflammatory disease, and the changes in an affected joint are apparently secondary to degenerative changes in the hyaline articular cartilage. The normally smooth white articular surface becomes irregular and yellow. In this joint, the articular cartilage is thinner than normal and its surface (top) is uneven and 'rough'. Several clefts extend deeply into the cartilage, one reaching as far as the underlying bone trabeculae (thin arrow). This process of fissuring of the articular cartilage is termed fibrillation. Fissuring exposes the chondrocytes in the cartilage and many have disappeared, leaving acellular matrix (thick arrows). Some of the remaining chondrocytes are however large and hypertrophic (double arrows). There are few changes in the deeply eosinophilic bone (bottom), but in severe osteoarthrosis the articular cartilage may be lost. Loss of articular cartilage stimulates new bone formation, the trabeculae of the exposed bone then tend to thicken, and nodules (osteophytes) usually form at the margins of the bone. HE ×55

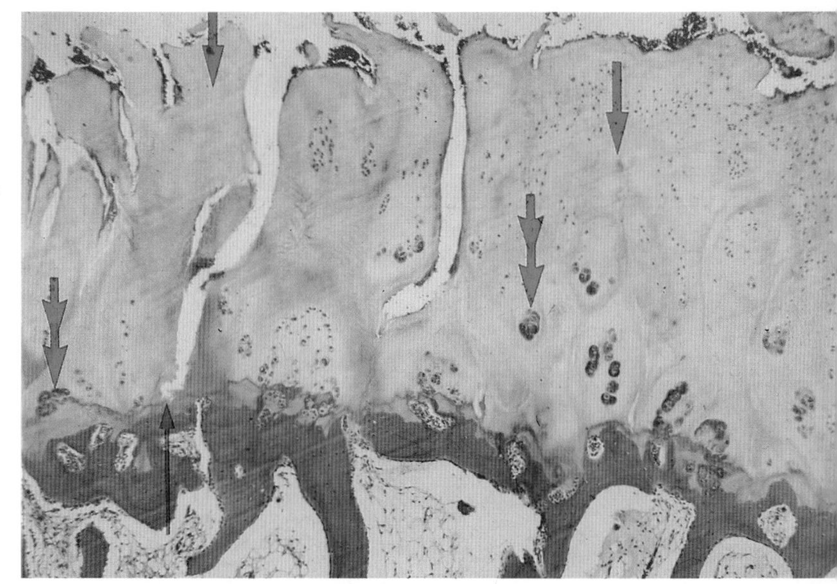

3.39 Fibromatosis (plantar fibromatosis)

Fibromatoses are one of the groups of locally aggressive soft tissue neoplasms intermediate in behaviour between benign and malignant, which are locally infiltrative and tend to recur after surgical excision. Despite their locally aggressive behaviour however, they do not metastasize and in this way differ from sarcomas. The term covers a wide range of types which differ markedly in structure and behaviour. They include keloid, nodular fasciitis, Dupuytren's contracture, juvenile aponeurotic fibroma, Peyronie's disease, proliferative myositis, myositis ossificans, congenital torticollis, retroperitoneal fibrosis, mediastinal fibrosis, nasopharyngeal angiofibroma and desmoid tumour. This lesion is not located in the palmar fascia of the hand but (unusually) in the plantar fascia in the sole of the foot of a man aged 30. It consists of a sheet dense collagenous tissue, with its scanty content of slender fibrocytes (thick arrow). The dense collagenous tissue is being eroded and replaced by highly cellular new connective tissue in which the numerous fibroblasts are much larger and active-looking (thin arrow). When the new connective tissue matures to become collagenous and scar-like fibrous tissue, it contracts and causes deformities of the toes. A similar lesion in the palms (palmar fibromatosis; Dupuytren's contracture) has the same effect on the fingers. HE ×360

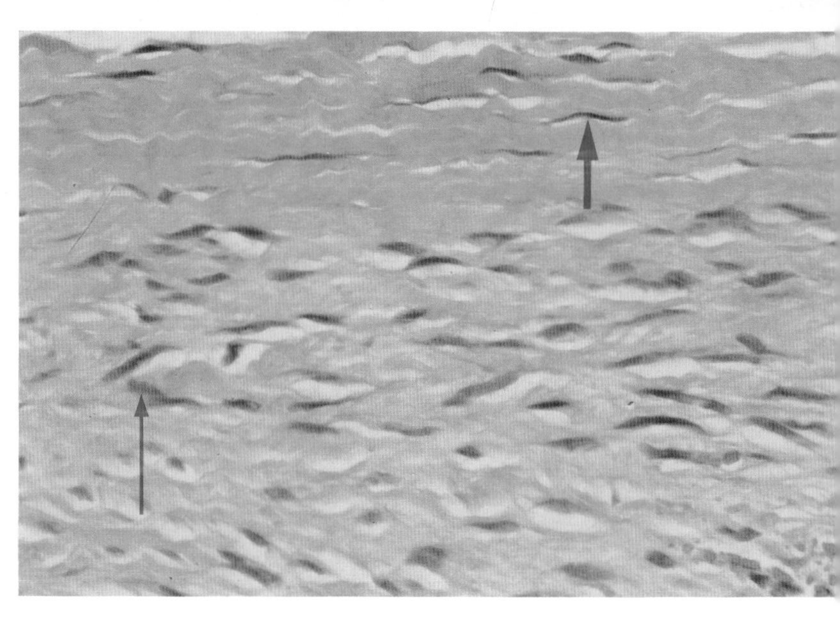

3.40 Fibromatosis (nodular fasciitis)

Fibromatoses are slow-growing lesions which form large tumour-like masses of collagenous fibrous tissue. Many of the lesions arise in the fascia of a muscle (musculo- aponeurotic fibromatosis), usually in skeletal muscle, most often in rectus abdominis muscle, and especially in women after pregnancy. The more aggressive types of fibromatosis infiltrate locally and may be confused with fibrosarcoma. They may also recur after excision but do not metastasize. This is an example of nodular fasciitis in a 46-year-old man who developed a subcutaneous lump on the medial aspect of his left arm 8cm above the elbow. It is an aggressive type of lesion which appears to be arising from a vertical aponeurotic band of fibrous tissue in the centre of the field. The lesion consists of cellular connective tissue (thin arrow) and large numbers of small blood vessels (thick arrows), with an appearance similar to that of granulation tissue. The vascular connective tissue is spreading from both surfaces of the fibrous tissue, more superficially into the overlying subcutaneous fat (double arrow) and more deeply towards the underlying muscle on the right (not visible). HE ×60

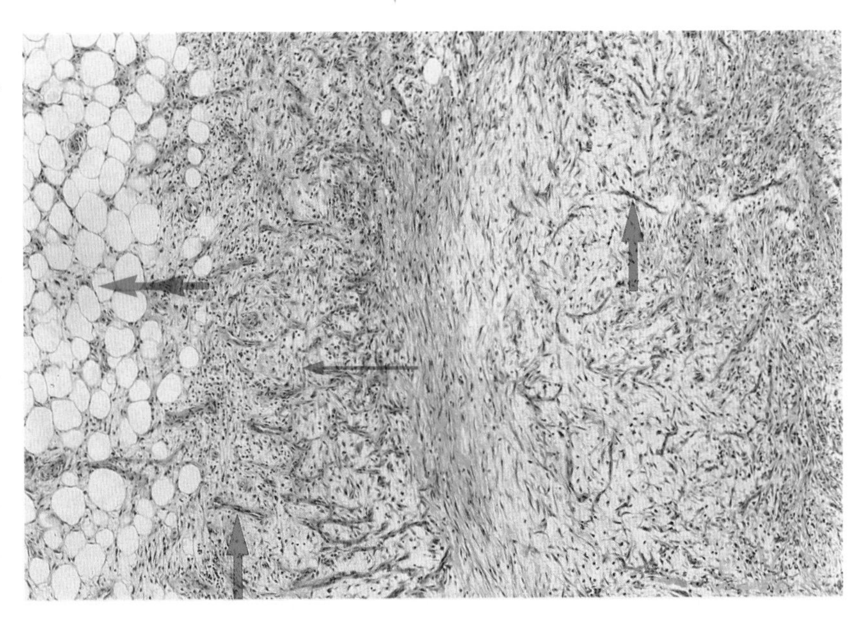

3.41 Fibromatosis (nodular fasciitis)

Nodular fasciitis is also called infiltrative fasciitis, proliferative fasciitis or pseudosarcomatous fasciitis. Most of the patients are between 20 and 35 years of age, and men and women are equally susceptible. The lesion is most often in the subcutaneous tissues and less often intramuscularly or adjoining a deeper fascial plane. This is part of the same lesion as in 3.40. The collagenous fibrous tissue of the aponeurosis (double arrow) is at the right edge of the field and the subcutaneous fat is on the left. In the centre there is a sheet of loose highly cellular connective tissue and large numbers of small blood vessels (thin arrow). This is new tissue, at the edge of the lesion (most of the lesion is out of sight elsewhere), and it is advancing from the surface of the mature fibrous tissue into the fat. Also present in the new tissue are macrophages (foamy from ingested lipid) (thick arrow), small lymphocytes and elongated fibroblasts. The fibroblasts, among which there is considerable mitotic activity, have already formed a considerable amount of collagenous tissue. HE ×150

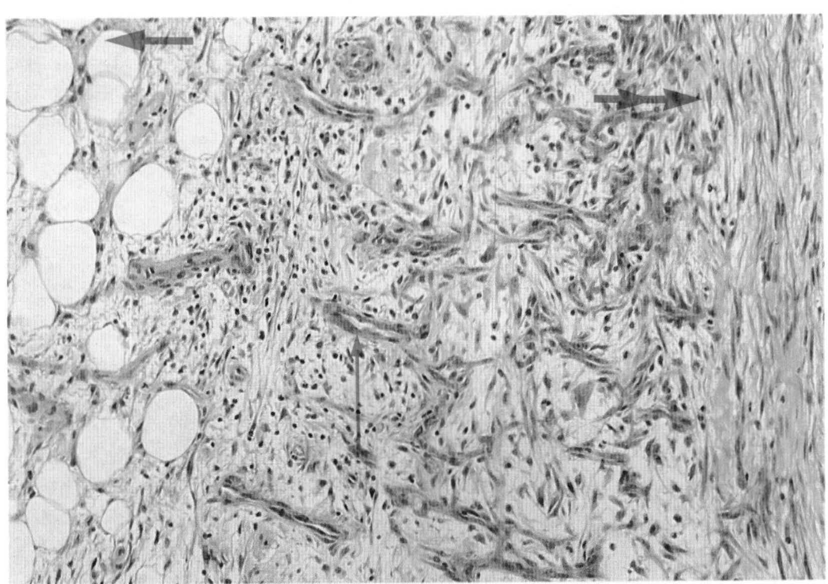

3.42 Fibromatoses

The majority of cases of nodular fasciitis are located in an upper limb (generally the forearm), and elswhere in the trunk, lower limb or head and neck. The lesion is generally ovoid, not encapsulated but freely movable, and composed of plump spindle-shaped or stellate fibrocytes in a loose (myxomatous) stroma. This is part of the same lesion as in 3.40 and 3.41. It is one of the more cellular 'fibroblastic' areas in the lesion, consisting of loose connective tissue in which there are numerous large and mostly very elongated fibroblast-like cells (thick arrow) with abundant eosinophilic cytoplasm and plump round-ended nuclei. The nuclei also show fairly considerable pleomorphism. The fibroblastic cells are forming strands of collagenous fibres in the connective tissue, the broad wavy band of dense fibrous tissue (thin arrow) being part of the aponeurosis. There are no mitoses among these cells but occasionally mitoses are present elsewhere. Despite these appearances, this type of lesion is benign and should not be mistaken for fibrosarcoma. HE ×360

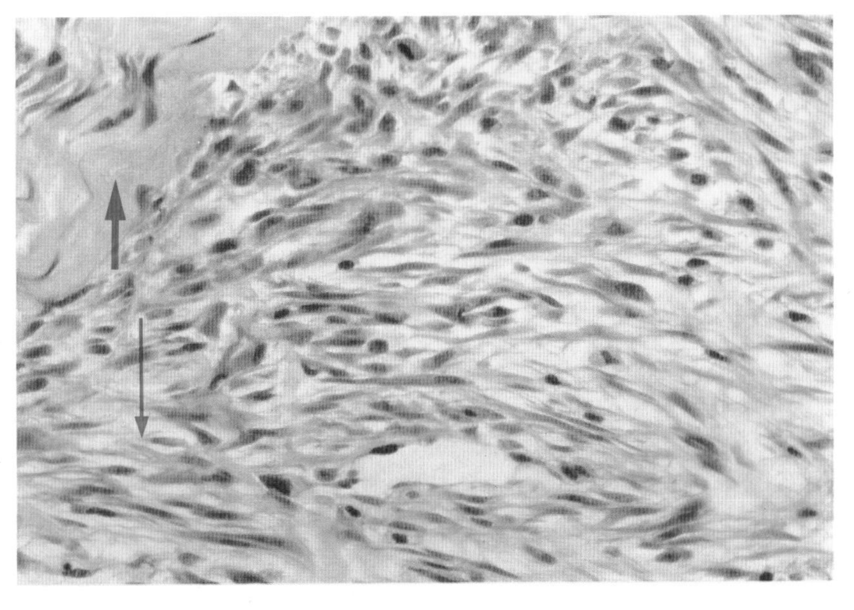

3.43 Synovial sarcoma

Synovial sarcoma is a rare neoplasm, arising from synovial epithelial cells, which may appear well-circumscribed but is malignant and prone to metastasize to the regional lymph nodes. It mainly affects young adults. Most examples are located around the knee- or ankle-joint but the tumour occurs occasionally in many other sites. This tumour has a biphasic pattern, consisting of two different types of malignant cell: firstly, large cells which resemble epithelial cells, and secondly basophilic spindle-shaped cells. The large epithelial cells have abundant deeply eosinophilic cytoplasm and pleomorphic round ovoid nuclei (thin arrow), most of which have one or more prominent nucleoli. These cells line elongated branching gland-like clefts, some of which contain amorphous materials. The basophilic spindle-shaped cells are very numerous and arranged in interlacing compact bundles (thick arrow) which form the stroma between the gland- like clefts. The stromal cells have elongated hyperchromatic spindle-shaped (fibroblast-like) nuclei and scant cytoplasm. At higher magnification, many mitotic figures were visible among both the spindle-shaped stromal cells and the epithelial cells lining the clefts.

HE ×150

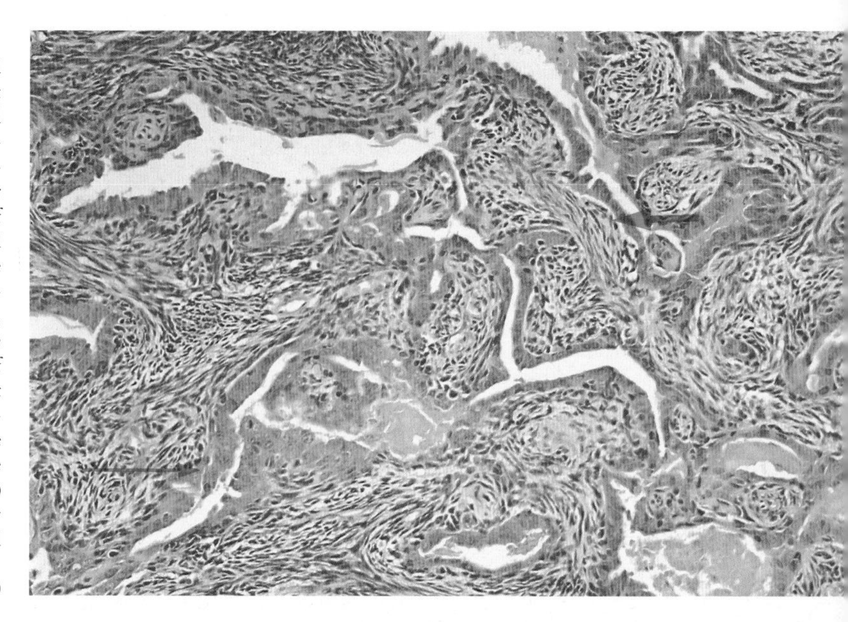

3.44 Synovial sarcoma

Synovial sarcomas are located more often in the vicinity of bursae and tendon sheaths than within joints. They therefore form extraarticular soft tissue masses, generally in the proximity of a joint in the extremities. They are high grade malignant neoplasm, with a high rate of recurrence and a tendency to metastasize. This lesion is part of the tumour in 3.43, at higher magnification. It consists of a large gland-like cleft, lined with several irregular layers of large epithelial cells (double arrow) with a fairly large amount of eosinophilic cytoplasm with ill-defined margins and large round or ovoid pale vesicular nuclei with coarsely granular chromatin and one or more prominent nucleoli. No basement membrane is present between these cells and the closely packed spindle-shaped cells (thin arrow) which form the stroma. The spindle-shaped cells have only a small amount of cytoplasm and the nuclei are elongated, spindle-shaped and very basophilic. There are mitotic figures (thick arrows) among the epithelial cells lining the clefts and also among the stromal cells. There is similar pronounced mitotic activity elsewhere throughout the tumour.

HE ×360

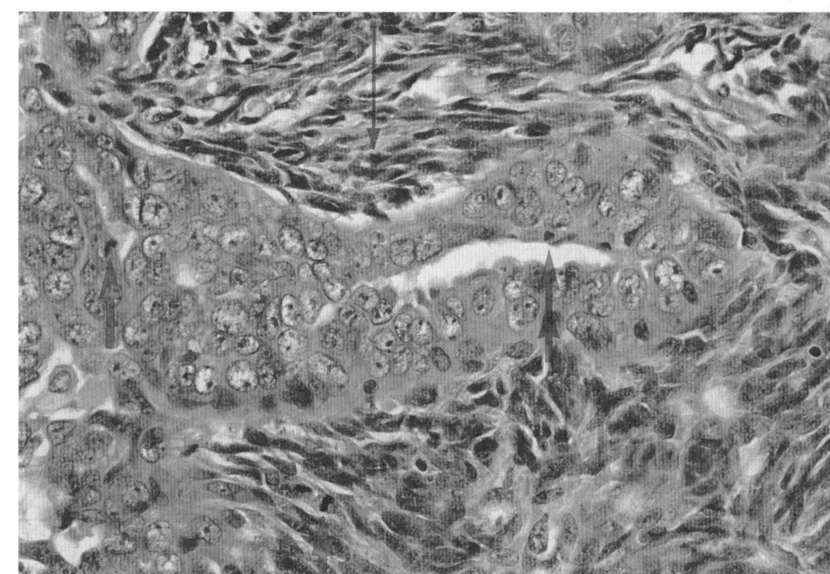

3.45 Musculo-aponeurotic fibromatosis (desmoid tumour): rectus abdominis

This lesion is a lobulated smooth surfaced mass (9.5 × 7 × 5cm) weighing 186g which was removed from the lower rectus abdominis muscle of a man aged 54. It is firm, and the cut surface is fibrous with a whorled pattern. This histological section has been stained by the van Gieson method which colours collagen fibres purplish-red and cytoplasm yellowish. The tumour consists of broad sheets of tightly packed interlacing bundles of purplish-red collagenous connective tissue (thin arrow), highly cellular and containing large numbers of uniformly distributed mature fibroblasts, very elongated and generally aligned in parallel, with elongated spindle-shaped nuclei. At higher magnification, scanty mitotic figures can be detected among these fibroblasts. Interspersed with the fibrous tissue there are broad strands of normal neutral fat, consisting of very large fat cells (adipocytes), each with a single large clear (empty) vacuole which contained fat (thick arrow). The lesion may be regarded as a benign fibrolipoma, but it is much more likely to be an example of musculo-aponeurotic fibromatosis (so-called desmoid tumour), particularly in view of its location. Such a lesion is liable to recur.

Van Gieson ×60

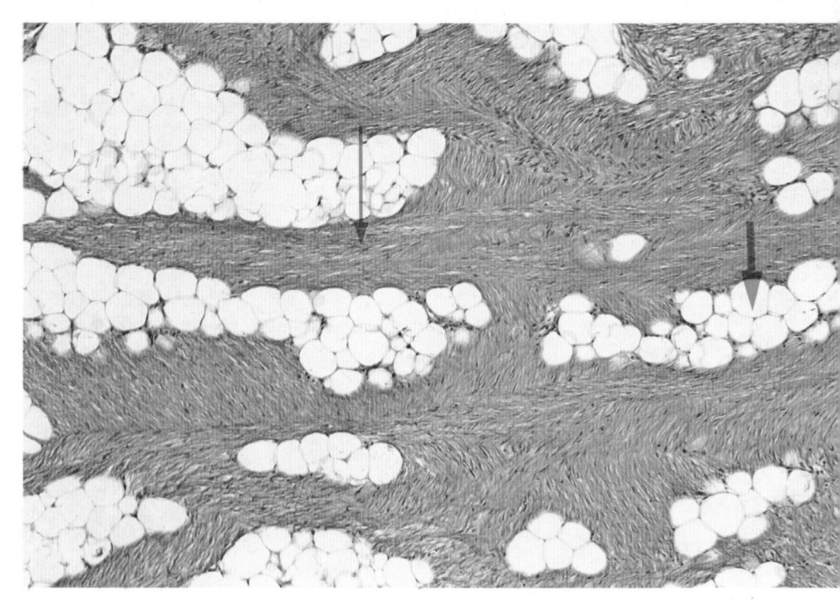

3.46 Elastofibroma: scapula

:lastofibroma is a distinctive lesion that is almost always onfined to the inferior angle of a scapula, generally in individuals more than 50 years of age who have worked as nanual labourers. It is not a neoplasm but a degenerative rocess caused by excessive repeated movements of the capula which forms an ill-defined mass (5-10 cm dia). The mass is usually attached to the scapula and also to the inderlying chest wall. This lesion is a mass of fibrofatty issue (8cm dia) and it was removed from the scapular region of a man of 60. There was no capsule around it. Histologically it consists of hyalinized collagen fibres (thin rrows) and very broad deeply eosinophilic fibres which esemble degenerate elastic tissue (thick arrows). The road eosinophilic fibres appear to be disintegrating, and longside them there are numerous small fragments and globules, of varying size, of the same material (double arow). Neutral fat is also present elsewhere in considerable mounts in the mass of tissue. HE ×360

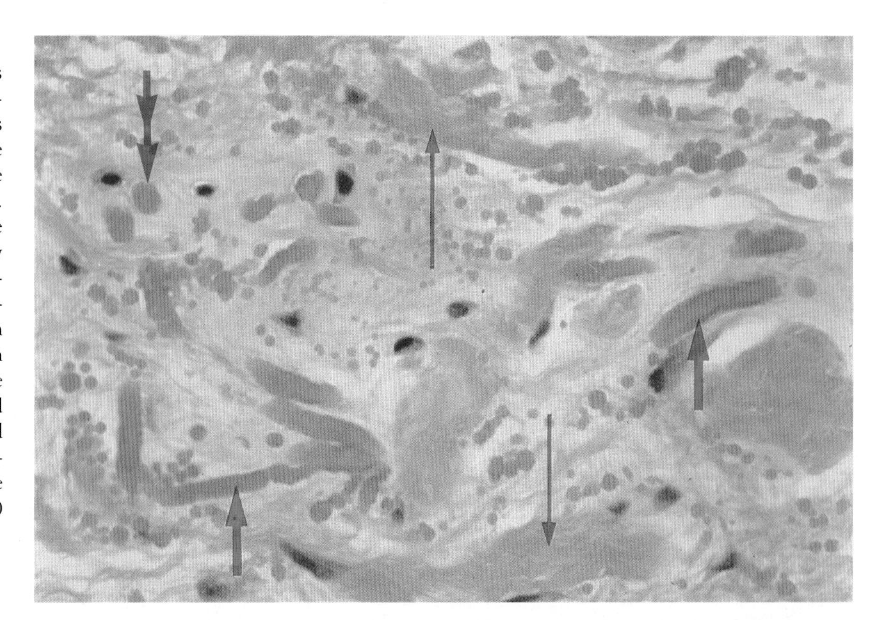

3.47 Elastofibroma: scapula

:lastofibromas are associated with recurrent bouts of eavy labour, but a response to injury rather than a neolasm has also been suggested. This is part of the same leion as in 13.46. The histological sections of the mass of legenerate tissue as been stained by a sequence which olours collagen purplish-red and elastic tissue black. The nass contains a considerable amount of mature deeply urplish-red collagen fibres (thin arrow), the most notale bundles being arranged along the bottom margin and n top left corner. Also present are elongated coarse ranching sinuous fibres and round or ovoid 'globular' odies, stained a dense black colour (thick arrow), preisely the same colour as that of normal elastic tissue. The lack 'elastic' fibres are in fact not parts of genuine elastic ibres but parts of degenerate collagenous tissue. The globular bodies are presumably fragments of the same ollagenous material

Elastic-van Gieson ×360

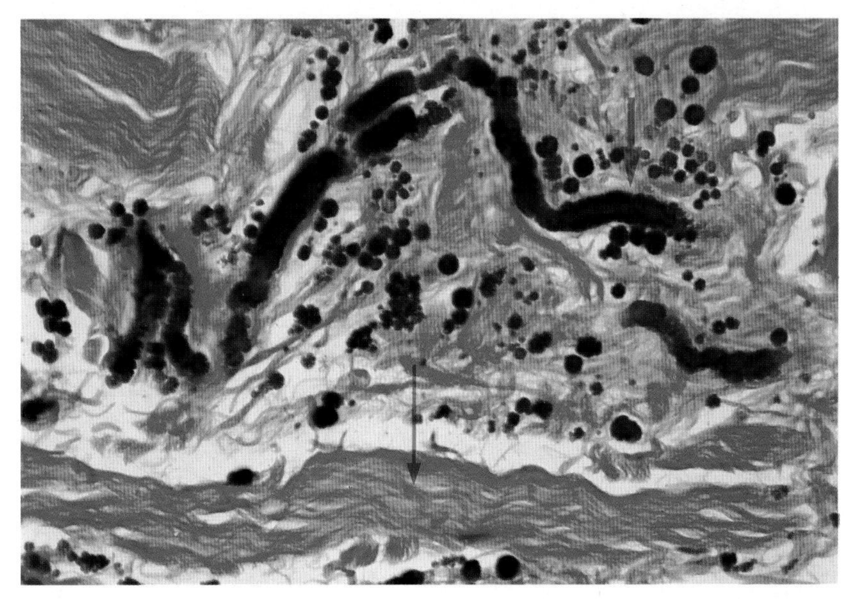

3.48 Intramuscular myxoma

ntramuscular myxomas tend to involve large muscle groups and also some in he head and neck. Other types of nyxomas tend to be subcutaneous or located alongside ascial planes and neuromuscular sheaths. Myxomas ppear to be sharply circumscribed, but intramuscular nyxomas are not encapsulated. Most myxomas are parsely cellular, and the widely separated neoplastic cells re stellate, oval or spindle-shaped in form, and their ytoplasm is ill-defined. In this case, a man 35 years of ge had a 'unilocular cyst' 4cm dia removed from his eck. It contained copious mucoid material. Histologically, it is a sheet of poorly cellular edematous issue, bounded at the right margin by eosinophilic triated muscle fibres (thin arrow). In the myxomatous issue (thick arrow) there are fairly numerous small blood essels and a sparse but evenly-distributed population of ibrocyte-like cells. No mitotic activity was detectable in hese at higher magnification. Most of the tumour is very ale, from the presence of much connective tissue mucin. There are also occasional collagen fibres, and a reticulin tain revealed a network of reticulin fibres throughout he tumour. Tumours of this type arise as a rule in skeletal nuscle, and although they may infiltrate neighbouring tructures, the prognosis is excellent after adequate esection. HE ×60

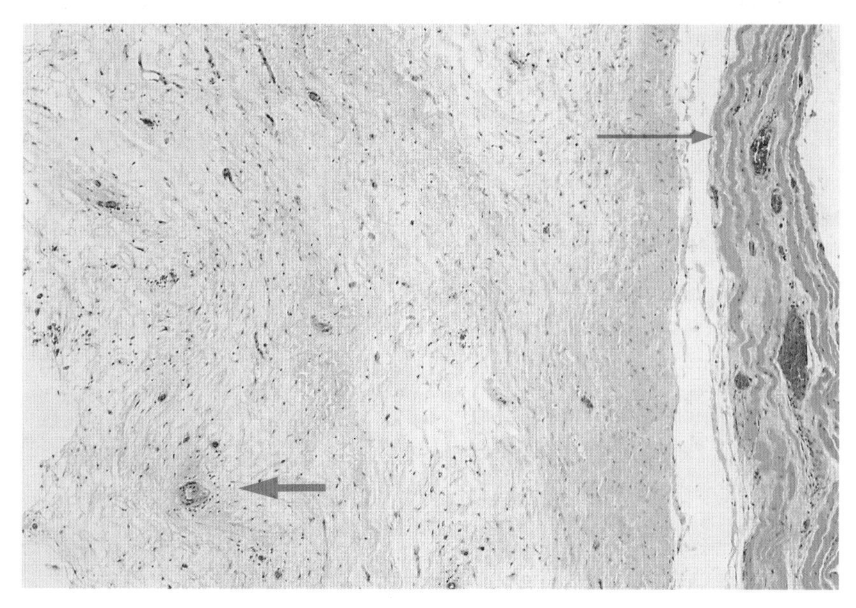

3.49 Lipomyxosarcoma: thigh

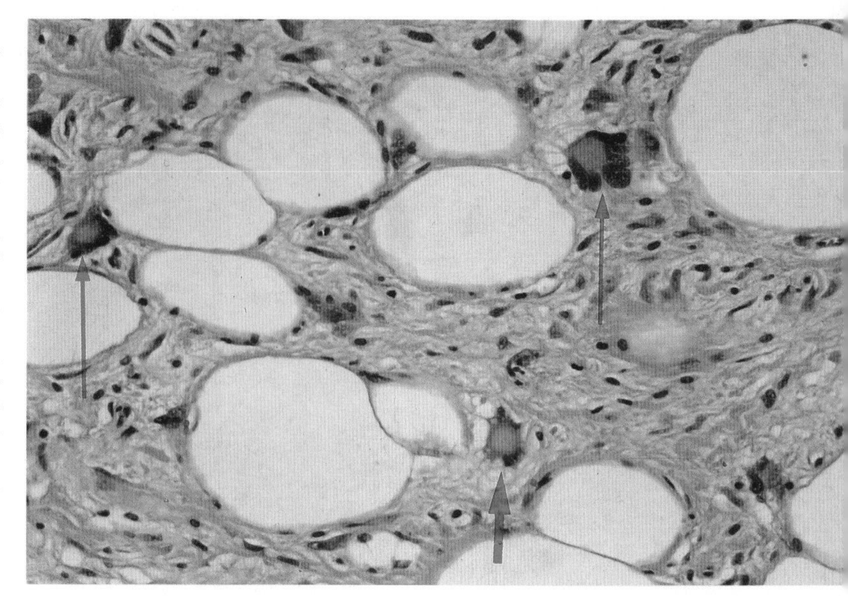

Low-grade sarcomas are better differentiated, less cellular and tend to resemble the tissue of origin to some extent. Cellular atypia is moderate and mitotic activity is usually low. Such tumours are generally slow-growing but there is a high risk of local recurrence after surgical excision and a relatively low risk of metastasis. This tumour, a mass (8 × 8 × 6cm), was removed from the thigh of a man of 70. It consists of firm white tissue, with areas of necrosis and calcification. Histologically it consists of connective tissue and fat cells of various types, including mature fat cells. Most of the cells of the connective tissue are spindle-shaped fibrocytes and fibroblasts, but various other forms are present, including small multinucleated giant cells (thin arrows). Some of the latter have very finely granular ('frosted-glass') cytoplasm (thick arrow). Mononuclear cells with finely dispersed fat in their cytoplasm elsewhere in the tumour are considered to be lipoblasts. The connective tissue is loose and special stains demonstrated much connective tissue mucin, and other parts of the tumour are myxomatous. The tumour was diagnosed as lipomyxosarcoma of low-grade malignancy.

HE ×325

3.50 Fibroliposarcoma: thigh

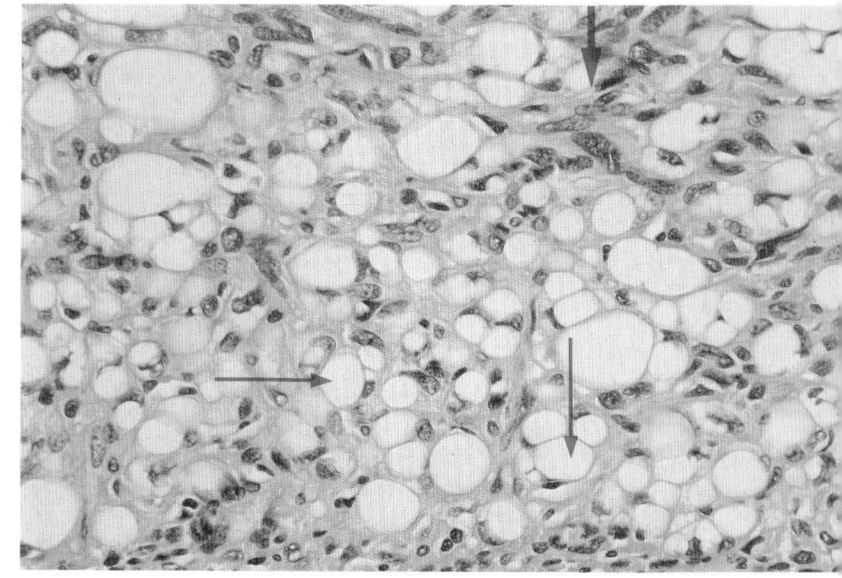

High-grade sarcomas are very cellular neoplasms, which grow rapidly, invade local tissues extensively and tend to metastasize early via the bloodstream. They are composed of poorly differentiated mesenchymal cells, and their nuclei are markedly abnormal. The rate of mitotic activity is high. Tumours of this type are frequently anaplastic and sometimes difficult to classify. The presence of lipoblasts (liposarcoma), cross-striations (rhabdomyosarcoma) or abnormal vascular channels (angiosacoma) may be helpful. A large tumour (3165g) was removed surgically from the right thigh of a woman 65 years of age. Its cut surface shows that it is composed of lobules of creamy-white partly necrotic soft tissue. On its deeper aspect it is attached to striated muscle. Microscopically the lesion is well-circumscribed but there is no true capsule. The neoplastic tissues are a mixture of pleomorphic spindle-shaped (fibroblastic) cells with elongated nuclei (thick arrow), and cells (lipoblasts) with one or more large or very large clear (previously fat-filled) vacuoles in their cytoplasm (thin arrows). In this part of the tumour the lipoblastic component predominates. Other parts of the tumour are more fibrosarcomatous.

HE ×360

3.51 Fibroliposarcoma: thigh

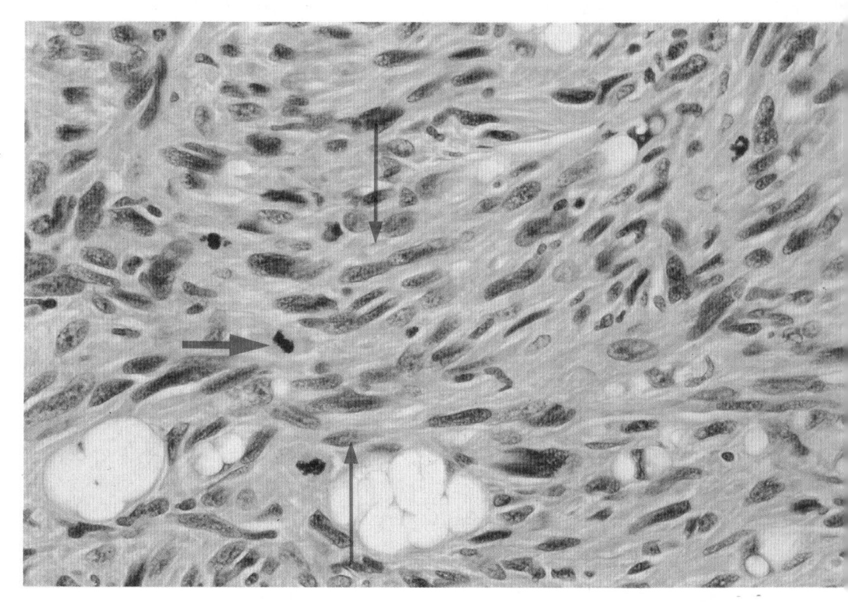

High-grade sarcomas generally metastasize early through the bloodstream but spread by the lymphatics is uncommon. They are usually fatal, and treatment is rarely successful. Identification of the cell of origin of a highly malignant tumour is sometimes very difficult, but it is now often possible to do so with the help of immunohistochemical methods. For example, factor VIII antigen is identifiable in angiosarcomas, keratin in synovial sarcomas, and myoglobin, actin and desmin in myosarcomas. Electron microscopy may also help, by demonstrating lipoblasts or Schwann cells or striated muscle fibres in the tumours. This is another part of the same tumour as in 3.50. It consists mainly of a sheet fibroblast-type cells (thin arrows) with plump elongated nuclei and abundant eosinophilic cytoplasm. Most of the nuclei have rounded ends but many are markedly pleomorphic and hyperchromatic. Numerous mitotic figures are present (thick arrow). Some of the cells have one or more large clear vacuoles (which contained fat) in their cytoplasm. The tumour was diagnosed as a high-grade (highly malignant) fibroliposarcoma of mixed fibroblastic and lipoblastic type.

HE ×360

3.52 Desmoplastic fibroma: femur

The behaviour of locally aggressive soft tissue neoplasms s usually somewhere between that of clearly benign neo- plasms and likewise that of frankly malignant tumours. Their behaviour is generally regarded as local infiltration .nd a tendency to recur after surgical excision but rarely o metastasize. One example of this type of tumour is des- noplastic fibroma. It is a rare tumour, derived from myo- ibroblasts but fibroblasts are also usually present in it. Despite the tumour's name, it may be locally destructive, .nd it often recurs if resection has not been truly ade- quate. It does not metastasize. This desmoplastic fi- oroma, in a woman 82 years of age, caused a pathological racture of her femur. The macroscopic appearance of the :ut surface of the tumour is that of firm white tissue which, histologically, consists of interlacing bundles of brightly eosinophilic dense collagenous fibrous tissue and elongated fibrocyte-like tumour cells (arrow). The neo- plastic cells scant ill-defined cytoplasm and slender hy- perchromatic nuclei which are only slightly pleomorphic .nd exhibit no mitotic activity. HE ×360

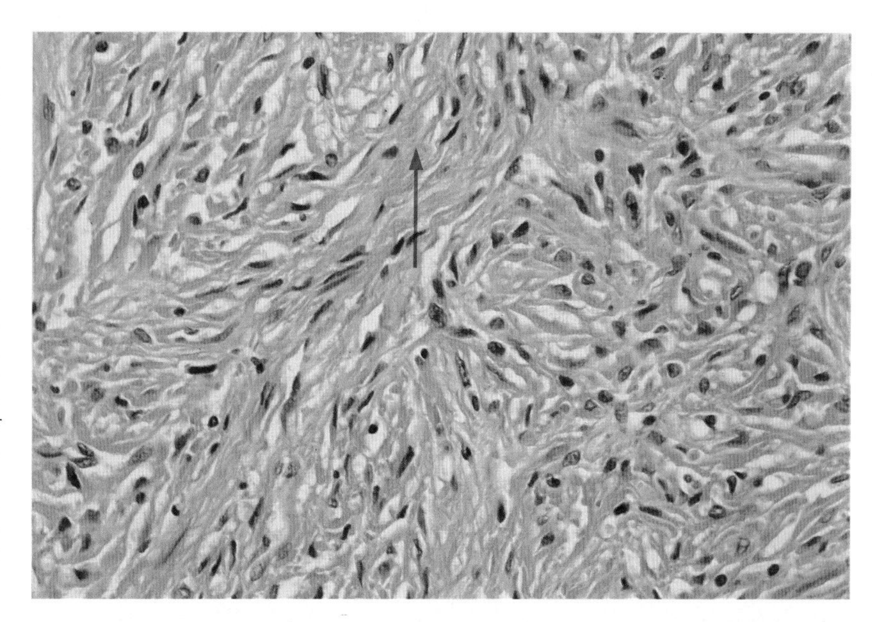

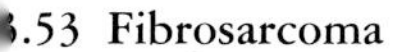

3.53 Fibrosarcoma

Sarcomas are malignant neoplasms derived from mesen- hymal cells, and they are classified according to the cell of origin. The most common types of sarcoma are malig- nant fibrous histiocytoma and liposarcoma, whereas habdomyosarcomas, leiomyosarcomas, fibrosarcomas, malignant neural neoplasms and angiosarcomas are rare. Fibrosarcoma may arise anywhere, but skin and fascia are avoured sites. It varies in malignancy from the 'desm- oplastic fibroma' to highly aggressive anaplastic tumours which rapidly metastasize by the bloodstream to the ungs. Collagen formation varies inversely with the de- gree of differentiation. This tumour was located at the origin of the pulmonary artery in a woman of 59. It is omposed of interlacing bundles of fibroblast-type cells thin arrow). Most of the nuclei are elongated and vesicu- ar and contain one or more prominent nucleoli. There is mitotic activity (thick arrows). The cells have a moderate .mount of cytoplasm but the cell boundaries are ill- defined. There is little evidence of collagen formation but . reticulin stain demonstrated many fibres. Small lym- phocytes are scattered throughout the tumour. HE ×235

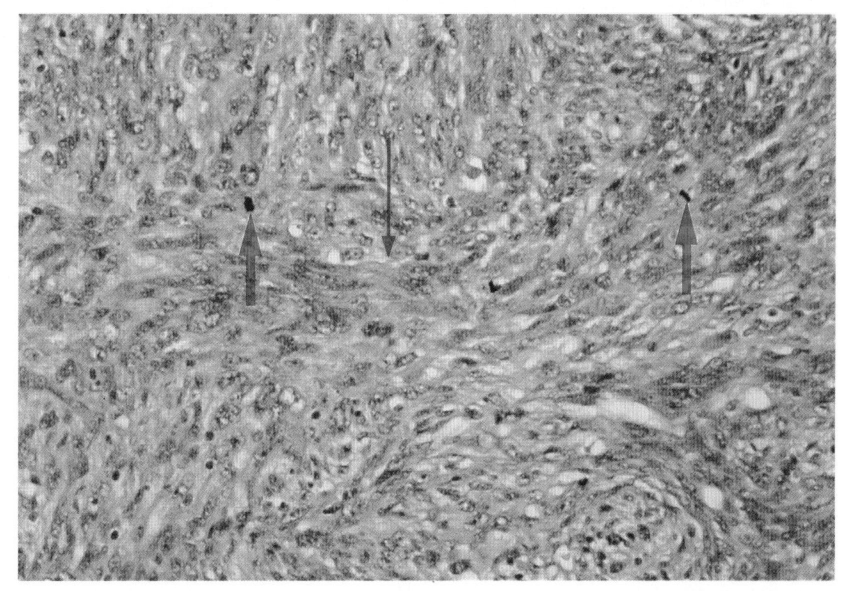

3.54 Fibrosarcoma: wrist

Sarcomas are generally much less common than arcinomas, and usually present as a soft tissue mass. Their behaviour is very variable. This tumour was on the dorsal aspect of the forearm of a woman of 63, just above he wrist, and it appeared to originate in the periosteum of a bone. Fibrosarcoma of bone is a rare tumour which generally starts in the endosteum rather than the periosteum; and the wrist is an unusual site for a ibrosarcoma arising in bone, since most arise around the nee-joint, in the femur or tibia. Fibrosarcoma of bone is osteolytic and may spread widely locally, in and around he bone. In this case, the tumour takes the form of a heet of diffusely distributed neoplastic cells with acuolated ill-defined cytoplasm and uniformly large ovoid vesicular nuclei with pale finely granular chromatin .nd inconspicuous nucleoli (thin arrow). The vacuoles probably contain connective tissue mucin, but formation of collagen is relatively slight. There is considerable mitotic activity (thick arrow). HE ×360

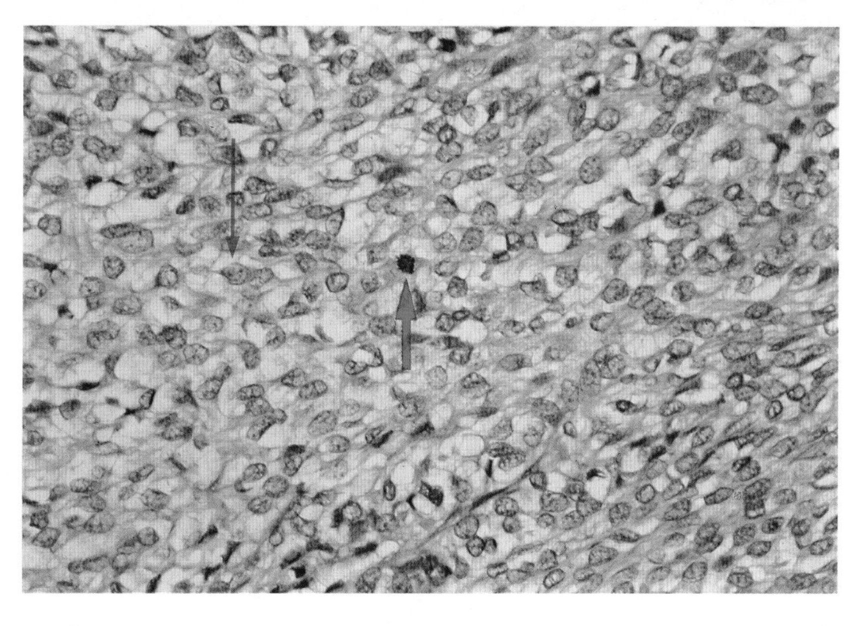

3.55 Malignant fibrous histiocytoma: scapula

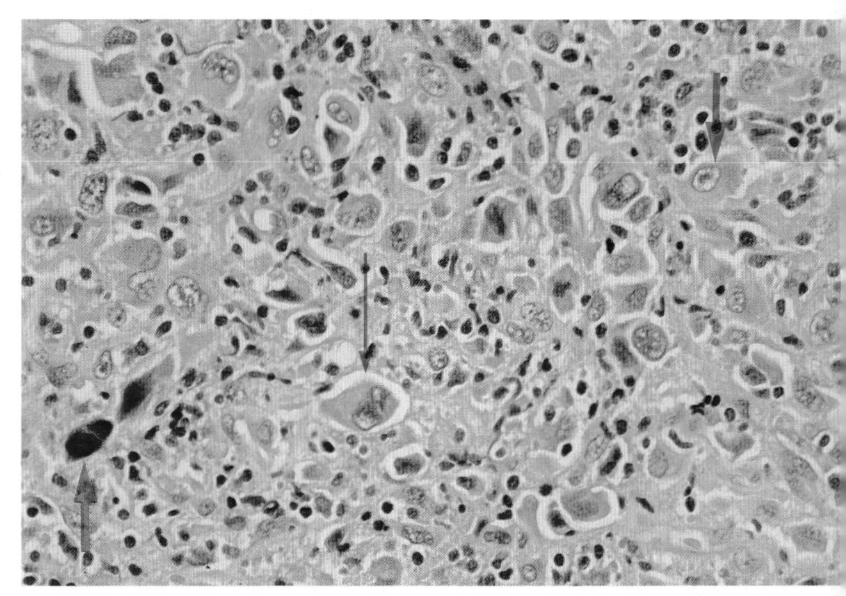

Malignant fibrous histiocytomas originate from fibrohistiocytes and are generally located in the limbs and retroperitoneum. They are mostly in individuals more than 50 years of age and more often in men than women. The tumour is a bosselated mass (5-10 cm dia) and the cut surface is fleshy, grey or yellowish, and often with areas of hemorrhage and necrosis. Histologically the fibroblast component of most malignant fibrous histiocytomas forms a storiform ('cartwheel' or 'spoke-like') pattern, with long spindle-shaped neoplastic radiating from a central focus. This tumour was located in the scapular region, and this part of it is composed of large or very large rounded histiocytes (thin arrows), with abundant eosinophilic cytoplasm and well-defined margins. These cells have extremely pleomorphic nuclei, containing one or more prominent nucleoli. Some of the histiocytes have two or more nuclei and many nuclei are hyperchromatic (thick arrow). Lymphocytes and plasma cells are present in moderate numbers throughout the tissues but there are only a few fibroblast-type cells. In other parts of the lesion the structure is that of a malignant spindle-cell tumour. HE ×360

3.56 Malignant fibrous histiocytoma: scapula

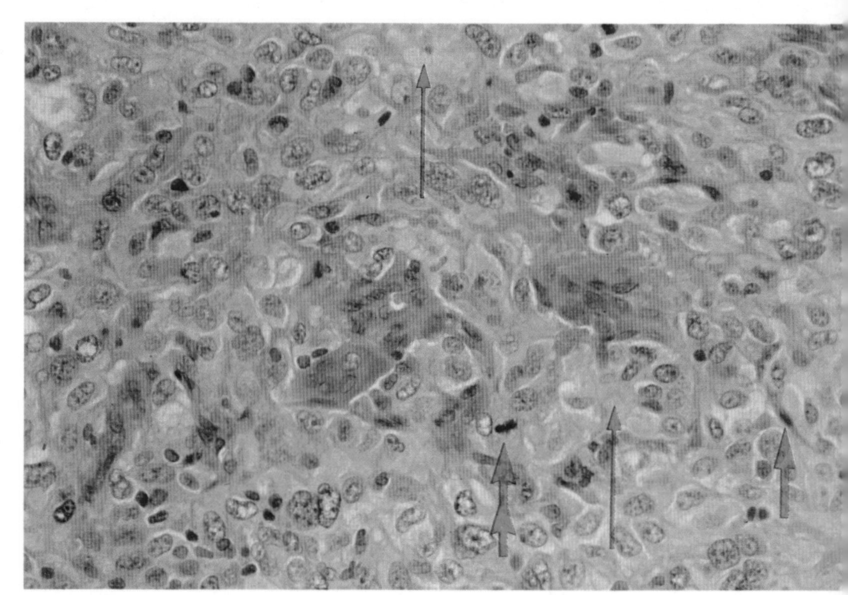

This is part of the same tumour as in 3.55. It consists of closely packed large pleomorphic histiocytes with a relatively large amount of weakly eosinophilic cytoplasm (thin arrows) and a network of elongated fibroblast-like cells with eosinophilic cytoplasm (thick arrow). Also present are very large (giant) cells (centre of field) with abundant deeply eosinophilic well-defined cytoplasm and numerous ovoid vesicular nuclei scattered throughout it. There is considerable mitotic activity among the histiocytes (double arrow). Elsewhere in the neoplasm the fibroblastic cells were the dominant component, but foci of lymphocytes, plasma cells and macrophages are also present. Some of the macrophages contain lipid or hemosiderin. Other parts of the tumour are myxoid in structure, and in the tissues the neoplastic cells are separated by mucoid intercellular substance. In the cytoplasm of some of the cells there are mucin-filled vacuoles. The grade of malignancy of malignant fibrous histiocytomas is generally low but they should be treated by radical excision, being liable to recur locally and sometimes metastasize to the regional nodes and lungs. HE ×360

3.57 Alveolar soft part sarcoma: thigh

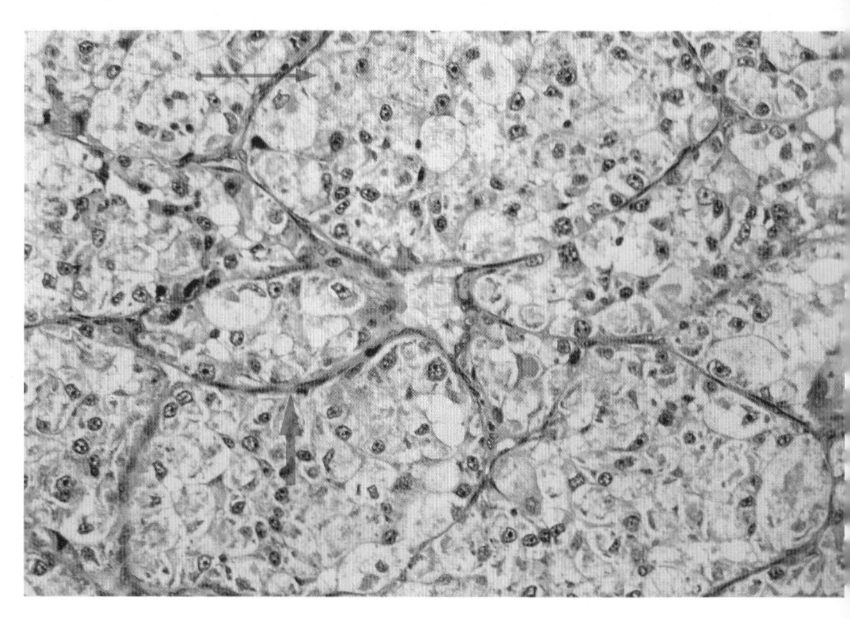

Alveolar soft part sarcoma is a malignant tumour of the deep soft tissues of the limbs, usually the thigh, of young adults and especially in women 20 to 40 years of age. It sometimes arises however in the abdominal wall or retroperitoneum. It tends to recur locally and may metastasize to the lung. It presents as a large fairly firm mass, apparently well-circumscribed and adjacent to a muscle. The cut surface is yellowish and firm, and histologically consists of lobules ('alveoli') of cells separated by fine vascular septa. This specimen was a lobulated mass (10.5 × 5 × 5.5cm) in the right thigh of a woman of 27. It was removed surgically, along with much adjacent skeletal muscle which it was invading. Histologically it consists of groups of large cells, bounded by a delicate fibrovascular stroma (thick arrow). The tumour cells have a considerable amount of pale granular cytoplasm (thin arrow) and round or ovoid pale vesicular nuclei which show considerable pleomorphism. There are no mitotic figures among these cells but there are occasional mitoses elsewhere in the tumour. HE ×235

3.58 Onchocerciasis: skin

Many different types of parasite may infest muscle, particularly in tropical countries where sanitation is unsatisfactory. The commonest parasites are worms. In this case the parasite is the filarial worm *Onchocerca volvulus*, and Onchocerciasis is a common cause of skin and eye disease in Africa and of blindness. The larvae are introduced into man by insect bites by the Simulium gnat, and the larvae mature in the dermis. They excite an inflammatory reaction which leads to the formation of subcutaneous nodules (onchocercomas), composed of a tangled mass of worms, surrounded by fibrous tissue and inflammatory cells, including large numbers of eosinophil leukocytes. When a fly bites someone with the parasites in the skin, the microfilarial larvae are ingested by the fly, and the larvae then undergo the next stage of their development. This shows part of a nodule in the subcutaneous tissues. It contains an adult female worm (in cross-section), enclosed in a capsule of dense but cellular fibrous tissue (thin arrow). The worm appears to have been fully viable and is full of small basophilic embryos (thick arrow).

HE ×120

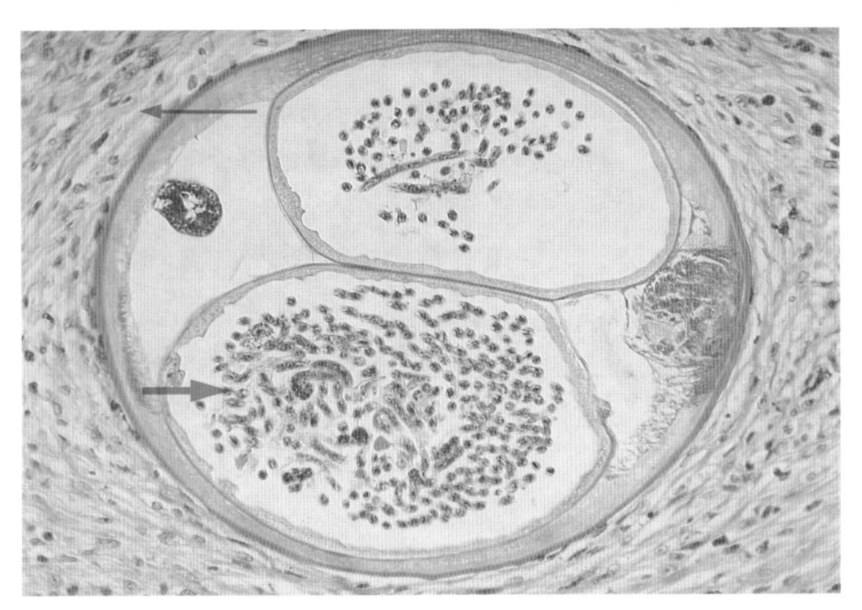

3.59 Cysticercosis: muscle

Cysticercosis s caused by the larval form of the pork tapeworm, T*aenia solium*, which lives in the small intestine of man. It occurs world-wide, and man is usually infected by eating 'measly' pork. The intermediate host is the pig, but when man ingests food contaminated with feces containing the ova of *Taenia solium*, the larvae are liberated in the stomach. They penetrate the stomach wall and travel by the blood to various tissues including the brain. In the tissues, each larva develops into a cysticercus, a small vesicle (5 × 10mm). When the cysticercus is alive, it evokes only a mild lymphocytic response, but when it dies an acute inflammatory reaction develops. In this example, the cyst has a thin membranous wall with a smoothly convoluted surface (thick arrows). The lumen of the cyst contains pale material including cell debris (thin arrow). The cysticercus has died, and external to and in contact with its wall there is a thick layer of basophilic pus-like exudate (double arrow). The exudate consists of large numbers of closely packed granular leukocytes and a smaller number of macrophages. Cysticerci can form in any organ and produce serious lesions.

HE ×200

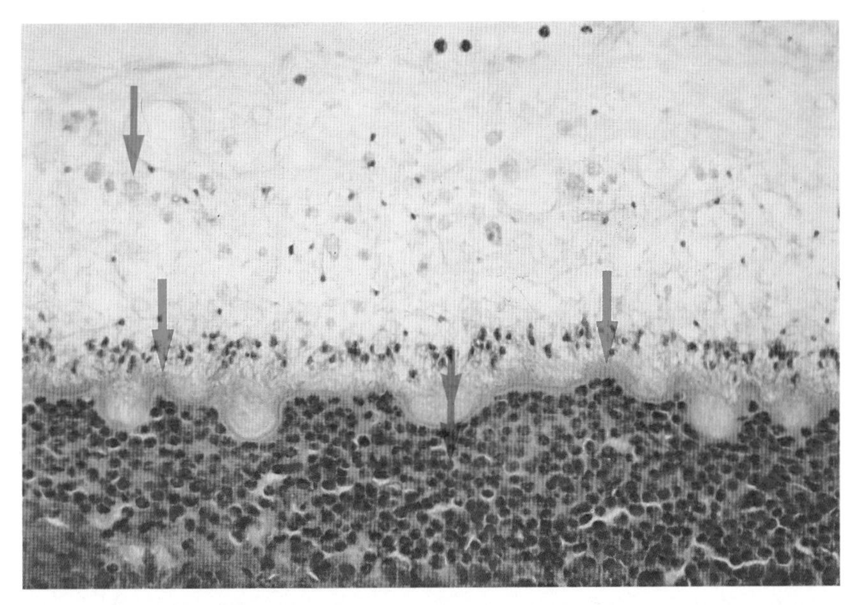

3.60 Trichinosis: muscle

The parasite is *Trichinella spiralis*, a common parasite of pigs in many countries, and a man is infected by eating raw or undercooked pork containing encysted larvae. The larvae are released by the digestive enzymes, attach themselves to the mucosa of the small intestine, and rapidly become sexually mature worms. The fertilized female penetrates the wall of the intestine and releases larvae which travel to all tissues. In muscle (but not in other tissues) the larva grows, coils in corkscrew fashion and forms a small cyst (about 1mm dia). This shows a larva (in two curved purple-stained parts (thin arrows), as a result of sectioning) in the centre of a small cyst (part of the lumen is empty and clear) and surrounded by a pale-staining capsule formed by muscle cells (whose nuclei are visible) (thick arrow) and a few compressed eosinophilic striated muscle fibres. In the interstitial tissues between the muscle fibres there is an infiltrate of small hyperchromatic chronic inflammatory cells. Larvae may remain alive for years in this state. HE ×110

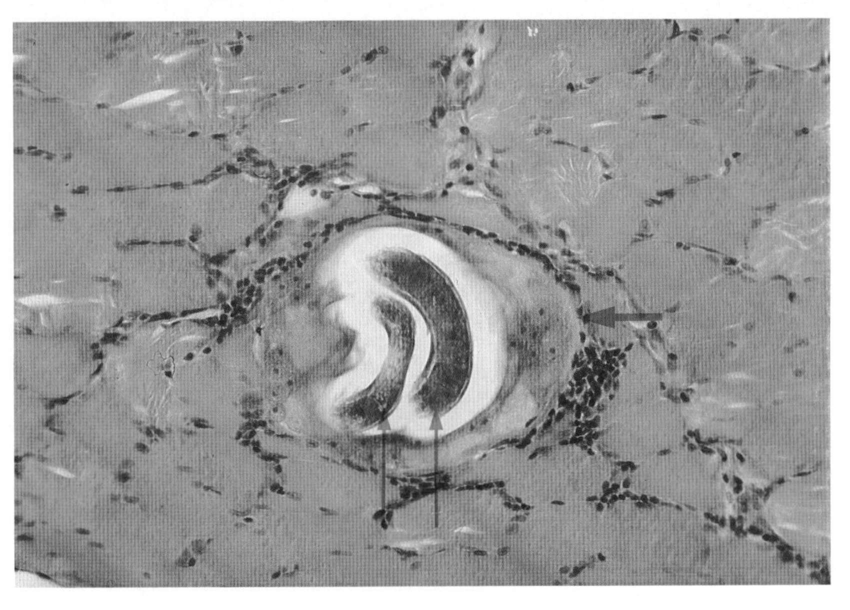

3.61 Infarct: muscle

Infarction, otherwise termed ischemic necrosis of tissue, is the development of an area of localized necrosis in a tissue which has had a sudden reduction of its blood supply. Total occlusion of all venous drainage from a tissue gives rise to venous infarction, the tissue hydrostatic pressure increasing sufficiently to obstruct arterial blood flow and cause infarction. Infarction of muscle can be caused in a variety of ways, sometimes on a massive scale, e.g. in the 'crush syndrome', where compression of a limb may cut off the blood supply for a considerable time; and the muscles of the forearm may lose their blood supply following injury to, and swelling of, the tissues round the elbow (Volkmann's ischemic contracture). In this case the affected muscle is the gastrocnemius. The fibres are swollen and have lost their striations and their nuclei (thin arrow). Macrophages are digesting the necrotic fibres, and fibrous tissue is forming (thick arrow). The fibrous tissue that replaces the dead muscle becomes densely collagenous, and considerable distortion of structure may result, with pressure on neighbouring structures such as nerves. HE ×270

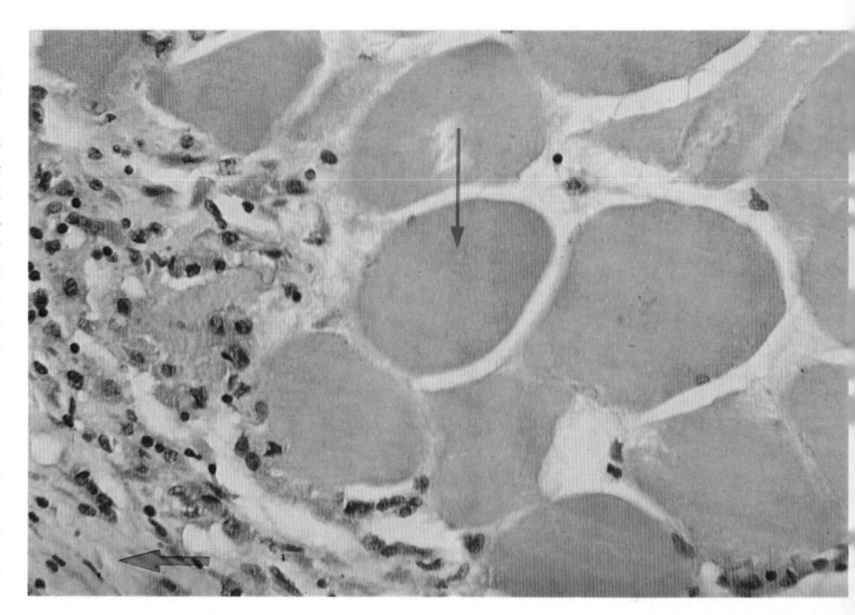

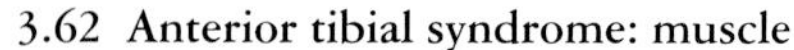

3.62 Anterior tibial syndrome: muscle

Anterior tibial syndrome is brought on by violent exercise, usually in untrained young men who are of condition, which can rupture muscle sheaths and cause hemorrhage and edema. The anterior tibial muscles, in the anterior tibial compartment, swell and ache within a few hours. If the syndrome becomes more severe, the skin overlying the muscles becomes erythematous, edematous and tense. When this happens in a rigidly confined space such as the anterior tibial compartment, the increase in volume can raise the pressure to a level which produces ischemia and degeneration of the muscles in the anterior tibial compartment. In this example of the syndrome, the more acute phase has passed, and although the eosinophilic muscle fibres have degenerated, there is evidence of regeneration, with large numbers of swollen sarcolemmal vesicular nuclei (thin arrow), each with a central prominent nucleolus (thick arrows). Some of the nuclei are in mitosis. Nevertheless there is a marked tendency for the muscle in this lesion to be replaced by fibrous tissue. HE ×270

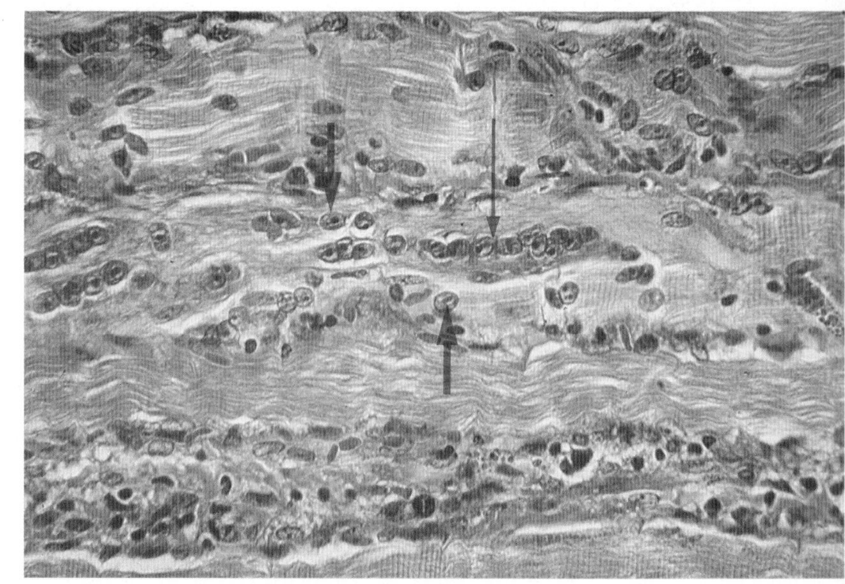

3.63 Progressive myositis ossificans: muscle

Myositis is a specific type of myositis, and it is characterized by formation of bone in the involved muscle. The condition usually appears as a hard mass in the muscle which is liable to be regarded, mistakenly, as a neoplasm. The tissue is osteogenic and bone is forming in it. In this example of the condition, alongside and spreading between deeply eosinophilic striated muscle fibres there is a sheet of pale edematous (myxoid) moderately cellular connective tissue (double arrow). In the connective tissue there is a scattered population of spindle-shaped fibroblast-like cells with elongated nuclei. Within this tissue there are two groups of large cells (thin arrows), some elongated, with abundant cytoplasm and ill-defined margins. The nuclei are round or ovoid and minimally pleomorphic, and the chromatin is very finely granular. The groups of cells have enlarged to become osteocytes, and some of them are surrounded with deeply basophilic (black) calcified matrix (thick arrows). These groups are, in effect, two small trabeculae of woven (coarse-fibred) bone. A similar process of bone formation sometimes occurs in the paralyzed muscles of paraplegic patients. HE ×200

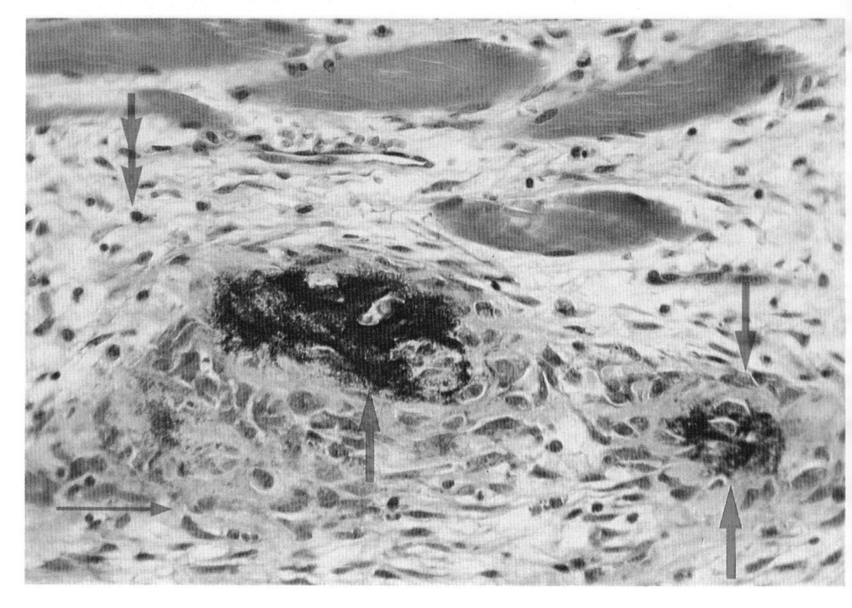

3.64 Rheumatoid arthritis: muscle

In rheumatoid arthritis the most common extra-articular lesions are subcutaneous nodules, which usually develop in areas close to the joints. Nodules may also form in bursae and tendon sheaths, and rheumatoid lesions sometimes develop in the heart muscle, pericardium or endocardium. Occasionally there is atrophy and wasting of skeletal muscles, particularly those muscles which are immobilized by inflammation and fixation of joints. Active polymyositis on the other hand is uncommon, but there is often an inflammatory reaction in the endomysium and between the fascicles of muscle fibres. The tissues in this lesion consist of pale loose connective tissue (double arrows) and a number of deeply eosinophilic striated muscle fibres (thick arrow). The delicate strands of interstitial connective tissue which surround the muscle fibres are being infiltrated by small lymphocytes, plasma cells and macrophages. The lymphocytes have only scant cytoplasm and an ovoid or round hyperchromatic nucleus. The various types of cells have infiltrated one or more muscle fibres, and the macrophages (thin arrow) are ingesting the probably-necrotic striated muscle tissue. The infiltrated fibres have also undergone floccular degeneration (fragmentation). HE ×335

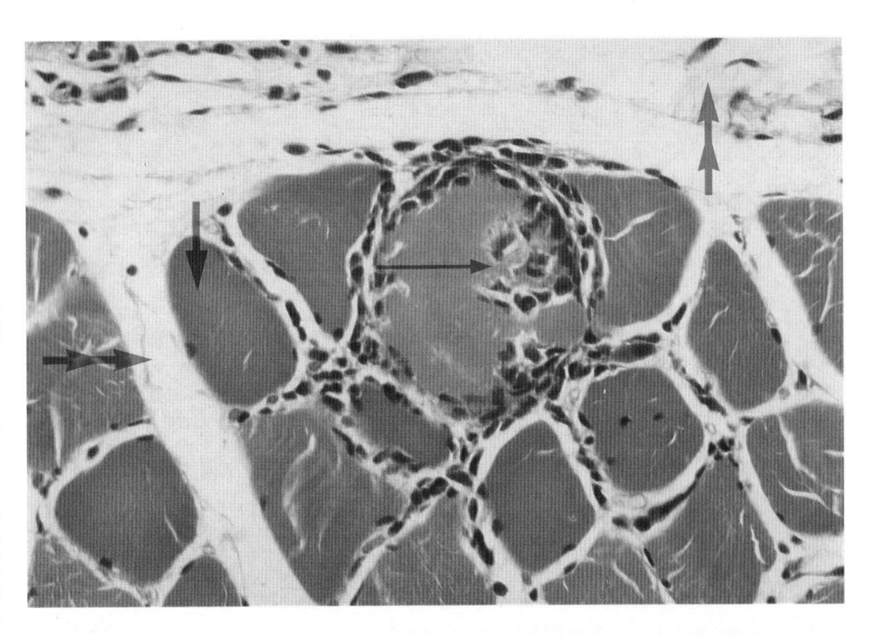

3.65 Polymyositis-Dermatomyositis: muscle

Polymyositis-Dermatomyositis is an uncommon disease of connective tissue, in which both skin and muscles are inflamed. Onset of the disease usually occurs between 40 and 60 years of age and women are affected twice as often as men. The cause of the disease is not known. Patients also risk developing a malignant neoplasm, especially when they are more than 60 years old. This is most often a carcinoma of lung but carcinomas of breast, kidney, stomach and uterus also occur. The disease may advance rapidly, and if heart and respiratory muscles are involved, may prove rapidly fatal. In most cases however remissions occur, followed by exacerbations. In this sheet of eosinophilic striated muscle fibres, cut longitudinally, the fibre in the centre (thin arrow) has undergone floccular degeneration (fragmentation) and is being ingested by macrophages, only an intensely eosinophilic fragment of the fibre remaining (thick arrow). Several of the other fibres are atrophic, and in some of them the sarcolemmal nuclei are large and increased in number. This may be an attempt at regeneration. Phagocytosis of degenerating muscle is more characteristic of myositis than of muscular dystrophy. HE ×335

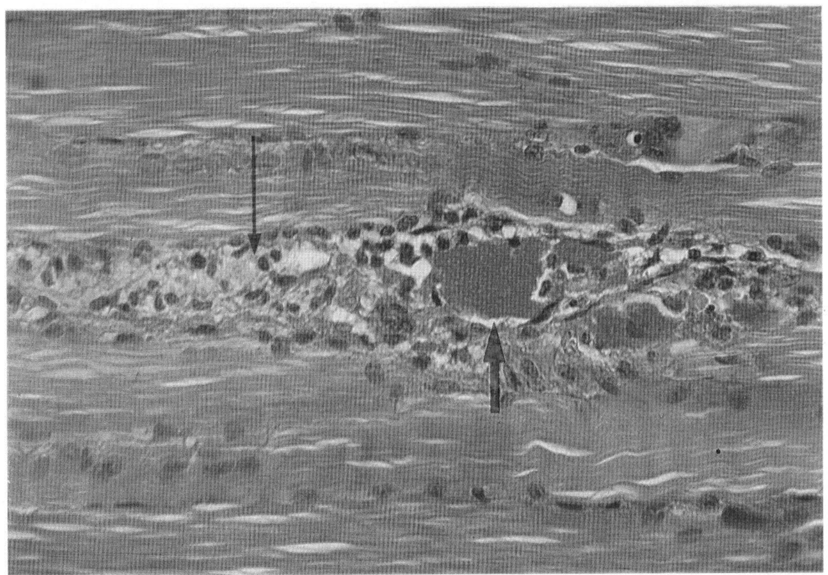

3.66 Polymyositis-Dermatomyositis: muscle

Polymyositis-Dermatomyositis is a chronic disease that affects striated muscle in all cases, and in individuals with dermatomyositis, the polymyositis element causes weakness and often also tenderness of the muscles. The proximal muscles of the limb girdles are often the first affected, and in severe cases the pharyngeal and respiratory muscles are also involved. The disease follows a chronic course, characterized by increasing disability from muscle wasting. There are also skin changes, caused by vasculitis and subsequently by dermal atrophy and calcification. The main danger however in polymyositis is the associated malignant disease. In this histological section of striated muscle from this case, there are a number of muscle fibres, cut in transverse section. The fibres are widely separated, shrunken and atrophied to varying degrees, and the myofibrils have retracted from the sarcolemmal sheaths. In the centre of each of several fibres there is a large 'empty' vacuole (arrow). A change of this type with in the fibres is virtually pathognomonic of polymyositis. HE ×335

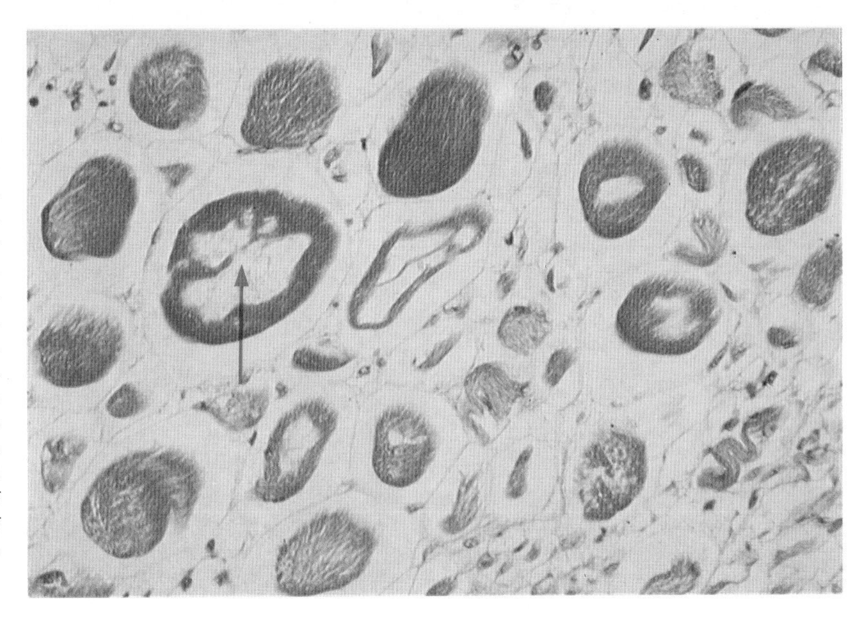

3.67 Muscular dystrophy: muscle

The muscular dystrophies are a group of rare inherited primary muscle diseases, which begin in childhood and follow a progressive course. They are characterized by distinctive distribution of involved muscles, but the histological appearances are similar in the various syndromes and differentiation between them is based on the clinical presentation. There is degeneration of skeletal muscle fibres and increasing muscle weakness. Each muscle fibre is affected individually, and fibres showing a variety of changes are found in close association. In this example, the muscle fibres are rounded (thin arrow) and vary considerably in size, most relatively large and several much smaller (atrophic). The fibres are cut in cross-section. In practically every muscle fibre the sarcolemmal nuclei have migrated from the periphery of the fibre into its substance (thick arrow). Inward migration of nuclei, particularly when widespread, is suggestive of muscle dystrophy and especially myotonic dystrophy, which is characterized by not by muscle weakness but by failure of relaxation of muscle after voluntary contraction

HE ×335

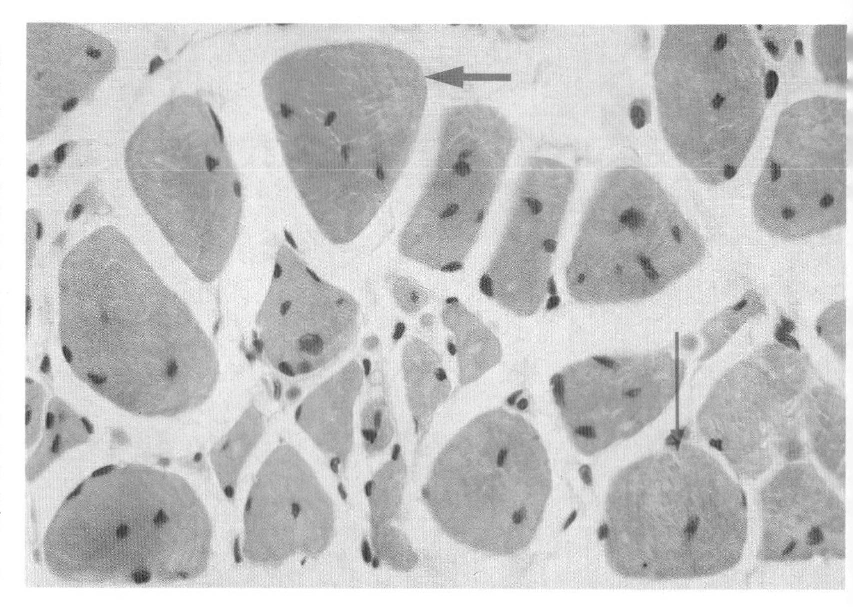

3.68 Muscular dystrophy: muscle

The onset of myotonic dystrophy is usually in adult life and it progresses very slowly. In contrast, Duchenne muscular dystrophy (pseudohypertrophic muscular dystrophy) is the commonest type, affected males being normal at birth and the condition manifest in early childhood. The disease progresses rapidly, the affected muscles being apparently larger than normal in the early stages, enlargement of muscle being caused by an increase in fat content. Pseudohypertrophy of this type is especially obvious in the calf muscles. Most children are functionally disabled within a few years, and generally die before the end of the second decade. Histologically, in this case there is considerable variation in the size of the muscle fibres, and several of them are degenerate, with ragged margins and vacuolated weakly eosinophilic cytoplasm (thin arrow). One fibre shows increased eosinophilia. Many sarcolemmal nuclei are enlarged and in places they form chains (thick arrow). Clumps of pyknotic nuclei are also present and there are nuclei within some fibres. Many myofibrils have disappeared completely and been replaced by very vascular fat (double arrow). HE ×150

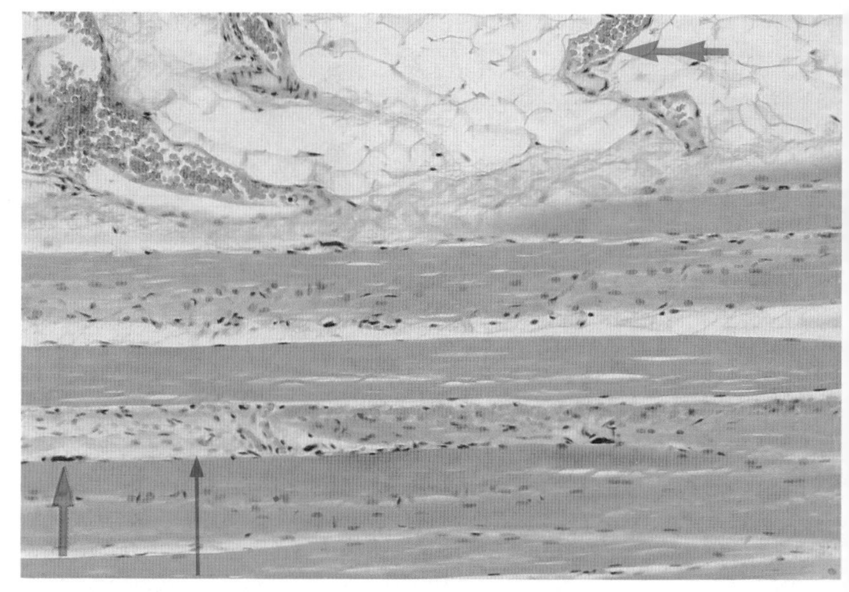

3.69 Muscular dystrophy: muscle

In addition to myotonic and Duchenne muscular dystrophies, there are many other types of dystrophy, recognized and characterized according to the distribution of initial weakness and observed patterns of inheritance. The time of onset and the rate of progression of muscular dystrophy differ markedly in the various entities. Most of the other dystrophies are less severe than Duchenne-type, but all are characterized by muscle weakness and atrophy, and the histological changes in biopsies of muscle are identical. The dystrophin gene is absent from both Becker's muscular dystrophy and Duchenne's disease, but the deficiency of dystrophin In Becker's disease results in a milder disease and a much longer life. In this histological section, there are several muscle fibres. One of the fibres has lost its eosinophilic myofibrils however and is now a very slender markedly basophilic fibre which is attempting to regenerate (thick arrow). In the adjacent eosinophilic muscle fibres the myofibrillary material appears normal, the 'waviness' being a processing artefact. The sarcolemmal nuclei are swollen and vesicular, and the chromatin in them is very finely granular. HE ×335

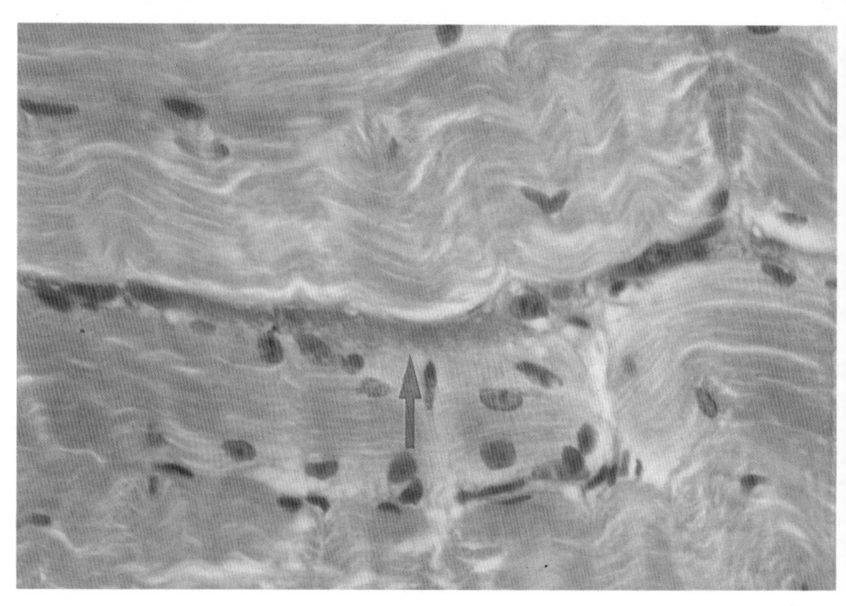

3.70 Neurogenic atrophy: muscle

When a muscle or part of a muscle is deprived of its motor nerves, the affected muscle fibres atrophy. The fibres shrink, and after a week or two the sarcolemmal nuclei of the affected muscle fibres swell, and some of them move to the centre, among the myofibrils. After a month he fibres are rounded and smaller than normal. After 4-6 months the shrunken fibres are only 10-15μm dia. Their staining qualities do not change however and the cross-striations remain. With loss of sarcoplasm, the sarcolemmal nuclei appear to increase in number. The fibres with an intact nerve supply do not hypertrophy. Fat may increase between the fascicles, and subsequently fibrous tissue may form. In this case, the bundle of eosinophilic muscle fibres (thin arrow) and that of the very atrophic and narrow denervated fibres (thick arrow) lie side by side and are separated by a band of pale loose connective tissue. Alongside the atrophic denervated fibres there is also an infiltrate of fat (double arrow). The number of sarcolemmal nuclei in the denervated fibres appears to be greatly increased, but in fact there is probably no absolute increase in their number. HE ×335

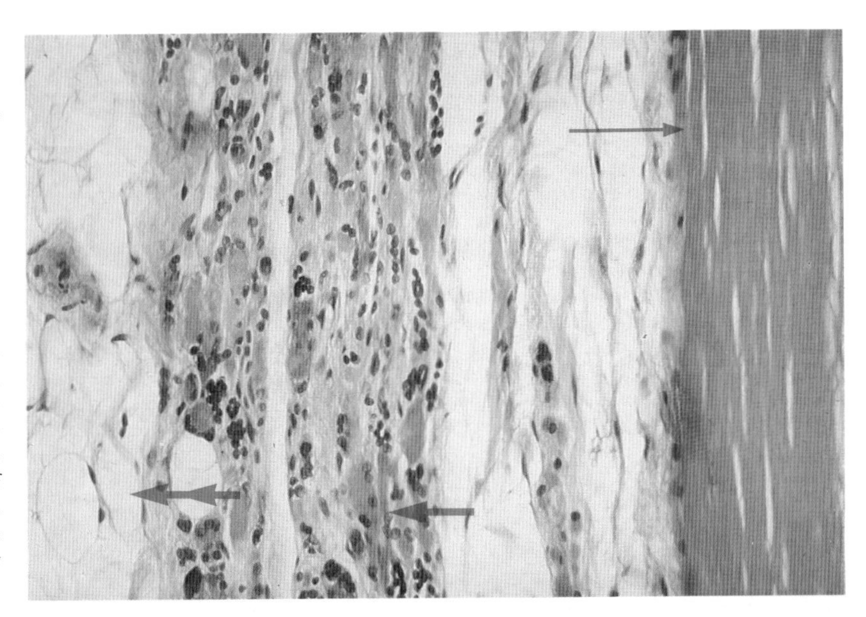

3.71 Neurogenic atrophy: muscle

If the denervation of muscle is not complete, the contrast between groups of shrunken denervated muscle fibres and plump normal or even hypertrophic muscle fibres is striking. As the denervated muscle fibres shrink, myofibrils are progressively lost from the periphery of the cells but cross-striations are preserved. After four months the rate of shrinkage of the denervated fibres slows, but the fibres continue to shrink and lose their myofibrils. The sarcolemmal nuclei form clumps, cross-striations are lost, and eventually only clusters of nuclei survive in a shrunken sarcolemma. In this case of neurogenic atrophy, three denervated fibres are undergoing atrophy. The sarcoplasm at the periphery of each fibre is spongy and loose-textured (thick arrow), with loss of myofibrils, but the dense band of eosinophilic myofibrils that remains in the centre of the fibre (thin arrow) still retains the cross-striations. The sarcolemmal nuclei are large, ovoid or round and more prominent than normal (double arrows). They appear to have increased in number because of the shrinkage of the fibres. HE ×335

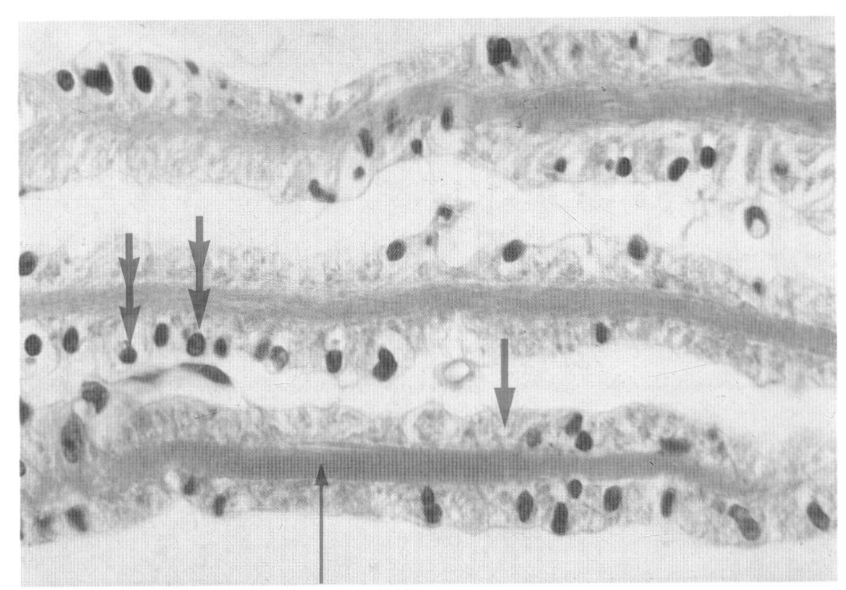

3.72 Idiopathic myoglobinuria: muscle

Myoglobinuria results from acute destruction of muscle (rhabdomyolyis) that sometimes occurs in acute toxic, metabolic, infectious or traumatic muscle disease. The low-molecular-weight protein myoglobin filters rapidly into the urine (myoglobinuria) and colours it red. The appearance of myoglobin in the urine is preceded by necrosis of muscle on a large scale and may occur in a wide range of disorders of muscle. After strenuous exercise, a person with idiopathic myoglobinuria feels weak, and the muscles are swollen and painful. The urine passed is dark-coloured from the presence of myoglobin. The urine contains no erythrocytes however, and this distinguishes myoglobinuria from hematuria, in which the urine does contain erythrocytes. The patient in this case was a boy of 5. In the centre of this sheet of eosinophilic striated muscle fibres, one fibre (above centre) has undergone floccular degeneration and necrosis (thin arrow), and the degenerate myofibrillary material is being ingested by macrophages (thick arrow). Although death may occur from renal failure after a severe attack, idiopathic myoglobinuria is a relatively benign condition, and since the basic structure of the muscles is maintained, recovery of muscle structure is usually complete. HE ×360

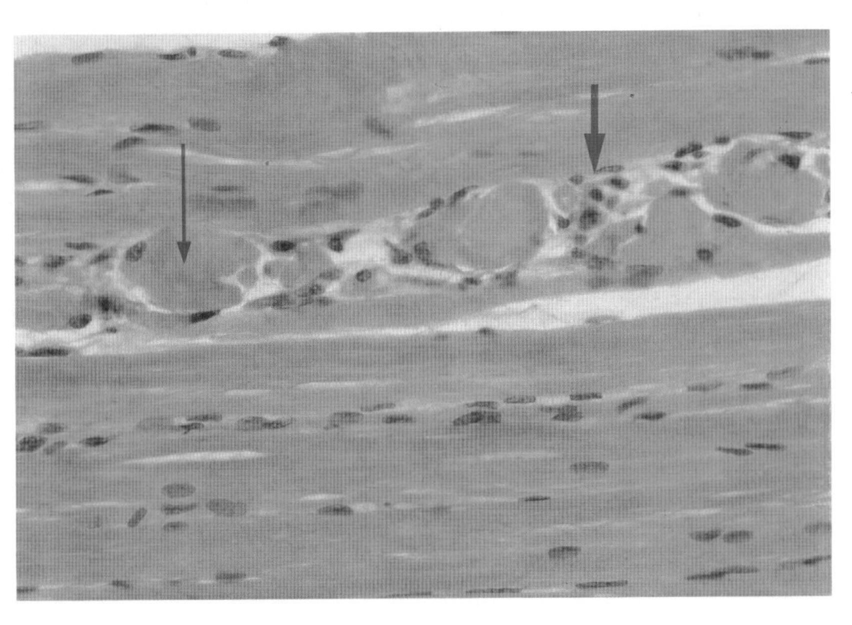

4.1 Chronic subdural hematoma

Chronic subdural hematoma is a common lesion, formed by the accumulation of blood in the subdural space, and it tends to occur in old people. Bleeding results from rupture of the many small communicating veins which traverse the 'space' between the arachnoid membrane (cerebral cortex) and the dura (superior sagittal sinus) and drain into the venous sinuses. After a head injury, usually slight, the veins bleed not infrequently, and although they do so slowly (days to months), a large subdural hematoma may form in the subdural space. Unusually, this chronic subdural hematoma was in a woman of 26. In this (subdural) space there is a 'membrane' which has two poorly-defined components: an upper layer (top of field), which consists of eosinophilic collagenous fibrous tissue (thick arrow), and a lower layer which consists of a looser more vascular connective tissue (a broader type of sterile 'granulation tissue') (thin arrow), the surface of which (double arrow) was in contact with the blood clot.

HE ×60

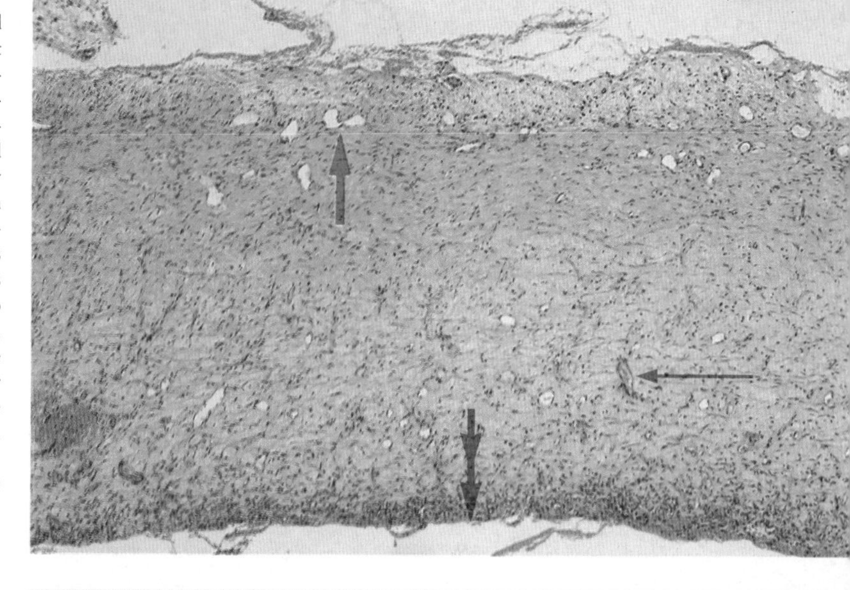

4.2 Chronic subdural hematoma

Rupture of the small veins occurs when the brain moves relative to the fixed superior sagittal sinus, and it is most likely when cerebral atrophy has previously developed. Although 'organization' of the subsequent blood clot takes place, recurrent bleeding may cause the mass of blood to increase in size. The clot breaks down, and then it expands slowly when fluid enters it from the adjacent subarachnoid space. This produces an increase in intracranial pressure, which compresses the brain and is life-threatening. This field is occupied by part of the 'membrane' present in 9.1. It is located in the subdural space and one (top) half consists largely of blood clot. The extravasated blood (double arrow) is being invaded and 'organized' by capillaries, fibroblasts and macrophages, forming a layer (on the leptomeninges) which consists of (sterile) granulation (organization) tissue, with many dilated capillaries (thick arrows), and maturing fibrous tissue (thin arrow) (lower half of field), with numerous fibrocytes and plump fibroblasts. Many of the macrophages in this tissue are siderophages, their cytoplasm being full of golden-brown hemosiderin.

HE ×150

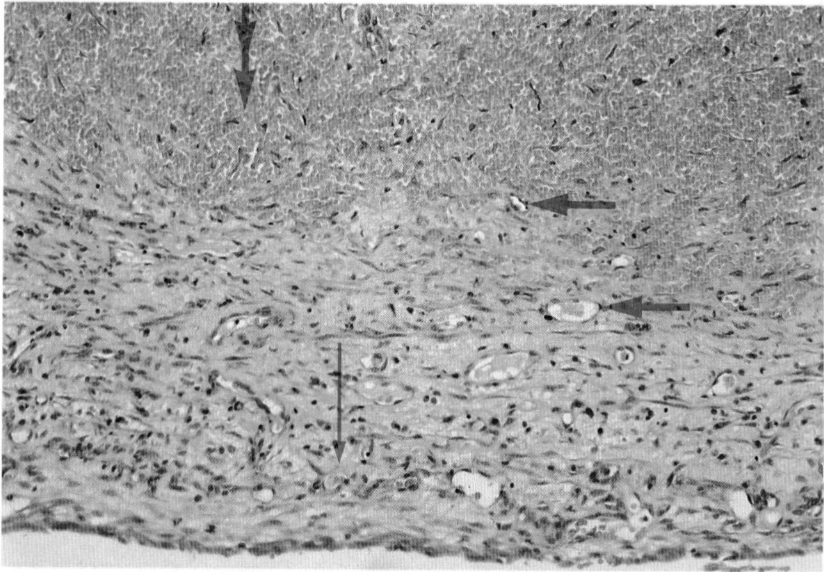

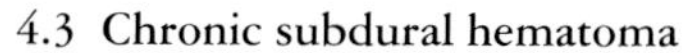

4.3 Chronic subdural hematoma

A chronic subdural hematoma contains brownish fluid, and is lined on one side by dura and by a ('new' or 'false') fibrous membrane on the leptomeningeal side. The thickness of the 'false' membrane is proportionate to the duration of the hematoma. This is part of the 'membrane' present in 4.1 and 4.2. It is composed, very largely, of granulation tissue in which there are large numbers of dilated capillary blood vessels (thick arrow), macrophages and elongated fibroblasts. Small numbers of lymphocytes are also present. The cytoplasm of most of the macrophages (siderophages) is dark brown (thin arrow) from the presence of hemosiderin from digested red blood cells. The many small blood vessels in this tissue are themselves liable to bleed in the event of mild trauma. The 'granulation tissue' (component of the membrane) is being formed by 'organization' of the more superficial aspect of the blood clot (double arrow), which consists of closely packed red cells and a sparse population of flattened macrophages and plump elongated fibroblasts.

HE ×360

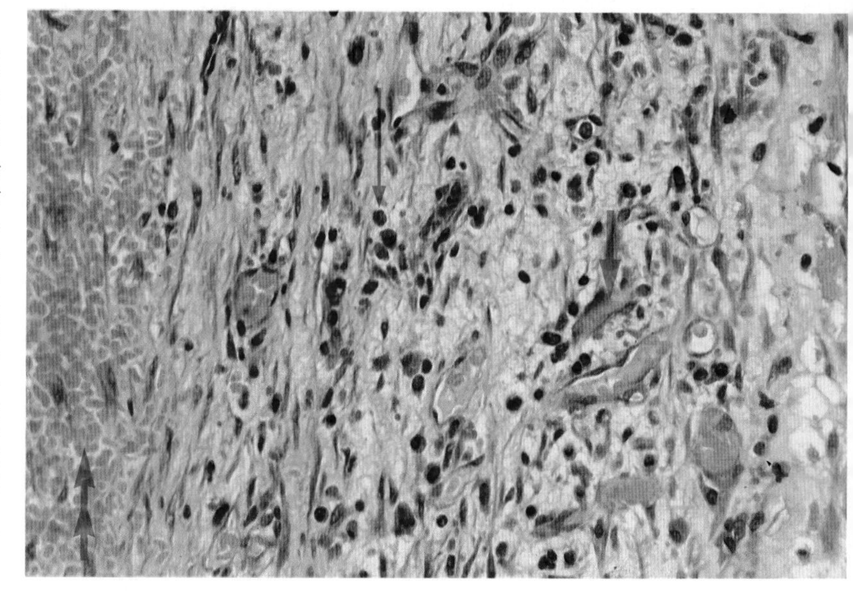

4.4 Infarct: brain

Infarction of the brain is caused by sudden reduction in the blood flow, for example by thrombotic occlusion of an atheromatous cerebral, internal carotid or vertebral artery. Severe ischemic (non-occlusive) damage and infarction may also occur in the absence of thrombotic occlusion or significant stenosis, as a result of a sudden reduction in blood flow, e.g. when severe hypotension develops. Within 72 hours the infarcted brain becomes a fully developed pale soft area (a 'softening') surrounded by edema. Some infarcts become hemorrhagic, possibly by restoration of the blood supply to the infarcted area; and occasionally a fluid-filled cystic cavity with a wall of reactive gliotic tissue forms. This infarct of white matter is of about 6 weeks' duration. The tissue has a spongy (vacuolated) structure, many of the myelinated fibres having undergone ischemic necrosis and disappeared. The large round cells with foamy cytoplasm (arrows) lying in the spaces between the surviving fibres are macrophages ('compound granular corpuscles') which have phagocytosed lipoproteins from the necrotic tissue. Also present are a number of astrocytes with small round basophilic nuclei and ill-defined cytoplasmic boundaries. HE ×335

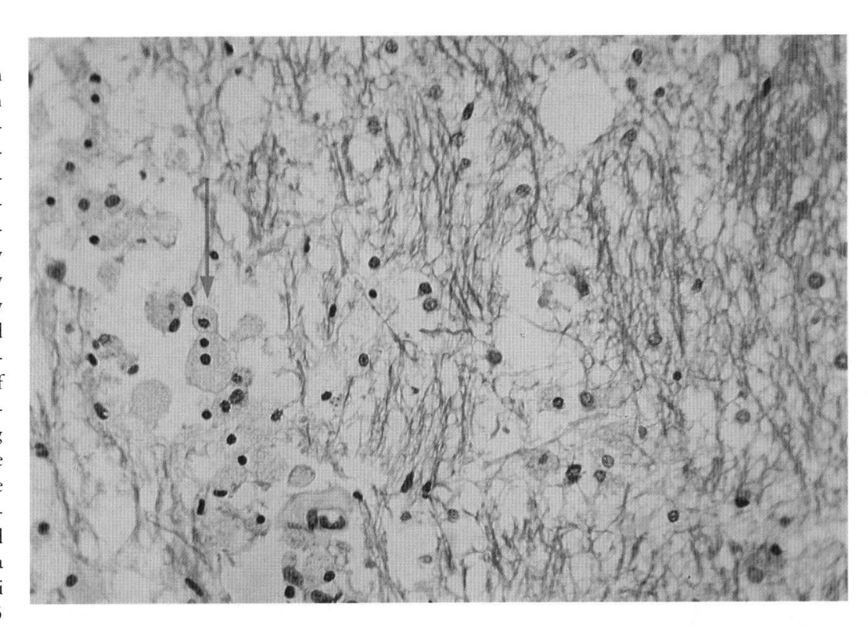

4.5 Cerebral hemorrhage: brain

Cerebral hemorrhage is the cause of about 90% of 'strokes', mostly in hypertensive individuals more than 40 years of age. The bleeding occurs around the basal ganglia and internal capsule, and its source is usually one of the multiple microaneurysms that form on the lenticulostriate arteries. The blood dissects and destroys brain tissue, forming a hematoma which expands and acts like a space-occupying tumour. Eventually the lesion may undergo cystic change and gliosis, coloured brownish-yellow by the presence of large numbers of hemosiderin-laden macrophages. This is the edge of a hemorrhage into the globus pallidus. The red zone of blood clot is on the left, and adjacent to the blood clot there is extensive pale patchy necrosis of the brain. The necrotic tissue is edematous and vacuolated (thin arrow), and many nerve cells and glial cells have disappeared. Scattered ischemic nerve cells survive as basophilic round bodies (thick arrow). The numerous vacuoles in the necrotic tissue contained watery fluid. HE ×135

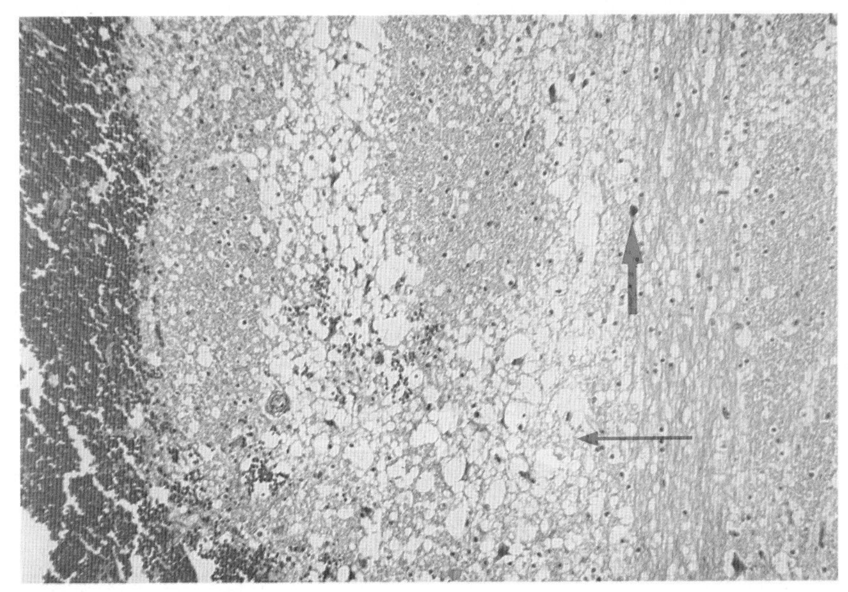

4.6 Fat embolism: brain

Recognizable cerebral emboli may come from fragments of thrombus, originating in the heart (mural thrombus) or from vegetations on cardiac valves. Small cerebral emboli are difficult to identify and may be classified as 'non-occlusive' infarction. When fatty tissue is traumatized or a large bone such as the femur fractures, globules of fat may enter the lacerated blood vessels and become emboli. The emboli are mostly retained by the lung capillaries, but sometimes they pass through, reaching the brain and producing small infarcts. If the infarcts are in vital centres death may result. In this case, there are multiple small (2-3mm dia) hemorrhagic foci in the brainstem, and this one is a circular ('ring') hemorrhage (thin arrow) around a dilated small blood vessel, blocked by red cells and polymorph leukocytes and probably thrombosed (thick arrow). The pale tissue between the vessel and the extravasated blood is necrotic. There is also necrotic tissue (double arrow) adjacent to another smaller blood vessel. Macrophages have infiltrated the extravasated blood and necrotic tissue. A frozen section showed fat globules in the lumen of the blood vessels. HE ×135

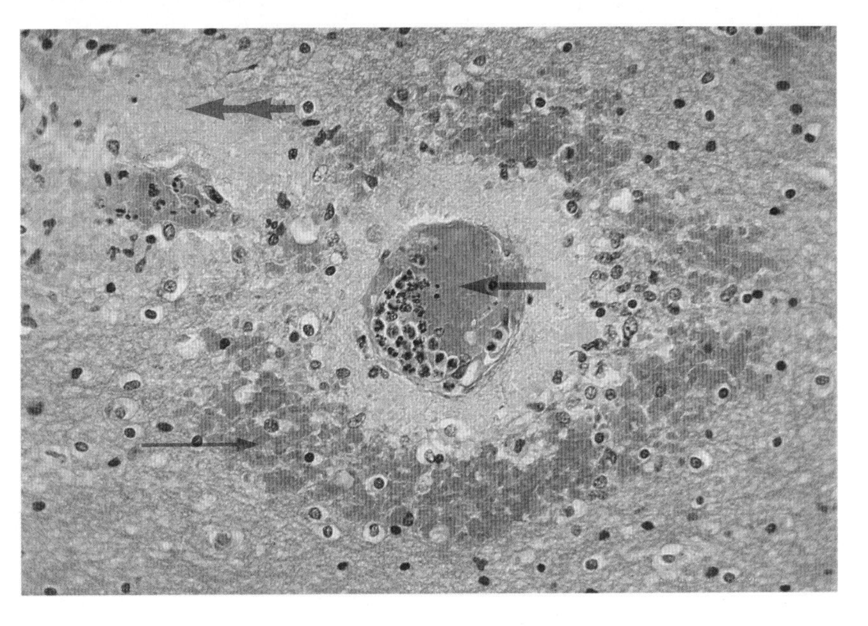

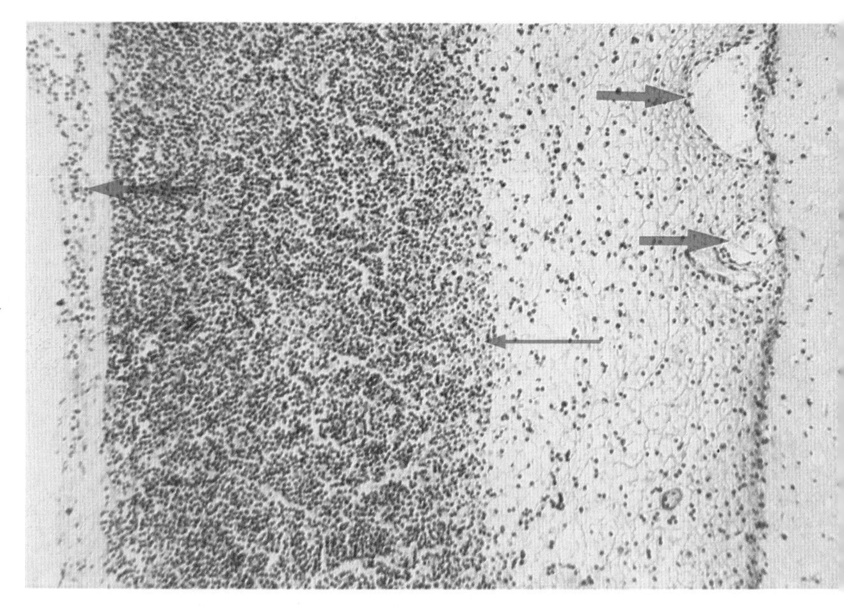

4.7 Acute bacterial (purulent) meningitis: brain

In acute bacterial meningitis, bacteria spread throughout the subarachnoid space. In children up to five years of age the most common pathogen causing acute bacterial meningitis is *Hemophilus influenzae,* but *Neisseria meningitidis* is the most common cause in adolescents. The pneumococcus *(Streptococcus pneumoniae)* causes meningitis in all age groups. The bacterial infection may spread very rapidly in the subarachnoid space and the patient may die within a few hours. The leptomeninges become hyperemic and opaque, an inflammatory exudate collects in the subarachnoid space, and greenish pus-like material quickly covers part or all of the surface of the brain. In this case, the surface of the brain is on the right. The small vascular channels (thick arrows) on the surface of the cerebral cortex are markedly dilated but there is no increase in the cellularity of the cortex. The thin delicate arachnoid membrane (double arrow) is infiltrated by a blue line of basophilic polymorph leukocytes, and the distended subarachnoid space is occupied by numerous thin strands of fibrin and a thick layer of loosely packed deeply basophilic polymorph leukocytes (thin arrow).

HE ×120

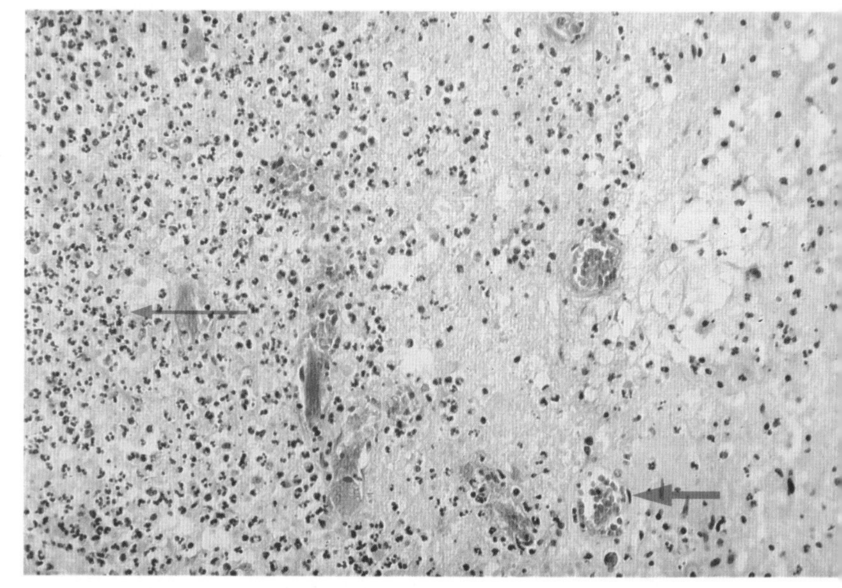

4.8 Cerebral abscess: brain

A brain abscess is a localized focus of bacterial (suppurative) encephalitis. Many types of microorganism may form an abscess in the brain, and more than one type may be present. *Streptococcus pneumoniae*, *Staphylococcus aureus* and anerobic bacteria play an important role. The infection reaches the brain by the bloodstream or by direct spread from a suppurative lesion in the adjacent tissues such as an infected middle ear or paranasal sinus. It may also be secondary to trauma, such as a fracture of the skull. This is part of an abscess which is developing in the white matter. The centre of the 'abscess' is out of the picture on the left, and the white matter adjoining it (left half of field) is necrotic and heavily infiltrated with polymorph leukocytes (thin arrow). The tissues on the right are pale, edematous and vacuolated, and there are relatively few polymorphs. There are many greatly dilated thin-walled blood vessels (thick arrow) in the 'wall' and some bleeding has occurred. If the focus of infection is localized, the brain tissue liquefies and forms pus. The pus is then enclosed within a fibrogliotic wall ('pyogenic membrane') which consists of connective tissue, glial cells, macrophages and capillaries. HE ×160

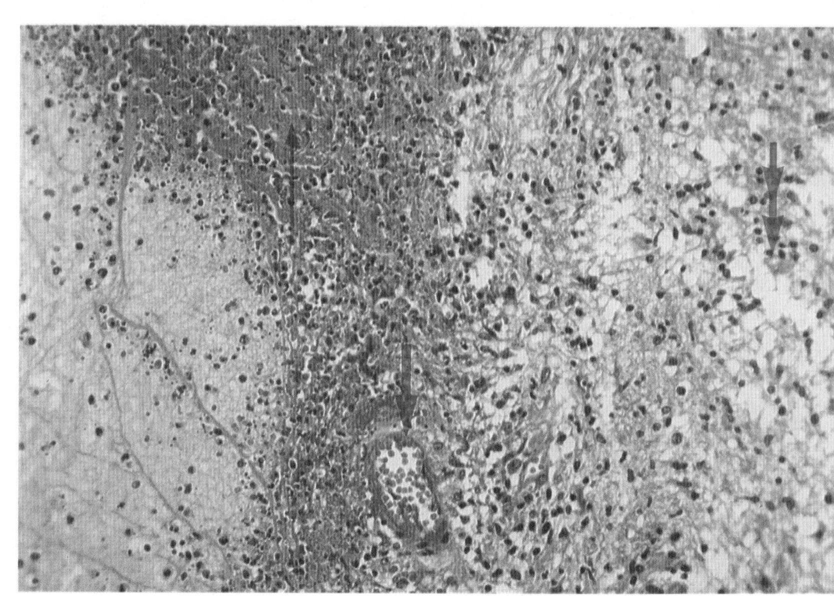

4.9 Tuberculous meningitis: brain

Tuberculous meningitis is typically chronic but in the early stages there may be an exudative phase which resembles acute meningitis. The tubercle bacillus (*Mycobacterium tuberculosis*) spreads to the brain via the bloodstream (tuberculous bacteremia), from sources such as miliary tuberculosis. A thick greyish-green gelatinous exudate forms in the subarachnoid space, and characteristic tubercles (1-3mm dia) are readily detectable (macroscopically) in the exudate. The subarachnoid space is full of inflammatory exudate (left half of field) which consists of fibrin and cellular debris (stained a deep purplish-red) (thin arrow). The cerebral cortex (right half of field) is edematous and extensively vacuolated (double arrow), and infiltrated by macrophages and lymphocytes. The exudate is adherent to the cerebral cortex and the boundary between the cortex and the exudate is blurred. There is a small intensely red blood vessel (thick arrow) at the junction between exudate and cerebral cortex, and it is probably necrotic and thrombosed. This superficial encephalitis has been caused by the inflammatory reaction in the meninges, but necrotizing arteritis is also an important factor. HE ×160

4.10 Aspergillosis: brain

Fungal infections of the brain are secondary to lesions elsewhere, usually in the lungs, and take the form of meningitis or multiple 'abscesses' which may resemble infarcts macroscopically. Frequently the patient's defences have been weakened, e.g. by drugs which depress immunity, and this patient was a girl of 13 who had received chemotherapy for Hodgkin's disease. Aspergillus is a branching filamentous organism, and there are many transverse septa in the hyphae (3-4μm dia). In this brain, elongated purplish-red filaments (hyphae) (thick arrow), cut in various planes, are growing alongside small blood vessels and penetrating the white matter. The hyphae may also have invaded the lumen of a venule. Parts of the hyphae are surrounded by a moderate infiltrate of polymorph leukocytes, and there are numerous small ill-defined deposits of purplish-red granular material in the immediate vicinity of the hyphae (thin arrow). The red material may be fibrin which has leaked from small blood vessels, but its granular texture suggests that it may be debris from necrotic polymorphs or degenerate hyphae.

HE ×200

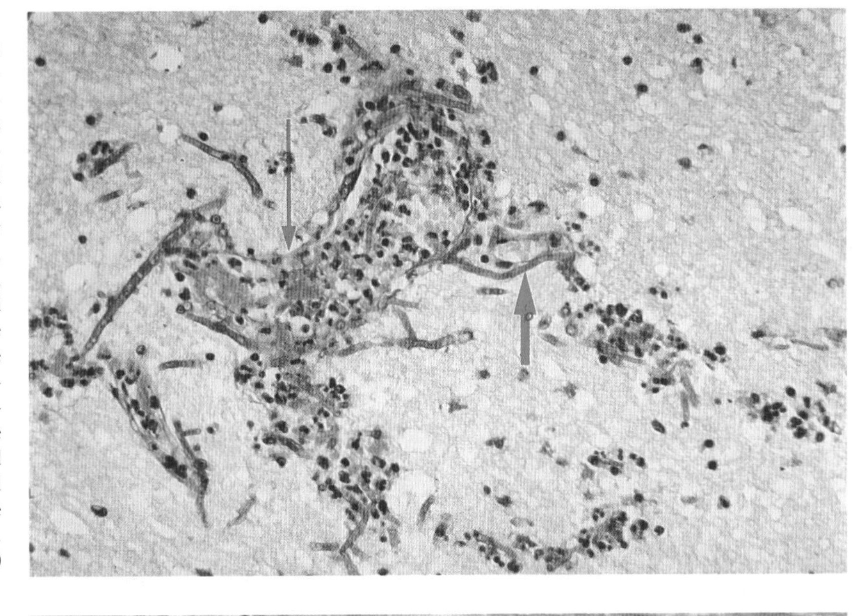

4.11 Cryptococcosis: brain

Depression of the immune system is often a predisposing factor with regard to fungal infections. The yeast *Cryptococcus neoformans* most often produces lesions in the lungs, by inhaling the fungus, common in the environment and especially from pigeon droppings. The infection may spread to the nervous system and cause subacute meningitis and lesions in the cerebral cortex (meningoencephalitis). The meninges are sometimes distended by a cloudy mucoid exudate. Cysts (1-2mm dia) often form in the dilated Virchow-Robin space on the surface of the brain and more deeply into its substance, and the macroscopic lesions have a mucinous (gelatinous) appearance from the presence of the large amount of capsular material in the very numerous organisms. This cyst in the eosinophil fibrillary superficial cortex is typically flask-shaped and contains large numbers of the microorganism. Each microorganism (5-20μm dia) is dark-coloured and enclosed within a thick pale grey mucoid capsule (thick arrow). The inflammatory response tends to be mild, There are small numbers of lymphocytes in the surrounding tissues but no macrophage or glial response.

HE ×360

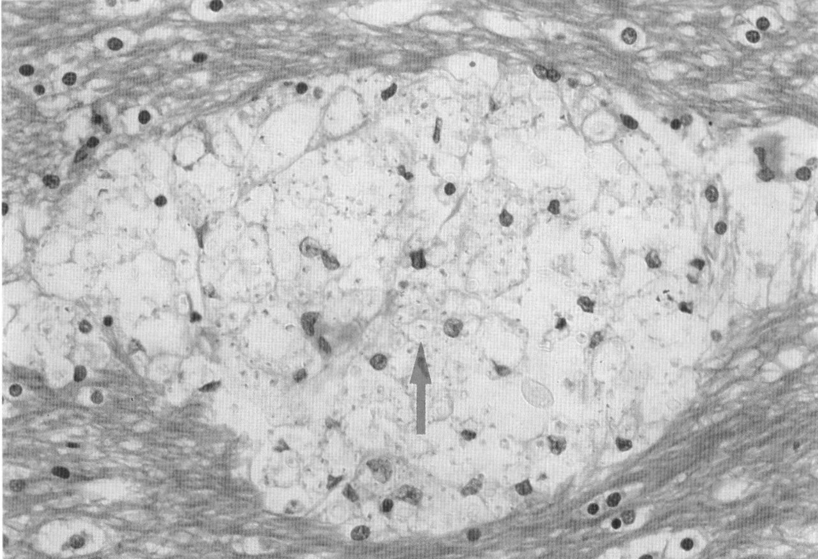

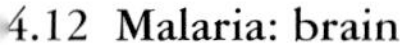

4.12 Malaria: brain

Malaria is caused by the Plasmodium species, and their vector is the Anopheles mosquito. *Plasmodium falciparum* causes subtertian malaria, which can affect many tissues and organs. In the blood, the erythrocytes are infected (and reinfected) by proliferating merozoites, which episodically release and lyse the erythrocytes. In addition, red cell membranes are altered (by an immune response) and adhere more tightly to the vascular endothelium of the small blood vessels in the brain. Many of these vessels are consequently blocked. This is a particularly important aspect of cerebral malaria, and the illness must be regarded as a very serious and often fatal condition. This picture shows one such small blood vessel in the brain of a fatal case. It is completely occluded by closely packed parasitized red cells, in which there are large numbers of the malaria parasite. These appear as very small deeply basophilic 'rings' (thick arrow). Around the blocked vessel there are very numerous extravasated red cells (thin arrows). Macroscopically, many similar petechial hemorrhages are visible throughout the brain.

HE ×580

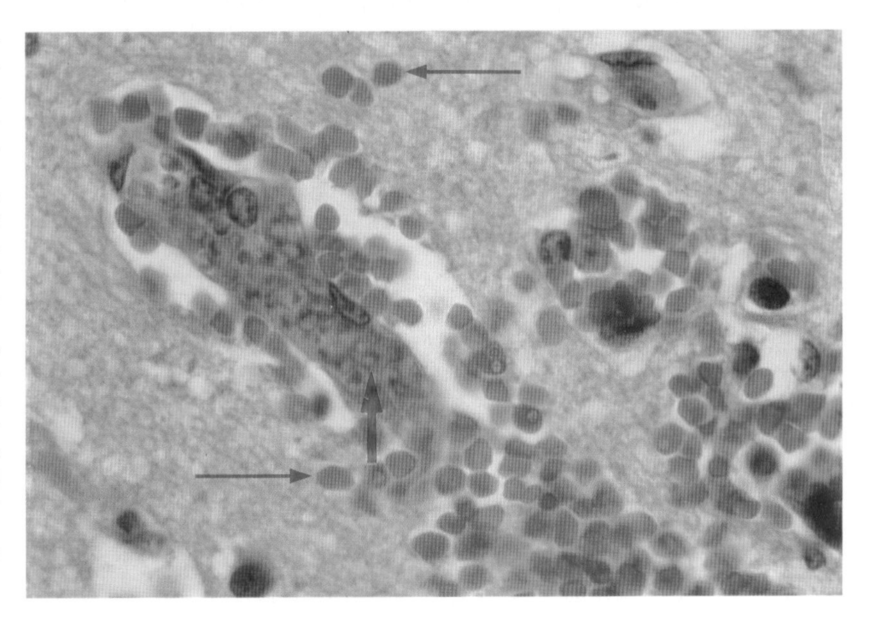

4.13 Tuberous sclerosis: brain

Tuberous sclerosis is a rare autosomal dominant disease which usually presents in young adults. Mental retardation and epilepsy are often present in the patients. In the cerebral hemispheres there are multiple benign hamartomas, composed of abnormal neurons and astrocytes. Macroscopically they are nodules which resemble raw potato tubers (hence the name). Sometimes, within the ventricles, there are tumour masses (subependymal giant cell ependymoma, composed of giant astrocytes) which may act as space-occupying lesions and block the cerebrospinal fluid (CSF), thereby causing hydrocephalus and increased intracranial pressure. This is part of a nodule in the cerebral cortex, bounded by a dilated thin-walled blood vessel (double arrow). The normal cortex has been replaced by tissue which consists of abundant glial fibres (thick arrows) and numerous bizarre giant cells (thin arrow) (apparently mononuclear and eccentric) with well-defined boundaries. Some of the giant cells, which are characteristic of tuberous sclerosis, have the features of neurons and others of astrocytes. There are also various lesions in other organs, including angiofibromatous papules in the skin of the face, rhabdomyoma of the heart, and angiomyolipomas of the kidneys.

HE ×150

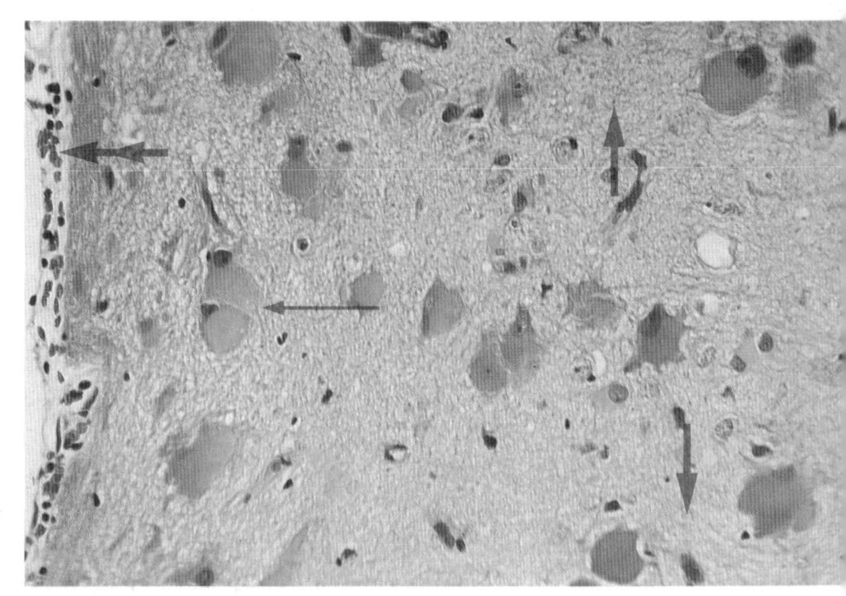

4.14 Gumma: brain

In the tertiary stage of syphilis, gummas may develop. They are characterized by extensive necrosis of tissue. Absorption of the necrotic tissue tends to take place relatively slowly and considerable scarring of the involved organ may result. This is a gumma of brain. The tissue on the left is part of the necrotic centre of the gumma. It consists of granular eosinophilic debris and sheets of closely packed large round macrophages with relatively small round or ovoid deeply basophilic nuclei. The macrophages have a large amount of granular weakly eosinophilic cytoplasm with well-defined boundaries (thick arrows), and they are distended with phagocytosed lipid-rich necrotic material. Peripheral to and surrounding the sheets of macrophages there are strands of fibrous tissue and elongated fibroblasts (double arrow). Small numbers of plasma cells, lymphocytes and macrophages are also present in the fibrous tissue, and to the right of this fibrous layer there is a highly cellular zone (thin arrow) which consists mainly of plasma cells and lymphocytes but also of occasional macrophages.

HE ×235

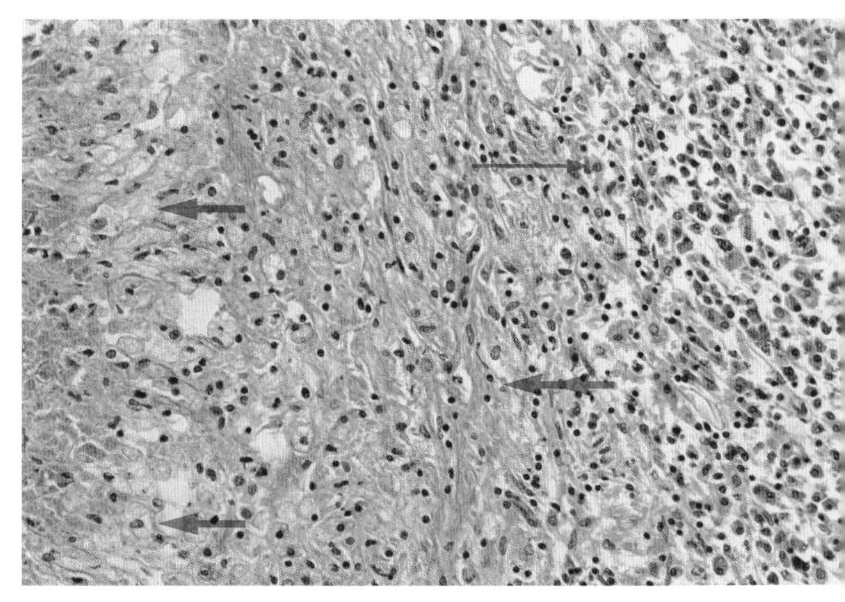

4.15 Tabes dorsalis: spinal cord

Tabes dorsalis is a late manifestation of syphilis, usually becoming evident only after 25 or more years have passed. The spinal cord is flattened, the posterior roots of the spinal nerves (particularly those entering the lumbar enlargement of the spinal cord and their upward extensions in the posterior columns) and dorsal ganglia have slowly and progressively degenerated. Demyelinization begins in the middle root zone of the cord close to the posterior horns and extends to destroy most of the posterior columns. Axons and myelin disappear and are replaced by gliosis. This is a section through segment L4 of the cord, stained by the Loyez method for myelin. There is an area of pallor in each of the posterior columns (thick arrows) in the middle root zone, caused by the loss of the myelinated fibres. These changes lead to loss of proprioceptor sense in the muscles and joints of the legs, as well as loss of pain sense. Similar changes are present in the affected roots (not shown here) and they may occur also in the sensory cranial nerves, including the optic nerves.

Loyez method ×11

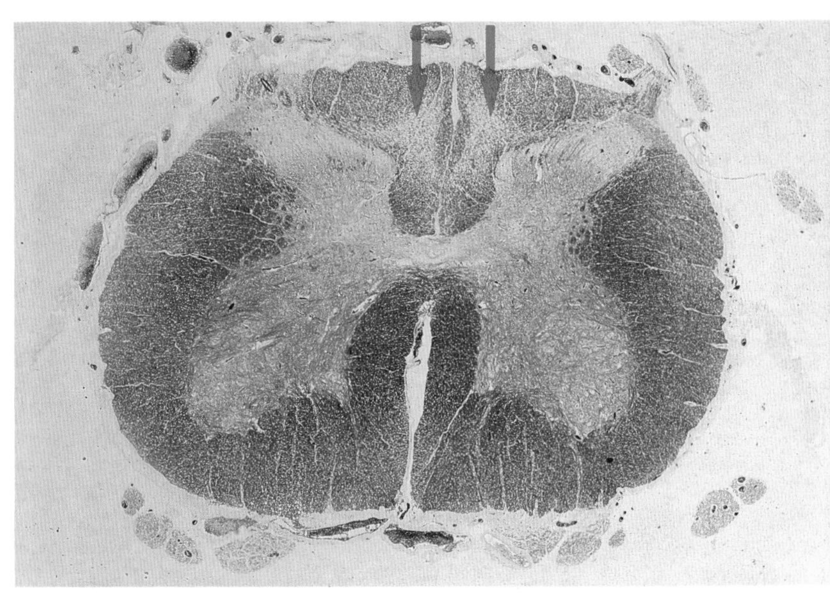

4.16 Creutzfeldt Jakob disease: brain

Creutzfeldt Jakob disease, in human brain, is characterized by a long latent period after infection, followed by a slow progressive degeneration of the brain which ends in death. In this case, the brain tissue shows spongiform changes, with confluent vacuolation of the cerebral substance ("neuropil") (thin arrows).

Initially the lesions in Creutzfeldt Jakob disease are small, 2-10 mm in diameter, with some neuronal loss. So-called "amyloid plaques" may also be seen. In addition, glial cells may increase in number, as a result of reactive change.

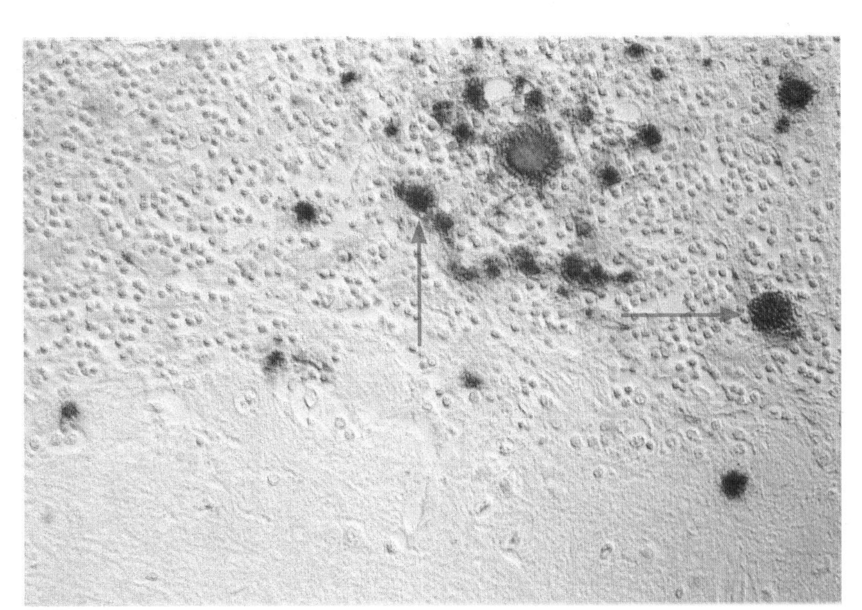

4.17 Creutzfeldt Jakob disease: brain

Creutzfeldt Jakob is a Prion (slow virus) infection, and this brain tissue has been stained by means of immunohistochemistry for Prion Protein (PrP). The amyloid plaques referred to above (4.16) are demonstrated by staining for PrP (thin arrows), which enables better recognition than in conventional sections.

In Creutzfeldt Jakob disease the main features are loss of neurons, demyelination and spongifrom change in the cerebral white matter. However there is no inflammatory reaction. The illness, which may occur in patients who received transplants of cornea and dura, mainly affects persons who are between 50 and 75 years of age, in all parts of the world. Recently however, younger persons (in the U.K.) have developed the condition, and it is supposed to be arising from an outbreak of Bovine Spongiform Encephelopathy (BSE) in cattle.

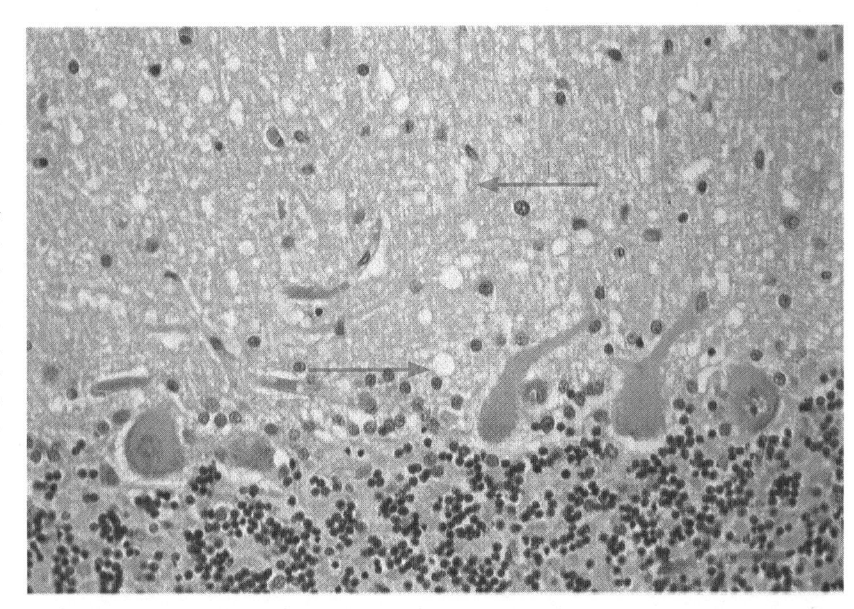

4.18 Alzheimer's disease: brain

Alzheimer's disease is similar to senile dementia but appears about a decade earlier ('pre-senile' dementia). The brain is small (often less than 1000g), and there is widespread shrinkage and atrophy of the cortex of the frontal and temporal lobes. The gyri are narrowed and the sulci widened. many neurons are lost, gliosis develops and their axons demyelinate. Neurofibrillary 'tangles' in the cytoplasm distort many of the affected neurons remaining in the cerebral cortex, the nucleus being pushed to one side by tangled bundles and loops of fibres. Also characteristic of the disease are large (150μm) neuritic plaques. This biopsy specimen from the cortex of a man of 63 has been treated by the periodic acid-silver method. The subarachnoid space and the surface of the cortex are at the top. Within the cortical grey matter there are many dark-staining (argyrophilic) round plaques (thin arrow) which consist of masses of small argyrophilic granules and filaments. The plaques are extracellular collections of degenerated cellular processes, arranged around a central mass of ß-amyloid protein material. Many small blood vessels (stained red) (thick arrows) are also shown, as well as larger vessels in the subarachnoid space. Periodic acid-silver ×90

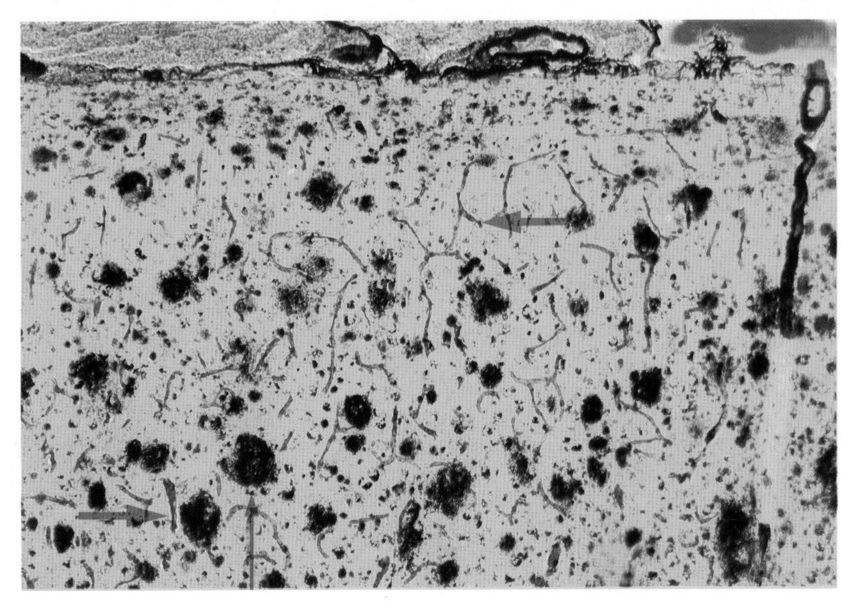

4.19 Poliomyelitis: spinal cord

Poliomyelitis is caused by the poliovirus, an enterovirus transmitted by the fecal-oral route, the virus entering the body through the intestine and infecting the spinal cord and brain via the bloodstream. Most infections with the poliovirus are clinically 'silent' and only a small minority (about 1%) get paralytic lesions from destruction of the lower motor neurons in the anterior (ventral) horn of the spinal cord and medulla oblongata. This is the anterior horn in a patient who died 6 days after the onset of the illness. The tissue is infiltrated with inflammatory cells, a mixture of polymorphs, lymphocytes and macrophages. All the neurons are degenerate, having no nucleus and containing little or no Nissl substance. The neurons are shrunken and occupy large vacuoles (double arrows). There are also numerous much smaller vacuoles in the surrounding edematous tissues. Several necrotic neurons are being phagocytosed by macrophages and polymorphs (neuronophagia); and in places where a neuron has disappeared, only swollen macrophages remain (thin arrow). The small blood vessels (thick arrow) are dilated and have a cuff of inflammatory cells. HE ×235

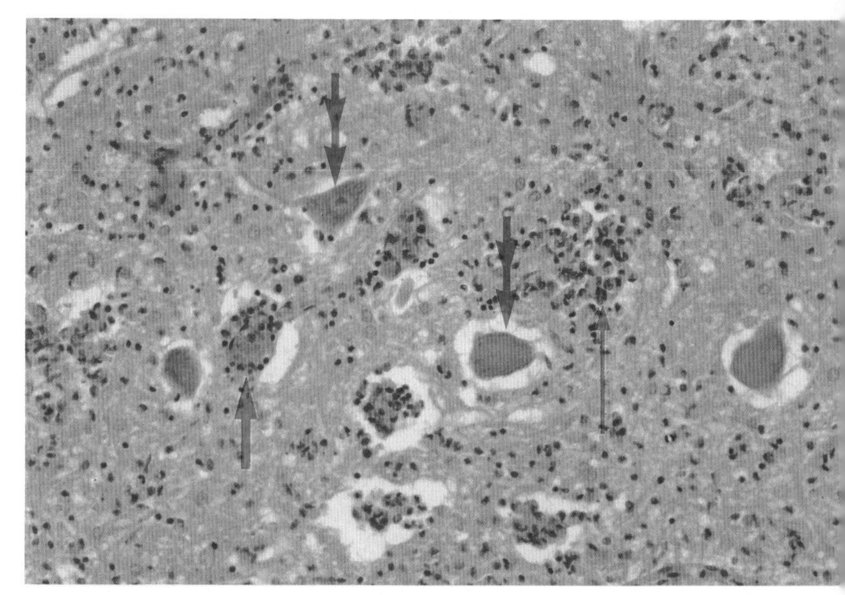

4.20 Poliomyelitis: spinal cord

Poliomyelitis is a very serious disease, with a significant mortality in the acute phase, generally because of paralysis of respiratory muscle, including the diaphragm. However, although once common, it has now become rare worldwide and is expected to be eradicated early in the next century. This is the ventral horn from a person who died one week after the onset of the illness. The inflammatory reaction is still acute and the small blood vessels are very widely dilated. There is a large amount of necrotic debris, resulting from very extensive destruction and disruption of tissue and cells. Apart from one degenerate and shrunken neuron (thick arrow), no neurons remain. The tissue is infiltrated with large numbers of lymphocytes, plasma cells and macrophages. In the lower left corner, most of the macrophages, having ingested the necrotic neurons and tissue, are greatly swollen, with a large amount of cytoplasm (thin arrows) and prominent sharply-defined margins. The macrophages are full of pale granular lipid which pushes the round deeply basophilic nucleus to one side of the cell. HE ×235

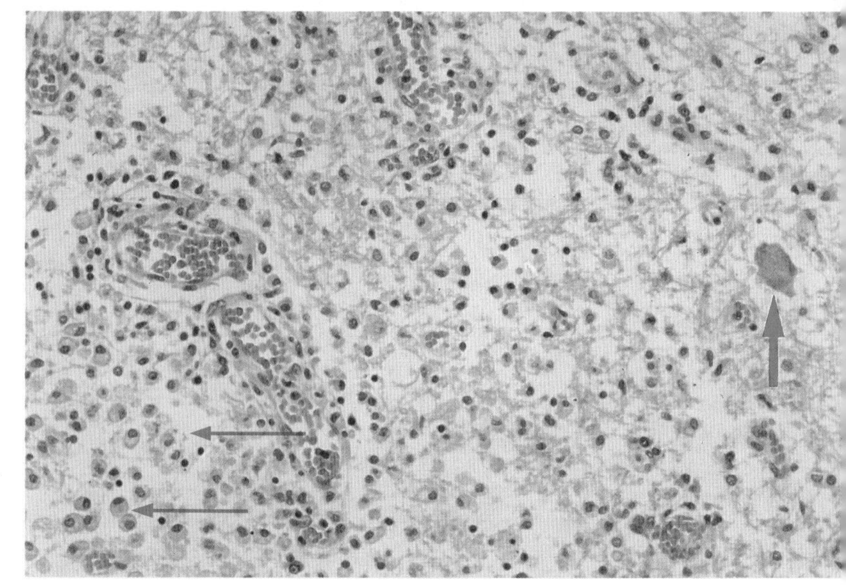

4.21 Multiple sclerosis: spinal cord

Multiple sclerosis is the most common demyelinating disease. Its etiology is uncertain, but it may be viral or immune-mediated. The incidence of the disease varies, progressively lessening from north to south. Exposure to environmental factors (such as an unidentified virus) in childhood may be responsible for multiple sclerosis. In the disease, parts of the nervous system undergo rapid loss of myelin (acute demyelination). Axons are preserved however and may function for a long time. The presence of these plaques of patchy demyelination causes increasing disturbance of both motor and sensory functions. This is a section of the cervical spinal cord stained by the Weigert-Pal method which colours myelin black. Two plaques of demyelination are present: a small round one in the ventrolateral part of the cord (thin arrow) and a much larger one (thick arrow) which affects most of the posterior columns. Notable features are the irregular shape of the large plaque, the lack of conformity it has with anatomical structure, the complete loss of myelin within the plaque, and the sharp line of demarcation between the plaque and the surrounding tissues. Weigert-Pal ×9

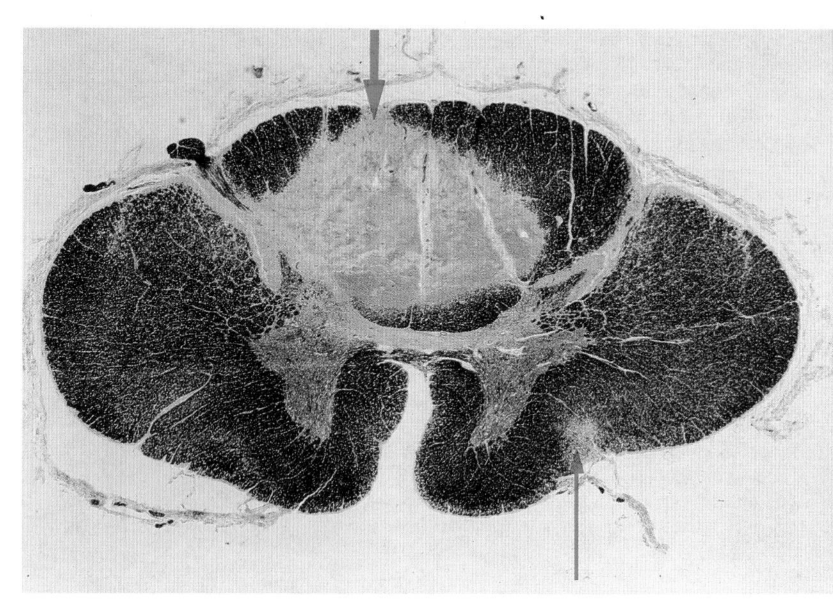

4.22 Multiple sclerosis: brain

The onset of multiple sclerosis is usually in individuals between twenty and forty years of age. The majority are female. The lesions in multiple sclerosis are thought to be foci of immunologically mediated demyelination, following damage to oligodendroglial cells (which then disappear). The lesions are randomly distributed and develop at irregular intervals. This is the edge of a plaque in the white matter in the brain. The plaque is on the left and the white matter on the right. There are only a few astrocytes (but no oligodendrocytes) in the plaque, and following complete loss of the eosinophilic myelin (the stain does not demonstrate axons), the plaque appears to be virtually structureless. It is very extensively 'vacuolated' and very pale (almost without colour) (thin arrow), whereas the white matter on the right is eosinophilic (thick arrow) and more or less normal in appearance. Most of the many cells in the eosinophilic white matter are small oligodendrocytes with a 'ring' of vacuolated cytoplasm and a round heavily stained nucleus. HE ×150

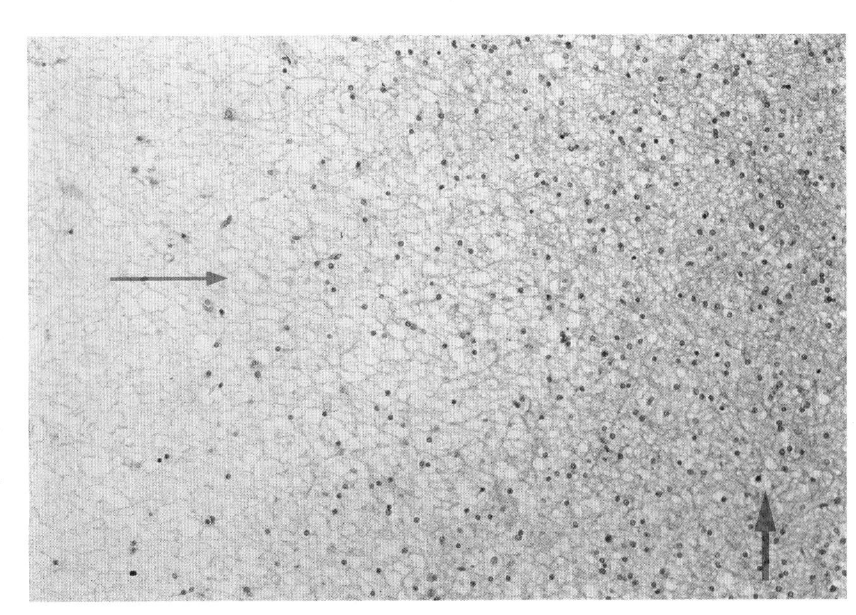

4.23 Multiple sclerosis: brain

Multiple sclerosis is characterized by the presence in the white matter of multiple plaques of demyelination (best demonstrated by stains for myelin), distributed widely throughout the central nervous system. The plaques are perivenular and take the form of irregular but well-demarcated translucent or grey lesions which vary in diameter from 0.1cm to several cm. This is a frozen histological section of a recent lesion in the cerebrum. It is stained with Sudan IV to show fat, and the plaque, located in the central white matter, is an orange-red colour (thick arrow), from the presence in it of much stainable fat. The fat has come from the breakdown of the complex lipids of the myelin of the medullary sheaths of the axons. Foci of active and recent demyelination are usually infiltrated by lymphocytes, but the cells are not visible at this low magnification. Above and to the left of the plaque there is a purplish-blue sheet of sub-cortical 'U' fibres (thin arrows) which have been spared by the demyelinating process. Sudan IV ×11

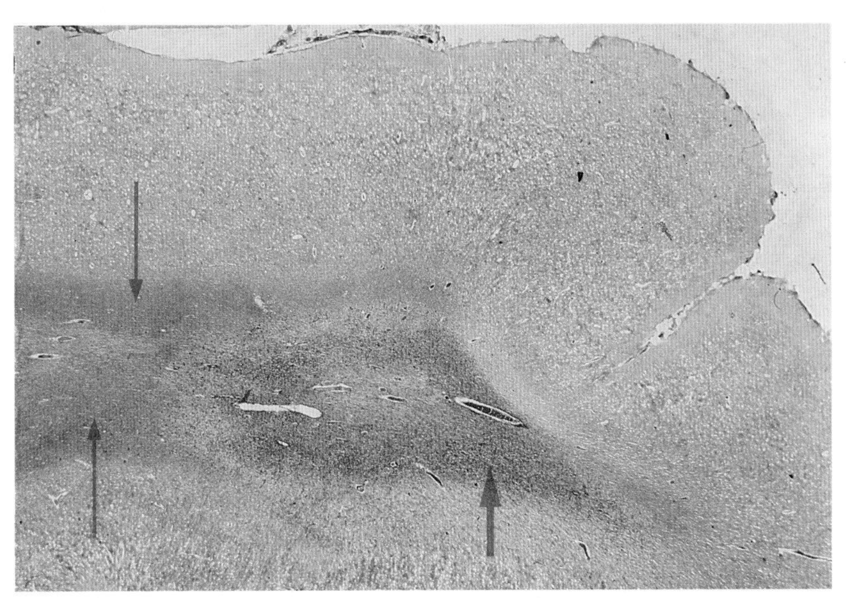

4.24 Multiple sclerosis: brain

In multiple sclerosis, there is reactive proliferation of astrocytes at the edges of the plaques, but typically oligodendrocytes are absent. After six months the quantity of fat in the plaque is greatly reduced, and fat-laden macrophages (lipophages) are present only around blood vessels. Gliosis of the plaques (unmyelinated axons in a mesh of glial fibres) develops slowly but steadily, eventually converting the plaques from soft translucent or yellowish areas to firm grey lesions which are particularly easy to see macroscopically. In this patient, the lesion is an old plaque in the wall of a lateral ventricle, a common site for the lesions, and at this stage the plaque consists entirely of diffusely scattered astrocytes. The astrocytes have round or ovoid or moderately pleomorphic nuclei and glial fibres but no visible cytoplasm. The ventricle is lined by single layer of plump cuboidal or flattened cells (arrows) with round or ovoid vesicular nuclei and fairly abundant eosinophilic cytoplasm. The chromatin is coarsely granular, as in nuclei of the astrocytes. HE ×200

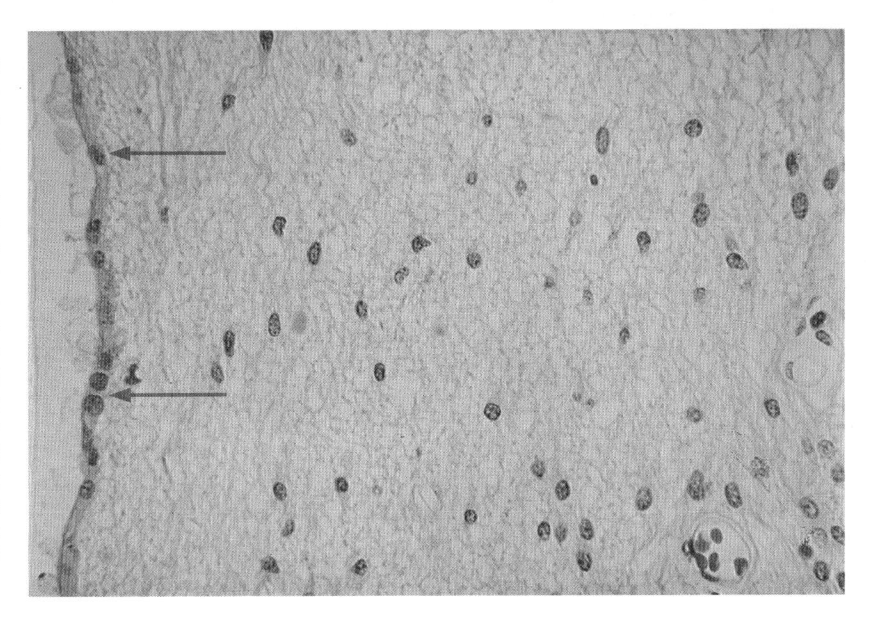

4.25 Motor neuron disease (amyotrophic lateral sclerosis): spinal cord

The etiology of motor neuron disease is unknown. The disease usually occurs sporadically, generally in individuals over 50 years of age. It is characterized by degeneration of both upper and lower motor neurons and the neurons degenerate spontaneously and progressively. If the affected neurons are in the spinal cord, the muscles supplied by them atrophy (progressive muscular atrophy), and when they are in the brainstem the condition is termed progressive bulbar palsy. When upper motor neurons in the brain are affected, fibres are lost from the corticospinal tracts and there is spastic paralysis (amyotrophic lateral sclerosis). This is the spinal cord from a patient with amyotrophic lateral sclerosis and it has been stained (deep blue) for myelin. There is loss of staining (pallor) in the lateral and anterior columns, affecting both the crossed cerebrospinal tracts (thin arrows) and the direct tracts (thick arrows). Loss of myelinated fibres is more pronounced in the crossed cerebrospinal tracts than in the direct tracts. Loyez method ×9

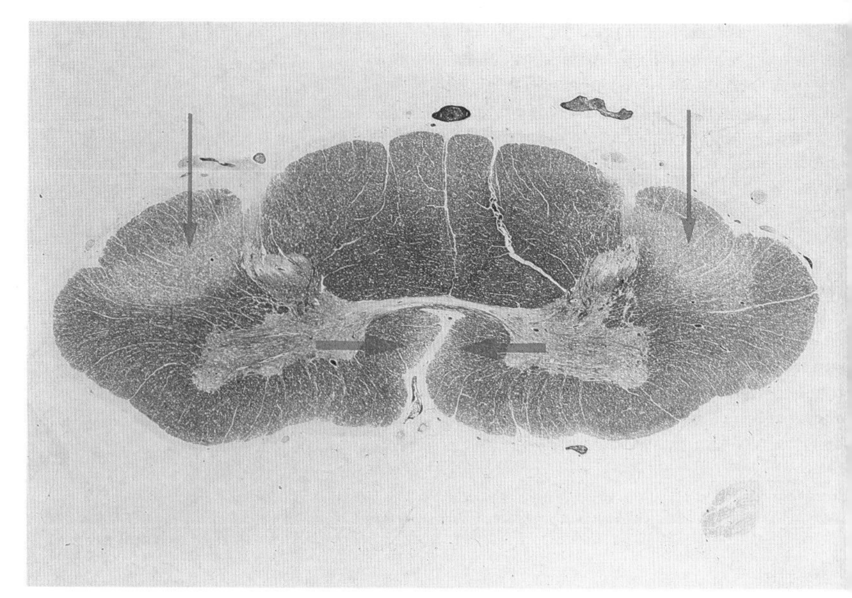

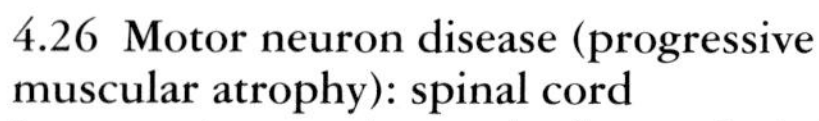

4.26 Motor neuron disease (progressive muscular atrophy): spinal cord

In progressive muscular atrophy the neurological deficit is purely motor, degeneration and loss of the motor neurons producing paralysis and atrophy (preceded by fasciculation) of the muscles which they supply. In this case there is preferential degeneration of motor neurons in the anterior (ventral) horn of the spinal cord, and the paralysis is in the extremities. This is a histological section of the anterior (ventral) horn of the spinal cord from a patient who had progressive muscular atrophy. The section has been stained (purple) with thionin to demonstrate the motor neurons selectively, and the number of motor neurons is much smaller than normal. The sparse neurons that remain are markedly degenerate and shrunken (arrows); and in the reduced amount of cytoplasm, much of the Nissl substance has disintegrated and disappeared (chromatolysis). In contrast, the nuclei are swollen and pale, from the (gradual) loss of chromatin (karyolysis). Thionin ×80

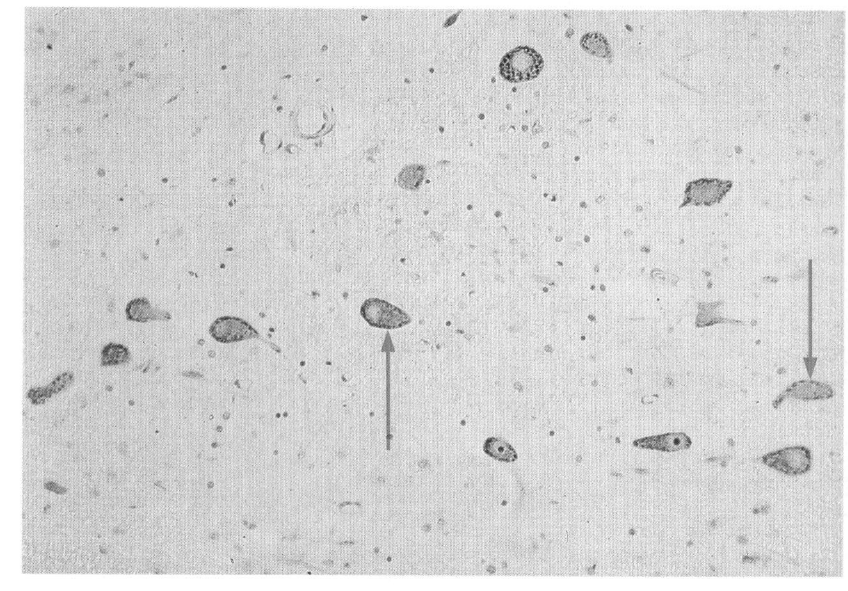

4.27 Subacute combined degeneration: spinal cord

Deficiency of vitamin B12 causes several components of the nervous system to degenerate, the most common lesion being subacute combined degeneration of the spinal cord. Myelinated fibres in the dorsal and lateral columns of the spinal cord disintegrate and disappear. In the dorsal (posterior) columns, demyelination leads to loss of position and vibration sense; in the lateral columns, it produces upper motor neuron paralysis. The lower thoracic region of the cord is most often involved, but degenerative changes spread upwards and downwards, as high as the cerebral cortex, from the affected part. Demyelination also affects peripheral nerves.

This section of the spinal cord (at level C2) has been stained (black) by the Weigert-Pal method for myelin. The nerve roots are unaffected, but the following tracts are degenerate and pale (unstained): the posterior columns (gracilis and part of cuneate) (thin arrows); the anterior (direct) cerebrospinal (thick arrows); and, on the lateral aspects of the cord, the anterior and posterior spinocerebellar and lateral (crossed) cerebrospinal tracts (double arrows). Weigert-Pal ×9

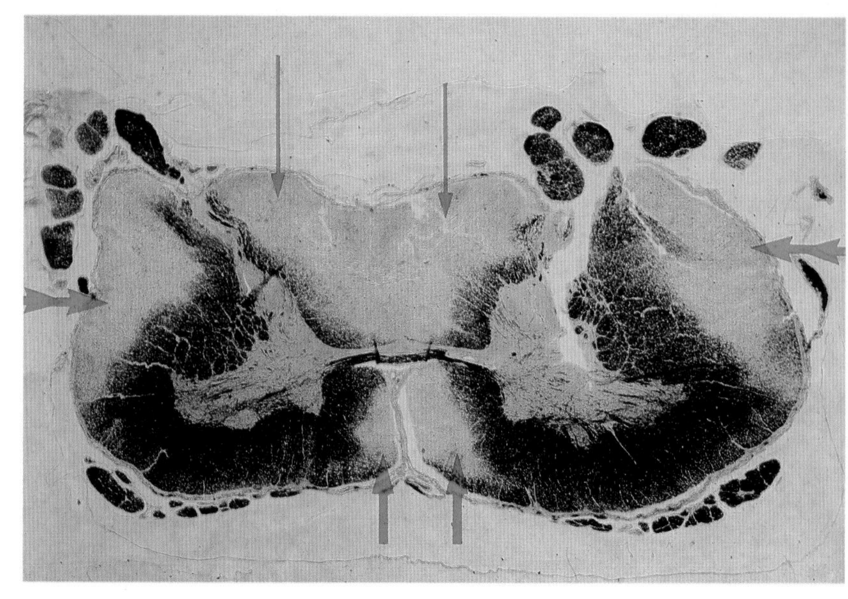

4.28 Peripheral neuropathy: sural nerve

Peripheral neuropathy is clinical term which denotes non-traumatic disease of the nerves. It includes two basic pathological lesions (in both of which nerve conduction fails), namely segmental demyelination and degeneration of axons. A man of 43 who had drunk 25 pints of beer a day for many years presented with the signs and symptoms of peripheral neuropathy, presumably the result of vitamin deficiency. A small portion of sural nerve was removed for diagnostic purposes. In this histological section, the myelin is coloured deep blue (arrow), which signifies marked demyelination of all the nerve fibres. Special stains showed however that the axons are intact. The pattern of breakdown of myelin in this case is typical of the segmental degeneration of Gombault in which the degeneration primarily affects segments of myelin lying between two nodes of Ranvier. If the etiological agent is removed, remyelination takes place with recovery of function. Gombault's segmental degeneration is found in other conditions, including the polyneuropathy of malnutrition and acute infectious polyneuritis (Guillain-Barré syndrome). Solochrome cyanin ×335

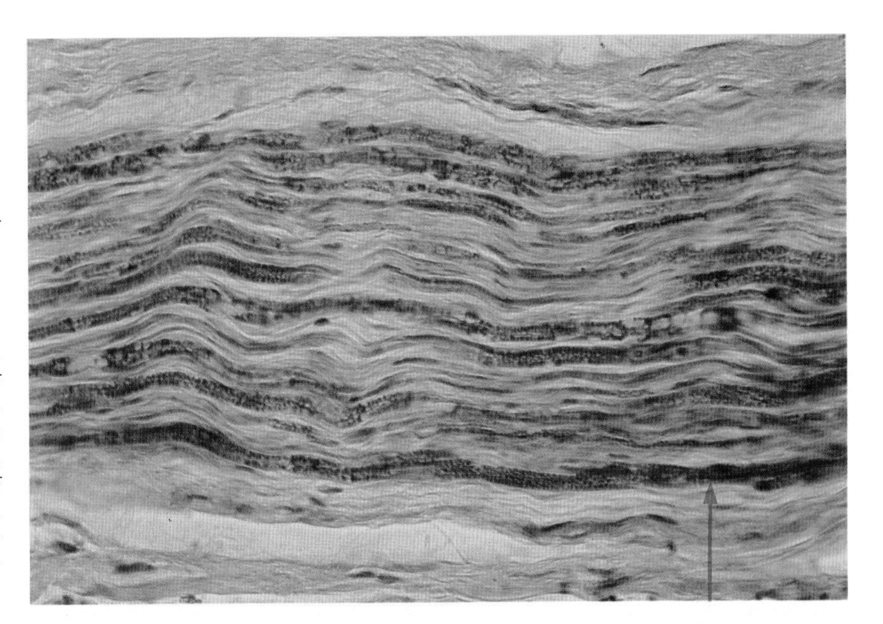

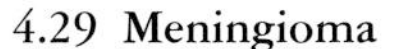

4.29 Meningioma

Meningiomas usually arise outside the brain substance and have an attachment to the dura, usually in the vicinity of the venous sinuses. They can occur at any age but predominantly in middle-aged women. They are firm lobulated encapsulated masses which may grow to a large size and compress adjacent neural structures but do not invade the brain. However they frequently infiltrate the dura, but this does not denote malignancy, and meningiomas are usually resectable. This is a cellular transitional meningioma. It consists of interweaving sheets of polygonal cells (thin arrows) with ill-defined eosinophilic cytoplasm and ovoid or round vesicular nuclei of fairly uniform structure. Many of the nuclei are pyknotic but there are no mitoses. There is also a very marked tendency for the cells to form whorls of various sizes. The cells at the centre of the whorls (thick arrows) are strongly eosinophilic, undergoing hyalinization and calcification (some of the whorls misleadingly look like blood vessels). Calcification which is just beginning in some of the whorls converts them into psammoma bodies. HE ×235

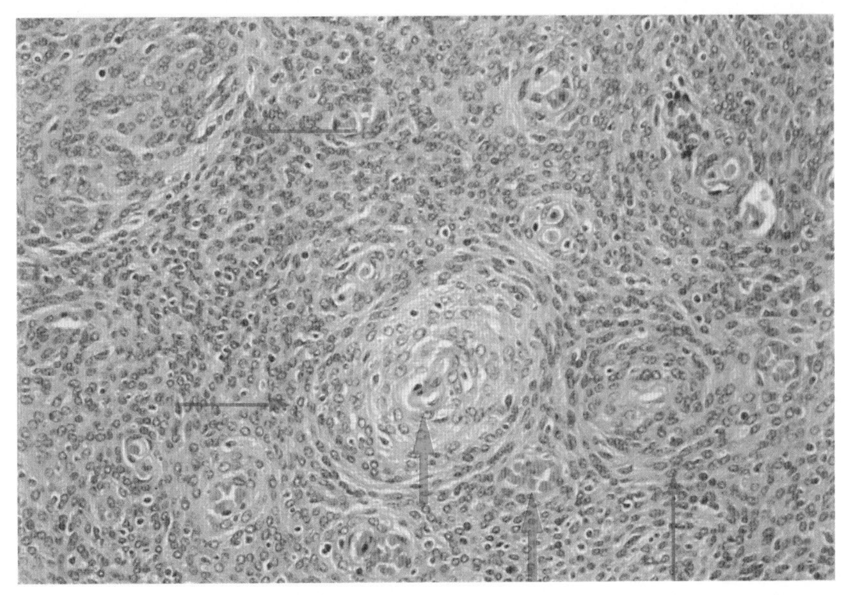

4.30 Meningioma

The skull bones which overly a meningioma are often associated with hypertrophy (hyperostosis) which may result in a palpable mass. Meningiomas may also infiltrate bone and invade the scalp, but a meningioma is termed malignant only when it infiltrates the underlying brain. This lesion, which arose in a woman of 59, invaded the dura which reacted and became much thicker. It is a transitional type of meningioma, and this part of it consists mainly of compact whorls of tumour cells (thin arrows). The cells have abundant eosinophilic cytoplasm, the boundaries of which are ill-defined. There are also small vacuoles in some cells. The nuclei are uniform ovoid and vesicular, and the chromatin is pale and finely granular. There is no significant pleomorphism of the nuclei, and no mitoses are present. There is a small cavity at the centre of the whorls of tumour cells (thick arrow), and the central cells eventually become hyalinized and may calcify to form 'psammoma' bodies. Sometimes there is a blood vessel at the centre of a cellular whorl. A meningioma with many psammoma bodies has a gritty texture when it is cut. HE ×360

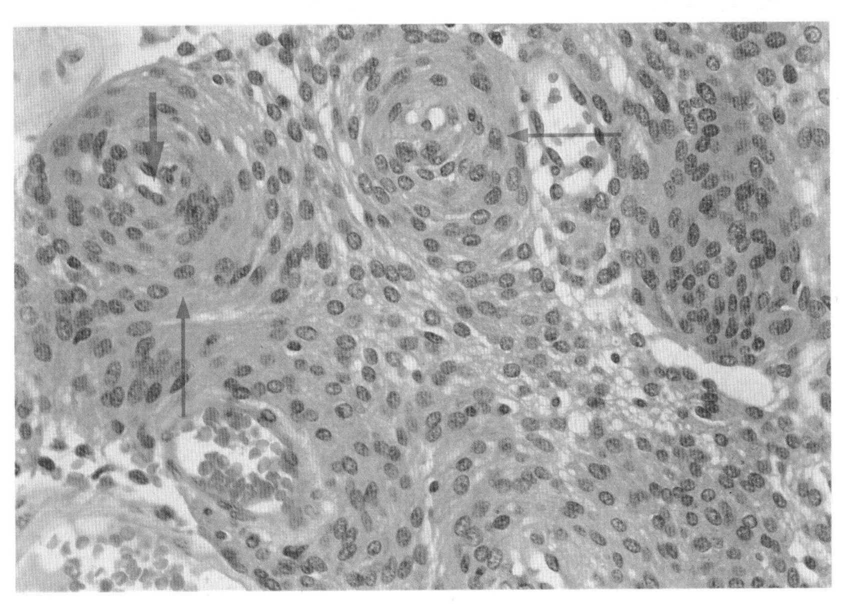

4.31 Oligodendroglioma: brain

Oligodendrogliomas generally arise the cerebral hemispheres of adults in the 30-50 age range. They are composed of oligodendrocytes, small glial cells with relatively few cell processes which play an important role in the maintenance of the myelin sheaths of the axons. In the majority of cases, the tumour is 'mixed', consisting of both astrocytes and oligodendrocytes. Oligodendrogliomas are slow-growing soft fleshy tumours, most often located in the white matter of the cerebral hemispheres. The prognosis is generally better than with astrocytomas, but a minority are aggressive in their behaviour. The histological structure of the tumour is characteristic. It is highly cellular, consisting of a population of small uniform neoplastic cell. Each cell has a moderate amount of eosinophilic cytoplasm, bounded by a well-defined cell membrane, and a small round very basophilic nucleus. In each cell there is a large clear perinuclear cytoplasmic vacuole (thin arrows) - an appearance termed 'boxing' of the nucleus. Mitotic activity is slight. There are also numerous small thin-walled blood vessels (thick arrow). Calcification (not evident here) is a frequent occurrence in oligodendrogliomas and is demonstrable in almost half of them radiologically. HE ×360

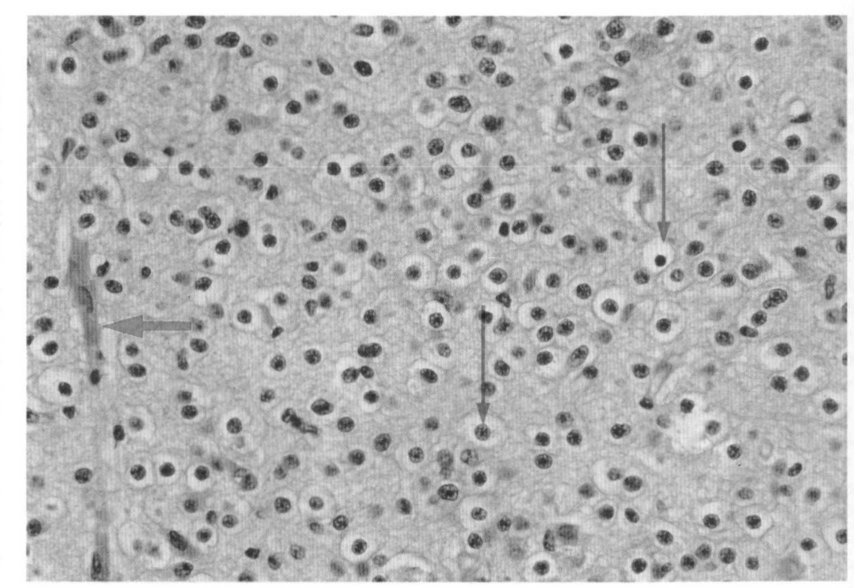

4.32 Astrocytoma: brain

Astrocytes are the predominant glial-forming cell, and astrocytomas are the most common form of primary neoplasm in the central nervous system. They vary considerably in malignancy, from Grade I, the well-differentiated, to Grade IV, the most malignant. It is often difficult however to allocate a tumour precisely to one grade, because of variations in its structure from one part to another. Astrocytomas are slow-growing firm masses which are not encapsulated. Resection of even a Grade I astrocytoma may be impossible if it is in a vital part of the brain. This is a fibrillary astrocytoma of Grade I (or possibly Grade II). It consists of a relatively small population of mature-looking neoplastic astrocytes with ill-defined cytoplasmic boundaries and pleomorphic ovoid or elongated basophilic nuclei. Their neurofibrillary processes are well-developed and abundant, and arranged in large eosinophilic bundles (thin arrows). Many of the astrocytes appear to be vacuolated, and there are collections of fluid (microcysts) in the interstices of the neurofibrillary processes. The dense red bodies (thick arrows) are Rosenthal fibres. HE ×200

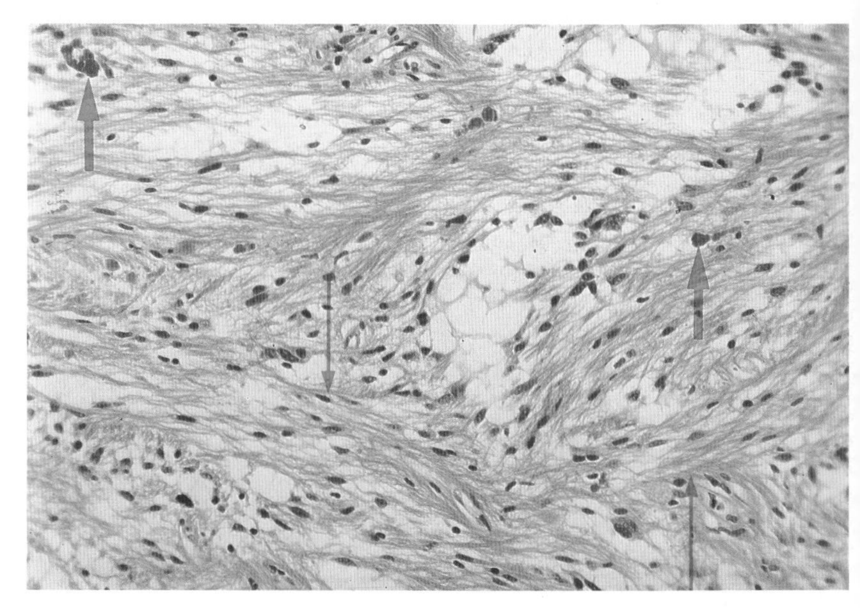

4.33 Astrocytoma: brain

Low grade well-differentiated astrocytomas are almost impossible to resect surgically, because neoplastic tissue generally extends well beyond the apparent margin of the tumour. This tumour was in the right frontal lobe of a man of 52. It is a fairly well-differentiated cellular astrocytoma (Grade II). The neoplastic cells have abundant eosinophilic cytoplasm, and most of them are closely packed. The individual tumour cells tend to be round, and the margins of their cytoplasm are well-defined. The nuclei of the tumour cells are large and moderately pleomorphic, with uniform finely granular basophilic chromatin (thin arrows). Some nuclei appear to have a nucleolus. There are no mitoses however. This form of astrocyte is a gemistocyte, and when it is the predominant form in an astrocytoma, the tumour is termed a gemistocytic astrocytoma. There are many vacuoles (thick arrow) between the neoplastic cells and they were filled with fluid. Sometimes fluid collects on a large scale in an astrocytoma, with the formation of a cyst into which neoplastic tissue projects. HE ×360

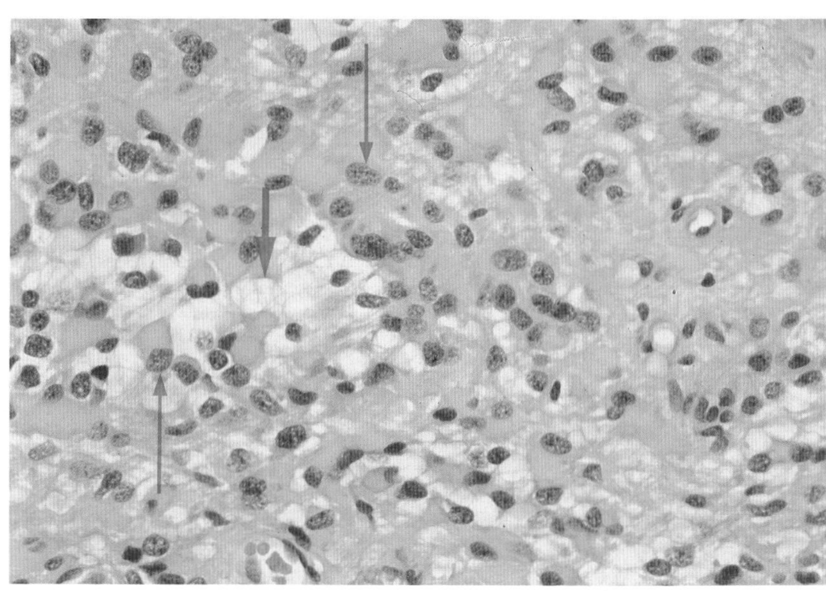

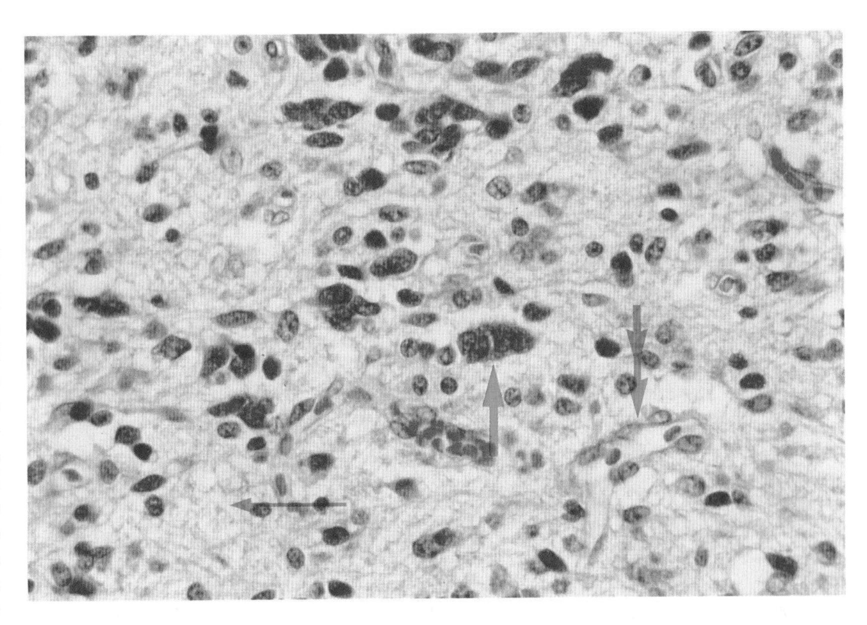

4.34 Astrocytoma: brain

Poorly-differentiated astrocytomas grow more rapidly then the better-differentiated tumours and generally form white infiltrative masses in the cerebral hemispheres. Their cellularity is greater, and the neoplastic cells are more pleomorphic.

A poorly-differentiated astrocytoma (Grade III) was removed from the left frontoparietal region of a man of 26 but recurred 4 years later. This is the recurrent lesion. The malignant astrocytes are markedly pleomorphic, and their nuclei vary greatly in size and shape, from small round forms to very large. The chromatin is granular and also deeply basophilic. Some tumour cells are multinucleated (thick arrow). There are no mitoses in this field, but elsewhere in the tumour there are moderate numbers of mitotic figures. The neoplastic astrocytes have abundant very pale cytoplasm, and in (or adjacent to) it there are large numbers of vacuoles (thin arrow). By means of special stains, the cytoplasmic processes were shown to be shorter and thicker than normal. Numerous small blood vessels are present, some lined by plump endothelial cells (double arrow). No necrosis is evident, but there are necrotic areas in other parts of the neoplasm. HE ×415

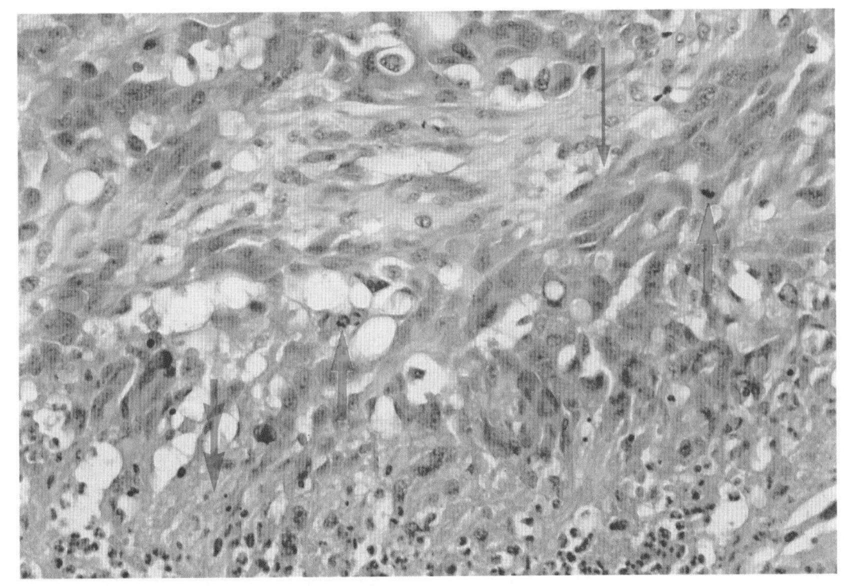

4.35 Glioblastoma multiforme: brain

Glioblastoma multiforme is the most common type of astrocytoma, and the term is sometimes still applied to Grade III or Grade IV tumours. It is one of the most malignant tumours, growing rapidly and forming a large infiltrative mass that typically extends across the midline, to be designated a so-called 'butterfly' tumour. The cut surface of the tumour is generally hemorrhagic and patchily necrotic. This lesion, a Grade IV astrocytoma, is a round (4cm dia) cream-coloured hemorrhagic mass in the left parietal lobe, composed of very pleomorphic neoplastic astrocytic cells which vary greatly in size and shape. Most of the tumour cells are elongated (thin arrow), with long fibrillary processes. The nuclei too are mostly elongated, with rounded (blunt) ends, but they are also pleomorphic and hyperchromatic, and many contain prominent nucleoli. Some of the tumour cells are multinucleated. There are many mitotic figures (thick arrows), some of abnormal form. Part of a large area of necrosis, in which much nuclear debris is just visible (double arrow). There are other extensive areas of necrosis elsewhere in the tumour. HE ×360

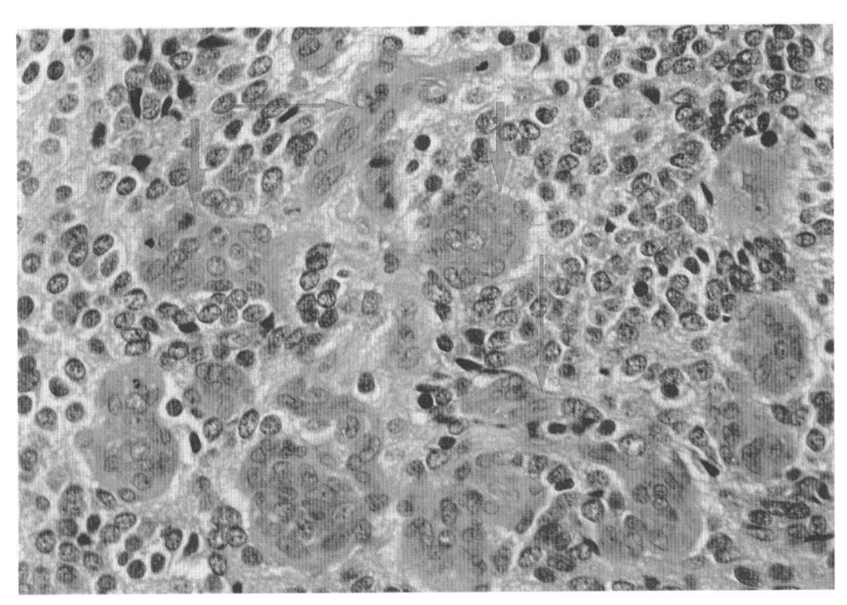

4.36 Polar spongioblastoma: brain

The term polar spongioblastoma has been applied to this lesion but is now regarded as unsatisfactory, the term glioblastoma (see 4.35) being more appropriate. Glioblastoma is one of the most malignant tumours of the brain, consisting of highly pleomorphic astrocytic cells, accompanied by large numbers of mitotic figures. This tumour is located in the right frontal lobe of a 16-year-old boy and the neoplastic astrocytic cells (e.g. right of centre) are primitive, with little cytoplasm and ovoid or round nuclei. The chromatin in the nuclei is moderately basophilic and granular. Many nuclei contain one or more nucleoli, and some nuclei are pyknotic. There are occasional mitoses. The tumour is very vascular, and the many small capillary-type blood vessels (prominent neovascularization) (thin arrows) are lined by large plump endothelial cells with abundant cytoplasm. 'Buds' of proliferating endothelial cells, which resemble miniature glomeruli (thick arrows), project from the surface of the blood vessels. Proliferation of the endothelial cells of small stromal blood vessels is often a prominent feature of poorly-differentiated astrocytomas (Grades III and IV).

HE ×360

4.37 Ependymoma: brain

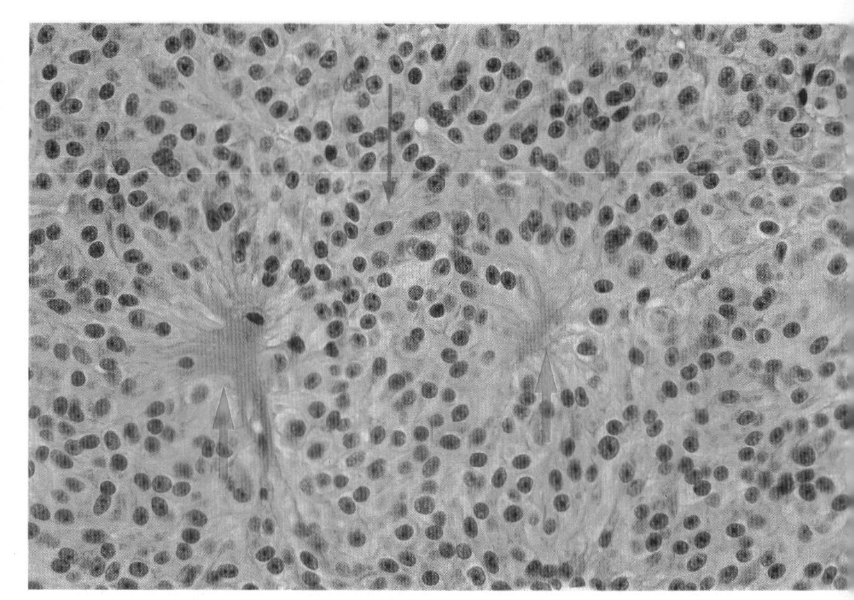

Ependymomas are uncommon tumours that arise at all ages but more often in children. They are generally reddish-brown nodular masses, most of which tend to be associated with the ventricular system of the brain. Many of them are located in the vicinity of the fourth ventricle. They are liable to block the flow of cerebrospinal fluid and also difficult to resect. This typically cellular ependymoma, with a delicate network of small blood vessels, is composed of closely packed polygonal cells with a moderate amount of eosinophilic cytoplasm (thin arrow). The cell boundaries are distinct and also eosinophilic. The nuclei are large and round or ovoid; and the chromatin is diffusely basophilic. In each nucleus there is a prominent nucleolus which tends to be located centrally, and some nuclei have more than one nucleolus. There are no mitotic figures in this field. Two blood vessels are encircled by the elongated strongly eosinophilic filamentous bases (thick arrows) of closely packed neoplastic cells. The tumour cells, orientated around and attached to the two central blood vessels, are arranged as pseudorosettes.

HE ×360

4.38 Ependymoma: brain

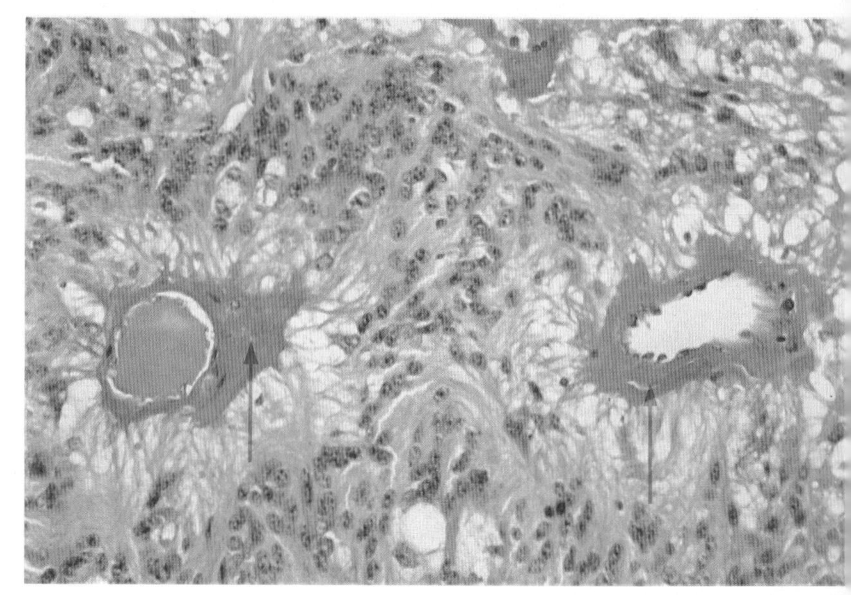

Most ependymomas are very cellular, and the neoplastic cells tend to spread readily in the cerebrospinal fluid. As with astrocytomas, the degree of malignancy of ependymomas varies widely. The better-differentiated tumours tend to grow slowly and have a good prognosis, after surgical resection. On the other hand, poorly-differentiated ependymomas grow rapidly and infiltrate, and their prognosis is poor. Typical ependymomas consist of small polygonal cells that form ependymal tubules and perivascular rosettes. This tumour is a circumscribed ovoid mass (2.8 × 1.5 × 1.5cm) attached to the cauda equina. The cells have a moderate amount of eosinophilic cytoplasm and round or ovoid markedly vesicular nuclei, in which there are one or more small but prominent nucleoli. Nuclear pleomorphism is slight and no mitoses are present. The neoplastic ependymal cells have formed large pseudorosettes, in the centres of which there are two widely dilated blood vessels with thick hyalinized deeply eosinophilic walls (arrows); and the cells are orientated around and attached to the walls by their elongated filamentous (and very vacuolated) bases. Elsewhere in the tumour there is extensive myxomatous change in the stroma.

HE ×360

4.39 Myxopapillary ependymoma: sacrum

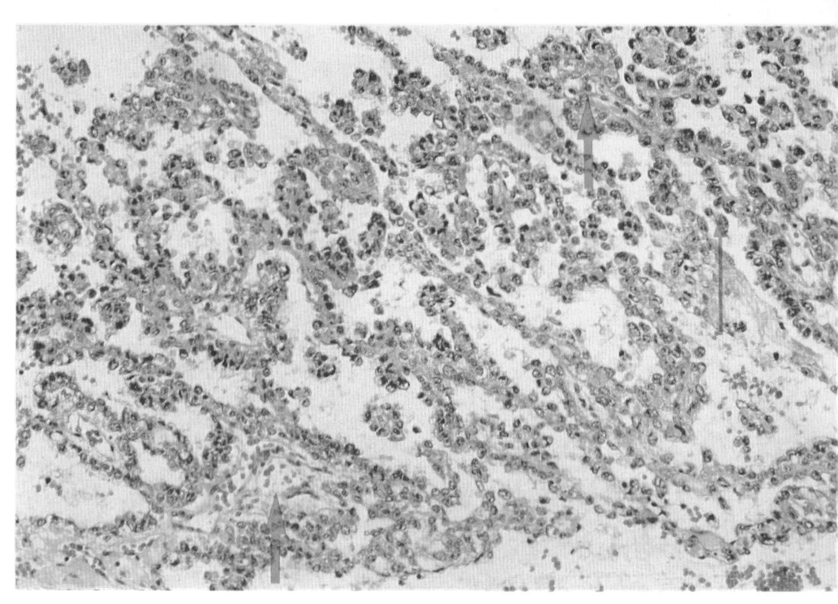

Myxopapillary ependymoma is a specific type of ependymoma which arises most often from the filum terminale of the spinal cord. It presents as a cauda equina tumour in young adults. Macroscopically this tumour, which had slowly enveloped the cord and nerve roots, has a gelatinous appearance. Histologically, this part of it has a highly developed papillary structure, consisting of numerous delicate papillae, each with a delicate core of connective tissue and inconspicuous thin-walled capillary-type blood vessels (thick arrows). The external surface of the papillae are covered by a single layer of small but prominent cuboidal or round epithelial cells (thin arrow), each of which has a small round vesicular nucleus and a moderate amount of well-defined cytoplasm. The spaces between the papillae are occupied by very pale (almost colourless) mucoid secretion and scant extravasated cellular debris (including red cells). This type of structure resembles normal choroid plexus, but the epithelial cells are slightly taller and more prominent than in the normal tissue. Elsewhere, in most of the tumour, the connective tissue of the papillae had undergone myxomatous change.

HE ×150

4.40 Capillary telangiectasis: bran

Telangiectases are common in the brain. Large vascular malformations occur infrequently but small vascular hamartomas are fairly frequently present in the central nervous system and often multiple. They vary considerably in their composition and complexity of structure, ranging from small lesions consisting of capillaries to large thick-walled vessels. Microscopically they are cavernous or capillary hemangiomas, similar to hemangiomas in other parts of the body. They rarely cause any dysfunction, but since they are mostly located on the surface of the brain, they tend to bleed into the subarachnoid space. They may also give rise to a large intracerebral hemorrhage. This was a solitary lesion. It consists of abnormal capillaries, each with a very thin wall (arrow), surrounding which there is an equally thin (external) layer of eosinophilic hyaline amorphous material. Some of the blood vessels are enormously dilated. The blood vessels of the lesion are separated by neural tissue and not fibromuscular tissue, as happens in an ordinary capillary or cavernous hemangioma. Complete resection of lesions of this type may be difficult or impossible. There is no evidence however of previous hemorrhage in this lesion.

HE ×80

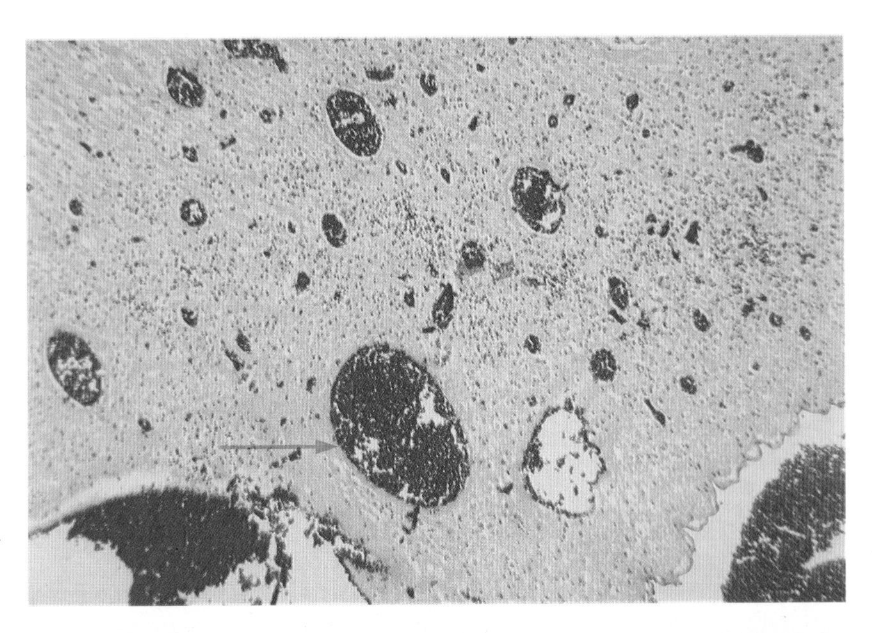

4.41 Medulloblastoma: brain

A medulloblastoma is a highly malignant cellular tumour, derived from primitive neurectodermal cells and occurring mostly in children. It is most often located in the midline cerebellar vermis, in the posterior fossa, and tends to invade the fourth ventricle. It generally appears as a greyish-white fleshy mass with irregular infiltrative margins, and the tumour cells spread readily via the cerebrospinal fluid to the surface of the brain and spinal cord, where they often form metastases, and to the other ventricles. The prognosis is poor but is now improved with treatment. This tumour is from a woman of 24. The malignant cells are remarkably uniform. Each cell has very scant cytoplasm and a round or ovoid basophilic vesicular nucleus. In some nuclei there is a prominent nucleolus. Many nuclei are shrunken and intensely basophilic (pyknotic). There are many small spaces and vacuoles between the malignant cells, but small rosettes of the type found in some medulloblastomas are lacking. The stroma consists largely of thin-walled blood vessels (arrow).

HE ×360

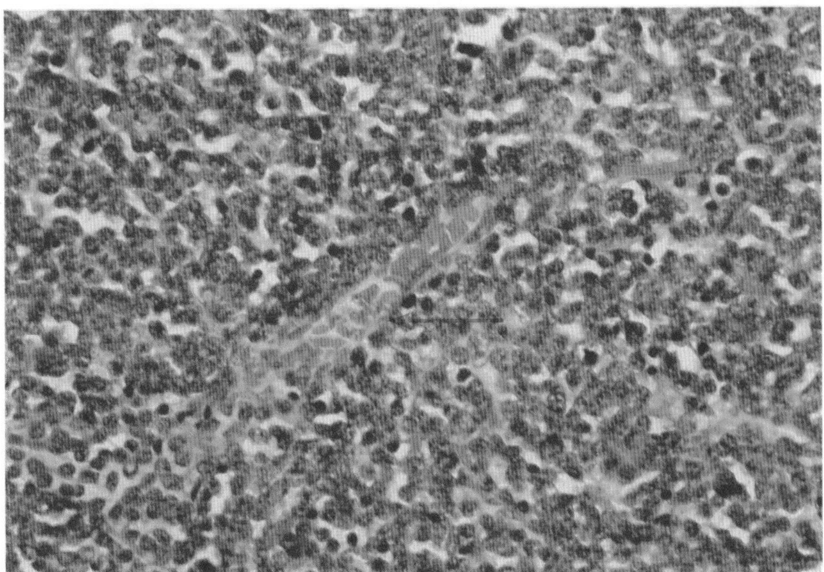

4.42 Retinoblastoma: eye

Retinoblastoma is a not uncommon tumour of early childhood (under five years of age). About one-third of the cases are inherited (familial) and the other two-thirds are sporadic. It is a malignant aggressive neoplasm, arising from primitive neural cells. It is very invasive locally, infiltrating the retina and the vitreous fluid, but it does not metastasize. In inherited cases, there are often tumours in both eyes, whereas in more than 90% of the sporadic cases there is only one (unilateral) tumour. Macroscopically, a retinoblastoma is a solid fleshy mass within the retina, and areas of necrosis and calcification are frequently present. Histologically, it is similar to neuroblastoma and medulloblastoma, consisting of small undifferentiated cells of uniform size and shape, with scant cytoplasm. The nuclei are deeply basophilic and round or slightly ovoid, and the nuclear/cytoplasmic ratio is high. Occasional mitoses are present. The tumour cells have formed 'rosettes' (thick arrows), of diagnostic significance, by arranging themselves round a central lumen full of eosinophilic fibrillary material. The fibrils are nerve fibrils, originating in the tumour cells. Small black deposits of melanin (thin arrow), spilled from the disrupted retina, are also present. HE ×360

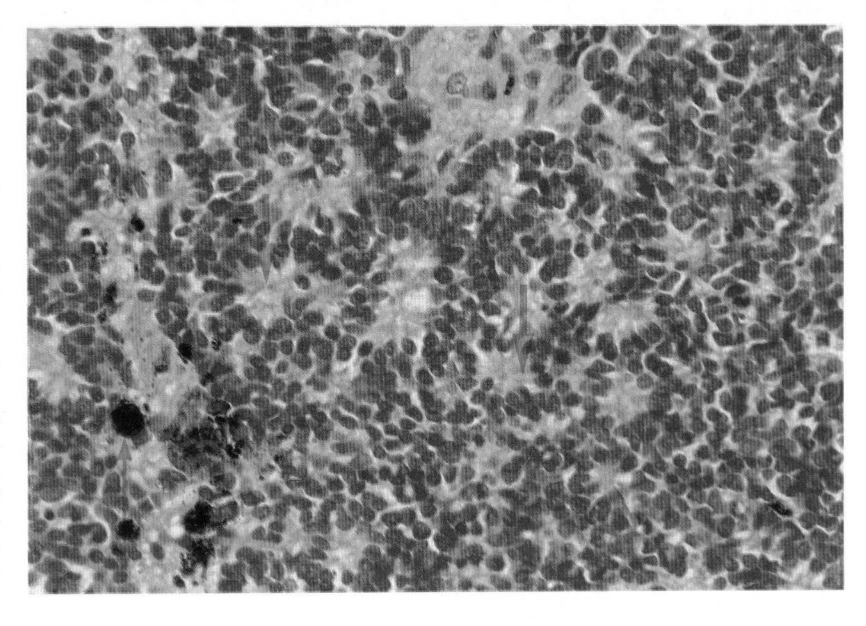

4.43 Cerebellar hemangioblastoma: cerebellum

Cerebellar hemangioblastoma is a benign neoplasm that occurs sporadically or as part of von Hippel-Lindau disease. The cerebellum is the commonest site for hemangioblastoma, although it may be found occasionally in the cerebral hemispheres. It is a true neoplasm of vascular origin and not a hamartomatous malformation. It may occur by itself or as part of Lindau's disease. It is a malignant tumour which appears grossly as a well-circumscribed mass with cystic and solid components, and when it is located in the cerebellum it is often resectable. However this lesion, a typical cystic hemorrhagic mass in the cerebellum of a 79-year-old woman, was not completely resectable. It consists of large numbers of extremely thin-walled dilated capillary-type blood vessels, many extravasating blood, and large round cells with abundant grey or weakly eosinophilic granular cytoplasm (thin arrow). Their nuclei are densely basophilic and many are very pleomorphic. The walls of the two larger blood vessels (thick arrows) are very thick, having been infiltrated by a large amount of eosinophilic amorphous hyaline material. HE ×150

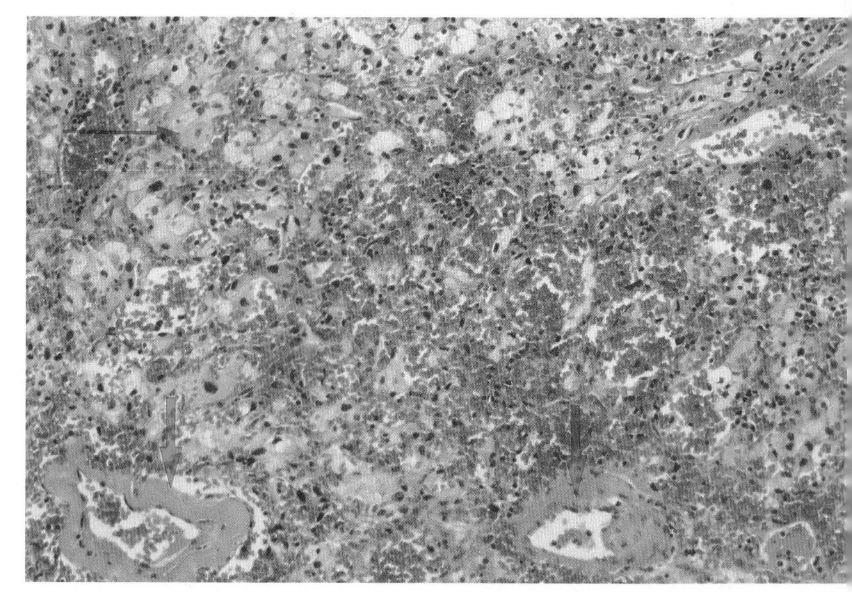

4.44 Cerebellar hemangioblastoma: cerebellum

A typical cerebellar hemangioblastoma consists of endothelium-lined vascular spaces, separated by trabeculae of cells with much lipid-laden cytoplasm. In contrast to the part of the same tumour in 4.43, the bulk of which consisted mostly of large numbers of capillary-type blood vessels, this part of the same tumour, at slightly higher magnification, consists of sheets of closely packed large cells. The cytoplasm of the cells has a well-defined cytoplasmic membrane and generally it has a finely granular pale 'frosted-glass' appearance (thick arrow). In some of the cells, however, the cytoplasm is eosinophilic. The nuclei are very pleomorphic, deeply and uniformly basophilic and varying greatly in size and in shape (from small to very large). However there is no mitotic activity. The cells are large macrophages, and the granular or foamy appearance of their cytoplasm is caused by the considerable content of lipid. The presence of these cells is characteristic of this type of tumour. A fairly large number of small lymphocytes is also present (thin arrow). HE ×235

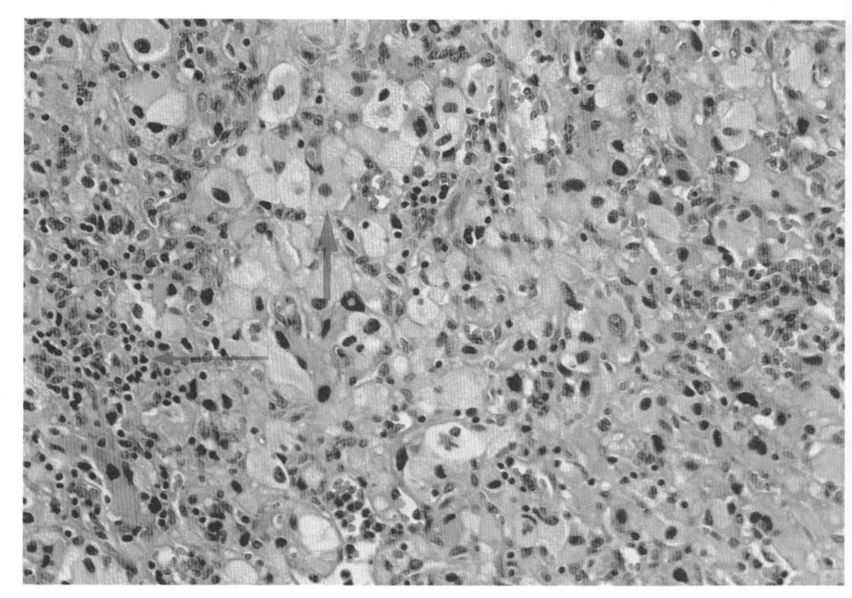

4.45 Schwannoma: cranial nerve

Schwannoma cells form the myelin sheaths, the neurilemma, around the axons in peripheral nerves, and a Schwannoma (neurilemmoma) is a slowly growing benign neoplasm which is generally associated with large nerve trunks. The tumour takes the form of a well-circumscribed round or lobulated mass which is often soft and even cystic. Resecting it may be very difficult however, because of its awkward location. This lesion has arisen from the vestibular portion of the 8th nerve, where it entered the internal auditory meatus (the 'cerebellopontine angle'), and it is accordingly termed an 'acoustic neuroma'. Histologically it contains two types of tissue. First, Antoni type A tissue, which consists of compact groups of spindle-shaped cells with spindle-shaped basophilic nuclei. The spindle-shaped cells surround an ovoid mass of strongly eosinophilic cytoplasm (ovoid bodies) (thick arrow) and tend to arrange themselves in parallel rows (palisades). Second, Antoni type B tissue, which consists of Schwann cells arranged haphazardly in very loose vacuolated reticular stromal tissue (thin arrow). The spaces in type B tissue contain watery fluid, and sometimes they are large and cystic. There is very little collagen in the tumour. HE ×150

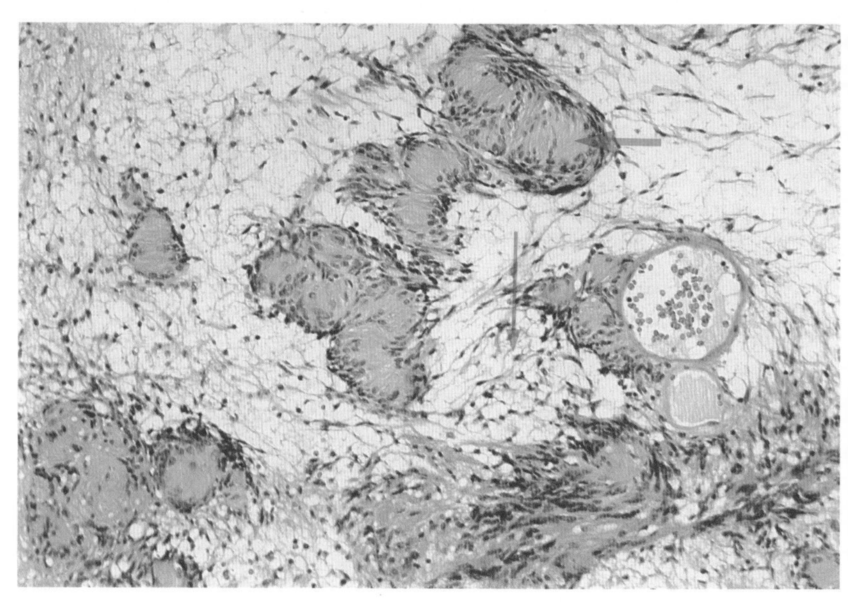

4.46 Schwannoma: spinal nerve

Schwannomas are usually solitary and appear as encapsulated masses which compress the nerve of origin and tend to compress surrounding structures. Multiple Schwannomas may be associated with von Recklinghausen's neurofibromatosis, and this tumour is from the spinal cord of a woman of 67 with neurofibromatosis. The Antoni type A tissue is highly cellular (arrows), consisting of elongated tumour cells arranged as long eosinophilic cords and compact ovoid bodies (Verocay bodies) (double arrows). The nuclei of the tumour cells are elongated and round- or blunt-ended. Most of them are palisaded and located at the periphery of the ovoid bodies, whereas the centres of the bodies are occupied by a mass of fibrillary eosinophilic cytoplasm. The Antoni type B tissue is very loose vacuolated myxomatous stromal tissue (thin arrow) (the vacuoles seem to be intracellular), and the lymphocyte-like nuclei of the stromal cells are small, very basophilic and round or ovoid. The walls of the blood vessels are very thick, from the presence in it of a layer of acellular hyaline material. Hyalinization of the blood vessels is a prominent feature of most Schwannomas. HE ×235

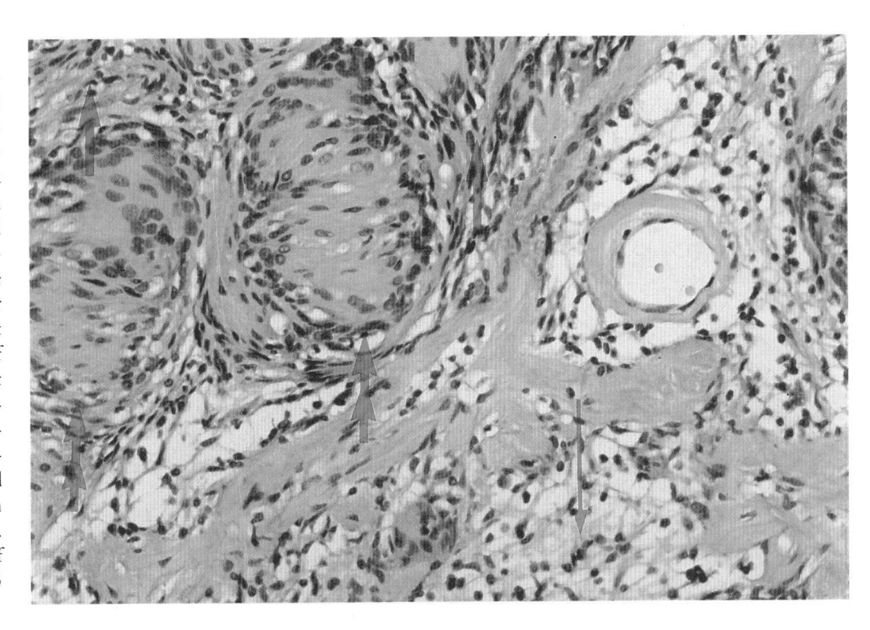

4.47 Secondary carcinoma: brain

The central nervous system is a common site of metastasis of malignant tumours. Generally there are multiple secondaries, characteristically round and apparently well-demarcated from the surrounding white matter. In this case, cords of malignant cells have invaded the white matter of the brain. The cords are papillary structures, each one consisting of a central core of connective tissue and a small thin-walled capillary-type blood vessels (thick arrow), covered with a single (outer) layer of uniform comparatively large cuboidal or low columnar epithelial cells (thin arrow). The epithelial cells have fairly abundant cytoplasm, and in many of the cells there is a large vacuole full of pale mucin. The nuclei of the tumour cells are round or ovoid and vesicular, and only slightly pleomorphic. Some of the nuclei have a prominent central nucleolus. There is also some mitotic activity. In the white matter there are a few small collections of small lymphocytes. Secondary tumours tend to have a histological structure similar to that of the primary, and the primary tumour in this case was a papillary adenocarcinoma of breast. HE ×150

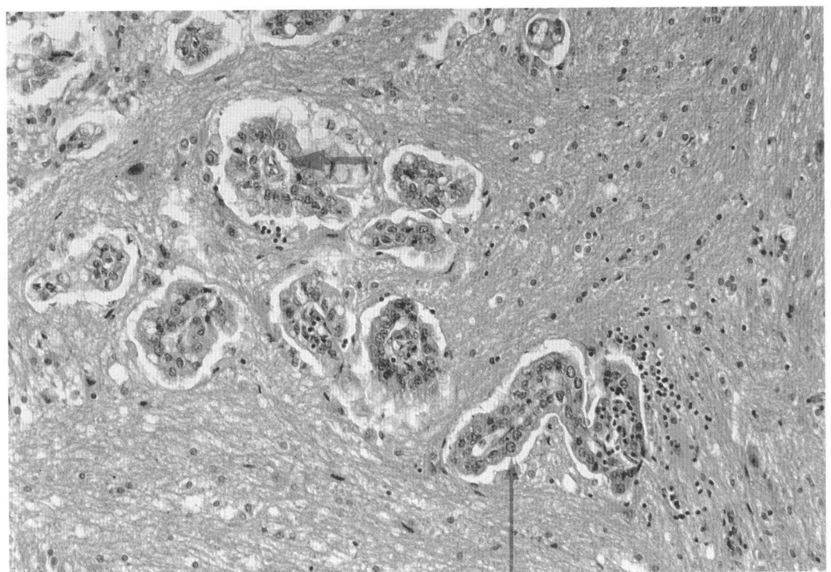

4.48 Secondary carcinoma: brain

Metastatic tumour is sometimes confined to the leptomeninges, the malignant cells growing in the subarachnoid space. The clinical signs and symptoms can be very suggestive of bacterial or fungal meningitis, and since the tumour cells metabolize the sugar in the cerebrospinal fluid, the fall in the sugar level in the CSF may increase the diagnostic difficulties, as happened in this case. The weakly eosinophilic cerebral cortex (thick arrow) is covered with a very thin layer of fibrous tissue, the pia mater (double arrow), and there is a similar thin layer of fibrous tissue (the arachnoid membrane) at the top of the picture. In the large (subarachnoid) space between the two membranes, there are small groups and single types of malignant cells which appear to be growing freely. The cells are very pleomorphic (thin arrow), and have a considerable amount of heavily vacuolated cytoplasm and large pale vesicular nuclei. In most of the nuclei there are one or more prominent nucleoli. A few of the tumour cells are shrunken and necrotic, but most are large or extremely large in comparison with the small lymphocytes adjacent to the fibrous membranes. The primary was a carcinoma of bronchus. HE ×160

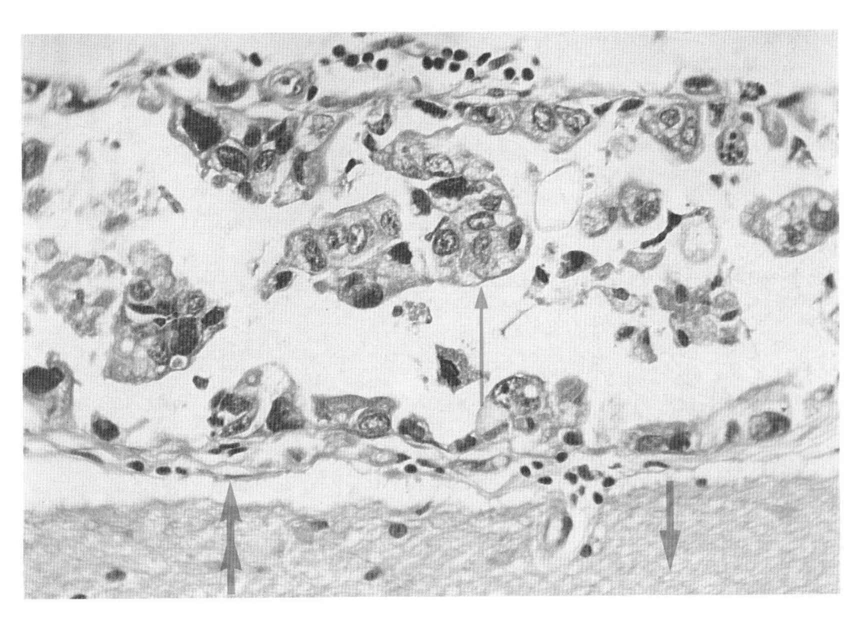

5.1 Branchial cyst

Lateral cervical cysts (branchial cysts) are located in the anterolateral part of the neck, and most commonly at the angle of the mandible, anterior to the sternocleidomastoid muscle. They are painless swellings which may originate in epithelial remnants of the cervical sinus, into which the second, third and fourth branchial clefts open in the embryo. An origin from epithelial inclusions within cervical lymph nodes has also been suggested. The cyst is lined by either stratified squamous epithelium or pseudostratified ciliated columnar epithelium. In this field the cyst is lined by stratified squamous epithelium (thin arrow) and it contains laminated keratin from stratum corneum (double arrow). The wall consists of lymphoid tissue in which there is a small pale-staining germinal centre and a layer of connective tissue (thick arrow). The epithelium lining the cyst is freely permeable to lymphocytes (like the epithelium of the tonsillar crypts) and the small dark-staining cells in the lumen mingling with the keratin are lymphocytes. HE ×120

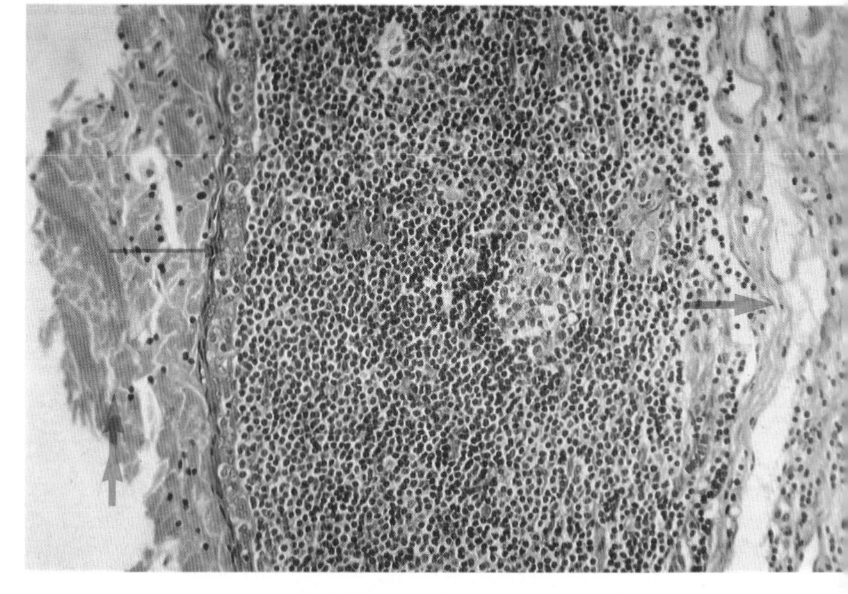

5.2 Branchial cyst

Branchial cysts are thought to develop from cystic degeneration of epithelium enclosed in cervical lymph nodes, and the cyst usually becomes apparent in the third decade. The contents of a branchial cyst are usually fluid or semifluid and cholesterol is generally present. The contents are sterile but infection may supervene, and pus may form. This is the same cyst as in 5.1. This part of it is lined by pseudostratified tall ciliated columnar epithelial cells (thin arrow), similar in appearance to the pseudostratified columnar epithelium that lines the respiratory tract. The columnar epithelium rests on a band of connective tissue, beneath which there is abundant lymphoid tissue. The lymphoid tissue, which forms part of the cyst wall, consists largely of small lymphocytes (thick arrow), but a much smaller number of larger paler histiocytes with large vesicular nuclei (double arrow) is also present. The lymphocytes do not penetrate the layer of columnar epithelial cells lining the cyst and there are no lymphocytes in the cyst lumen (left margin). HE ×200

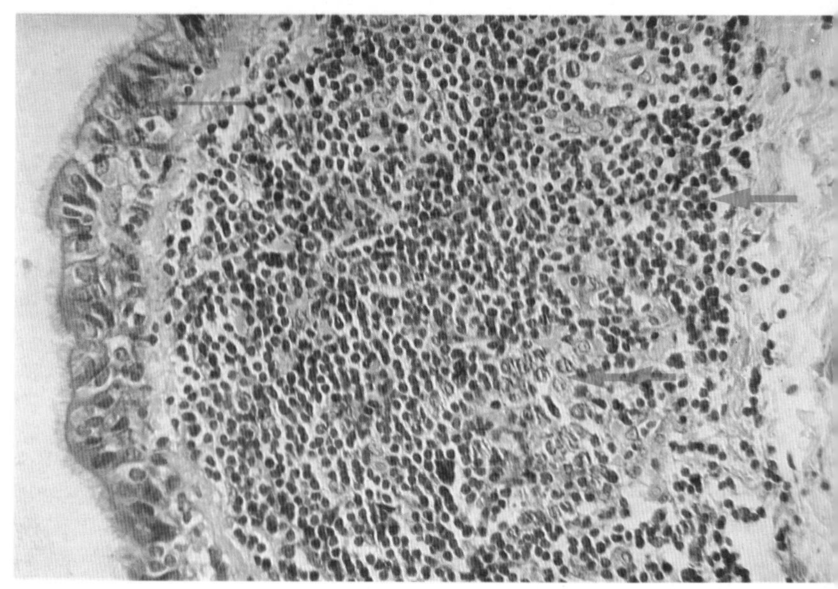

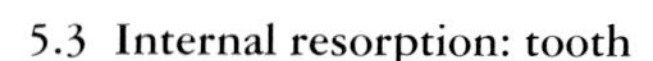

5.3 Internal resorption: tooth

Carious destruction of dental hard tissues frequently produces pulpitis, an inflammatory lesion of the pulp which may be acute or chronic. The lesion may be non-infective, as a result of trauma or very marked changes in temperature, but more often it is caused by infection. This shows the inner (pulpal) surface of the eosinophilic acellular dentine, the characteristic uniform structure of which is evident (thin arrow). The surface of the dentine is covered by a layer of vascular connective tissue (left) and large numbers of chronic inflammatory cells (upper right). The connective tissue appears to be extending into the dentine and eroding it extensively (double arrow). Most of the chronic inflammatory cells are plasma cells, and among them there are Russell bodies, large plasma cells with much intensely eosinophilic cytoplasm (thick arrows). Resorption of dentine may continue until both the dentine and enamel of the crown of the tooth are absorbed. HE ×150

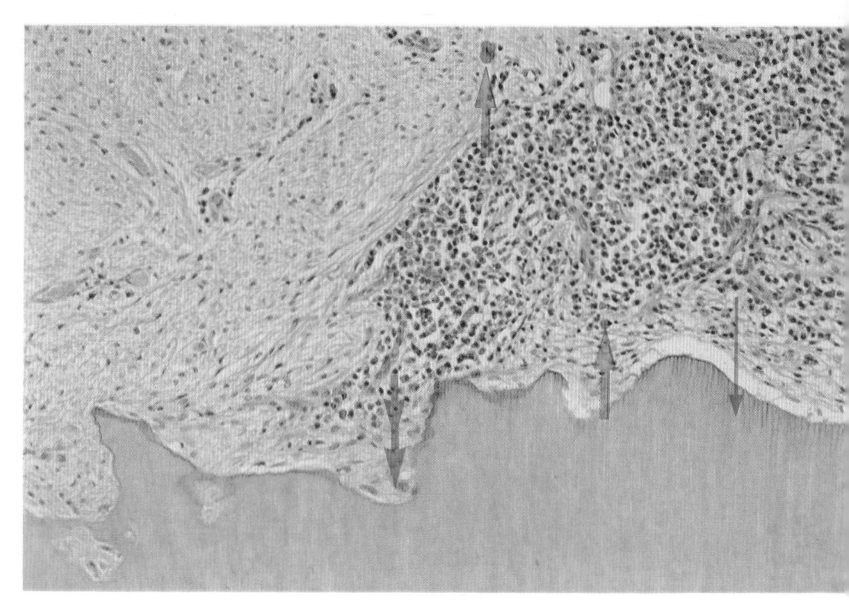

5.4 Radicular (periapical) cyst

The most common odontogenic cyst is the periodontal cyst, and most often it is located at the apex of an erupted tooth. It is designated as a radicular (periapical) cyst and is accepted as the commonest cyst of the jaws. The origin of this radicular cyst appears to be in the cystic degeneration of epithelialized granulomas, at the apex of a tooth, which have resulted most often as sequelae to dental caries and pulpitis; and the stratified squamous epithelium which lines the cyst arises from the epithelial rests of Malassez (in the periodontal ligament). The cyst is usually symptom-free, although it may expand slowly to distort the jaw. The lumen of this cyst is on the left (thin arrow). The wall of the cyst consists of a layer of vascular fibrous connective tissue (thick arrow) and it is lined by a thick sheet of non-keratinized strongly eosinophilic stratified squamous epithelial cells (double arrow).

HE ×150

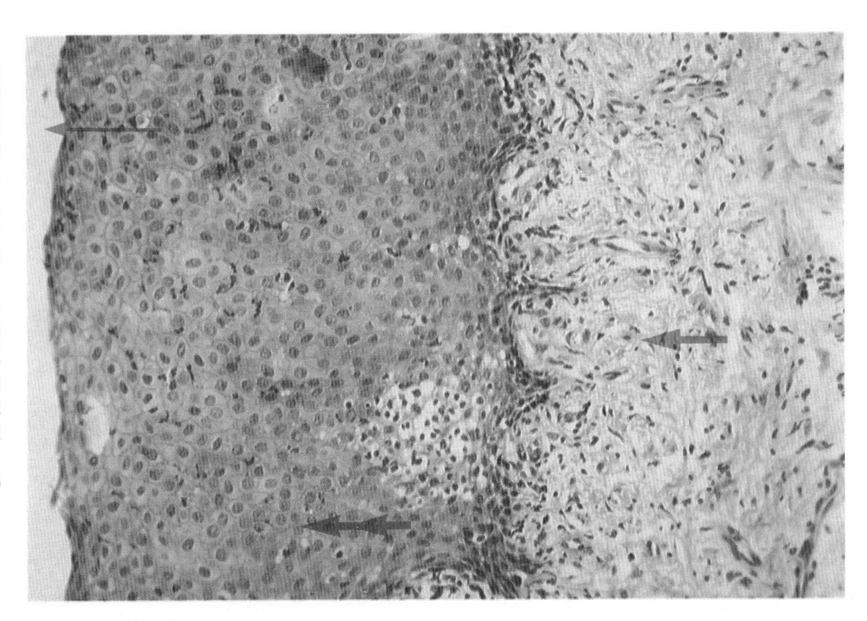

5.5 Giant-cell granuloma: mandible

Giant-cell granuloma is found at all ages and is more common in females than males (2:1 ratio). It is not a neoplasm but an inflammatory reaction to injury and hemorrhage; that is, it is a 'reparative' granuloma of the gingiva. It is usually a single lesion and may be situated within bone (either in the maxilla or, more often, in the mandible) or in the soft tissues of the gingiva. Giant-cell granulomas destroy bone, and it may be difficult to distinguish one of them from true giant-cell tumour, which also may occur in the same sites. Macroscopically, the tissue is generally reddish-brown or black, as a result of hemorrhage. This particular lesion was within the mandible. It consists of a cellular stroma of connective tissue (double arrow) in which there are many giant multinucleated cells of osteoclast type (thick arrow). The stromal connective tissue is relatively mature-looking but within it there are large numbers of elongated plump fibroblasts with fairly pleomorphic basophilic nuclei (thin arrow). They show no mitotic activity in this field.

HE ×135

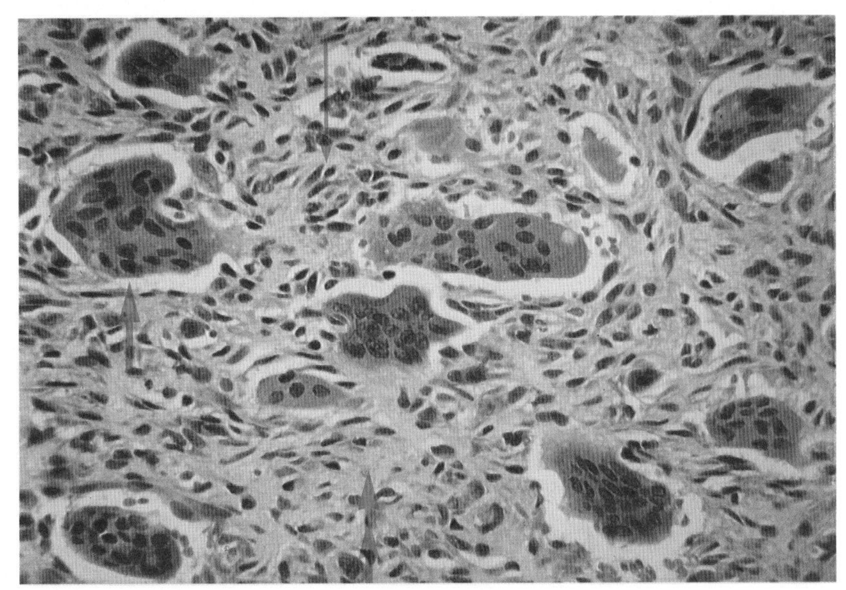

5.6 Calcifying epithelial odontogenic tumour

Calcifying epithelial odontogenic tumour is a rare neoplasm which generally arises in the fourth and fifth decades. Most of the tumours originate in the mandibular premolar-molar region, in association with an embedded tooth. They behave like ameloblastomas, tending to be invasive and recur locally after removal, but they do not metastasize. There is no sex predilection. The tumour consists of closely packed polyhedral cells with abundant eosinophilic cytoplasm and large fairly pleomorphic basophilic oval or round nuclei (thin arrow). There are no mitotic figures. The stroma is scant. There is however intracellular degeneration in the polyhedral cells, taking the form, in the cytoplasm, of vacuoles of various sizes, full of pale-staining amorphous material in which there are numerous clear spaces (thick arrow). A large purple (densely-calcified) laminated body (double arrow) is present on the left. Laminated bodies stain blue only after they have become calcified, and other laminated bodies, elsewhere in the tumour, are still eosinophilic.

HE ×135

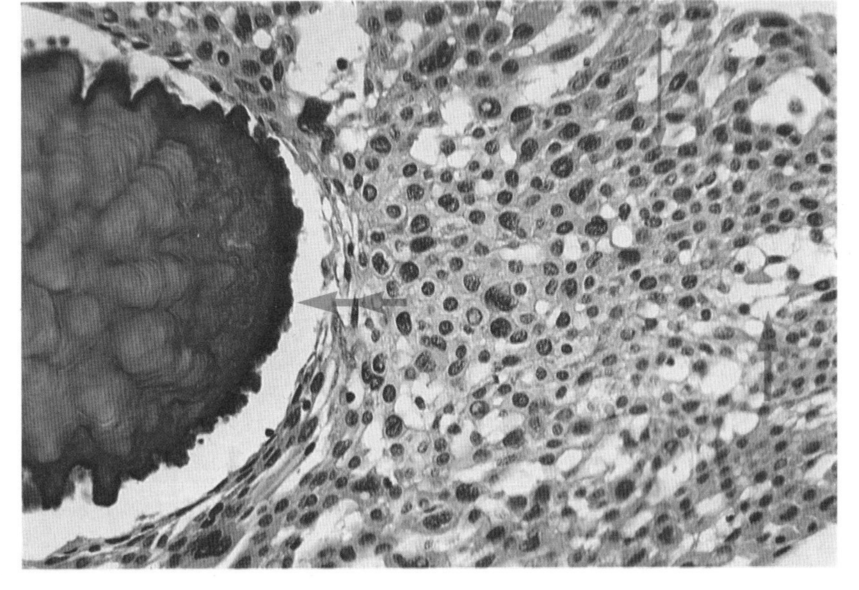

5.7 Nasal polyp

Nasal polyps are not true neoplasms but polypoid thickenings of the nasal mucosa, usually associated with chronic recurrent inflammation. The causes are mainly allergy and infection. The polyps may be large rounded or elongated masses of stromal connective tissue covered with respiratory epithelium. They are often bilateral. This polyp, a soft piece of greyish-white tissue 1cm dia, is from a man of 43. The surface of the polyp is covered with a fairly thick layer of transitional epithelium (thin arrow). The rest of the polyp consists of delicate edematous 'loose' connective tissue, heavily vacuolated, and many dilated small blood vessels (thick arrow), more numerous in the more superficial parts of the polyp. There are many plasma cells, eosinophil leukocytes and lymphocytes in the connective tissue, particularly towards the surface of the polyp. A small duct containing deeply eosinophilic secretion and lined with cuboidal epithelium is present (double arrow). HE ×150

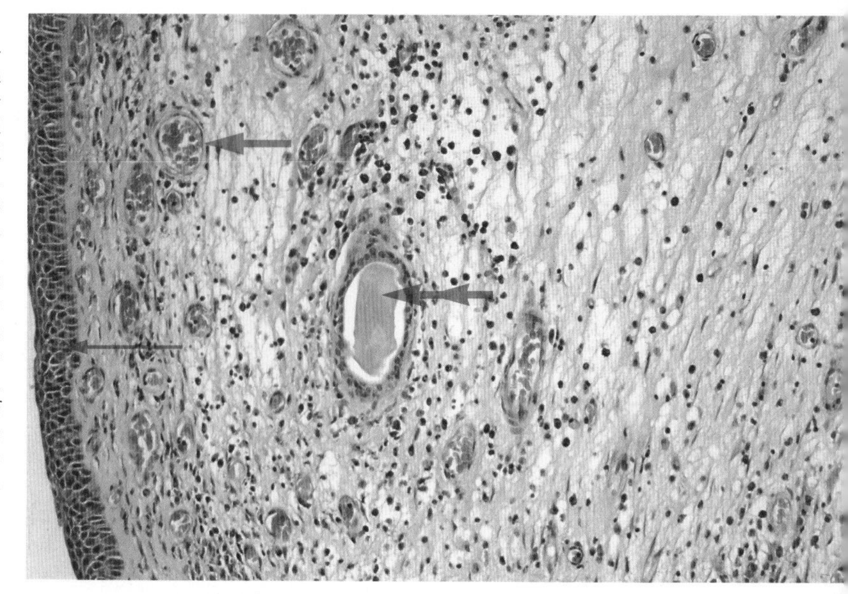

5.8 Nasal polyp

Nasal polyps usually have a gelatinous texture, and their surface is smooth and shiny from the presence of mucoid secretion, from the surface epithelium or from occasional mucous glands in the edematous stroma. The surface epithelium is often normal ciliated respiratory-type epithelium, but the surface of this polyp, from a woman of 53 and measuring 2.5cm in its long axis, is covered with pseudostratified tall columnar epithelial cells and a large number of tall mucin-secreting goblet cells (thin arrow). The surface epithelium, vacuolated in its basal layers (thick arrow), rests on a thick hyaline basement membrane (double arrow), a common feature of nasal polyps. The stroma consists of edematous and extensively vacuolated connective tissue. The weakly eosinophilic and unstained parts (vacuoles) of the connective tissue contain edema fluid. The stroma is also vascular, and in it there are large numbers of inflammatory cells, including lymphocytes, plasma cells and eosinophil leukocytes. HE ×360

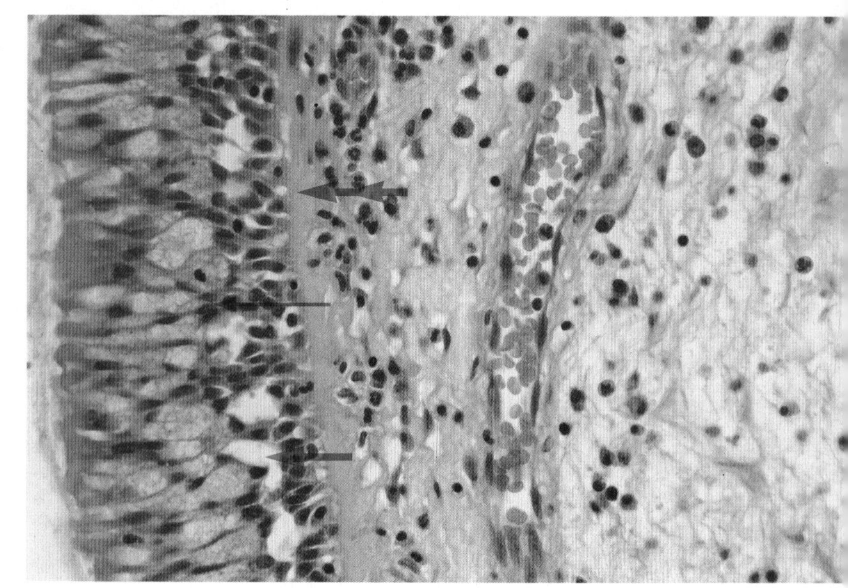

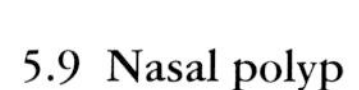

5.9 Nasal polyp

Squamous metaplasia of the epithelium covering nasal polyps is a common occurrence, and the epithelium on the surface of this polyp has undergone metaplasia, becoming a squamous or very thick transitional form of epithelium. The epithelium is remarkably thick but it is not forming keratin. It has a thin surface layer of small flat epithelial cells (double arrow) but the others are very numerous closely packed large elongated epithelial cells with large hyperchromatic nuclei (thin arrow). Their nuclei show considerable pleomorphism and dysplasia, many being elongated or ovoid. Nucleoi are also present in some of the nuclei, but they are prominent and visible only at higher magnification. Several mitotic figures are present (thick arrows). These appearances suggest malignancy. However, the underlying stroma, consisting of vacuolated connective tissue (bottom of field), is infiltrated by a moderate number of inflammatory cells (polymorphs and plasma cells). Sometimes the stroma in a polyp undergoes changes similar to those in the epithelium in this polyp, but malignant change is very rare in a nasal polyp, and such a diagnosis is usually erroneous. HE ×110

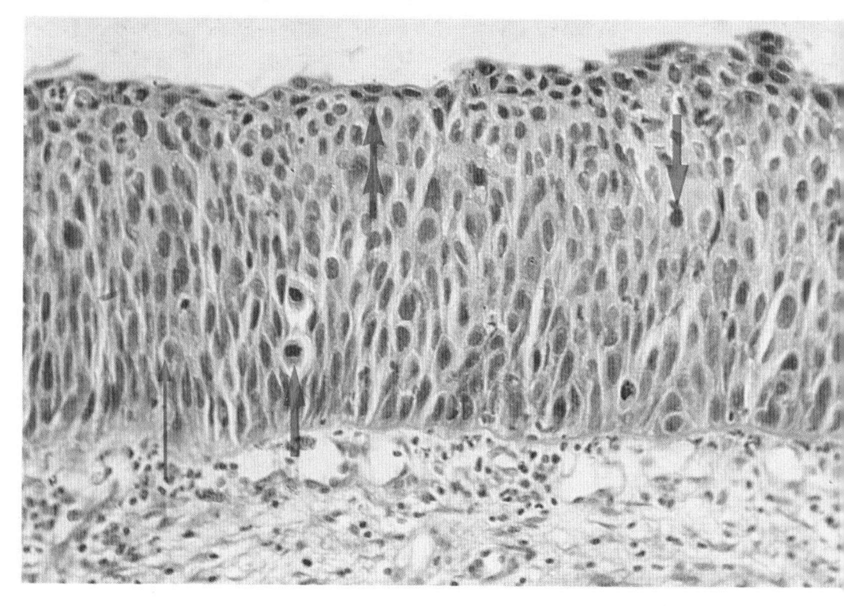

5.10 Inverted papilloma: nose

Inverted papilloma is a true papilloma of the mucosa of the nasal cavity. It is a benign neoplasm but it is generally bulky and friable when first seen and tends to recur, about 30% of inverted papillomas doing so after excision. The ill-defined margins of the tumour can be misleading however and only about 2% undergo malignant change. This specimen, from a man of 63, has an edematous sparsely cellular connective tissue stroma covered by thick layer of squamous epithelial cells (thick arrow). Beneath the surface epithelium there is a much thicker layer of non-keratinizing squamous epithelial cells (not visibly connected to the surface epithelium) which has invaginated the stroma and formed large clefts or pits, one of which is at the top right corner (thin arrow). Apart from the smaller basophilic basal cells, all the cells in the upper layer have a very large clear cytoplasmic vacuole. Occasionally the invaginations are lined in part by a singe layer of ciliated columnar cells instead of a layer of squamous epithelium. Inversion of the epithelial covering can be readily mistaken for invasion and malignancy. The edematous fibrous stroma contains a moderate number of chronic inflammatory cells. HE ×60

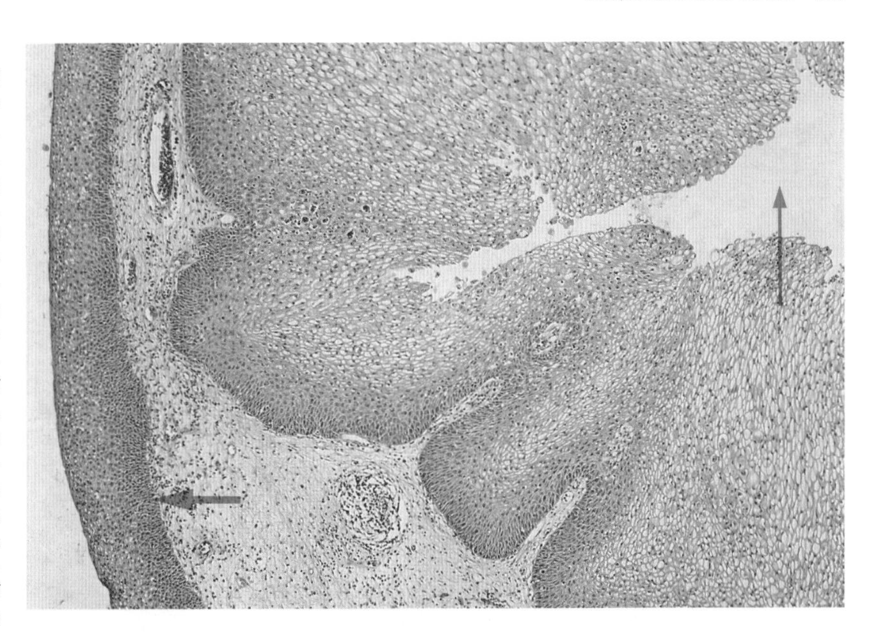

5.11 Inverted papilloma: nose

Most inverted papillomas of the nose arise from the lateral wall of the nasal cavity. Sometimes the tumour is highly vascular, edematous and translucent. Although the epithelium lining the clefts is generally regarded as non-keratinizing, there are foci of keratinization in about 10% of tumours. This shows the structure of the papilloma in **5.10** in more detail. The layer of epithelial cells on the surface of the papilloma is thick and intensely cellular, and the cells are squamous epithelial-type cells (thin arrow). Most of the epithelial cells lining the cleft are greatly swollen and vacuolated (thick arrow), but some of them are pleomorphic. The compact cells of the basal layer are basophilic and not vacuolated (double arrow), and some show dysplasia. There is an area of hemorrhage in the stroma. The number of chronic inflammatory cells in the stroma is small, although elsewhere there are numerous plasma cells. Inverted papillomas are occasionally called transitional papillomas because the non-keratinizing squamous epithelium resembles the transitional epithelium of the urinary tract. HE ×150

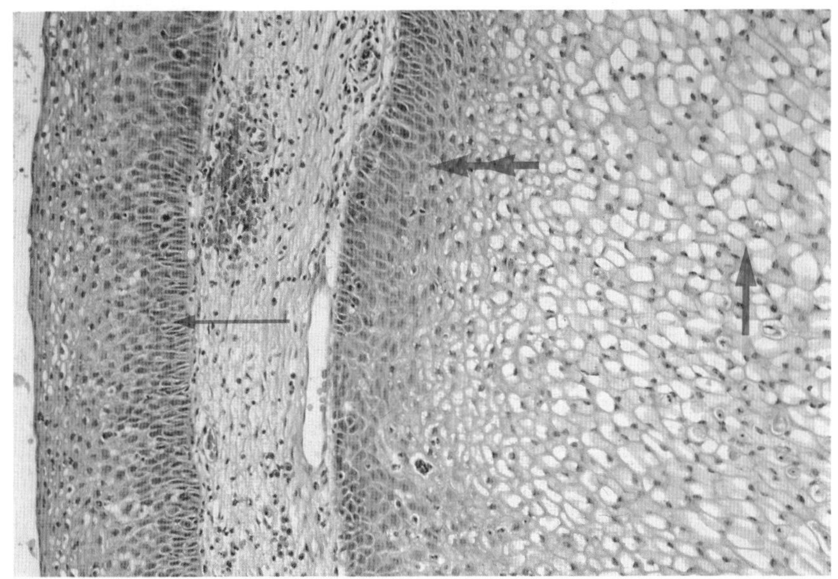

5.12 Lichen planus: mouth

Lichen planus affects mucous membranes as well as skin. The mouth is frequently involved, with irregular lace-like whitening of the oral mucosa, sometimes in the absence of cutaneous lesions. The lesions generally take the form of flat violaceous shiny plaques, often polygonal. They generally involve only a small area of skin or mucous membrane. Lichen planus may be mistakenly diagnosed as leukoplakia but it shows no evidence of epithelial atypia. In this lesion there is irregular thickening of the epidermis, but the granular layer is just detectably thickened. Unlike the changes in the skin (**14.20**), there is only a thin layer of keratin on the epidermal surface. There is moderate hyperplasia of the keratinocytes (acanthosis) but there is a marked change in the rete ridges, which are short and pointed like the teeth of a saw (thick arrows). The epidermal basement membrane is prominent and intact (thin arrow). A dense infiltrate of small round deeply basophilic cells (double arrow), mainly lymphocytes (mostly helper T cells), occupies the submucosa and extends up to the epidermal basement membrane. A few lymphocytes are also present within the basal layers of the epithelium. HE ×190

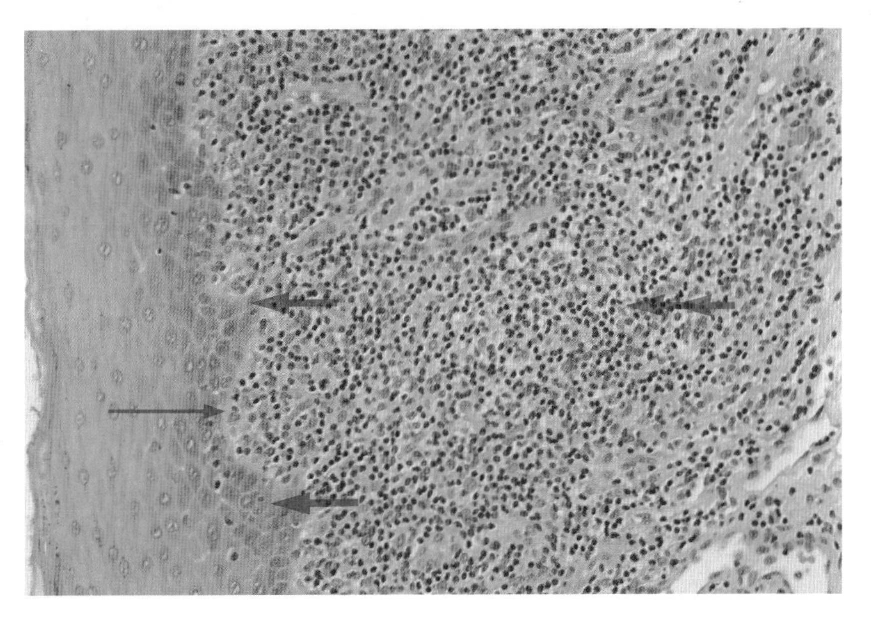

5.13 Leukoplakia: tongue

Leukoplakia is a clinical term which means 'white plaque'. White plaques are not uncommonly present on the oral mucosa, particularly in the floor of the mouth and lateral margins of the tongue of older people. In simple leukoplakia, the lesions generally consist of thickened keratotic epithelium which obscures the normal red colour of the underlying vascular tissues of the submucosa. In atypical leukoplakia, the epithelium is thickened, often keratinized and the cells in the deeper (basal) parts of the epithelium are dysplastic and markedly atypical. The significance of leukoplakia lies in the fact that it predisposes to malignancy. This shows a rete ridge of the mucosa of the tongue of an elderly man. It is enlarged, and the numerous keratinocytes are hyperplastic and dysplastic. They show some loss of cell polarity, and among them there are many mitotic figures (thick arrows). The submucosa (right) is heavily infiltrated with small lymphocytes and larger plasma cells with typical eccentric nuclei (thin arrow).

HE ×360

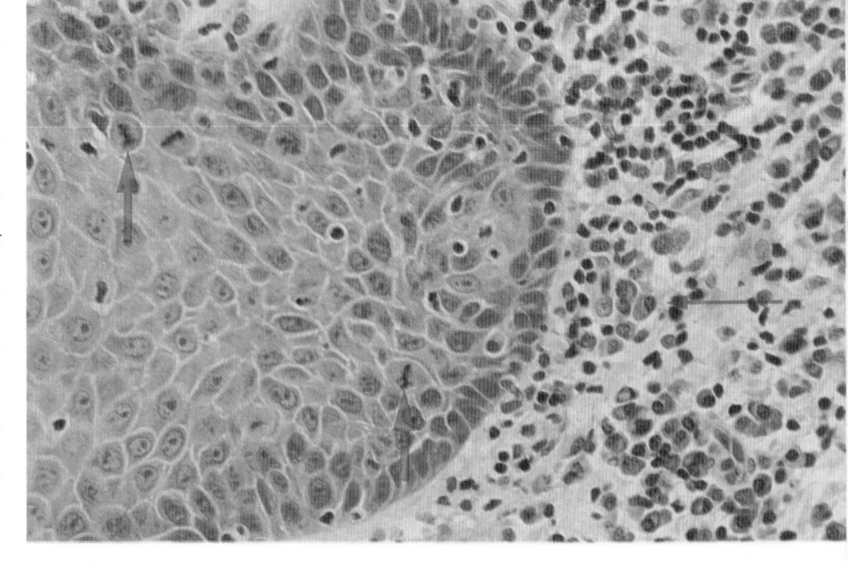

5.14 Granular cell tumour: tongue

Granular cell tumour (myoblastoma) is uncommon and occurs in a variety of sites, including breast, larynx and particularly tongue. In the tongue, the tumour forms nodule (usually less than 1cm dia) beneath the epithelium. This tumour arose in the tongue. The submucosa is occupied by a sheet of eosinophilic tumour cells (right margin of field) which extend up to the epidermis. The neoplastic cells are closely packed large cells with abundant granular cytoplasm and a (relatively) small round or ovoid nucleus. The squamous epithelium overlying the tumour (it is out of the field on the left) is strikingly hyperplastic, with greatly elongated rete ridges (thick arrows) advancing downwards into the submucosa and sheet of eosinophilic tumour cells. Some of the rete ridges, cut in cross-section, simulate the cell nests of squamous cell carcinoma. The change is termed pseudoepitheliomatous hyperplasia and it is a more or less constant feature of granular cell tumours. It is readily mistaken for squamous carcinoma, the underlying tumour being overlooked, particularly in the tongue.

HE ×150

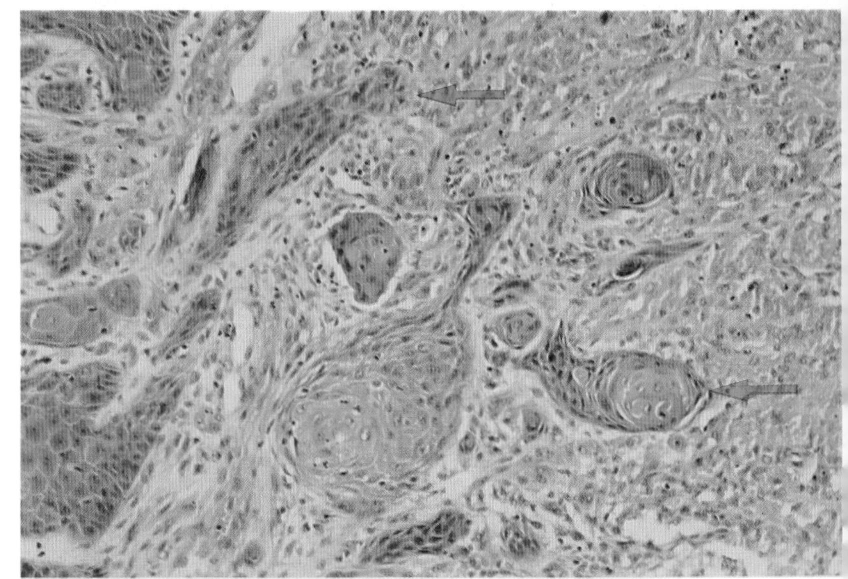

5.15 Granular cell tumour: tongue

Granular cell tumour is a benign lesion which grows very slowly and seldom recurs. Its nature and histogenesis are uncertain. The neoplastic cells are large and very distinctive in appearance, with a large amount of cytoplasm (double arrow) rather like degenerate or embryonic muscle cells with densely eosinophilic granules filling their cytoplasm, which is the reason for devising the term myoblastoma (granular cell tumours however are not derived from striated muscle cells but probably come from Schwann cells). Some of the cytoplasmic granules are large (up to 5μm dia). The cell borders of the tumour cells are generally well-defined but indistinct in this field, and this gives the tumour structure an almost syncytial form. The nuclei are (relatively) small round or ovoid and very uniform in structure (thin arrow). There is no mitotic activity. The blood vessels (thick arrows) are thin-walled and sinusoidal, with occasional foci of hyaline thickened basement membrane.

HE ×360

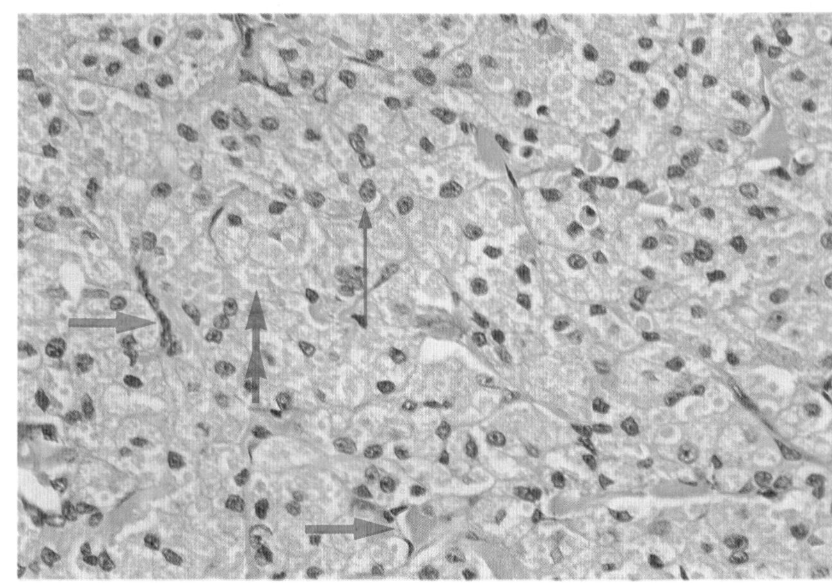

5.16 Squamous carcinoma: tongue

Squamous carcinoma of the tongue constitutes over 90% of the malignant tumours of the oral cavity. The majority are on the lateral margins of the tongue or on the lower lip. Carcinoma of the tongue has a poor prognosis, tending to invade the muscles of the tongue or spread to the regional lymph nodes. This part of the tumour consists of several clusters of very atypical (malignant) squamous epithelial cells (thin arrows), invading the elongated eosinophilic (striated) muscle fibres of the tongue. At the periphery of each group of tumour cells there is a thin layer of small basophilic squamous epithelial cells, and the centre of each group is occupied by a sheet of large and very large eosinophilic keratinocytes. The large keratinocytes have formed masses of intensely eosinophilic keratin (thick arrows) which lie within large vacuoles. There are moderate numbers of chronic inflammatory cells, mostly small lymphocytes, in the vicinity of the advancing edge of the tumour (centre right). HE ×135

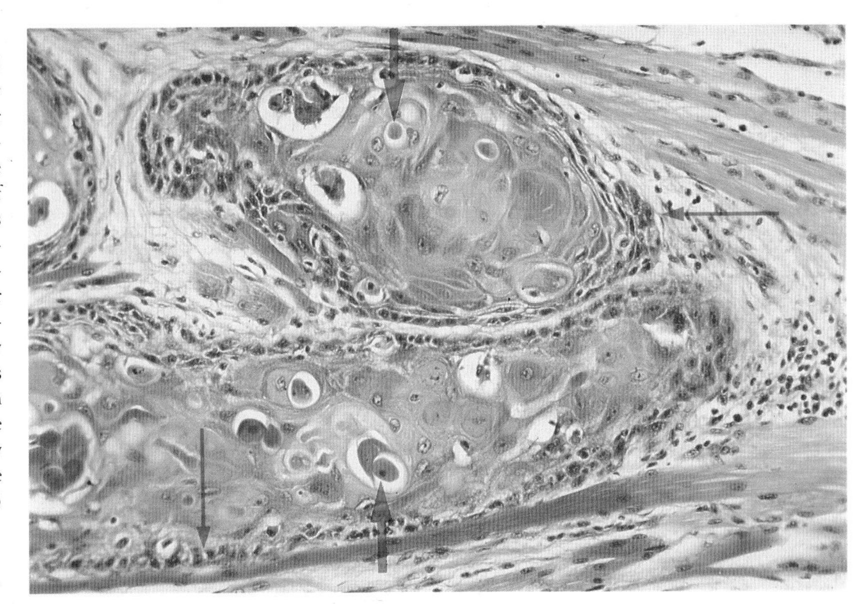

5.17 Verrucous (buccal) carcinoma

This is a well-differentiated squamous carcinoma of the mucosa of the buccal cavity and lower gingiva. Leukoplakia is usually present and the lesion mainly affects men who chew tobacco. It is a large soft papillary growth which grows slowly, invading the adjacent tissues. It has a distinctive structure and clinical behaviour and may cause extensive destruction. It rarely metastasizes to lymph nodes and never to distant sites. The buccal mucosa (thin arrow) is thick and hyperplastic. The tumour forms a large broad rounded and apparently well-circumscribed sheet which bulges from the overlying epithelium into the underlying tissue, invading the submucosa on a broad front and pushing aside the muscles of the cheek rather than penetrating them (thick arrows). A small mucus-secreting salivary gland is present (double arrow). HE ×20

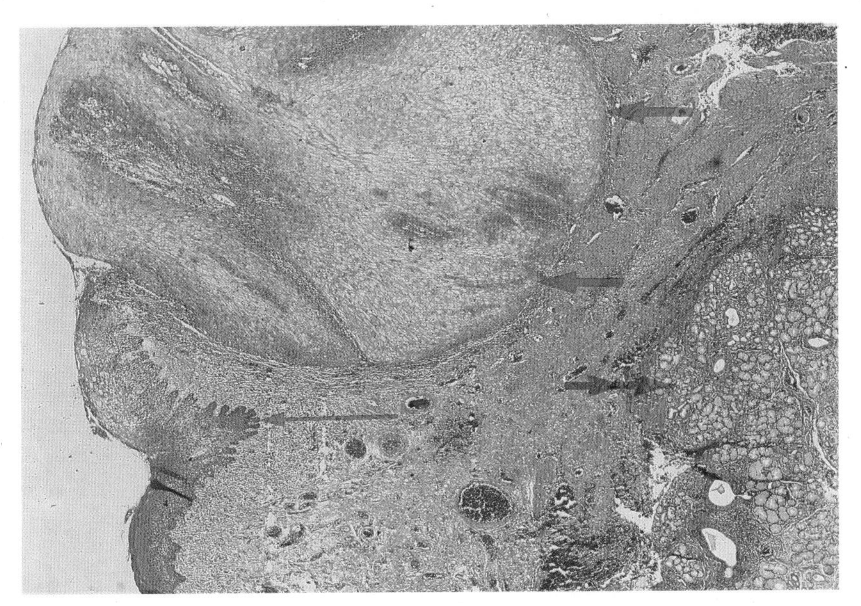

5.18 Verrucous (buccal) carcinoma

The epithelium overlying a verrucous carcinoma is often extensively hyperkeratotic. Most of the same sheet of large vacuolated tumour cells as in 5.17 are out of sight on the left. The remaining (visible) part of the sheet (at high magnification) is the invading edge of the tumour (centre & left), consisting mainly of large squamous epithelial cells with abundant pale or clear (foamy and vacuolated) cytoplasm (thin arrows). Whereas in most of the more-superficial large vacuolated neoplastic cells there are no visible nuclei, in the more compact cells closer to the invading edge there are large pale vesicular nuclei which contain a prominent nucleolus (thick arrows). These nuclei exhibit little or no atypicality. There are no mitoses. Polymorphs, many degenerate, are present among the large neoplastic cells, and there is an infiltrate of all deeply basophilic chronic inflammatory cells in the tissues close to the invading edge of the tumour. The tissue on the right, which is being invaded on a broad front by the tumour, is part of a cheek muscle. HE ×215

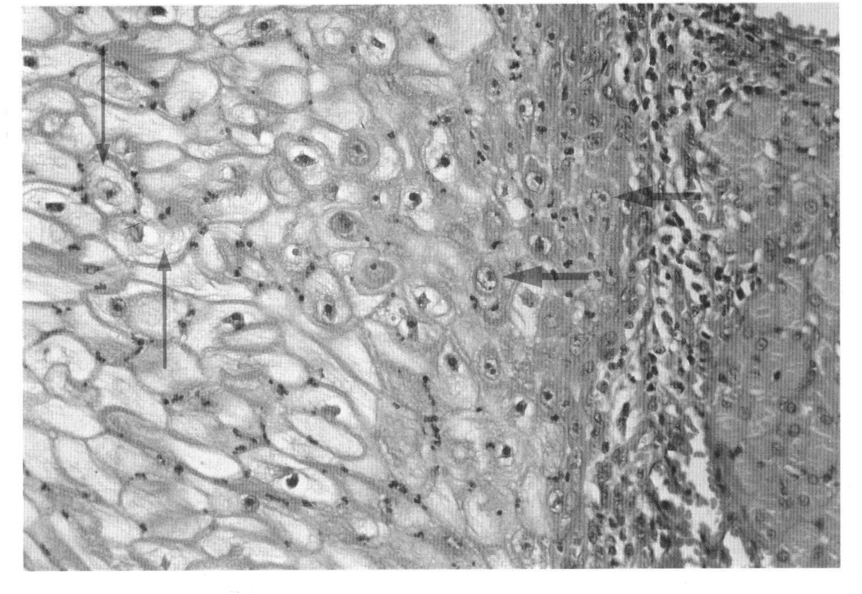

5.19 Nasopharyngeal carcinoma

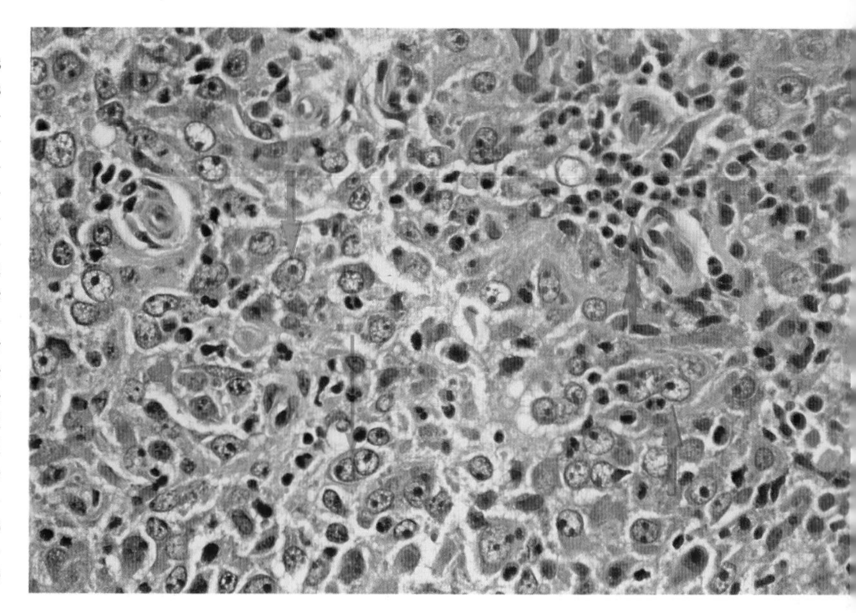

Carcinoma of the pharynx is uncommon in some countries and common in others such as China. Epstein-Barr virus (EBV) is strongly associated with nasopharyngeal carcinoma (as well as nasal T- & NK-cell lymphomas). The tumour is a poorly-differentiated or undifferentiated squamous cell carcinoma, the malignant cells generally arranged in small groups and syncytial sheets. Large numbers of lymphocytes and eosinophil leukocytes are also often present. The age range varies, and this tumour is from the nasopharynx of a girl aged 11 years. It consists of large anaplastic epithelial cells with a considerable amount of cytoplasm and large vesicular nuclei in which there are one or more very prominent central nucleoli (thick arrows). Some of the tumour cells are binucleated (thin arrow). The large size of the tumour cells is obvious when they are compared with the lymphocytes and the numerous heavily stained eosinophil leukocytes (double arrow). There is considerable mitotic activity elsewhere in the tumour. Sometimes lymphocytes are the predominant inflammatory cell (tumours with this structure are sometimes termed lymphoepitheliomas). HE ×360

5.20 Nasopharyngeal carcinoma

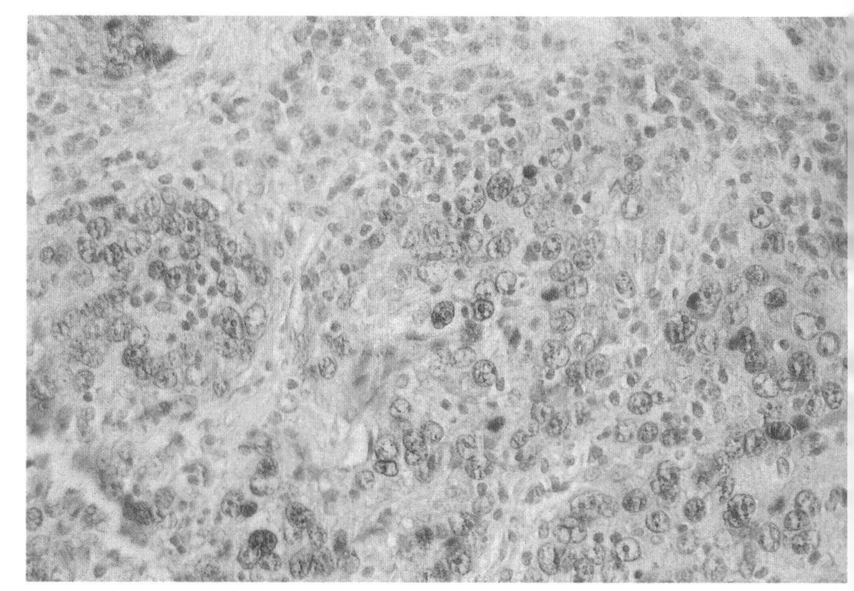

Nasopharyngeal carcinoma, stained for Epstein-Barr virus, showing a positive brown reaction product in the large malignant cells. In the Far East, the EMV has a strong and frequent association with this malignancy.

Nasopharyngeal carcinoma originates in squamous epithelium overlying the lymphoid tissue of the nasopharynx. The tumour is closely associated with Epstein-Barr virus (EBV), with multiple copies of the EBV genome in all the tumour cells. Carcinoma develops however in only a small minority of infected people and after a very long latent period. It is usually a squamous cell carcinoma, poorly differentiated or anaplastic, and there is a prominent infiltrate of lymphocytes in the stroma of the tumour, often giving the carcinoma the name of lymphoepithelioma.

5.21 Plasmacytoma: palate

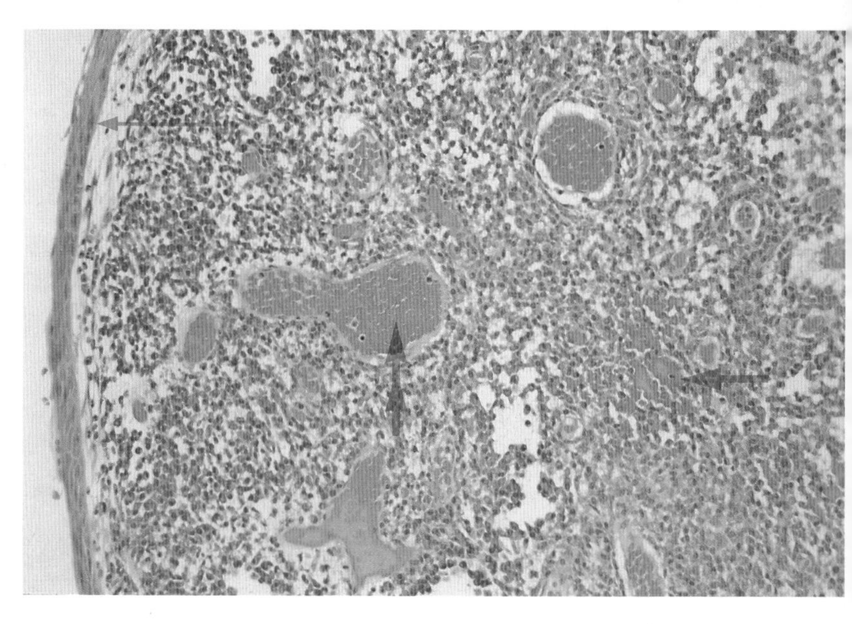

Plasmacytomas usually arise in marrow and rarely in lymph nodes. Extramedullary plasmacytomas are most common in paranasal sinuses, nasopharynx, oropharynx and upper respiratory tract. Solitary plasma cell tumours occur occasionally in the soft tissues. The lesion may consist of one or more round nodules. It is important to distinguish plasmacytomas from plasma cell granulomas (inflammatory lesions rich in non-neoplastic plasma cells). The onset is as a rule insidious and the behaviour of the lesion is unpredictable. Some behave in benign fashion but the majority, cytologically identical, recur locally and eventually become widely disseminated. The stratified squamous epithelium of the palatal mucosa (thin arrow), attenuated but intact, is stretched over an extremely vascular and extensively vacuolated sheet of moderate-sized neoplastic cells. The population of cells is uniform and mature but those nearer the surface are more heavily stained than those deeper in the submucosa (right). Several of the plasma cells are distended with strongly eosinophilic amyloid-like material and there are also extracellular deposits (thick arrow). The blood vessels are thin-walled and greatly dilated (double arrow). HE ×150

5.22 Plasmacytoma: palate

Paraproteinemia less common in extramedullary plasmacytoma than in multiple myelomatosis. This is the same lesion as in 5.21, at higher magnification. The plasma-cell nature of the cells of the tumour is clearly evident. The cytoplasm is abundant (and pyroninophil) and the nuclei are round and of moderate size. However the nuclei are eccentrically located at one pole of many of the cells. Adjacent to the eccentric nuclei in many cells, there is generally a clear halo in the cytoplasm which represents the Golgi apparatus (thick arrow). Within the nuclei, the chromatin is distributed as granules which are arranged in a coarse clock-face or cart-wheel pattern (thin arrow), and a single nucleolus in some nuclei. Several of the plasma cells are greatly distended with amorphous eosinophilic amyloid-like material (double arrow). There are many small blood vessels, but no lymphocytes or blast cells. Inflammatory cells such as polymorph leukocytes are also absent, a feature which helps to distinguish solitary plasmacytoma from inflammatory lesions. Multinucleated plasma cells do not necessarily indicate malignancy. HE ×360

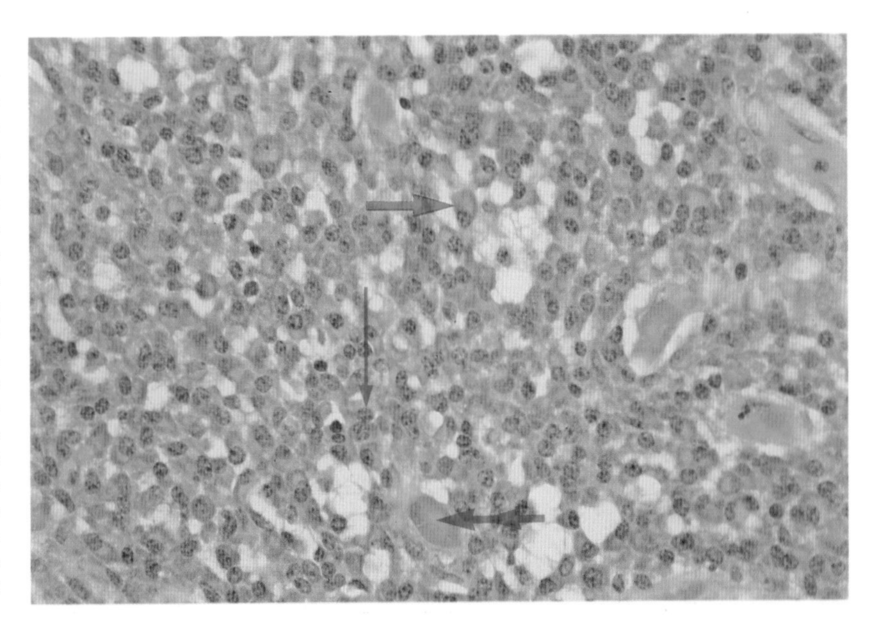

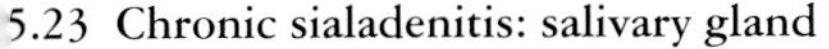

5.23 Chronic sialadenitis: salivary gland

Chronic inflammation of a salivary gland is often associated with obstruction of the duct, usually by a calculus (sialolithiasis). A calculus may form in a previously non-inflamed gland but bacterial infection predisposes to its development. The submaxillary gland is more liable to be affected by calculus formation than the parotid, because of the calcium-rich nature of its secretion. This is a submandibular gland from a woman of 67. There is a follicular collection of small lymphocytes in a band of eosinophilic fairly dense fibrous tissue (thick arrows), but the broad bands of dense fibrous tissue which divide the affected gland into multiple lobes are not visible in this field, the most obvious feature being the extensive loss of acini in the gland. Only small ducts with their characteristic double layer of lining cells remain (thin arrow), and they are surrounded by a considerable amount of pale (vacuolated) cellular connective tissue and a scanty infiltrate of chronic inflammatory cells (double arrow).
HE ×150

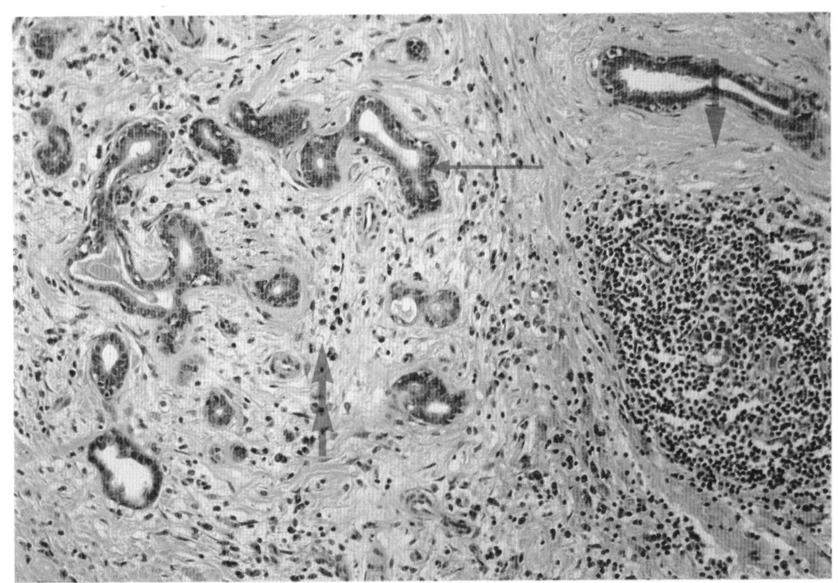

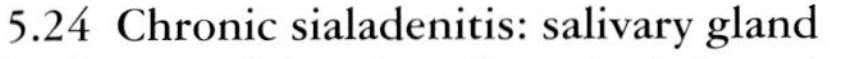

5.24 Chronic sialadenitis: salivary gland

In this part of the submaxillary gland shown in 5.23, some glandular acini (thin arrows), surrounded by loose pale connective tissue and a moderate number of chronic inflammatory cells, have survived. They are degenerate however and show no secretory activity. In contrast, the small ducts are markedly dilated and lined by a single thin layer of flat (attenuated) epithelial cells (thick arrows) The lumen of each dilated duct is filled with pus-like material which consists largely of polymorph leukocytes. This is evidence of previous acute inflammation. The connective tissue which surround the ducts and acini is densely fibrous in places, and in the looser tissues there are elongated fibroblasts, lymphocytes, plasma cells and a few polymorphs. Eventually, if obstruction of the duct system of the gland persists, the gland or part of it is likely to be replaced by scar-like tissue and fat cells. HE ×235

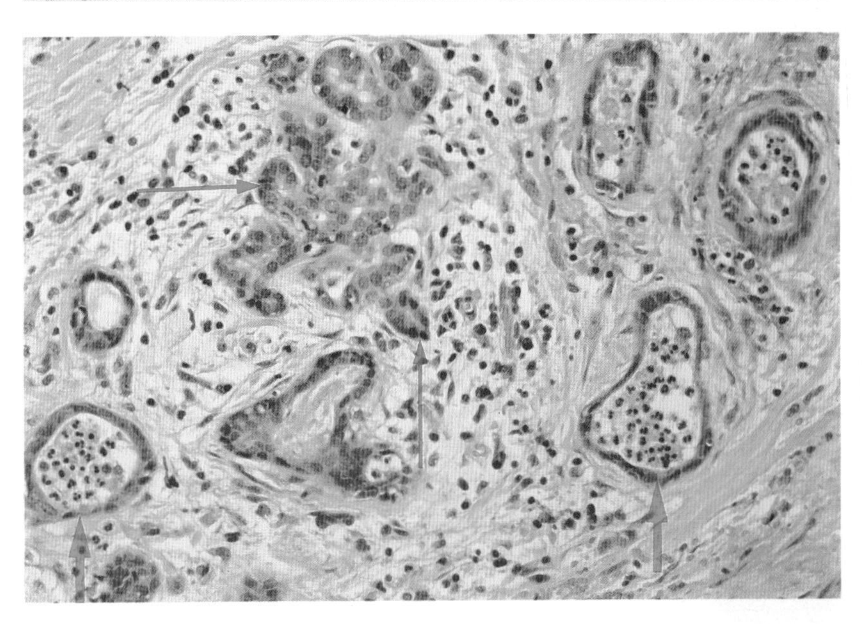

5.25 Mumps: parotid

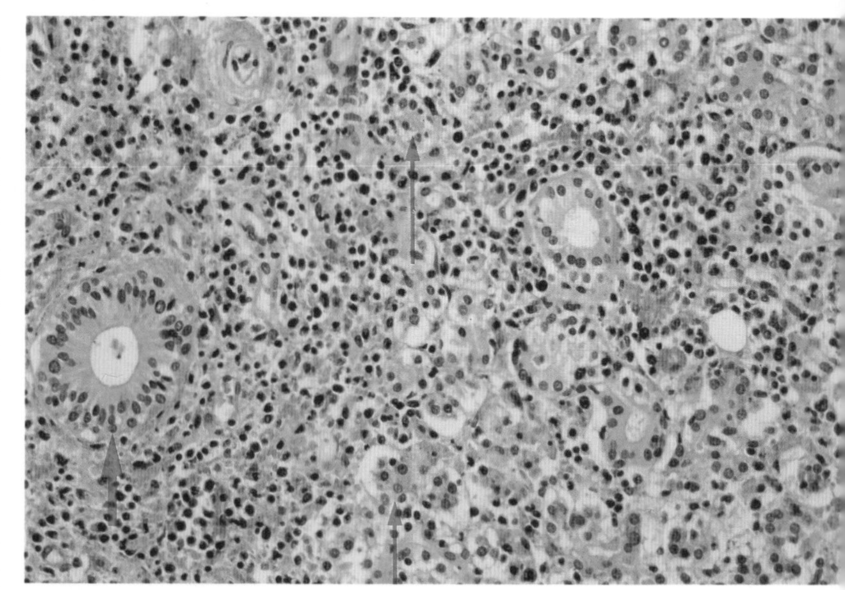

Mumps is an acute inflammatory lesion of the salivary glands caused by the mumps virus, more common in children. The parotid glands are the most vulnerable salivary glands and most commonly attacked. The testes may also be involved, notably in men but rarely in boys, and so may the pancreas. This is a section of an inflamed parotid gland which became tense, swollen, acutely tender and painful; there is extensive destruction of the parenchymal (acinar) structure, and many acini (thin arrows) are small and disorganized. Many of the small intensely basophilic nuclei are the pyknotic nuclei of necrotic epithelial cells. The columnar epithelium lining the small ducts (thick arrow) appears to be less affected than the acinar epithelium. There is a fairly dense diffuse infiltrate of lymphocytes, plasma cells and macrophages. No polymorph leukocytes are visible however. Despite the marked intensity of the inflammatory reaction in this disease, repair appears to be effective, and significant permanent damage to the glands is uncommon. HE ×235

5.26 Sjögren's syndrome: salivary gland

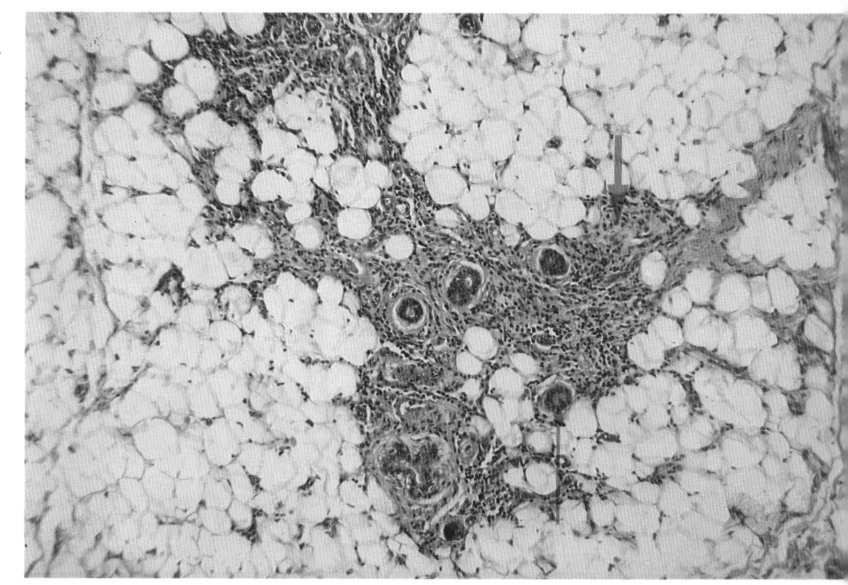

The precise nature of Sjögren's syndrome (benign lymphoepithelial lesion) is uncertain, since the systemic features, including the polyarthritis, are lacking. Occasionally non-Hodgkin's lymphoma develops in an affected gland, which suggests that the condition is sometimes pre-lymphomatous. It is a systemic disorder and, as part of this, the secretory cells of the lacrimal, conjunctival and salivary glands degenerate. Patients tend to get conjunctivitis (keratoconjunctivitis sicca) and a dry mouth from lack of saliva. The syndrome affects mainly middle-aged women and it is often accompanied by chronic polyarthritis of the rheumatoid type. The affected salivary glands are swollen, and part or all of the glands may be involved, involved parts being sharply demarcated from uninvolved parts by the interlobular septa. Histologically the glandular acini have disappeared and the gland now consists of fat and fibrous tissue in which only small ducts (thin arrow) survive. The connective tissue around the ducts is heavily infiltrated with a uniform population of lymphocytes (mostly helper T cells) and plasma cells (thick arrow). Similar cells are present in smaller numbers in the fatty tissue. HE ×80

5.27 Sjögren's syndrome (benign lymphoepithelial lesion): parotid

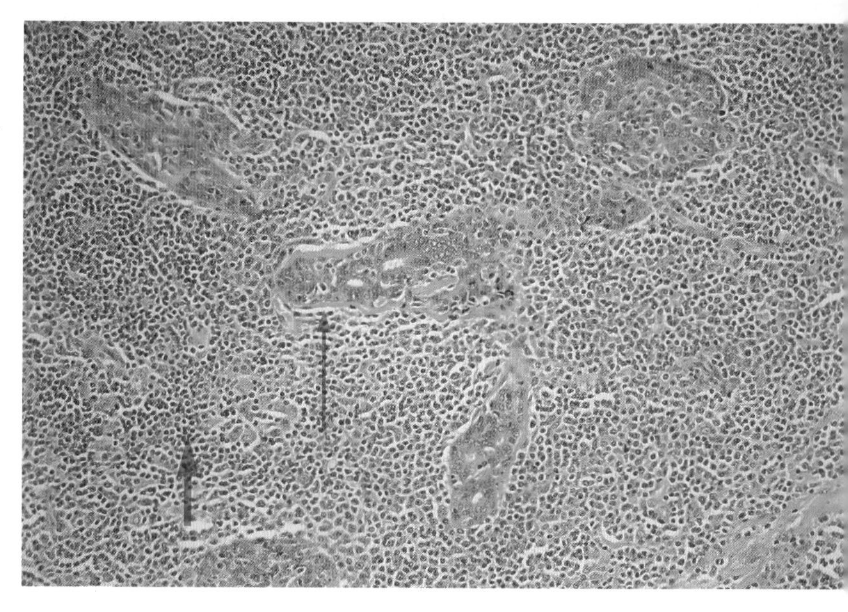

Benign lymphoepithelial lesion is an asymptomatic swelling of the salivary glands which is bilateral and symmetrical and may be very pronounced. The parotid seems to be affected more severely than the other salivary glands. This specimen was an irregular lobulated greyish-white mass of tissue (8 × 5 × 3cm) from the right parotid of a 46-year-old woman. It lacked a capsule. Histologically, in the parotid there is initially a periductal mononuclear cell infiltrate, mostly of small lymphocytes (thick arrow). Later the acinar structure is replaced by a dense infiltrate of large lymphocytes and also histiocytes; and within the infiltrate there are scattered large groups of epithelial cells, sometimes with a central lumen. The proliferating cells are eosinophilic myoepithelial cells and they fill the lumen of the ducts. Along with deposits of hyalinized basement membrane they form so-called 'myoepithelial islands' (thin arrow). These 'islands' are important diagnostic features. No germinal centres are present in the lymphoid tissue in this field but they were present elsewhere. The precise nature of the lymphoepithelial lesion is uncertain, since the systemic features of Sjögren's syndrome, including the polyarthritis, are lacking. Occasionally non-Hodgkin's lymphoma develops in an affected gland, which suggests that the condition is sometimes pre-lymphomatous. HE ×150

5.28 Papillary cystadenoma lymphomatosum: parotid

Papillary cystadenoma lymphomatosum (also called adenolymphoma) rarely involves glands other than the parotid, and it may originate from excretory salivary gland ducts within an intraparotid lymph node (*see* **5.30**). It takes the form of an ovoid or round mass, often flattened and sometimes bilateral. It is benign, usually being encapsulated and easily excised. It affects men much more often than women. On section, the stroma contains a considerable amount of lymphoid tissue and there are many irregular cystic spaces into which papillary structures project. In this field, there is a capsule of dense eosinophilic fibrous tissue and, external to it, acini lined by large deep blue mucus-secreting epithelial cells of the normal parotid (double arrow). Just inside the capsule there is fibrous stroma, heavily infiltrated by small lymphocytes (thick arrow), and a cystic space (containing cell debris) into which a bulbous papilla (left half of field) projects. The epithelial cells on the surface of the papilla and lining the cystic spaces are large, very eosinophilic, non-ciliated and multilayered (thin arrow). Their nuclei are large, pale, round or ovoid and vesicular, and they contain a prominent nucleolus. The core of the papilla is distended by small mature lymphocytes.

HE ×200

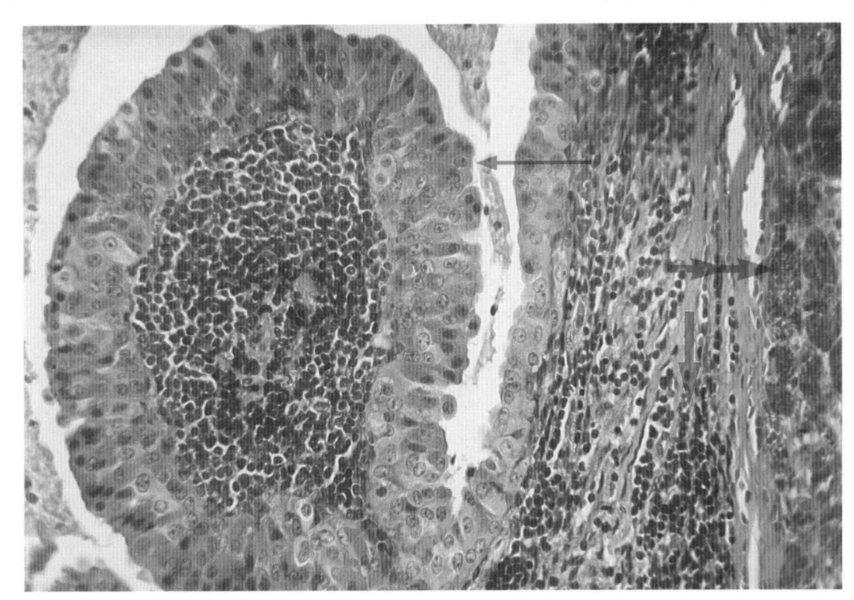

5.29 Pleomorphic adenoma: parotid

Pleomorphic adenomas are the commonest tumours of salivary glands. The tumour is generally a moderately firm nodule, round or bosselated and occasionally multiple. It is benign, but encapsulation is not always complete and tends to recur. The cut surface is lobulated, semi- translucent and bluish in some areas (pseudocartilage). Inside the fibrous capsule (double arrow) of this tumour, there small groups and cords of compact epithelial cells with a moderate amount of cytoplasm and a round or ovoid deeply basophilic nucleus (thin arrow). These neoplastic cells seem to be invading a sheet of pale-staining richly-mucoid connective tissue (thick arrow). This myxoid tissue, which is often accompanied by cartilage-like tissue, consists of individual cells with numerous large vacuoles containing very pale bluish mucinous secretion. These cells have a stellate appearance and ill-defined cytoplasmic boundaries. Epithelial mucin and acinar structures are generally also present in the tumour. Pleomorphic adenoma has been regarded as a 'mixed' tumour, and there is good evidence that both epithelial and myoepithelial cells contribute to its formation.

HE ×200

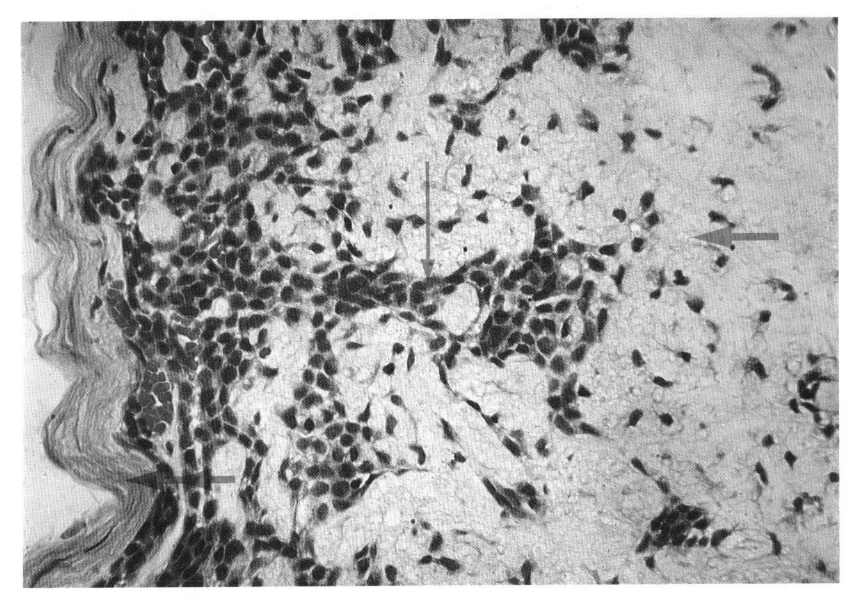

5.30 Oxyphil adenoma: parotid

Oxyphil adenoma (oncocytoma) is a benign slow-growing well-circumscribed smooth-surfaced neoplasm which arises from the epithelium of the excretory ducts. It is generally found in the parotid but may occur in other salivary glands. There is no lymphoid tissue in the tumour. Recurrence is extremely rare. The cut surface is tan-coloured and fairly uniform in appearance. This lesion was removed from the parotid of a man of 59. It measured 4.5 × 2.7 × 2.3cm and weighed 30g. It consists of closely packed well-formed acini, lined by uniform tall plump or polygonal columnar epithelial cells with a large amount of granular pink cytoplasm (thin arrows) (loaded with mitochondria). The nuclei of these oxyphilic cells are large round pale and vesicular, and each has a prominent (often central) nucleolus (thick arrow). The nuclei are not pleomorphic however and there are no mitoses. There are occasional lymphocytes in the very thin band of fibrovascular stroma which encircles the acini (double arrow).

HE ×270

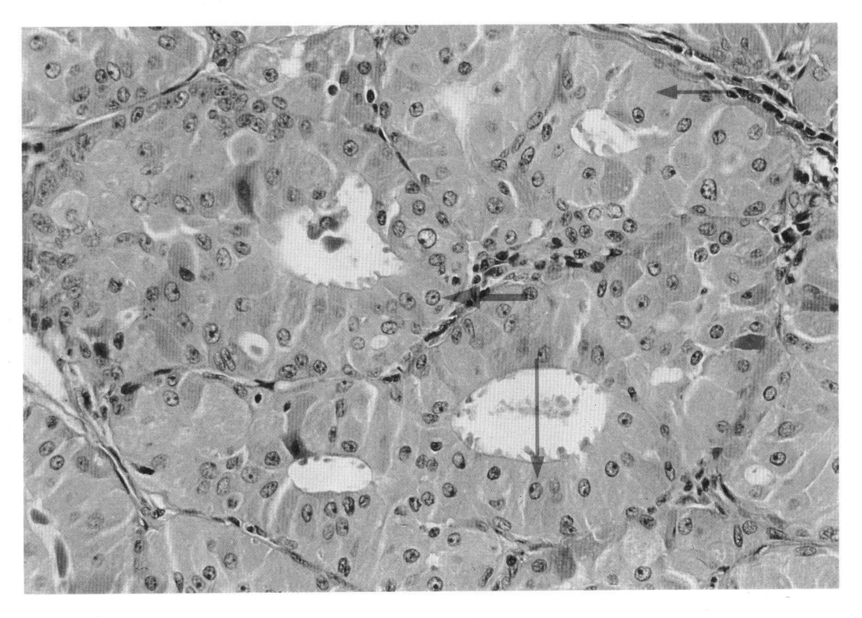

5.31 Acinic cell tumour : parotid

Acinic cell tumour is a rare slow-growing tumour of low-grade malignancy which generally presents, in the third and fourth decades, as a round apparently encapsulated mass. It probably represents a variant of the pleomorphic adenoma. It is encapsulated (in a minority of cases) and tends to recur unless adequately resected (about 90% have a 5-year survival rate). Most arise in the parotid gland, and this lesion is from the right parotid of a man of 50. It consists of closely packed anastomosing cords of mucus-secreting polygonal epithelial cells, with small densely-staining round or ovoid nuclei at the bottom of the very abundant faintly basophil (bluish) cytoplasm (thin arrows). The cytoplasm contains large numbers of vacuoles and secretory granules (resembling the serous cells of the normal gland), and sometimes the cytoplasm is so extensively vacuolated as to appear as 'clear', simulating clear-cell carcinoma. There are no mitotic figures. The stroma consists almost entirely of thin-walled blood vessels (thick arrow). HE ×270

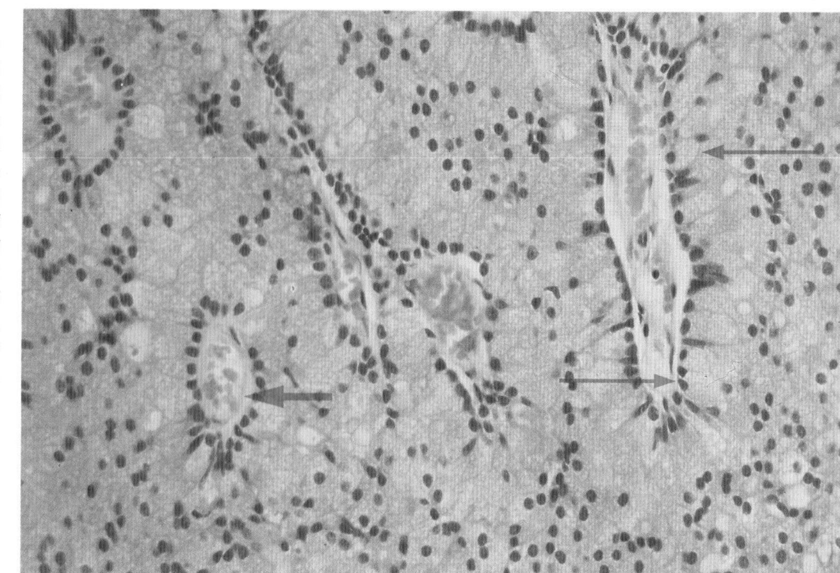

5.32 Adenoid cystic carcinoma: parotid

Adenoid cystic carcinoma, also called cylindroma, is usually a small white firm mass, usually poorly encapsulated, arising mostly in middle age, with slight female predominance. It is of moderate or low grade malignancy, but its clinical behaviour is often misleading, the tumour showing a marked tendency to recur or invade perineural lymphatics and metastasize to the lungs. The tumour has various patterns: cribriform (sieve-like) or solid (anaplastic) or ductular (tubular). This lesion is from the right parotid of a man of 41. It had infiltrated the parotid extensively. This shows several nodules of tumour, surrounded by fibrous tissue. Each nodule consists of clusters of small basaloid cells (thick arrow) with a small amount of cytoplasm and uniform ovoid or round deeply basophilic nuclei exhibiting only slight atypia, separated by thick strands of homogeneous hyaline eosinophilic basement membrane-like material (thin arrow). There are many round or ovoid 'clear' vacuoles or gland-like spaces (double arrows) between the tumour cells. HE ×150

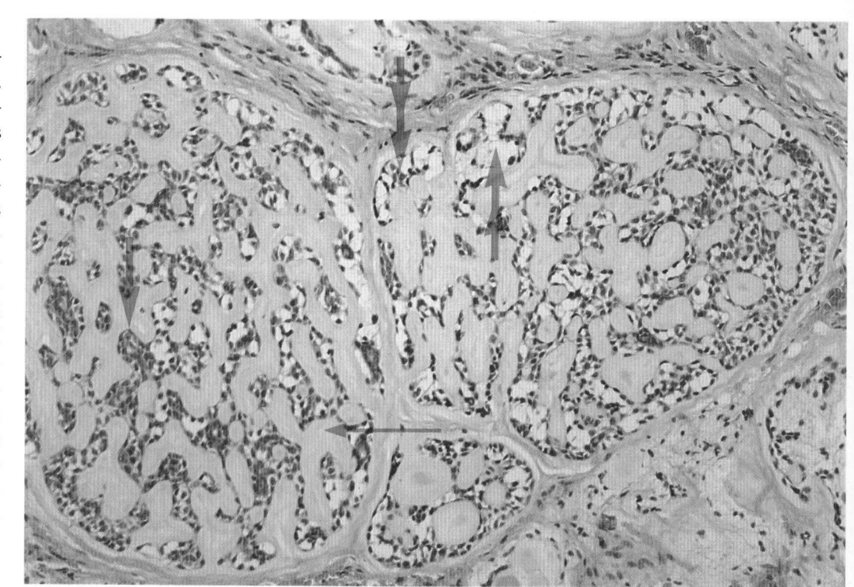

5.33 Adenoid cystic carcinoma: parotid

The tumour in 5.32 recurred, and this is part of one of the nodules that developed. At the left margin of this field there are several normal compact deep blue mucin-secreting parotid acini and large (clear) fat cells, as well as much dense eosinophilic fibrous tissue in which there are plump fibroblasts and slender fibrocytes. The rest of the field is occupied by a round (circular) cribriform sheet (nodule) of neoplastic (malignant) cells of moderate size, surrounded by a thick band of basement membrane and collagenous fibrous tissue, somewhat hyalinized (thin arrow). The neoplastic cells (thick arrows) have a small amount of vacuolated cytoplasm and round or ovoid strongly basophilic nuclei of regular form. There is very little nuclear pleomorphism and no evidence of mitotic activity. Within the circular sheet of tumour cells there are relatively large areas (mostly round) full of weakly eosinophilic amorphous basement membrane-like material (double arrow). Despite its usually somewhat bland histological structure, adenoid cystic carcinoma is a highly invasive tumour. HE ×360

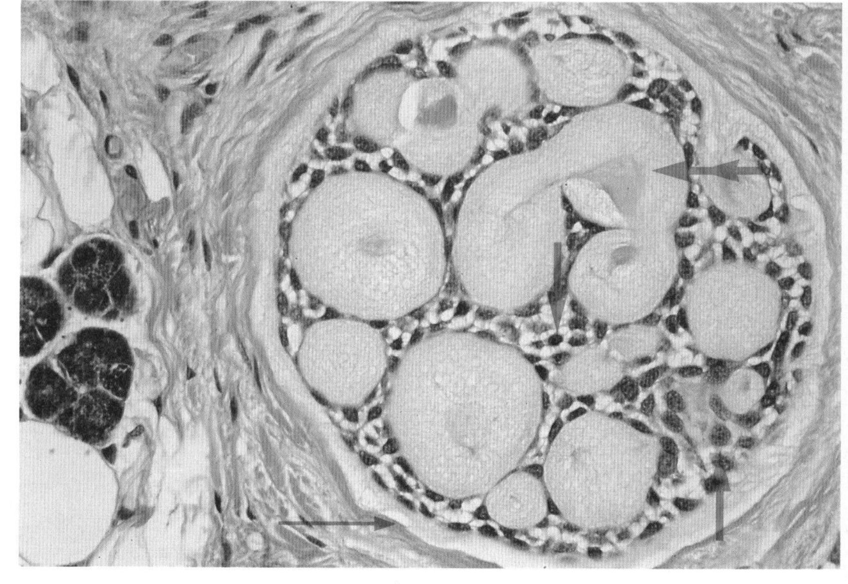

5.34 Mucoepidermoid carcinoma: parotid

Mucoepidermoid carcinoma is thought to arise from the epithelial cells lining the ducts of the salivary glands. Some of them are of low-grade malignancy but others are highly malignant. A low-grade lesion presents as a well-circumscribed mass which is not encapsulated, tending to infiltrate locally and eventually to metastasize. This field is part of a well-defined nodule (4 × 3 × 3cm) which is a local recurrence in the submandibular gland of a man of aged 88. The centre of the field is occupied by a sheet of extremely atypical squamous epithelial cells. The malignant epithelial cells have a large amount of deeply eosinophilic cytoplasm and very large extremely pleomorphic nuclei (thick arrows) which contain prominent nucleoli. Within the sheet of tumour cells, which is traversed by a greatly dilated thin-walled blood vessel, there are also several small round cysts, full of pale (epithelial-type) mucin (thin arrow). Despite the microscopic appearances, the tumour was invading the surrounding tissues and perineural lymphatics. HE ×235

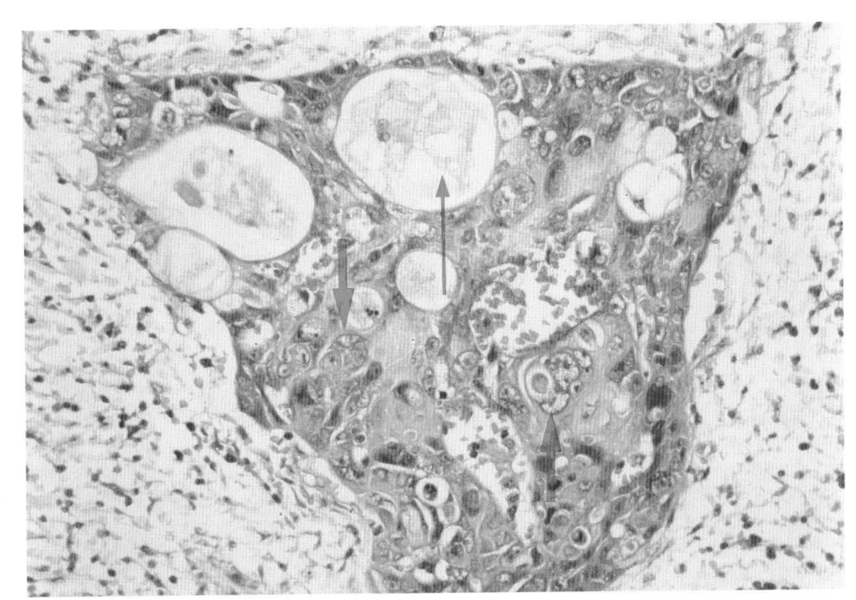

5.35 Adenocarcinoma: parotid

Adenocarcinoma may arise from a pleomorphic adenoma but this happens infrequently. Others arise *de novo*. There is no age or sex predilection. The tumour, which is generally firm, tends to infiltrate blood vessels, lymphatic channels & perineural spaces. The prognosis is determined by the degree of differentiation. This tumour did not appear to be associated with a pleomorphic adenoma. In this field, there is a considerable amount collagenous stroma, which surrounds small clumps and irregular gland-like structures of widely varying sizes, lined by malignant epithelial cells. The cells lining the glandular structures show considerable pleomorphism, some being small and flattened (thin arrow), and others large and cuboidal or columnar (double arrow). The large cells have round or ovoid nuclei, which are large pale and vesicular and occasionally contain a prominent nucleolus (thick arrow). There is much debris, densely eosinophilic and keratin-like, in most of the glandular structures. Mitotic figures are not visible among these epithelial lining cells but there are some elsewhere in the tumour.

HE ×200

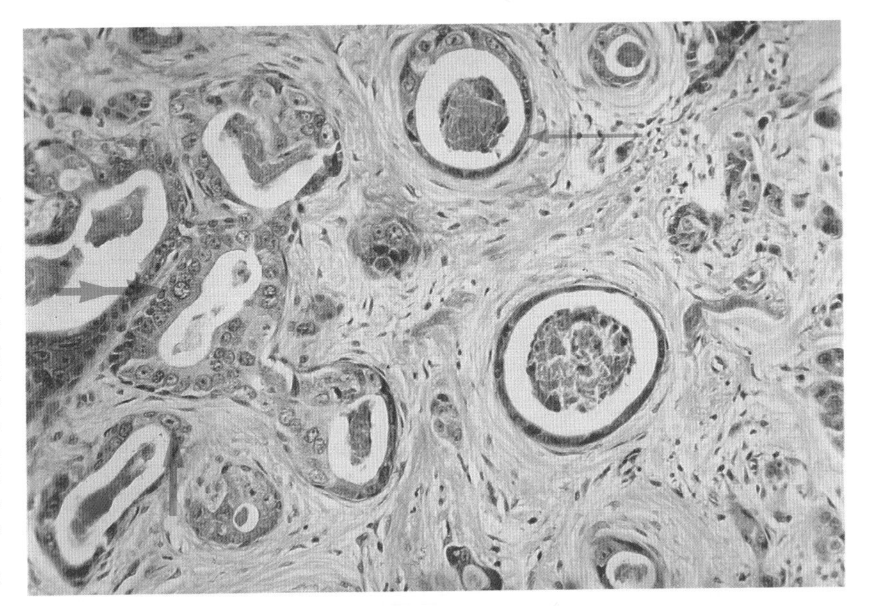

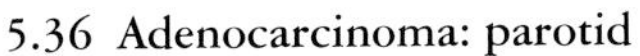

5.36 Adenocarcinoma: parotid

A small minority of salivary gland tumours are highly malignant, poorly-differentiated lesions. Such tumours often take the form of a large firm mass, sometimes with areas of hemorrhage and necrosis in the cut surface, and histologically composed of sheets and cords of undifferentiated (malignant) epithelial cells. This is an anaplastic tumour, at high magnification, consisting of closely packed polyhedral cells with very little cytoplasm and large round or ovoid nuclei (thick arrow). The nuclei are fairly basophil but vesicular in appearance, and in a minority of them there is a nucleolus. Several mitoses are visible and are numerous in the remainder of the tumour. The malignant cells do not form glands or tubules but among them there are elongated well-defined spaces (thin arrow) which contain a little debris. The stroma consists mainly of small blood vessels (double arrow) but little or no connective tissue. The histogenesis of this type of tumour is not known but an origin from the epithelium of the ducts is possible. HE ×335

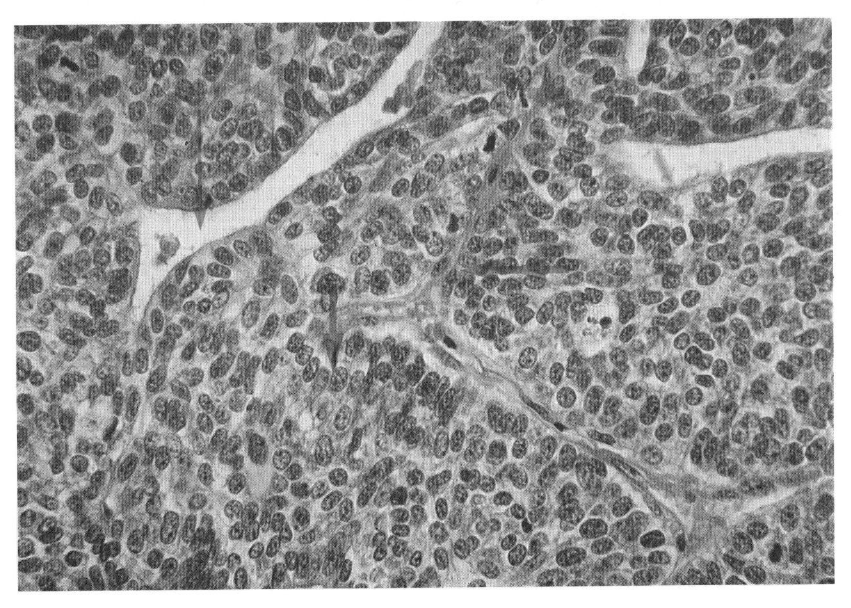

6.1 Infarct (+Sheehan's syndrome): pituitary

Hypopituitarism in adults (Simmond's disease) is rare. Previously the most common cause was ischemic necrosis of a gland that had undergone hyperplasia and enlarged during pregnancy. Should the trauma and post-partum hemorrhage of childbirth precipitate shock and hypotension, the pituitary's blood supply is liable to fail and cause extensive ischemic necrosis of the gland; and when more than 90% of it is necrotic, hypopituitarism (Sheehan's syndrome) may develop. Hypopituitarism in female adults causes amenorrhea and infertility, but Sheehan's syndrome is now uncommon in developed countries. Histologically, more than half of the tissue is intensely red and necrotic, consisting of large numbers of extravasated red cells and dilated blood-filled sinusoids (double arrow), as well as necrotic pituitary cells (thick arrow), some with pyknotic nuclei and others anucleate. The viable pituitary tissue consists of groups of closely packed small basophilic round cells (pituicytes) (thin arrow), surrounded by vascular septa of fibrous tissue. The pituicytes have deeply basophilic compact round nuclei but only a moderate amount of ill-defined cytoplasm. HE ×150

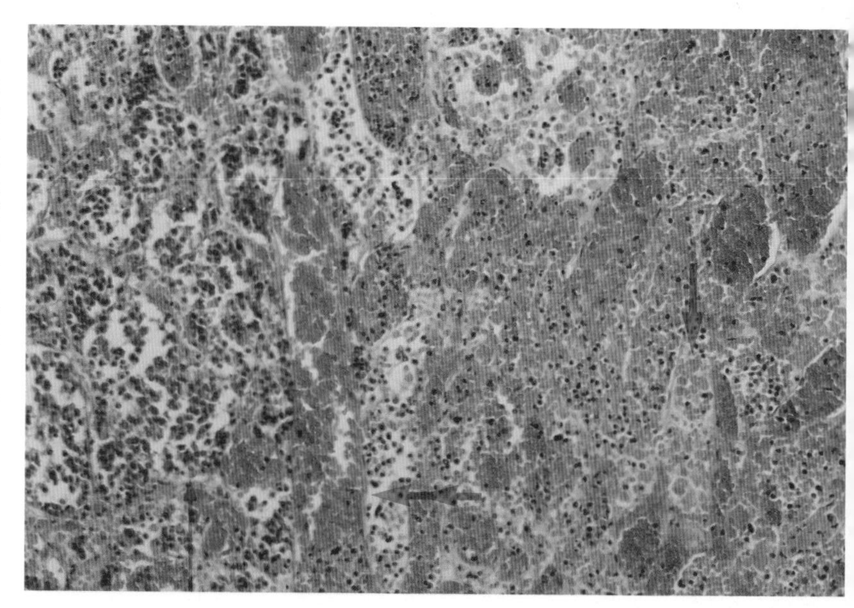

6.2 Chromophobe adenoma: pituitary

Cut sections of pituitary adenomas are generally fleshy and red to grey in colour. Histologically, most of the cells are of one type and structurally uniform. They form groups (nests) and trabeculae, separated by sinusoidal blood vessels. The terms basophil (ACTH, TSH), acidophil (GH, prolactin) and chromophobe (non-functional) are now of little value, whereas chromophobe adenomas have been frequently shown immunohistochemically to produce hormones. This patient was an 81-year-old man who died of coronary artery disease and heart failure. Although a pituitary tumour had been resected 24 years previously, a lobulated mass (3 × 3 × 4cm) was found protruding from the pituitary fossa. It had compressed the anterior cerebral artery and caused infarction of part of the right frontal lobe of the brain. Histologically the tumour consists of groups of closely packed polygonal cells (thin arrow), separated by delicate vascular septa (thick arrow). The tumour cells have a fairly large amount of eosinophilic cytoplasm and round central nuclei which vary in slightly in size. There are no mitoses. With the use only of special stains, the tumour was classified as a chromophobe adenoma. HE ×235

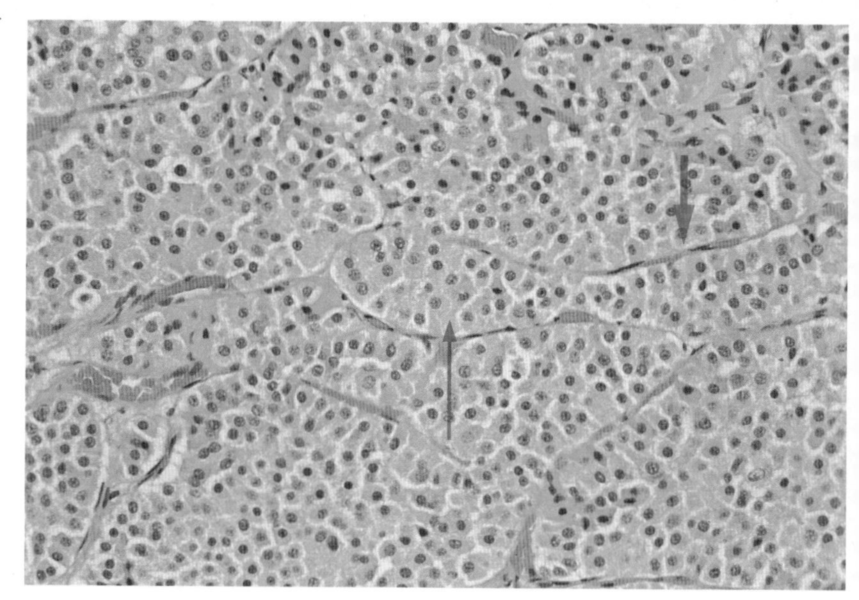

6.3 Acidophil adenoma (+ acromegaly): pituitary

Acidophil adenomas secrete growth hormone (GH) and prolactin. The effects of prolactin are mainly proliferation of ductal tissue in the breast (and initiation of milk secretion), whereas growth hormone stimulates the growth of all body tissues andproduces acromegaly and gigantism. Growth hormone also antagonizes the action of insulin, which occasionally leads to diabetes mellitus. Acidophil adenomas are usually large and may destroy much of the tissue around the pituitary fossa. This acidophil adenoma of pituitary, removed surgically from a man of 43 with acromegaly, consists of compact well defined trabeculae (two cells thick) (thin arrow) of neoplastic cells (pituicytes) of uniform size and shape, separated by dilated thin-walled blood vessels (thick arrow) and a small amount of connective tissue. The neoplastic cells have abundant eosinophilic cytoplasm, and each has a round vesicular nucleus in the base of the cell. There is no nuclear pleomorphism and no mitotic activity. Special stains showed sparse granules in the cytoplasm of the tumour cells, and immunohistochemistry confirmed the presence growth hormone (somatotropin). HE ×360

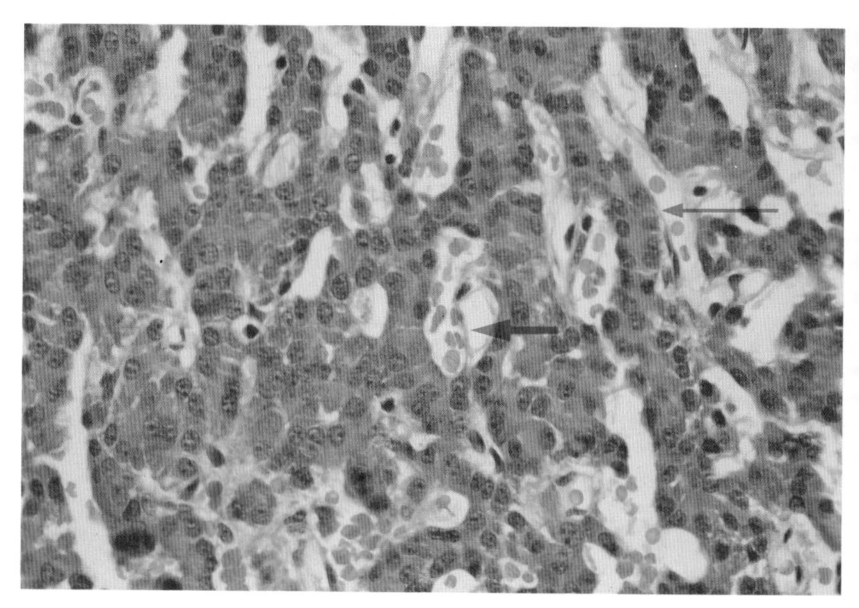

6.4 Acidophil adenoma (+acromegaly): pituitary

The effect of increased levels of growth hormone (somatotropin) depends on the age of the patient. In children there is excessive uniform bone growth at the epiphyses, and a great but proportionate increase in height (gigantism). In adults however, the epiphyses are fused and the bones are generally enlarged (acromegaly). An acidophil adenoma was removed surgically from a 44-year-old man who had suffered from acromegaly for many years. This is a thin 'plastic' section (1μm thick) of an acidophil adenoma of pituitary, stained HE. The tumour consists of sheets of round neoplastic cells (somatotrophs) with abundant eosinophilic cytoplasm and well defined boundaries (thin arrows). The cytoplasm is finely granular and in some cells there is a pale-staining juxtanuclear halo (thick arrow). The nuclei are ovoid or round and vesicular, and some are especially large and moderately pleomorphic. The chromatin is finely granular, and in many of the nuclei there is a prominent nucleolus. There is no mitotic activity. The stroma consists of small thin-walled blood vessels, lined by large cells with very pale cytoplasm. HE ×860

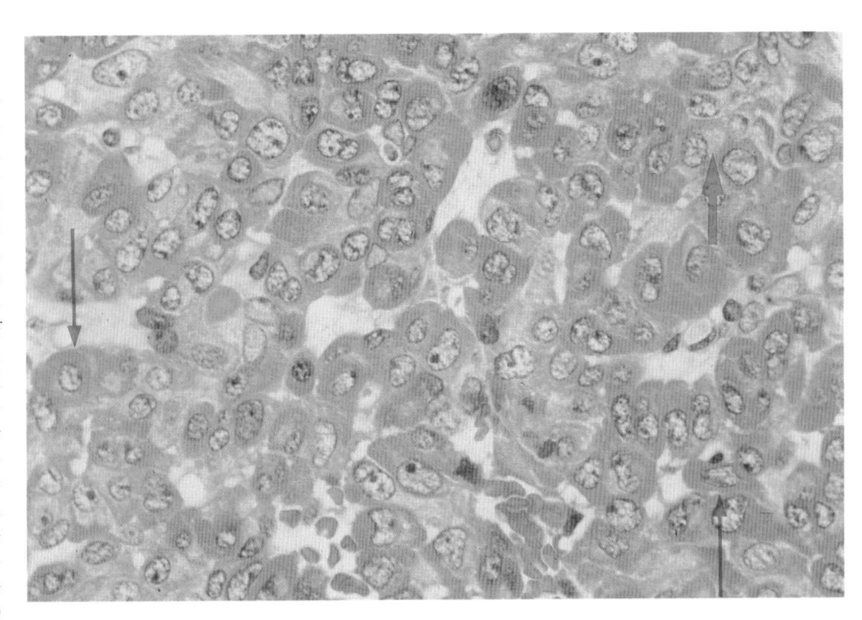

6.5 Acidophil adenoma (+acromegaly): pituitary

In many patients with acromegaly, the normal pituitary cells are compressed by the adenoma and undergo atrophy, with the result that secretion of other pituitary hormones decreases. However, histological sections stained by hematoxylin and eosin (HE) are usually of very limited value in distinguishing the various types of pituitary cells, and special techniques are required. As a rule, Brooke's stain colours the cytoplasm of acidophil cells brownish yellow, and Brooke's stain has now been applied to a section of the same adenoma as that shown in 6.4. With few exceptions, the cytoplasm of the cells of the adenoma is likewise brownish yellow (thin arrow), confirming that the adenoma is of the acidophil type (and that the neoplastic cells are somatotrophs). Other structures which are well demonstrated in this section are the pale vesicular moderately pleomorphic greyish nuclei containing a fairly prominent red nucleolus (thick arrow). The stroma consists almost entirely of delicate connective tissue fibres (stained blue) and small thin-walled blood vessels full of brilliantly red erythrocytes (double arrow).

Brooke's stain ×860

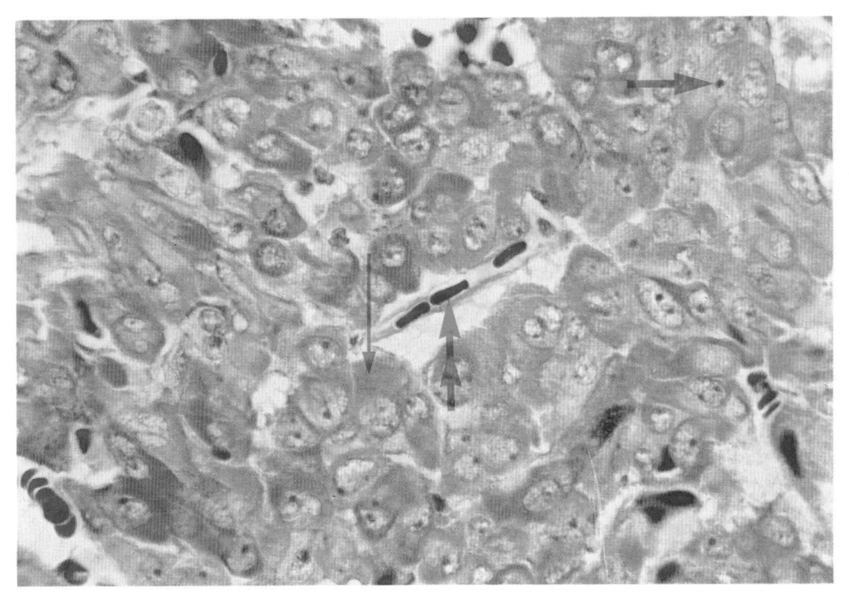

6.6 Acidophil adenoma (+acromegaly): pituitary

Immunogistochemical methods are usually highly specific and capable of identifying the various cells of the pituitary and those in pituitary adenomas. This is a histological section of the same adenoma as that shown in 6.4 and 6.5 and it has been subjected to the indirect immunoperoxidase method. In this method, a specific antibody is applied to a histological section which (presumably) contains a particular hormone. In this case it is growth hormone (somatotropin). In the histological section there are small clusters and groups of neoplastic cells, separated by pale (almost colourless) connective tissue and thin-walled blood vessels. In the cytoplasm of most of the neoplastic cells in the section, the reaction between the antigen (growth hormone) and antibody is strongly positive, colouring the cytoplasm brown (thin arrow) and signifying the presence of growth hormone. The cytoplasm of a small minority of similar cells is pale grey and non-reactive (thick arrow).

Indirect immunoperoxidase method for growth hormone ×360

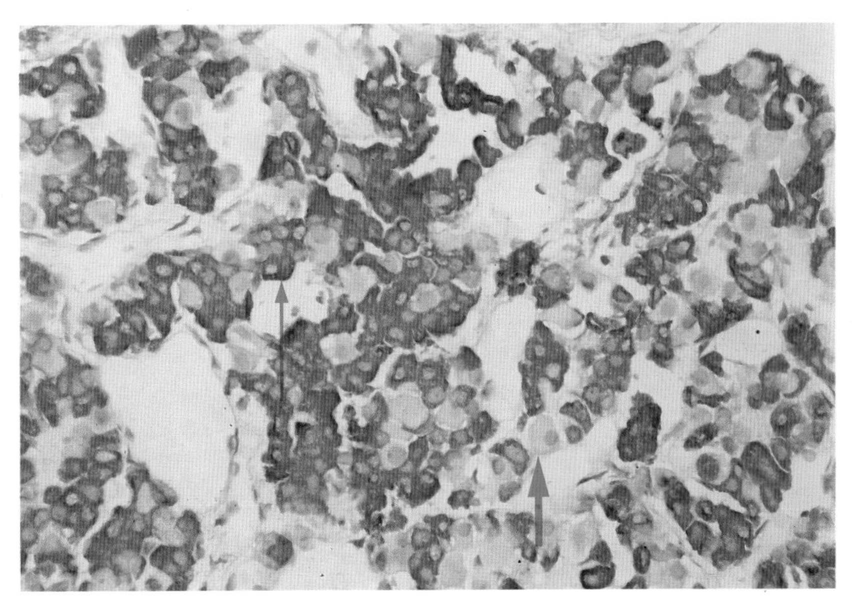

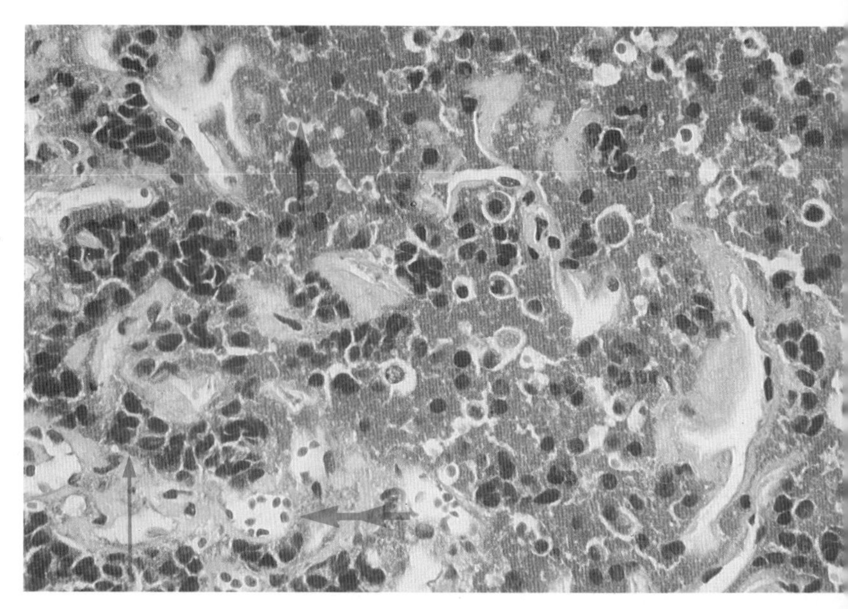

6.7 Secondary small cell carcinoma (oat cell): pituitary

Undifferentiated small cell carcinoma probably arises from neuroendocrine cells in the bronchial mucosa and is highly malignant. Neuroendocrine immunological markers such as chromogranin and neuron-specific enolase are usually identifiable in the cytoplasm; and neurosecretory granules may be visualized by electron microscopy. Secondary deposits of small cell carcinoma of bronchus are occasionally found in the pituitary, generally from primary carcinoma of bronchus or breast. This is a metastasis of small cell carcinoma in the anterior pituitary. Most of the pituitary cells are necrotic, consisting of intensely eosinophilic granular cytoplasm but lacking nuclei (thick arrow). Infiltrating the necrotic tissue there are irregular cords and small groups of compact cells with no visible cytoplasm (thin arrow) with no cytoplasm but deeply basophilic fairly pleomorphic round-to-ovoid nuclei, solid- and viable-looking. There are no mitotic figures in this field but they are numerous elsewhere. The stroma consists mainly of sinusoidal blood vessels with thick hyaline walls (double arrow). HE ×270

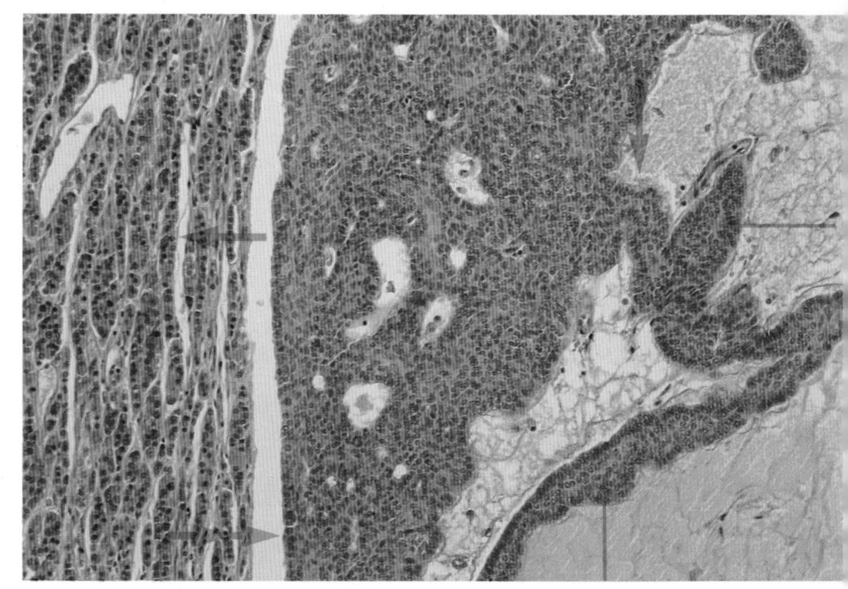

6.8 Craniopharyngioma: pituitary

Craniopharyngiomas arise from epithelial 'rests' derived from the pars tuberalis (Rathke's pouch) which also gives rise to the hypophysis. They tend to be located above the sella turcica, and consist of cystic and solid components (suprasellar cysts) which compress adjacent tissues but are well demarcated and generally appear to be encapsulated. This specimen is from a man of 87 who developed hypopituitarism shortly before his death. His pituitary had been largely replaced by a multicystic tumour, with only a thin rim of pituitary remaining. The remaining pituitary is severely compressed, consisting of cords of flattened atrophic cells (thick arrow). The edge of the tumour is sharply demarcated, with a cleft between it and the pituitary. The tumour consists of sheets and trabeculae of fairly large epithelial cells (thin arrows) with prominent round-to-ovoid basophilic nuclei and a moderate amount of strongly eosinophilic cytoplasm, surrounded by a single layer of cuboidal or columnar epithelial cells similar to the other epithelial cells but arranged in an irregular palisade (double arrows). The palisaded cells also line the 'spaces' in the stroma. The stromal 'spaces' vary widely in size and shape and contain a considerable amount of amorphous material and also eosinophilic fibrils. HE ×150

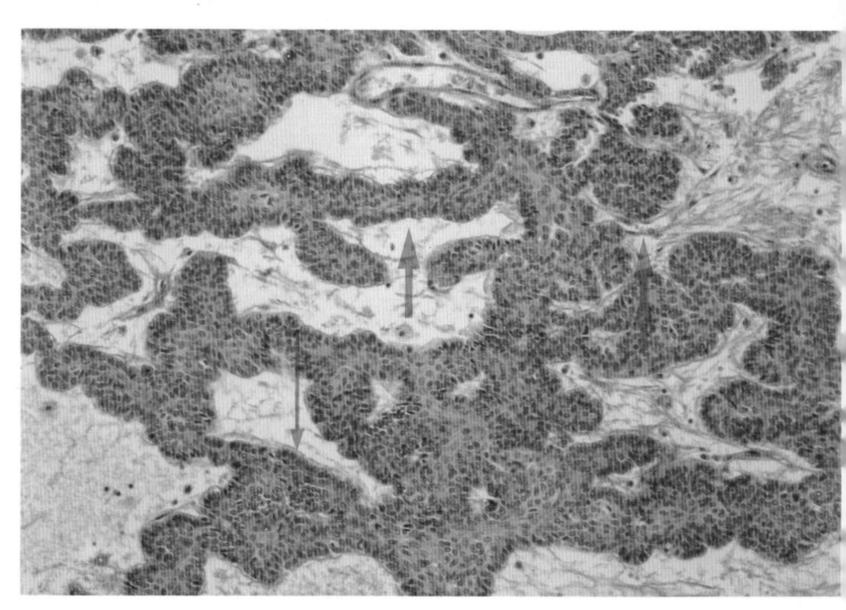

6.9 Craniopharyngioma: pituitary

This is part of the same tumour as in 6.8. Keratin 'pearls' may form in the sheets of well-differentiated squamous epithelial cells but there are no 'pearls' in this lesion. The neoplastic epithelial cells, which are arranged in long irregular trabeculae (thick arrow), have ovoid-to-round nuclei and a moderate amount of eosinophilic cytoplasm. The periphery of the trabeculae is demarcated by a palisaded layer of cuboidal or columnar epithelial cells (thin arrow) with round-to-ovoid vesicular basophilic nuclei. There is no mitotic activity in this field. The palisaded epithelial cells also line and simultaneously enclose the large stromal 'spaces'. The 'spaces' are in fact extremely edematous stroma, consisting of much amorphous material (extremely vacuolated in places) and many very elongated eosinophilic fibres (double arrow), some of them collagenous. Along with small numbers of indeterminate cells, there are a few thin-walled blood vessels in the stromal spaces. HE ×150

6.10 Thyroglossal duct cyst

The isthmus of the thyroid gland is derived from a tube of epithelium that grows down from the base of the tongue, in the region of the foramen caecum. Above the hyoid bone the tube is lined by squamous epithelium, and below the bone by ciliated columnar epithelium. If the tube fails to involute, cysts may form in the midline of the neck and they may rupture. Above the hyoid bone the cyst is a 'lingual dermoid' and below it a thyroglossal cyst. The cyst is usually lined by respiratory epithelium and sometimes there are lymphoid follicles and thyroid remnants in the cyst wall. However this cyst (with the lumen on the left) is lined by stratified squamous epithelium (thin arrow), and its wall consists of collagenous fibrous tissue and dilated thin-walled blood vessels (double arrow). Also present is a narrow band of inactive-looking thyroid tissue (thick arrow), consisting of thyroid follicles, mostly small, which contain weakly eosinophilic secretion. If there are large amounts of thyroid tissue in the cyst wall, the cyst is termed a 'lingual thyroid'. HE ×135

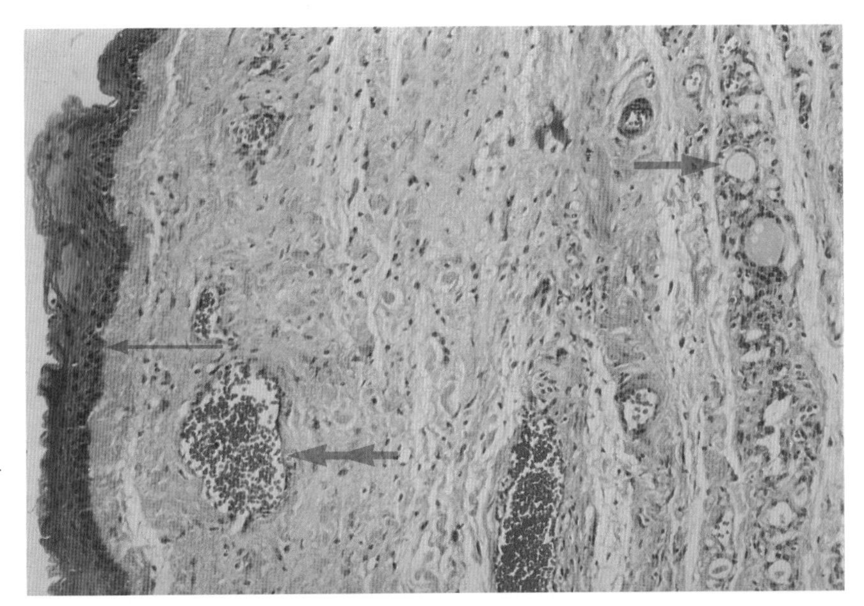

6.11 Thyroglossal duct cyst

Thyroglossal duct cysts present in late childhood or early adult life, and are commonly found between the hyoid bone and the isthmus of the thyroid gland. Thyroid tissue tends to be found in the walls of thyroglossal cysts. In a significant number of cases, the thyroglossal cyst may communicate with the pharynx at the foramen caecum, and it may also become infected. Abscesses tend to form and then drain externally via a (thyroglossal duct) fistula. The lumen of this cyst (at the top) is lined by a single layer of epithelial cells, essentially respiratory-type. The respiratory-type cells are closely packed ciliated columnar or cuboidal epithelial cells (thin arrow), and their ovoid basal deeply stained nuclei appear to be pseudostratified. Mucin-containing (goblet) epithelial cells are also present. The wall of the cyst consists of an inner layer of eosinophilic collagenous fibrous tissue and many fibrocytes (thick arrow), lightly infiltrated with plasma cells and lymphocytes. There is also an external layer of looser connective tissue, in which there are numerous dilated thin-walled blood vessels (double arrow). HE ×235

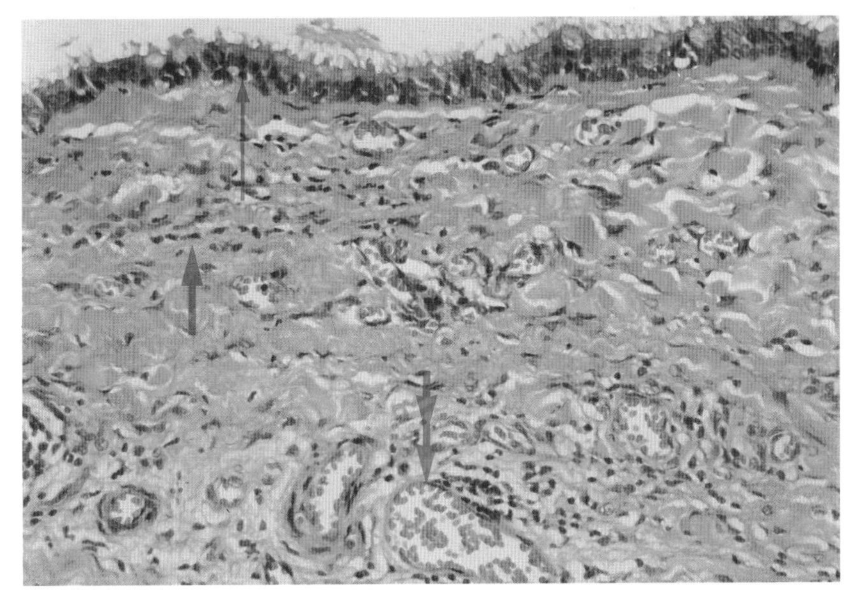

6.12 Endemic goitre

Endemic goitre is the result of chronic deficiency of iodine in the diet. The iodine-deficient parts of the world are mainly inland mountainous regions, and up to 5% of the population there may have thyroid enlargement, sometimes massive. The enlargement of the thyroid is initially parenchymatous; that is, the thyroid tissue is markedly hyperplastic. The number of follicles is increased and the epithelial cells are enlarged and columnar. Later, focal changes occur, with some parts of the gland becoming hyperactive in their uptake of iodine and other parts becoming atrophic. In this way the gland becomes nodular, and its histological structure varies considerably from one part to another. This thyroid is from a colloid-rich area. Most of the thyroid follicles are distended with deeply eosinophilic colloid, and lined by a very attenuated layer of small flat epithelial cells (thick arrow). The epithelial cells are very uniform, and there is no tendency to form papillae. Hemorrhage has occurred into an extremely large follicle, in the form of small collections of erythrocytes in the colloid (thin arrow). Sometimes the whole of a goitrous thyroid has a structure similar to that shown here: a colloid goitre. HE ×60

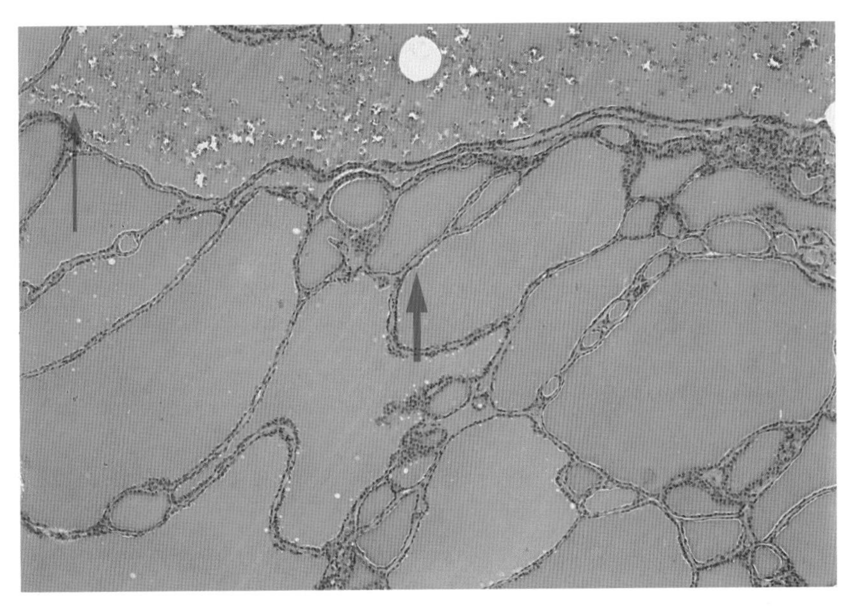

6.13 Graves' disease: thyroid

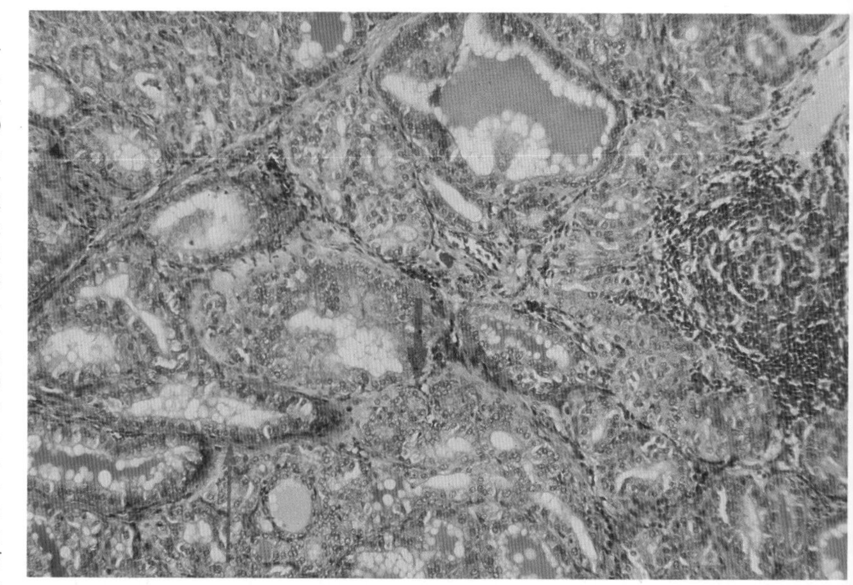

Graves' disease is an autoimmune disease, and responsible for the great majority of cases of hyperthyroidism. Autoantibodies (in the serum) of the IgG class are directed against the thyroid-stimulating hormone (TSH) receptor on the surface of the thyroid epithelial cells. When the antibody combines with the receptor, the thyroid epithelial cells are stimulated to produce thyroid hormone. The thyroid secretes excess of hormone, which has widespread effects on many tissues. In this untreated case of Graves' disease, the cut surface of the thyroid was fleshy and a pale greyish-pink colour instead of the glistening reddish-brown colour of a normal gland. Histologically, this gland is diffusely hyperplastic and contains little colloid. Most of the follicles are small (thick arrow) but others are fairly large (thin arrow) and lined by fairly large cuboidal cells with ovoid or round vesicular nuclei. Several follicles contain strongly eosinophilic colloid, vacuolated at the periphery, probably the effect of preoperative treatment of the patient with iodine. In the larger follicles the epithelium tends to form papilliform processes. The colloid is vacuolated at the edges, a sign of active resorption. There is a lymphoid follicle in the stroma (double arrow). HE ×95

6.14 Graves' disease: thyroid

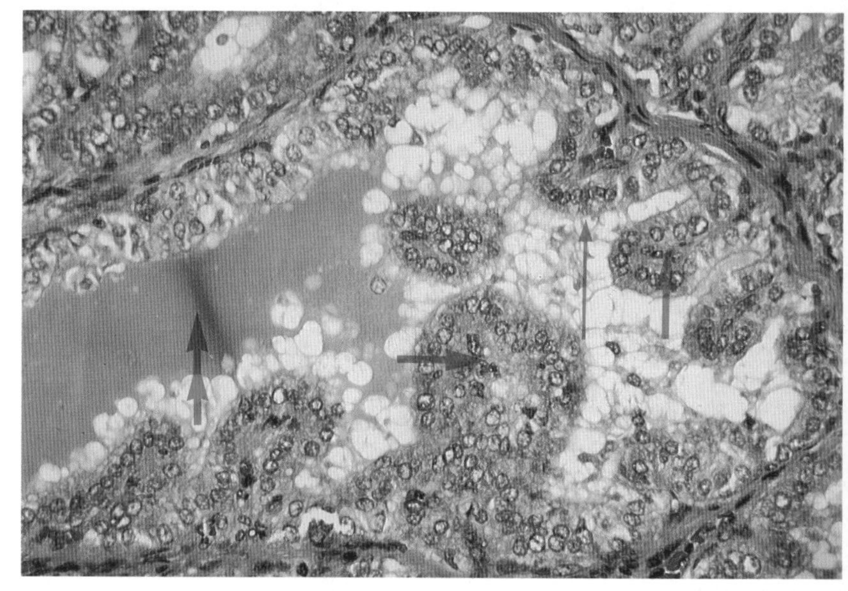

This histological section is from the same tissue as in 6.13. Some relatively small thyroid follicles, which were very numerous elsewhere in the gland, are visible at the top of this field. The centre of the field is occupied by part of a very large follicle, lined by intensely hyperplastic columnar or cuboidal epithelial cells (thin arrow). The lining cells have a fairly large amount of pale vacuolated cytoplasm and prominent round or ovoid pale vesicular nuclei which contain granules of chromatin. The lining epithelial cells show a marked tendency to form papilliferous projections (thick arrows) of various sizes into the lumen. There is a sheet of eosinophilic colloid in the lumen (double arrow), but the secretion in the remainder of the lumen is excessively vacuolated (the result of proteolysis of thyroglobulin) and almost colourless (probably the result of tangential sectioning). The large follicle is surrounded by a prominent eosinophilic strands of fibromuscular stroma. The stroma is very vascular but the vascularity is not obvious, since the small vessels tend to collapse during tissue processing. HE ×360

6.15 Graves' disease: thyroid

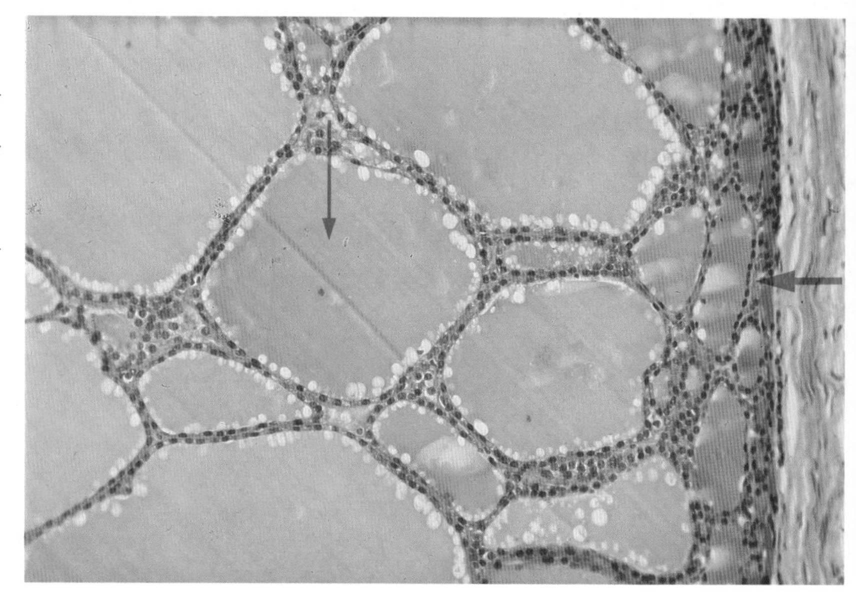

In Graves' disease the thyroid gland is diffusely and symmetrically enlarged and extremely vascular. This case had been treated with iodine prior to surgical resection of the thyroid, and involution of the gland is now almost complete. The thyroid is enclosed by a capsule of eosinophilic collagenous fibrous tissue (right margin). At the periphery of the gland, close to the densely fibrous capsule, there is a slender layer of slightly flattened small thyroid follicles (thick arrow). The follicles are full of strongly eosinophilic colloid, at the periphery of which there are a few clear vacuoles. However, almost all of the thyroid gland now consists of medium-sized and large follicles (thin arrow). These follicles are lined by a single layer of very flat epithelial cells and full of uniformly eosinophilic colloid. However, at the periphery of the colloid (and in contact with the surface of lining epithelial cells) there are fairly numerous small round clear (empty) vacuoles, demonstrating that resorption of colloid continues. HE ×135

6.16 Riedel's thyroiditis: thyroid

Riedel's thyroiditis is a rare lesion which usually affects only part of the gland. It is a sclerosing 'inflammatory' process which is sometimes associated with similar fibrosing lesions in the retroperitoneum and mediastinum. The gland is usually slightly enlarged, and replaced, partly or wholly, by stoney-hard greyish fibrous tissue and termed 'woody' or 'ligneous' thyroiditis). The adjacent muscles are often involved and the condition may be mistaken for an invasive neoplasm, particularly since the affected part of the gland feels very hard. This lesion was painless and typically limited to one pole of the thyroid, which was adherent to the surrounding tissues of the neck. Apart from several small follicles lined by atrophic epithelial cells (thick arrows), no other thyroid epithelial cells can be identified, the tissue consisting mainly of thick bands of scar-like eosinophilic collagenous fibrous tissue (thin arrow), in which there are many plasma cells and lymphocytes. Hypothyroidism is not usually present in Riedel's thyroiditis, presumably because it is a focal lesion. HE ×235

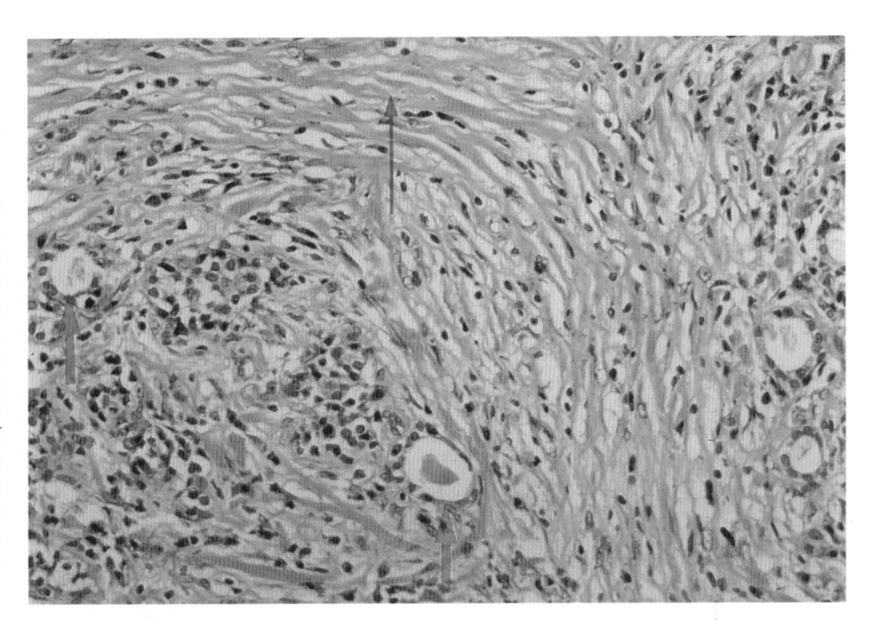

6.17 Granulomatous (de Quervain's) thyroiditis: thyroid

Granulomatous thyroiditis (also termed de Quervain's or subacute or giant cell thyroiditis) is an uncommon self-limiting inflammatory condition which is probably caused by a virus infection. The thyroid gland is diffusely enlarged, firm and often adherent to adjacent structures. It becomes painful and tender, and fever is often present. Most patients are euthyroid, but occasionally the thyroiditis is accompanied by transient hyperthyroidism. In this case the patient was a woman of 38. Part of the isthmus of the gland was removed surgically. Much of the gland's architecture had been destroyed, and replaced by clusters of epithelial cells and small follicles, irregular in size and shape. Only a few larger follicles, including one filled with colloid (thin arrow), have survived. The small follicles are surrounded by sheets of eosinophilic strands of collagenous fibroblast/fibrocytic tissue. The fibrous tissue is diffusely infiltrated with lymphocytes, and a small collection of giant multinucleated cells (giant-cell granuloma) (thick arrow) is also present in the stroma.
HE ×150

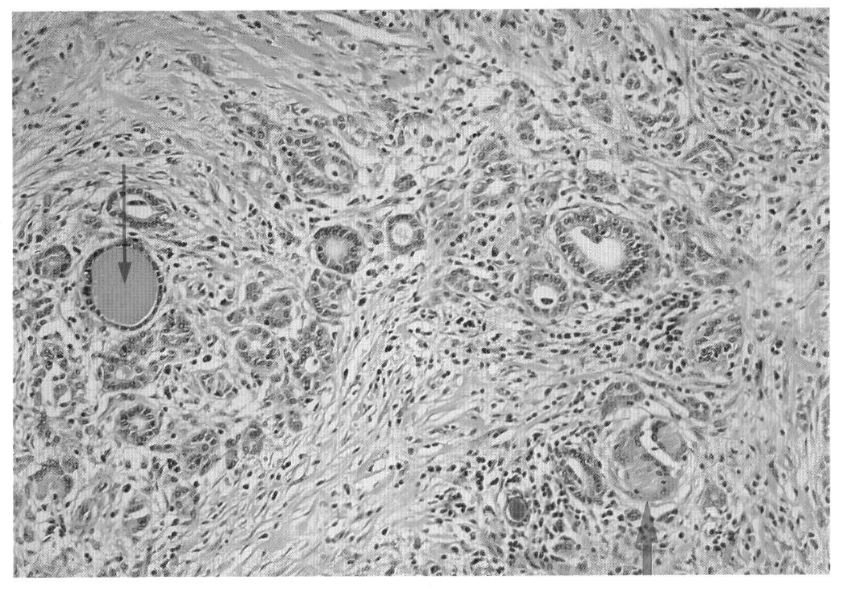

6.18 Granulomatous (de Quervain's) thyroiditis: thyroid

Although the enlargement of the thyroid gland may be symmetrical, the inflammatory reaction is often confined to one side of the gland and sometimes only to a localized area in one lobe. This is a histological section of the same tissue as in 6.17, at higher magnification. Destruction of the normal thyroid follicles is more obvious than in 6.17, and the follicles are now mostly small and very irregular in shape (thin arrows). The follicles are also greatly reduced in number, and those present are lined by cuboidal or flattened epithelial cells with uniformly round or ovoid vesicular nuclei. In most of the follicles the epithelial lining is disrupted (thick arrow), often only partly but occasionally severely or almost completely. Most of the eosinophilic colloid in the lumen of the follicles has been digested by macrophages. These features are particularly obvious in large follicles. The stroma consists of loose connective tissue and it is abundant. Numerous lymphocytes, macrophages and plasma cells are scattered throughout the stromal fibrous tissue and they are even more numerous in the lumen of follicles which have been markedly disrupted.
HE ×235

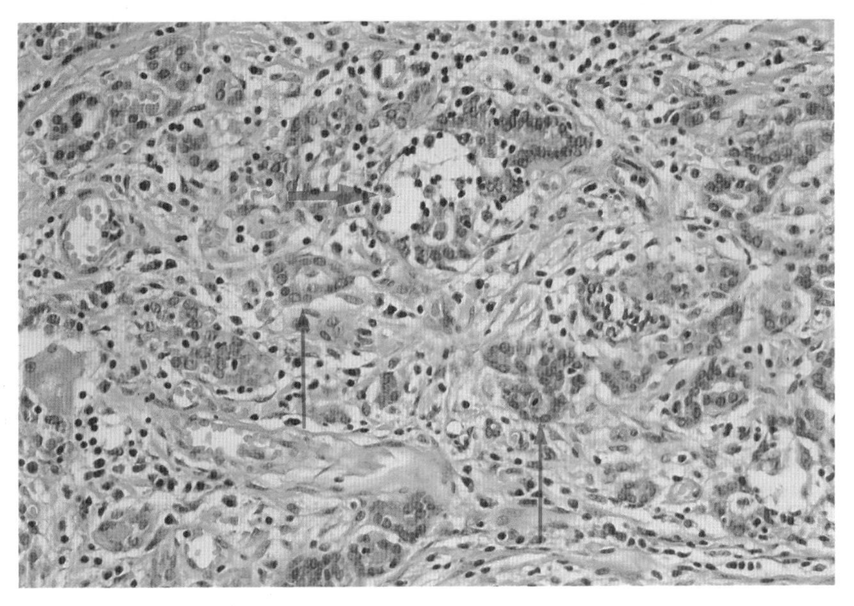

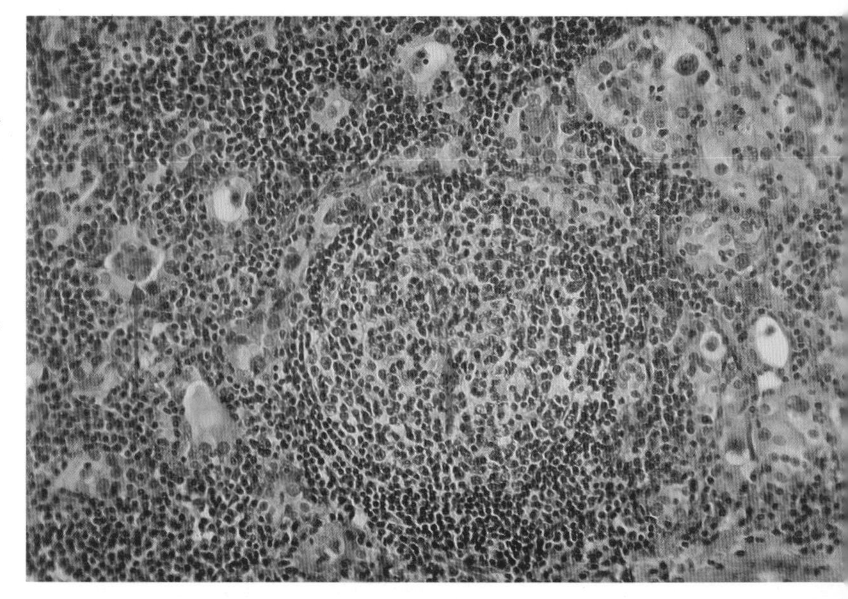

6.19 Hashimoto's thyroiditis: thyroid

Hashimoto's thyroiditis is thought to be an autoimmune response against the thyroid. Several different IgG autoantibodies are generally present in the serum, but serum levels of the antibodies do not correlate with severity of the disease. The thyroid cells are probably destroyed by a cytotoxic T cell-mediated hypersensitivity mechanism. Destruction of epithelium generally leads to hypothyroidism. Sometimes goitre does not develop, but destruction and shrinkage of the thyroid progress until the gland is largely functionless (primary myxedema). In this field, many follicles have disappeared, and those remaining are very irregular in size and shape, some consisting only of tight clusters of epithelial cells (thin arrows). Most of the epithelial cells, including those lining the glandular structures, have markedly pleomorphic nuclei and varying amounts of eosinophilic cytoplasm. There is also a mature-looking lymphoid follicle with a pale germinal centre (thick arrow), and it is surrounded by a heavy infiltrate of plasma cells and small lymphocytes with round deeply stained nuclei. Very little colloid is present in the thyroid gland. HE ×200

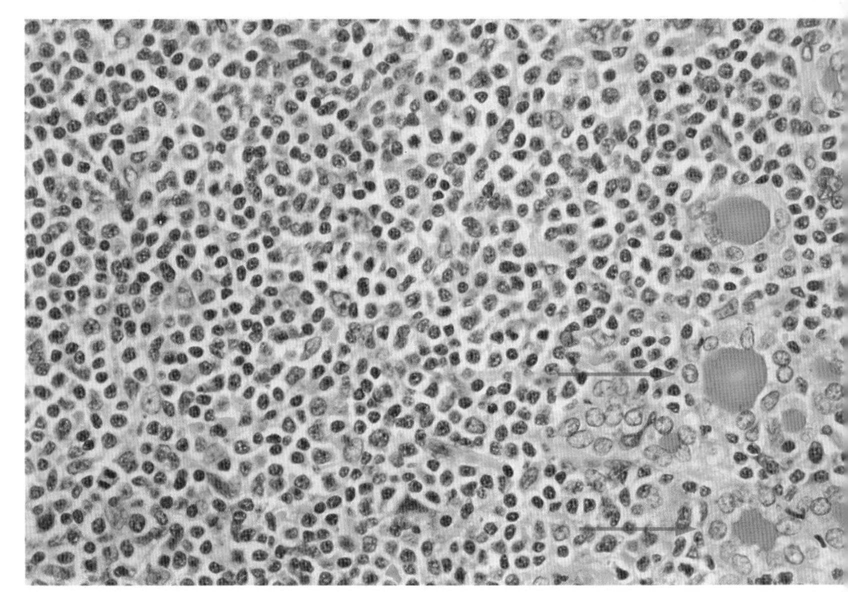

6.20 Hashimoto's thyroiditis: thyroid

Most patients with Hashimoto's thyroiditis present with gradual diffuse enlargement of the thyroid. The gland is firm and rubbery, with a coarsely nodular appearance. The gland becomes smaller as the disease progresses. Large lymphoid follicles with germinal centres are often present, along with lymphocytic infiltrate. Surviving follicular epithelial cells often acquire a considerable amount of eosinophilic cytoplasm and in this way transform into large cells termed Hürthle cells. In this case the thyroid was markedly enlarged. The few thyroid follicles that survive in this field are full of strongly eosinophilic colloid and lined by cuboidal epithelial cells with a pale round vesicular nucleus (arrows). The follicles are surrounded by a dense infiltrate of closely packed small lymphocytes and histiocytes; and the remainder of this field (and of the thyroid gland) consists mainly of sheets of similar cells. There is some mitotic activity. The monomorphic nature of the lymphocytic infiltrate suggested that lymphocytic lymphoma had developed in the gland, but the cervical lymph nodes were not involved. HE ×360

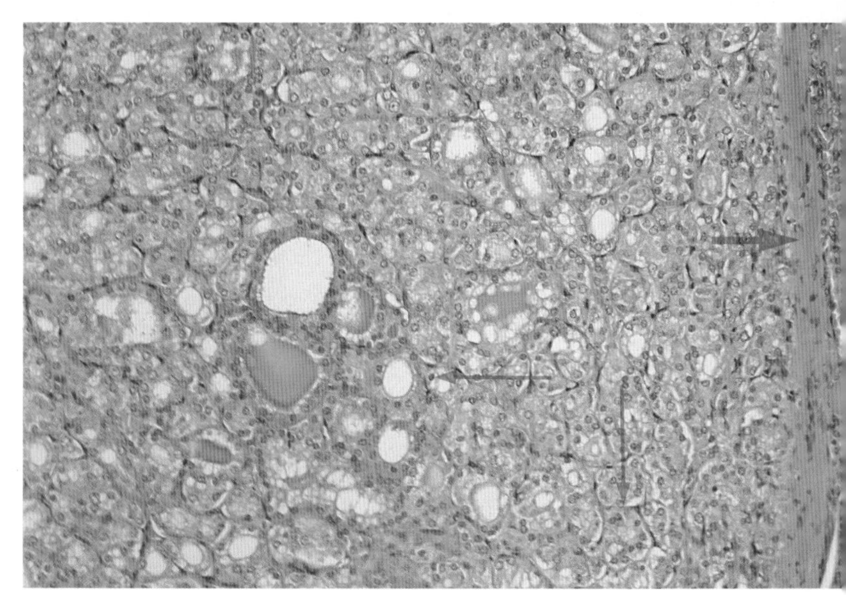

6.21 Microfollicular adenoma: thyroid

Follicular adenomas of thyroid are common lesions and usually composed of follicles of various sizes. The adenomas are generally surrounded by a complete fibrous capsule of variable thickness but, nevertheless, it is difficult and very occasionally impossible to distinguish between a true neoplasm and a localized hyperplastic nodule in e.g. a nodular goitre. It may also be difficult to distinguish a benign lesion from carcinoma. In this gland, from a woman of 35, there were multiple well-circumscribed nodular lesions. This one is a microfollicular adenoma (a so-called fetal adenoma). It is enclosed within a fairly broad band of eosinophilic fibrous tissue (thick arrow) and, apart from one decidedly larger follicle, consists of closely packed small and very small follicles (thin arrows). The follicles are lined by cuboidal epithelium, and only a few of them are filled with colloid. The colloid is vacuolated at the periphery, and close inspection reveals the presence of numerous small and very small vacuoles in the cytoplasm of the epithelial cells which line many of the follicles. In contrast, the smallest follicles lack a lumen and look 'solid'. The epithelial cells exhibit no nuclear pleomorphism or mitotic figures. HE ×235

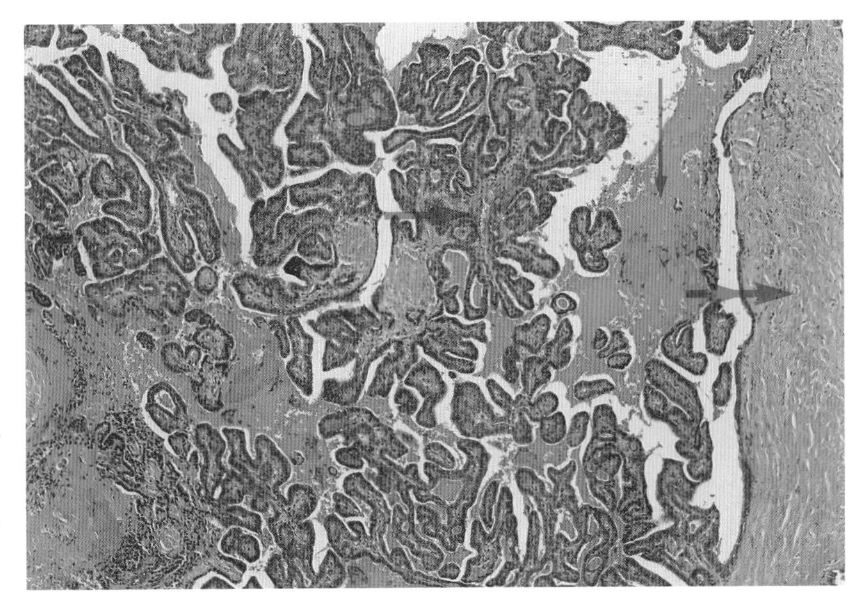

6.22 Papillary adenocarcinoma: thyroid

Papillary adenocarcinoma is the most common type of carcinoma of thyroid. It varies considerably in size, from microscopic lesions to large masses. It arises mainly in the 15-35 age group, and females form the large majority. A small minority of papillary adenocarcinomas appear to be encapsulated but, despite the relatively benign appearance of the neoplastic epithelium, they are usually infiltrative and metastasize readily to the adjacent lymph nodes. Distant metastases are infrequent. This tumour is from a man aged 70. It is a well-differentiated extremely papilliferous mass, occupying a large cystic space. Each of the very numerous branching papillary structures has a core of vascular connective tissue (thick arrow) and the surface is covered with a single layer of basophilic cuboidal epithelial cells with a small amount of cytoplasm. Within the cystic space there is a considerable amount of eosinophilic secretion and many desquamated epithelial cells (thin arrow). The cystic space is enclosed within a thick capsule of eosinophilic collagenous fibrous tissue (double arrow), but elsewhere the capsule is incomplete.

HE ×30

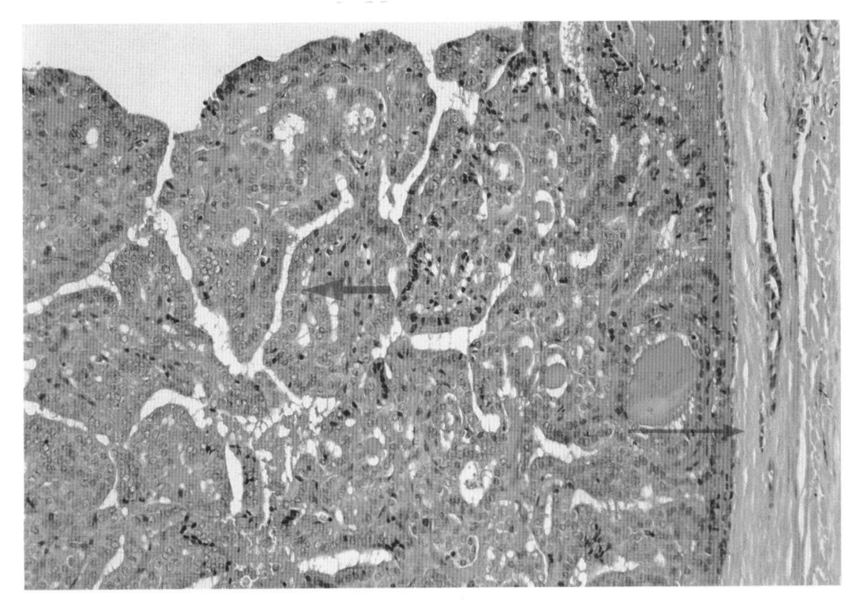

6.23 Papillary adenocarcinoma: thyroid

The incidence of thyroid cancer has increased greatly in the last 50 years, probably because of increased exposure to radiation. Radiation-induced cancers are mostly papillary- or follicular-type lesions, and young people with a history of X-irradiation to the neck are particularly liable to develop a papillary adenocarcinoma. This nodule is one of a number of nodules in the left lobe of the thyroid of a man of 47. Histologically, it has a thick 'pseudocapsule' of eosinophilic collagenous fibrous tissue (thin arrow) which was incomplete elsewhere. The tumour consists of closely packed convoluted papillae, their surfaces covered with a single layer of palisaded cuboidal or low columnar epithelial cells (thick arrow). The nuclei of the epithelial cells are relatively large, oval or round, and the chromatin is diffusely pale blue. Some of the nuclei appear 'clear' or 'empty', their appearance being artefactual but diagnostic. The papillae have a complex structure, with follicles lined with similar cells in their 'cores', and there are many papillae of this type in other parts of the tumour. Only one follicle contains colloid. Occasional mitotic figures were detectable elsewhere in the lesion, particularly in the follicular areas.

HE ×150

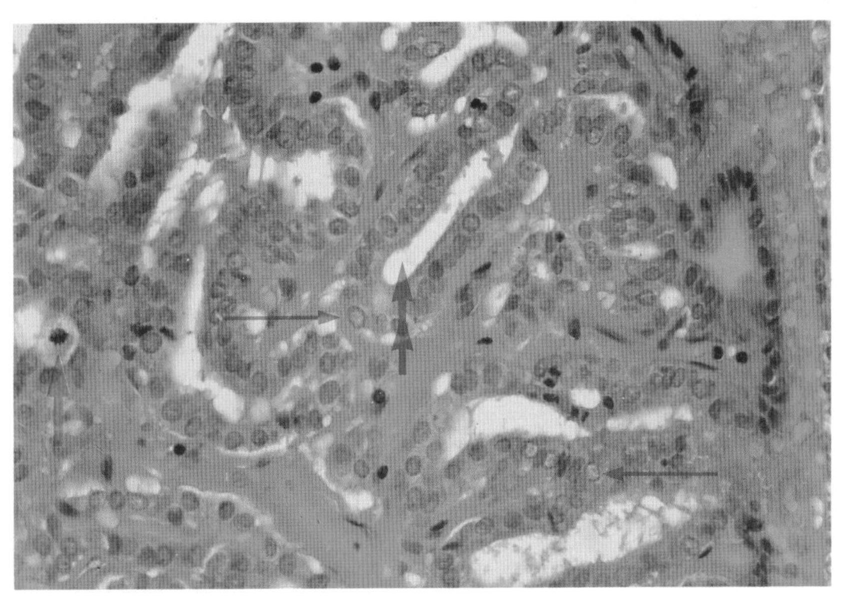

6.24 Papillary adenocarcinoma: thyroid

Papillary cancers grow very slowly and generally spread by local invasion. There are metastases in the cervical lymph nodes in about 40% of cases at presentation, and often previously misdiagnosed as 'congenitally aberrant thyroid'. Blood-borne metastasis is uncommon. This is part of the tumour in 6.23, at higher magnification. The structure appears to be follicular but its has this appearance because of the close apposition of the complex papillae. The 'follicles' (double arrow) are lined with cuboidal epithelial cells, each containing a large ovoid or round basally-located nucleus. The nuclei are of uniform size and shape, and in some of them there is a nucleolus. The nuclei are also characteristically pale-staining and 'empty-looking' (thin arrows), an appearance identical to those in the more obviously papillary areas elsewhere in the tumour. Sometimes there are nuclear grooves in the nuclei, but there are none in this field. There are several mitotic figures (thick arrow). Several nuclei are pyknotic but most of the small densely-stained nuclei are in lymphocytes. There is eosinophilic amorphous material in the stroma but no colloid within the follicles. HE ×360

6.25 Follicular carcinoma: thyroid

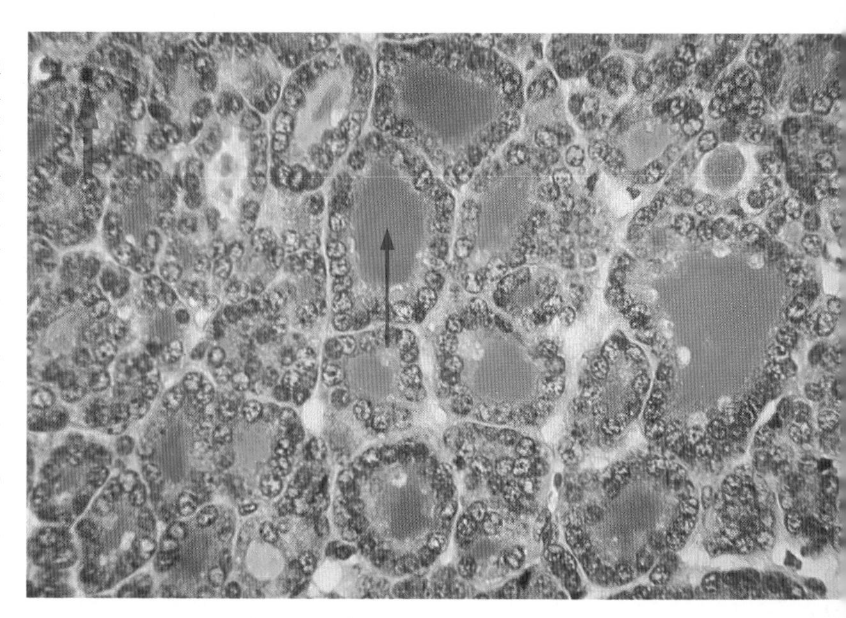

Histologically, follicular adenocarcinomas of the thyroid may be well-differentiated and difficult to distinguish from 'adenomas' (encapsulated follicular carcinoma), or it may be a large grossly infiltrative mass. Undifferentiated forms of thyroid adenocarcinoma can easily be confused with lymphomas. Follicular adenocarcinoma may arise at any age, and the survival rate is approximately 65%. This was a large locally invasive thyroid cancer in an 11-year-old girl who had had X-irradiation to her neck in infancy. It was locally invasive and recurred several times after resection. Histologically, it is well-differentiated, consisting of follicles of fairly uniform shape and variable size, filled with deeply eosinophilic colloid (thin arrow) and lined with a single layer of cuboidal epithelial cells that resemble normal thyroid cells. The lining cells have relatively large ovoid or round vesicular nuclei with a coarsely granular pattern, apart from occasional 'clear' ('empty') nuclei (clear cell variant). Although the nuclei are only slightly pleomorphic, there are scattered mitoses (thick arrow) in this field and elsewhere in the tumour.

HE ×360

6.26 Follicular carcinoma: thyroid

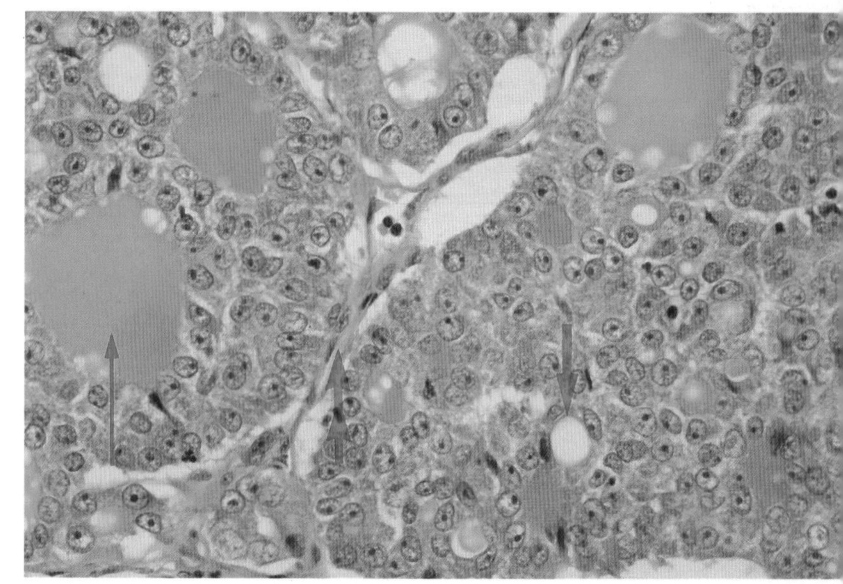

The diagnosis of follicular carcinoma depends on the presence of invasion of the capsule or vascular structures. In some tumours there are solid sheets of neoplastic cells which are pleomorphic and exhibit cytological atypia. They are also generally accompanied by increased mitotic activity. A woman of 35 had a subtotal thyroidectomy for carcinoma of the thyroid. Macroscopically there were many fleshy nodules throughout the gland, as well as areas of hemorrhage and necrosis. This is part of a nodule. The relatively large well-formed follicles are filled with fairly pale-staining colloid (thin arrow) and lined with epithelial cells which have only a small amount of cytoplasm. Each epithelial cell however has a relatively large vesicular nucleus and a prominent central nucleolus. There are also very small follicles (thick arrow) containing no colloid. To the right the very small follicles there are also solid sheets of epithelial cells. There is one mitosis in this field but others were present in considerable numbers elsewhere. A few epithelial cell nuclei are pyknotic. A delicate fibrovascular stroma is present (double arrow). Elsewhere the tumour was enclosed in a fibrous 'pseudocapsule' but it was invading a vein. HE ×360

6.27 Hürthle-cell carcinoma: thyroid

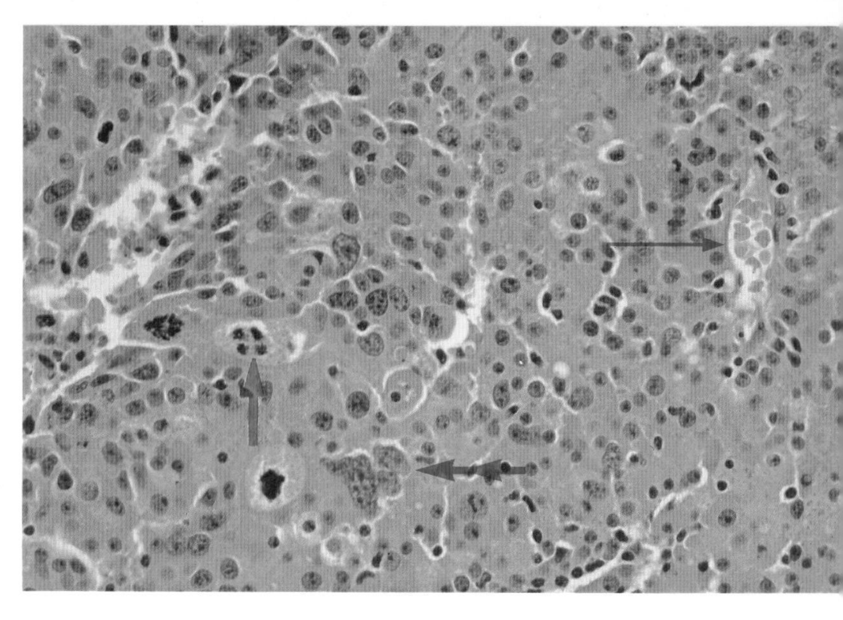

Hürthle-cell carcinoma is a rare variant of follicular carcinoma. It tends to be regarded as a highly malignant tumour but it has the same prognosis as follicular carcinoma. This tumour was an encapsulated nodule (4 × 3 × 3cm) in the right lobe of the thyroid of a woman aged 65. The cut surface showed that it was lobulated and foci of necrosis were present. Histologically, it is a solid poorly differentiated carcinoma of Hürthle-cell type, composed of sheets and trabeculae of large polyhedral epithelial cells which have very variable amounts of deeply eosinophilic cytoplasm. The cytoplasmic boundaries are ill-defined and some cells appear to be very large. The nuclei of the epithelial cells are very pleomorphic, varying greatly in size and to lesser extent in shape (double arrow). There is much mitotic activity, and some of the mitoses are abnormal (thick arrow). There is a small group of necrotic epithelial cells at the left margin. The stroma consists mainly of thin-walled blood vessels (thin arrow). HE ×360

6.28 Medullary carcinoma: thyroid

Medullary carcinoma is rare. It originates in the parafollicular cells (C cells) which usually secrete calcitonin. About 10% of the tumours are familial and may form part of the multiple endocrine adenomatosis (MEA type II) syndrome (concurrence of medullary carcinoma of thyroid, pheochromocytoma of adrenal medulla and parathyroid adenoma). It does not produce a characteristic clinical syndrome. It grows slowly but progressively, forming a solid greyish-white infiltrative mass which appears well-demarcated but often invades adjacent tissues in the neck. Histologically, it consists of sheets and clumps of compact cells (thin arrow) with small round or oval nuclei and very scant cytoplasm with ill-defined boundaries. The nuclei are only slightly pleomorphic and the texture of the chromatin is fairly smooth. No mitotic figures are present in this field. Dilated small blood vessels are also present. The most prominent feature in this field however is the presence of a large amount of amorphous weakly eosinophilic stroma (thick arrow) which contains fibrillar amyloid. The amyloid consists of calcitonin fragments (identifiable by appropriate staining methods); and there are membrane-bound dense-core neurosecretory granules (demonstrated by electron microscopy) in the cytoplasm of the tumour cells.

HE ×235

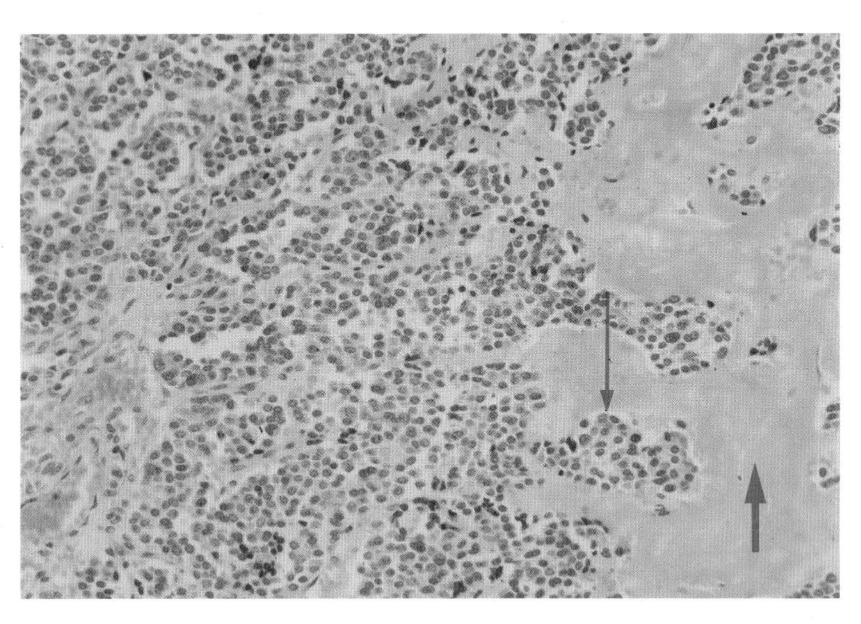

6.29 Medullary carcinoma: thyroid

Medullary carcinoma of the thyroid immunostained for calcitonin. This hormone is very frequently produced by these tumours and is used immunohistochemically to confirm the diagnosis of these carcinomas.

Medullary carcinoma of thyroid consists of solid irregular small groups and cords of neoplastic cells, and calcitonin is demonstrable in all cases. Amyloid is thought to be derived from the calcitonin precursor and detectable in about 50% of cases. The tumour spreads via both vascular and lymphatic channels, into lymph nodes and by distant metastasis.

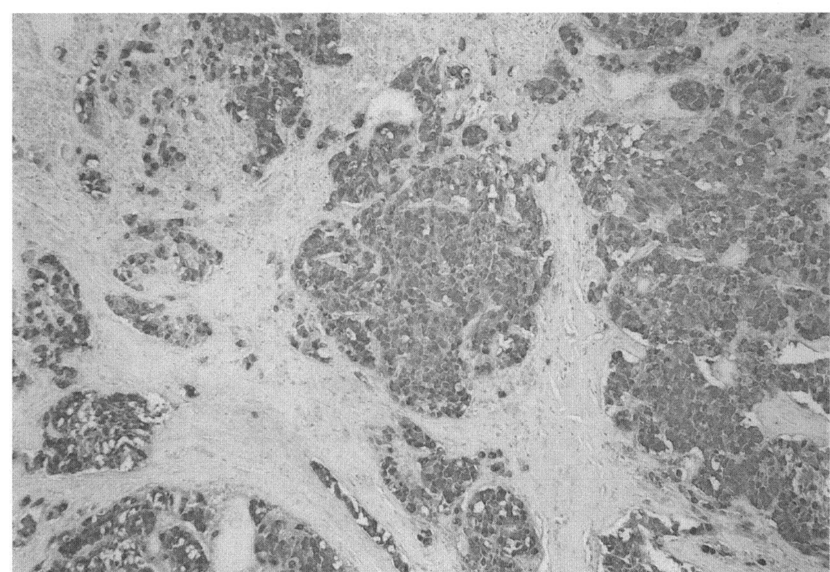

6.30 Adenoma: parathyroid

Parathyroid adenomas are yellowish-brown (tan-coloured) encapsulated ovoid nodules. They secrete parathyroid hormone (PTH), and increased secretion (the result of an intrinsic abnormality in one or more of the four glands) gives rise to primary hyperparathyroidism. Care has to taken to distinguish adenomas from hyperplasia, and the presence of normal parathyroid tissue at the periphery of an adenoma is a helpful distinguishing feature. This adenoma, with an inconspicuous fibrovascular stroma, consists of a deeply eosinophilic sheet of large neoplastic cells with round pleomorphic deeply basophilic nuclei and much strongly eosinophilic cytoplasm (thin arrow). These are oxyphil cells, and they are present in adenomas but not in hyperplastic parathyroids. Nuclear pleomorphism is very marked but of little significance. The periphery of the sheet of large neoplastic cells is sharply defined and separated from normal parathyroid tissue by a capsule of loose connective tissue. The normal parathyroid tissue consists of chief cells, small compact cells with round basophilic nuclei and a moderate amount of cytoplasm (thick arrow). HE ×150

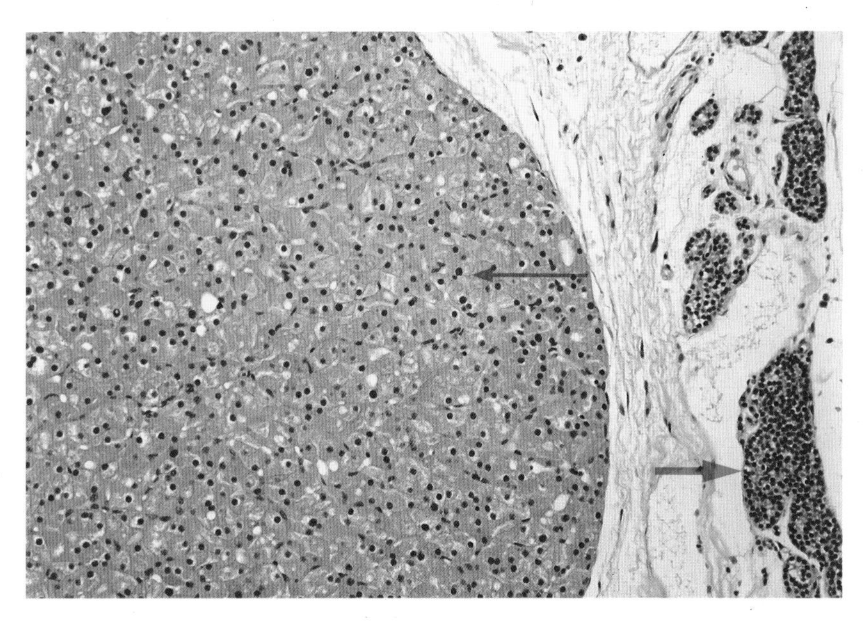

6.31 Adenoma: parathyroid

Primary hyperthyroidism is most often caused by a solitary adenoma in one parathyroid gland, and secondary hyperthyroidism (compensatory hyperplasia of all four glands) is caused by lowered serum calcium. Parathyroid adenomas are usually small (1-2cm dia) and sometimes difficult to locate. This was an ovoid mass (2.5 × 2cm) in the right lower parathyroid of a woman of 75. The cut surface was tan-coloured. The predominant cell is the oxyphil cell. Oxyphil cells have abundant deeply eosinophilic cytoplasm (thin arrow) and form sheets or cords. The cells are closely apposed, and the cytoplasmic boundaries, although they appear to be ill-defined, can be identified. The nuclei are basophilic and show a striking degree of pleomorphism, ranging from small round nuclei to extremely large hyperchromatic forms (double arrows). There is no mitotic activity in this field however and little elsewhere in the tumour. Nuclear pleomorphism in lesions of this type does not denote malignancy. The stroma consists of delicate connective tissue and thin-walled blood vessels (thick arrow). Adenomas composed entirely of oxyphil cells (oxyphil adenomas) do not as a rule secrete a significant excess of parathyroid hormone. HE ×235

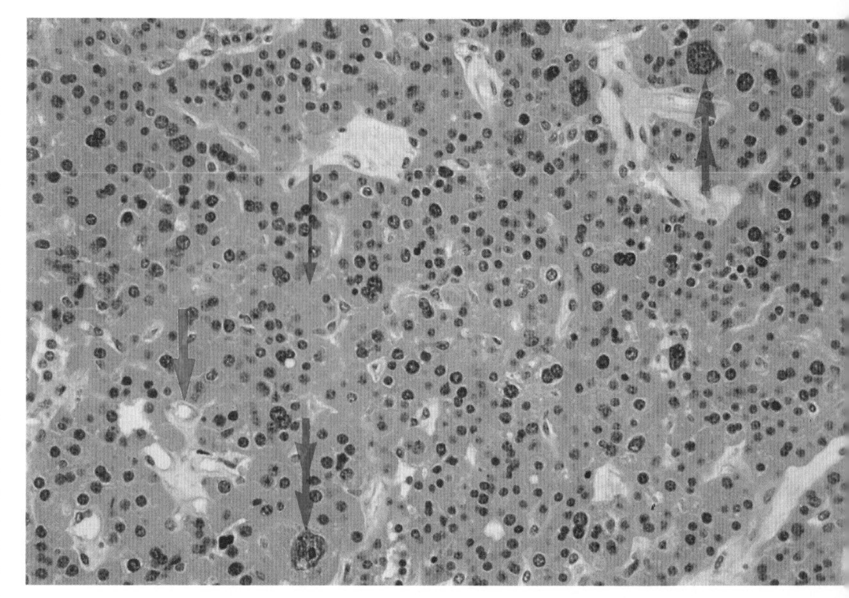

6.32 Adenoma: parathyroid

Parathyroid adenomas are composed of a mixture of chief cells, water-clear cells and oxyphil cells which form sheets, trabeculae and/or glandular structures. The cells are, as general rule, fairly small and uniform in size and shape. Hormone levels do not always correspond with the predominant type of cell. Mitotic activity is very uncommon. A parathyroid adenoma can be differentiated from a normal parathyroid gland by its increased size and the absence of fat. This was an ovoid nodule (1 × 1.5cm) in the right upper parathyroid of a woman of 46. The cut surface was dark brown, and histologically it consisted mainly of chief cells with occasional groups of oxyphil cells and 'water--clear' cells. This part of the adenoma however is a chief cell region. The tissue consists of closely packed chief cells, arranged in a solid mass (thin arrow) and forming no acini. The cells have a moderate amount of cytoplasm and uniformly round nuclei with finely granular chromatin. The stroma is inconspicuous, consisting of delicate connective tissue and small blood vessels. There is a mitotic figure (thick arrow) but the tumour is benign, carcinoma of parathyroid being extremely rare. HE ×360

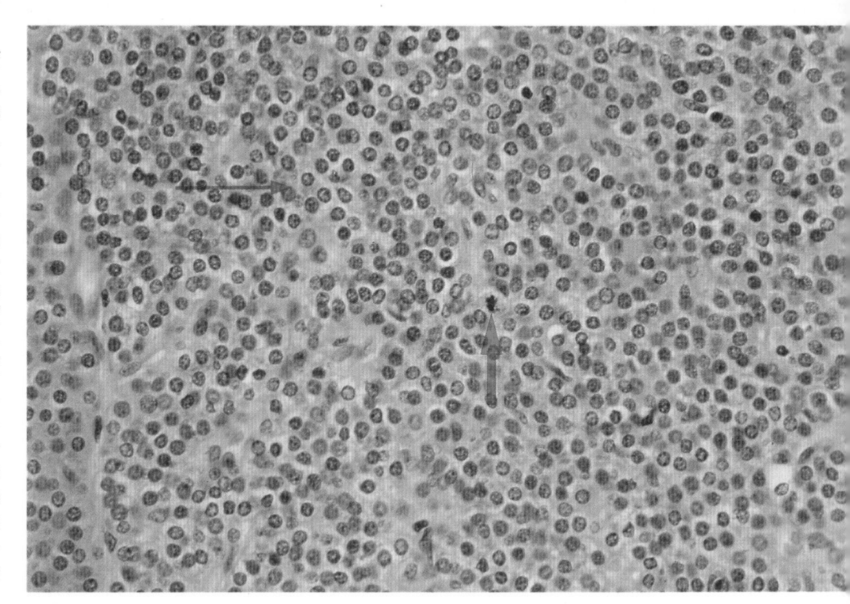

6.33 Adenoma: parathyroid

It is often difficult to differentiate between hyperplasia of a parathyroid gland from an adenoma of parathyroid. If a second parathyroid gland is biopsied and found to be histologically abnormal, the (first) gland is hyperplastic. If however the second gland is normal, the lesion in the first gland is a parathyroid adenoma. This is part of the same adenoma as in **8.31**. The tissue consists of closely packed neoplastic cells with uniformly compact round nuclei, similar to those of chief cells. The cells have abundant cytoplasm and prominent well-defined cytoplasmic membranes. The cytoplasm of almost all the neoplastic cells is 'water-clear', from the presence in it of several large ('empty') vacuoles (thick arrow). 'Water-clear' cells are rarely the major component of a parathyroid adenoma. The stroma is inconspicuous, consisting mainly of a delicate network of small inconspicuous blood vessels. One of the blood vessels however (presumably a vein) is greatly dilated (thin arrow) and lined with large elongated endothelial cells with vesicular nuclei. HE ×360

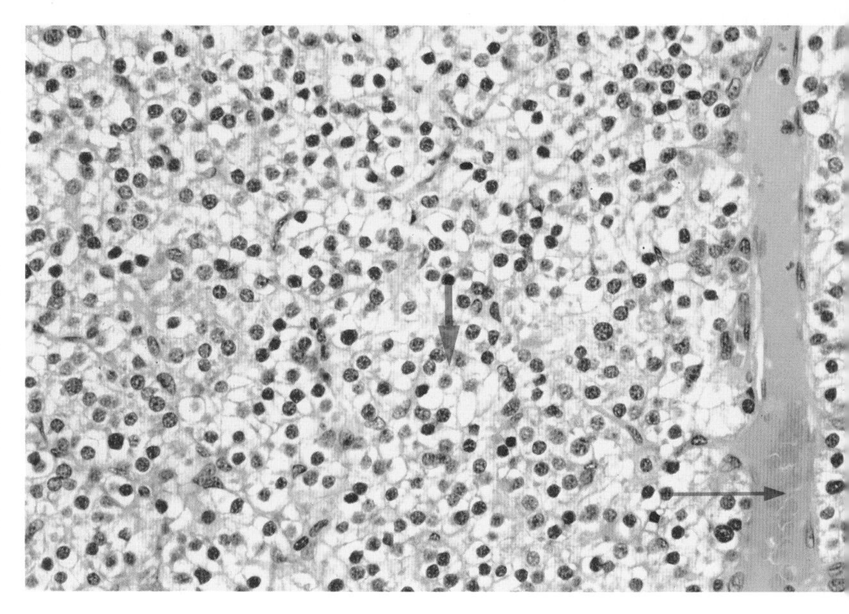

6.34 Adenoma: adrenal cortex

Adenomas of the adrenal cortex form well-circumscribed nodules, which are usually less than 5cm dia (a cortical nodule more than 1cm dia is probably an adenoma). The nodules are a bright yellow colour from their content of lipid and steroid hormones, and sometimes develop foci of cystic degeneration. The tumour cells secrete hormone(s), and if the amount is sufficient, clinical signs and symptoms are produced. This tumour is from a woman of 53 on whom it had a virilizing effect. It was a firm apparently-encapsulated yellowish mass 1.5cm dia. It is cortical adenoma, composed of small groups and trabeculae of large neoplastic cells (thin arrows), separated by hyalinized stroma. The neoplastic cells have varying amounts of eosinophilic cytoplasm, occasionally vacuolated, with well-defined boundaries. Their nuclei are moderately pleomorphic but there are no mitoses. The neoplastic cells in some groups are arranged in a pseudoglandular pattern. At the right margin there is a thick capsule of eosinophilic collagenous fibrous tissue, and between the capsule and the adenoma there is a thin layer of compressed normal (non-neoplastic) adrenocortical cells with vacuolated (mostly clear) cytoplasm (thick arrow) and round deeply basophilic nuclei. HE ×150

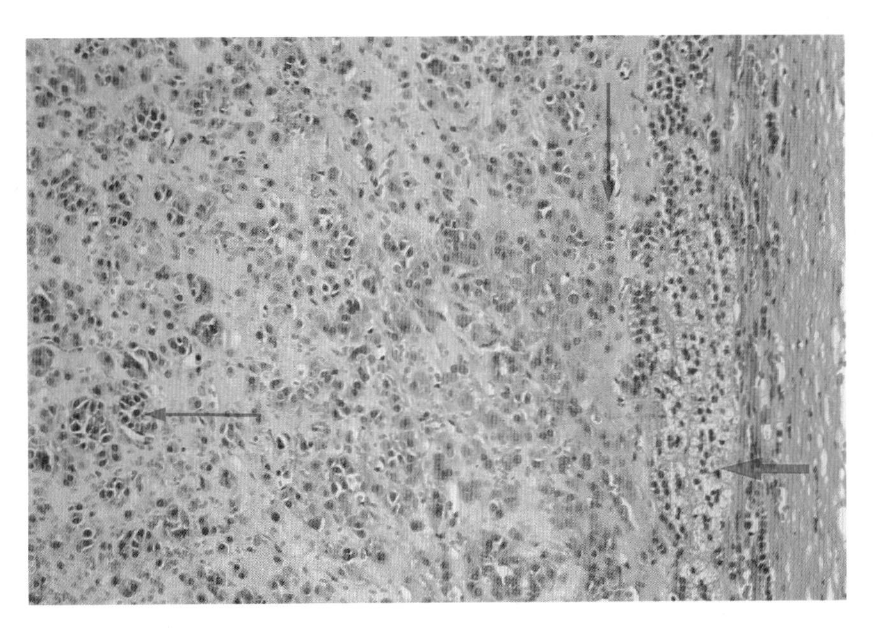

6.35 Carcinoma: adrenal cortex

Carcinoma of the adrenal arises from the cortex and is generally highly malignant. Lymphatic and hematogenous spread readily occurs. It is usually a large (more than 20cm dia) mass at the time of diagnosis. The tumour is poorly circumscribed, often infiltrating the perinephric fat and kidney and metastasizing to the lymph nodes and via the bloodstream. It may secrete hormones, sometimes non-steroidal, but some neoplasms are non-secretory. The cut surface is characteristically yellow, but necrosis and hemorrhage are generally prominent. Histologically, as in this lesion, the neoplastic cells are extremely pleomorphic, the amount of granular eosinophilic cytoplasm ranging from a large amount to enormous (thin arrow). The cells are closely packed and tend to be ovoid or elongated in shape. The nuclei of the tumour cells vary greatly in size and shape, from small round nuclei to very large hyperchromatic forms (double arrow). Some cells are multinucleated. Many nuclei have prominent nucleoli, and in the largest nuclei the chromatin is very coarsely granular. In this nucleus there is an eosinophilic cytoplasmic inclusion (thick arrow), and there are similar inclusions of various sizes in other nuclei. HE ×235

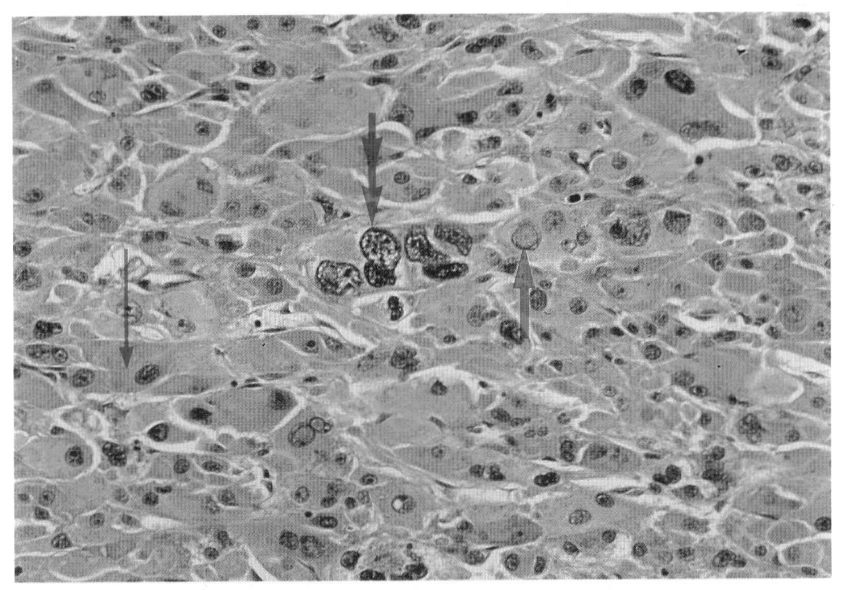

6.36 Pheochromocytoma: adrenal medulla

Although pheochromocytomas usually arise sporadically, from the chromaffin cells of the adrenal medulla and uncommonly from chromaffin cells elsewhere (extra-adrenal paraganglia), a small minority give a positive family history for a wide range of other diseases. A similar percentage of other patients have multiple pheochromocytomas. Most pheochromocytomas are benign but about 10% are malignant, with local invasion and metastasis. The high levels of catecholamines secreted by the tumour cells give rise to a variety of signs and symptoms, most notably systemic hypertension. This tumour was a bosselated mass (5 × 4 × 3.5cm), cystic and with a firm capsule, in the right adrenal of a woman of 56. It consists of a sheet of large closely packed polyhedral cells, arranged around small inconspicuous stromal blood vessels (thick arrows). The tumour cells have a large amount of granular strongly eosinophilic cytoplasm, apparently with well-defined cytoplasmic boundaries, and a large round or ovoid nucleus in which there is (occasionally) one or more nucleoli. There is slight nuclear pleomorphism, but a pleomorphic appearance may be more pronounced without signifying malignancy. HE ×360

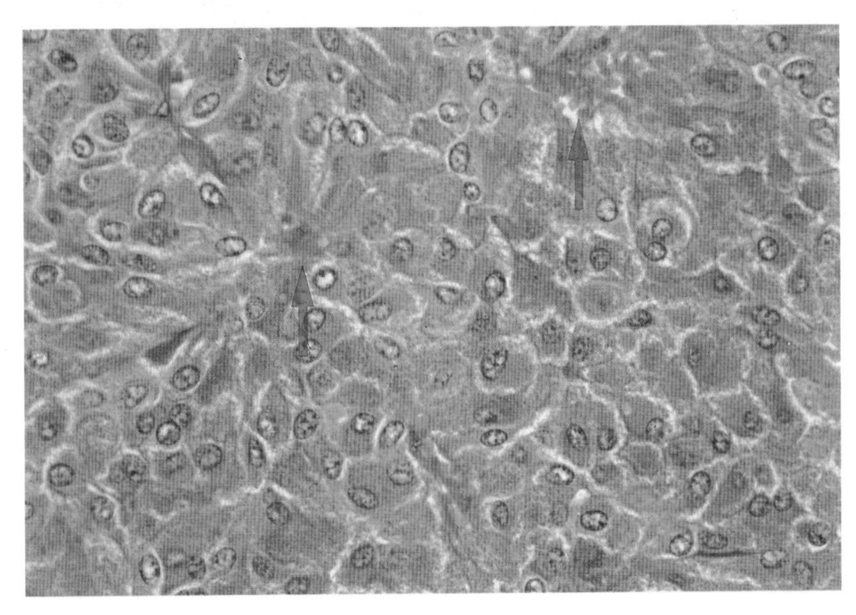

6.37 Neuroblastoma: adrenal medulla

Neuroblastomas are highly malignant, arising most often in the adrenal medulla and less often in neural crest derivatives in the retroperitoneum. It is composed of primitive neural crest cells - neuroblasts - and mainly affects infants and very young children. It tends to form a large soft hemorrhagic mass, often accompanied by widespread secondaries in lymph nodes, liver and bones. Slightly increased amounts of catecholamines may be secreted, and their metabolites such as VMA (vanillyl mandelic acid) and HVA (homovanillic acid) may be excreted in the urine. This tumour, a secondary deposit in skeletal muscle, consists of a sheet of malignant cells with very little cytoplasm and round or ovoid nuclei (the heavily stained chromatin tends to obscure mitotic activity). There are numerous circular rosettes of uniform size, consisting of a central eosinophilic mass (thin arrow), surrounded by closely packed tumour cells. The mass consists of fine filaments which originate in the tumour cells, and the nuclei of the innermost tumour cells are irregularly palisaded. Several small stromal blood vessels are visible (thick arrow). HE ×360

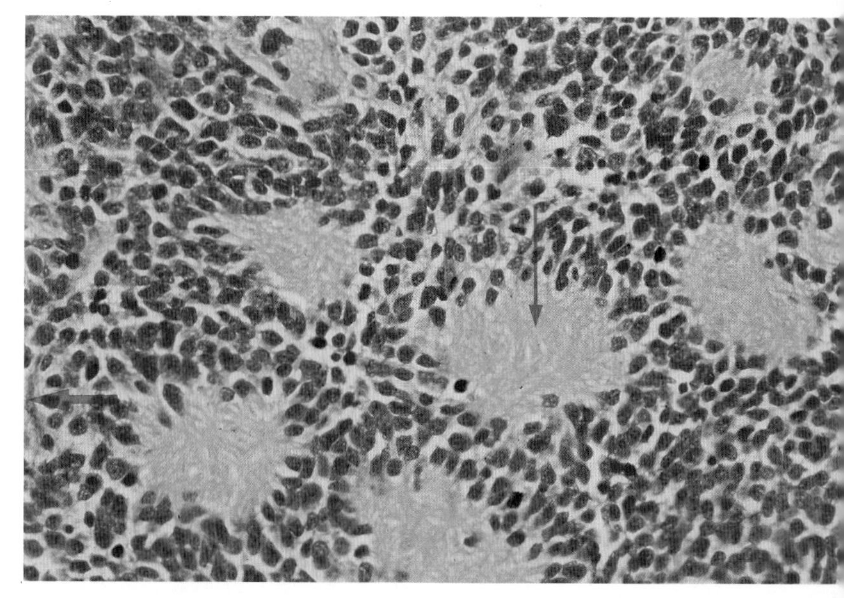

6.38 Islet cell hyperplasia: pancreas

Islet cell hyperplasia is often seen in fetuses born of diabetic mothers as a response by the fetal pancreas, during the pregnancy, to the high glucose environment in the mother. The infant may suffer from severe hypoglycemia. Islet cell hyperplasia sometimes occurs in adults, and if the increase is mainly in B (beta) cells, enough insulin may be secreted to produce hypoglycemia. This is the pancreas of an adult who presented with the signs of hypoglycemia. Two compact islets are shown (thin arrows), both increased in size, that on the left 265μm dia and the other on the right 465μm dia. They are surrounded by strands of eosinophilic collagenous fibrous tissue. The islets are vascular, being traversed by a complex inconspicuous network of capillaries. The islet cells range from small to very large. Likewise their nuclei, mostly round and vesicular, vary greatly in size and shape. Most of the islets elsewhere in the pancreas are similarly enlarged. The exocrine tissue is normal, consisting of compact acini lined by epithelial cells with a considerable amount of eosinophilic cytoplasm and small round basal nuclei (thick arrow). HE ×150

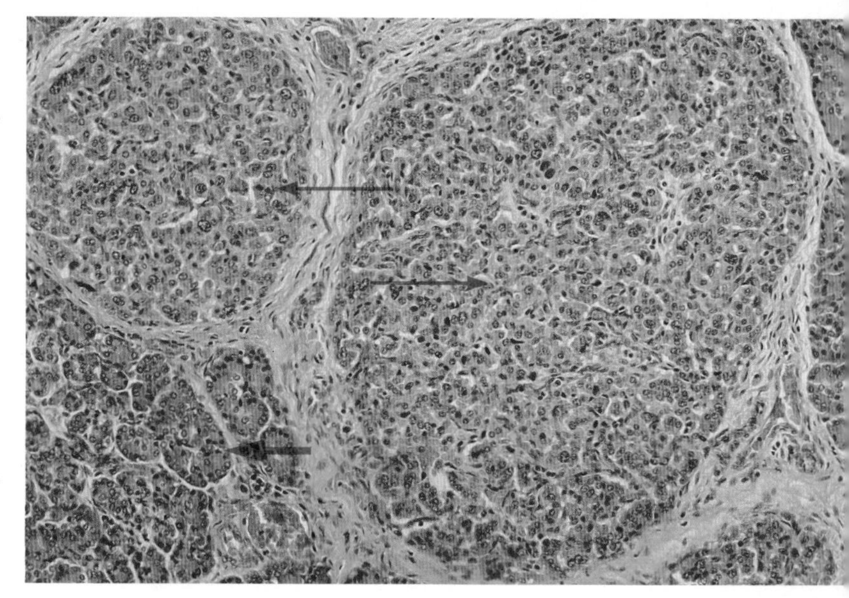

6.39 Islet cell adenomatosis: pancreas

Adenomas derived from islet cells are relatively common and islets of Langerhans more than 700μm dia are microadenomas. Islet cell tumours can secrete a variety of hormones in addition to insulin and produce a range of clinical syndromes. When there are hyperplastic islets in a resected pancreas, a careful search for an adenoma should be made in the remaining pancreas. A soft tumour 2cm dia in the head of pancreas, not encapsulated, was resected. It consists of pleomorphic groups of cells, surrounded by vascular connective tissue and fat and heavily infiltrated by small lymphocytes. There is no fibrous capsule. The groups of cells are well-defined (thick arrow) and intersected by large thin-walled blood vessels (thin arrow) and numerous small lymphocytes. The tumour cells have fairly uniform ovoid or round nuclei and a moderate amount of eosinophilic cytoplasm. Multiple other groups of cells, varied in size and poorly-defined, were found in the surrounding pancreatic tissue and considered to be multiple primary tumours. Special stains gave results consistent with a B (beta) cell origin. The patient suffered from hypoglycemic episodes. HE ×235

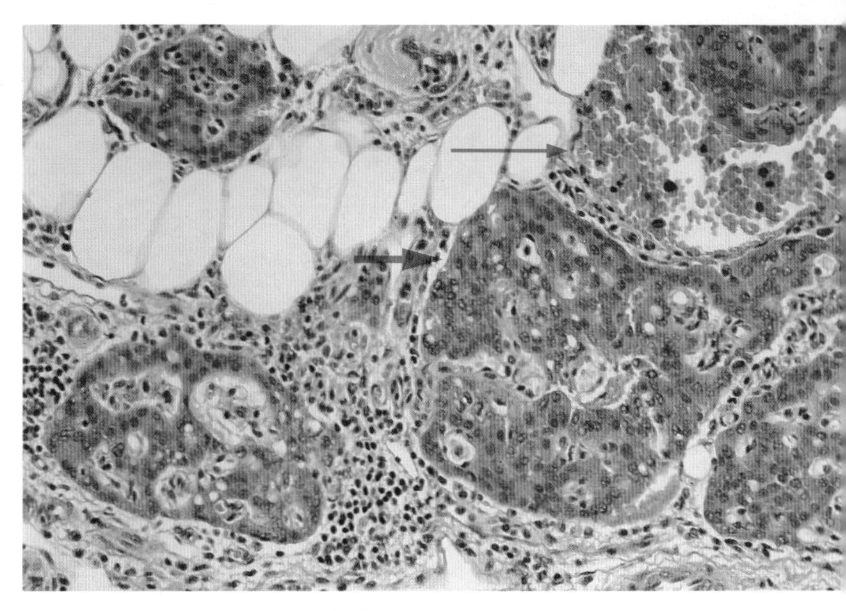

6.40 Islet cell carcinoma: pancreas

Islet cell carcinomas do occur, but less frequently than islet cell adenomas. About 10% of islet cell tumours metastasize and are regarded as carcinomas. This patient suffered from hypoglycemia. An ill-defined mass (approximately 1cm dia) was found within the head of pancreas. The tumour consisted of fairly well-demarcated nodules of neoplastic cells, and in this field the histological structure of part of one of the nodules is shown. The neoplastic tissue consists of sheets and cords (thin arrow) of neoplastic cells, and is traversed by numerous bands of hyalinized connective tissue and blood vessels (thick arrow). The neoplastic cells are fairly uniform in size and shape, with relatively large ovoid or round basophilic nuclei and a very moderate amount of cytoplasm. This nodule looks round and well-defined, but it is surrounded by an incomplete 'capsule' of fibrous tissue and extravasated blood (double arrow). The nodules of tumour elsewhere are similarly not encapsulated, and the tumour mass was found to invade adjacent tissues. HE ×150

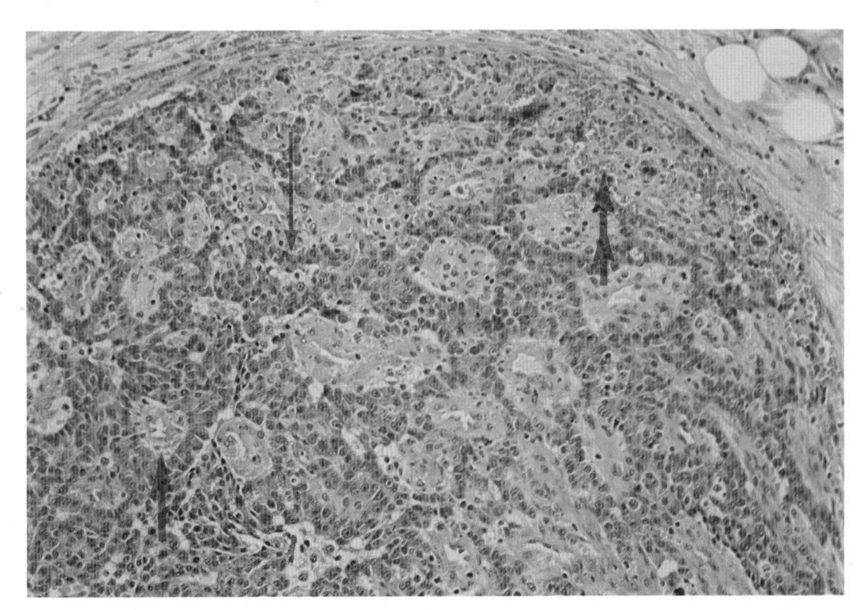

6.41 Islet cell carcinoma: pancreas

This is part of the same tumour as in 6.40, at higher magnification. It consists of cords and sheets of tumour cells (thin arrows), intersected by vascular stroma (thick arrow), the fibrous tissue of which is hyalinized and eosinophilic. The neoplastic cells have a very moderate amount of faintly basophilic cytoplasm and their nuclei are relatively large and moderately pleomorphic. They are also round or ovoid and, although the chromatin is coarsely granular, there are prominent nucleoli in many of the nuclei. There are no mitotic figures in this field but they are numerous elsewhere in the tumour. The cytoplasm of the tumour cells gave a positive argyrophil reaction, but it is difficult to predict the clinical behaviour of an islet cell tumour solely from its histological structure (unaided otherwise). In this case however a lymph node had been almost entirely replaced by metastatic tumour, and metastases were also present in the liver. HE ×360

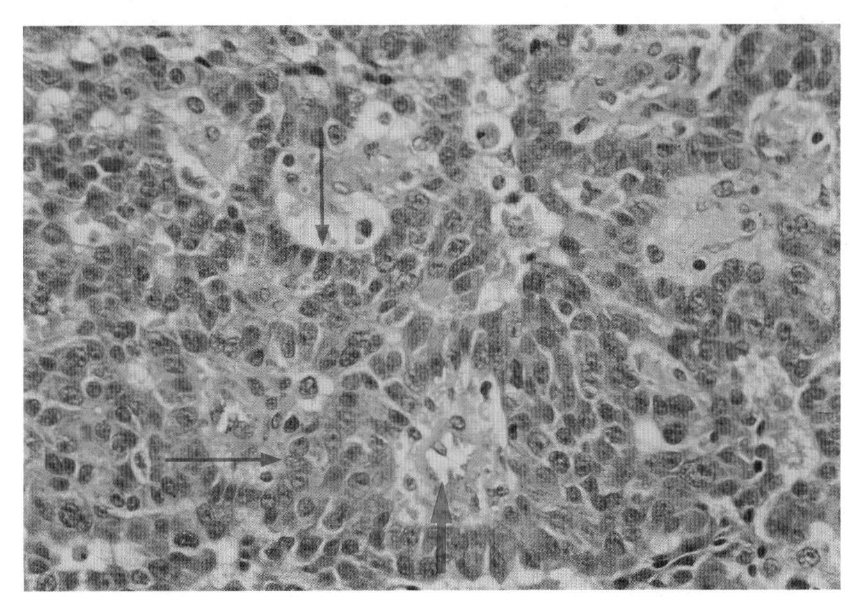

6.42 Islet cell carcinoma: pancreas

This is part of the same tumour as in 6.40 and 6.41. To identify the hormone secreted by the tumour cells, paraffin sections of the tumour were treated by the indirect immunoperoxidase method with antibodies against insulin, glucagon and somatostatin. The sections treated with anti-glucagon and anti-somatostatin gave a negative result. However, in this section, treated with the antibody against alpha-insulin, granular brown reaction product is present in the basal region of the tumour cells (thin arrow). This confirms that they are B (beta) cells. The abundant stroma consists mainly of hyaline, pale and amorphous (amyloid-like) material (double arrow) but also of small inconspicuous blood vessels (thick arrow). The pale finely granular vesicular structure of the nuclei of the tumour cells is well shown. There are also several nucleoli in many of the nuclei.

Indirect immunoperoxidase method for alpha-insulin ×470

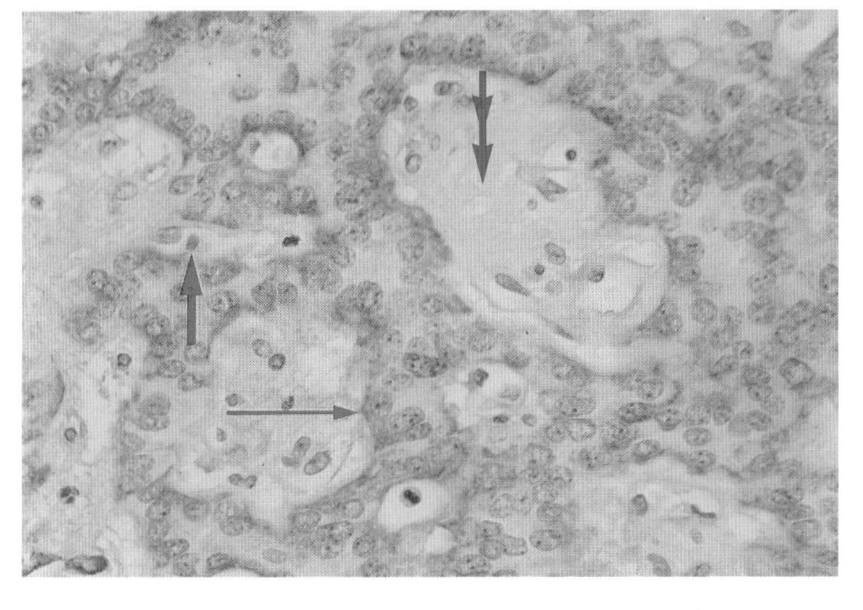

7.1 Fat necrosis: breast

Fat necrosis is an uncommon but important disease of the breast, occurring on a scale large enough to produce a firm but not stony-hard mass which may simulate carcinoma. Its etiology is unknown. It occurs more often in pendulous breasts, and there is some association with trauma. However the role of physical trauma to the breast is now thought to be relatively insignificant. Fat released from necrotic fat cells provokes a vigorous reaction which soon becomes more chronic and granulomatous. The lump is often attached to the overlying skin but not to the deeper tissues and it does not cause retraction of the nipple. Differentiating fat necrosis from carcinoma requires histological examination. This lesion (1.5cm dia) was in the axillary tail of the breast of a woman of 76. It is a granulomatous mass, consisting of sheets of histiocytes, lymphocytes and plasma cells. Among them there are also many large vacuoles and smaller cysts (thick arrows) which contained extracellular neutral fat. The fat had been released from necrotic fat cells, but it was dissolved by processing reagents and the spaces are now clear (empty). Several multinucleated giant cells are also present, as well as hyaline areas of necrosis (thin arrow). HE ×150

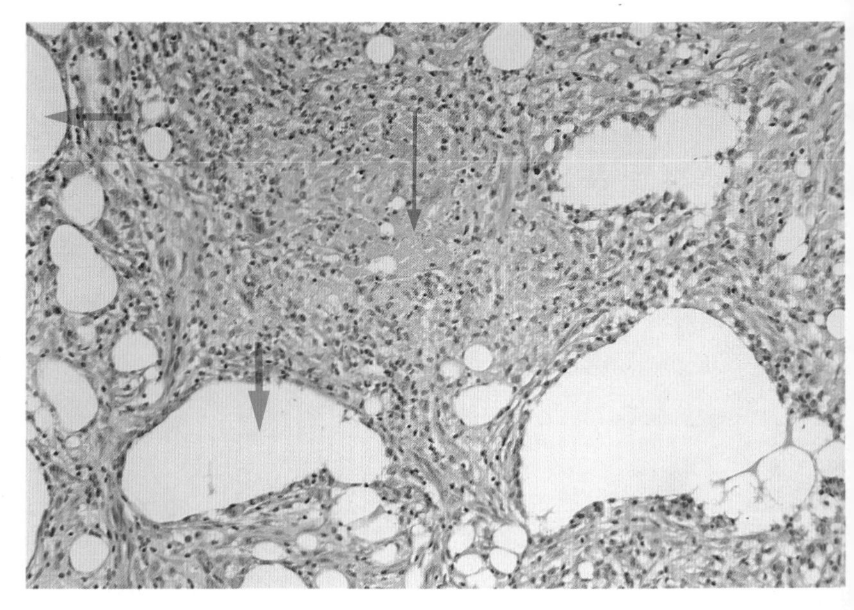

7.2 Fat necrosis: breast

The early stage of fat necrosis is characterized by clusters of neutrophil leukocytes and histiocytes around necrotic fat cells (adipocytes), and the necrotic tissue is subsequently replaced by granulation tissue and collagenous tissue. Calcification also may occur. This is part of the same lesion as in 7.1, at higher magnification. In it there are several large empty (clear) vacuoles, spaces which contained droplets of extracellular fat (but dissolved by tissue-processing reagents). The flat-surfaced cells in close contact with the extracellular fat are mostly macrophages with much eosinophilic cytoplasm (thin arrows) and some of them have a large pale vesicular nucleus with finely granular chromatin. In the surrounding tissues there are also many fairly similar but more rounded macrophages with foamy (lipid-laden) cytoplasm (thick arrows). Considerable numbers of plasma cells (double arrows) are present, as well as occasional small lymphocytes. Elongated fibroblasts are starting to lay down fibrous connective tissue, with many small vacuoles. HE ×360

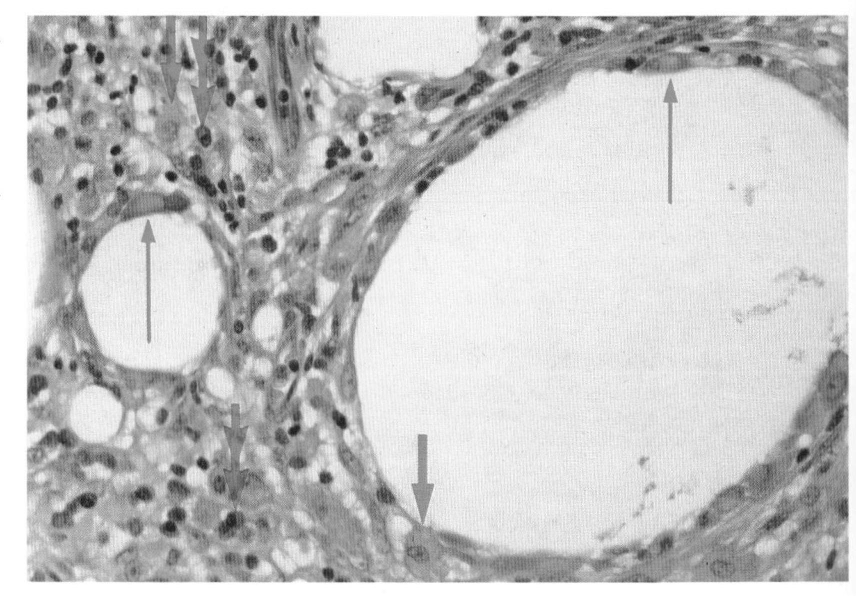

7.3 Fibroadenoma: breast

Fibroadenomas of the breast are 'mixed' tumours which are composed of both epithelial and connective tissue components. They are very common benign tumours which tend to be found in younger women (20-35 years) but occur at all ages. They increase in size in pregnancy but often regress with age and may calcify. They are generally encapsulated and firm, with a uniformly greyish-white cut surface. They very rarely become malignant. In this case, the fibroadenoma takes the form of a firm well-defined mass, up to about 3cm dia. Some compressed normal breast is visible on the right, and between it and the fibroadenoma there is a well-formed capsule which consist of collagenous fibrous tissue (thick arrow) and a small number of fibrocytes. The fibroadenoma has a well-developed pericanalicular pattern, i.e. it consists of elongated sinuous ducts (thin arrow), surrounded by myxomatous but uniformly cellular connective tissue (double arrow). These neoplastic ducts are larger and more basophilic than those in the normal breast tissue, and they are lined by a single layer of cuboidal epithelial cells with scant cytoplasm and a round hyperchromatic nucleus. The lumen of most of the ducts contains eosinophilic secretion. HE ×95

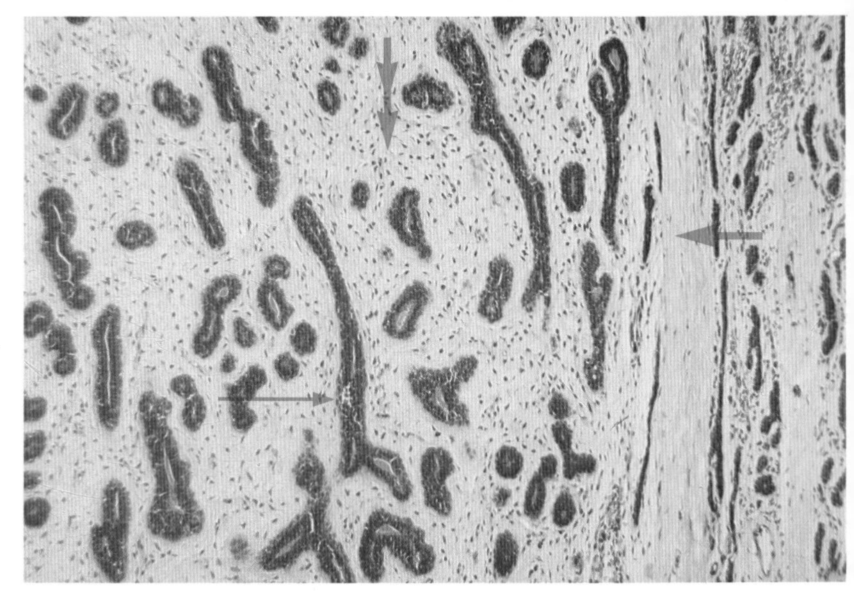

7.4 Fibroadenoma: breast

The relevant amount of each component (glandular and stromal) caries from case to case. In 'pericanalicular' fibroadenomas the glandular component is dominant, whereas the stroma dominates in 'intracanalicular' fibroadenoma. In the latter the connective-tissue element proliferates more actively than the epithelial component, and in effect 'grows into' the ducts, which then appear to be stretched out over the lobules of connective tissue, thereby creating an 'intracanalicular' pattern, as clearly evident in this fibroadenoma. The connective-tissue component (thin arrow) forms lobular masses of myxomatous pale-staining myxomatous tissue, intersected by greatly elongated slender ducts (thick arrow). The lobular masses are large and mutually compressed. The ducts are lined by a single blue-stained epithelial cells, but some of them are relatively wide and moderately distended by collections of proliferated epithelial cells. The nodules of intracanalicular fibroadenomatous tissue are surrounded by bands of dense eosinophilic collagenous fibrous tissue (double arrow). Both intracanalicular and pericanalicular patterns are not uncommonly present in the same fibroadenoma. The different patterns have no clinical significance. HE ×38

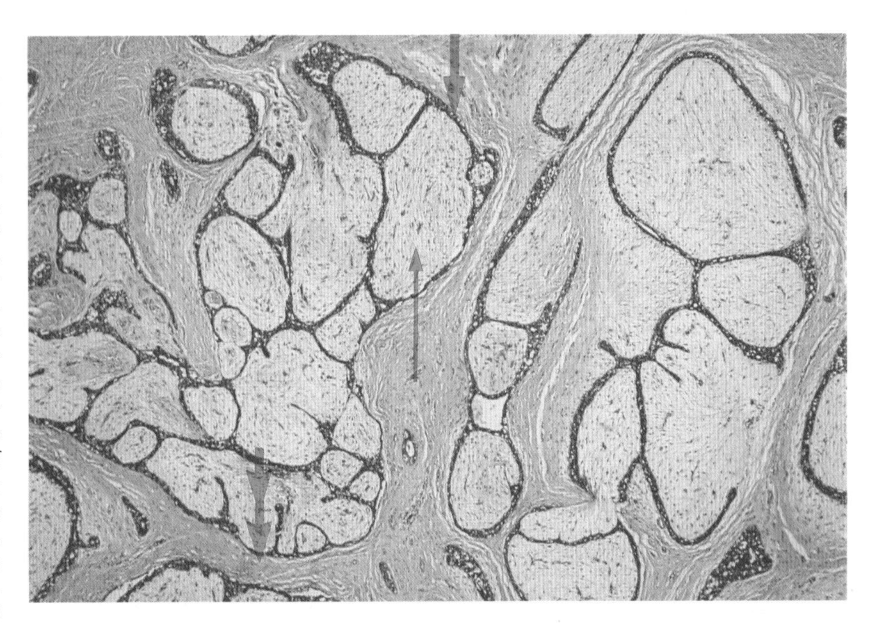

7.5 Ductal papilloma: breast

Ductal papillomas of the breast are benign neoplasms but vary considerably in their structure, from obviously benign lesions to malignant growths. They often arise in a major lactiferous duct near the nipple, and may be multiple or single (an 'isolated' or 'solitary' lesion). The larger tumours take the form of a subareolar mass and are palpable. Single papillomas are usually small however (not more than 1cm dia) and generally present with bleeding from the nipple, as happened with this benign lesion in a dilated duct in the breast of a woman of 61. The wall of the duct consists of dense hyalinized fibrous tissue (double arrow) and the duct is lined by a single layer of flattened epithelium. The surface of the intraductal papilloma is smooth and covered with a single layer of very attenuated epithelial cells which is deficient in places. The papilloma consists of numerous small irregular glands (thin arrows) and a large amount of moderately cellular fibrous stroma (thick arrow). Some of the glands are lined by cuboidal epithelial cells and others by atrophic epithelium. There is no nuclear pleomorphism or mitotic activity in the epithelial cells. HE ×150

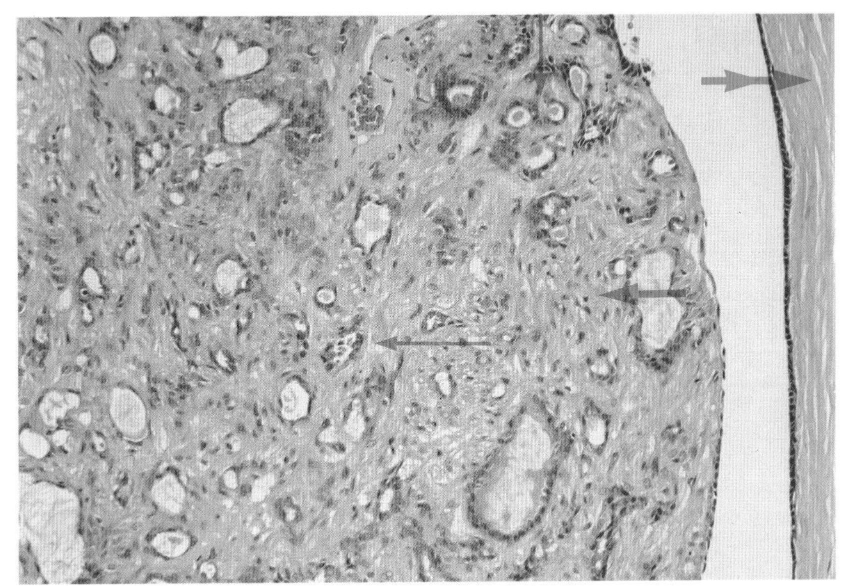

7.6 Ductal papilloma: breast

A typical ductal papillomas is a papillary mass which projects into the lumen of a large duct, consisting (histologically) of numerous papilliform processes. The processes have a core of fibrovascular tissue and are covered with a layer of epithelial and myoepithelial cells. This papilloma is from a woman of 61. The duct is cystic and lined by a single layer of flat epithelial cells, and it has a wall of hyalinized fibrous tissue (double arrow). The papilloma consists of elongated slender papilliform processes, with a core of connective tissue and delicate thin-walled blood vessels (thick arrow) and a layer of epithelial cells on the surface. The surface of the papilloma (and where the papilliform processes are probably compressed) is lined a single layer of flattened (compressed) epithelial cells. In contrast, most of the surfaces of the papilliform processes are covered with a layer of tall columnar epithelial cells and beneath it a layer of myoepithelial cells (thin arrows). The presence of the double layer of cells indicates that the lesion is benign. The thin-walled blood vessels in the stroma of the papilliform processes tend to bleed, bleeding from the nipple being a common presenting sign. HE ×150

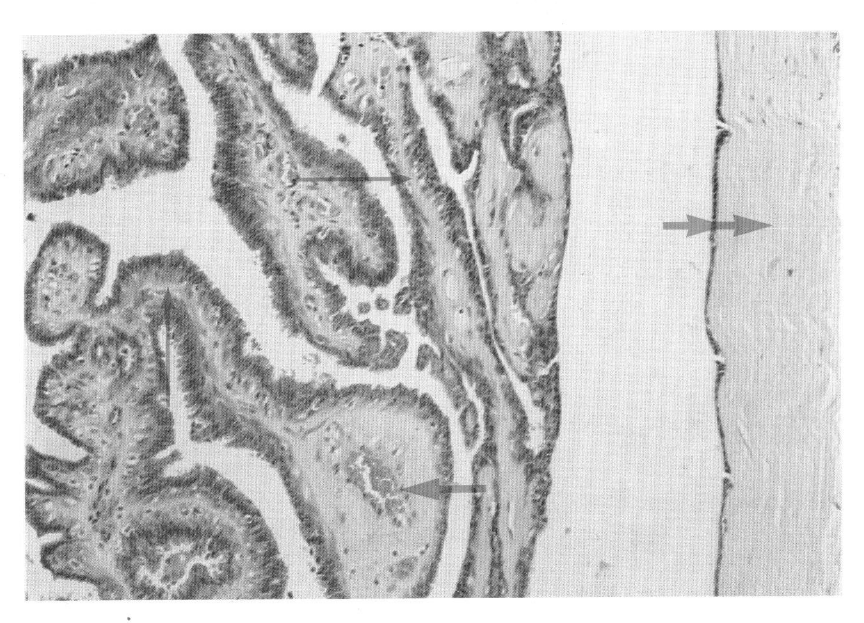

7.7 Phyllodes tumour (Cystosarcoma Phyllodes): breast

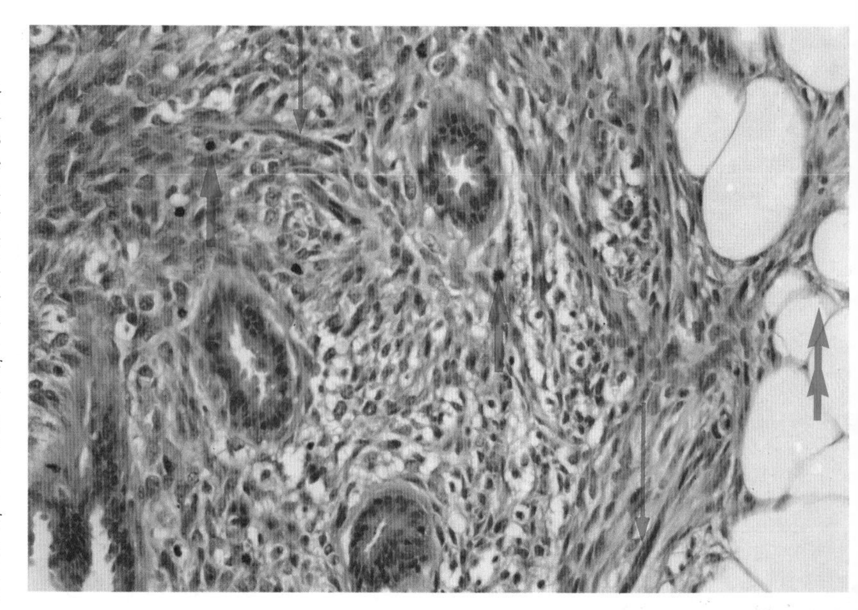

Cystosarcoma phyllodes is an imprecise term based on a particular ('leaf-like') naked-eye appearance. A typical tumour occurs in middle-aged women and it often forms a large mass with areas of cystic degeneration. In a large majority of cases it is a low-grade malignant neoplasm which infiltrates locally and has tendency to recur locally after simple excision. In a minority of cases however, it behaves as a high grade neoplasm, metastasizing to distal sites and particularly to the lungs. Histologically it is a mixture of abundant sarcomatous connective tissue and benign ductal structures. This tumour was a well-circumscribed nodular white mass 5cm dia in a woman of 61. Characteristically the predominant element is highly cellular connective tissue, composed largely of interlacing bundles of fibroblast-like cells (thin arrows) among which there are numerous mitoses (thick arrows). The connective tissue is invading adjacent fatty tissue (double arrow). The epithelial element of the neoplasm consists of small ducts lined by plump cuboidal epithelial cells. The epithelial cells lining ducts are well-differentiated and show no mitotic activity. HE ×235

7.8 Fibrocystic disease of breast

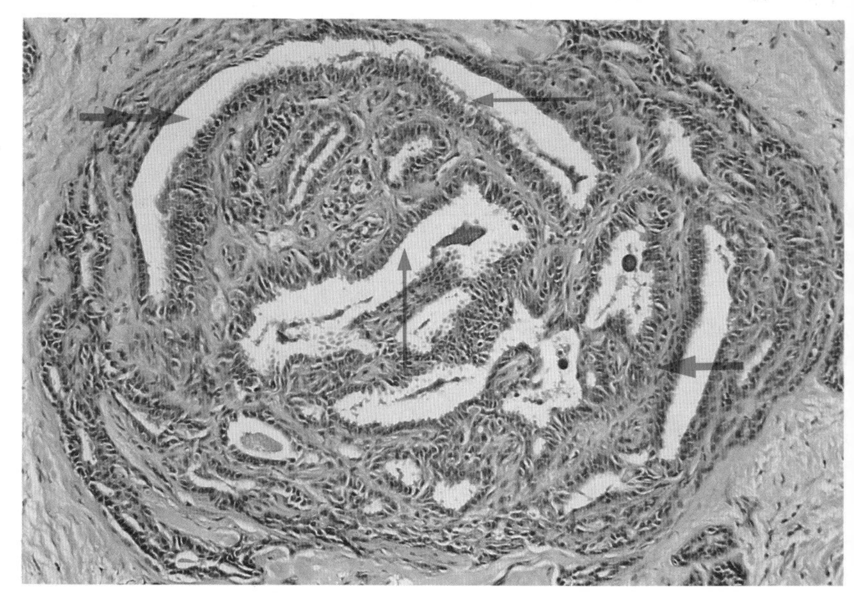

Fibrocystic changes in the breast (cystic mastopathy) are considered to be the result of cyclical changes in the levels of female sex hormones, mainly estrogens, but no constant endocrine abnormality has been identified. The hyperplastic epithelium takes a variety of forms, one of which is papilliform ingrowth of epithelium into the ducts, producing duct papillomatosis. The patient in this case was a woman of 21 who already had florid fibroepithelial hyperplasia of the breast, including duct papillomatosis. This duct is filled with papillary ingrowths which merge to form a kind of cribriform structure, consisting of elongated glandular spaces (double arrow), lined by epithelial cells (thin arrows) and supported by thick cords of eosinophilic fibrous tissue (thick arrow). The glandular spaces are mostly lined with a double layer of epithelial cells, but in some of the spaces parts of the lining consist of only a single layer of low cuboidal or flat epithelial cells. There are small round basophilic (calcified) bodies and cellular debris in the lumen of the glandular spaces. At a higher magnification, no mitoses or nuclear pleomorphism could be identified among the epithelial cells. HE ×150

7.9 Fibrocystic disease of the breast

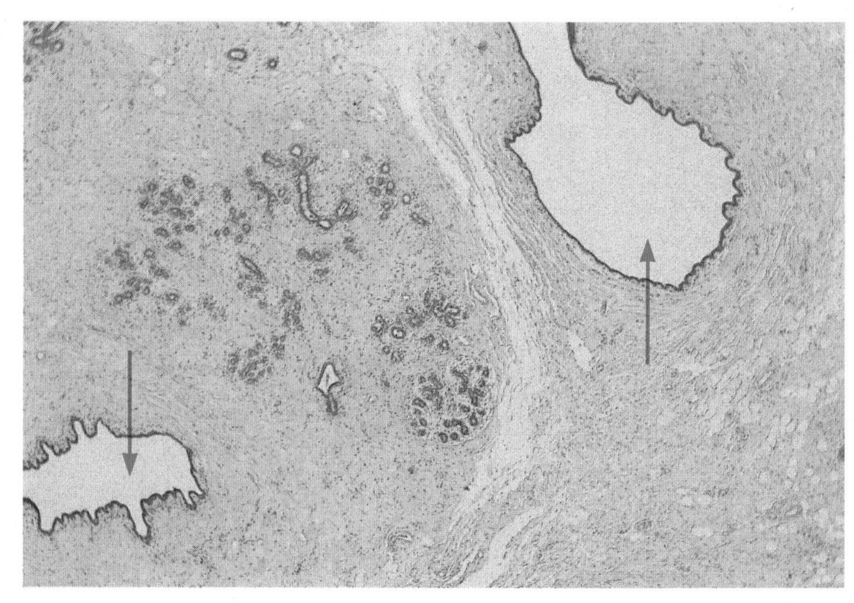

This is an example of fibrocystic disease of the breast. It is the commonest of all breast conditions, and the incidence is highest in the decade preceding the menopause. The lesion can be mistaken clinically for cancer but it is entirely benign. Centrally, there is some relatively normal breast tissue but on both sides there are cystically dilated glands (arrow), surrounded by fibrotic tissue. The cysts arise, in large numbers, from localized dilatation of lobular and terminal ducts. The cysts are mostly less than 1cm dia but occasionally some are larger. They are thin-walled, containing clear or watery or mucinous fluid and lined by flat epithelial cells. Apocrine metaplasia may occur, the cells becoming columnar, with strongly eosinophilic cytoplasm.

7.10 Fibrocystic disease of breast

This is another example of ductal papillomatosis in the same breast. The papilliform structures are larger and more cellular than those shown in 7.8, and appear to be fused or linked together. They are attached to the wall of the duct and project into its lumen. At the bases of some of the papilliform structures, there is a short thick core of eosinophilic fibrous tissue (thin arrow), but the central and more distant parts of the papilliform structures are composed largely of sheets and interlinked trabeculae of relatively small hyperplastic epithelial cells (thick arrow). The hyperplastic epithelial cells show some variation in size and shape, but most of them appear to be closely packed and slightly spindle-shaped. They have a moderate amount of eosinophilic cytoplasm, with poorly-defined boundaries, and small pleomorphic elongated or round deeply basophilic nuclei. There is no mitotic activity among the epithelial cells, and the lesion is considered to be benign. HE ×150

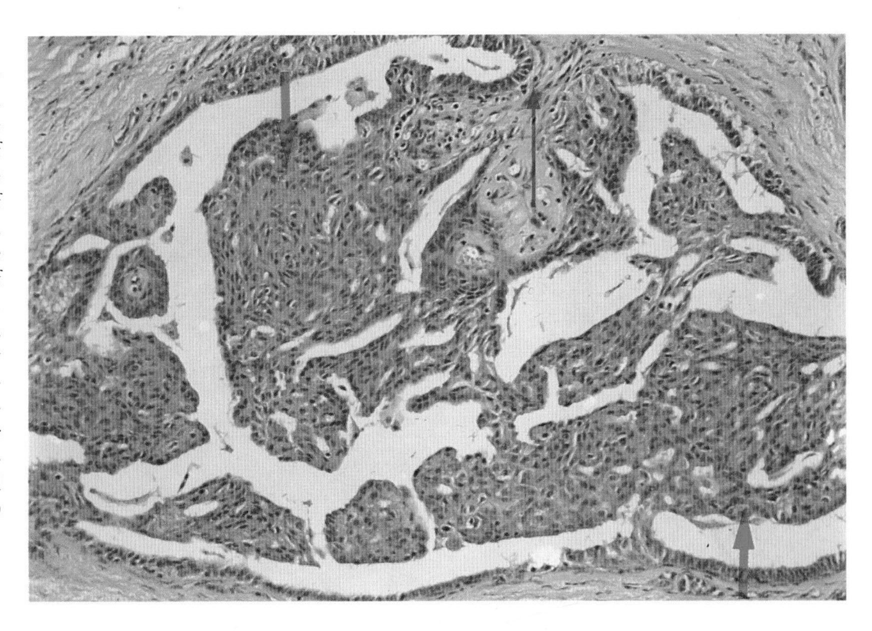

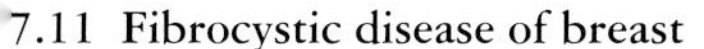

7.11 Fibrocystic disease of breast

Another feature of generalized cystic mastopathy is dilatation of ducts (duct ectasia). Dilatation may be great, with production of multiple cysts, sometimes of considerable size. The dilated ducts and cysts are filled with clear fluid or more turbid material. A piece of tissue measuring 4 × 2.5 × 2cm was removed for diagnostic purposes from the breast of a woman of 46. On section it was fibrofatty in nature, with 'flecks' of white cheesy material. This shows two ducts, both greatly dilated and cystic (thin arrows), and full of eosinophilic amorphous material. Each duct is lined mostly with a single layer of flat or cuboidal extremely basophilic cells (double arrow), but other parts of the ducts are lined two layers of cells. The underlying layer of epithelial cells is incomplete but in few areas it is several cells thick. In one of the two dilated ducts there are also a few small papilliform ingrowths of the basophilic epithelial cells (thick arrow). Both ducts are surrounded by sheets of collagenous fibrous tissue, in which there are collections of small lymphocytes. HE ×60

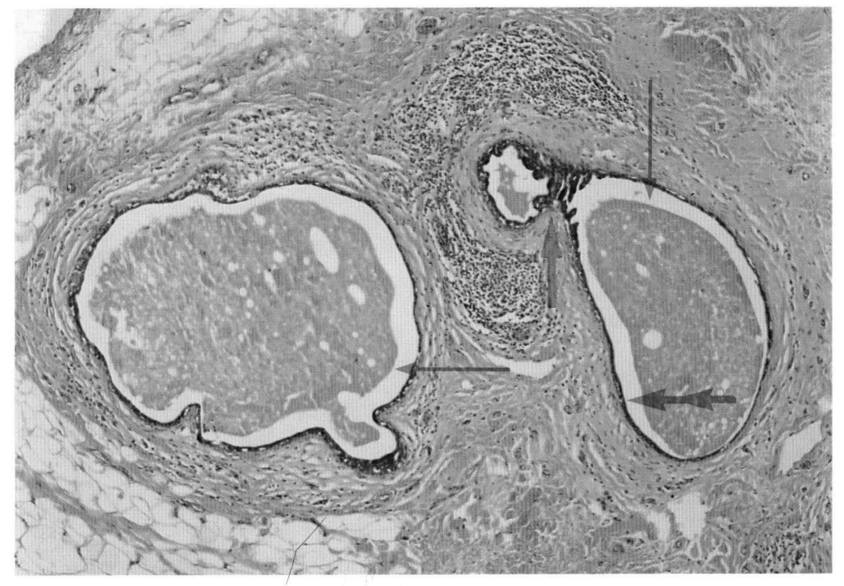

7.12 Fibrocystic disease of breast

An increase in stromal fibrous tissue is often frequently present, and may take the form of ill-defined rubbery masses. The term fibrous mastopathy is sometimes applied when fibrosis is predominant. Cysts often form in the breast, and vary in size from small (microcysts) to several centimetres dia, probably as the result of obstruction of ducts. This is the same breast as in 7.11. In this part of the breast there is a small cystic duct (microcyst) full of deeply eosinophilic amorphous granular debris and lined by several layers of epithelial cells (double arrows). The predominant layer of cells consists of closely packed and palisaded tall columnar epithelial cells; and beneath is an incomplete layer of small basophilic cells with vacuolated cytoplasm. Broad bands of hyalinized fibrous tissue (thick arrow) form a wall around the cyst, but it has ruptured at one point (thin arrow) and allowed the cyst contents to spill into the surrounding stroma. In response there are many macrophages, including a multinucleated giant cell (bottom left), in the stroma. The hyalinized fibrous tissue in the wall reacts positively with special stains for elastic tissue and is termed 'elastosis'. Peripheral to the elastotic material the breast tissue is fibrous and infiltrated with lymphocytes. HE ×150

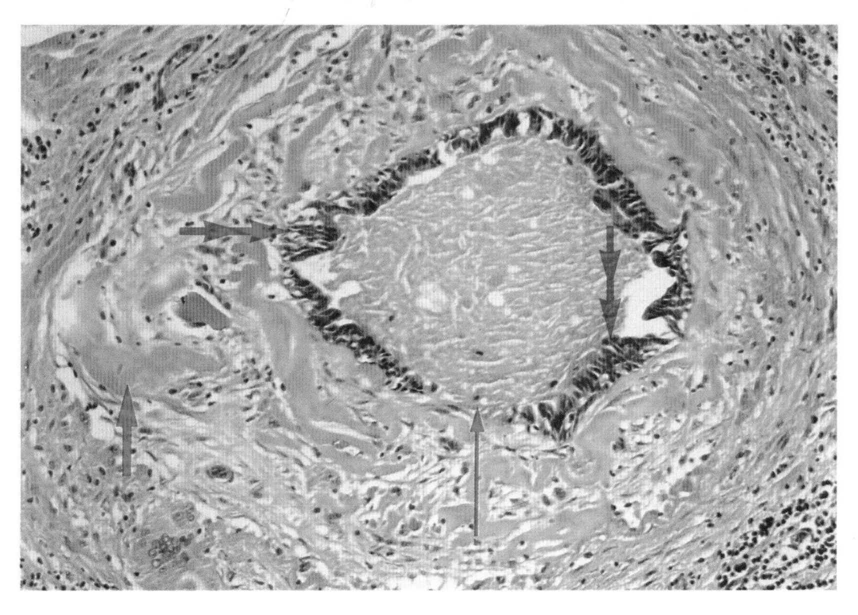

7.13 Fibrocystic disease of breast

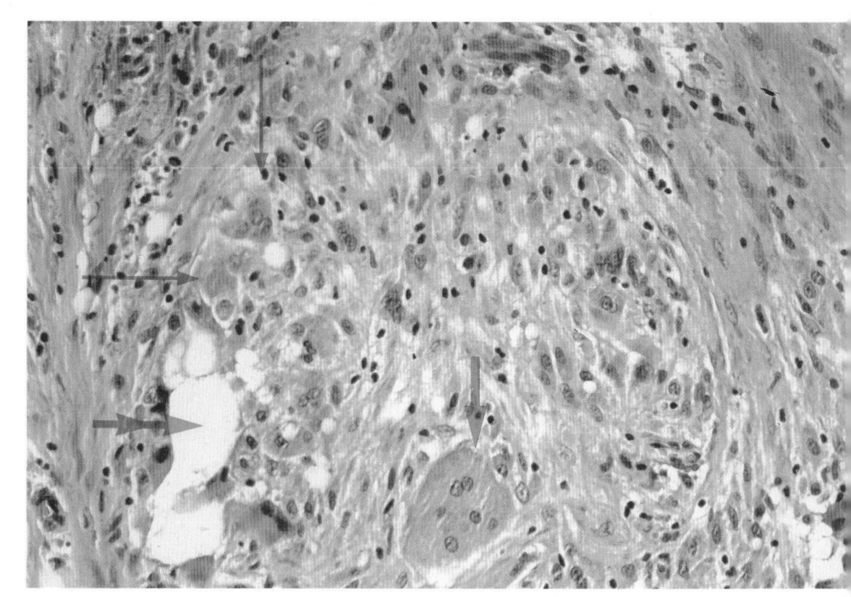

In cystic mastopathy, the cysts are generally lined by flattened or apocrine epithelium and contain a turbid 'glairy' fluid. Some cysts, with a translucent wall, are a bluish colour and are occasionally called blue-domed cysts. The wall is very thin and easily aspirated. Rupture of a cyst often evokes a histiocytic reaction which resembles granulomatous mastitis. This is part of the same lesion as in 7.12, at higher magnification. The extravasated material, leaking from the cyst, has provoked a vigorous cellular response which is surrounded by broad eosinophilic bands of connective tissue and elongated fibroblasts with plump vesicular nuclei. The granulomatous inflammatory focus consists mainly of macrophages (thin arrows) with a considerable amount of eosinophilic cytoplasm in which there is much ingested material. The nuclei are large ovoid or round and vesicular, and the nuclear chromatin is finely granular and pale. Some of the macrophages are binucleated and others are very large (foreign body) multinucleated giant cells (thick arrow). Lymphocytes and plasma cells are also present The (empty) vacuoles of various sizes (double arrow) contained lipoid material which dissolved during processing of the tissue. HE ×235

7.14 Fibrocystic disease of breast

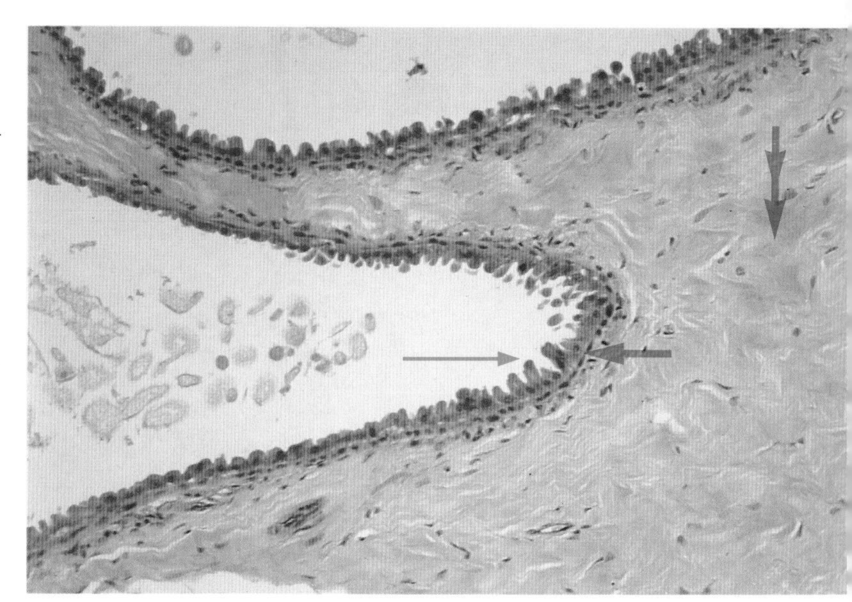

In cystic mastopathy the epithelium of dilated ducts frequently undergoes 'apocrine metaplasia', in which the ducts are lined with large cells with relatively small nuclei and abundant deeply eosinophilic cytoplasm and decapitation-type secretion. In this tissue from the breast of a woman of 30 there are parts of two large dilated (cystic) ducts which show apocrine metaplasia. The ducts are lined by single layer of large eosinophilic epithelial cells. The cells have much strongly eosinophilic cytoplasm and protruding 'secretory snouts' of various sizes (thin arrow), the 'snouts' being the apical part of the cytoplasm which buds off into the duct lumen in the same way as apocrine glandular epithelial cells secrete. The eosinophilia of the cytoplasm is caused by the presence of large numbers of mitochondria. Beneath the apocrine-type epithelial cells there is also a single continuous layer of much smaller flatter myoepithelial cells with small elongated basophilic nuclei (thick arrow). The stromal connective tissue around and between the two ducts is densely fibrous and hyalinized (double arrow). There is no evidence that so-called apocrine metaplasia is linked with carcinoma of the breast. HE ×150

7.15 Fibrocystic disease of breast

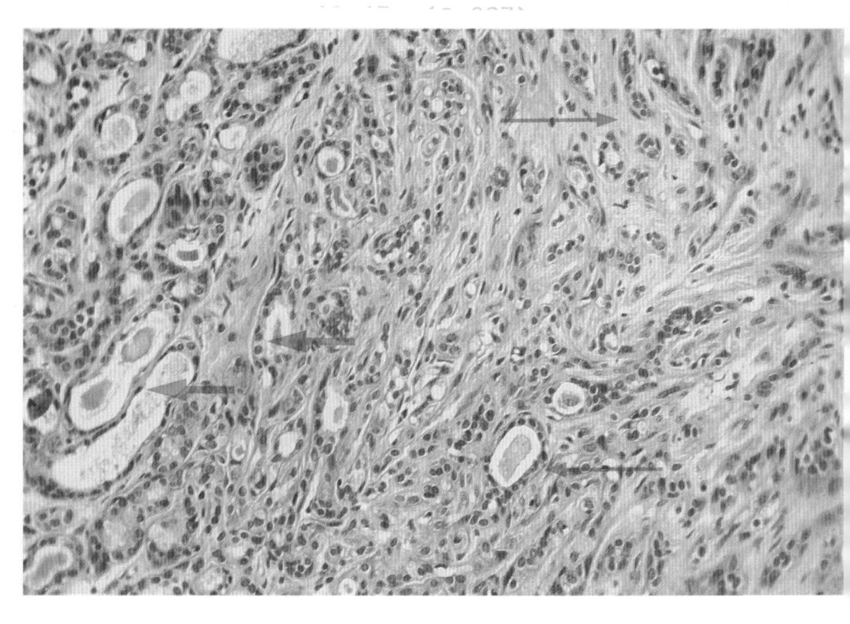

Mild hyperplasia of lobules (adenosis) or of epithelium within ducts is very common and is sometimes accompanied by marked fibrosis (sclerosis). The normal lobular pattern is markedly distorted as a result, and the histological appearance is termed sclerosing adenosis or microglandular adenosis. This variant of cystic mastopathy may be very difficult to distinguish the appearance from carcinoma. This is an example of sclerosing adenosis of the breast, the lobular pattern of which is distorted by proliferating connective tissue stroma. The numerous ductules vary considerably in size and shape and are lined by a single layer of epithelial cells which range from cuboidal to very flat (thick arrows). The ductules are surrounded by abundant very cellular fibrous tissue (thin arrows) which appears to compress and distort them. In the fibrous stromal tissue there are also many individual cells and groups of cells, most of which are probably myoepithelial cells. There is no nuclear pleomorphism or mitotic activity. At very low magnification it was possible to see that the glandular elements had retained a lobular pattern, and this is the single most important feature that helps to distinguish this condition from carcinoma. HE ×135

7.16 Fibrocystic disease of breast

Undoubtedly the most important change in cystic mastopathy is the epithelial hyperplasia (epitheliosis) that is almost invariably present in the ducts and ductules, since it may be linked with the development of carcinoma. The change is characterized by marked atypical proliferation of ductal epithelial cells, which undergo stratification and often fill the lumen of the distended duct. The change is also associated with a four-to-five times increase in the risk of cancer. A notable feature in this breast from a woman of 30 with generalized cystic mastopathy is the very active atypical proliferation of the ductal epithelial cells. Several ducts are cystic and lined (more or less) by a single layer of flat epithelial cells (thin arrow), whereas in almost all the other ducts and ductules the degree of the hyperplasia varies considerably. In most of the ducts the epithelium is very hyperplastic and thick. In some of the larger ducts however the rate of proliferation of the atypical epithelial cells is enough to fill the lumen. The pattern in these larger ducts tends to be cribriform (thick arrows). The amount of connective tissue between the ducts is considerable and more fibrous than normal (double arrow). HE ×60

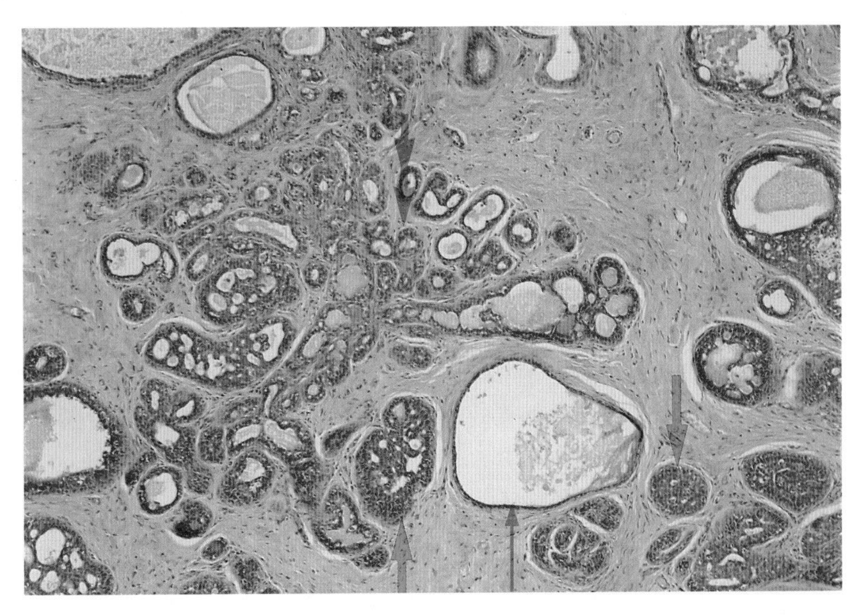

7.17 Fibrocystic disease of breast

This is part of the same lesion as in 7.16, at higher magnification. In the distended duct on the left, epithelial hyperplasia is relatively slight but the lumen is full of large foamy macrophages with abundant well-defined finely granular cytoplasm and uniform small round nuclei. Epithelial hyperplasia (epitheliosis) is much more marked in the duct on the right (thin arrow). The duct is partly lined with several layers of epithelial and myoepithelial cells and there is some eosinophilic secretion in its lumen. In contrast, the remainder of the lumen is filled with a sheet of hyperchromatic epithelial cells, in which there are numerous small gland-like spaces. The small duct at the top of the picture (thick arrow) and the duct in the centre shows a similar degree of epitheliosis. The epithelial nuclei are basophilic but not pleomorphic and there are no mitotic figures. There is also evidence of epitheliosis (thin arrow) in the dilated duct at bottom centre. The stroma between the ducts and ductules is consists of broad strands of dense poorly cellular fibrous tissue (double arrow). HE ×150

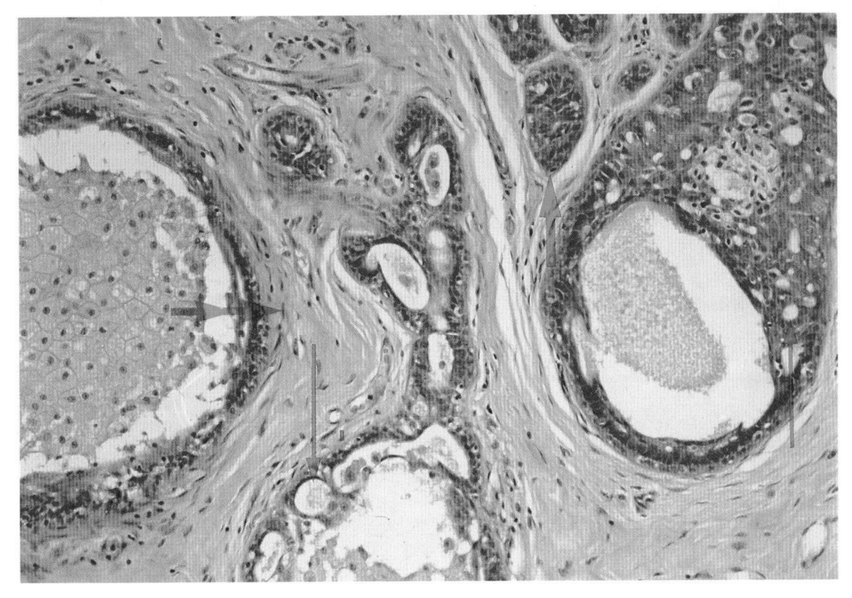

7.18 Fibrocystic disease of breast

If atypical ductal hyperplasia is present in patients with a family history of breast cancer, the risk of cancer is twice as great, the term 'borderline lesion' is sometimes applied to the lesion. This is the breast of a woman of 45. Two distended smaller ducts and part of a much larger duct are shown. The lumen of all three ducts is full of proliferated epithelial cells which exhibit only slight atypia. The nuclei of the epithelial cells are fairly uniformly round or ovoid and the chromatin is finely granular but not hyperchromatic. There are nucleoli in many of the nuclei and they are small and relatively inconspicuous. There is no mitotic activity. There is a continuous thin layer of flat myoepithelial cells with small elongated very basophilic nuclei (thick arrows) around each duct. The ducts are also surrounded by a thick (prominent) eosinophilic basement membrane but there is no periductal 'elastosis'. Nor is there any cellular necrosis. The stroma between the ducts consists of loose fibrous tissue and a few lymphocytes. This is an example of marked but wholly benign epithelial hyperplasia (benign epitheliosis). HE ×360

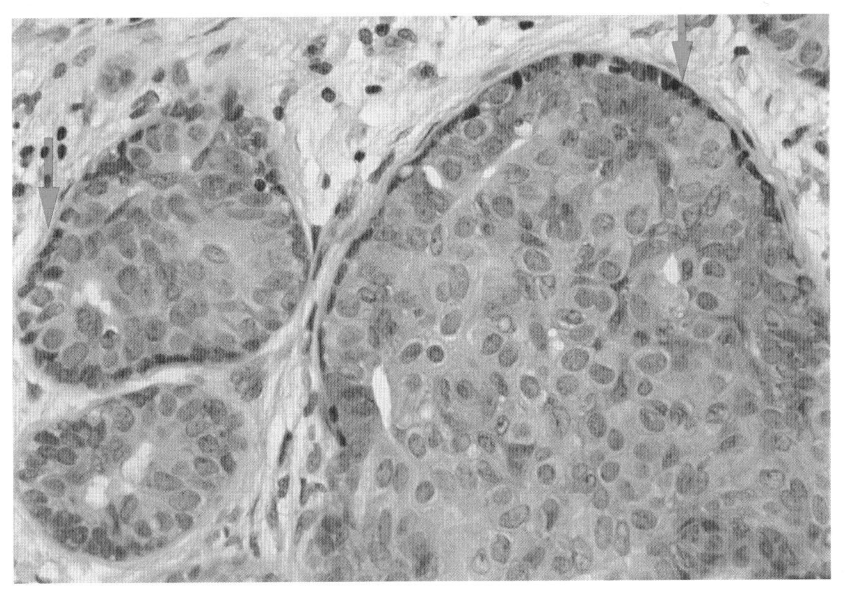

7.19 Ductal carcinoma in situ (DCIS): breast

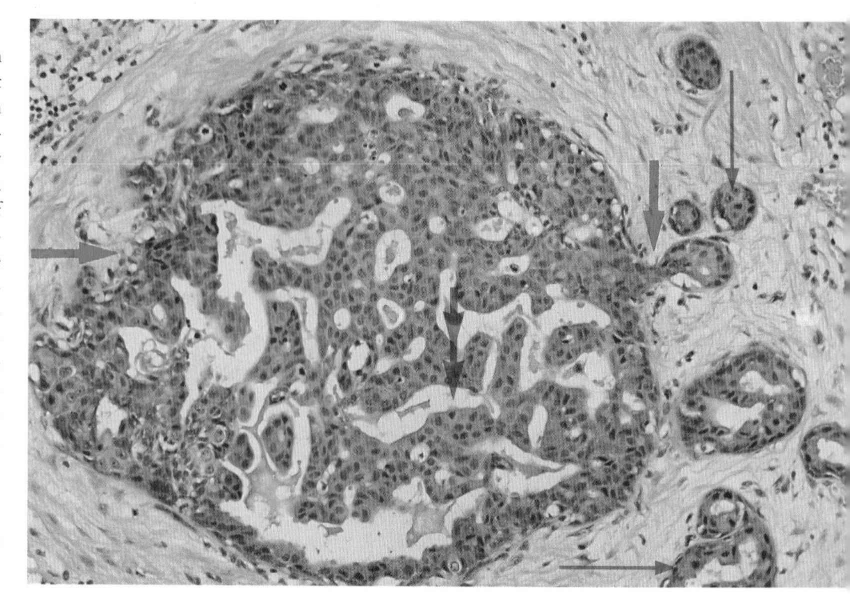

Intraductal carcinoma of breast is a relatively uncommon form of breast cancer. It is a proliferation of neoplastic ductal epithelial cells, filling the duct and confined within the basement membrane. The lesion is multifocal and bilateral in about 20% of cases, and it is detectable by mammography. The in situ phase is generally short. In this part of a DCIS lesion there is a distended duct, full of malignant epithelial cells, arranged in well-defined anastomosing trabeculae (double arrow). The trabeculae are separated by irregular spaces and form a cribriform structure (cribriform structures tend to be associated with carcinoma). The spaces contain small amounts of eosinophilic secretion. The tumour cells have a moderate amount of eosinophilic cytoplasm and moderately pleomorphic round or ovoid vesicular nuclei. Many nuclei are also hyperchromatic, and in some of the larger nuclei there is a nucleolus. There are numerous mitotic figures. The wall of the duct is irregular in outline, the myoepithelial layer is indistinct, and the basement membrane appears to have been breached by protruding tumour cells at several points (thick arrows). The surrounding tissues are fibrous but there is no elastosis. Several small ducts (thin arrows) also contain malignant cells.
HE ×150

7.20 Ductal carcinoma in situ (DCIS): breast

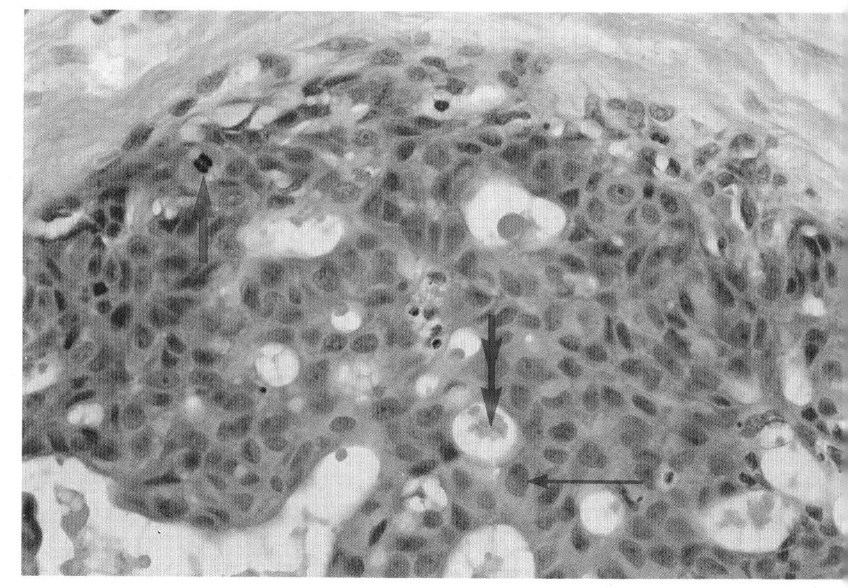

Ductal carcinoma in situ (DCIS) is the type of carcinoma most often associated with Paget's disease of the nipple. Pure DCIS is also frequently associated with infiltrating ductal carcinoma but it does not metastasize. This shows part of the lumen of large duct shown in 7.19. Within the lumen there are cords and sheets of malignant epithelial cells. The neoplastic cells enclose numerous gland-like spaces which contain a small amount of eosinophilic secretion (double arrow). The cells have abundant eosinophilic cytoplasm but the cell margins are indistinct. The nuclei are ovoid pleomorphic and vesicular. The nuclear chromatin is finely granular and relatively pale-staining (thin arrow), and in most of the nuclei there is a small often-central nucleolus. There is considerable mitotic activity (thick arrow) The periphery of the duct is ill-defined, with only a small population of spindle-shaped (probably myoepithelial) cells with elongated vesicular nuclei at the top. There is no basement membrane and also no evidence of elastosis in the fibrous tissue around the duct. HE ×360

7.21 Ductal carcinoma in situ (DCIS): breast

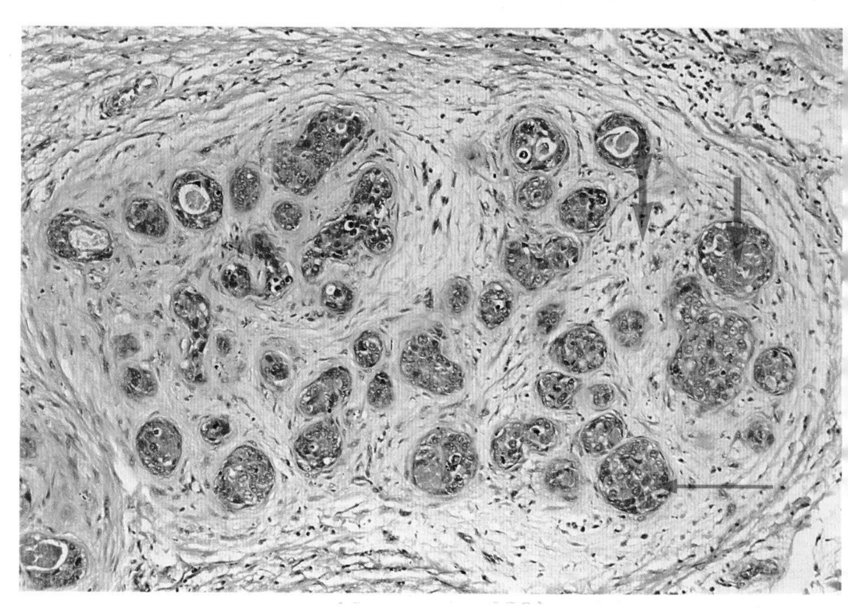

Grossly, ductal carcinoma in situ (DCIS) tends to produce a hard mass in the breast which is composed of thick cord-like structures. Histologically, these cord-like structures are full of proliferating malignant cells which may be arranged in cribriform, papillary or solid patterns and may eventually convert many ducts and ductules into tubes full of cancer cells. When the distended ducts are cut, the malignant cells can be squeezed out like toothpaste. The expressed material has been compared to a 'comedo' (a 'blackhead') and the condition is sometimes called comedo carcinoma. This is an example of a 'comedo' carcinoma from a woman aged 42 whose left breast was removed because of the presence of several hard irregular nodules which were thought to be malignant. In this part of the breast, all the ducts are filled with extremely atypical cells (thin arrow), many of which have large pleomorphic vacuolated nuclei but very little cytoplasm. The nuclei are hyperchromatic and the chromatin is very coarse. Importantly, in most of the ducts large numbers of the neoplastic cells have undergone eosinophilic necrosis (thick arrow). The stroma around the ducts consists of loose (myxoid) connective tissue (double arrow). HE ×95

7.22 Ductal carcinoma in situ (DCIS): breast

In a typical ductal carcinoma in situ (DCIS), the closely packed neoplastic epithelial cells which distend the ducts are large and uniform, with round non-overlapping nuclei and well-defined cell membranes, and the basement membrane is intact. This shows two ducts from the lesion in 7.21, at higher magnification. The walls of the ducts are intact (double arrow), and the ducts are full of closely packed tumour cells (thin arrows). The cytoplasm of the tumour cells is vacuolated and the cell boundaries are indistinct. The nuclei are ovoid or round and very pleomorphic, and several nuclei are hyperchromatic. The nuclei are also vesicular and pale, and in some of them there are one or more prominent nucleoli. In the larger duct, all the neoplastic cells appear viable, but in the smaller duct most of the cells are necrotic, and the sheet of cells which distends smaller duct has undergone extensive central eosinophilic necrosis (thick arrow). The stroma surrounding both ducts is loose myxoid connective tissue. No tumour was found in the axillary lymph nodes. HE ×415

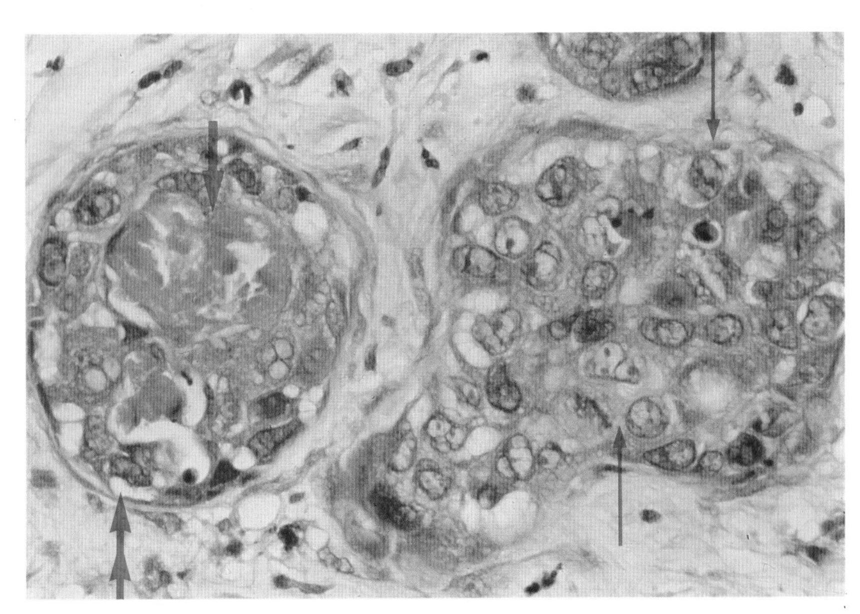

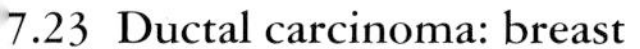

7.23 Ductal carcinoma: breast

Invasive ductal carcinoma has its origin in the epithelium lining the ducts of the breast and is the most common type of breast cancer (about 75%). It forms a very firm, sometimes hard, ill-defined infiltrating lump in the breast, the cut surface of which has a greyish-white colour and a gritty texture. In the later stages, the tumour becomes fixed to the chest wall and skin, but variant forms of the carcinoma (medullary, tubular, mucinous or papillary) may have a better prognosis than the usual infiltrating ductal carcinoma. This tumour was in the breast of woman of 36. The neoplastic cells form irregular duct-like spaces, and long narrow cords of similar cells are also present (thin arrow). The malignant cells have abundant eosinophilic cytoplasm and large moderately pleomorphic round or ovoid vesicular nuclei. A few nuclei are pyknotic but most are also very pale (vacuolated), and contain one or more large nucleoli. There is considerable mitotic activity (thick arrows). The stroma is fibrous and infiltrated with lymphocytes and plasma cells. The connective tissue around the two normal ducts (double arrow) is hyalinized. In undifferentiated ductal carcinomas there are no duct-like structures. HE ×150

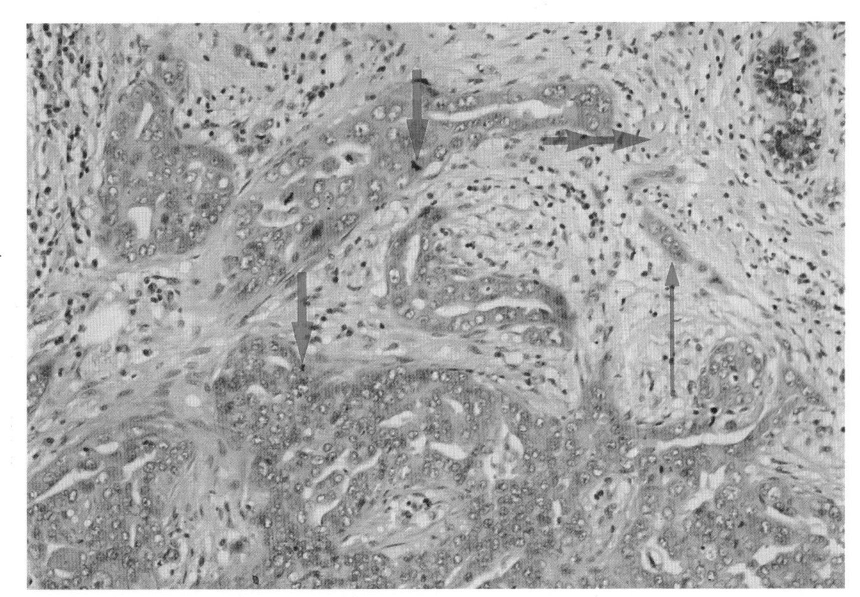

7.24 Ductal carcinoma: breast

In the cut surface of invasive ductal carcinomas of breast, there are frequently characteristic yellowish-white chalky streaks which correspond to an unusual deposition of elastic tissue around non-malignant ducts in the vicinity of the tumour. Histologically the deposits consist of thick bands of eosinophilic hyaline tissue, and since the altered fibrous tissue stains with elastic-tissue stains, the condition is termed 'elastosis' of the ducts. It is not specific for carcinomatous lesions however but may be seen in association with benign lesions. This shows a normal duct from the breast in which there was a mucin-secreting carcinoma. The duct is lined with a single layer of brownish-yellow plump cuboidal epithelial cells (thin arrow) and surrounded by a thin band of collagenous fibrous tissue (stained purplish-red). Outside the fibrous tissue layer there is a much thicker band of closely packed wavy black elastic fibres. In the adjoining sheet of dense purplish-red collagenous fibrous tissue there is an infiltrate of brownish-yellow single (individual) forms and clusters of carcinoma cells (thick arrows). Elastic-van Gieson ×360

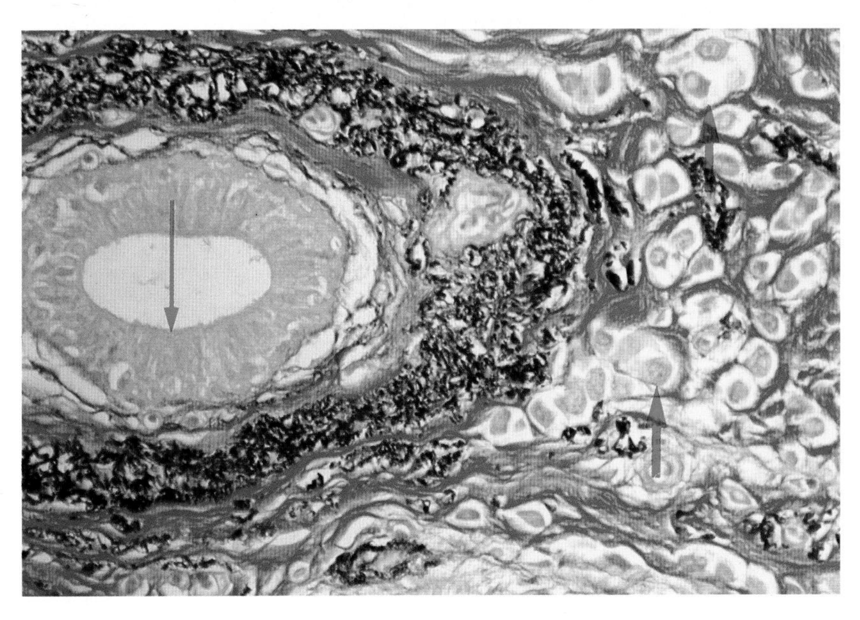

7.25 Mucinous carcinoma: breast

The malignant cells in breast carcinomas not infrequently contain droplets of mucin in their cytoplasm. The term mucinous carcinoma is however reserved for those carcinomas of breast in which the malignant cells produce mucin in such large quantities that it makes up a significant part of the bulk of the neoplasm. Mucinous carcinoma is an uncommon type of breast carcinoma, and it is reputedly less liable to metastasize by the lymphatics than other types of ductal carcinoma. This type of behaviour is unproven however. In this example, large compact clusters of malignant cells float in large quantities of mucin (almost colourless) secreted by the tumour cells. The neoplastic cells have pleomorphic (round or ovoid) deeply basophilic nuclei and a fairly large quantity of eosinophilic cytoplasm (thin arrow). In the cytoplasm there are large numbers of small spherical vacuoles which presumably contain a droplet of epithelial mucin. The stroma consists entirely of a sheet of pale blue mucin (double arrow), and in which a thin-walled blood vessel floats (thick arrow). The vessel is lined with large endothelial cells with elongated nuclei, most of them vesicular.

HE ×135

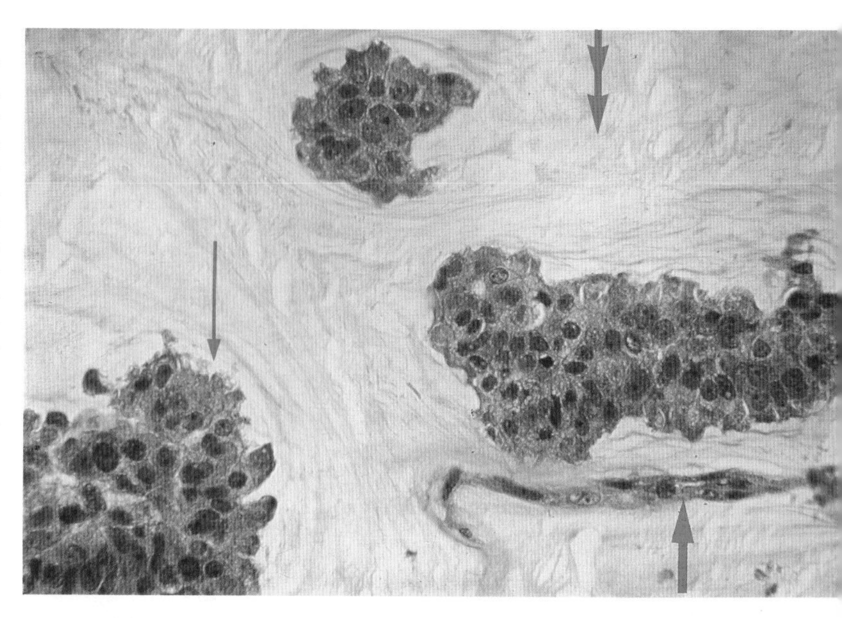

7.26 Lobular carcinoma in situ (LCIS): breast

Carcinoma in situ (LCIS) starts within the lobules in the breast and is often discovered incidentally in a breast biopsy. The disease is multifocal and bilateral in 70% of cases. The neoplastic epithelial cells proliferate sufficiently to fill and distend all the acini of at least one complete lobular unit. The lumens of the acini are thereby obliterated. However, so long as the basement membrane of the acini remains intact, there is no risk of disseminating the lesion. A woman of 45 developed a lump in her right breast and it was resected. The tumour consists of ducts which are completely filled with small polygonal cells with round or ovoid nuclei (thin arrow).The nuclei show little pleomorphism, and in some of the nuclei there is a small nucleolus. The cells have a moderate amount of cytoplasm but the cell boundaries are indistinct. There is no necrosis or mitotic activity. A few lymphocytes are also present in the ducts. The ducts are surrounded by loose fibrous tissue, and each duct has a complete well-defined basement membrane (thick arrow). All the ducts of the lobule are similarly affected. There is no evidence of invasion, and the diagnosis is lobular carcinoma in situ.

HE ×360

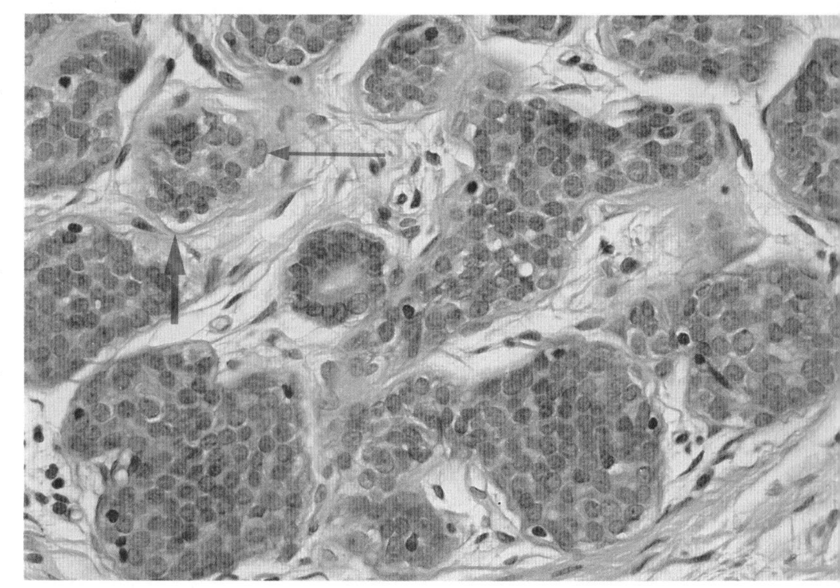

7.27 Invasive lobular carcinoma: breast

In lobular carcinoma, the terminal ducts are filled with closely packed malignant cells which eventually, perhaps after many years, break out. The result is an invasive (infiltrating) carcinoma. Invasive lobular carcinoma is more frequently bilateral than infiltrating ductal carcinoma, but the prognosis is the same for both types of tumour. A woman of 50 had the left breast removed for suspected malignancy. A very firm mass (8.5 × 6 × 2cm) in the upper and outer quadrant proved to be an invasive lobular carcinoma, with massive involvement of the axillary nodes. This part of the breast lesion consists of a large numbers of neoplastic cells, with pleomorphic nuclei and considerable eosinophilic cytoplasm, and a small non-neoplastic duct heavily infiltrated with small lymphocytes (thick arrow). The tumour cells, as single cells and small clusters, are lined up one behind the other in rows (Indian files) which are arranged in concentric circles (a targetoid or dartboard pattern) around the duct (thin arrows), in a cuff of loose connective tissue. Cords of malignant cells are also invading adjacent fatty tissue.

HE ×150

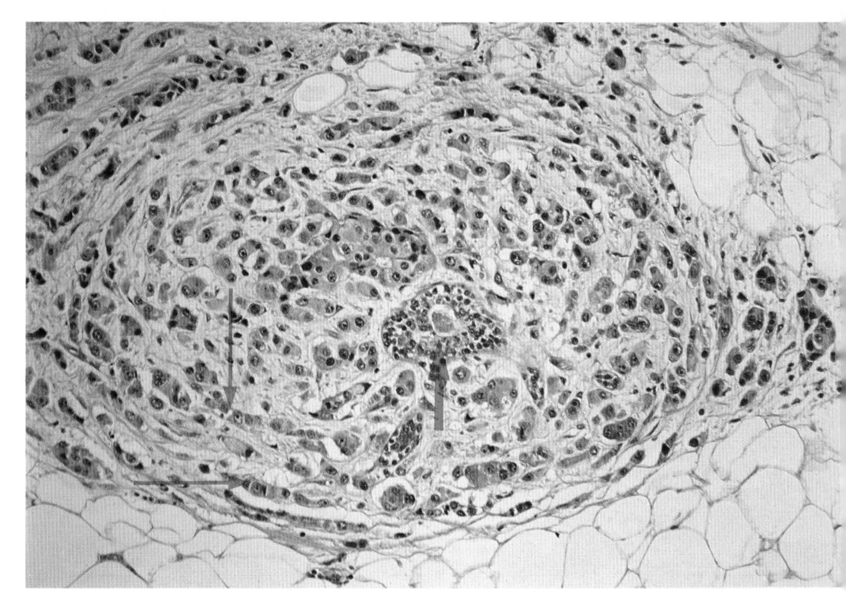

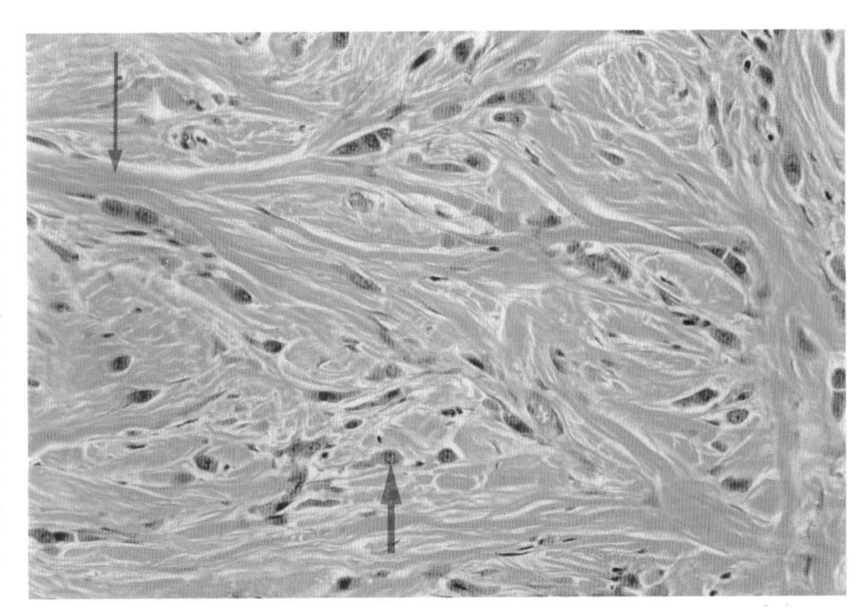

7.28 Invasive lobular carcinoma: breast

About 5-10% of all breast carcinomas are infiltrating lobular carcinomas, and they are similar to infiltrating ductal carcinomas apart from a different histological pattern of infiltration and a slightly higher incidence of bilaterality. This is part of the same invasive lobular carcinoma as in 7.27. It consists of a sheet of interlacing collagenous fibrous tissue, infiltrated by a relatively sparse population of neoplastic cells. The collagenous fibres are deeply eosinophilic (hyalinized) and most of them broad (thin arrow). The infiltrating tumour cells are relatively small (thick arrow) but very variable in size and shape. Most of them have only a very moderate amount of cytoplasm and a round or ovoid vesicular nucleus. In some of the nuclei there is an inconspicuous nucleolus. Nuclear pleomorphism is moderate and no mitoses are present. The neoplastic cells do not attempt to form glands but, as individual cells and small clusters, they have a distinct tendency to lie one behind the other in a single row; that is, as Indian files. Invasive lobular carcinomas form no glands. HE ×235

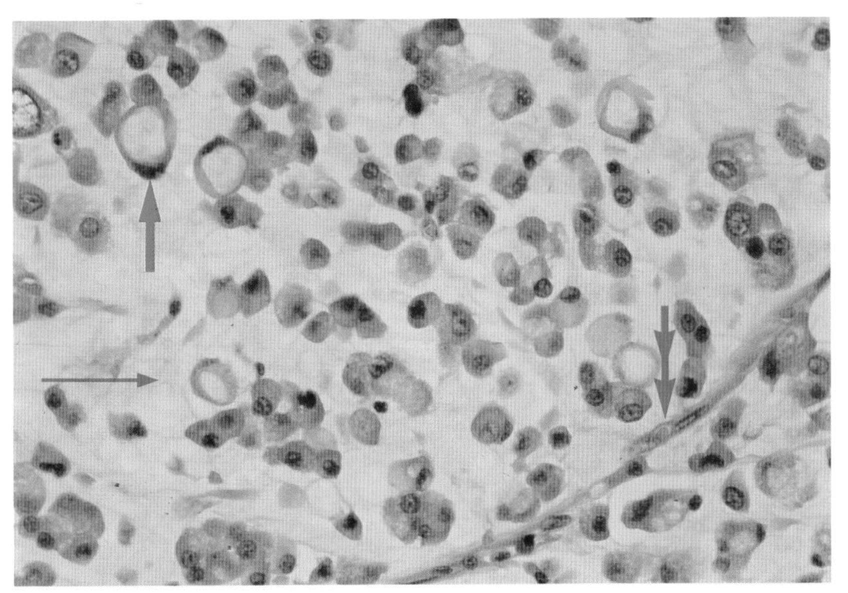

7.29 Invasive lobular carcinoma: breast

Intracellular mucin is detectable in most cases of intralobular carcinoma, as demonstrated in this invasive (infiltrating) lobular carcinoma from a woman of 57. The tumour cells vary in size, but they have a relatively large amount of eosinophilic cytoplasm which appears 'granular' from the presence of large numbers of very small vacuoles which presumably contain droplets of epithelial mucin. In some cells there is a large pale cytoplasmic vacuole which gives them a signet-ring appearance (thick arrow). The nuclei are mostly small round and only moderately pleomorphic. A few of them are very small and pyknotic, but the chromatin in most of the nuclei is diffusely pale and a prominent nucleolus is clearly visible in it. The stroma around the cells is pale, almost colourless, consisting almost entirely of mucin (thin arrow). Mucin stains confirmed that the tiny vacuoles in the tumour cells do contain mucin and that the stromal sheet of extracellular mucin also is epithelial mucin, presumably secreted by the tumour cells. A small capillary-type blood vessel (double arrow) is also present in the 'stroma'. HE ×360

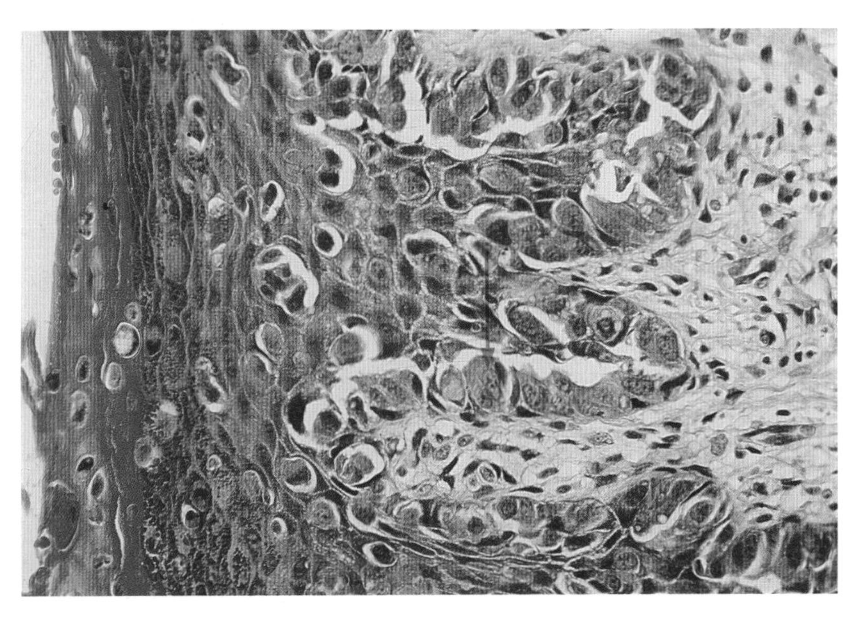

7.30 Paget's disease: breast

Paget's disease of the breast arises when malignant cells migrate to the nipple via the ducts of the breast and infiltrate the stratified squamous epithelium (epidermis) of the nipple, where they become Paget's cells. Paget's disease of the breast may be an early sign of a carcinoma that is still confined within the ducts (intraduct carcinoma). In this case however, at the time of clinical presentation of Paget's disease of the breast, the carcinoma of breast was found to be already invasive. In this case, an ellipse of skin 7 × 2.5cm bearing the nipple, along with a wedge of underlying breast 5cm deep, was resected from a woman of 64 who had suffered from red painful left nipple for some months. This is a histological section of the squamous epithelium of the nipple. There are large numbers of markedly atypical epithelial cells with pale ovoid or round nuclei and a moderate amount of slightly basophilic cytoplasm (arrow) (Paget's cells) in the basal layers of the stratified squamous epithelium, and in smaller numbers throughout the more superficial layers. The Paget's cells are not an integral part of the squamous epithelium, and they are displacing and causing pressure atrophy of the adjacent epithelial cells. There is mild lymphocytic infiltration of the underlying dermis but there are no malignant cells in the dermis. The cells which comprise the stratified squamous epithelium of the nipple show no signs of being tumorous, in contrast to Bowen's disease. HE ×200

7.31 Condyloma acuminatum: vulva

Condyloma acuminatum is a common benign verrucous lesion, caused by the papillomavirus, of which there are many types. The infection is usually transmitted sexually. It takes the form of soft polypoid wart-like masses in moist regions and particularly on the vulva or penis or in the anal region. It is characterized by hyperplasia of the squamous epithelium, with marked cytoplasmic vacuolation (koilocytosis) and condensation of the nuclear chromatin. Atypia of the nuclei is also often present. This shows the top of one of the papillary structures. The sheet of stratified squamous epithelial cells on the surface of the papilla is very thick (thin arrow), but there is no hyperkeratosis (left margin). There is however some parakeratosis. The squamous epithelial cells are well-differentiated, and the most striking features are the enormous hyperplasia of the keratinocytes (acanthosis) and elongation of the rete ridges (thick arrow). Many of the keratinocytes are swollen and vacuolated. The dermal papillae have responded to the changes in the rete ridges and are greatly increased in length. In the dermis (double arrow) there is an extremely dense infiltrate of lymphocytes and plasma cells. HE ×80

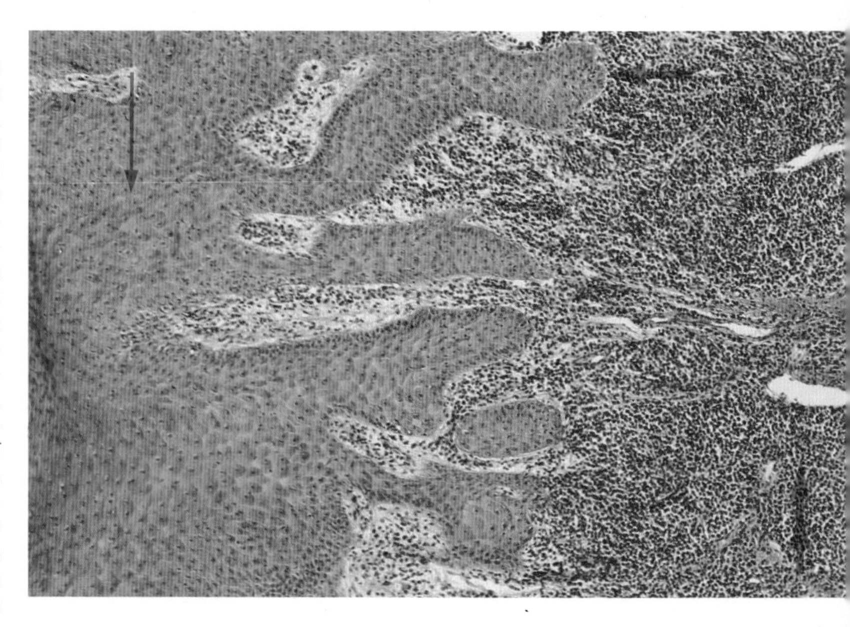

7.32 Bartholin's cyst: vulva

If the excretory duct of one or both the Bartholin's glands is blocked, the gland becomes dilated by its mucoid secretions and may form a cyst. A cyst full of inspissated secretion may measure up to 5cm dia, and if the contents of the cyst get infected, a Bartholin's abscess forms. This cyst, which was in a 24-year-old woman, measured 2.5 × 1.5 × 1.0 cm and was not acutely inflamed. It is lined by transitional epithelium (thin arrow) which consists of closely packed epithelial cells with large pleomorphic vesicular nuclei but only a small amount of cytoplasm. The nuclear chromatin is coarsely granular but relatively pale. There is a thin layer of numerous flat macrophages laden with dark brown pigment within the epithelium and close to its surface (thick arrow). The pigment is a mixture of hemosiderin and lipofuscin. The wall of the cyst consists of loose fibrous tissue and dilated capillaries. Large numbers of mature plasma cells and smaller numbers of small lymphocytes (double arrow) have infiltrated the fibrous wall and also the basal layer of the epithelium. HE ×360

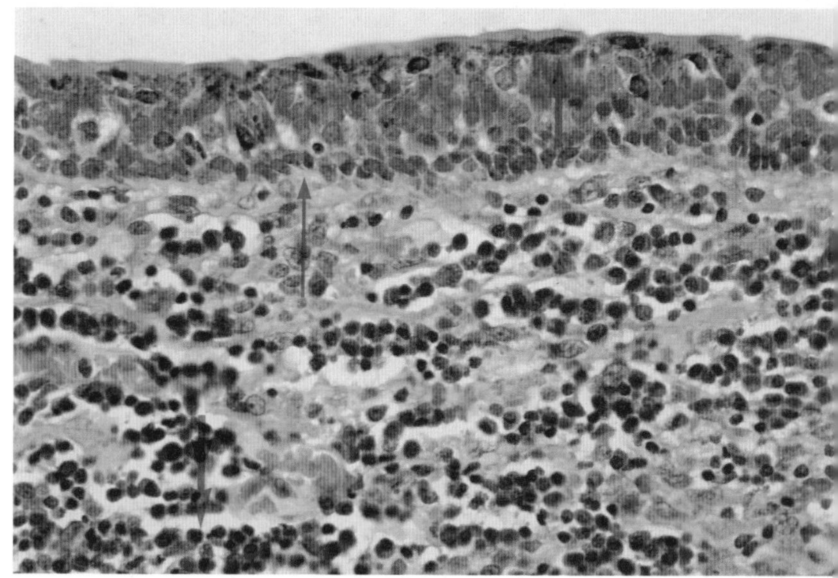

7.33 Hidradenoma papilliferum: vulva

Hidradenoma papilliferum is a neoplasm of the apocrine sweat glands of the vulva, not present before puberty. It takes the form of a small well-defined subcutaneous nodule, usually located on or near the labia majora. It is benign and curable by excision. Occasionally red tumour tissue prolapses through an opening on the skin. Histologically, the surface of the skin is on the right, and the stratified squamous epithelium (double arrow) stretched over the well-circumscribed papilliferous mass in the dermis is intact. The tumour occupies a large round cystic space, demarcated from the adjoining dermal connective tissues by a 'capsule' of markedly compressed connective tissue (thin arrow). The tumour consists of large numbers of elongated slender branching complex fronds (thick arrows), each branch having a well-formed core of fibrous tissue and an irregular layer (double in places) of basophilic cuboidal or columnar epithelial cells on its surface. The structure of the lesion is similar to that of an intraduct papilloma of breast. HE ×55

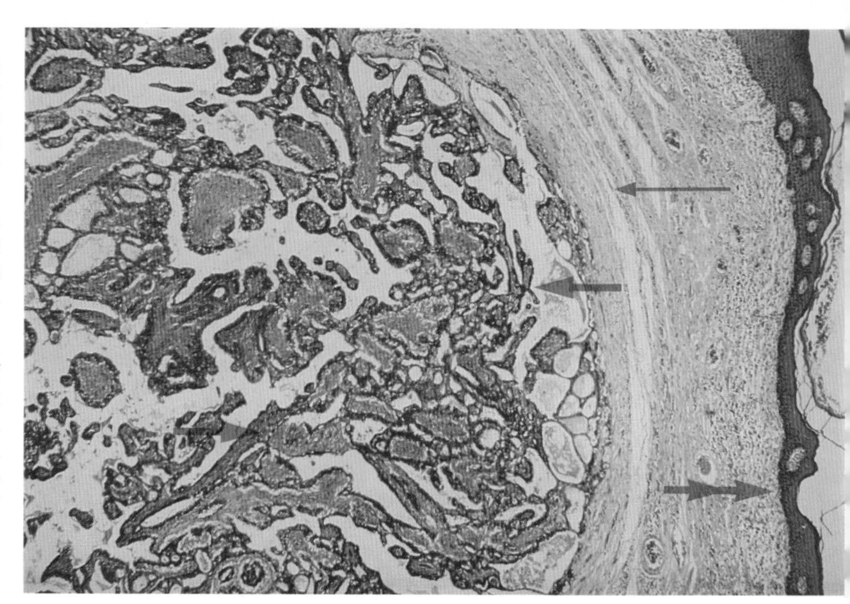

7.34 Cervical intraepithelial neoplasia (CIN): cervix

Cervical intraepithelial neoplasia (CIN) is the term used to describe malignant changes in the squamous epithelium of the cervix, and it has the same significance as dysplasia. CIN I is equivalent to mild (minimal) dysplasia, CIN II to moderate dysplasia, and CIN III to severe dysplasia or carcinoma-in-situ. Dysplasia affects surface epithelium and also extends well down into endocervical glands. Macroscopically, dysplastic epithelium lacks glycogen and looks pale, whereas normal epithelium stained with iodine is brown. This lesion (CIN II) is from the cervix of a woman aged 34. The stratified squamous epithelium is hyperplastic and much thicker than normal (thick arrow). There is a layer of flattened nucleated epithelial cells on the surface (thin arrow) but the polarity of the epithelial cells is fairly well-preserved. The nuclei are relatively large and show moderate pleomorphism. There is also increased mitotic activity in the basal layers of epithelial cells. There are moderate numbers of small lymphocytes in the connective tissues beneath and within the squamous epithelium. HE ×235

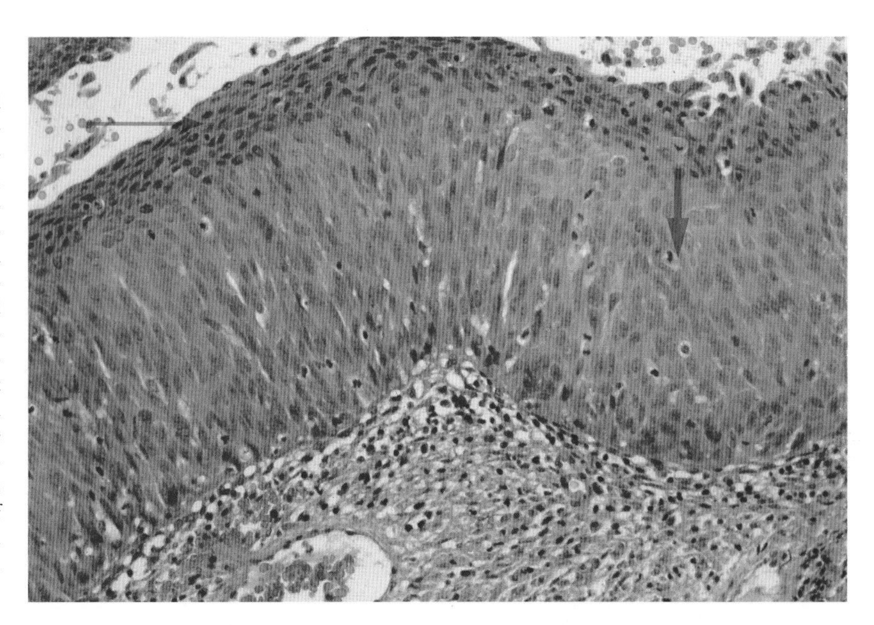

7.35 Cervical intraepithelial neoplasia: cervix

Dysplasia often occurs at the squamocolumnar cell junction. Mild dysplasia (CINI) is typified by a slight increase in nuclear:cytoplasmic ratio, hyperchromasia and an abnormal chromatin pattern. Maturation of the epithelial cells is disorderly, and there are mild cytological changes. However, in severe dysplasia (CIN III), the criteria are a high nuclear:cytoplasmic ratio in basal-type cells, marked hyperchromasia and abnormal chromatin. The epithelial cells fail to mature, there are marked cytological changes, and mitotic activity occurs near the surface of the epithelium. The three grades of CIN do not imply inevitably progress from CIN I to CIN III or from CIN III to invasive carcinoma. In this lesion, the features are those of CIN III (carcinoma-in-situ). The epithelium is distorted, and loss of polarity of the epithelial cells of the basal layer is more or less complete. The epithelial cells have scant cytoplasm and large very pleomorphic vesicular nuclei, among which there is active and frequently atypical mitotic activity (thick arrows) at all levels in the epithelium. A few epithelial cells have shrunken pyknotic nuclei, and there are small numbers of polymorphs in the epithelium, most of them near the surface. HE ×255

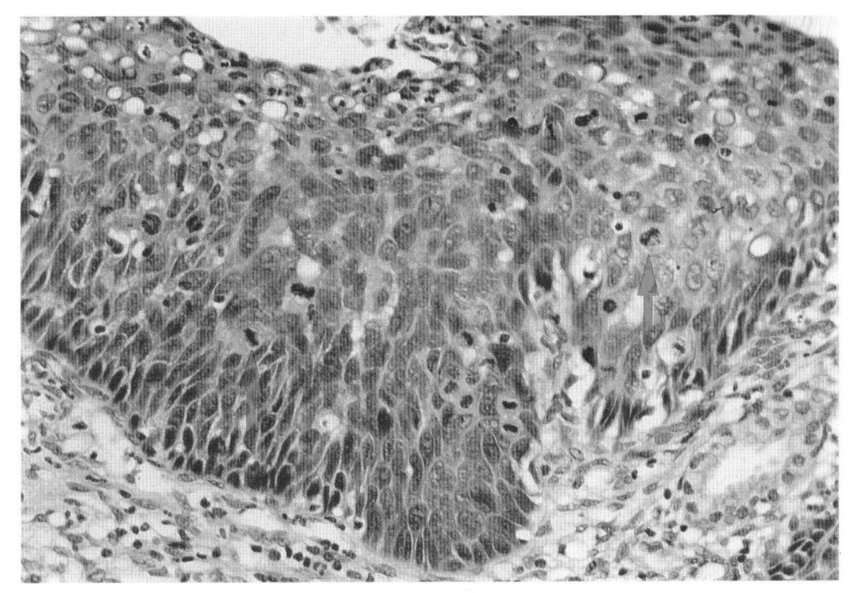

7.36 Cervical intraepithelial neoplasia (CIN): cervix

In the same way as dysplasia, squamous carcinoma tends to arise at the junction of the stratified squamous epithelium of the ectocervix and the columnar epithelium lining the endocervix. Carcinoma-in-situ may thus extend down into glandular structures. The lumen of the cervical canal is at the top but not visible. In this CIN III lesion, several of the cervical glands (bottom left) are lined by normal palisaded tall columnar epithelial cells with a large amount of pale mucin-containing cytoplasm (thin arrow). However, a sheet of atypical hyperchromatic squamous epithelial cells (double arrow), heavily infiltrated with polymorph leukocytes, has displaced the columnar epithelium which normally lines the endocervix. The atypical squamous cells also fill the lumen of the underlying branching glands (thick arrow). The atypical squamous cells have large hyperchromatic vesicular nuclei, and there are many mitoses at all levels. The basement membrane beneath the sheets of atypical squamous cells is still intact and the lesion is not invasive carcinoma. HE ×80

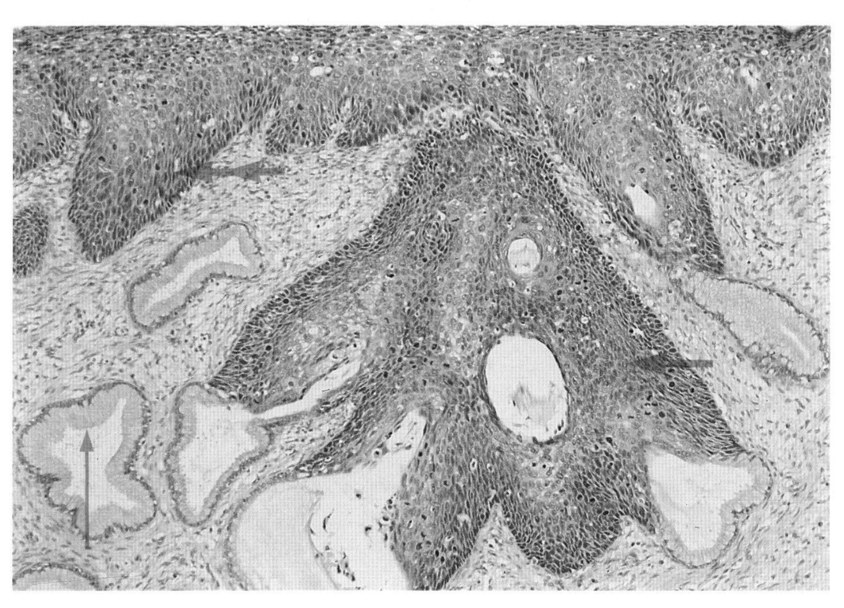

7.37 Cervical Intraepithelial Neoplasia (CIN)

Tripolar mitosis (arrow), surrounded by eosinophilic neoplastic squamous epithelial cells (CIN)

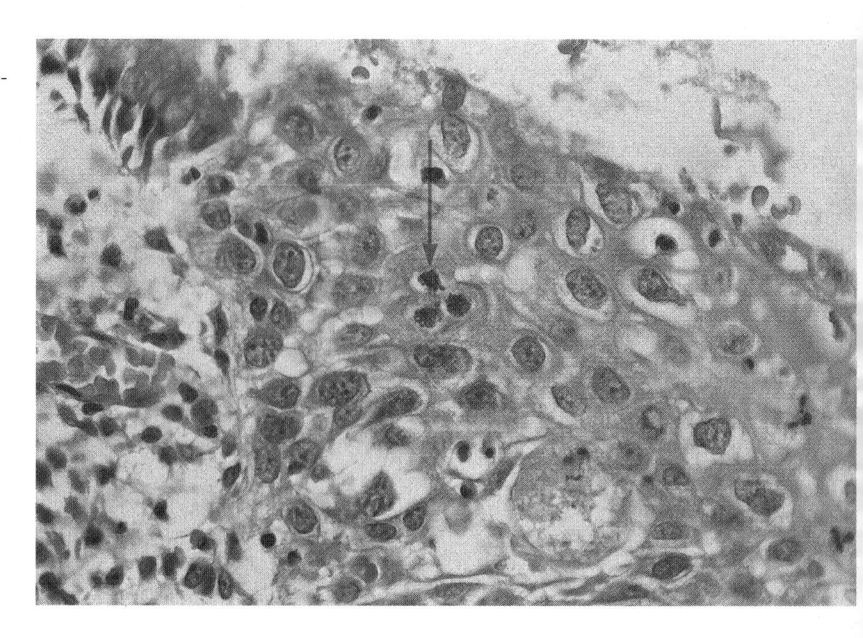

7.38 Cervical intraepithelial neoplasia (CIN)

Human Papilloma Virus (HPV), type 31, has been demonstrated by means of in-situ DNA hybridisation in many of the cells (arrow). Several types of HPV are known to be the causative agents in CIN and carcinoma of cervix, and elevated flat areas or wart-like papillomatous growths tend to form. The risk of cervical carcinoma increases greatly, whereas the incidence of cervical carcinoma in patients infected with Herpes Simplex Virus type 1 (HSV-2) is low, which indicates that the carcinogenic potential of the virus is not great.

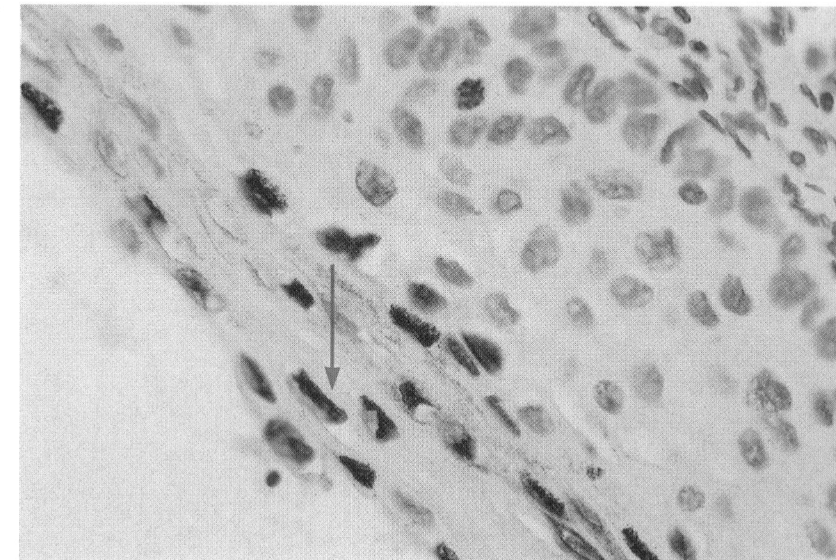

7.39 Cervix - high-grade glandular in-situ neoplasia

Cervical glandular epithelium is showing severe dysplasia of the non-squamous part of the epithelium (Cervical Glandular Intraepithelial Neoplasia, CGIN). Bizarre cells (arrow) are seen high up in the epithelial layer. This change is often associated with Cervical Intraepithelial Neoplasia (CIN) as a result of infection with Human Papilloma Virus (HPV).

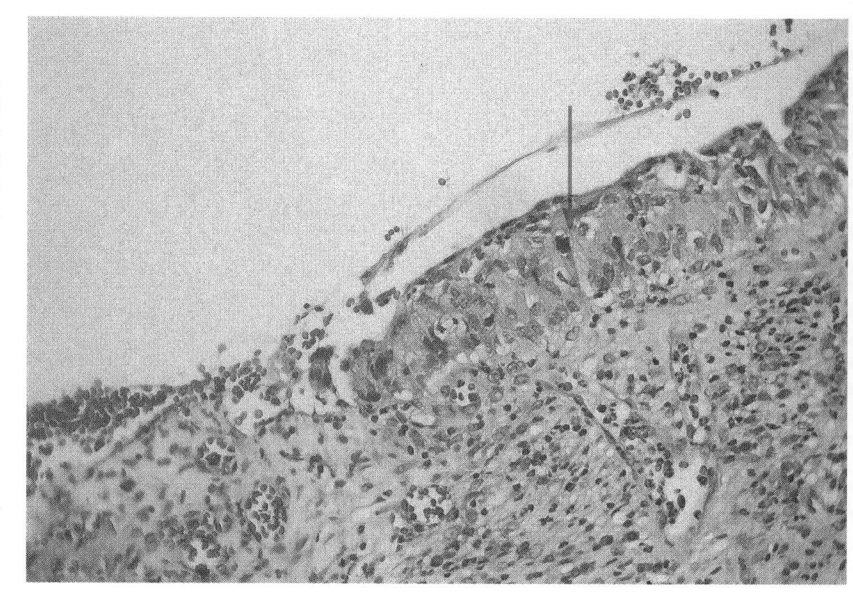

7.40 Squamous carcinoma: cervix

Squamous (epidermoid) carcinoma of the cervix is a fairly common tumour, which tends to occur in middle-aged women (40 years and more). Human papillomavirus, particularly types 16 and 18, is regarded as an important etiological agent. The mortality rate has been falling, partly because of the early detection of premalignant dysplasia of the squamous epithelium by routine cytological screening of cervical smears. Many cases are detected in the preinvasive stage and resected. In contrast to carcinoma however the incidence of dysplasia persists and appears to be occurring in younger women. In this lesion, the tumour cells are arranged in clumps, and characteristically show no tendency to keratinization or cell nest formation. They have abundant eosinophilic cytoplasm and large moderately pleomorphic nuclei, most of them round; and in the centre of the nuclei there is a prominent central nucleolus (thin arrow). No mitotic figures are visible, and mitotic activity is moderate elsewhere. The scant stroma which separates the groups of tumour cells consists mainly of thin-walled blood vessels and is infiltrated with small lymphocytes (thick arrow). HE ×270

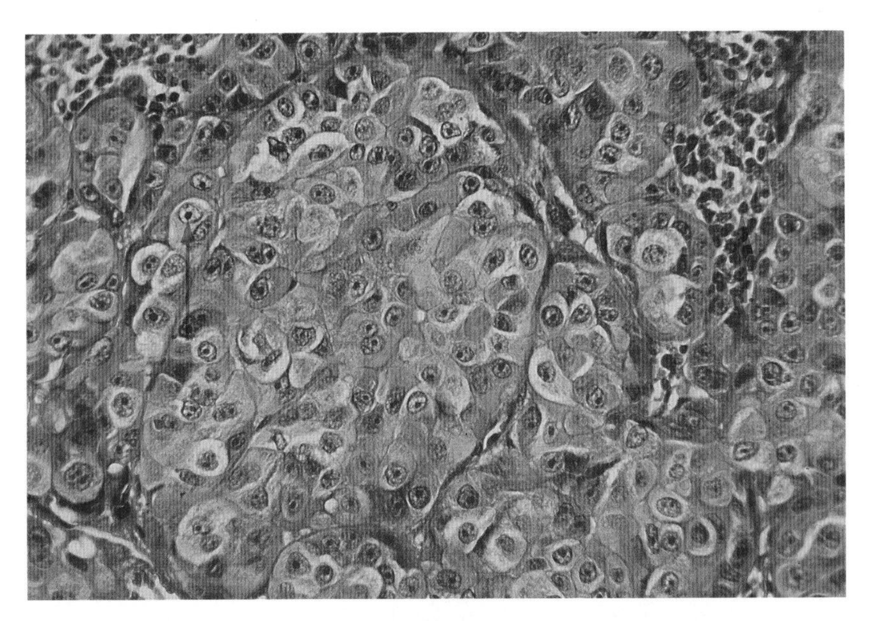

7.41 Endocervical polyp

Polyps of the cervix are common lesions, usually occurring about the time of the menopause. They originate in the endocervical canal, which is lined with mucus-secreting columnar epithelial cells, and form pedunculated smooth-surfaced benign neoplasms which may be several cm in diameter. An unusually large polyp may protrude through the external os. A typical endocervical polyp consists of hyperplastic glands of various sizes in highly cellular connective tissue. This shows part of one polyp. It consists of glandular spaces which vary in size from small to dilated and occasionally to very large (cystic) forms. The glands are lined with a single layer of cuboidal or tall columnar mucus-secreting epithelial cells which are closely packed and palisaded (thin arrows), with small basal nuclei and a large amount of pale mucin-containing cytoplasm. The vascular fibrous tissue between the glands is heavily infiltrated with chronic inflammatory cells. The surface of the polyp is not ulcerated, but undergoes metaplasia. Instead of being covered with conventional columnar epithelial cells, the polyp has a single layer of flat atrophic non-mucin-secreting cells on its surface (thick arrow).

HE ×120

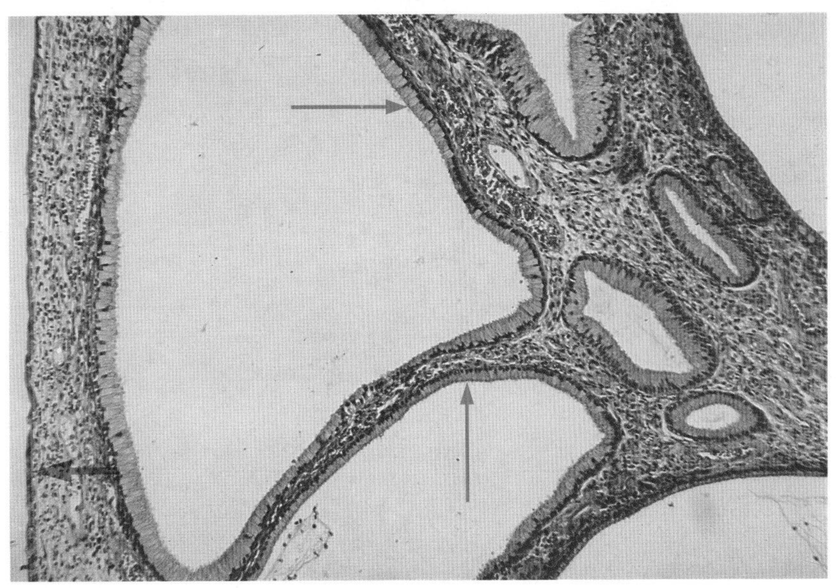

7.42 Endometrial polyp: uterus

Most endometrial polyps are not neoplasms but polypoid smooth-surfaced fleshy masses (0.5 - 3cm dia) which project into the uterine cavity. They are covered with endometrial epithelium and composed of hyperplastic endometrial glands. They may be asymptomatic or cause excessive bleeding from the uterus. In this polyp, both the glandular elements and the cellular stroma are clearly recognizable as endometrial in origin. Apart from a few cystic types, most of the glands are of moderate size. They are arranged irregularly however and are lined with very closely packed columnar cells with hyperchromatic ovoid nuclei which tend to overlap (thin arrow). Although endometrial polyps may ulcerate and bleed, the surface of this polyp is covered with an intact layer of flattened epithelial cells (thick arrow). The epithelial cells lining the glands in this polyp are non-secretory (the glands of an endometrial polyp are often unresponsive to progesterone). The stroma is cellular but edematous and pale (double arrow). There is also no evidence of inflammation, and the vascularity of the polyp is slight.

HE ×120

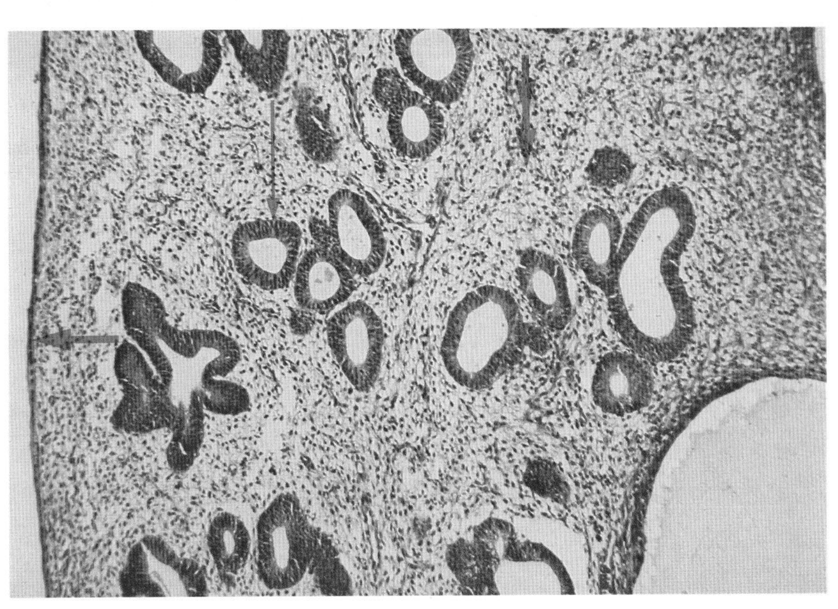

7.43 Effect of contraceptive: endometrium

In this biopsy of the endometrial tissue lining the uterus, the effect of a contraceptive on the structure of the endometrium is evident. The few endometrial glands that are visible here are small simple structures lined by cuboidal or flat (hypoplastic) non-secretory cells (thick arrow). In the stroma surrounding the few glands, there is a fairly well-developed pseudodecidual reaction. It consists of a moderate population of uniformly scattered cells with abundant edematous well-defined cytoplasm and round or ovoid nuclei, most of them located in a large clear vacuole and giving the stroma a 'chondroid' appearance (thin arrow). The amount of connective tissue in the stroma is minimal. After prolonged use of the pill, the stroma tends to lose the pseudodecidual reaction and become more compact and atrophic. When the woman stops taking the contraceptive, the endometrium soon resumes its normal cycle of activity. HE x235

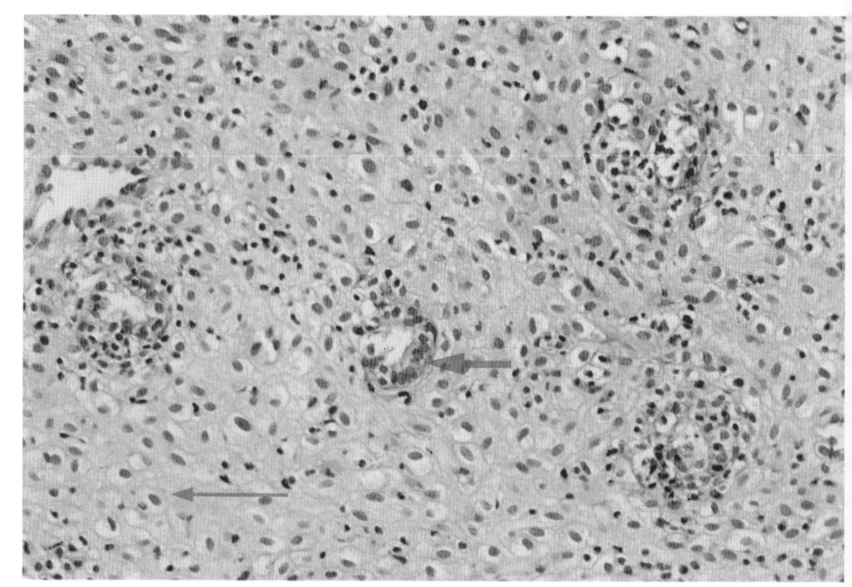

7.44 Endometrial hyperplasia: uterus

Endometrial hyperplasia is a premalignant lesion, caused by unopposed stimulation by estrogen, the risk of malignancy varying proportionately with the intensity of the hyperplasia. At its most extreme (atypical hyperplasia), it is a focal lesion. It is most common around the menopause. The risk of malignant change is significant, and since it is difficult to distinguish hyperplasia from adenocarcinoma, it is probably better to regard atypical hyperplasia as intraendometrial carcinoma rather than hyperplasia. In this example, the endometrium is moderately hyperplastic (complex hyperplasia without atypia). The glands are crowded (slightly back-to-back), moderately dilated and lined with a single layer of closely packed palisaded tall columnar epithelial cells with a small amount of cytoplasm (thick arrow). The nuclei are elongated and markedly hyperchromatic, and although they are only moderately pleomorphic they often overlap. The cells show no evidence of secretory activity. Elsewhere the glands were more dilated and cystic. The stroma also is intensely cellular, consisting of very large numbers of cells (thin arrow) with basophilic ovoid or fusiform nuclei and a relatively small amount of cytoplasm. Numerous mitoses are present among both the epithelial and stromal cells. HE ×135

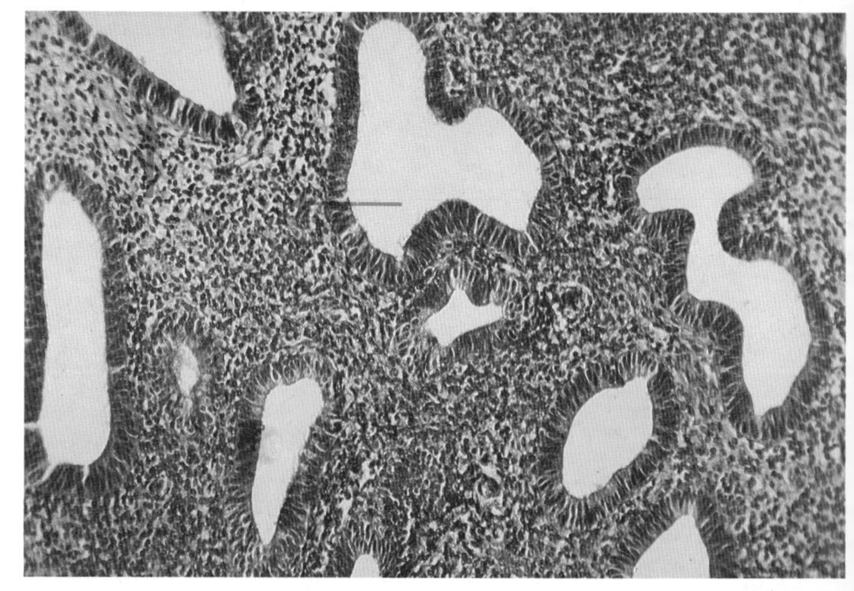

7.45 Adenomyosis (endometriosis interna): uterus

In adenomyosis, islands of endometrial tissue (endometrial glands and stroma) are abnormally deep in the myometrium, more than 3mm from the base of the endometrium but in direct continuity with it. It is common in older women (more than 40 years of age). Diffuse adenomyosis involves most of the uterus, diffusely thickening its wall, whereas focal adenomyosis forms a nodular mass resembling a leiomyoma ('adenomyoma'). This lesion is part of a nodule of ectopic endometrial tissue (focal adenomyosis). The muscle coat, a band of intensely eosinophilic smooth muscle cells, is visible at the right margin (thin arrow). There is no fibrous capsule around the nodule of endometrial tissue, which consists of a sheet of cellular stroma and glands, clearly of endometrial origin, lined with overlapping cuboidal and columnar cells (thick arrow). There is dense eosinophilic secretion in some glands but no sign of previous hemorrhage in or around the lesion, perhaps because the glands are basal. The stroma is unusually fibrillary (double arrow) and most of the cells are elongated and spindle-shaped. HE ×80

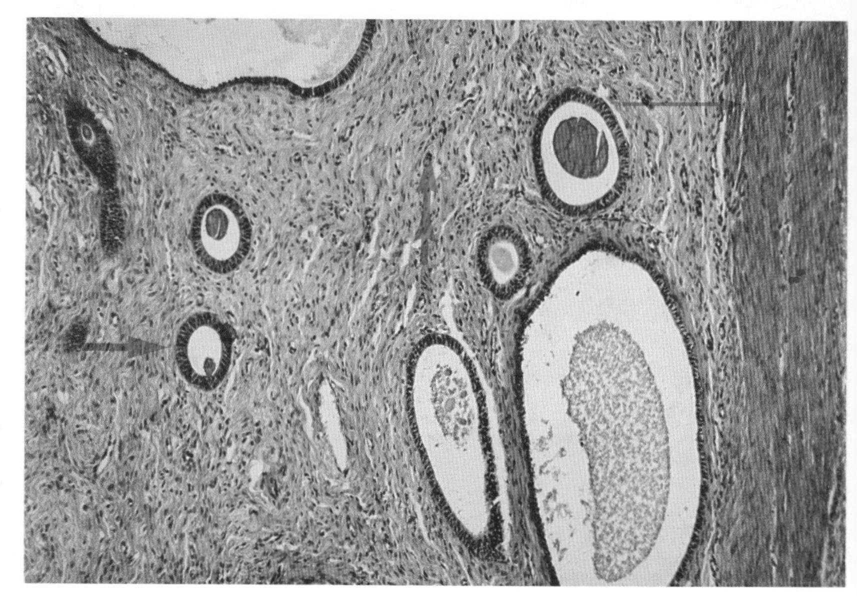

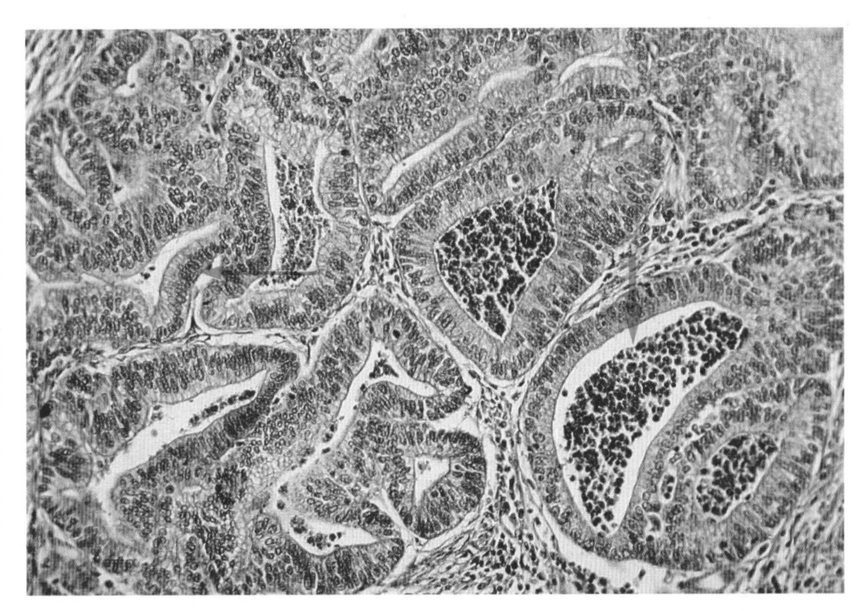

7.46 Endometrial carcinoma: uterus

Endometrial carcinoma occurs mainly in post-menopausal women, and nulliparous women have a greater tendency to develop the tumour than parous women. It is usually preceded by endometrial hyperplasia. The tumour may be localized to one part of the uterine cavity but more often the whole of the cavity contains a polypoid rather nodular fungating mass which enlarges the uterus. The tumour tends to bleed and there may be considerable necrosis. In this case, a bulky mass of tissue fills the uterine cavity, and this part of it consists of very abnormal glands, nearly all arranged closely 'back-to-back'. The glands vary greatly in shape and are lined with a thick layer, usually single but sometimes seemingly multiple, of very tall columnar epithelial cells (thin arrow). There is considerable mitotic activity in the columnar epithelial cells that line the glands, and some glands contain a considerable amount of necrotic cell debris (thick arrow). The relatively scant stroma between the glands is heavily infiltrated with inflammatory cells. HE ×120

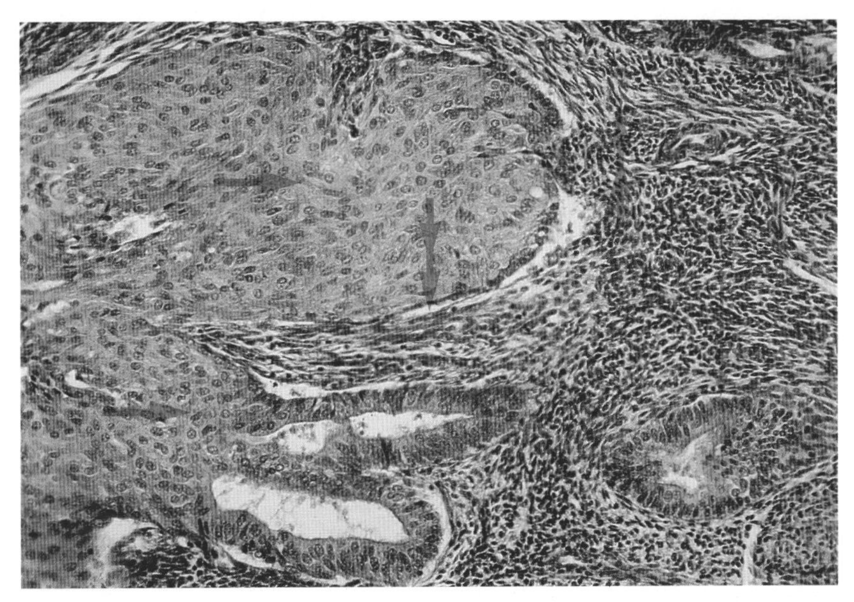

7.47 Adenosquamous carcinoma (adenoacanthoma): uterus

In about a quarter of the cases of endometrial carcinoma, the malignant columnar epithelial cells that line the carcinomatous glands undergo metaplasia to form sheets of squamous epithelium. In this example of adenosquamous carcinoma, the very cellular myometrium, consisting of large interlacing bundles of spindle-shaped cells (double arrows) with minimal cytoplasm and intensely hyperchromatic elongated nuclei, is infiltrated by well-differentiated adenocarcinomatous glands (thin arrow). The adenocarcinomatous glands are relatively small and lined with closely packed malignant columnar epithelial cells with overlapping ovoid vesicular nuclei. Adjoining the adenocarcinoma, and fusing with two of the malignant glands, there are sheets, with rounded well-defined margins, of eosinophilic squamous epithelial cells (thick arrows). The squamous epithelial cells have pale ovoid vesicular nuclei, uniformly distributed. The nuclei lack hyperchromasia and do not look unduly malignant. Nor is there any obvious mitotic activity. The prognosis of adenosquamous carcinoma is the same as that for the adenocarcinomatous component and is not influenced by the presence of the metaplastic squamous epithelium. HE ×135

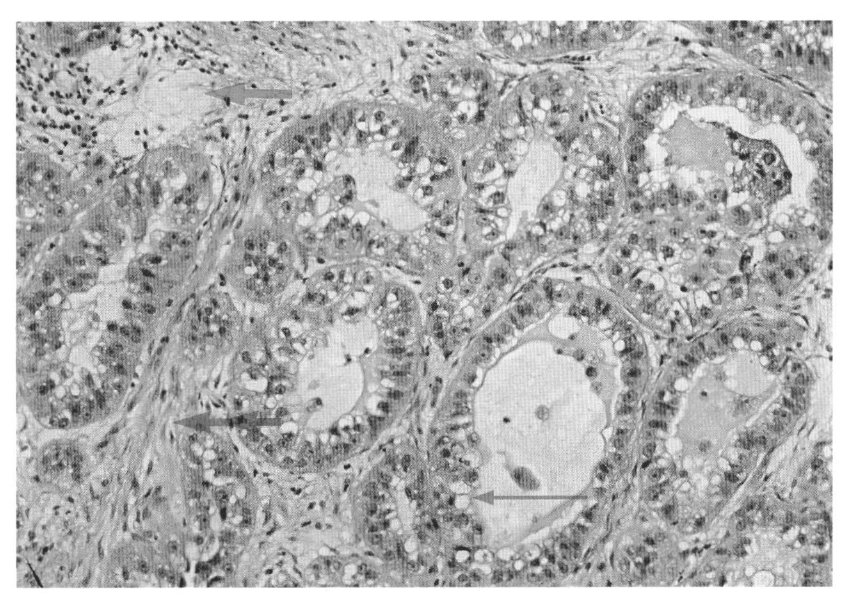

7.48 Clear cell carcinoma of endometrium: uterus

About 5% of endometrial carcinomas resemble clear cell carcinoma of ovaries. The term clear cell carcinoma is applied only if a major portion of the endometrial carcinoma is of clear cell type but not when the foci of clear cell carcinoma are small. Despite a superficial resemblance histologically to the mesonephric carcinomas of ovary, cervix and vagina, the endometrial tumour is unlikely to arise in mesonephric remnants, and a Müllerian origin is more probable. This tumour consists of closely packed slightly irregular malignant glands. Most of the glands are arranged 'back-to-back' but the others are separated by thick strands of eosinophilic fibrillary connective tissue and elongated fibrocytes (double arrow). The malignant glands are lined by tall columnar epithelial cells, with ovoid or elongated vesicular nuclei and, in many cells, a large clear (empty) supranuclear vacuole (thin arrow) (vacuolation of the cytoplasm is caused by the presence of much glycogen). The nuclei of the tumour cells are moderately pleomorphic and some contain a large central nucleolus. Many nuclei are pyknotic. Pale-staining mucoid secretion fills the lumen of most of the glands. and there is a small quantity of mucin in the stroma (thick arrow). HE ×150

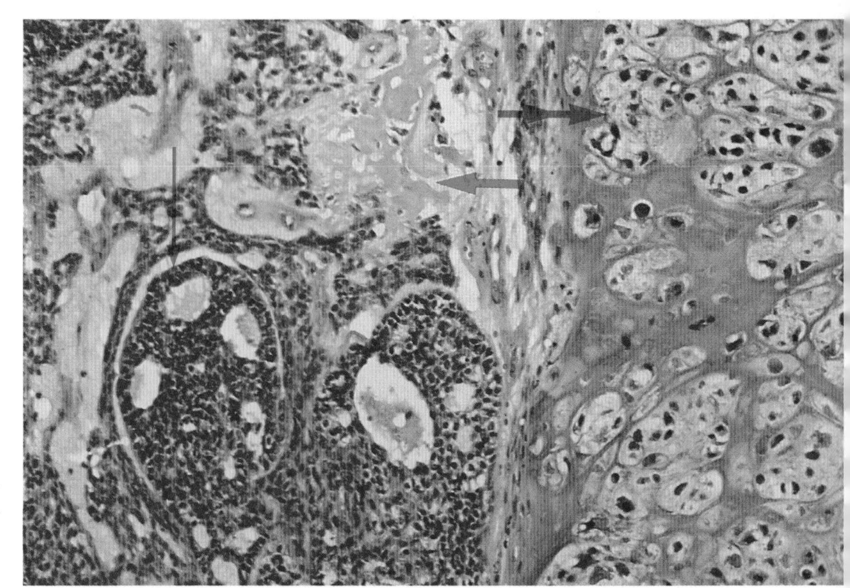

7.49 Mesodermal mixed tumour: uterus

Mesodermal mixed tumour contains both a malignant epithelial component (usually and adenocarcinoma) and a malignant mesenchymal component. It is a very rare tumour, and usually occurs in women more than 55 years old. It arises in residual Müllerian cells in the endometrium and usually forms a bulky fleshy (soft) mass. It often fills the uterine cavity and may protrude through the cervical os. In the cut surface of the tumour there is often extensive necrosis and hemorrhage. The carcinoma is generally an adenocarcinoma. The tumour is radioresistant and tends to spread by the lymphatics or bloodstream. The prognosis is poor. This tumour consists of a sheet of chondrosarcomatous tissue (double arrow), separated by thin strands of collagenous fibrous tissue (right of centre) from cords and sheets of epithelial cells with round hyperchromatic nuclei (left), and also irregular fragments of weakly eosinophilic cartilage-like tissue (thick arrow). In the bluish deeply basophilic matrix of the chondrosarcomatous tissue there are large clusters of very atypical chondrocytes, with extremely pleomorphic nuclei. In the sheets of basophilic epithelial cells (thin arrow) there are small gland-like spaces, some containing eosinophilic secretion. HE ×150

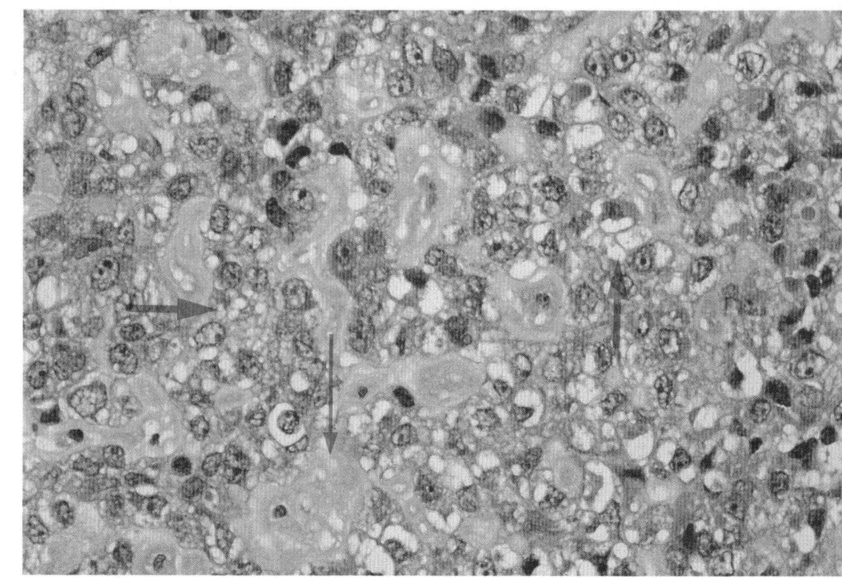

7.50 Mesodermal mixed tumour: uterus

Mesodermal mixed tumour is highly malignant, with a survival rate of about 20%, and tends to metastasize early. The sarcomatous component of the tumour is generally less conspicuous than the epithelial element, often resembling leiomyosarcoma or fibrosarcoma, but rhabdomyosarcomatous cells and other malignant mesenchymal tissues (including chondro- or osteosarcoma) may be present. In this mesodermal mixed tumour, which arose in a woman of 69, there was extensive necrosis. This part of the tumour consists of groups and cords of cells, separated by hyaline amorphous bluish-pink material (thin arrow) not unlike cartilage matrix. The neoplastic cells have an ill-defined amount of cytoplasm, with indistinct cell boundaries and in which there are large numbers of small vacuoles (thick arrows). The nuclei are large round and pleomorphic and contain one or more prominent nucleoli. Many tumour cell nuclei are pyknotic. There are no mitotic figures in this field but many were present elsewhere in the tumour. In the matrix between the cords and groups of cells there are many pale vacuoles, and the tissue in general has a chondroid appearance.

HE ×360

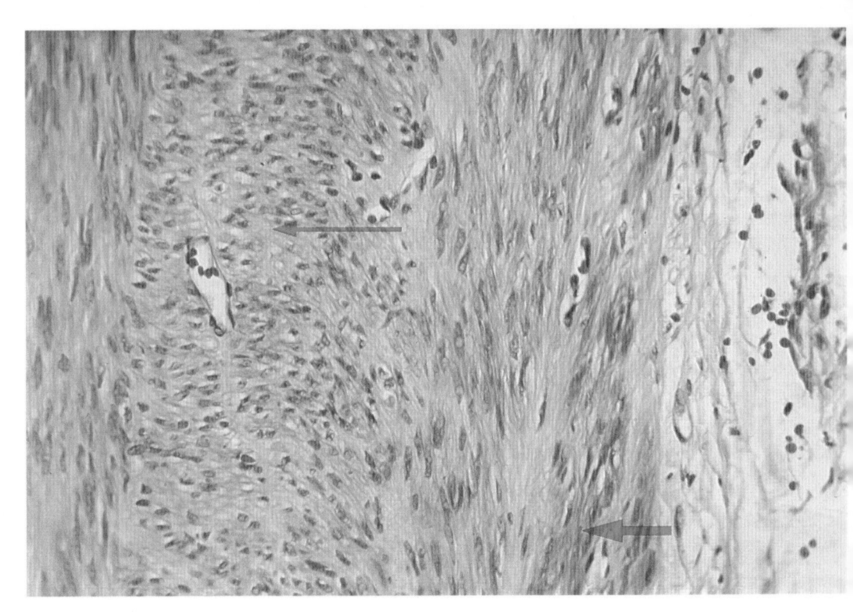

7.51 Leiomyoma: uterus

Leiomyoma is a benign neoplasm of uterine smooth muscle. It is one of the commonest tumours, being found in the majority of women. It generally arises between 20 and 40 years of age, and tends to stop growing actively after the menopause. A large tumour may have significant mechanical effects, whereas a small lesion projecting into the lumen of the uterus may interfere with conception or become ulcerated and cause heavy bleeding. Malignant change is very rare. The edge of this tumour is on the right. Although typically well-defined, the tumour lacks a fibrous capsule but there are dilated small thin-walled blood vessels and some loose fibrous tissue on its surface. The tumour consists of broad bundles of mature smooth muscle cells that run at various angles, so that some bundles are visible in longitudinal section (thick arrow) and others in cross-section (thin arrow). There is some fibrous tissue between the bundles of muscle cells and it usually increases. As a result, older tumours become hard and fibrous (fibromyomas or 'fibroids'). Some tumours eventually calcify. HE ×200

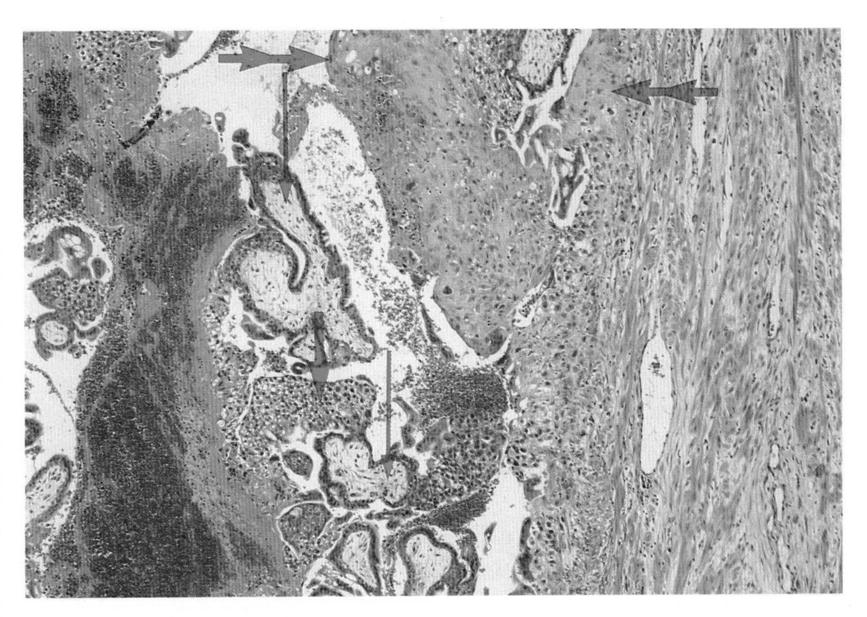

7.52 Tubal (ectopic) pregnancy: Fallopian tube

An ectopic pregnancy occurs when the fertilized ovum is implanted at a site other than uterine cavity, and Fallopian tubes which are fibrosed as a result of chronic inflammation or which are congenitally abnormal may delay or prevent the passage of the ovum. The retained ovum may implant itself in the wall of the tube and become an ectopic (tubal) pregnancy. This tubal pregnancy was diagnosed in a woman aged 22, and consequently a portion of her left Fallopian tube, 5cm long, was resected surgically. The resected part of the tube was found to be expanded by blood clot. Histologically, the wall of the tube on the right consists of interlacing bundles of very elongated smooth muscle cells, and the epithelium that normally lines the tube has been replaced by a broad sheet of well-developed decidua (double arrows). In the lumen of the tube there is a mass of deep red clotted blood (left), alongside which there are numerous pale chorionic villi (thin arrows). The core of the villi consists of edematous (myxoid) connective tissue, and the surface of the villi is covered with a layer of basophilic trophoblast. There are also sheets of trophoblast, lying free in the lumen (thick arrow). HE ×60

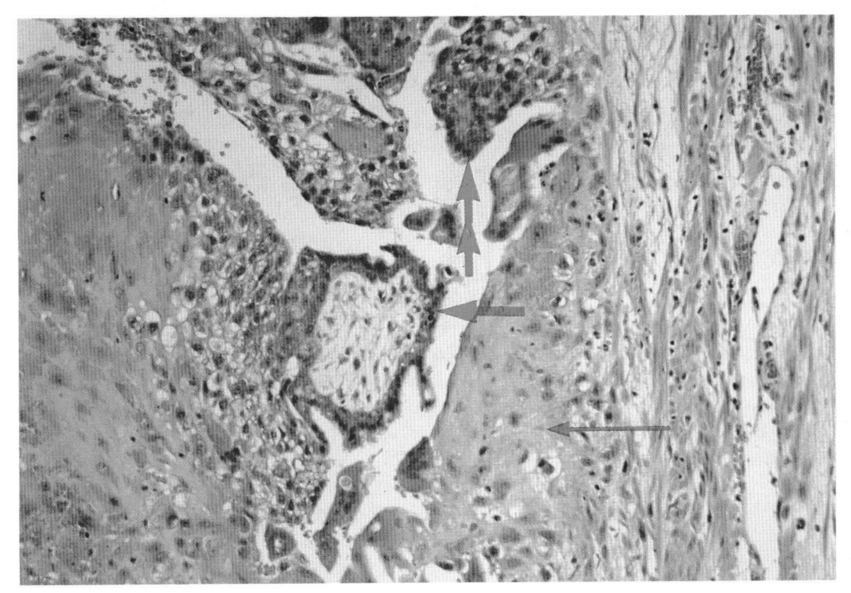

7.53 Tubal (ectopic) pregnancy: Fallopian tube

Endometriosis involving the uterine tube is also liable to cause an increased risk of tubal pregnancy, but in many cases no etiological factor can be identified. This is the same lesion in 7.55, at higher magnification. The sheet of smooth muscle cells in the wall of the Fallopian tube (right margin) is vascular and edematous. The lumen of the tube is partly lined with eosinophilic decidua (thin arrow). There is also a sheet of similar decidual tissue lying free within the lumen (left margin) and, alongside it, a sheet of basophilic cytotrophoblast. The cytotrophoblast consists of cells with a considerable amount of vacuolated cytoplasm, with very well-defined cell boundaries, and adherent to it is a chorionic villus (thick arrow). The villus has a pale-staining core of myxoid tissue, covered with a thin (outer) layer of syncytiotrophoblast and (inner) cytotrophoblast. Other fragments of trophoblast are attached to the tube lining (double arrow) or lie free in the lumen. No fetal elements were found among the contents of the tube. A decidual reaction usually develops simultaneously in the uterus. Only a very small proportion of ectopic pregnancies go on to term. HE ×150

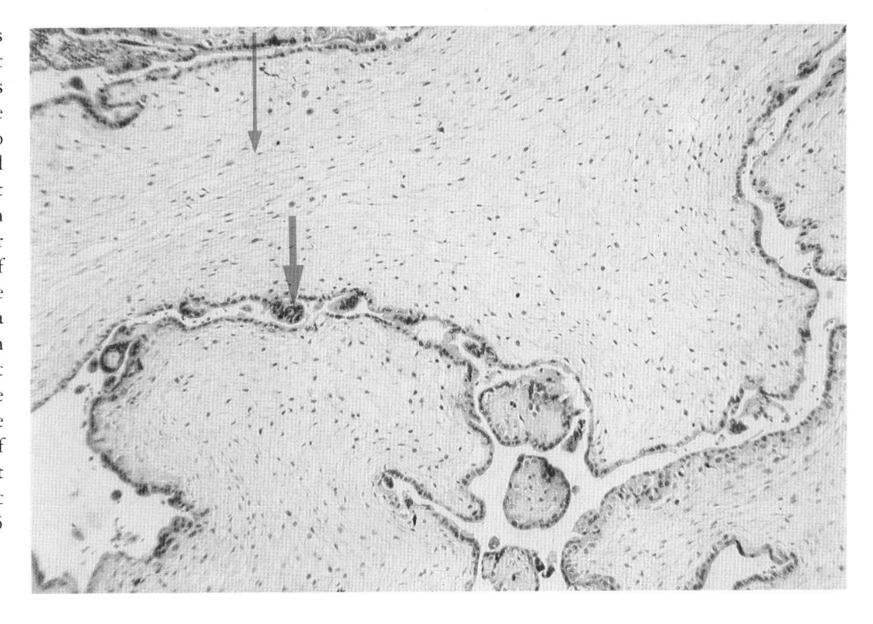

7.54 Hydatidiform mole: uterus

A hydatidiform mole arises in the placenta (the embryo is usually absent) and forms a large numbers of cystic grape-like structures (up to 2cm dia) which fill the uterus and cause it to enlarge beyond the size appropriate for the stage of pregnancy. In most cases these cystic structures do not invade the muscular wall of the uterus, but in a small minority of 'invasive' moles the villi and trophoblast penetrate extensively into the myometrium and may even 'metastasize'. The 'metastases' regress however after removal of the mole. This is part of a mole, consisting of hydropic dilated avascular chorionic villi. The villi are greatly expanded and their core of each villus consists of a large sheet of pale edematous connective tissue (thin arrow), throughout which a sparse population of fibrocytic cells with pleomorphic nuclei are widely distributed. There are no fetal blood vessels in the cores of the villi. The surface of each villus is covered with a thin layer of trophoblast from which small nodules of cytotrophoblast project (thick arrow). The extent of trophoblastic proliferation is often considerable. HE ×55

7.55 Gestational choriocarcinoma: uterus

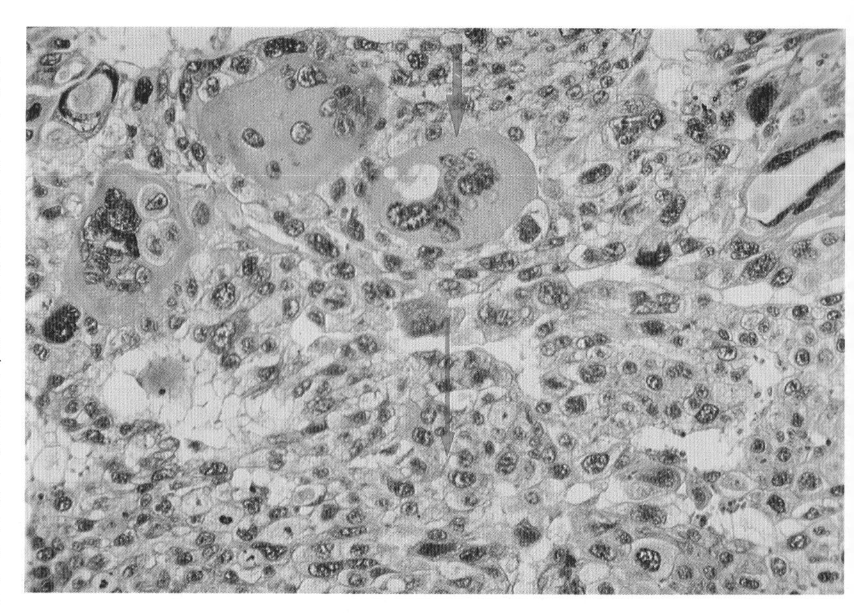

Gestational choriocarcinoma of the uterus is a rare highly malignant neoplasm of trophoblast and therefore of fetal origin. It is identical to ovarian or testicular choriocarcinoma. About half of the gestational choriocarcinomas follow a hydatidiform mole, and the others occur after an abortion. Chorionic villi are not present in choriocarcinoma. The tumour presents as a friable mass of round hemorrhagic nodules in the uterine cavity. It infiltrates the myometriun extensively, tending to invade blood vessels early, and is prone to metastasize by the bloodstream to various organs. This tumour consists of sheets of cells derived from the cytotrophoblast (lower half). The cells have pleomorphic vesicular nuclei and a considerable amount of clear cytoplasm with well-defined cytoplasmic boundaries (thin arrow). The upper half of the picture consists (largely) of syncytiotrophoblast, which consists of sheets (of various sizes) of multinucleated cytoplasm (thick arrow). The tumour produces chorionic gonadotropin (hCG), and the levels of this hormone in the serum are extremely useful for monitoring treatment. Elevated levels indicate persistence of trophoblastic tissue and the need for further treatment. HE ×135

7.56 Polycystic ovary syndrome: ovary

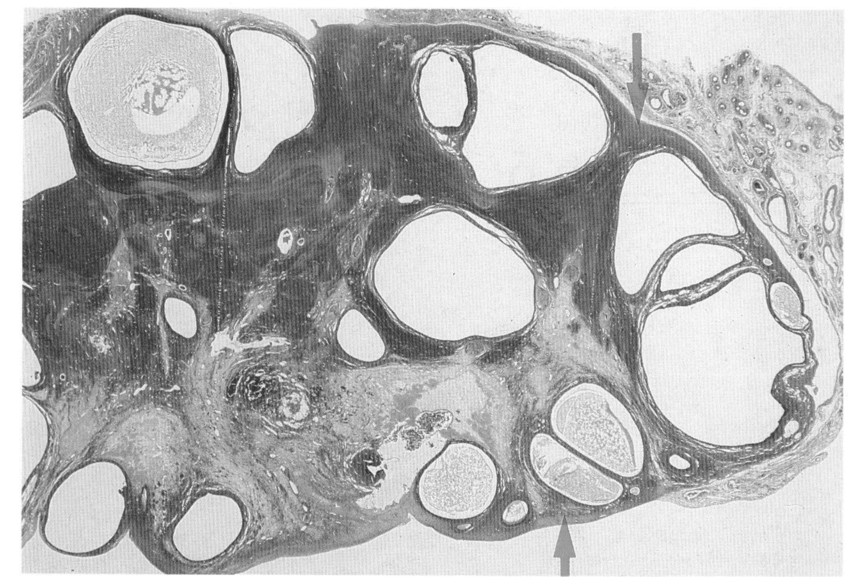

Polycystic ovary syndrome is characterized by a) bilaterally enlarged ovaries; b) multiple follicular cysts in the outer subcapsular region; c) absence of corpora lutea (failure of ovulation); and d) hyperplastic ovarian stroma with thickening of the capsule. The patient is associated with amenorrhea, infertility and virilism, and is usually sterile. The cause of polycystic disease is probably abnormal secretion of pituitary gonadotropins. The various abnormalities include the Stein-Leventhal syndrome. Both ovaries are enlarged, from the presence of multiple follicular cysts. Numerous atretic follicles are also present, but corpora lutea and corpora albicantia are absent. Wedge resection of the ovary usually restores the menstrual cycle. This shows part of one ovary, cut in longitudinal section. The most superficial layer of the ovarian cortex (thick arrows) is fibrous, and the ovary is enclosed in a thick so-called 'capsule' of stromal fibrous tissue. Within the ovary there are multiple large round follicular cysts, distributed throughout the cortex. These are simple follicular cysts and lined with a single layer of flattened cells. Several of the cysts contain eosinophilic fluid. HE ×5

7.57 Polycystic ovary syndrome: ovary

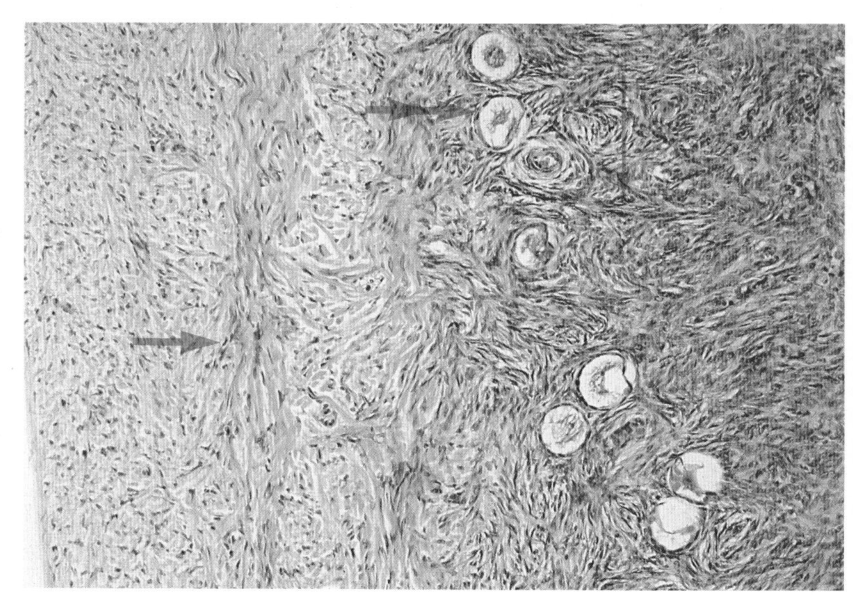

In polycystic ovary syndrome both ovaries are about twice their normal size, and their smooth greyish-white surfaces are studded with small blue cysts. The outer part of the cortex is collagenized and sometimes hyalinized, and the stroma in the deeper part of the ovaries is increased and sometimes luteinized. This is part of the same lesion as in 12.56, at much higher magnification. This shows the cortex between two of the cysts in the ovary. The surface of the ovary is just visible at the left margin, and beneath its surface the most superficial part of the cortex takes the form of a 'capsule' of interlacing bundles of fibrocyte-type cells and strands of eosinophilic collagenous fibrous tissue (thick arrow). Deep to this collagenous tissue there is a layer of highly cellular basophilic stroma (thin arrow), in which there are also a small number of round (atretic) follicles (double arrow). This basophilic stroma consists of interlacing bundles of closely packed elongated fibrocyte-type cells with elongated spindle-shaped basophilic nuclei. Large numbers of similar follicles were present in both ovaries. HE ×150

7.58 Corpus luteal cyst: ovary

Corpus luteal cysts are derived from the corpus luteum of pregnancy. A normal corpus luteum is itself slightly cystic, but occasionally a much larger solid cystic structure (up to 6cm dia) develops at the end of the menstrual cycle or in pregnancy. Macroscopically the wall of this cyst has a yellow-brown colour. Histologically the wall of the cyst is composed of broad folded sheets of large luteinized cells with abundant well-defined granular or vacuolated (lipid-rich) cytoplasm (thin arrow). The cells are arranged in clusters and trabeculae, separated by delicate stromal fibres. There has been bleeding into the lumen of the cyst, above the sheets of luteinized cells, and a considerable amount of extravasated blood has collected in the cyst and distended it (thick arrow). A corpus luteum cyst may also bleed into the peritoneal cavity. Corpus luteal cysts produce estrogens and occasionally androgens, but the cysts disappear spontaneously. HE ×55

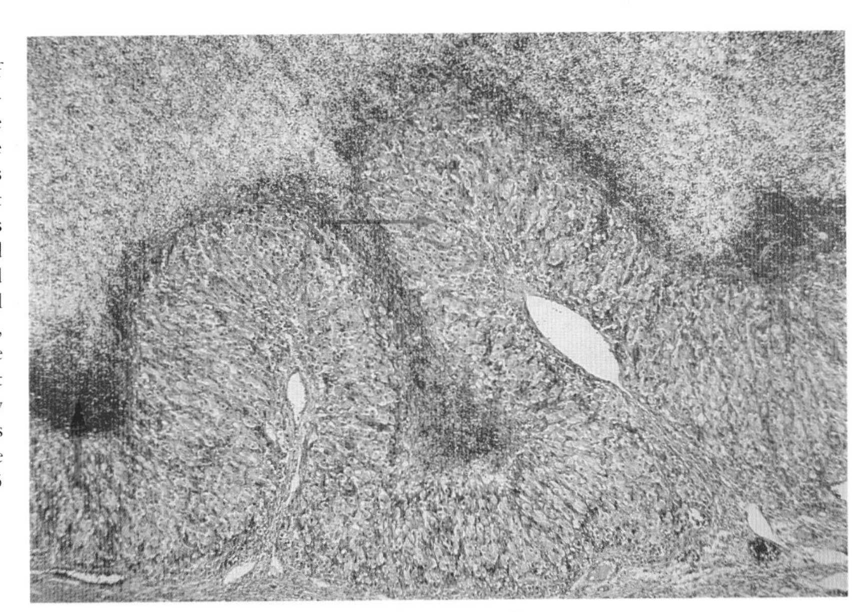

7.59 Endometriosis: ovary

Not infrequently endometrial tissue is found in sites other than the uterus (extrauterine endometriosis), and it is usually composed of both epithelial and stromal cells. The sites tend to be in the pelvis, and include the ovaries and peritoneal cavity. Foci of endometrial tissue and the associated hemorrhage usually provoke a fibrous reaction, and appear as cysts or fibrous nodules. The nodules may interfere with the functioning of adjacent organs, but in the ovaries a cyst filled with brown debris from previous hemorrhages tends to develop. The ovarian cysts are sometimes called chocolate cysts. This shows part of a cystic lesion in the ovary. The cystic space on the left, possibly a very dilated gland, is lined with cuboidal or low columnar epithelial cells (thick arrow), and in the sheet of very cellular endometrial stroma there is a moderately-sized endometrial gland lined by closely packed columnar epithelial cells with large elongated basophilic nuclei (thick arrow). There is (fresh) bright red hemorrhage around the gland in the stroma (thin arrow), and in the cystic space there is a large amount of brown debris (double arrow), the product of old hemorrhage.

HE ×200

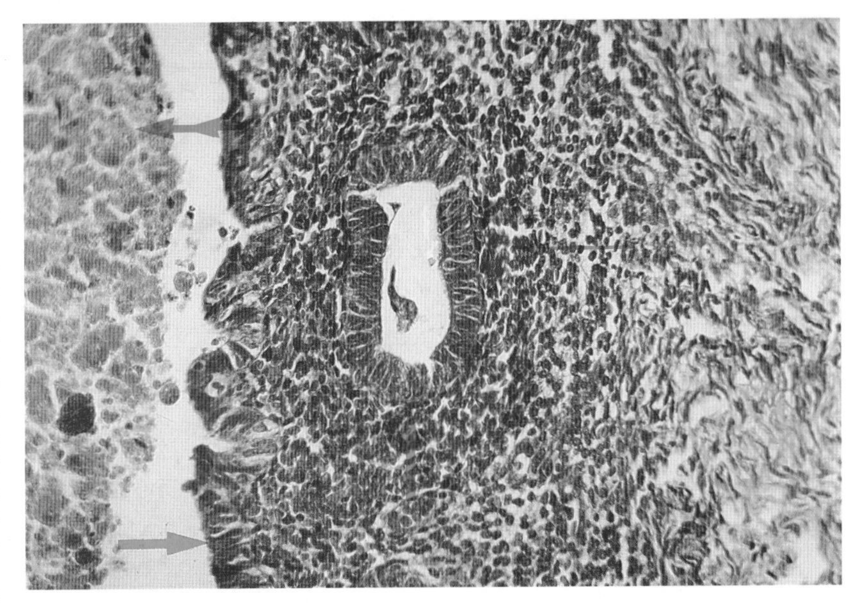

7.60 Endometriosis: skin

Spontaneous endometriosis of the skin is found only at the umbilicus and in the inguinal regions, although it may develop in surgical scars in many other sites, particularly after caesarean section. This lesion presented as a firm nodule at the umbilicus in a woman of 25. It is enclosed in atrophic very eosinophilic striated muscle fibres (double arrow), and consists of a small number of glands of various sizes and different forms of stroma. In the more extensive sheet of pale edematous (myxoid) spindle cell stroma on the left (thin arrow) there are several glands lined by cuboidal or flat epithelial cells. On the right however the glands are lined by a single slightly papilliform layer of fairly large cuboidal or columnar epithelial cells (thick arrow) and are surrounded by a dense infiltrate of chronic inflammatory cells. There are also thick strands of dense fibrous tissue around the glands. Some glands contain a small amount of secretion, mostly pale but strongly eosinophilic in one gland. Elsewhere in the lesion there is a considerable amount of hemorrhage but only small amounts of hemosiderin.

HE ×60

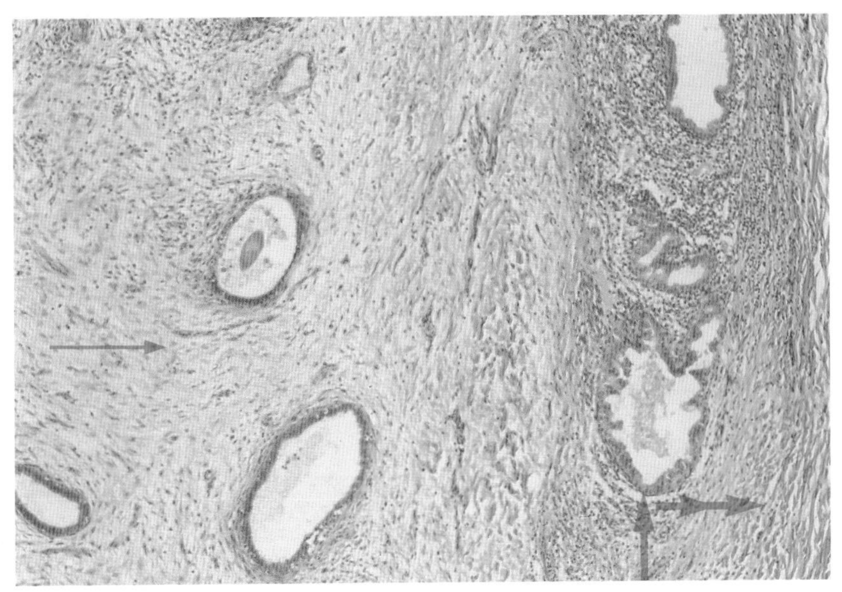

7.61 Benign cystic teratoma (dermoid cyst): ovary

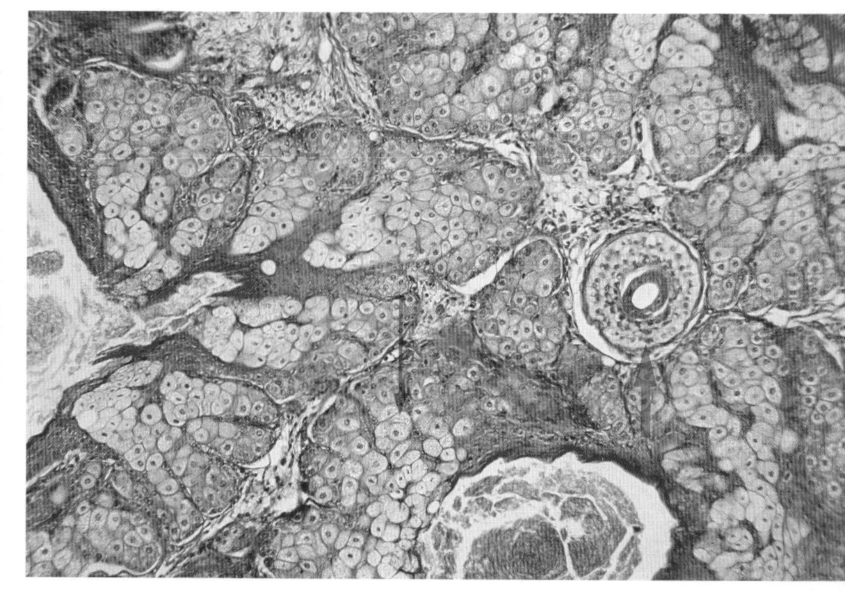

A teratoma contains a wide range of tissues in a disorderly arrangement. 80% of germ cell tumours of the ovary are teratomas. They are similar in derivation from their counterparts in the testis but there are however striking differences. Mature teratomas of the ovary, but not teratomas of the testis, are benign at all ages.

The ovary and testis are the commonest sites, but teratomas occur in other sites (retroperitoneal, mediastinal, etc.). In mature ovarian teratomas, skin and its appendages are usually the dominant tissue and the product is a cyst full of sebaceous debris. This teratoma was a large unilocular ('dermoid') cyst full of sebaceous material and hair. Most of the this part of the wall consists of mature sebaceous glands, lined by large epithelial cells with abundant pale cytoplasm and a small round central nucleus (thin arrow). The glands open into numerous ducts and discharge secretion on to a 'surface' covered with stratified squamous epithelium (left). A hair follicle is also present, cut in cross-section (thick arrow). Elsewhere in the wall of the cyst there are various other tissues, all fully differentiated. HE ×55

7.62 Struma ovarii: ovary

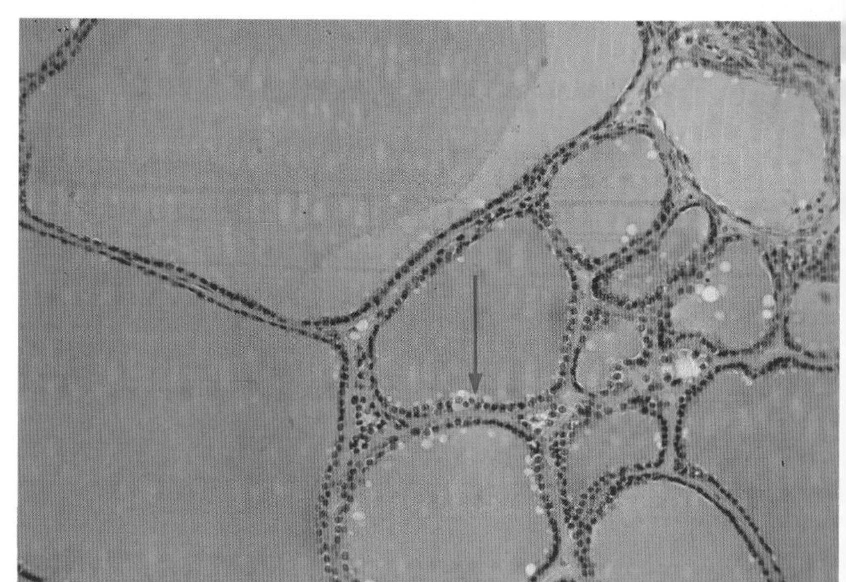

Rarely, in a benign cystic teratoma, one type of tissue may outgrow the other tissues and become completely predominant. Thyroid tissue is present in about 10% of cystic teratomas of ovary, but less than 3% of ovarian teratomas consist largely or entirely of thyroid tissue, as happened in this case. Most ovarian strumas (strumata ovarii) are benign, but the thyroid tissue in struma ovarii can undergo any or all of the pathological changes that affect the normal thyroid gland, such as hyperplasia, thyrotoxicosis, etc. Malignant change may also (rarely) develop and lead to metastasis in pelvic and abdominal lymph nodes or occasionally to more distant metastases. In this part of the (struma ovarii) tumour, the tissue consists of well-formed thyroid acini, small to very large and full of eosinophilic colloid. The acini are lined with a single layer of low cuboidal or flat epithelial cells with uniformly round or slightly ovoid nuclei (arrow), none of which is mitotically active. HE ×135

7.63 Benign cystic teratoma of ovary: malignant change

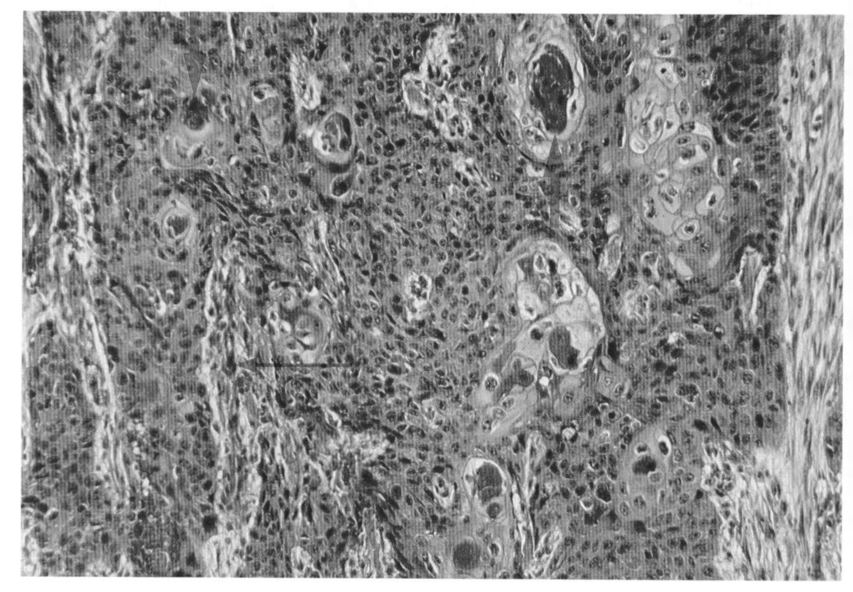

Very rarely malignant transformation occurs in one type of tissue in 2% of benign teratomas, generally in patients over 40 years of age and most often in the squamous epithelium. The malignant change then gives rise to squamous cell carcinoma or, less often, to an adenocarcinoma or to a sarcoma or to a melanoma. When metastases develop, they too consist of the same type of tissue. In this benign cystic teratoma, a squamous cell carcinoma has developed in the epithelial elements. The malignant tissue sometimes forms a warty mass which thickens the wall of the cyst diffusely or projects into the cyst. In this case, the sheets of malignant squamous epithelial cells have large and very basophilic nuclei which show considerable pleomorphism, but the tumour is well-differentiated, with numerous cell nests, with clusters of deeply eosinophilic keratinized epithelial cells in the centre (thin arrows). There is abundant vascular fibrous stroma (thick arrow) between the sheets of malignant cells. HE ×120

7.64 Immature teratoma: ovary

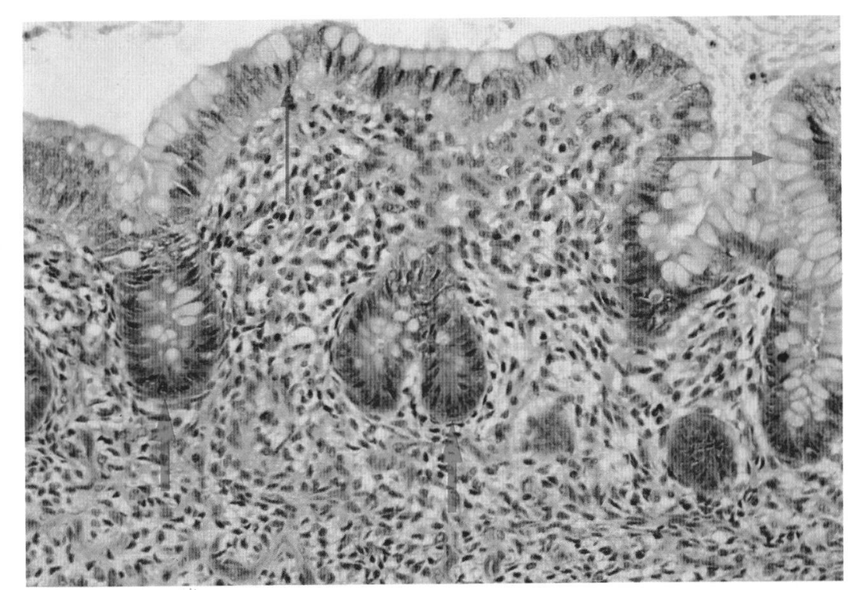

Immature teratoma of ovary is a rare malignant variant that generally occurs in children and adolescents, and the prognosis is poor. Tumours of this type are composed of immature (poorly differentiated) elements and contain a mixture of embryonic and adult tissues, derived from all three germ layers. Primitive neuroectodermal (neuroblastic) elements are especially common. This teratoma is from a 13-year-old girl. The tumour contains few mature tissues, and the tissue in this part resembles small intestine fairly closely. The cystic space at the top is lined with a single layer of tall columnar mucin-secreting goblet-type epithelial cells with basal ovoid nuclei (thin arrows), and beneath the layer there is a sheet of loose extremely cellular connective tissue. Within the connective tissue there are small tubular glands which open on to the layer of epithelial cells on the surface of the connective tissue. The crypts of the glands are lined by closely packed columnar cells with vary basophilic nuclei (thick arrows). The layer of epithelial cells on the surface undulates and tends to form rudimentary villi. HE ×200

7.65 Immature teratoma: ovary

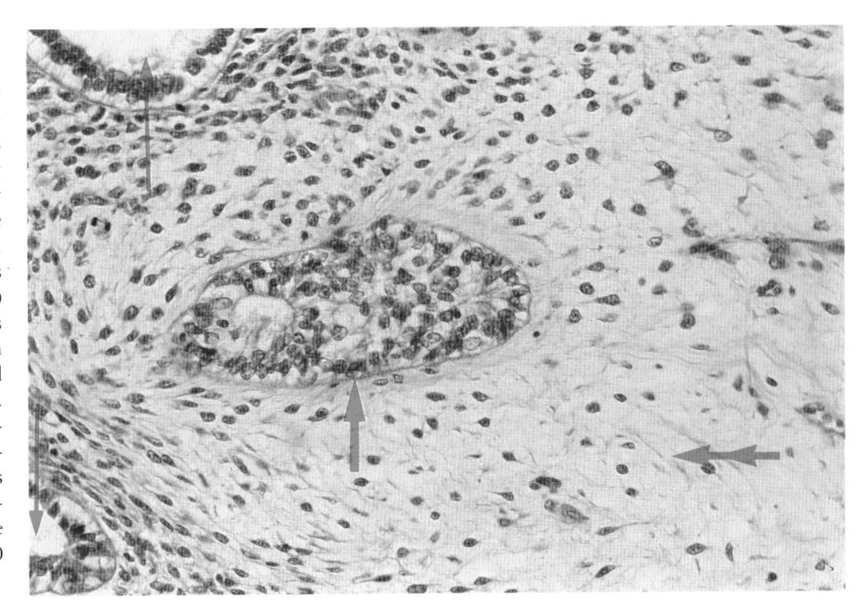

Immature teratomas are usually solid neoplasms with minimal cystic change. There may be many small cysts (microcysts) however. The more-malignant types of immature teratoma may contain few or no mature tissues and vice versa. They are graded histologically according to the amount of primitive neuroectodermal tissue they contain. Tumours with large areas of neuroblast are the highest grade (grade 3) and have the worst prognosis. The tissue from part of this immature teratoma consists of a sheet of loose (myxomatous) embryonic (immature) connective tissue, throughout which numerous large cells with ovoid or elongated hyperchromatic nuclei and much pale (vacuolated) cytoplasm. The cells have well-defined cell margins and are distributed more or less uniformly. Within the sheet there are glandular structures (thin arrows) lined by columnar cells each with a large infranuclear vacuole. Also present in the sheet of myxomatous tissue (double arrow) there is a compact group of vacuolated polyhedral cells, bounded by a basement membrane (thick arrow). HE ×270

7.66 Immature teratoma: ovary

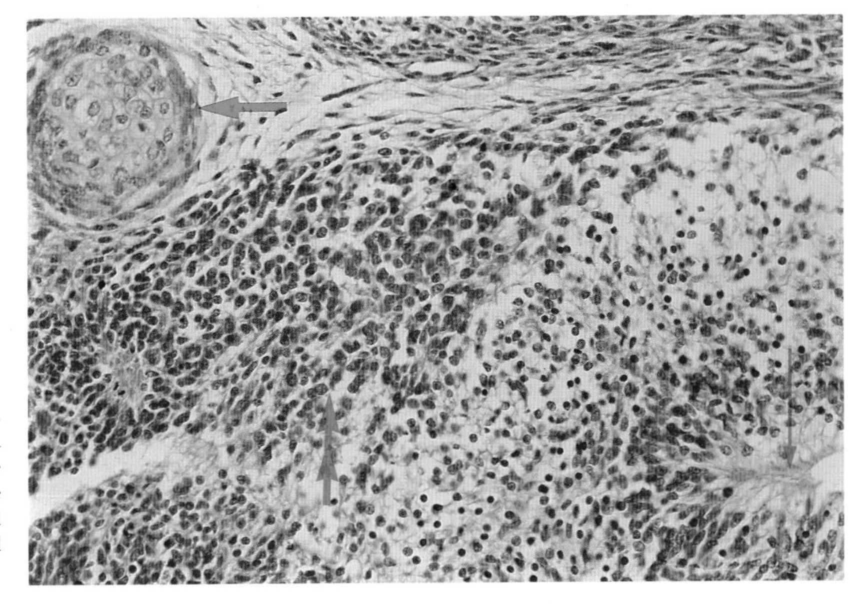

In immature teratomas of ovary there may be one or more large cysts. The main component however is generally neurogenic tissue, but usually there are also foci of immature cartilage or muscle and tubules lined by undifferentiated cells. This shows part of the same teratoma as in 7.65. It consists mostly of cells of very primitive appearance (double arrow), with very little cytoplasm and round deeply basophilic nuclei which exhibit considerable mitotic activity. Cells with similar but more elongated nuclei surround clefts that contain bundles of very fine eosinophilic fibrils (thin arrow), in an arrangement suggestive of embryonic neural tissue. There is also a sheet of similar cells which are distended by the presence of a large clear cytoplasmic vacuole. These primitive cells are separated by a bundle of fibrils and cells with elongated fibroblast-like nuclei from a solid cord of tissue which closely resembles primitive cartilage (thick arrow). The cord of cartilage-like tissue consists of cells with round or ovoid pale vesicular nuclei and a moderate amount of bluish cytoplasm and prominent cell membranes. HE ×215

7.67 Serous cystadenocarcinoma: ovary

Serous cystadenomas and serous cystadenocarcinomas are the most common neoplasms of the ovary, arising from surface (celomic) epithelium of the ovary. They occur in individuals who are in the 15-50 age group, but those with a benign tumour tend to be younger. The smaller lesions tend to be unilocular, but as they enlarge they generally become multilocular. The epithelium lining the cysts varies from a single layer of flat inactive cells (cystadenomas) to a thick lining of highly malignant cells which form innumerable papillomatous outgrowths into the cystic spaces (cystadenocarcinomas). The majority of malignant serous tumours are bilateral. The cystic cavity shown here is part of a large tumour with many cystic cavities full of watery fluid. This cavity contains a large number papilliferous processes (thin arrows), some very short and others elongated and complex. The surface of the papilliferous processes is covered, usually, with a single of deeply basophilic epithelial cells. The processes have also grown outwards and penetrate the fibrous wall of the cyst (bottom margin) to reach the serosa (thick arrow). The contents of the cavity are very pale and probably serous. HE ×55

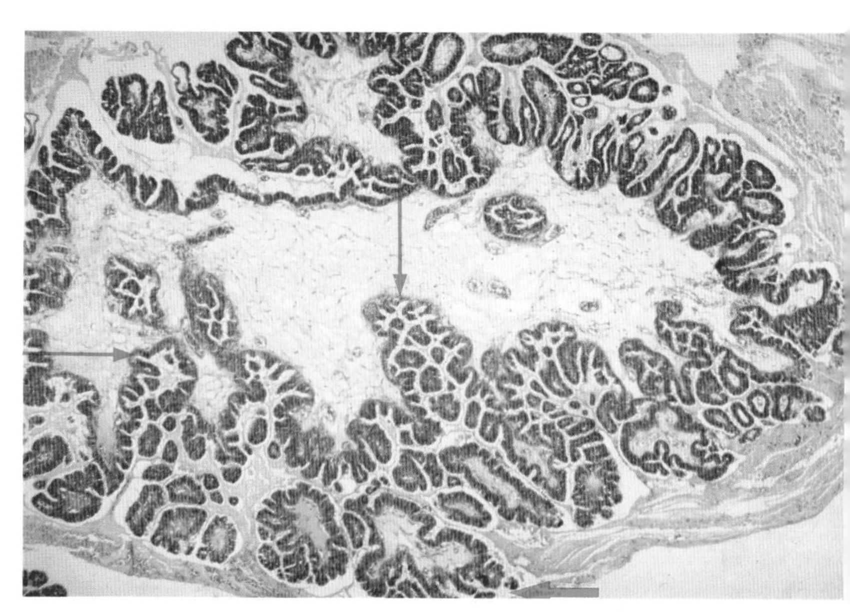

7.68 Serous cystadenocarcinoma: ovary

In serous cystadenocarcinomas there are irregular solid areas and also cystic structures. This is the same tumour as in 7.67, at higher magnification. The wall of this large cystic cavity consists of collagenous fibrous tissue (double arrow). The cavity is lined with an apparently single layer of very tall columnar pleomorphic epithelial cells (thin arrow) which form long papilliform processes. The papilliform processes have a delicate core of vascular connective tissue (thick arrow), and the epithelial cells on their surface have a moderate amount of eosinophilic cytoplasm and large vacuolated vesicular ovoid nuclei. The nuclei are crowded and often overlapping, and most of them are located at the base of the cell. There is considerable mitotic activity among them. The epithelial cells do not contain large droplets of mucin, and the contents of the cavity are pale and very weakly basophilic. Many serous cystic tumours are difficult to categorize as benign or malignant, about one-third being of low malignant potential and regarded as borderline lesions.

HE ×270

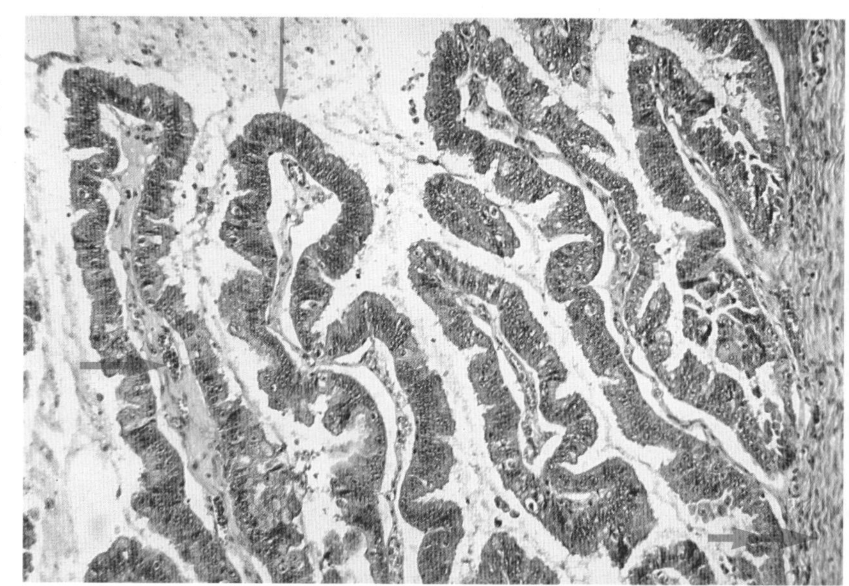

7.69 Mucinous tumour of low malignant potential: ovary

Mucinous cystadenomas and cystadenocarcinomas are less often bilateral than serous tumours. Mucinous tumours of low malignant potential (borderline mucinous tumours) are distinguished from benign tumours by the presence of complex papillary projections (less papilliferous than in serous tumours) and (compared with carcinoma) milder cellular atypia and reduced stratification of cells. The epithelial cells lining the cysts secrete much mucus and they vary from a single layer of tall cells filled with mucin to a thick layer of anaplastic cells. This shows part of a smooth-surfaced multiloculated ovarian cyst (15 × 12 × 10cm) which weighed 990g and was removed from a woman of 28. The walls of the loculi consist of connective tissue and numerous fibroblast-like cells (thick arrows) and are lined by single layer of columnar mucin-filled epithelial cells. The lining cells are highly papilliferous and form multiple short intracystic papilliform structures (thin arrows). The epithelial cells do not invade the wall and the serosa (bottom) is intact. Each loculus is filled with pale mucus and much eosinophilic cell debris. There is no firm evidence of malignancy in this tumour and it is considered to be a 'borderline' mucinous cystadenoma/cystadenocarcinoma. HE ×60

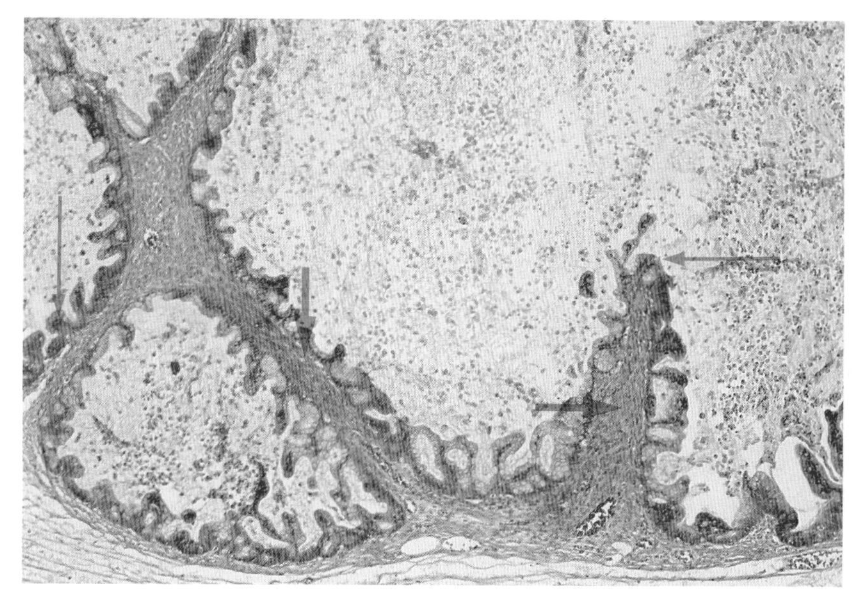

7.70 Mucinous cystadenocarcinoma: ovary

This is an ovarian cyst measuring 15 × 11 × 9cm which was removed by surgical operation from a woman of 65. It is multilocular, the walls of the loculi varying in thickness from 0.1cm to 1cm. There is also a polypoid gelatinous mass 5cm dia which projects into one loculus. In this part of the tumour there are three loculi, separated by bundles of cellular fibrous tissue. One loculus is lined by a single layer of mucin-secreting cuboidal or columnar cells (thin arrow) with eosinophilic cytoplasm and basal nuclei, and another loculus is lined by similar but much taller columnar cells (thick arrow). Epithelium of this type is sometimes called 'picket-fence' epithelium. The third loculus (below left) contains a large amount cell debris and mucin and is lined by a single layer of epithelial cells larger than those lining the other loculi. These epithelial cells also form many short papillae (double arrow) which project into the loculus, and their nuclei are markedly layered. They also show moderate basophilia and pleomorphism. HE ×150

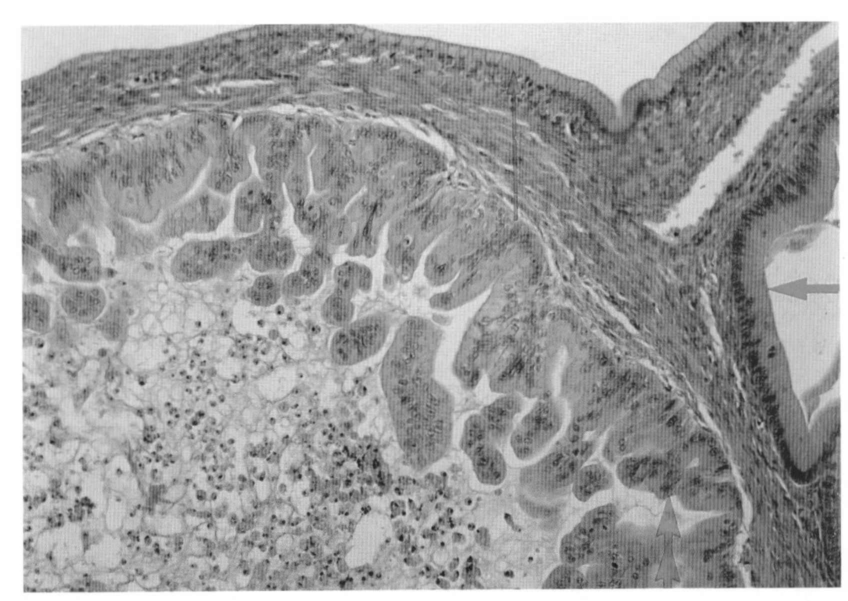

7.71 Mucinous cystadenocarcinoma: ovary

Mucinous cystadenocarcinoma is a highly malignant type of tumour which can be recognized by the presence partly of solid and partly of cystic areas. Generally, numerous papillary structures project into the cysts, and there is also evidence of extensive infiltration. The tumour invades locally and also metastasizes to the peritoneal cavity, lymph nodes and more distant sites. The prognosis is poor. This is part of the same tumour as in 7.73, at higher magnification. It consists of several loculi, some large and others smaller (gland-like) loculi. All the loculi are lined by closely packed very tall columnar cells, with a large amount of deeply eosinophilic cytoplasm (thin arrows). The nuclei are ovoid, hyperchromatic and vesicular, and most of them are located in the bases of the epithelial cells. In several places the nuclei are stratified and appear to be arranged in several layers. They also show considerable mitotic activity (thick arrows). There are no droplets of mucin in the cytoplasm of the large epithelial cells. The stroma consists of fibrous tissue in which there are many elongated fibroblasts (double arrow). HE ×235

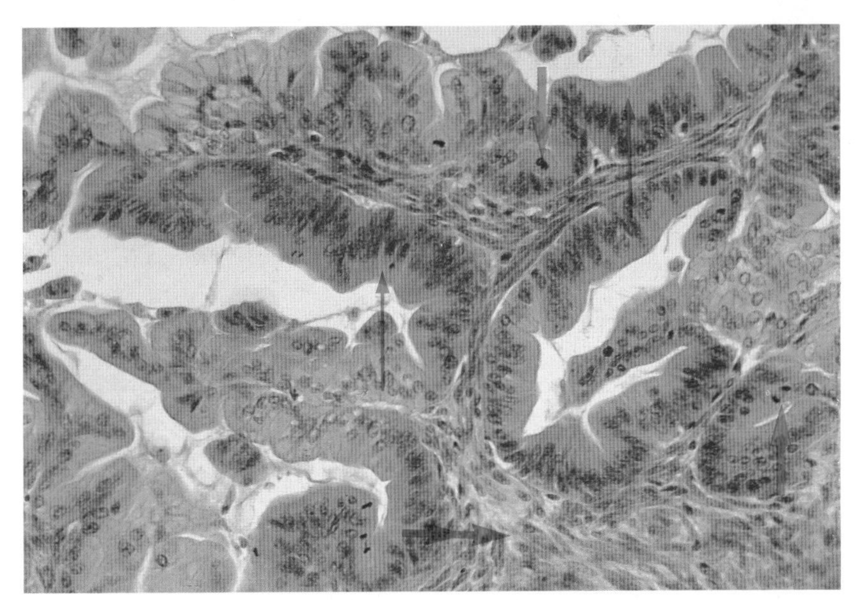

7.72 Clear cell carcinoma: ovary

Clear cell carcinoma of ovary, a rare tumour, is characterized histologically by large cells with clear cytoplasm, arranged in solid, glandular, tubular or papillary patterns. It was originally called mesonephric carcinoma, because of its presumed origin from mesonephric rests and the large vacuoles in the cytoplasm of the malignant cells. The cytoplasmic vacuoles are caused by glycogen and give the tumour a distinctive histological appearance reminiscent of carcinoma of kidney. Clear cell carcinoma has no link with mesonephric structures however and originates from the surface epithelium of the ovary. In this example, the sheets of clear malignant cells are separated by scanty strands of fibrous stroma (thick arrow). The cells are polyhedral and have abundant clear cytoplasm (thin arrows). Most of their nuclei are round but others are extremely pleomorphic. They are all markedly hyperchromatic but there are no mitoses in this field. The carcinomatous clear cells may also arrange themselves in tubules, and when they do so they may be 'peg-shaped'. HE ×335

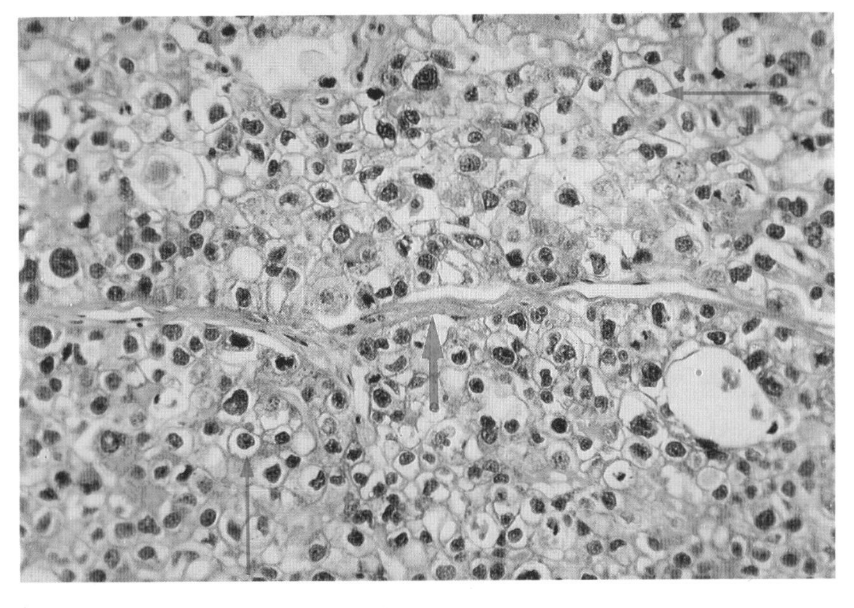

7.73 Brenner tumour: ovary

The Brenner tumour is an uncommon lesion which is derived from the celomic epithelium covering the ovary. It is usually a single firm mass with a white cut surface and is almost always benign. It is solid but within it there are usually small cysts containing mucinous material. The tumour occurs at all ages but is most often incidental discovery in older patients. It is associated with endometrial hyperplasia (hyperestrinism) and uterine bleeding in post-menopausal women. Histologically the tumour pattern unmistakable. It consists of a large sheet of interlacing bundles of collagenous fibrous stroma (thin arrow), in which there are islands ('nests') of uniformly benign-looking cells (thick arrows) which resemble transitional (or sometimes squamous) epithelial cells. The cytoplasm of the epithelial cells is pale, with a large 'clear' perinuclear vacuole, from the presence of glycogen. The clear cells are also occasionally accompanied by mucin-secreting cells. There are numerous elongated fibroblast-like cells in the dense stroma. Rarely the transitional epithelium in a Brenner tumour shows evidence of proliferation, and the tumour is then regarded as of low malignant potential.

HE ×120

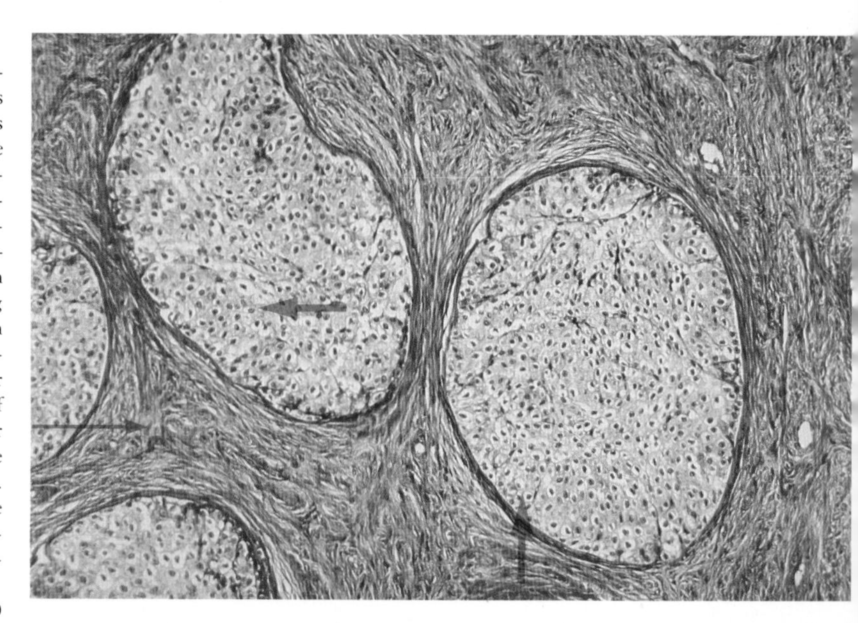

7.74 Granulosa-theca cell tumour: ovary

Granulosa-theca cell tumours arise in ovarian mesenchymal stroma and originate from the follicular epithelium of primordial follicles. A small minority are bilateral. They may occur at any age but are present most often in post-menopausal women. In adults, endometrial hyperplasia and excessive bleeding occur, and in children, precocious puberty may be induced. In young women a variant (juvenile granulosa cell tumour) occurs. Granulosa-theca cell tumours are usually solid fleshy smooth-surfaced masses, in which hemorrhage and cystic change are frequently evident, and histologically they are composed of a variable mixture of granulosa and theca cells. This tumour consists of a sheet of closely packed polyhedral granulosa cells (thin arrow) with a moderate amount of cytoplasm and uniformly round or ovoid nuclei. Among the granulosa cells there are several small round spaces ('follicles') (thick arrows) which contain one or more cells with very pale cytoplasm (abortive graafian follicles or Call-Exner bodies). The presence of the 'follicles' makes the diagnosis of granulosa-theca cell tumour easier. Another feature which helps is the presence in the tumour cells of nuclear folds or grooves (just visible in this tumour).

HE ×335

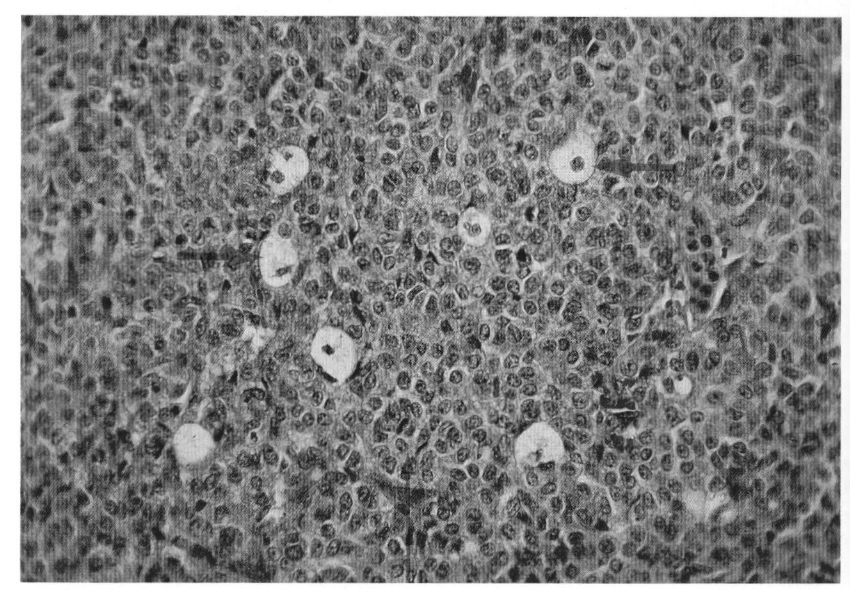

7.75 Granulosa-theca cell tumour: ovary

The composition of granulosa-theca cell tumours may range from pure granulosa cell tumour with few thecal elements through thecomas to luteinomas. They are usually benign, but their behaviour cannot be predicted accurately on the basis of their histological features. A minority (about 25%) behave in a locally aggressive way and tend to recur, and 10-15% form distant metastases. This granulosa cell tumour consists of a fairly uniform population of small ovoid or elongated cells (thin arrow) (probably theca-type) with scant cytoplasm and round or ovoid moderately basophilic vesicular nuclei. In some of the larger paler nuclei there is an inconspicuous nucleolus. The cells show only slight nuclear pleomorphism and there is no mitotic activity. The neoplastic cells are arranged in mostly elongated bundles, but alongside they also form very elongated very slender trabeculae (only one or two cells thick), separated by narrow (empty) clefts (thick arrow). There is also an inconspicuous network of small capillary-type blood vessels.

HE ×335

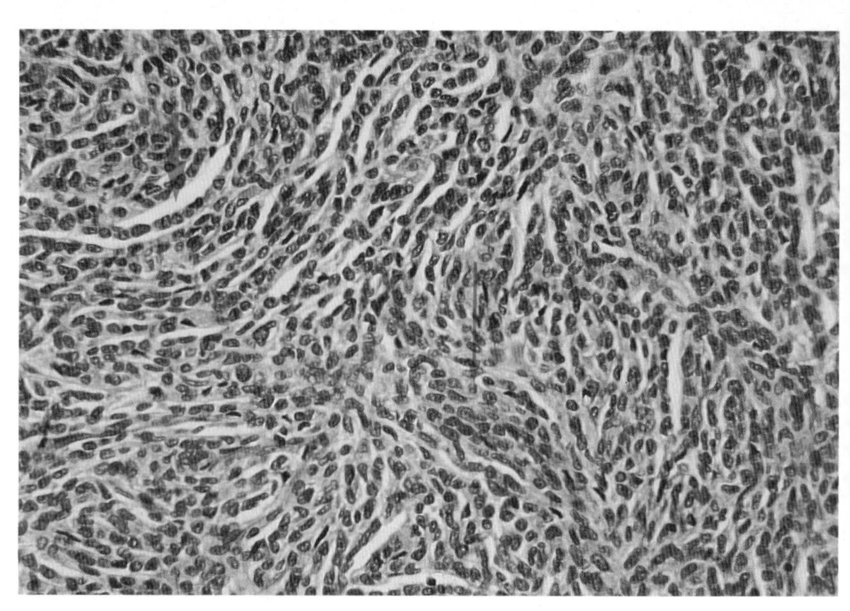

7.76 Fibroma (fibrothecoma): ovary

Fibroma (fibrothecoma) of ovary also is derived from the mesenchymal stromal tissue of the ovary. It is an encapsulated benign neoplasm of older women (the large majority are post-menopausal), and usually single. It is usually a combination of fibroblasts and theca cells. This tumour is from a woman aged 70 years. Although fibrothecomas are usually white, those that have a significant theca cell component are yellow, and the cut surface of this tumour is distinctly yellow. The tumour is composed of broad strands of dense eosinophilic fibrous tissue (thick arrows) and large numbers of elongated cells with abundant pale finely granular or vacuolated cytoplasm and elongated moderately pleomorphic vesicular nuclei (thin arrow). The appearance and texture of the cytoplasm is produced by the relatively large content of lipid (steroids). A reticulin stain usually reveals delicate connective tissue fibres around individual tumour cells. Deposits of hyaline material are also found occasionally in thecomas.

HE ×235

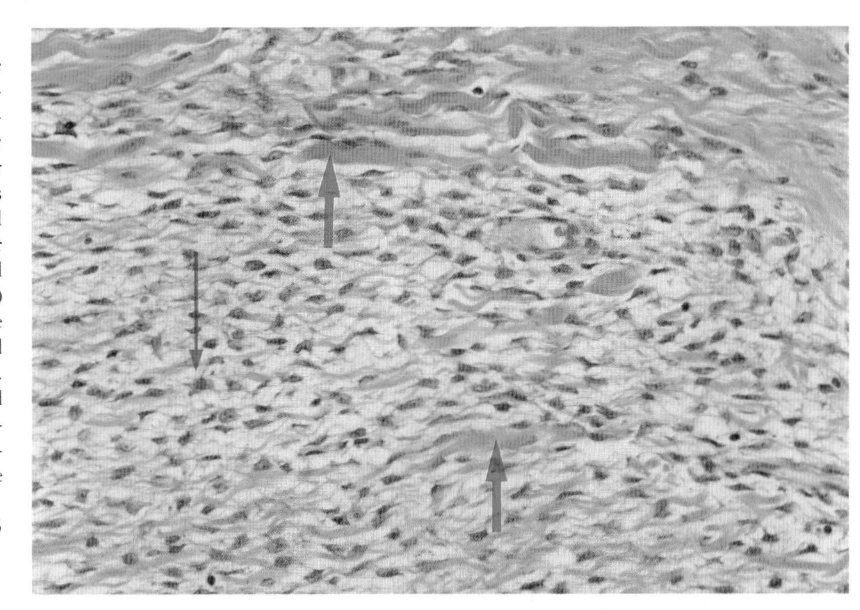

7.77 Fibroma (fibrothecoma): ovary

Many ovarian fibromas are undoubtedly inactive fibrothecomas, and it may be difficult to differentiate a 'pure' fibroma from an ovarian fibroma (fibrothecoma). An ovarian fibroma is generally a solid white mass, but myxomatous change is occasionally present. About 1 in 5 patients with an ovarian fibroma have marked abdominal ascites and also, very occasionally, a pleural effusion on the same side as the tumour (Meig's syndrome). The extravasated fluid disappears after removal of the tumour, which is usually large. This tumour (13 × 10 × 6cm) weighed 650g and is (macroscopically) a smooth bosselated mass. Its cut surface is yellowish-white and the pattern is whorled. Histologically the tumour consists of interlacing bundles of very cellular connective tissue. The neoplastic connective-tissue cells are spindle-shaped fibroblasts (arrows), uniformly distributed in the connective tissue, with plump spindle-shaped nuclei and a fairly large amount of pale cytoplasm and well-defined cell margins. The cytoplasm is also vacuolated and weakly eosinophilic. Elsewhere there is no evidence of malignancy and the serosal surface is intact.

HE ×235

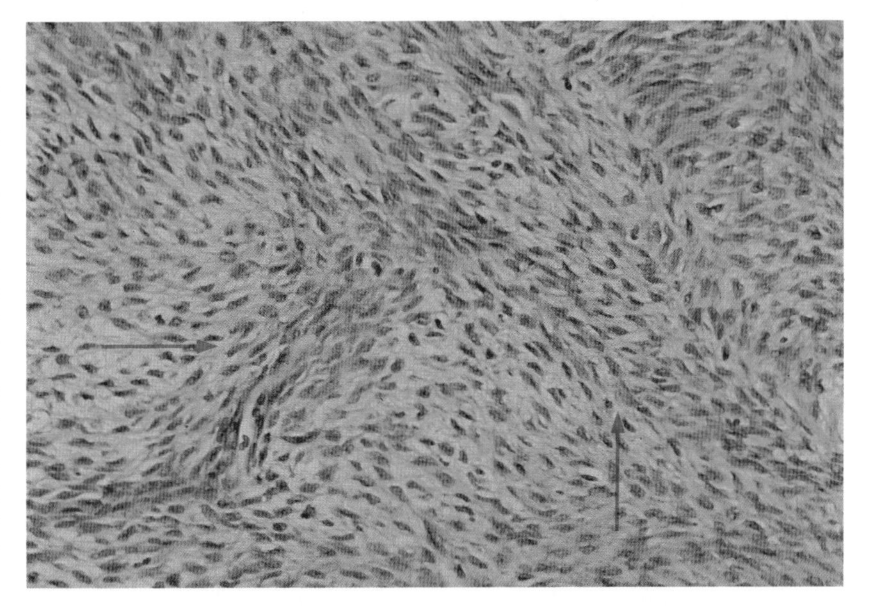

7.78 Luteoma of pregnancy: ovary

Luteoma of pregnancy is an extreme form of luteal hyperplasia which produces a nodular mass (unilateral or bilateral) in the ovary in the last trimester of pregnancy. It may reach a large size. Luteomas are often encountered during caesarean section and should not be mistaken for neoplasms. They are solid yellowish-brown masses and they consist of sheets of large luteinized cells. In general, the cells resemble epithelial cells and contain so much lipid (steroids) that they resemble the lutein cells of the mature corpus luteum. In this case, the cells are large and round, and have a considerable amount of very pale granular (foamy) cytoplasm with well-defined cell margins (thick arrow). The nuclei are round and very uniform and they exhibit no mitotic activity. The sheets of luteinized cells are separated by a thick band of eosinophilic fibrous stroma (thin arrow). Luteomas of pregnancy involute spontaneously within a few weeks of delivery. Rarely, they produce androgens and cause virilization.

HE ×335

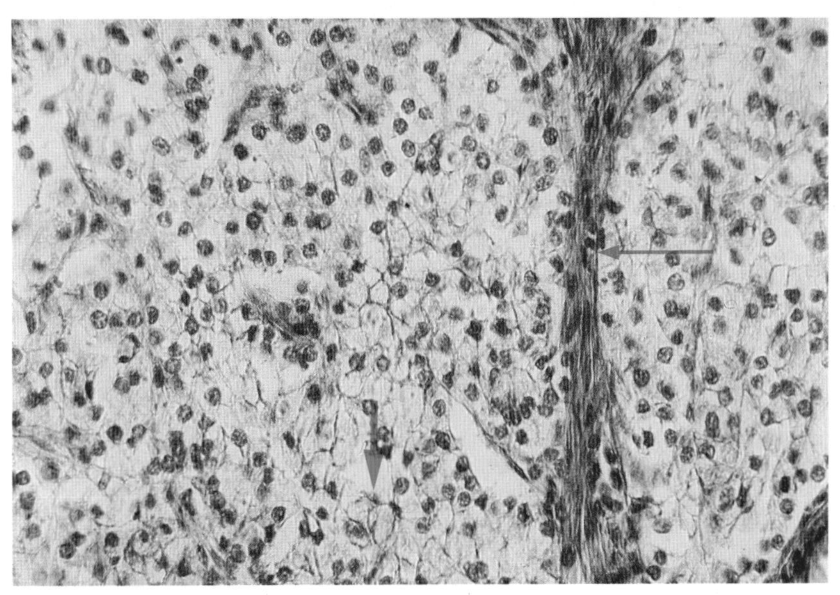

7.79 Sertoli cell tumour: ovary

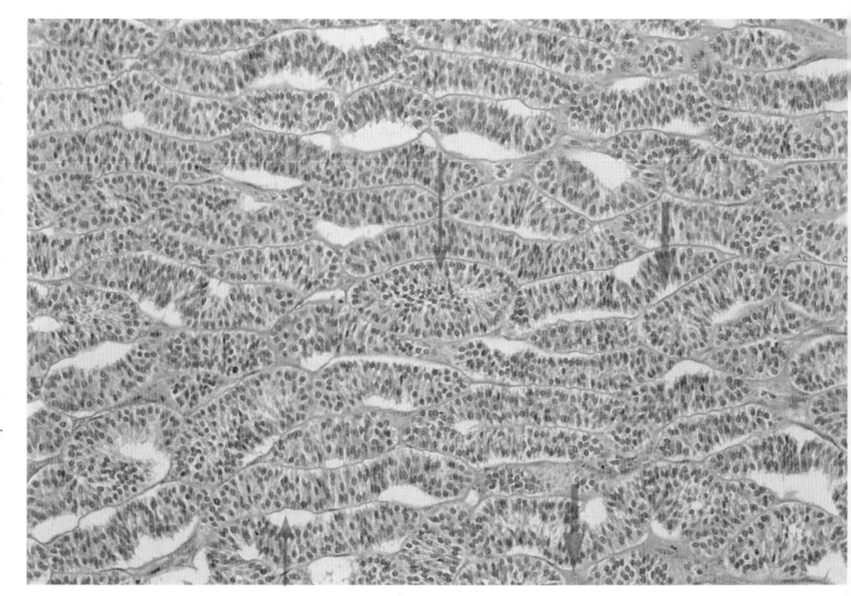

Rarely, an ovarian tumour consists of tubules (resembling seminiferous tubules) or columns of Sertoli cells but does not have Leydig cells in the stroma. In some tumours, fat is abundant in the cytoplasm of the neoplastic cells. Generally, Sertoli cell tumours do not secrete significant amounts of steroid hormones, and the small minority that do so may secrete estrogens or androgens. Tumours of this type are exceptionally rare in testis. This tumour is composed of long well-formed tubules which have little or no lumen and look 'solid'. They are lined with several layers of closely apposed well-differentiated cells (thin arrows), bounded by a thick eosinophilic basement membrane (thick arrows) (the empty spaces between the tubules are artefactual). The neoplastic cells are palisaded and arranged with their long axes at right angles to the basement membrane. They have a moderate amount of eosinophilic cytoplasm and uniform ovoid nuclei. The nuclei show no pleomorphism and the chromatin in them is very finely granular. HE ×150

7.80 Sertoli cell tumour: ovary

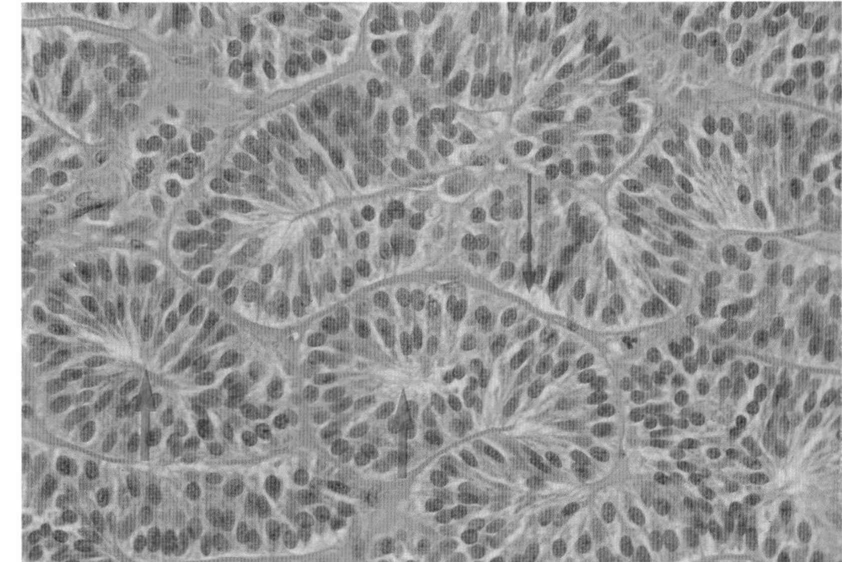

This is part of the same tumour as in **7.82**, at higher magnification. The tubules are lined with tall columnar cells which are closely packed, with considerable 'layering' of their nuclei. The apices of the neoplastic cells are tapered (thick arrows) and drawn out into short 'fibrils' which project into the very small lumen of the tubules (only a few tubules have a lumen, the large minority of tubules appearing 'solid'). The tumour cells have uniform ovoid nuclei with very finely granular chromatin, and in many of them there are one or more inconspicuous nucleoli. The tubules are bounded by a thick well-formed eosinophilic basement membrane (thin arrow), reinforced in places by small amounts of connective tissue and an inconspicuous network of capillary-type blood vessels. There is no mitotic activity in this field but occasional mitoses were present throughout the tumour. Sertoli cell tumours are relatively benign lesions however and rarely recur after surgical excision. HE ×360

7.81 Sertoli-Leydig tumour (arrhenoblastoma): ovary

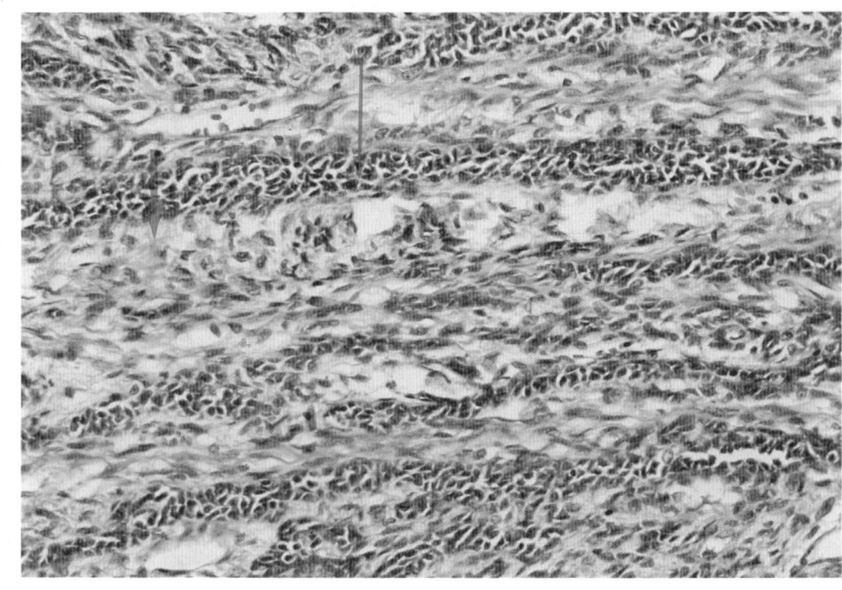

Sertoli-Leydig tumours are rare and resemble the corresponding testicular tumours. They occur at all ages but usually between 10 and 30 years of age. They usually produce androgens and cause virilization, but rarely secrete estrogens. Macroscopically Sertoli-Leydig tumours look like granulosa cell tumours. Generally they are solid neoplasms, with foci of necrosis, hemorrhage and cystic degeneration. Some of the cysts may be large and full of blood. Histologically they consist of islands of tumour cells which contain tubules lined by Sertoli cells or cords of similar cells. Leydig cells are usually numerous in the collagenous septa between the tubules and cords of Sertoli cells. In this case the tumour consists of long branching cords (thin arrow) which resemble the sex cords of the embryonic testis before they acquire a lumen. The cells in the cords have minimal cytoplasm and round or ovoid very basophilic nuclei. Between the cords there are vascular trabeculae of eosinophilic spindle-shaped Leydig (interstitial) cells (thick arrow) with elongated nuclei and a moderate amount weakly eosinophilic cytoplasm. The Leydig cells are relatively inconspicuous in the stroma in this field but more obvious elsewhere in the tumour. HE ×235

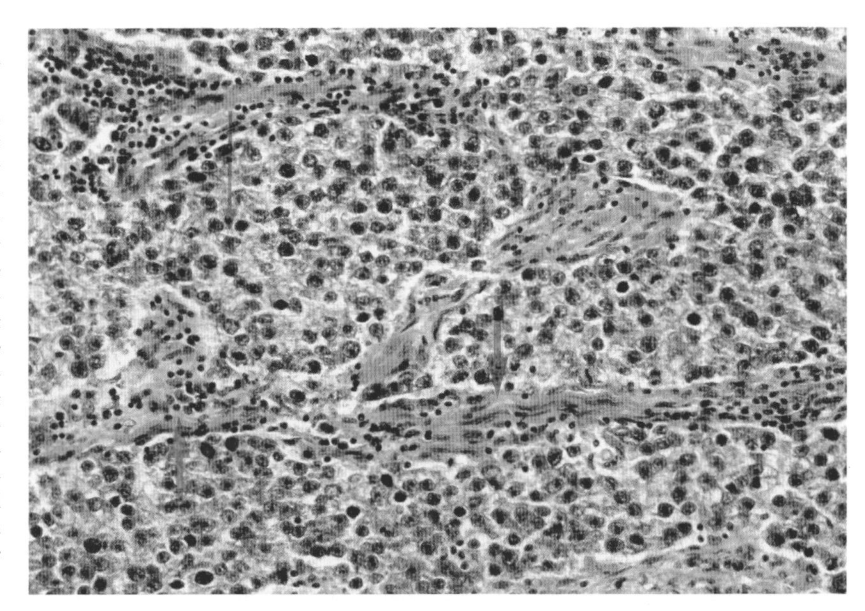

7.82 Dysgerminoma: ovary

Dysgerminoma is an undifferentiated germ cell tumour which is histologically identical with seminoma of testis. It usually occurs in individuals between 10 and 30 years of age. Dysgerminomas are generally solid, and the cut surface is a homogeneous yellowish-white colour. They vary in size from very small to enormous and are rarely bilateral. Like seminomas, they spread readily to the regional lymph nodes and are very radiosensitive. They consist of large round germ cells, with abundant pale granular cytoplasm (thin arrow), and they resemble primordial germ cells of the sexually indifferent embryonic gonad. They are arranged in groups and cords, and in the cytoplasm the round or slightly ovoid nuclei are moderately pleomorphic and usually contain a very prominent and mostly central nucleolus. The groups and cords of tumour cells are separated by thick bands of elongated fibroblastic cells and eosinophilic fibrous tissue (thick arrow), heavily infiltrated with lymphocytes with small round deeply basophilic nuclei. No mitoses are present in this field but there are scattered mitotic figures elsewhere in the tumour. HE ×235

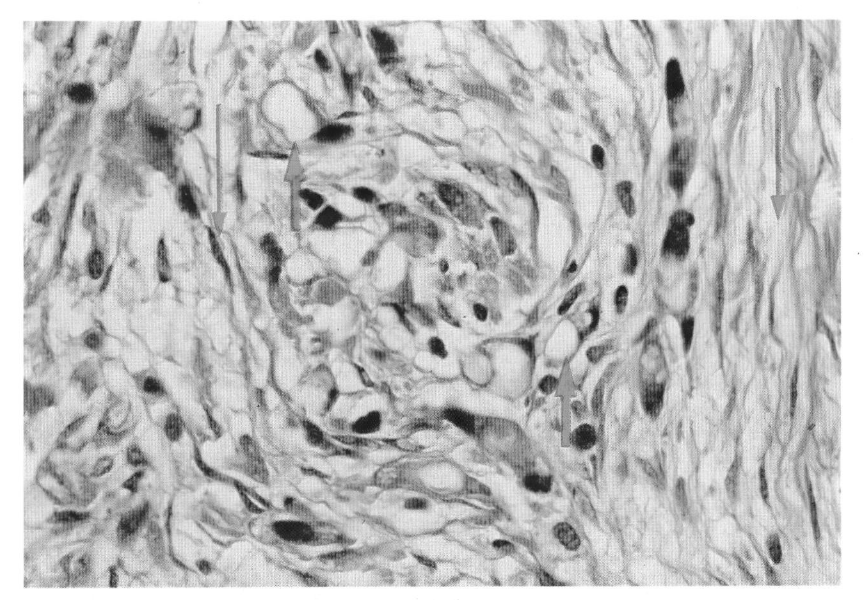

7.83 Krukenberg tumour: ovary

The ovaries are a common site for metastatic deposits from tumours in the alimentary tract or the pelvic organs, and Krukenberg tumours are metastatic desmoplastic signet-ring mucin-secreting adenocarcinomas, of gastric origin, in the ovaries. Both ovaries are enlarged and solid. Occasionally the term Krukenberg is misapplied to any metastatic adenocarcinoma of the ovary. In this case, a woman of 61 presented with obstruction of the large intestine, and at operation both ovaries were found to be enlarged and they were resected. One (6 × 6 × 4cm) weighed 35g and the other measured 7 × 4.5 × 4cm. The cut surfaces were white, homogeneous and slightly whorled. In this histological section of one of the tumours, the malignant (carcinomatous) epithelial cells are scattered throughout an abundant spindle-cell fibroblastic stroma (thin arrows). The malignant cells have hyperchromatic pleomorphic nuclei and very large amounts of pale (epithelial) mucin in the very abundant vacuolated cytoplasm (thick arrows). Some of the malignant cells have only large vacuole and look like signet ring cells. There are no mitoses in this field and few could be detected elsewhere in the ovaries. HE ×540

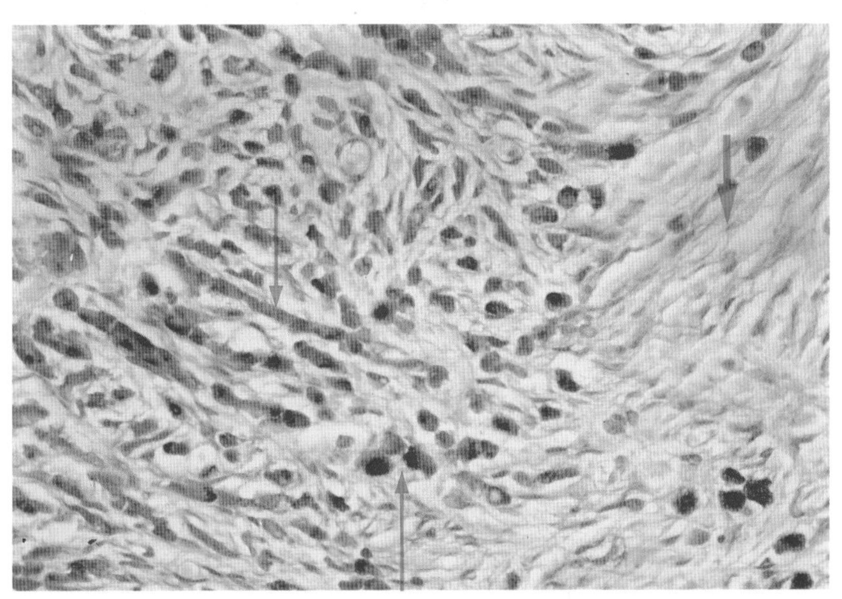

7.84 Krukenberg tumour: ovary

This histological section is from one of the ovaries in **7.86**. It has been stained by the periodic acid-Schiff (PAS) method which colours epithelial mucin purplish-red. The stroma consists of relatively pale spindle-shaped fibrocytic and fibroblastic cells (thick arrow) with elongated nuclei. Within the stroma there are large numbers of mucin-containing malignant epithelial (carcinomatous) cells, some of them lying singly and others arranged in cords. The tumour cells vary greatly in size and shape, from small round forms to large and very elongated types (thin arrows). The cytoplasm in each of them however is full of deep purplish-red epithelial mucin. The term Krukenberg was originally applied to secondaries from a gastric carcinoma, but has been extended to include other primary sites; and the carcinoma of colon, resected at the same time as the ovaries, was assumed to be the source of the Krukenberg tumours in this case. It was also believed that the tumour cells crossed the peritoneal cavity to reach the ovaries (transcelomic spread) but this view is not now generally accepted. PAS ×360

8.1 Gynecomastia: breast

Gynecomastia is an uncommon condition, characterized by proliferation of the ducts of the breast. It is generally benign however and carries no increased risk of malignancy. At puberty the male breast often enlarges moderately. The lesion may present as a firm nodule or plaque beneath the nipple and it may be unilateral or bilateral. A man of 65 developed a 'lump' in the right breast (6 × 4 × 1.5cm) was removed surgically. This shows several small ducts. The ducts proliferate and are lined by several layers of markedly hyperplastic epithelial cells (thin arrow). The epithelial cells show considerable nuclear pleomorphism, with scant cytoplasm and relatively large ovoid or elongated basophilic nuclei. There is no mitotic activity however. The ducts are surrounded by edematous myxoid stromal connective tissue (thick arrow), similar to that in a fibroadenoma, and the structural appearance is similar to that elsewhere in the resected tissue. These changes are typical of simple gynecomastia. Sometimes the epithelial hyperplasia is even more marked than in this case and more liable to be mistaken for carcinoma. HE ×360

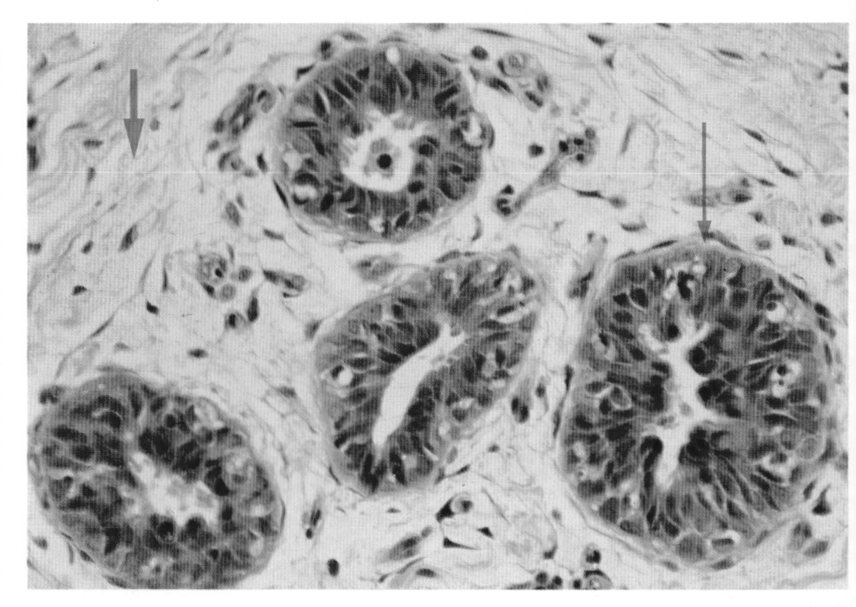

8.2 Erythroplasia of Queyrat (Bowen's disease): penis

Queyrat's erythroplasia is an area of squamous cell (epidermoid) carcinoma-in-situ and it takes the form of a bright red velvety plaque on the glans or inner surface of the prepuce. The risk of developing invasive carcinoma is high, and after a long quiescent phase, in a small minority of cases, the lesion becomes invasive. In this example, the squamous epithelium of the penis is greatly thickened. On its surface (left margin) there is a very thick layer of eosinophilic keratin (hyperkeratosis), beneath which there is a sheet of markedly acanthotic squamous epithelial cells (thick arrow). The epithelial cells show some loss of stratification but nuclear pleomorphism is slight. In the basal layers of the epithelium, there are scattered individual large black cells (thin arrow), laden with melanin pigment. The rete ridges are greatly elongated (double arrow), but there is no evidence of invasion of the dermis. The underlying dermal connective tissues are occupied by a very intense diffuse infiltrate of chronic inflammatory cells (right). Some of the inflammatory cells are lymphocytes but the great majority are larger slightly paler plasma cells. HE x85

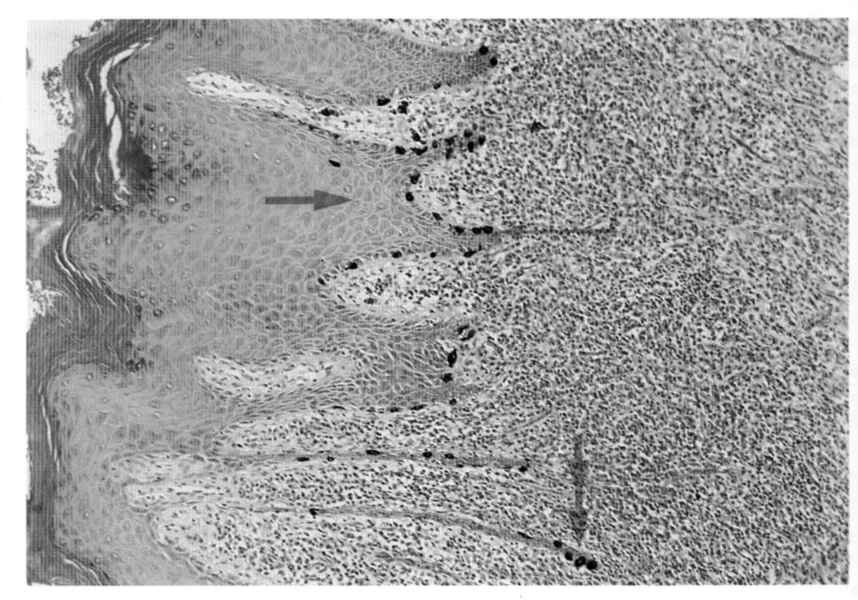

8.3 Primary syphilitic chancre: penis

Syphilis is caused by the spirochete Treponema pallidum. The incubation time 9-90 days, the spirochetes multiplying and then spreading to lymph nodes and blood. The first visible lesion is the primary chancre, an ulcerated papule with an indurated base at the site of initial invasion by the spirochete, usually on the penis, vulva or cervix. The chancre may be 2 or 3cm dia but it is often smaller. If untreated, the ulcer heals and the induration disappears in 6-8 weeks, leaving no scar or only a small scar. A man of 19 had an ulcer on his foreskin which was biopsied. The surface of the chancre (left) is ulcerated, the stratified squamous epithelium having been replaced by a thick network of strands of eosinophilic fibrin. In the meshes of the network there are polymorphs, lymphocytes and macrophages. Beneath the fibrin there is a layer of granulation tissue with thin-walled blood vessels, as well as a large sheet of fibrous connective tissue and thick-walled small blood vessels (arrows) lined by plump endothelial cells. There is an intense infiltrate of chronic inflammatory cells, mostly plasma cells, in the connective tissue. HE ×60

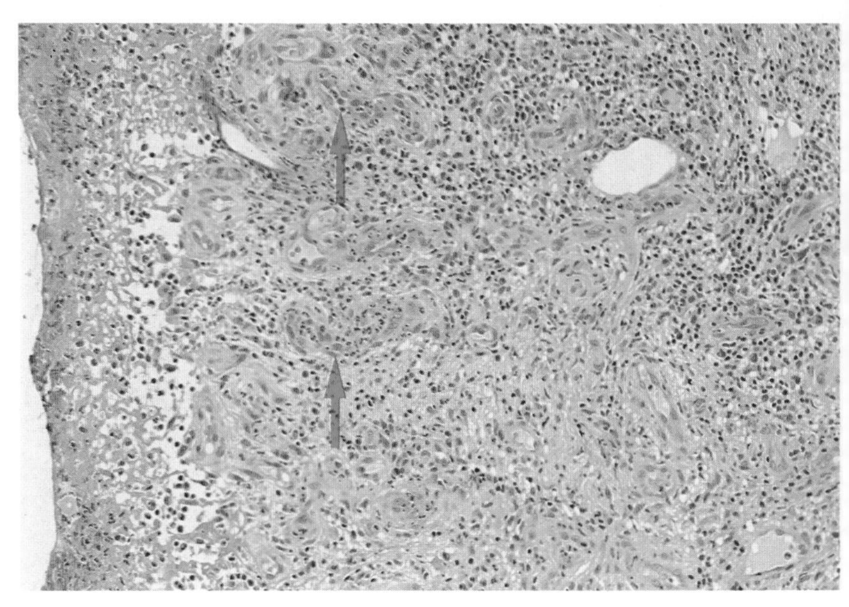

.4 Primary syphilitic chancre: penis

iagnosing syphilis at this early stage is not best achieved y tissue biopsy but by identifying spirochetes in the erous exudate from the chancre, by means of dark-field nicroscopy. This lesion is part of the chancre shown at .3, at higher magnification. It consists of chronically inlamed very vascular connective tissue. The small blood essels in the chancre are very prominent, thick-walled nd lined by large plump cuboidal endothelial cells (thick rrows). The endothelial cells have only a moderate mount of cytoplasm but the lumen of each vessel is very mall and inconspicuous. The nuclei of the endothelial ells are ovoid and vesicular; and the nuclear chromatin is iffusely and very finely granular. In some of the nuclei here is a prominent nucleolus. The inflammatory infilrate in the connective tissue is highly cellular and polynorphic (thin arrow), consisting of plasma cells, lymphoytes, macrophages and polymorph leukocytes. Elonated fibroblast-like cells are also present, around the lood vessels. A silver stain demonstrated many spirohetes in the tissue. HE ×360

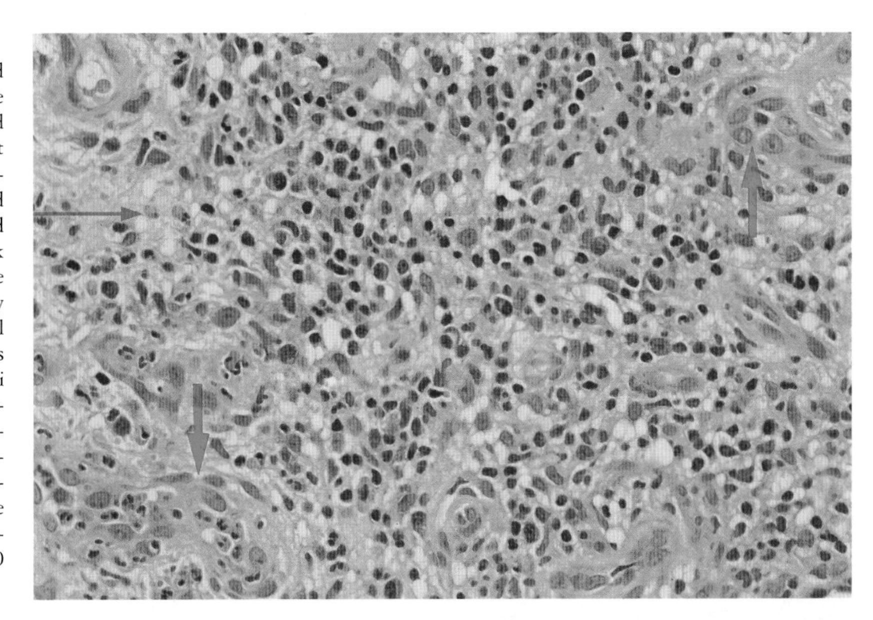

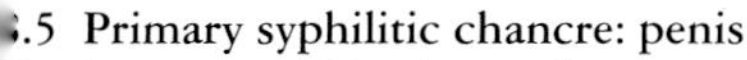

.5 Primary syphilitic chancre: penis

This lesion is part of the chancre shown at 8.3, at higher nagnification. Deeper in the chancre, the chronic inflamnatory cells tended to be located in the adventitia of the lood vessels, 'cuffing' them, but in some vessels there are ery marked changes in the intima and elsewhere. In this ield the blood vessel is a venule, and a very pronounced ndophlebitis (and phlebitis) has developed in it. The intima of the vessel is very thick and edematous (thin arow), and the lumen of the vessel is much reduced. The ntima contains a large population of small chronic inlammatory cells, and these are predominantly plasma ells and lymphocytes. There is also a similar but much ess cellular inflammatory exudate between the smooth nuscle fibres in the media (thick arrow) and other coats f the vessel. When many vessels are affected in this way, nd especially when thrombus completely occludes the tenosed lumen, the tendency to necrosis and ulceration f the chancre is much increased. HE ×135

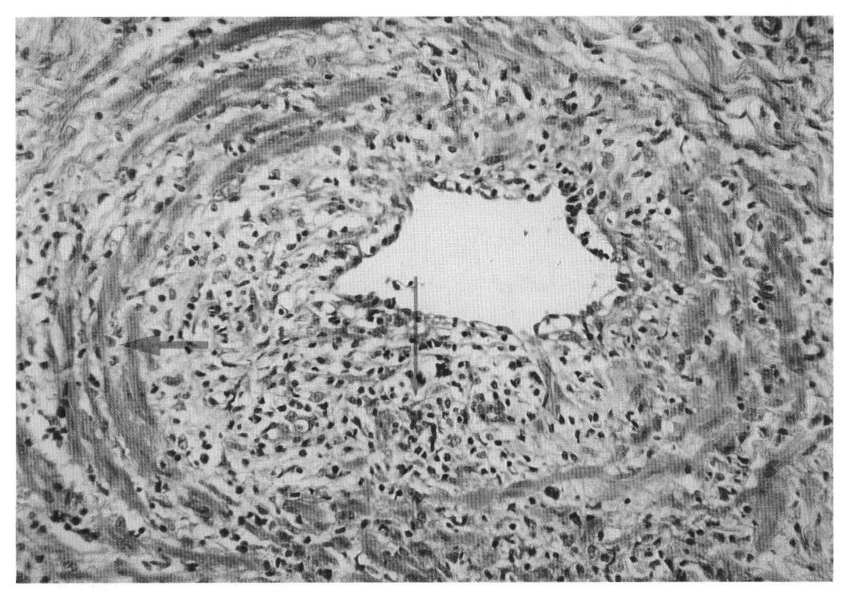

.6 Lichen sclerosis: penis

ichen sclerosis is a chronic progressive disease of nknown etiology, but probably not associated with utoimmune phenomena. In addition to affecting the kin, it may involve the vulva or penis but it is not a remalignant lesion. It is characterized, mainly, by hinning of the epidermis and formation of dense hyaline ollagen in the upper dermis. This lesion was on the oreskin of a man of 23. On the surface of the stratified quamous epithelium there is a thick layer of intensely osinophilic keratin (thick arrow) (lamellar yperkeratosis). There are occasional small lymphocytes vithin the epithelium. The rete pegs are flattened, and here are relatively small vacuoles in the dermis beneath nd very close to the basement membrane. Liquefaction egeneration of this layer often occurs but in this case the asal cells of the epithelium are intact. In the upper lermis, and closely apposed to the epithelium, there is a road sheet of eosinophilic hyalinized and poorly-cellular lense collagenous tissue (thin arrow). This tissue appears o be amorphous, but the deeper collagenous tissues are learly fibrillary (double arrow) and moderately nfiltrated with chronic inflammatory cells. The dermal lood vessels are thin-walled and markedly dilated. HE ×150

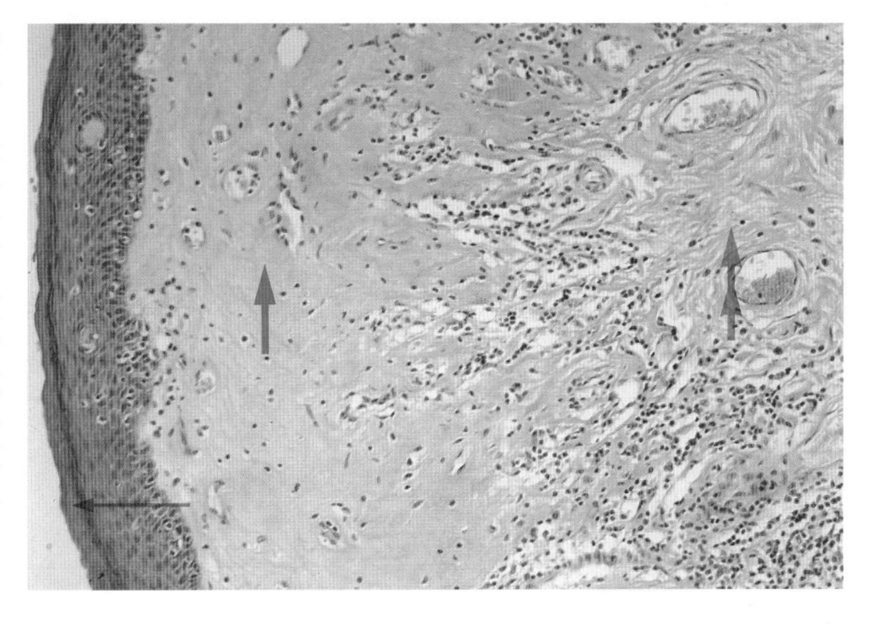

8.7 Benign nodular hyperplasia: prostate

Hyperplasia of the prostate is common in older men, and its enlargement is caused by hyperplasia of both the glandular and the stromal elements. The prostate consists of yellowish nodules of firm rubbery glandular tissue which may weigh several hundred grams. The condition tends to affect the central (periurethral) parts of the prostate and thereby cause obstruction to the outflow of urine. The risk of infection of the renal tract is then greatly increased. Bilateral hydronephrosis and renal failure are possible complications. This is one of the nodules from the enlarged prostate of a man aged 71. The prostatic tissue consists of abundant fibromuscular stroma and numerous acini. The acini, which tend to arrange themselves in groups (arrow), are lined with cuboidal or columnar epithelial cells with a considerable amount of eosinophilic cytoplasm and small basophilic nuclei. The lining cells proliferate and tend to form papilliform structures which project into the lumen of the acini and give them a tortuous shape. Some of the acini are surrounded by a mild infiltrate of chronic inflammatory cells and a few contain weakly eosinophilic secretion. HE ×60

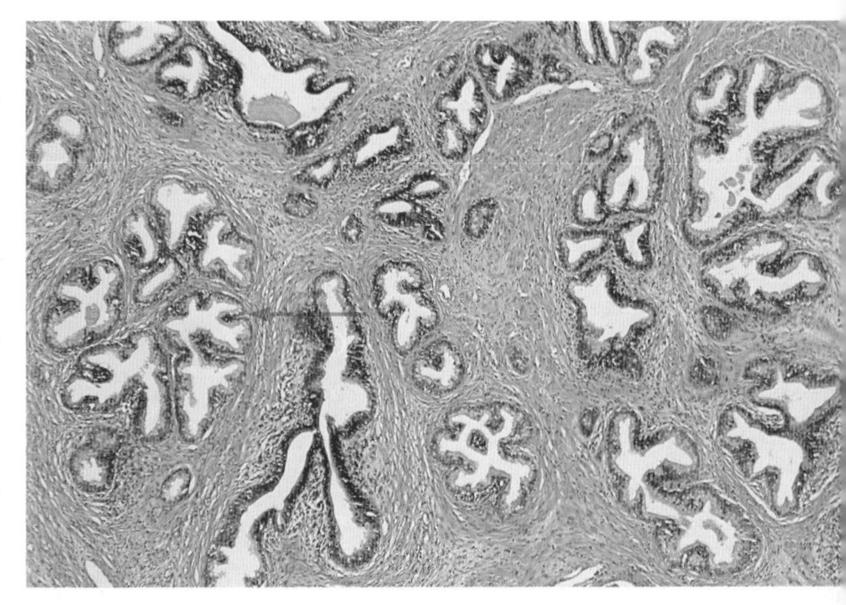

8.8 Benign nodular hyperplasia: prostate

Prostatic hyperplasia occurs in nearly all men over seventy years of age but it is symptomless in most of them. The etiology of the condition is unknown but declining levels of androgen (perhaps relative to estrogen levels) may play a part. This is part of the lesion in 8.7, at higher magnification. The glandular acini are hyperplastic and larger than normal, and lined with a single layer of palisaded tall well-differentiated columnar epithelial cells. Each cell has abundant eosinophilic cytoplasm, markedly vacuolated ('foamy') (thin arrow), and a compact round vesicular nucleus in the cell base. There is no mitotic activity. The lining cells are similar to the normal prostatic epithelium but show little evidence of secretory activity. They show, however, a tendency to proliferate and form intaluminal papillary structures. One acinus (thick arrow) is occupied by a round laminated deeply eosinophilic corpus amylaceum and accompanying fragments. Between the glandular acini is there bundles of eosinophilic smooth muscle fibres (likewise hyperplastic) and paler-staining fibrous connective tissue. HE ×150

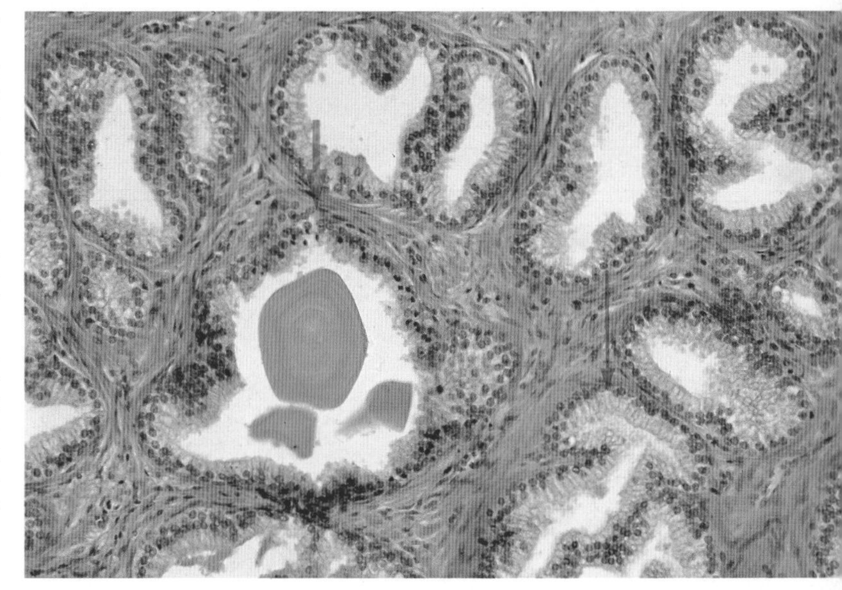

8.9 Infarct and squamous metaplasia: prostate

Catheterization (often associated with infection) is liable to cause occlusion of blood vessels and infarction of a nodule in an enlarged hyperplastic prostate. Acute swelling of the gland may occur, leading to acute pain and retention of urine. This is the edge of an infarcted area of prostatic tissue. The thin-walled blood vessels are dilated, some greatly (thick arrow), and there is considerable hemorrhage into the stromal connective tissue. The two larger acini are lined by a thick layer of large squamous epithelial cells with very pleomorphic nuclei (thin arrow). These cells closely resemble stratified squamous epithelium. In several (smaller) acini, similar squamous epithelial cells have proliferated so actively as to fill the lumen completely (double arrow). In the lumen of the two larger acini there are deeply eosinophilic corpora amylacea and necrotic cell debris. Squamous metaplasia occurs not uncommonly around infarcts of prostate, and care must be taken not to confuse the change with carcinoma. Although the metaplastic epithelium resembles squamous epithelium, intercellular bridges are not usually present and keratin is not formed. HE ×120

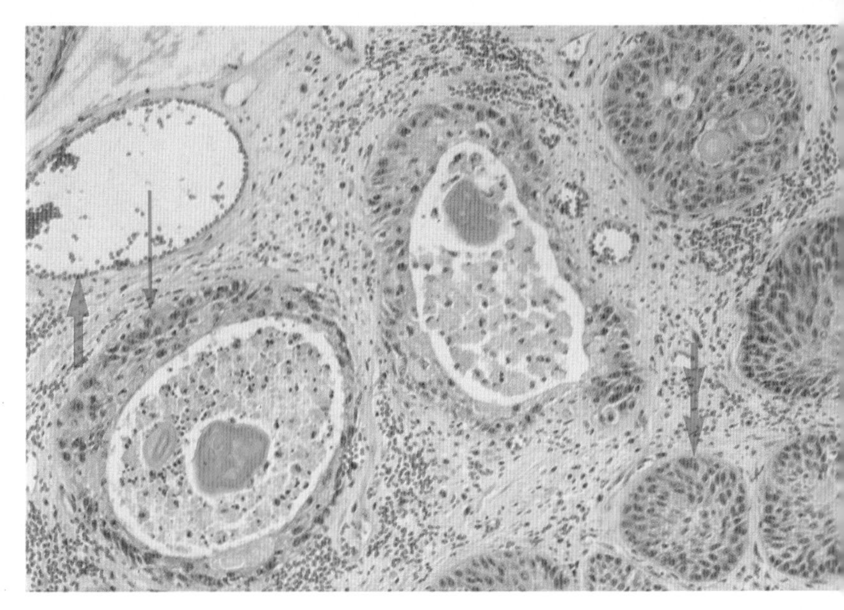

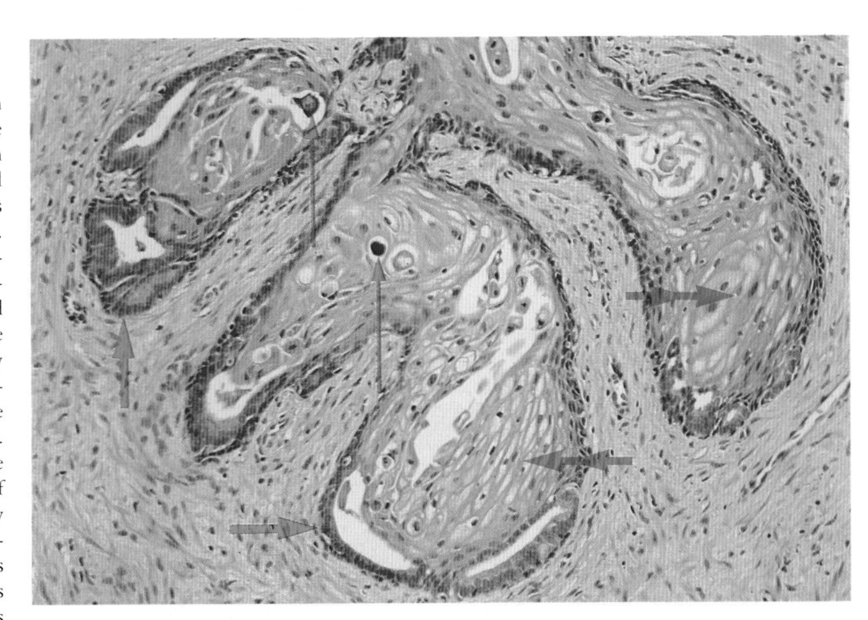

8.10 Squamous metaplasia and carcinoma: prostate

Carcinoma of prostate is a common finding at autopsy. In life, the vast majority are not detected and are therefore 'occult' cancers. Nearly all prostatic cancers are in men over fifty years of age, and there is a moderate familial tendency. The etiology is unknown, although androgens are involved in some way. often treated with estrogens. The therapy tends however to cause squamous metaplasia in the normal glandular epithelium. A man of 72 developed a carcinoma of prostate, for which he was treated with stilbestrol. A year later fragments of the prostate were removed *per urethram*. This shows several acini. They are very large and completely filled with sheets of stratified squamous epithelial cells (double arrows), with large amounts of eosinophilic and often vacuolated cytoplasm. Small round heavily stained deposits of keratin have formed (thin arrows). The nuclei of the basal layer of squamous epithelial cells are basophilic and moderately pleomorphic. There is however no evidence of malignancy. In several places normal columnar epithelium has survived (thick arrows). The fibromuscular stroma is abundant, probably with an increased content of fibrous tissue. HE ×150

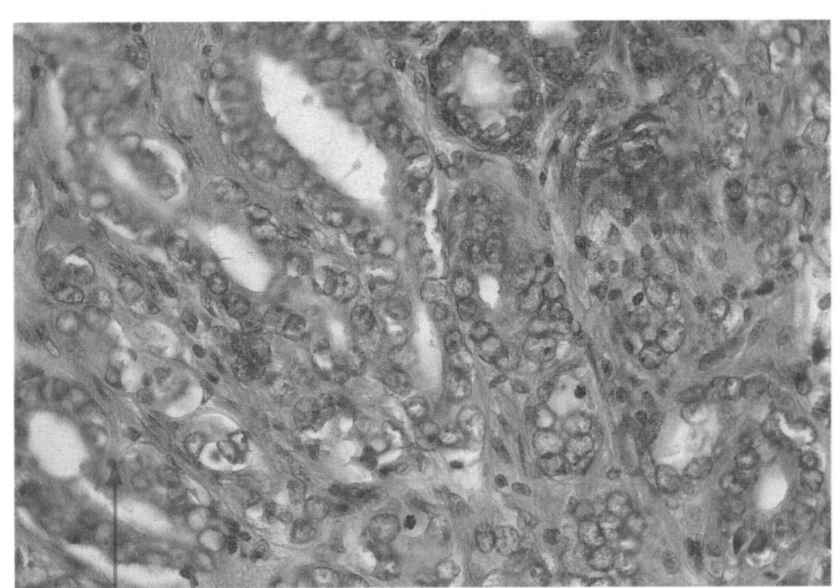

8.11 Prostatic intraepithelial neoplasia (PIN)

Prostatic tissue showing intraepithelial neoplasia (PIN). The epithelial cells have prominent nucleoli (arrow) in pale nuclei but no evidence of invasive carcinoma. This phenomenon is recognized increasingly and is very often associated with invasive carcinoma in the same gland. PIN precedes development of invasive cancer. High grade PIN, in a gland that has normalarchitecture, is characterized by nuclear changes: stratification of nuclei; enlargement of nuclei; hyperchromasia; and the presence of large nucleoli. The highest grade is PIN3. It is almost invariably associated with carcinoma and regarded as equivalent to carcinoma-in-situ. Prostate specific antigen (PSA) in PIN appears to be intermediate between carcinoma of prostate and normal level.

8.12 Carcinoma: prostate

Prostatic carcinoma, which has been immunostained with an antibody to Prostate Specific Antigen. This protein is measured in the serum to detect and monitor prostatic carcinoma and is frequently used histochemically to diagnose the disease. Prostate-specific Alkaline Phosphatase is used similarly. Both Prostate Specific Antigen and Prostatic Acid Phosphatase can be demonstrated by microtechniques which confirm that metastatic carcinoma is of prostatic origin.

8.13 Carcinoma: prostate

After stilbestrol therapy for carcinoma of prostate, the carcinomatous cells often show marked regressive changes, and they may take the form of collections of small cells with pyknotic nuclei and not detectable cytoplasm. In this case however, in addition to the squamous metaplasia in the non-neoplastic acini (as in **8.10**), there were also small cords of malignant cells which still looked fully viable. One of these cords of tumour cells is shown here. The cells are large, with fairly abundant cytoplasm, and are arranged in small very irregular groups (thin arrows), in some of which a small primitive lumen seems to be forming. The nuclei of the tumour cells are pleomorphic but mostly round or ovoid and full of uniformly diffuse moderately basophilic chromatin. In a few of the nuclei there is a small nucleolus. The stroma consists of large bundles of strongly eosinophilic smooth muscle fibres with large elongated basophilic nuclei (thick arrow), and also many fibrocytes in paler moderately vacuolated fibrous tissue. HE ×360

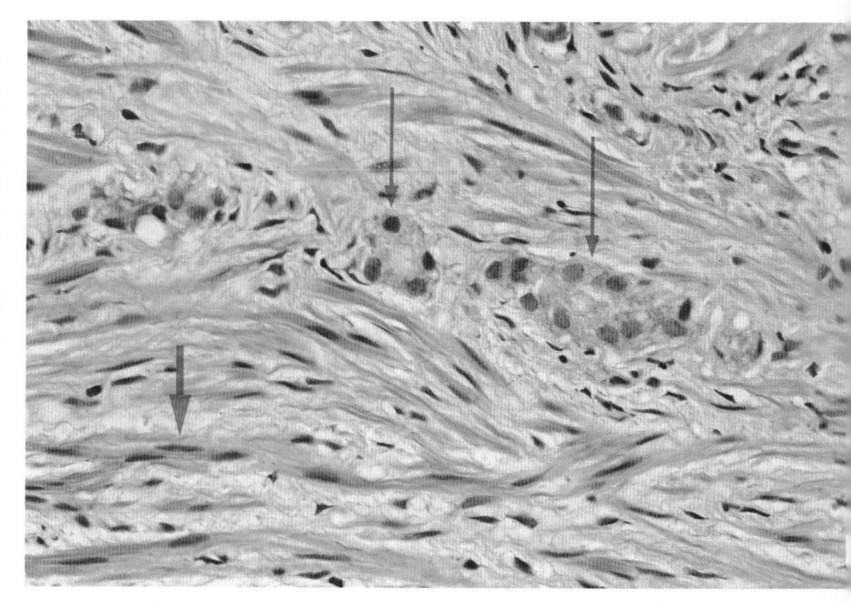

8.14 Carcinoma: prostate

In contrast to benign hyperplasia, the growth of prostatic carcinoma is androgen-dependent; and, significantly, most carcinomas of prostate arise in the subcapsular peripheral area of the posterior lobe of the organ, the region most sensitive to changes in androgen levels. The tumour often presents with symptoms and signs (including hematuria), caused by local growth and invasion of adjacent tissues. Tissues removed via the urethra are not ideal for early diagnosis, and cytology is of little value. Transrectal biopsy specimens are often used with success. The tumour is an adenocarcinoma, consisting of closely packed irregular acini, lined by a single layer of cuboidal epithelial cells (thin arrows). The cells are fairly uniform, with a very moderate amount of cytoplasm and a large round pale vesicular nucleus, each containing a strikingly large (prominent) central nucleolus. Some of the acini are unusually small and there are groups of malignant cells which are probably not parts of acini (they may be acini cut in cross-section). Mitotic figures are present. The stroma is highly cellular, consisting of a mixture of paler fibrous tissue and eosinophilic smooth muscle fibres (thick arrow). HE ×360

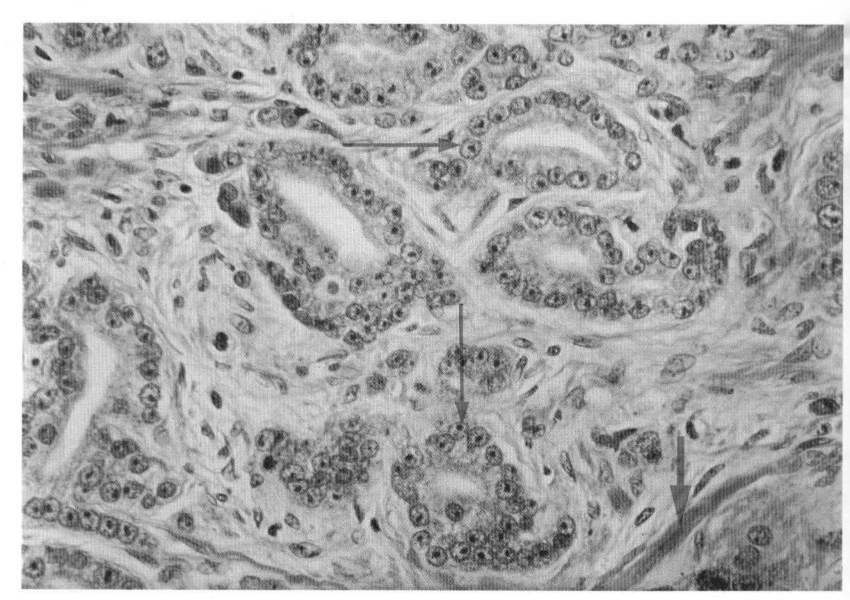

8.15 Carcinoma: prostate

Carcinoma of prostate may be well-differentiated and resemble normal prostate fairly closely. In a prostatic gland (acinus) with normal architecture, prostatic intraepithelial neoplasia (PIN) (otherwise dysplastic changes in the epithelial cells) is characterized by stratification, enlargement and hyperchromasia of nuclei, and the presence of large nucleoli. This type of lesion precedes the development of invasive cancer and if it is the highest grade, it is almost invariably associated with the cancer. This malignant tumour, from a 68-year-old man, does not form acini however. Instead, it forms solid cords of large swollen malignant cells (thick arrow) which are infiltrating sheets and bundles of large eosinophilic smooth muscle fibres (thin arrow). The swollen cells have abundant pale finely vacuolated (foamy) cytoplasm with well-defined boundaries, and their nuclei are small round or ovoid and deeply basophilic. They are also uniform in size and shape. A nucleolus is visible in only a few of them. There are no mitotic figures. Local extension of carcinoma of prostate through the prostatic capsule into the pelvic fat occurs early. It may also spread rapidly to regional lymph nodes and the bone marrow, and multiple metastases in the skeleton may be the first clinical sign.

HE ×360

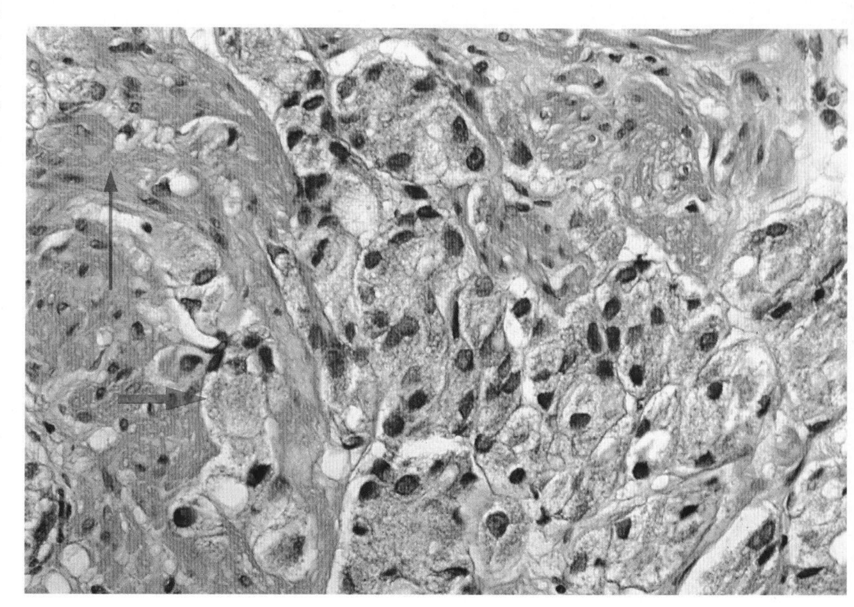

8.16 Carcinoma: prostate

A man aged 80 had a prostatectomy for benign hyperplasia. Histology confirmed the diagnosis but it also revealed a small carcinomatous focus adjacent to the hyperplastic nodules. This is the carcinomatous focus, and it consists of several irregular cords and clusters of large malignant cells (thick arrows). The tumour cells have scant cytoplasm, which is ill-defined and sometimes vacuolated. The cells are infiltrating sheets of eosinophilic fibrous tissue and smooth muscle cells (thin arrow), and their nuclei are relatively large. In several of the largest neoplastic nuclei there is one or more prominent nucleolus. One rudimentary malignant acinus is also present. There are no mitotic figures in any of the neoplastic cells. Careful examination of tissues removed for benign hyperplasia of the prostate often demonstrates small foci of carcinoma, and the incidence of these small tumours increases with the age of the patient. Such lesions should therefore be regarded as latent microcarcinomas and of no clinical significance for the individual concerned. Treatment for carcinoma is not indicated. HE ×360

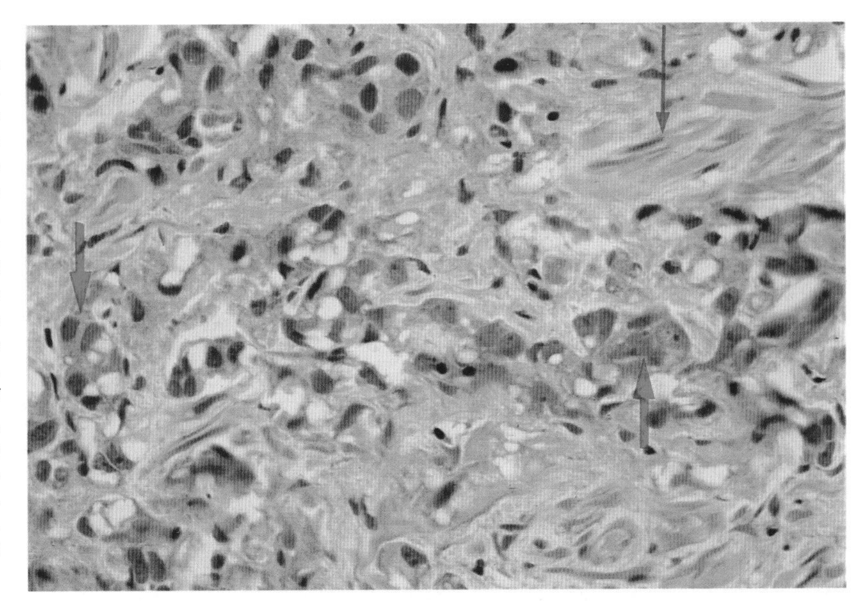

8.17 Cryptorchid (undescended) testis

Arrest of testicular descent is common, occurring in about 3% of full-term male infants. Normally, the testes should be in the scrotum by the age of 4, and if a testis is still extrascrotal (inguinal region or abdomen) at 6 years of age, treatment should be given. Otherwise irreversible atrophy will take place in the testis after puberty; and the risk of developing a malignant germ cell neoplasm later in life is greatly increased (30-50 times). This is an undescended testis that was removed surgically. It is smaller than normal (2.5 × 2 × 0.5cm), and histologically many seminiferous tubules have been lost. The small number of tubules that survive are markedly atrophic. Their basement membranes are completely hyalinized (thick arrow) and much thicker than those in normal tubules. The larger tubules contain Sertoli cells, with large pale vesicular nuclei and heavily vacuolated cytoplasm. There are no germ cells within the tubules however. The spaces between the tubules are filled with sheets of hyperplastic interstitial (Leydig) cells with a considerable amount of deeply eosinophilic cytoplasm (thin arrows). HE ×150

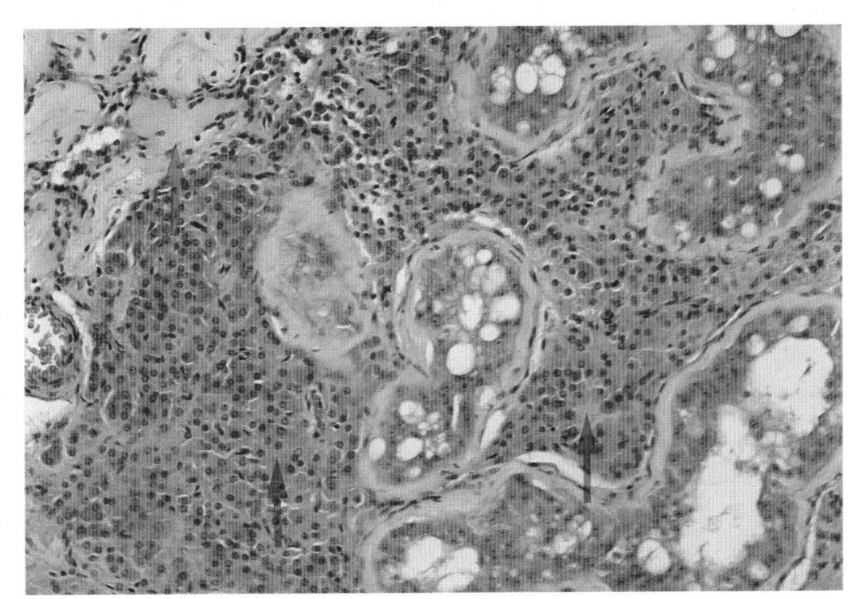

8.18 Cryptorchid (undescended) testis

In individuals with undescended testes, the risk of developing a malignant germ cell tumours is much greater if the maldescent is not corrected. This shows part of **8.17**, at higher magnification. The tubular atrophy is striking. The basement membrane is very thick and hyaline (thin arrow), and the cells in the lumen are Sertoli cells. They are large cells, with much ill-defined strongly eosinophilic vacuolated cytoplasm (thick arrows). Some of the vacuoles are large and empty (clear). The nuclei are vesicular and more or less uniformly round or slightly ovoid, and in some of them there is a prominent nucleolus. The nuclear chromatin is moderately basophilic and finely granular. There are no germ cells and no evidence of spermatogenesis in the tubules. The tissues around the tubules are packed with interstitial (Leydig) cells (double arrow). The cytoplasm of the Leydig cells is characteristically deeply eosinophilic, and uniform round vesicular nuclei contain finely granular chromatin. The apparent hyperplasia of the Leydig cells is undoubtedly greater because so many tubules have been lost from the testis. HE ×360

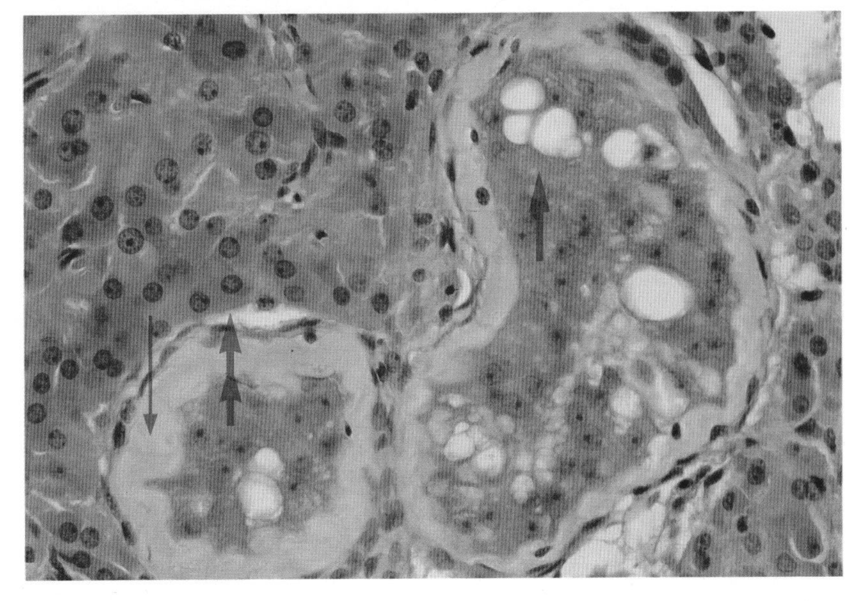

8.19 Klinefelter's syndrome: testis

Klinefelter's syndrome is an infertile male with gynecomastia and small testes and is often mentally retarded. It occurs fairly frequently (about 1 in 600 live births). The disorder is chromosomal in origin, usually caused by non-disjunction of the X chromosome in the mother of the affected child. The result is an extra X chromosome (47,XXY). Less often there are more than two X chromosomes (48,XXXY or 49,XXXXY). In Klinefelter's syndrome, interstitial (Leydig) cells form much of the tissue in the atrophic testes, and this group consists of large interstitial cells with finely granular deeply eosinophilic cytoplasm (thin arrow) and round vesicular nuclei. The chromatin is oderately granular, and in some of the nuclei the extra X chromosome is visible as a sex chromatin (Barr) body (thick arrow). Characteristically, the sex chromatin body differs from a nucleolus in being smaller and attached to the nuclear membrane. It is also basophilic, whereas nucleoli are eosinophilic. The small very basophilic nuclei at the periphery of the group of interstitial cells are lymphocytic. HE ×940

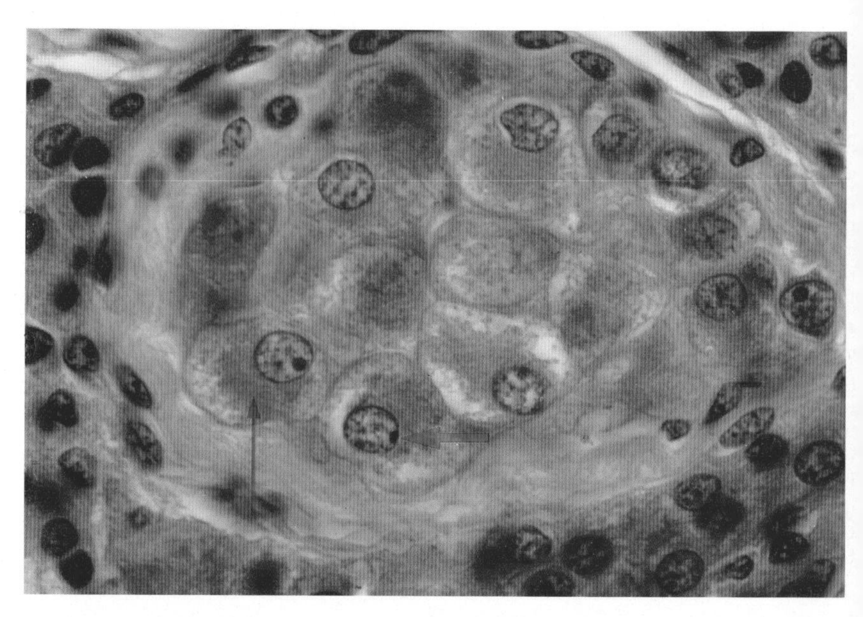

8.20 Idiopathic granulomatous orchitis: testis

Idiopathic granulomatous orchitis is an uncommon lesion of the testis which tends to occur in middle-aged men. Some affected individuals have autoantibodies to testicular antigens, which may give rise to an autoimmune (and still unconfirmed) disease. The condition usually presents as a painful enlarged testis, encased in a smooth capsule. The swelling gradually subsides, to leave a testis that is firmer than normal and less sensitive to pressure. Its normal cut surface is replaced by multiple firm greyish-white nodules. Histologically, there is an intense granulomatous reaction in the testis, centred on the seminiferous tubules and giving it a follicular distribution which is liable to be mistaken for tuberculosis. This lesion was in the left testis of a man of 42. Three seminiferous tubules and the peripheral parts of two others are shown. The seminiferous tissue has been destroyed, and each tubule is distended with closely packed epithelioid cells with abundant eosinophilic cytoplasm. There are also very large (giant) multinucleated cells of the Langhans type (thick arrows). The interstitial tissue of the testis is heavily infiltrated with chronic inflammatory cells (thin arrow), most of them plasma cells. HE ×150

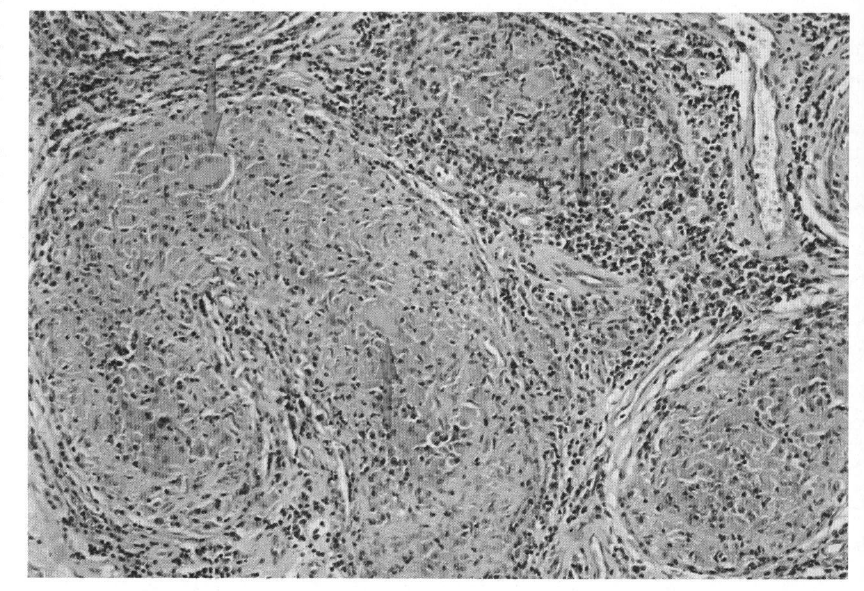

8.21 Granulomatous orchitis: testis

This is the same lesion as in **8.20**, at higher magnification. This is a seminiferous tubule, in cross-section, which has been destroyed by an intense granulomatous reaction. The cells normally present in the lumen of the tubule have been completely destroyed, as has the tubule's basement membrane; and both have been replaced by an ovoid mass of large epithelioid cells (arrows) with a large quantity of pinkish cytoplasm. The nuclei in the epithelioid cells are vesicular and also relatively large. The nuclear chromatin is weakly basophilic (pale) and very finely granular. There are no very large (giant) Langhans-type cells in this tubule, but they are frequently present elsewhere in the testis. The group of pink-stained epithelioid cells is surrounded by a cuff of small chronic inflammatory cells, nearly all of them plasma cells, each with relatively abundant cytoplasm and an eccentric nucleus. The resemblance of the granulomatous lesion, which replaced the seminiferous tubule, to a tuberculous follicle is close. However there is no necrosis, and tubercle bacilli are never been demonstrated. The etiology of granulomatous orchitis is still uncertain. HE ×360

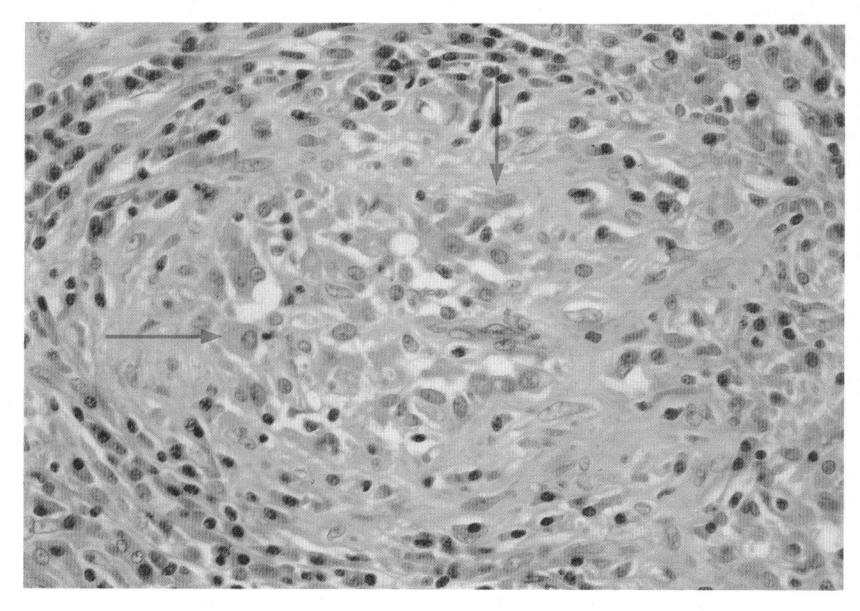

8.22 Seminoma: testis

Seminoma of testis is a firm solid tumour, which originates from the germinal (seminiferous) epithelium of the mature testis. The tumour tends to appear in early middle age (around 40 years of age), and with early diagnosis and adequate treatment including radiotherapy, the prognosis is very good. Macroscopically, the cut surface is usually a uniform yellowish-white colour, with occasional areas of necrosis. The histological structure is characteristic. The tumour consists of groups of closely packed swollen round or polyhedral cells, which resemble primary spermatocytes in the seminiferous tubule, with much clear or foamy cytoplasm (containing a large amount of glycogen) and distinct cell membranes. The nuclei are large, round or ovoid, and mostly in the centre of the cell (thin arrow). In almost all of the nuclei there is at least one prominent nucleolus (double arrow), usually located in the centre of the pale finely granular chromatin. The delicate fibrous trabecula (thick arrow) which separates the groups of tumour cells is heavily infiltrated with small basophilic lymphocytes. HE ×335

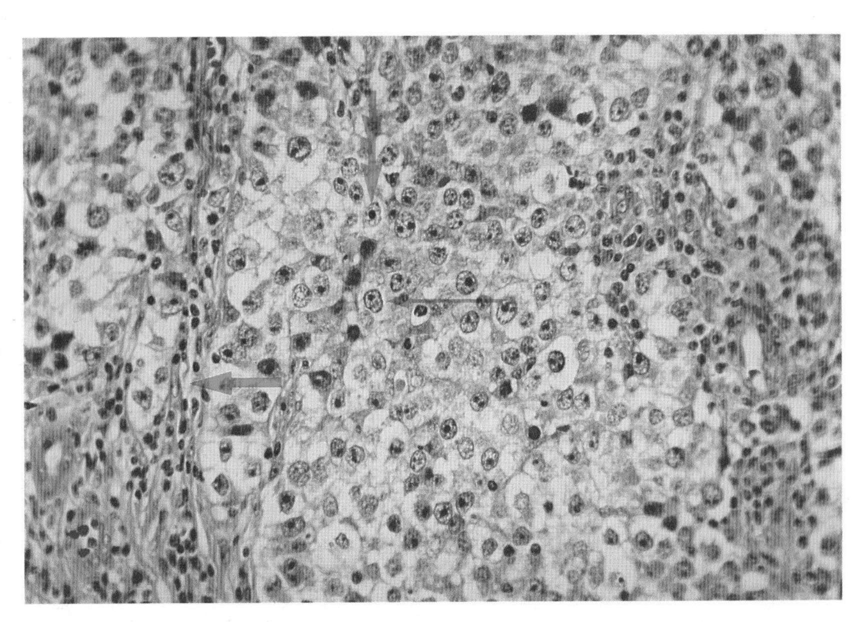

8.23 Seminoma: testis

There are granulomatous foci in about 50% of seminomas, and they consist largely of giant cells and necrotic cells. In this seminoma, the spematogonia-like malignant cells are arranged singly or in very small clusters, which are surrounded by a very extensive infiltrate of chronic inflammatory cells. Only a small amount of cytoplasm with its characteristic foamy texture surrounds and clings to the nucleus in each large neoplastic cell, its remaining cytoplasm having been almost completely replaced by a very large empty (clear) vacuole. The nuclei of the tumour cells are almost all located in the centre of the large cytoplasmic vacuole (thin arrow) (the vacuole is almost certainly caused by abundant glycogen in the cytoplasm). The inflammatory cell infiltrate in the stroma is remarkably intense, consisting of large clusters of epithelioid histiocytes (thick arrow), lymphocytes and plasma cells. The epithelioid cells have abundant ill-defined eosinophilic cytoplasm and pleomorphic vesicular nuclei. The nuclear chromatin is pale and very finely granular, and in many of the nuclei there is a prominent nucleolus. Langhans-type giant cells are present elsewhere in the tumour.
HE ×150

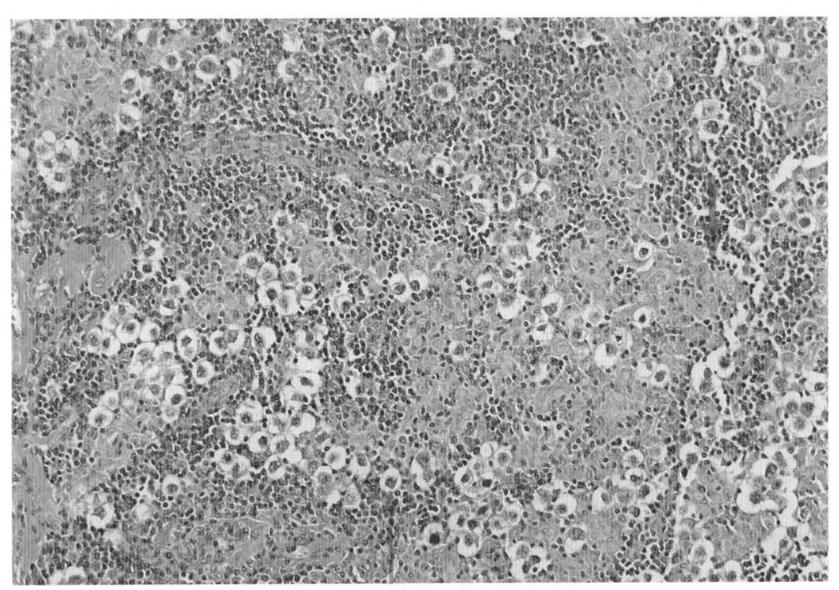

8.24 Seminoma: testis

Variants of seminoma include spermatocytic seminoma, characterized by tumour cells which mature enough to resemble secondary spematocytes; and anaplastic seminoma, the cells of which are more pleomorphic and mitotically more active than usual. This is part of the lesion in **8.23**, at higher magnification. The tumour cells (thick arrows) have large nuclei and vacuolated 'clear' cytoplasm, with only wisps of cytoplasm adherent to the nucleus. The epithelioid histiocytes (thin arrow) have eosinophilic slightly granular cytoplasm and pale-staining ovoid or elongated vesicular nuclei. They are closely packed and the cell boundaries are indistinct. The cells with small deeply-staining nuclei are lymphocytes and plasma cells. The presence of a large population of lymphocytes in seminomas suggests a strong defensive reaction on the part of the host to the tumour; and this view is strengthened by the presence in many seminomas of the epithelioid histiocytes, a reaction similar to that seen in tuberculous or sarcoid follicles. The combination of lymphocytes and epithelioid cells is suggestive of a delayed hypersensitivity type of reaction.
HE ×360

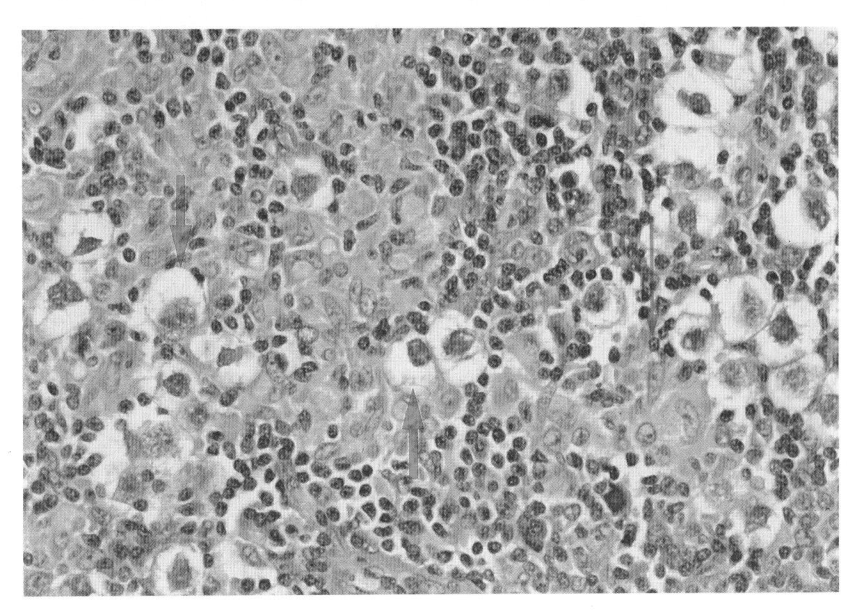

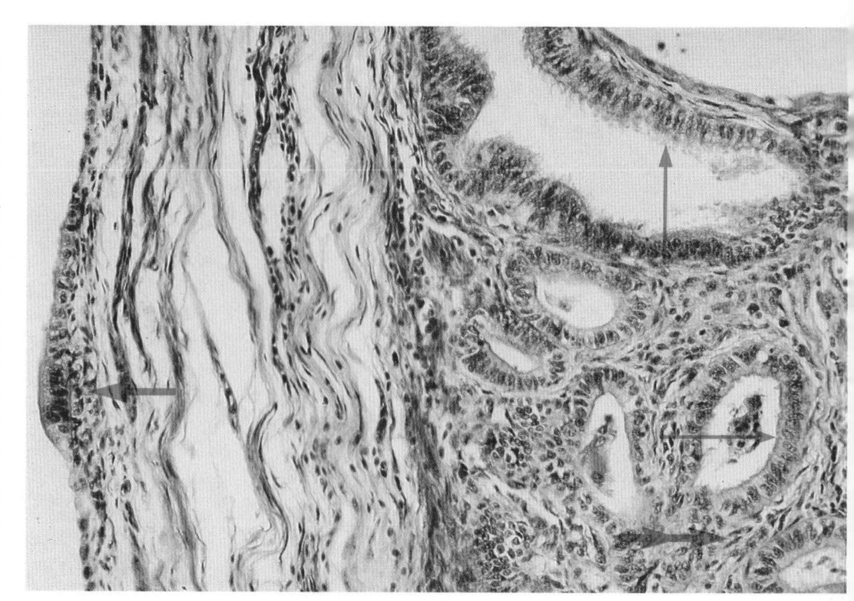

8.25 Teratoma: testis

Teratomas of testis are rare and characterized by somatic differentiation, all three germ layers being represented. That is, they are true 'mixed' tumours, containing all types of tissue in varying proportions and degrees of differentiation. Occasionally the tissues adopt an organoid arrangement. Teratomas of testis are invariably malignant, unlike their ovarian counterparts which in a high proportion of cases are benign 'dermoids'. All teratomas in adults are biologically malignant, whereas teratomas in children under 12 years of age behave as benign neoplasms. This lesion is a differentiated ('mature') teratoma which consists of mature-looking tissues. The large cyst, part of it just visible at the left margin, is lined by epithelial cells of widely varying height (thick arrow), from flat to tall columnar. The smaller cysts and ducts on the right are lined by columnar epithelial cells (thin arrows). The stroma is a mixture of dense fibrous tissue and highly cellular connective tissue (double arrow), e.g. around the small ducts. The mixture of cystic glands and fibrous tissue gives a teratoma a characteristic naked-eye appearance (fibrocystic disease).

HE ×135

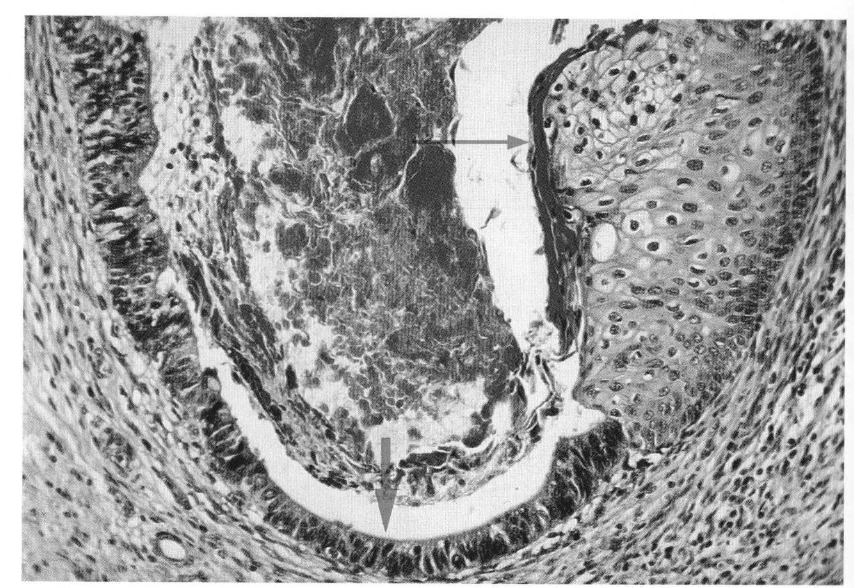

8.26 Teratoma: testis

Teratomas of testis generally occur between 10 and 30 years of age, and they contain elements of all three germ-cell layers, most notably glandular epithelium (endoderm), squamous epithelium (ectoderm) and cartilage (mesoderm). Teratomas are usually solid, with cystic areas which tend to be located centrally. This lesion also is a differentiated (mature) teratoma, similar to **8.25**. In the centre there is a large cyst, lined partly with tall columnar epithelial cells (thick arrow) and partly with a thick layer of large stratified squamous epithelial cells (thin arrow). Squamous epithelium is often abundant in differentiated teratomas, and the cyst is full of deeply eosinophilic keratinous squames which have been desquamated from the squamous epithelial cells. The cyst is surrounded by a wall of fibrous tissue and elongated fibrocytes, and infiltrated by a moderate number of small lymphocytes. Differentiated teratomas of the testis may appear to be composed of mature-looking tissues but it should not be assumed that they will behave like a benign neoplasm, since malignant areas are readily overlooked during histological examination; and a proportion of differentiated (mature) teratomas of testis do metastasize.

HE ×150

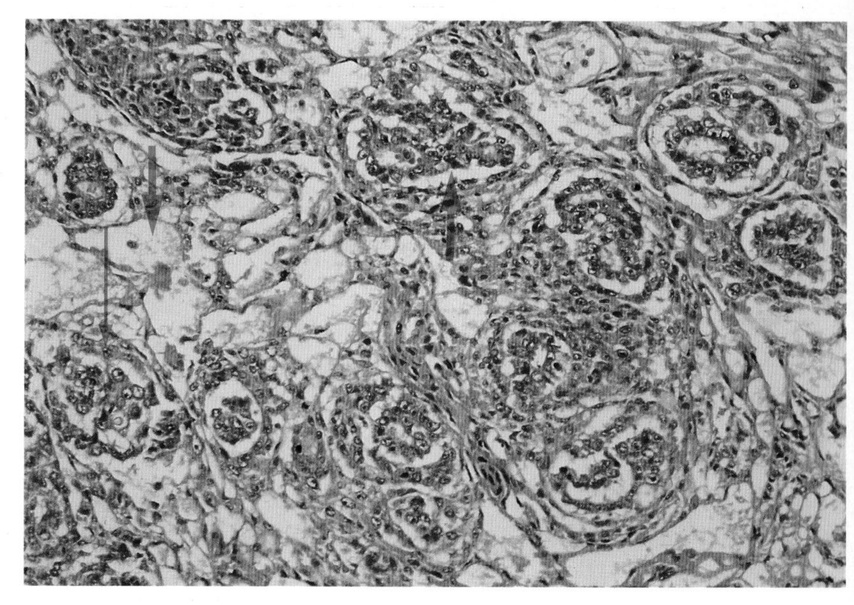

8.27 Yolk sac tumour: testis

Yolk sac (endodermal sinus) carcinoma is a malignant teratoma in which embryonal yolk sac tissue predominates. It is rare and generally occurring in individuals between 10 and 30 years of age. A typical tumour of this type is solid, fleshy and soft but also friable. This lesion presented as a lump in the left testis of a man of 20. The testis was enlarged (8 × 4 × 3cm) and it was resected. The testicular tissue had been almost entirely replaced by highly vascular tissue in which there was extensive necrosis. Histologically it consists of an extremely 'loose' (very edematous) mesenchymal stroma with many clear (microcystic) spaces (thick arrows), in which there are complex tubular structures (thin arrow). The tubular structures are lined with malignant cuboidal cells which have a moderate or minimal cytoplasm and large vacuolated nuclei in each of which there is a very prominent nucleolus. The malignant cells also tend to form large papillary projections into the lumen of the tubules, thereby producing structures which vaguely resemble glomeruli. These are Schiller-Duval bodies and are a diagnostic feature of yolk sac tumours. HE ×150

8.28 Choriocarcinoma: testis

Choriocarcinoma of testis is a rare highly malignant tumour, characterized by trophoblastic differentiation. It is assumed to develop in a teratoma. It is a solid tumour, and it is usually very hemorrhagic. A man of 29 presented with a swollen left testis which was removed surgically. It measured 9 × 6 × 5cm and within it there was a tumour, the cut surface of which was light brown and faintly lobulated. Histologically the neoplasm is composed of both cytotrophoblast (thin arrow) and syncytiotrophoblast (thick arrow), and they arranged in a pattern that reflects their relationship in chorionic villi. The cytotrophoblast consists of cells with clear or vacuolated cytoplasm and well-defined cell boundaries; and syncytiotrophoblast consists of sheets of eosinophilic cytoplasm in which there are very large nuclei. There are prominent nucleoli in both types of malignant cell, but many of those in syncytiotrophoblast are relatively enormous. Individual (single) giant multinucleated cells (syncytiotrophoblastic) are also present (double arrow). There is also abundant eosinophilic fluid (e.g. bottom left), containing fairly numerous polymorph leukocytes, between the sheets of neoplastic cells. HE ×150

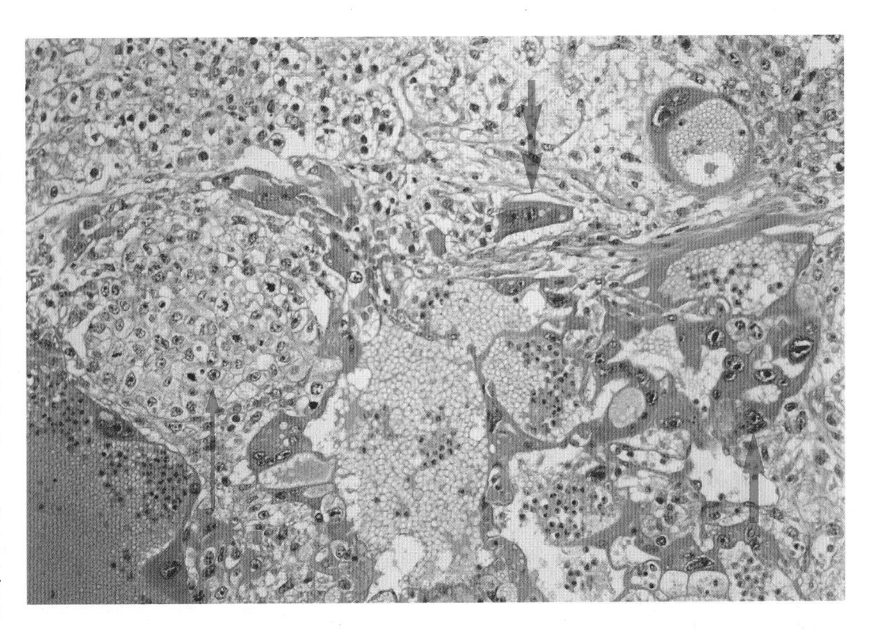

8.29 Lymphoplasmacytic lymphoma: testis

Lymphoplasmacytic lymphoma of the testis (also termed LP immunocytoma) is rare. It occurs most often in men over 60 years of age, and is the commonest type of neoplasm in this age group, accounting for 2% of all testicular tumours. This lesion was in a man of 64. The testis was greatly enlarged (7 × 5 × 4cm), weighing approx. 110g. Its cut surface was firm and creamy-white, with flecks of hemorrhage. Histologically, non-neoplastic atrophic thick-walled seminiferous tubules, containing only Sertoli cells (arrows) (no germinal cells) and cell debris, are surrounded by a diffuse dense neoplastic infiltrate of closely packed small basophilic cells with deeply basophilic nuclei. Scattered among the small neoplastic cells there is a much smaller number of large histiocytes with much pale cytoplasm. At higher magnification, the neoplastic cells are recognizable as plasmacytic cells, among which there are numerous mitoses. The whole of the testis has the same structure. The diagnosis is lymphoplasmacytic lymphoma but the prognosis of testicular lymphoma is poor, since lesions are usually present elsewhere. HE ×60

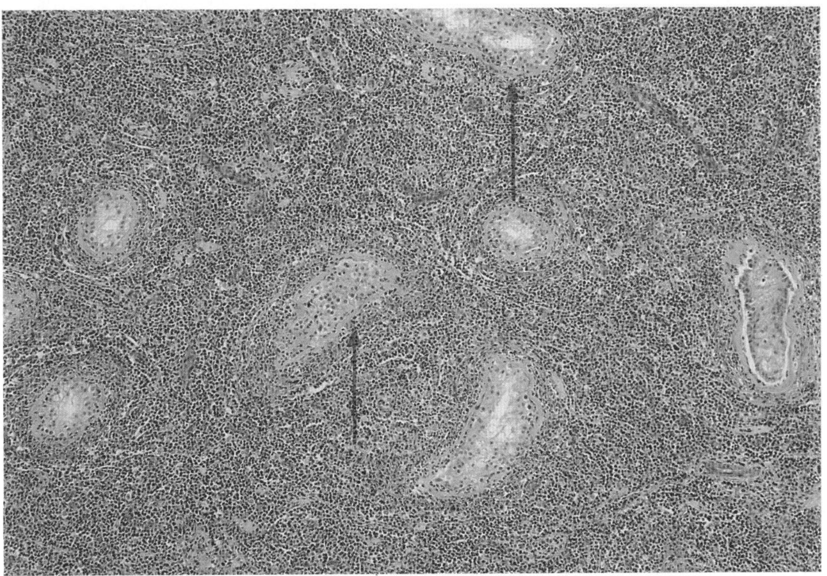

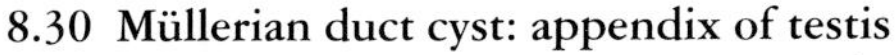

8.30 Müllerian duct cyst: appendix of testis

The appendix of the testis is a remnant of the paramesonephric duct (Müllerian duct) and it is located between the top of the testis and the head of the epididymis. It corresponds to the fimbriated end of the Fallopian tube. It is sometimes pedunculated and may undergo torsion. A man of 47 developed a swelling in his scrotum, and a cyst filled with clear fluid and attached to the testis was removed surgically. The cyst is lined by a single layer of uniform very closely packed tall columnar cells (arrow) with a very moderate amount of eosinophilic cytoplasm (some of the cells are ciliated) with large elongated nuclei with rounded (blunted) ends. The chromatin in the nuclei is very basophilic and very finely granular. There is no mitotic activity. The wall around the cyst consists of loose strands of collagenous connective tissue and small thin-walled blood vessels. The lesion was diagnosed as a Müllerian duct cyst of the appendix of the testis. HE ×360

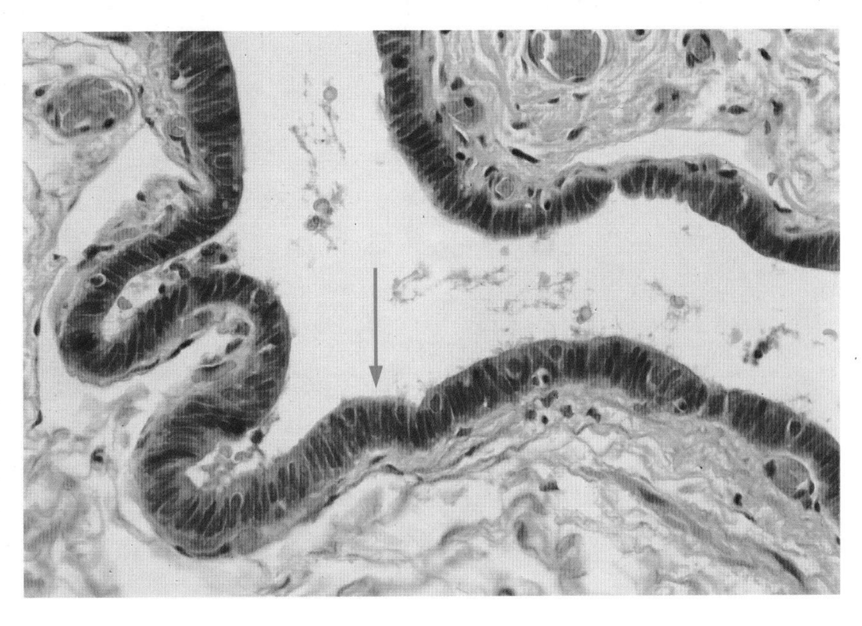

8.31 Adenomatoid tumour: epididymis

Adenomatoid tumours are benign encapsulated neoplasms that usually arise in the epididymis, probably from mesothelial cells in the tunica vaginalis (a similar tumour occurs also in the pelvic cavity in females, on the external surface of the uterus and fallopian tubes). The tumour usually occurs in men in their twenties and thirties, and taking the form of a relatively small circumscribed nodule with a greyish-white cut surface. This lesion however is a firm smooth-surfaced mass (3cm dia) in a 42-year-old man, with a cream-coloured cut surface. Histologically it is composed of a complex arrangement of thin-walled gland-like spaces or slit-like clefts (thick arrow), surrounded by abundant eosinophilic stroma. Most of the spaces and clefts are lined with flat mesothelial cells, but occasionally they are lined (in parts) with low cuboidal mesothelial cells (thin arrow). Some of the spaces contain small clusters of desquamated lining cells, and other (larger) spaces seem to lack any lining of mesothelial cells. The stroma consists of collagenous fibrous tissue, smooth muscle cells and fibroblasts.

HE ×150

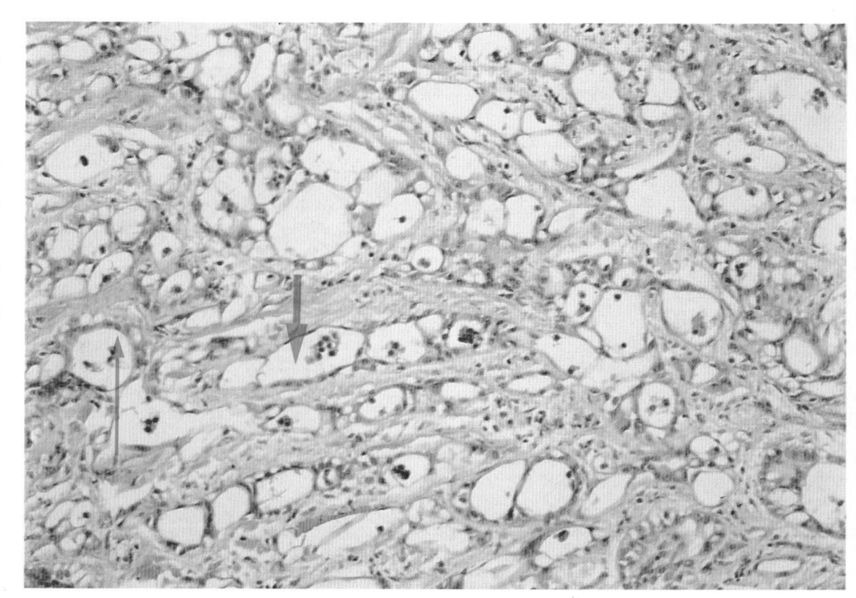

8.32 Adenomatoid tumour: epididymis

This is the same lesion as in **8.31**, at higher magnification. There are numerous gland-like spaces and clefts in this part of the tumour, lined (almost completely) by very flat mesothelial cells (thin arrow) with a large amount (thin sheets) of extremely attenuated cytoplasm. Within some of the spaces and clefts there are desquamated single (individual) cells and small clusters of cells (double arrow). The desquamated cells vary considerably in size, and the larger cells have fairly abundant eosinophilic cytoplasm and a relatively large round vesicular nucleus, the chromatin of which is pale and very finely granular. Apart from the desquamated cells, the spaces appear empty, but mucinous secretion can be demonstrated in them in sections of appropriately-fixed tissue. The stroma consists of fibrous connective tissue but there are smooth muscle cells in other parts of the tumour. The large elongated cells (thick arrow) with pale vesicular nuclei lying between the spaces are probably neoplastic, and so (almost certainly) are the cells within the spaces.

HE ×360

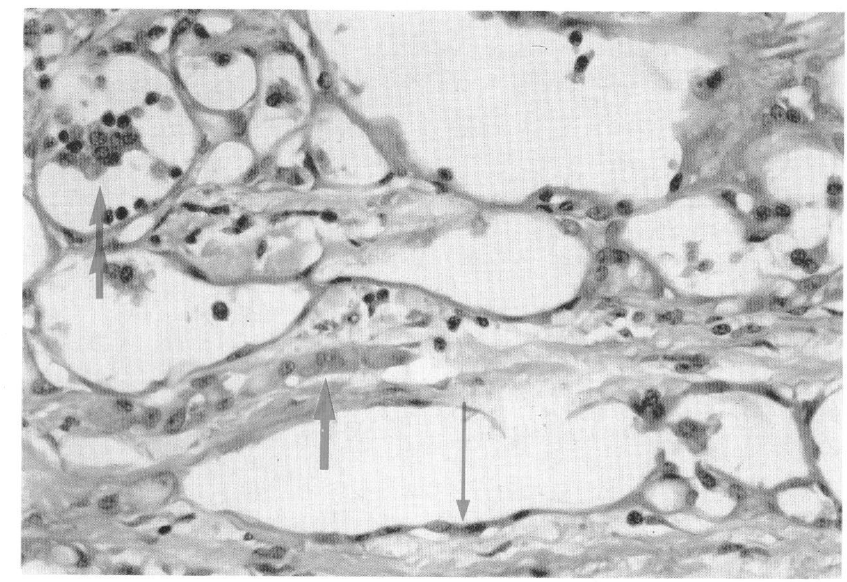

8.33 Paratesticular leiomyosarcoma: testis

Paratesticular malignant tumours of non-germinal cell origin in children are generally rhabdomyosarcomas, but in adults other types of tumour are more likely. This tumour (7 × 5 × 5cm) was located in the spermatic cord of a man of 52 and appeared to arise from the upper part of the epididymis. It proved to be a leiomyosarcoma. The cut surface was lobulated and greyish-white, with areas of necrosis and hemorrhage. Histologically it is a spindle-cell sarcoma, consisting of interlacing bundles of very elongated neoplastic smooth muscle cells (thin arrow). The neoplastic cells have a large amount of strongly eosinophilic cytoplasm, in which special stains demonstrated myofibrils. The nuclei are hyperchromatic and moderately pleomorphic. Most of them are elongated, some extremely. Many of the nuclei have tapering ends, but a small minority of them have round (blunted) ends. There are numerous mitotic figures (more than 10 per 10 HP fields) (thick arrows). Leiomyosarcomas tend to recur, even when they appear to be well-differentiated.

HE ×360

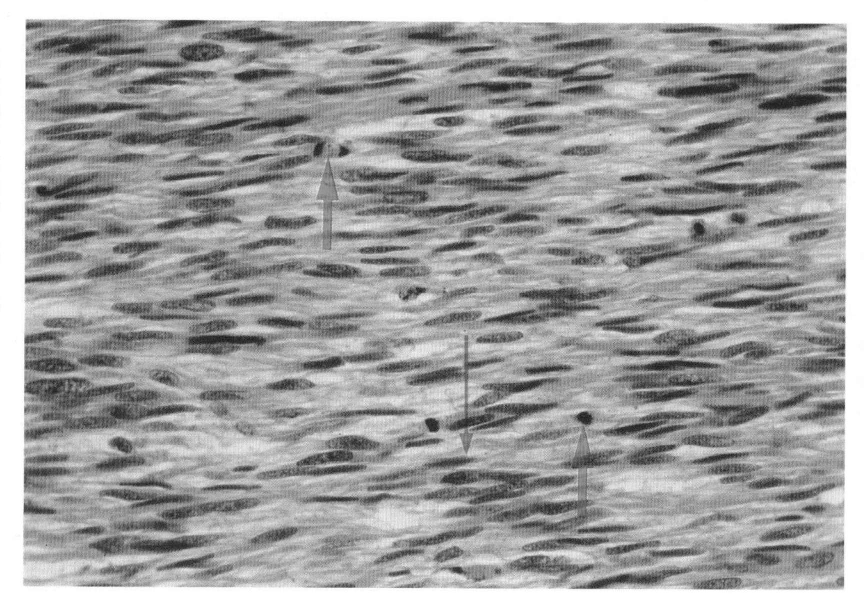

8.34 Embryonal rhabdomyosarcoma: spermatic cord

Rhabdomyosarcoma is an uncommon soft tissue sarcoma, and there are three types of it : embryonal, alveolar and pleomorphic. Embryonal rhabdomyosarcoma is a highly malignant tumour of the first two decades of life but most occur before the age of 5. It presents as a rapidly growing neoplasm in various sites. It is extremely infiltrative and tend to metastasize via the bloodstream at an early age. This tumour, unusually, was in the spermatic cord of a man of 21. It was a large lobulated homogeneous mass 7cm dia and it was compressing the testis. On section, it was of firm consistency and cream-coloured, but one area was gelatinous and spongy. The cells show very considerable pleomorphism of both nucleus and cytoplasm. Most cells are round (thin arrow), with basophilic nuclei. Others are fusiform (thick arrow), with large nuclei; and some are very large and strap-like (double arrow), with a large amount of solid-looking deeply eosinophilic cytoplasm. The cytoplasm of most of the cells is highly vacuolated. There is abundant loose fibrillary stroma between the tumour cells. HE ×150

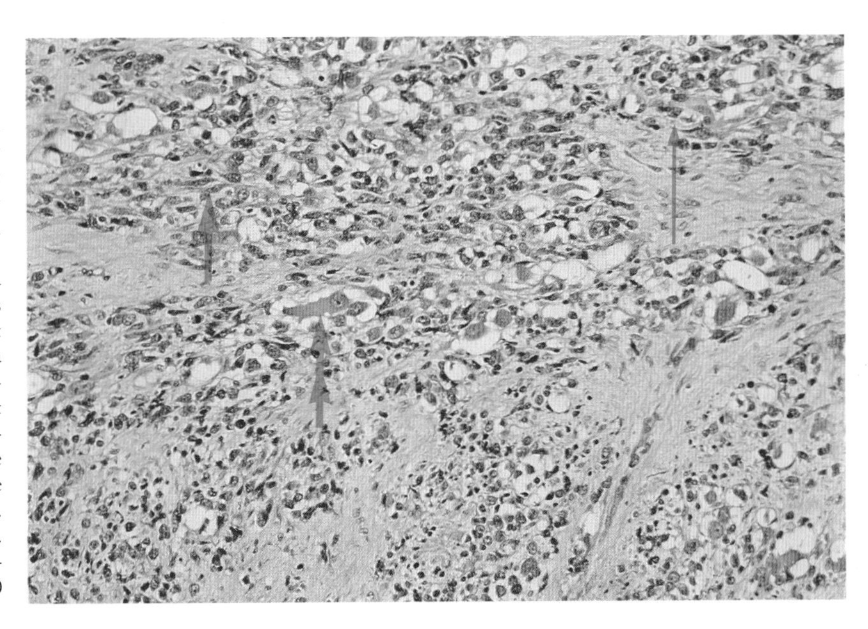

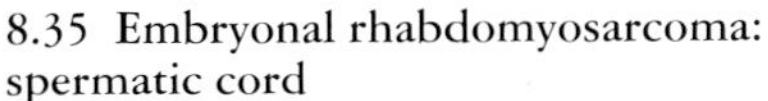

8.35 Embryonal rhabdomyosarcoma: spermatic cord

Embryonal rhabdomyosarcoma is highly cellular, and the nuclei of the extremely pleomorphic tumour cells generally appear primitive and hyperchromatic. This is part of the same tumour as **8.34**, at higher magnification. The extreme pleomorphism of the tumour cells, both nuclear and cytoplasmic, is evident. The nuclei are deeply basophilic (hyperchromatic) and most are large; and although the majority are round or ovoid, others are elongated. There are nucleoli in some of the nuclei, and a few of the nucleoli are very large and prominent (thin arrow). There are many large clear (empty) vacuoles, varying greatly in size and shape, and most of them are apparently intracytoplasmic. Several tumour cells are very elongated and strap-like, with abundant cytoplasm which is strongly eosinophilic (thick arrow). The appearance of these cells suggests that they are neoplastic muscle cells, and their identity can be confirmed by demonstrating either cross-striations in the cytoplasm or the presence of muscle proteins such as myoglobin. The stroma consists of pale loose fibrillary connective tissue (double arrow). HE ×360

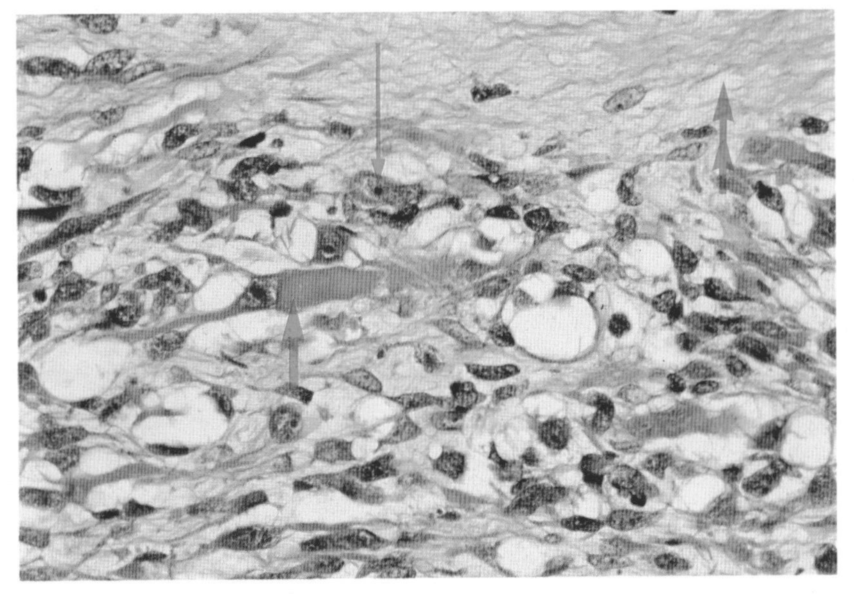

8.36 Embryonal rhabdomyosarcoma: spermatic cord

This is a section of the same tumour as in **8.34** and **8.35**. It has been stained with toluidine blue, a dye which demonstrates the cross-striations in muscle fibres much more effectively than hematoxylin and eosin. The stain also emphasizes the basophilia and pleomorphism of the nuclei of the tumour cells. The neoplastic cells are large, and both the cytoplasm and the (particularly) nuclei very heavily stained and opaque. However some of the large nuclei are much paler, with finely granular chromatin, and in one of them there is a large central nucleolus (bottom right corner). Likewise the very abundant cytoplasm of several of the elongated 'strap-like' cells is translucent; and within the cytoplasm there is a long series of parallel blue bands (thick arrow). These are cross-striations in the cytoplasm, and they appear identical to those in striated muscle fibres, confirming that the tumour is a rhabdomyosarcoma. Within and between the tumour cells there are many large clear (empty) vacuoles. Toluidine blue ×800

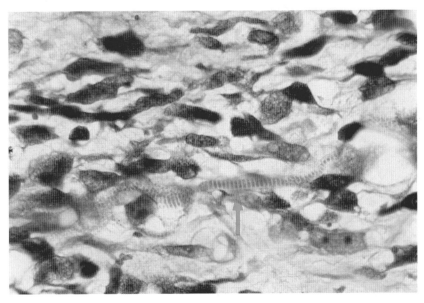

9.1 Atheroma: coronary artery

Atheroma is a patchy thickening of the intima of arteries, caused mainly by the deposition of lipid and fibrous tissue. When it narrows the artery, ischemia develops and is a major cause of disease and death. This is a coronary artery from a middle-aged man who suffered from severe angina pectoris. The lumen of the artery, encircled by extremely thick, is reduced to less than half the normal diameter. The layer of intimal tissue nearest the lumen consists of dense fibrous tissue, apart from one area rich in lipid-filled macrophages (thin arrow). On the right, deep in the intima and pressing on an atrophic media (extreme right) are a crescent-shaped mass of eosinophilic material and a large number of small clefts (thick arrow) which contained cholesterol crystals. On the left, the (clear) gap deep in the fibrous intima contained similar material. The dense (blue) fibrous tissue beneath the gap is patchily calcified (double arrow), and external to it is a thin layer of atrophic media. HE ×15

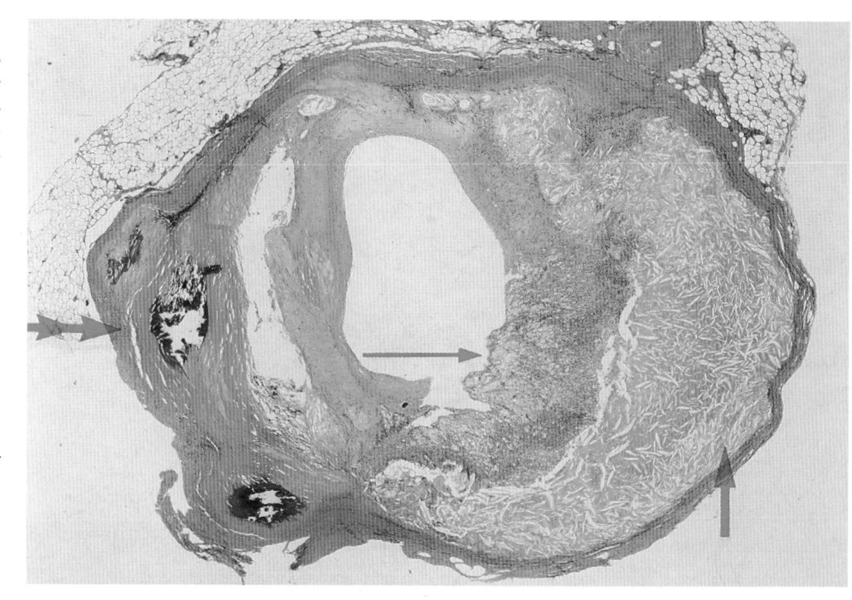

9.2 Atheroma: coronary artery

Atherosclerotic plaques are focal and scattered throughout the aorta and arteries. The intervening parts of the intima are normal. The severity of atherosclerosis is very variable. The condition may be mild even in the elderly but severe in much younger individuals. When plaques form in arteries, they are usually pearly-white but may appear yellowish. The surface is lined initially be smooth shiny endothelium. The plaques generally contain lipoid material and fibrous tissue, in widely differing amounts. This is the same coronary artery as in 9.1, at higher magnification. The lumen of the artery is at the top right corner, and the band of smooth muscle (thin arrow) is the atrophic media. The intima is enormously thickened, by the presence deep in it of amorphous material containing large numbers of cholesterol crystals (initially in large clefts) (double arrow). There are also very many foamy (lipid-filled) macrophages and chronic inflammatory cells in this zone, which is separated from the lumen of the artery by a thick layer of densely collagenous fibrous tissue (thick arrow). HE ×60

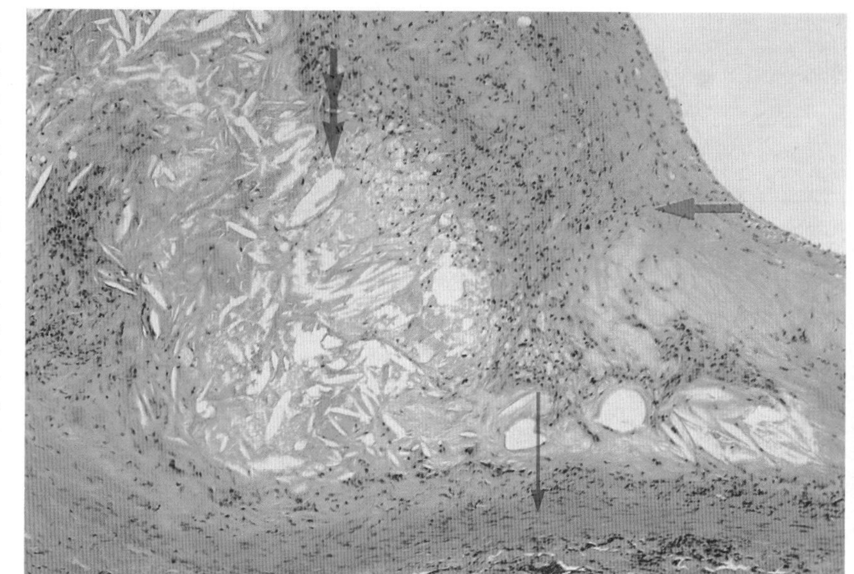

9.3 Atheroma: coronary artery

Atherosclerosis frequently narrows or occludes coronary arteries. The most common and dangerous effect is ischemia, which causes infarction of parts of the myocardium. The extent of myocardial ischemia and infarction has widely varying effects, which may range from mild angina to sickness and ultimately to death. This field shows part of the same coronary artery as in 9.1, at higher magnification. In 9.1 the artery is lined for the most part by dense fibrous tissue, but in this part of the vessel the tissue lining the lumen (which is just visible on the right) consists almost exclusively of large or very large closely packed macrophages (arrow) with abundant pale granular or finely vacuolated (foamy) cytoplasm and small basophilic nuclei (similar cells are present elsewhere, in the cholesterol-rich material deep in the intima). This sheet of foamy macrophages is also traversed by a few slender strands of fibrous tissue. The origin of the lipids of atheromatous plaques and their mode of entry into the intima are uncertain but their composition suggests an origin from the plasma.

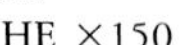

HE ×150

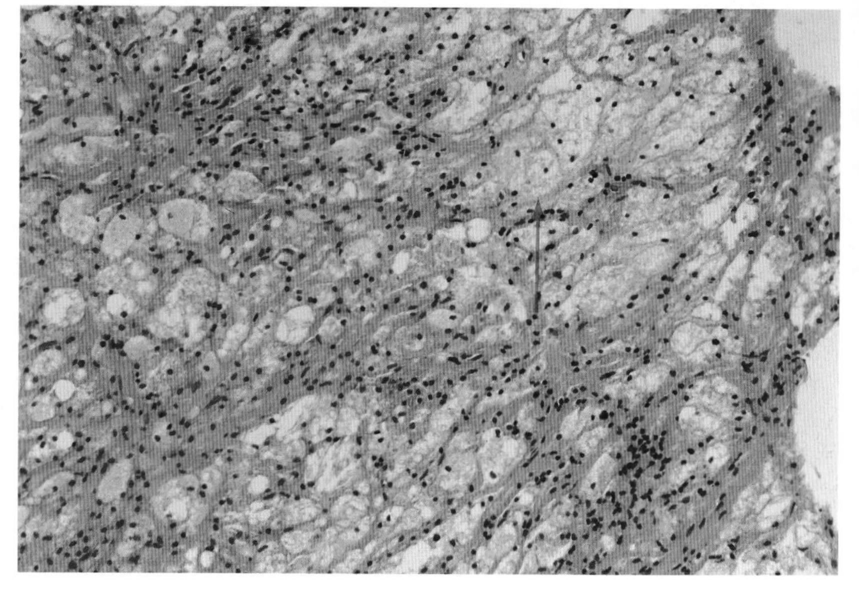

9.4 Atheroma: coronary artery

In this coronary artery, the junction of the intimal plaque (left) and the media (right) is clearly demarcated by the internal elastic lamina (thick arrows). The brightly eosinophilic elastic lamina is wrinkled, and although broken in many places elsewhere, it is intact. It has also reduplicated to form a second thinner elastic lamina. Fibrous tissue has replaced much of the muscle in the media. The intimal plaque consists of dense fibrous tissue (thin arrow), much of it acellular and hyaline. Special stains would reveal the presence of both fibrin and lipid. The atherosclerotic plaques in arteries are often vascularized by capillaries, and in this field there are thin-walled widely dilated capillaries (double arrow) in the fibrous plaque. Capillaries in the media come from the vasa vasorum, and it is likely that the vessels in the plaque are extensions of these. It has been suggested that capillaries also enter the intima directly, from the lumen of the artery. Hemorrhages from small blood vessels in intimal plaques can cause the size of the plaque to increase rapidly and consequently reduce the lumen of the vessel. This sequence can simulate thrombotic occlusion of the artery. HE ×235

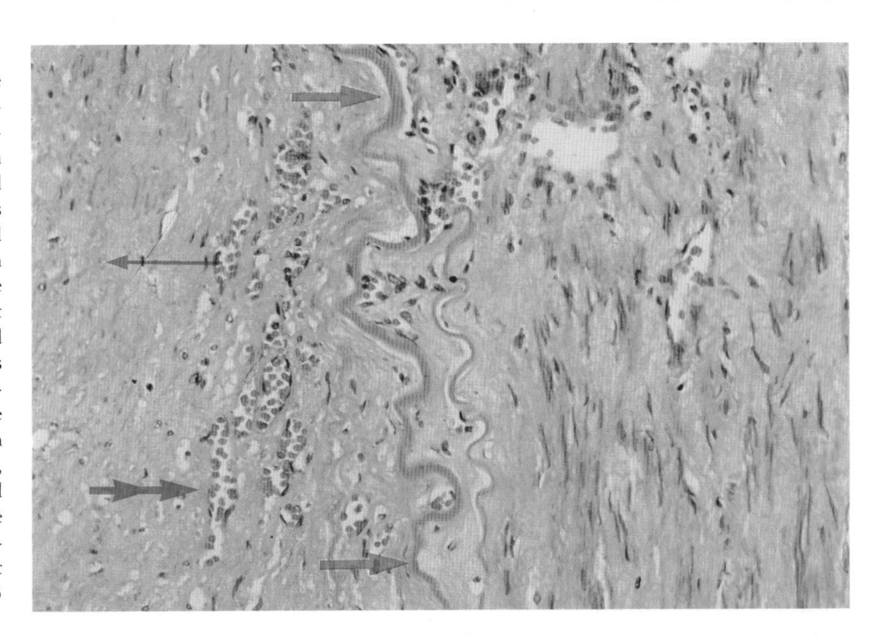

9.5 Aneurysm: femoral artery

Atheromatous plaques tends to cause atrophy of the underlying muscular media (9.1, 9.2) of an artery, and the media of a severely atheromatous artery may be so weakened by the plaques as to produce aneurysmal dilatation of the artery. The aorta is similarly affected, and atheroma is now the commonest cause of aneurysm of aorta in many countries. Aortic aneurysms are usually fusiform. Aneurysms may develop in various large arteries and this aneurysm has formed in a femoral artery near its origin. The muscle fibres of the medial coat have disappeared, and are now completely replaced by poorly cellular collagenous fibrous tissue (thin arrow). Small blood vessels, accompanied by many small basophilic lymphocytes, lie between the coarse collagenous fibres. In the lumen of the aneurysm, there is a layer of deeply red-stained thrombus (double arrow) (with numerous vacuoles) which reputedly has a large content of fibrin. Between the red thrombus and the fibrous wall of the aneurysm there is a lipid-rich zone in which there are many empty (cholesterol-containing) clefts (thick arrow). This lipid-rich zone is probably the remnant of a large atheromatous plaque. HE ×135

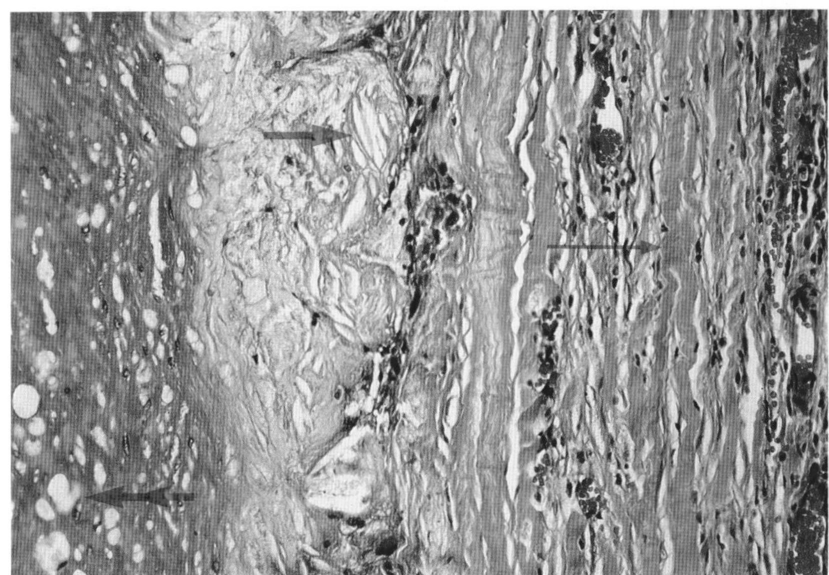

9.6 Congenital ('berry') aneurysm: cerebral artery

'Berry' aneurysms are small spherical lesions, about 1cm dia, which protrude from one side of an artery. The aneurysm is often located in the Circle of Willis, near the bifurcation of an artery. Aneurysms of this type are not congenital, but there is probably a defect in the medial coat of the artery at the site which, if the internal elastic lamina degenerates, leads to aneurysm formation. This aneurysm and the associated vessels were removed surgically from man of 23. It was a saccular aneurysm 2cm dia, the lumen of which is full of eosinophilic thrombus (double arrow). The thrombus is adherent to a thick inner layer of paler hyaline acellular fibrous tissue (left of centre) in which there are black deposits of calcium salts. There is no endothelial lining. The outer part of the aneurysmal wall consists of a broad layer of loose collagenous tissue (thin arrow) and numerous small thin-walled blood vessels (thick arrow). There are also small numbers of chronic inflammatory cells (mostly small lymphocytes). Granules of hemosiderin were demonstrated in the arterial wall, but no medial muscle fibres or elastic laminae remain in the wall. HE ×150

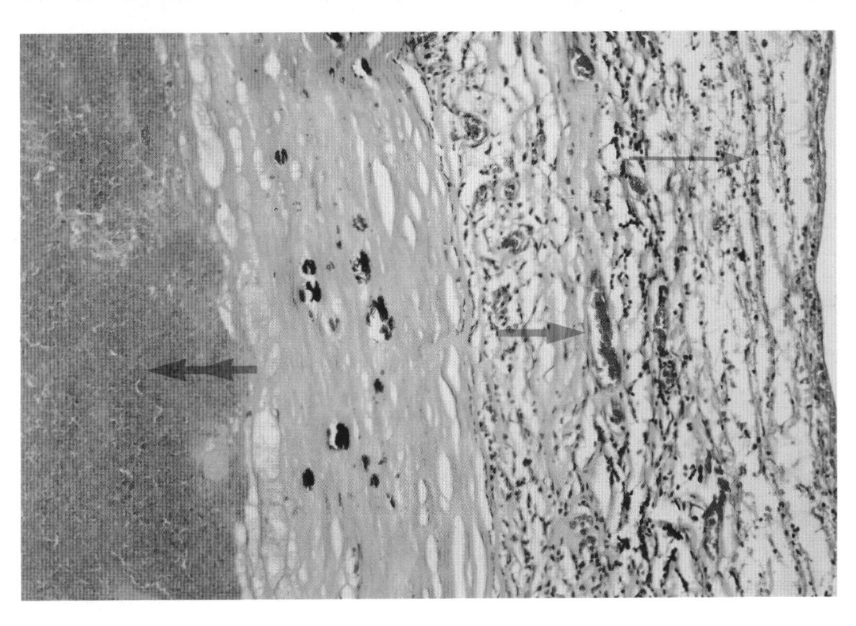

9.7 Arteriolosclerosis: spleen

Arteriolosclerosis occurs in arterioles and small muscular arteries. It tends to affect older people but develops earlier and the lesion is more advanced when systemic hypertension is present. It is often particularly severe in individuals with diabetes mellitus. The organs most affected are kidney, pancreas, liver and spleen, but with increasing age the arterioles of the spleen and to a lesser extent of the renal glomeruli are liable to undergo hyaline thickening of their wall, even in the absence of systemic hypertension. In this spleen, a large amount of deeply eosinophilic acellular hyaline material (thin arrow) has been deposited beneath the endothelium of several arterioles (possibly one tortuous vessel cut three times). Consequently the lumen of the vessels is now very small, although it still has an endothelial lining, and the flow of blood to the tissues is correspondingly reduced. The few smooth muscle fibres (thick arrow) in the medial coat of the arterioles are thin and atrophic. The tissue (white pulp) surrounding the arterioles consists of closely packed small basophilic lymphocytes. HE ×250

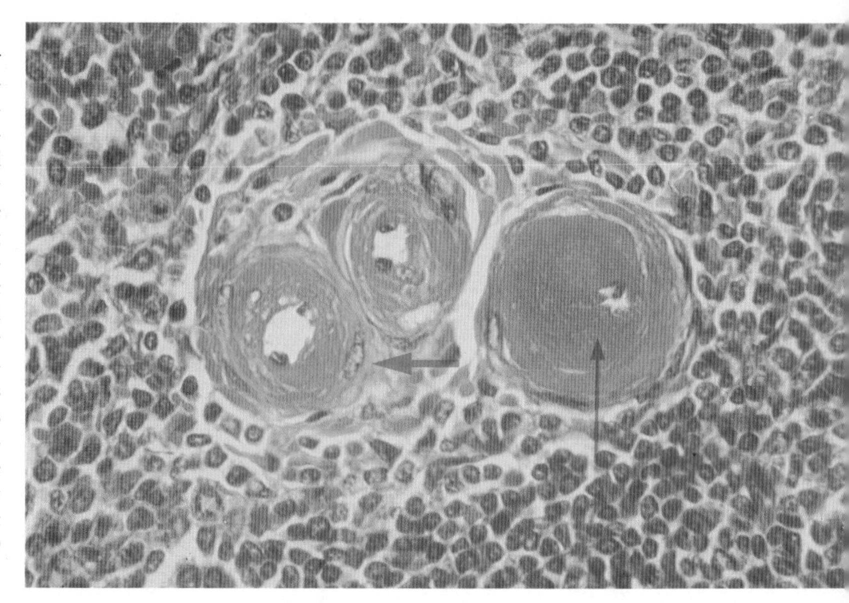

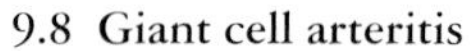

9.8 Giant cell arteritis

Giant cell arteritis is focal granulomatous inflammatory lesion of a segment (a few cm long) of the wall of a medium-sized muscular artery, with destruction of the muscular and elastic tissues. The temporal arteries are the commonest site, and the femoral artery is an uncommon site for the condition. The patient is usually over 50 years of age. This is the temporal artery from a man of 65 who complained of headaches and tenderness in the temporal region. The lumen was full of thrombus which was being organized. The intima and tunica media of the artery fill this field, the lumen being out of the field at the top. The elastic laminae and most of the smooth muscle fibres of the media have been destroyed, and only a few eosinophilic smooth muscle fibres (cut in longitudinal section) survive (thin arrow). In their place is a highly cellular granulomatous tissue which consists of histiocytes (thick arrow), giant multinucleated macrophages (double arrows), lymphocytes and plasma cells. Fragments of elastic laminae were detectable at higher magnification. HE ×235

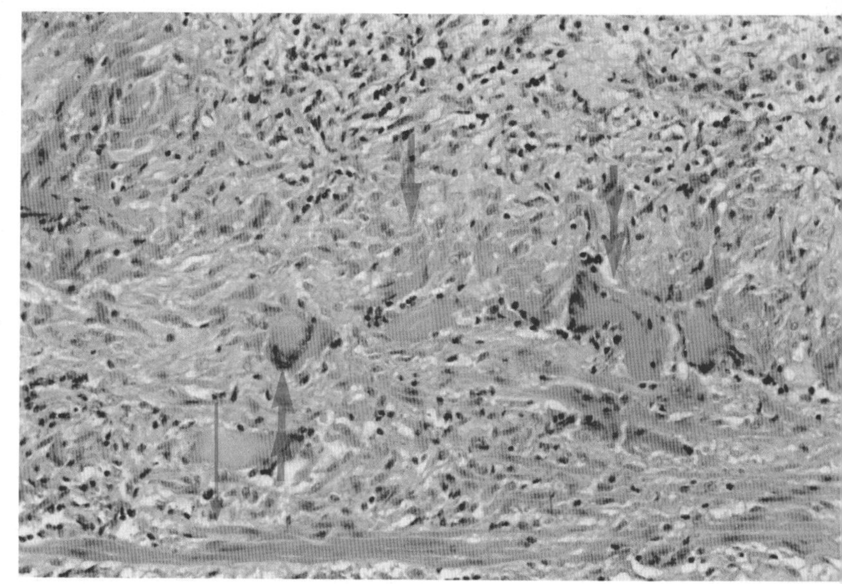

9.9 Polyarteritis nodosa: artery

Polyarteritis nodosa (necrotizing arteritis) affects medium-sized muscular arteries, often at a bifurcation. Well-demarcated short segments (1cm or less) of the artery become acutely inflamed. All layers of the tissues (intima, media and adventitia) are edematous and heavily infiltrated by neutrophil leukocytes. The inflammatory reaction may also penetrate for a short distance into the adjoining tissues, to form a palpable 'node'. Thrombosis and vascular occlusion often occur, producing ischemia and frequently infarction of the related tissues. The vessel may rupture, with severe hemorrhage. This artery is in the healing phase. The inflamed vessel has thrombosed, and organization of the thrombus has filled the original lumen with loose connective tissue. The small channel in the centre (double arrow) is the result of partial recanalization. Inflammatory cells, mostly lymphocytes, are still numerous in the adventitia. Necrotic remnants of the smooth muscle fibres in the arterial wall have been removed by phagocytes (lower right), but parts of the media (thin arrow) and of the brightly eosinophilic corrugated internal elastic lamina (thick arrow) have survived. HE ×270

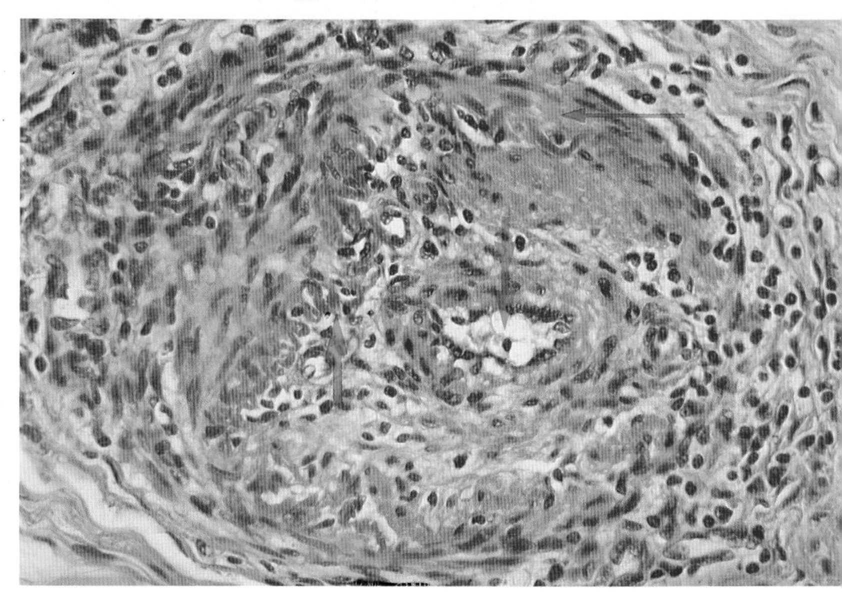

9.10 Thrombotic thrombocytopenic purpura: heart

Anything that causes fibrin to deposit in the blood vessels but does not prevent blood flow will probably cause microangiopathic anemia. In the deposits of fibrin in small blood vessels, the strands of fibrin form a mesh through which the red cells are forced. The red cells are thus damaged and fragmented. The platelets are used up in the thrombi, and thrombocytopenia often develops. A girl of 16 suffered from fever, purpura, hemolytic anemia and vague neurological signs. This is the myocardium, consisting of eosinophilic muscle fibres (thick arrows), some with a large nucleus and others seemingly necrotic. Between the fibres there are numerous red cells, hemorrhage (thin arrow) having occurred into the edematous interstitial tissues. Notably, the two small blood vessels (double arrows) are full of deeply eosinophilic amorphous material; that is, they contain fibrin thrombi. There is no inflammatory reaction in the vicinity. Similar microthrombi were present in small vessels in other organs but not in large vessels. HE ×135

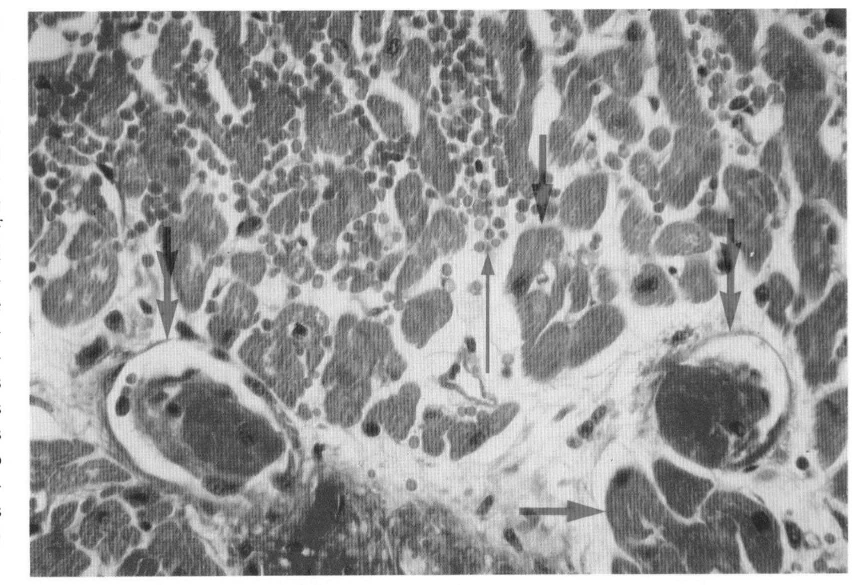

9.11 Progressive systemic sclerosis (scleroderma): artery

Progressive systemic sclerosis, a rare disease of unknown etiology, invariably involves small and medium-sized muscular arteries and arterioles. The intima is thickened, with concentric layers of intimal cells and abundant intercellular material. The flow of blood is reduced, causing atrophy and loss of specialized tissues, with replacement by fibrous tissue. In older lesions, the intima becomes increasingly fibrotic. In this case, a finger was ulcerated and gangrenous at its tip, and this is a section of a digital artery from the finger. The lumen of the artery is blocked by dense hyaline collagenous tissue, acellular apart from a few elongated cells entering from the media. The weakly eosinophilic internal elastic lamina is very convoluted (thick arrow), which suggests that the artery is markedly contracted. The elastic lamina is also broken at several points. The media, lightly infiltrated by lymphocytes, is thin (atrophic), consisting of bands of slender elongated smooth muscle cells (thin arrow). The eosinophil adventitia is extremely thick and densely fibrous (double arrow), with only few small blood vessels and a small number of chronic inflammatory cells. HE ×120

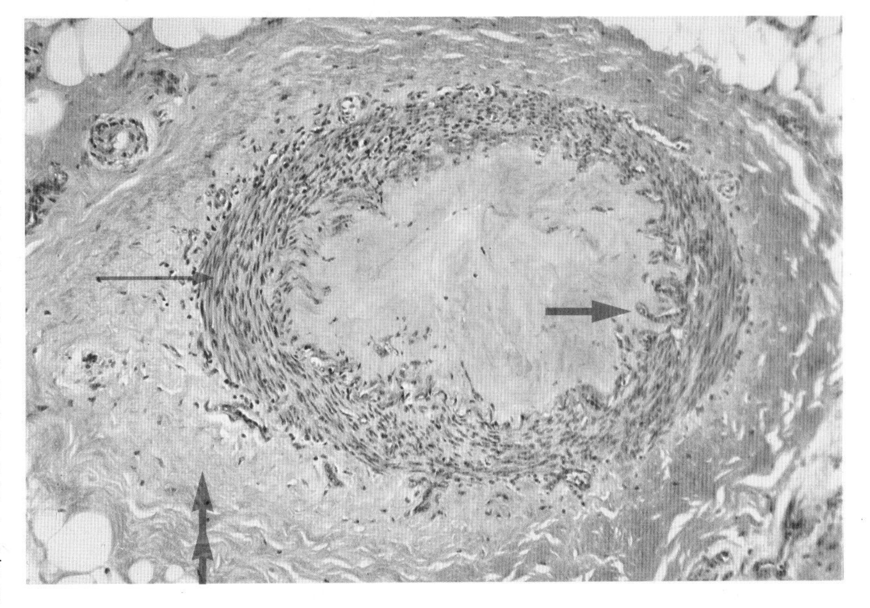

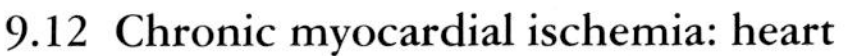

9.12 Chronic myocardial ischemia: heart

Myocardial ischemia is usually caused by narrowing or occlusion of one or more arteries supplying the heart, and atherosclerosis, thrombosis or embolism are the most common causes. Not uncommonly, when narrowing of an artery occurs, parts of the myocardium are found in which the muscle fibres have been partly replaced by fibrous tissue, and, as shown here, the surviving muscle fibres (thin arrow) are located mainly around blood vessels. Characteristically, some of the myocardial fibres are thin and atrophic (diameter smaller in cross-section), whereas some of the other fibres appear to be hypertrophied (thicker than normal in cross-section). Further from the main blood supply there is a considerable amount of pale poorly cellular fibrous tissue (thick arrow). In cases like this the coronary arteries are invariably severely atheromatous, with the lumen much reduced in size. It is assumed therefore that the changes are the result of chronic ischemia. However it is difficult, if not impossible, to exclude the possibility of a previous undetected infarction as the cause of the changes.

HE ×150

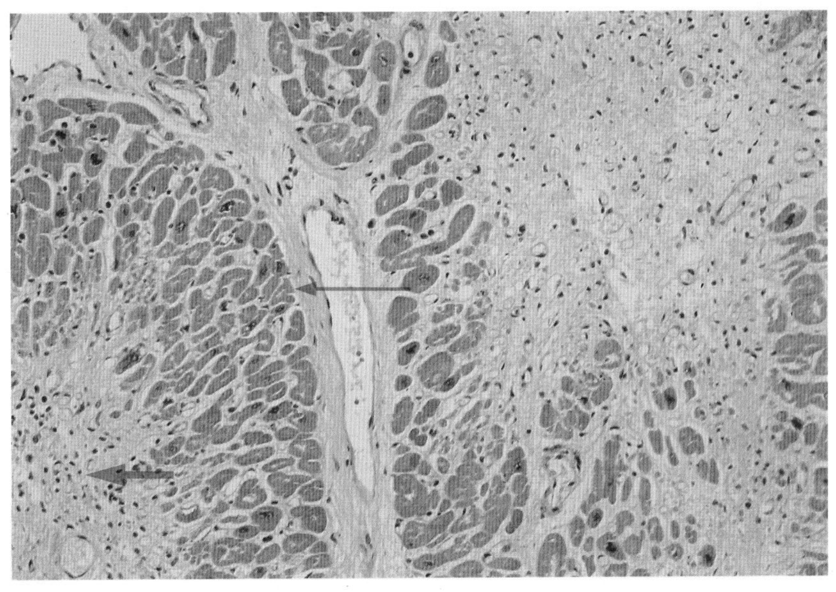

9.13 Thrombosis: coronary artery

Thrombosis occurs only in vessels in which blood is flowing, and it is initiated by endothelial injury or destruction. Platelets adhere to the damaged endothelium and form an aggregate (a white thrombus). Fibrin binds the platelets together and to the vessel wall, and a layer of red clot forms on the surface of the platelet thrombus. This sequence is followed by deposition of alternating layers of platelets and red clot. The right main coronary artery of this patient was suddenly blocked by thrombosis, and he died 4 hours later. The artery is atheromatous and its lumen (only partly visible) is occupied by thrombus (centre and top). The thrombus consists of pale-staining finely granular sheets of fused platelets (thick arrows) and eosinophilic strands of fibrin. Trapped leukocytes are present throughout the thrombus, along with collections of erythrocytes. The thrombus is firmly adherent at one point to the intima of the coronary artery (thin arrows). The intima (bottom margin) is a thick layer of fibrous tissue (double arrow).

HE ×150

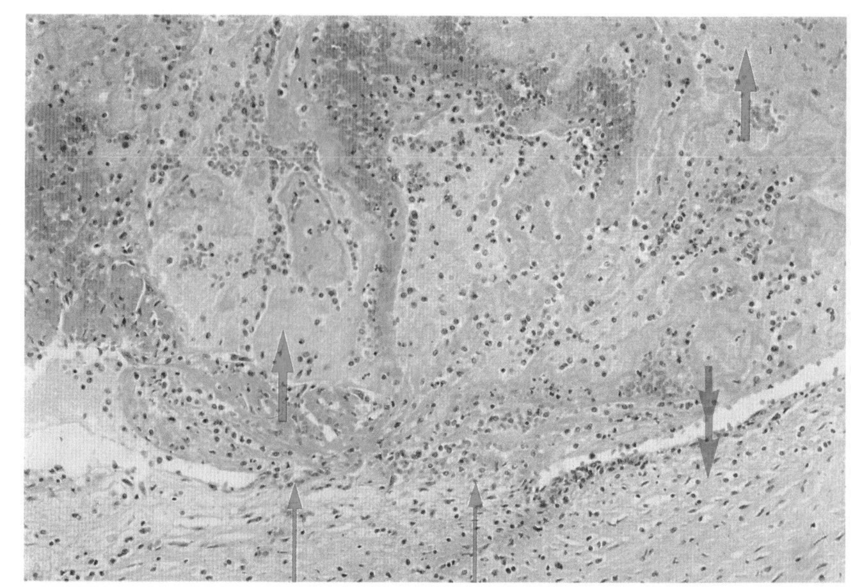

9.14 Thrombosis: coronary artery

A thrombus that forms in an artery is usually firm and 'dry' and securely attached to the vessel wall. Macroscopically it consists of alternating layers of yellowish platelets and red clot. Platelets are a major component of thrombus and they initiate the process of thrombus formation. Fibrin strands however usually form alongside the aggregates of platelets. The resulting thrombus is pale. Only when the blood flow slows does the content of red cells increase to significant proportions. This is part of the thrombus that occupied the lumen of the coronary artery in 9.13, at higher magnification. In the thrombus there are considerable amounts of pale-staining granular material (thin arrow) and tortuous strands of eosinophilic fibrillary material. The pale granular material consists of fused platelets, and the fibrillary material consists of fibrin (thick arrows). Also in the thrombus there are modest populations of large mononuclear cells (monocytes), lymphocytes and polymorphs. Clusters of red cells are also present (double arrow), and there is a sheet of deeply eosinophilic fused red cells at the left margin.

HE ×360

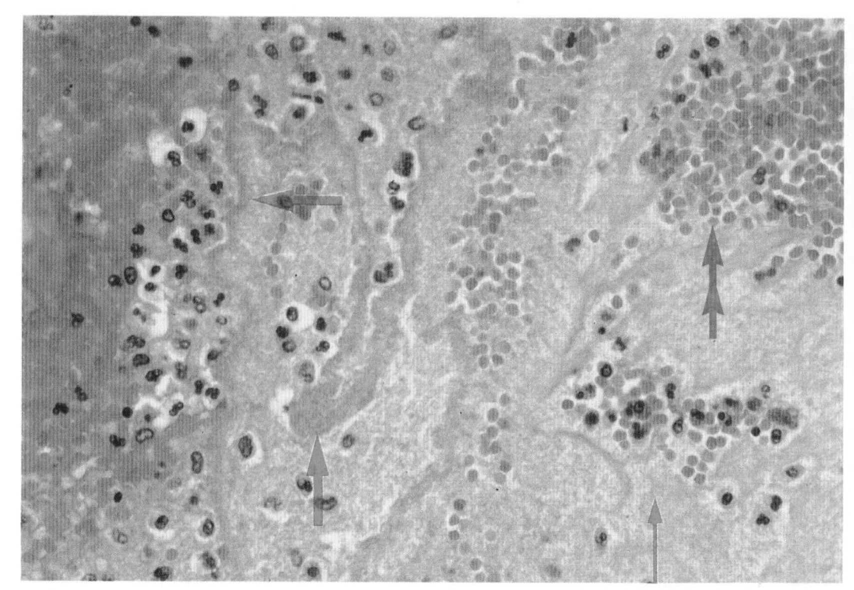

9.15 Infarct: heart

Infarction of the myocardium is caused by acute ischemia, the result (generally) of sudden narrowing of a coronary artery. In most cases the artery is blocked by occlusive thrombus which has formed on the surface of an atheromatous plaque. Myocardial infarcts are usually located in the lateral wall of the left ventricle or in the interventricular septum (or both). In this case the infarct was one week old, as estimated from the clinical history. This shows the edge of the infarct. The necrotic muscle fibres (thick arrow) stain a denser red than the bands of eosinophilic viable muscle fibres on the right. The necrotic muscle fibres have retained their shape but their nuclei no longer stain and are not visible. The sheets of living muscle fibres and necrotic muscle fibres are separated by a richly cellular and vascular tissue (thin arrow) which contains many polymorphs, macrophages and fibroblasts. If the patient had survived, the dead muscle would have been digested by the macrophages and the fibroblasts would have formed a fibrous scar.

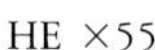

HE ×55

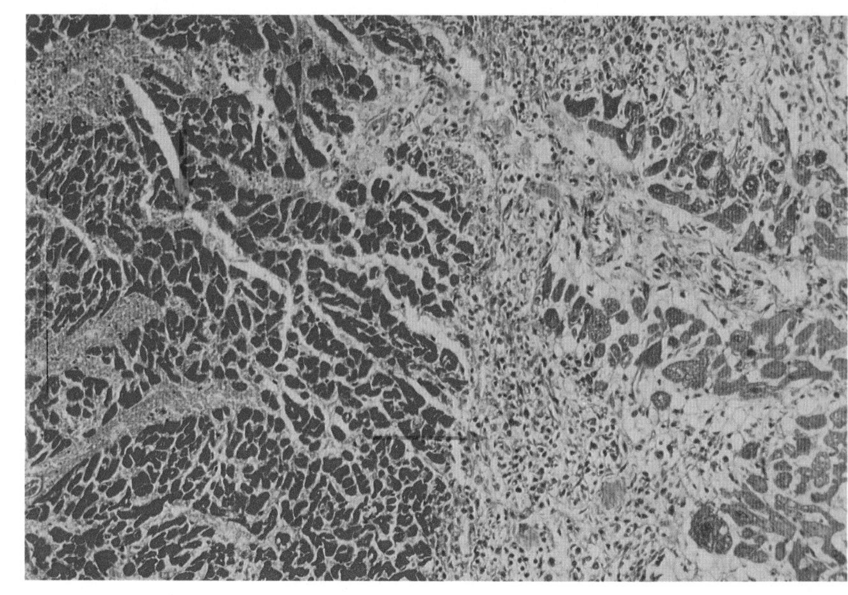

9.16 Infarct: heart

Infarcts confined to the right ventricle or the atria are rare, for no obvious reason. In the large majority of myocardial infarcts, the whole thickness of the wall of the left ventricle is necrotic, only a small percentage of infarcts being confined to the subendocardial part of the wall. This is the same infarct as that in 9.15, at higher magnification. In this part of the infarct, the myocardial muscle fibres are elongated, necrotic and aligned in parallel (thin arrow). The nuclei in the muscle fibres are not visible, having been dispersed by karyolysis. The muscle fibres themselves are more deeply eosinophilic (almost brick-red) than normal myocardial muscle fibres, but the staining is patchy, with areas of pallor. The striations can still be detected however in the myocardial muscle fibres. In the pale interstitial tissue there are, in addition to some nuclear fragments, macrophages which have migrated into the sheet of dead muscle (thick arrows). If the patient survives long enough, all the necrotic muscle (even in a large infarct) is removed by phagocytosis. HE ×135

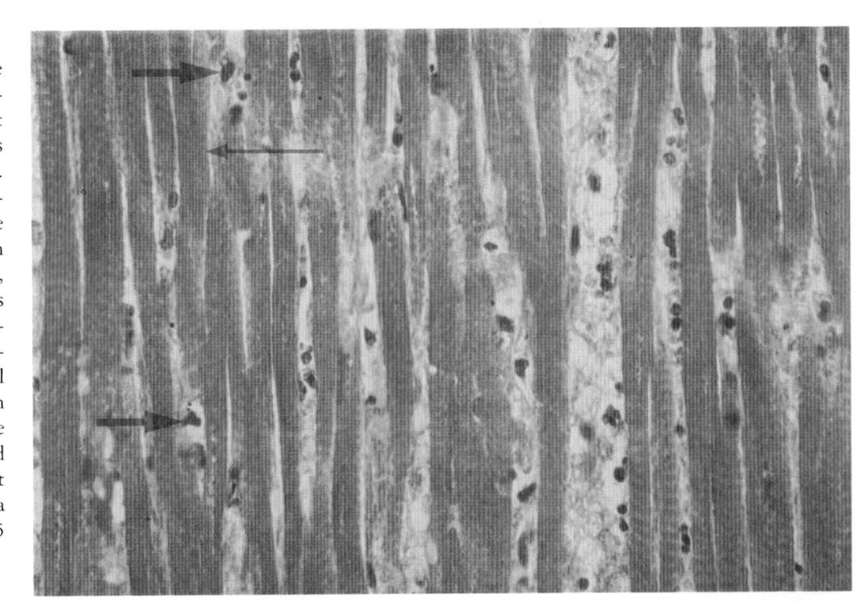

9.17 Myocardial infarction (early stage)

Damaged myocardial fibres are stained brown because they have reacted with an antibody to complement fraction 9. This would not be apparent on an HE-stained section.

Myocardial infarction is generally caused by fissuring or ulceration of an atheromatous plaque, followed by penetration of blood into the plaque. The plaque rapidly enlarges and thrombus may form in the lumen of the artery and occlude it.

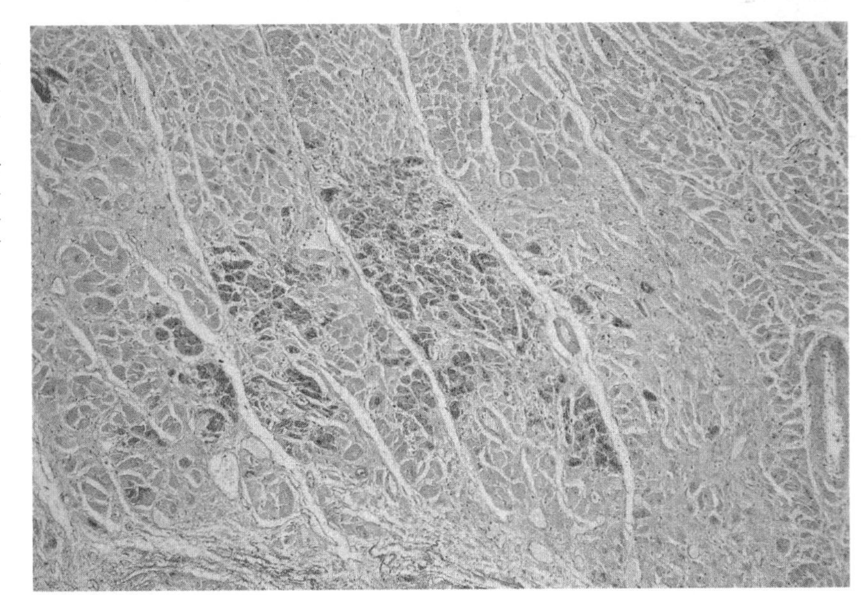

9.18 Aneurysm: heart

When an infarct of myocardium heals, the necrotic muscle is digested by macrophages and replaced by fibrous tissue. Sometimes the fibrous tissue is unable to withstand the high pressure of the blood in the left ventricle and it stretches eventually to form an aneurysm. A man aged 42 developed an aneurysm of the left ventricle 6 months after coronary thrombosis and infarction of the myocardium. Two elliptical pieces of the wall of the aneurysm were removed surgically, one 7 × 3.5cm and the other 7 × 2cm. The endocardial surface of both pieces appeared white and fibrosed. In this field, the lumen of the aneurysm (just visible at the left margin) is lined by a fairly broad eosinophilic layer of poorly cellular fibrous tissue (thin arrow). Deep to this layer there is a sheet of pleomorphic eosinophilic (very atrophic) smooth muscle fibres (thick arrow) separated by pale fibrous tissue. Some of the muscle fibres are cut in cross-section and the others are arranged longitudinally. The remainder of the wall of the aneurysm consists of collagenous fibrous tissue (double arrow) (similar to the lining layer) and several dilated thin-walled blood vessels. HE ×60

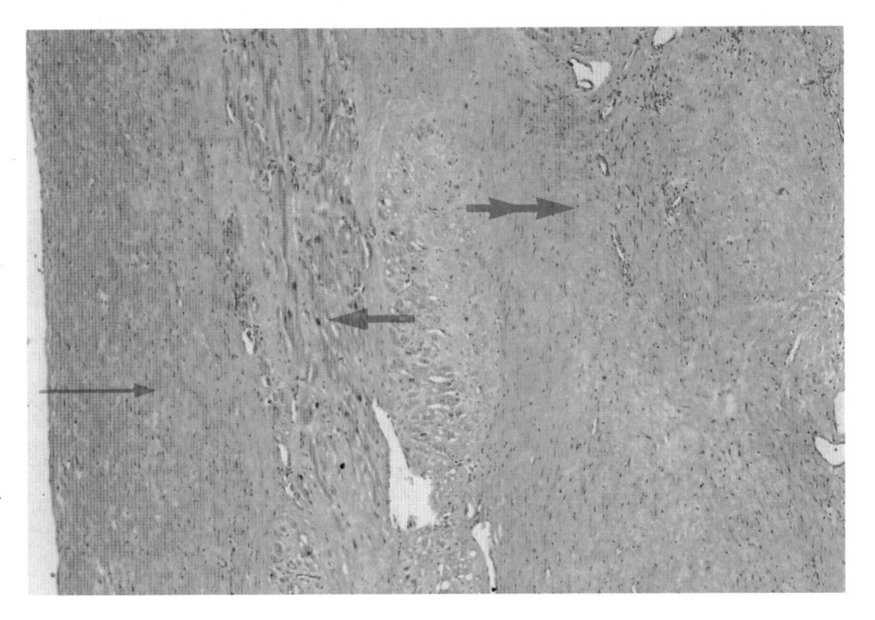

9.19 Organization of thrombus: renal artery

Thrombosis of a renal artery is uncommon. Atheroma is an important predisposing factor, and in diabetes mellitus atheroma of the renal arteries and their main branches is often severe. An atrophic right kidney was removed surgically from a man aged 53 with systemic hypertension. This is part of the inner media in the wall of the attached renal artery. The tissue consists of widely separated elongated eosinophilic smooth muscle cells, in pale edematous connective tissue (thin arrow) closely apposed to an extremely wrinkled brightly eosinophilic internal elastic lamina. These tissues show little or no abnormality, and there is no intima or lining of endothelial cells. The lumen however is distended by extremely loose pale myxoid connective tissue (double arrows), in which there are widely dispersed cells with small elongated basophilic nucleus and large clear ('empty') vacuoles in ill-defined cytoplasm. In the myxoid tissue there are thin-walled blood vessels and irregularly shaped fragments of eosinophilic amorphous material, probably fibrin (thick arrow). HE ×150

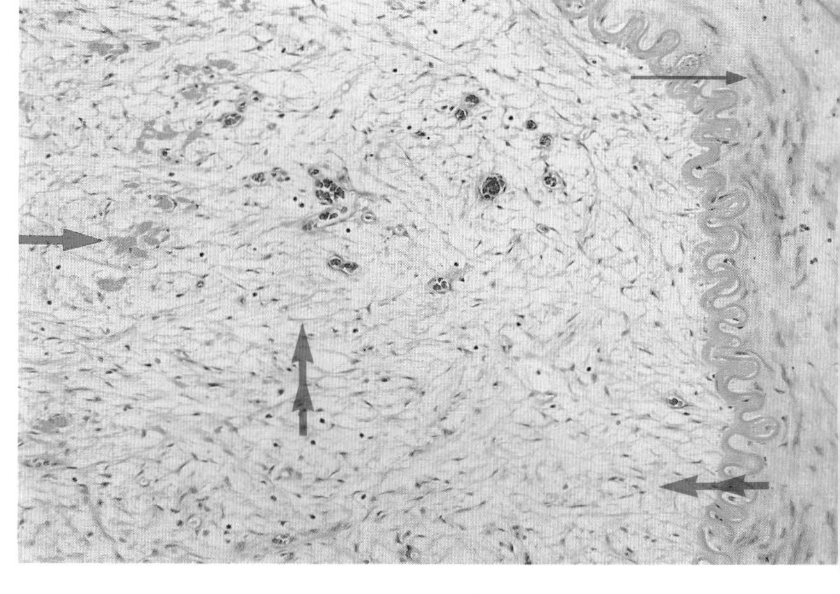

9.20 Organizing thrombus: renal artery

This is part of the same renal artery in 9.19, at higher magnification. The small section of inner media (at the right margin) contains elongated smooth muscle cells, widely separated by pale myxoid connective tissue. The internal elastic lamina is reduplicated (thick arrow) but not broken. There is no distinct intima or endothelial lining. The lumen however is full of pale-stained myxoid extensively vacuolated connective tissue (double arrows) which rich in connective tissue mucin. The cells in the connective tissue are a mixture of elongated fibroblasts and round macrophages. Abundant reticulin is demonstrable by special stains but only relatively few mature collagen fibres. In the myoid tissue there are fairly numerous thin-walled blood vessels (thin arrow), some widely patent, and a small amount of hemosiderin (top left). This renal artery had thrombosed some months prior to the removal of the kidney, and the connective tissue in the lumen has been produced by organization of the thrombus. HE ×235

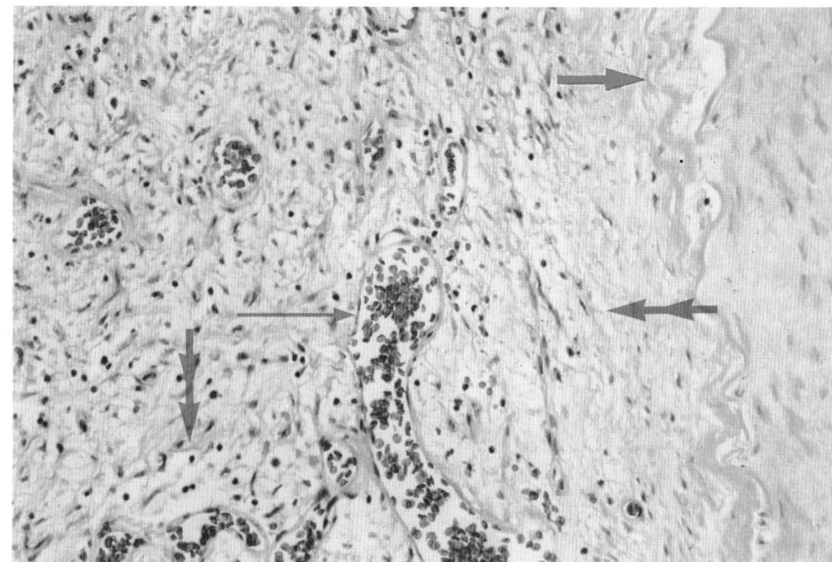

9.21 Rheumatoid arthritis: aorta

Rheumatoid arthritis is a systemic disease, one of the group of connective tissue diseases. There is much evidence that rheumatoid arthritis frequently co-exists with rheumatic cardiovascular disease. Frequently, in some members of this group, acute necrotizing arteritis, which tends to cause thrombosis of the vessel and possibly infarction, occurs. In this case, a man of 38 with a history of rheumatoid arthritis, had his aortic valve removed surgically because of aortic incompetence. The tissue consists of the inner half of the media of the aorta and part of the intima. The intima is thick and fibrous (thin arrow), and in it there are elongated fibrocytes, chronic inflammatory cells and small capillary-type blood vessels. In the slightly more eosinophilic media, consisting of eosinophilic musculo-elastic laminae, there is a much denser infiltrate of small basophilic chronic inflammatory cells (thick arrow), surrounding thin-walled blood vessels. There is extensive destruction of the medial tissues in the vicinity of the inflamed vessels. HE ×150

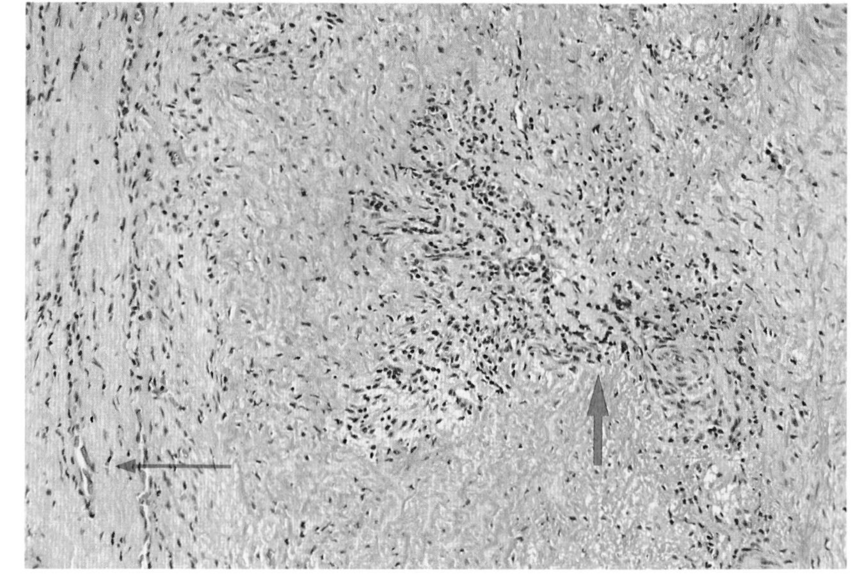

9.22 Rheumatoid arthritis: aorta

This shows, at higher magnification, part of the same inflammatory reaction as that in 9.21, around small blood vessels (periarteritis) in the media of the aorta. The reaction is granulomatous, consisting of mononuclear cells of various types, including large cells (thin arrows) (probably histiocytes and smooth muscle cells) with ill-defined cytoplasmic boundaries and a large pale vesicular nucleus (a few very large and very pleomorphic) lacking nucleoli, small lymphocytes with very little cytoplasm and a round deeply basophilic nucleus, and relatively few plasma cells and polymorph leukocytes. At the centre of this destructive granulomatous inflammatory reaction there are a number of small thin-walled blood vessels but no larger muscular vessels. A large number of short curved segments of eosinophilic elastic tissue (thick arrows), fragments of the disrupted musculo-elastic laminae in the medial coat, are visible in vacuolated connective tissue. There were similar lesions in the outer half of the aortic media. HE ×360

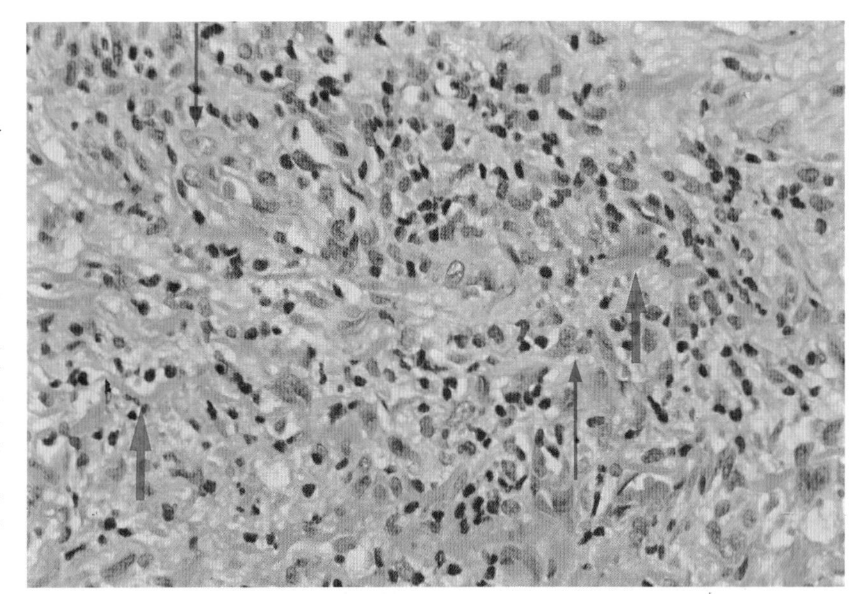

9.23 Rheumatoid arthritis: aorta

This is the same inflammatory reaction as that illustrated in 9.21 and 9.22, but the section has been stained to show elastic fibres (black) and collagenous tissue (purple-red) in the outer two-thirds of the medial coat of the aortic wall, where the inflammatory reaction, including numerous small blood vessels, are centred. The granulomatous reaction surrounding the small blood vessels in the media (periarteritis) and around the larger muscular arteries in the adventitia (endarteritis) are having a destructive effect (similar to that in syphilitic mesaortitis) on the musculo-elastic laminae in this part of the medial coat of the aorta. All the wavy elastic laminae in this area have been broken into small wavy black fragments (thin arrows) and the intervening gaps are filled with pale purple-red collagenous fibrous tissue (thick arrows). Elastic-van Gieson ×150

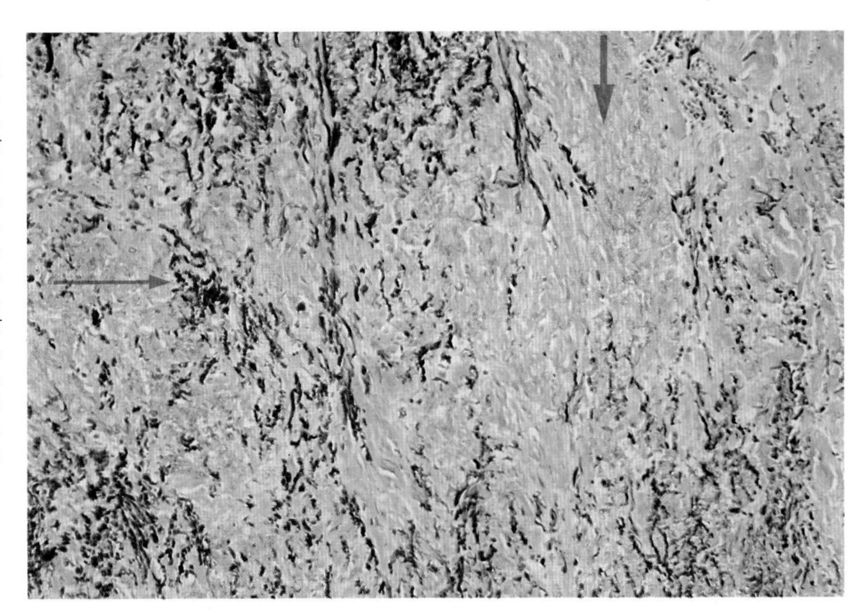

9.24 Syphilitic mesaortitis: aorta

Cardiovascular syphilis causes inflammation of small muscular arteries, especially the small nutrient arteries in the adventitia (vasa vasorum) which supply the small blood vessels in the media of the ascending part of the aorta and its arch. The adventitia is chronically inflamed and fibrotic, and the obliterative endarteritis of the vasa vasorum which develops destroys parts of the media. However the damaging effect diminishes gradually in the more distal aorta. This shows the outer half of the media of the aorta, the adventitia being just out of sight on the right. Between the eosinophilic musculo-elastic laminae (thin arrow) of the wall of the media, there are numerous thin-walled small blood vessels (thick arrow), some of them greatly dilated. Most of the thin-walled vessels are surrounded by a cellular infiltrate which consists almost exclusively of mature plasma cells, and the perivascular inflammatory reaction (double arrow) has disrupted many of the adjacent musculo-elastic laminae. Obliterative endarteritis of the vasa vasorum reduces the blood supply to the media and consequently greatly weakens the wall of the aorta. HE ×235

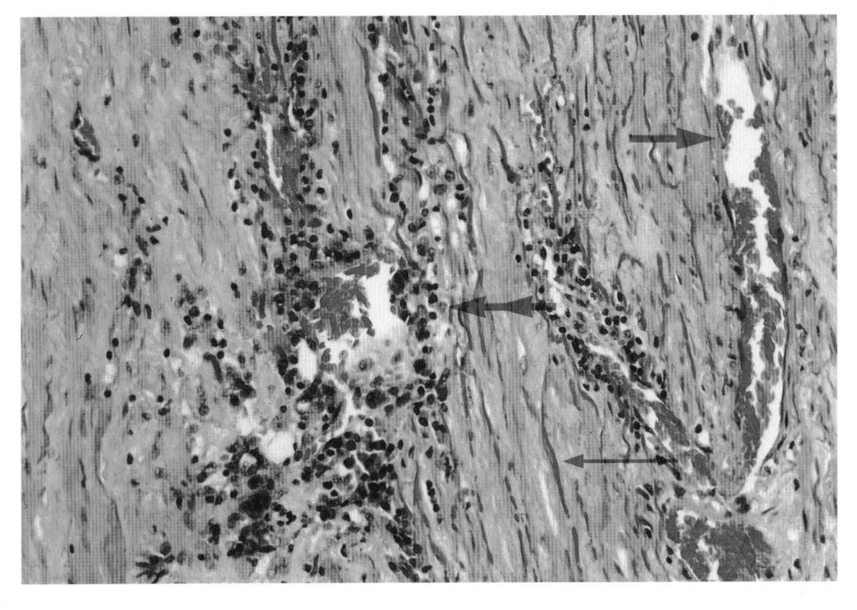

9.25 Medial degeneration and dissecting aneurysm: aorta

In middle-aged and elderly people, degenerative changes, with loss of elastic tissue and muscle, are often present in the media of the aorta. An aorta affected in this way is liable to rupture and allow the blood to enter the media and track within it,. The blood splits the media into an outer and inner layer, to form a 'dissecting' aneurysm. In this case, the blood had entered the aortic wall, of a man aged 50, through a slit-like opening 5cm above the aortic valve, and then formed a dissecting aneurysm in the thoracic aorta. The pale adventitia of the aorta is just visible at the top of the field, and the inner media occupies the remainder. The media has been split by the blood (double arrow), and its lumen is partly empty. Blood is also tracking beyond the lumen and separating the elastic laminae of the media (thin arrows). Significantly there is abnormal amount of basophilic connective tissue mucin (thick arrows) in the inner media, a sign of degenerative change in the aortic wall.

HE ×60

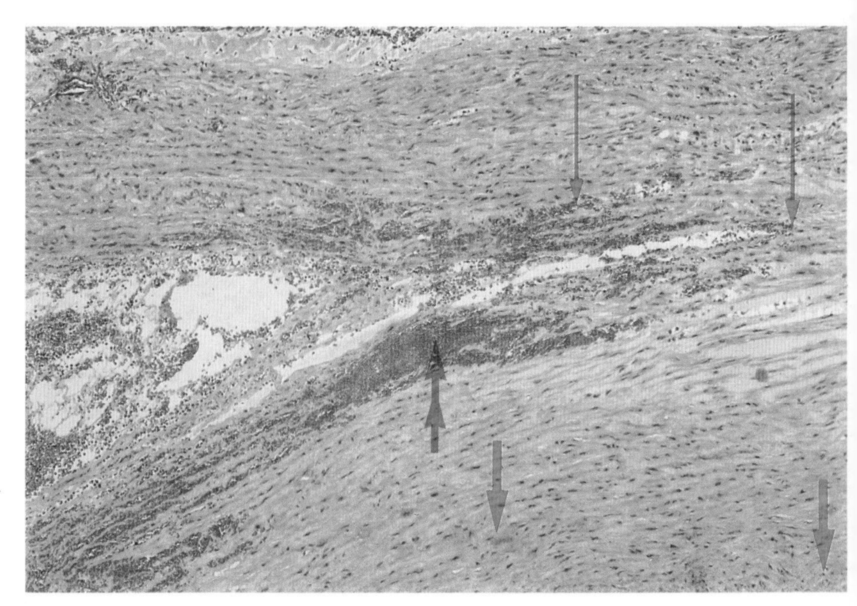

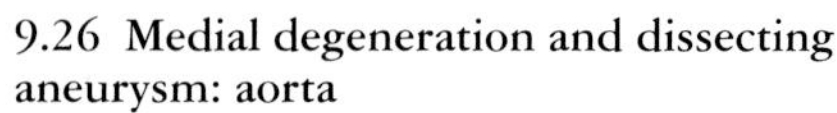

9.26 Medial degeneration and dissecting aneurysm: aorta

This is the same dissecting aneurysm as that in 9.25, at higher magnification. The lumen of the aneurysm is on the right, and it is lined by a layer of eosinophilic thrombus, consisting of platelets, fibrin and red cells, which is firmly adherent to the musculo-elastic media (inner layer) of the aorta. Just beneath the thrombus in the lumen, there is also a thin track of 'fresh' blood in the media (double arrow). Generally, the media (centre and left) shows reduced cellularity, consisting a decreased number of smooth muscle cells and an increased amount of pale bluish (basophilic) connective tissue mucin. The pale weakly-stained elastic laminae are also fewer and more widely separated than normal (thin arrow) by the mucin; and in some parts of the media there are small pools of connective tissue mucin (thick arrows). This is mucoid medial degeneration of the aortic wall, and these changes are accompanied by some disruption and loss of the musculo-elastic laminae. Loss of elastica and smooth muscle fibres from the media and increase of connective tissue mucin is sometimes called Erdheim's medial degeneration.

HE ×150

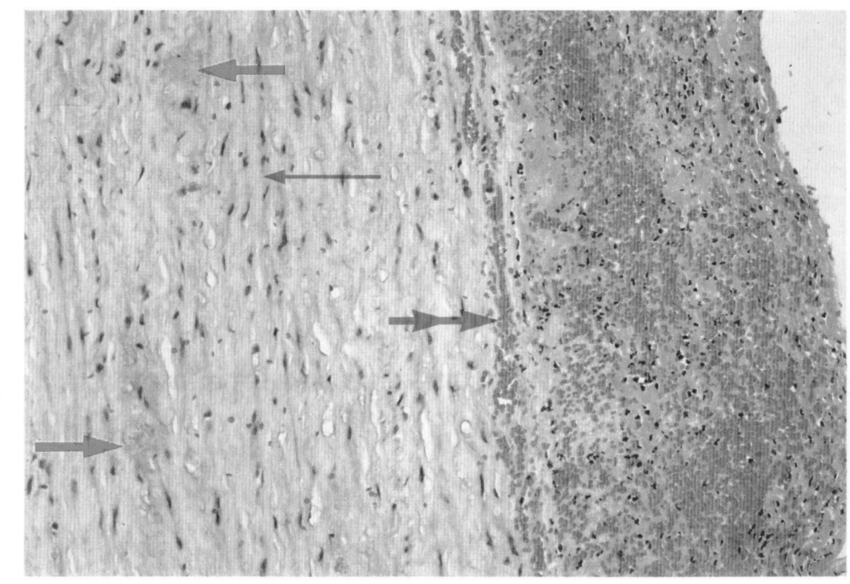

9.27 Medial degeneration and dissecting aneurysm: aorta

In medial degeneration of the aorta, excessive quantities of mucoid 'ground substance' (connective tissue mucin) accumulate in the media of the aorta, especially in its outer third, the pools of mucin separating the muscle and elastica of the media. The term medionecrosis is applied occasionally to this type of lesion, but the term 'true necrosis' is rarely encountered. This is part of the same lesion as in 9.25 and 9.26, at higher magnification, showing the inner media of the aorta. There are relatively fewer eosinophilic smooth muscle fibres with elongated deeply stained nuclei (some round-ended and others spindle-shaped) and their associated weakly-stained laminae of elastic tissue. Some of the musculo-elastic laminae are fragmented. The smooth muscle fibres are also atrophic and thin (double arrow), and between the diminished population of laminae there are considerably increased amounts of connective tissue mucin. Most of the mucin is pale bluish (basophilic) and extensively vacuolated (thin arrow), but some of it is almost unstained (thick arrow).

HE ×235

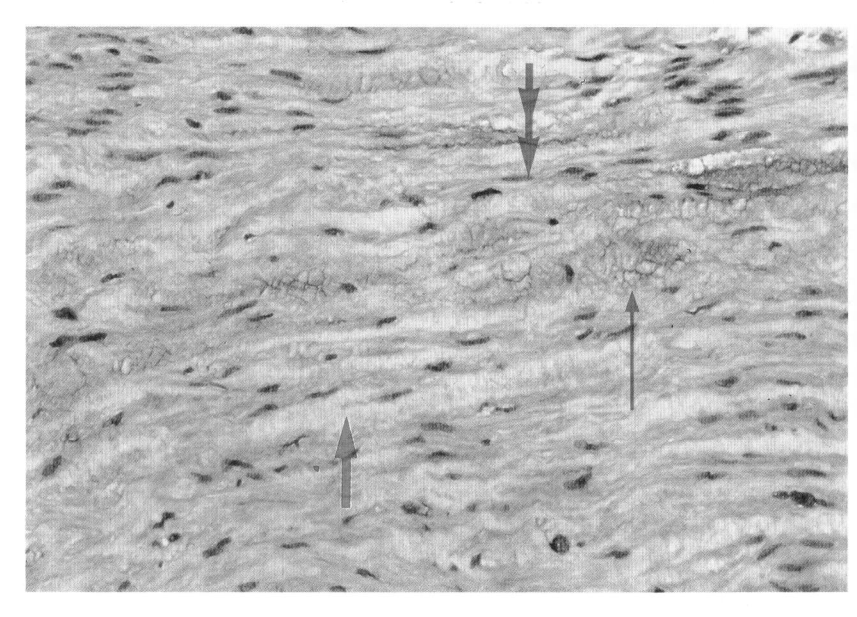

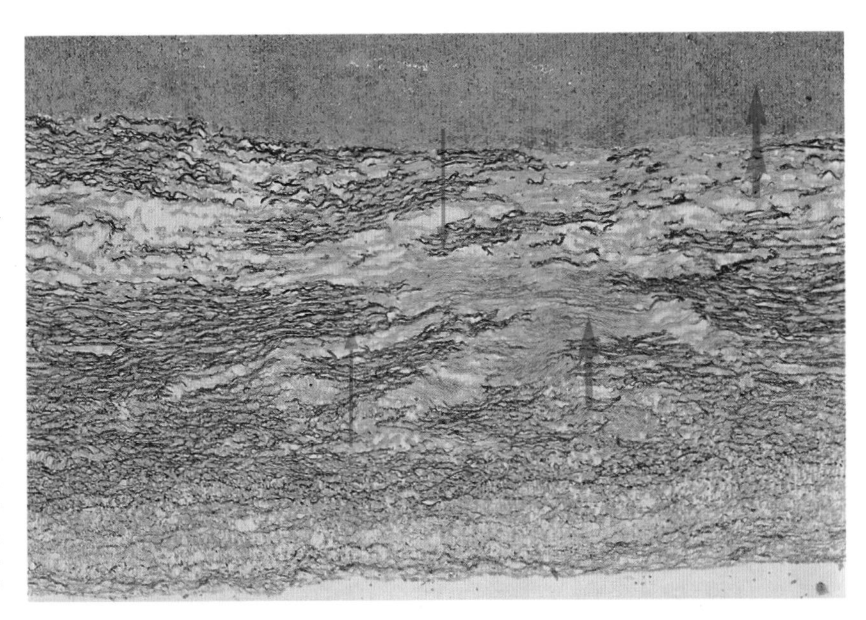

9.28 Medial degeneration and dissecting aneurysm: aorta

It is often difficult to delineate, with accuracy, foci of medial degeneration of the musculo-elastic laminae of the medial coat of the aorta. Determining the amount of degeneration and loss of the elastic tissue can be made easier by the use of specific stains, and particularly for elastic tissue. Results by this method show that the exact loss of elastic tissue is invariably greater than that visible in HE-stained histological sections. In this section, the elastic-van Gieson method has been used to demonstrate elastic fibres (as grey-black tissue) in the inner half of the aortic wall (the lumen of the aorta is at the bottom), including the part of the inner media adjacent to the lumen of the dissecting aneurysm which is full of brownish-yellow blood and thrombus (double arrow). The grey-black musculo-elastic lamellae are extensively fragmented (thin arrows), and a considerable amount of elastic tissue has disappeared, as shown by the areas of pale (unstained) tissue in the media (thick arrow) in which there is only mucinous material, the elastic laminae having disappeared. Elastic-van Gieson ×60

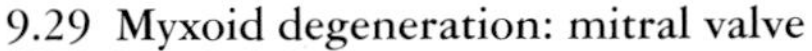

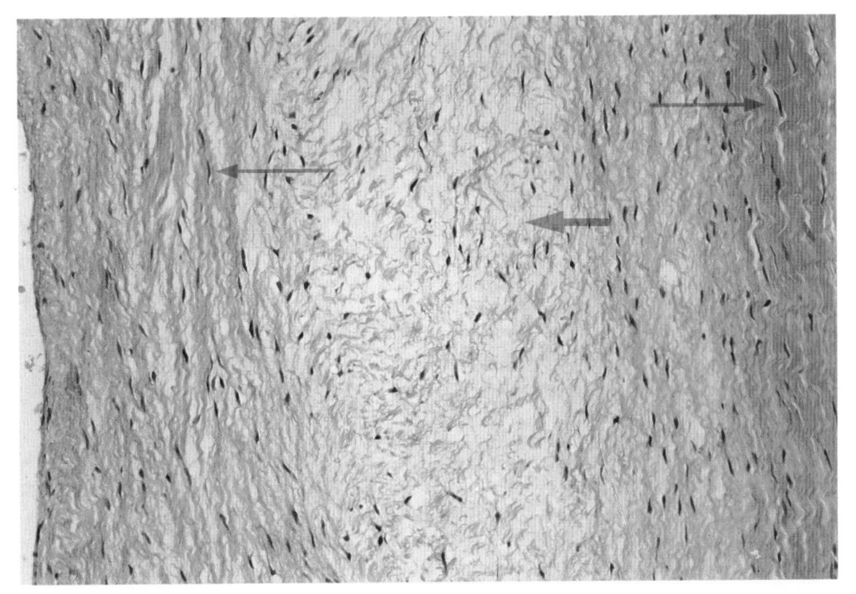

9.29 Myxoid degeneration: mitral valve

Myxoid degeneration occasionally occurs in the cusps of the mitral valve. Cusps affected in this way are liable to stretch and become 'floppy'. As a result, they may prolapse during ventricular systole and render the mitral valve incompetent. Older people are generally affected, but younger individuals with a defect in collagen synthesis such as Marfan's syndrome may undergo similar changes. A man aged 57 was diagnosed as having the floppy valve syndrome affecting his mitral valve. The valve was removed surgically. Part of the cusp is illustrated in this field, with the edge of the cusp at the left margin. The cusp is thicker than normal, consisting of a thick layer of eosinophilic collagenous fibrous tissue and elongated fibrocytes (thin arrows); and in the centre of the cusp there is abundant pale-staining myxoid (mucin-rich) connective tissue (thick arrow). A modest population of elongated fibrocytes with poorly-defined cytoplasmic margins is scattered uniformly and widely throughout the myxoid tissue. There is also an increase of myxoid tissue in the chordae. HE ×150

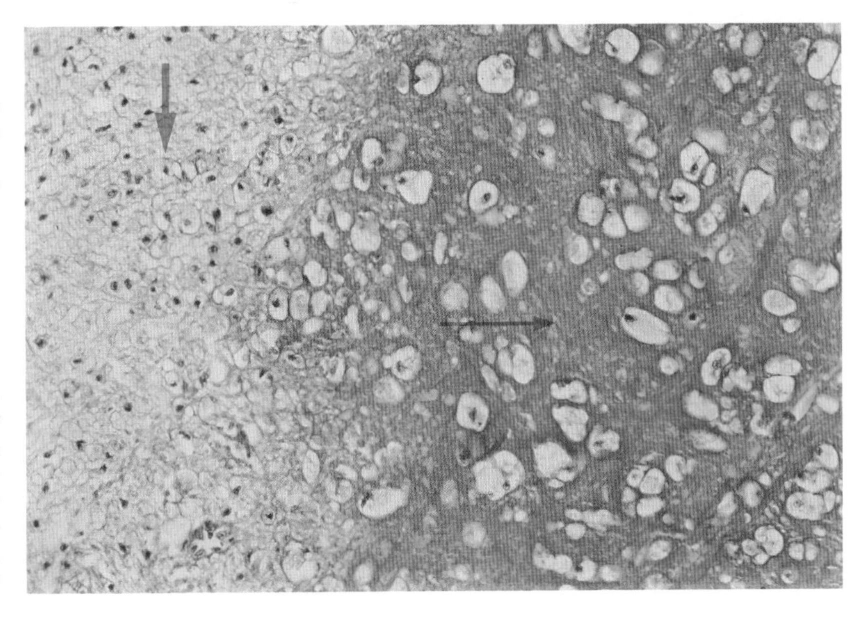

9.30 Mucopolysaccharidosis (Hurler's syndrome): mitral valve

In this condition, also known as gargoylism, there is a defect of mucopolysaccharide metabolism, a deficiency of the lysosomal enzyme alpha-L-iduronidase. As a result of the deficiency of the enzyme, mucopolysaccharides are not broken down, and excessive amounts of mucopolysaccharide accumulate in various types of cell in many tissues. The most striking changes are in the valves of the heart, which are irregularly thickened. Similar change sometimes occurs in the chordae tendineae. This is a small part of a greatly thickened fibrosed mitral valve cusp. The cusp consists mostly of very loose connective tissue, in which there are fairly numerous round, swollen and widely scattered cells, usually with a small round or ovoid basophilic nucleus (thick arrow). The cytoplasm of the connective tissue cells is very pale or clear. It is also well-defined and greatly distended. In the connective tissues of the deeper parts of the cusp there is a massive accumulation of purplish-red (PAS+ve) mucopolysaccharide in the intercellular matrix (thin arrow). PAS ×120

9.31 Brown atrophy: heart

Phagolysosomes containing the indigestible remnants of cell organelles and cytoplasmic materials are called residual bodies, which appear as brown granules (also called lipofuscin or lipochrome) by light microscopy. When the parenchymal cells of an organ have atrophied, because of increasing age or the presence of a wasting disease, yellowish-brown lipofuscin (residual bodies) tends to accumulate in many of the tissues. The condition is termed 'brown atrophy'. In this case, death of an individual followed prolonged cachexia caused by malignant disease. At necropsy the heart found to be small and lacking epicardial fat, and compared with a normal heart it looked dark brown. Microscopically the muscle fibres are atrophic and narrow (thin arrow) (fragmentation of the fibres is artefactual), and collections of pale golden-brown (lipofuscin) granules (thick arrow) are present at the poles of most of the large blunt-ended nuclei in the myocardial muscle fibres. HE ×850

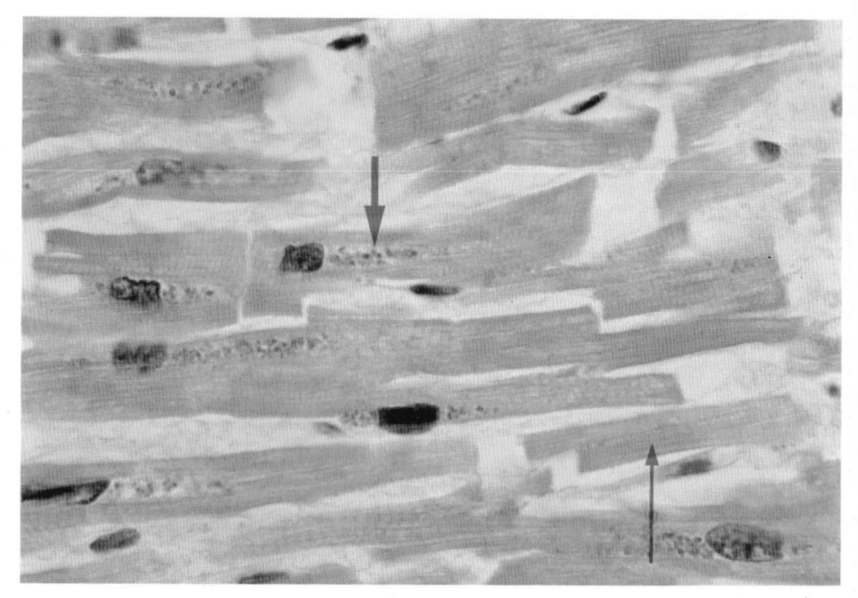

9.32 Viral myocarditis: heart

Many viral diseases, including influenza, poliomyelitis and infectious mononucleosis, occasionally cause inflammatory changes in the myocardium (myocarditis). However Coxsackie viruses (groups A and B) are the most common cause of significant disease and particularly important because it mainly affects children (including infants) and young adults. These viruses produce a diffuse inflammatory reaction in the interstitial tissues throughout the heart. In this example, several strongly eosinophilic elongated myocardial muscle fibres, with very large pleomorphic nuclei, seem (probably) to be viable (thin arrow), but the other muscle fibres are mostly necrotic and fragmented (thick arrows). Between the elongated muscle fibres and among the fragments of necrotic muscle there is a fairly intense infiltrate of small lymphocytes with deeply-stained round nuclei and macrophages with larger paler vesicular nuclei, in a considerable quantity of pale edematous interstitial tissue (double arrow). There are also occasional plasma cells and very eosinophilic leukocytes. The inflammatory changes in Coxsackie myocarditis are considered to be reversible, but occasiomally they are regarded as liable (perhaps) to cause diffuse interstitial fibrosis. HE ×360

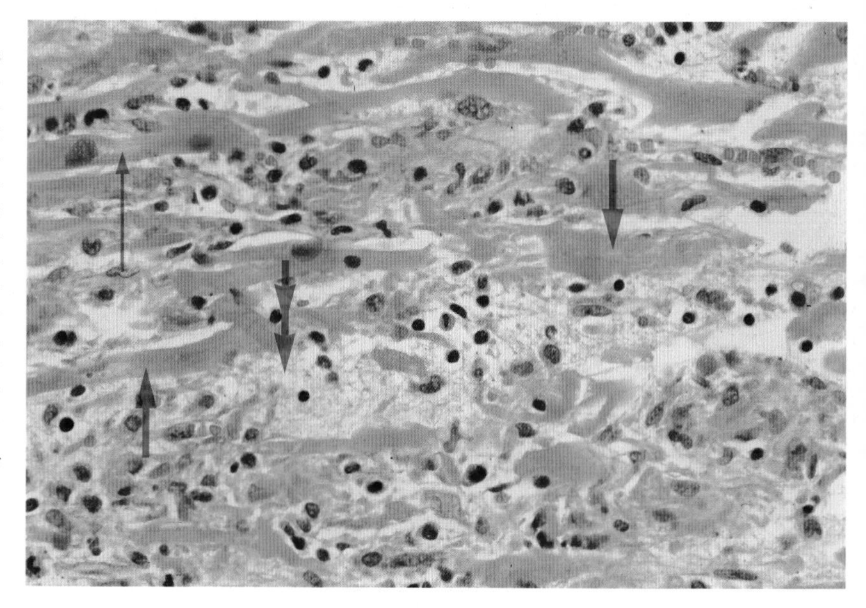

9.33 Toxic (diphtheritic) myocarditis: heart

The diphtheria bacillus does not invade the tissues but forms a toxin which is absorbed into the bloodstream. The toxin is injurious to the nervous system and the cardiovascular system. The myocardium becomes inflamed, and damage to (particularly) the conducting system of the heart is often prominent. In this section of heart, the brightly eosinophilic myocardial muscle fibres show varying degrees of degeneration, ranging from loss of striations to complete necrosis and fragmentation of fibres (thick arrow). Between the muscle fibres, which contain large elongated pale-staining round-ended nuclei, there is a considerable amount of pale edematous (interstitial) connective tissue and a moderate infiltrate of inflammatory cells (thin arrow). Most of the cells in the inflammatory infiltrate are lymphocytes with a small round deeply stained nucleus, but they are accompanied by larger macrophages with paler vesicular nuclei. Diphtheria toxin can also cause fatty change in the heart muscle. HE ×200

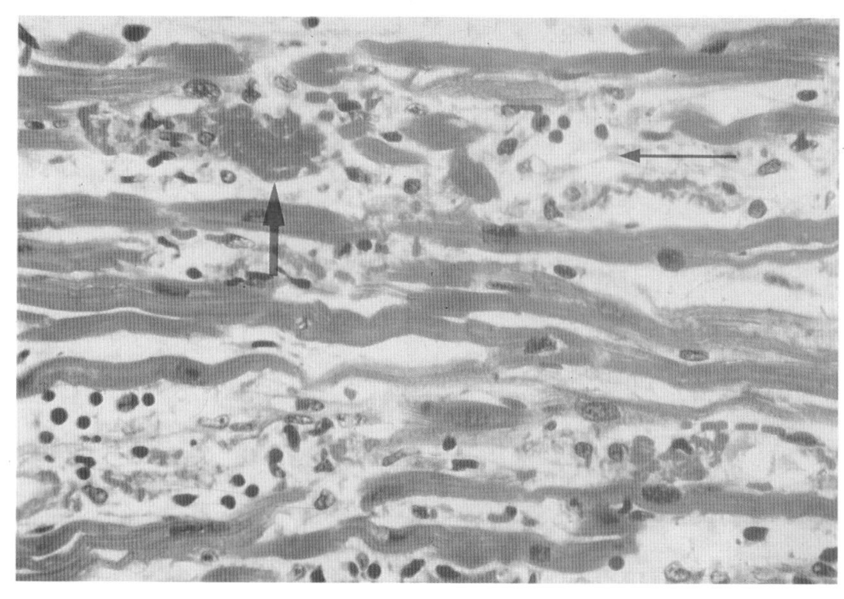

9.34 Acute rheumatism: heart

Acute rheumatism (rheumatic fever) causes a pancarditis, affecting all parts of the heart and other organs such as brain and joints. In the myocardium the pathognomonic lesion is the Aschoff body, one of which is shown here. It begins to appear after a few weeks after the onset of pancarditis, and consists of a collection of closely packed large histiocytes (thin arrows) with large very pleomorphic basophilic nuclei, in most of which a very prominent nucleolus is visible. The presence of a nucleolus gives the cell an 'owl-eye' appearance. Several of the cells are binucleated. The cytoplasm is fairly abundant and slightly basophilic. In the centre of an Aschoff body there is often necrotic collagenous tissue. Aschoff bodies are characteristically located near a small blood vessel, and at the left margin of this body there are two capillary-type vessels (thick arrows), containing erythrocytes and lined by endothelial cells with large elongated nuclei. The cells which form the Aschoff body could be myogenic but are more likely to be histiocytic in origin. Aschoff bodies heal by fibrosis but the function of the myocardium is not generally permanently affected. HE ×580

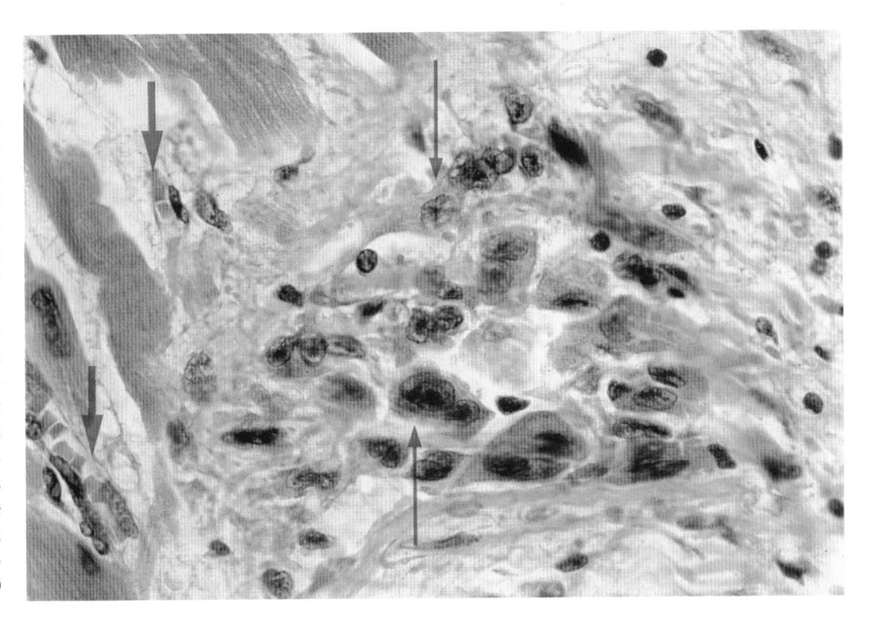

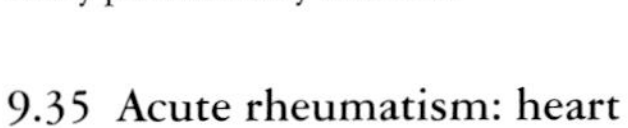

9.35 Acute rheumatism: heart

In rheumatic fever, the endocardium is inflamed and small thrombi form along the lines where the valve cusps come into firm contact during closure. These small thrombi (termed vegetations) initially consist mainly of fused platelets, but the fibrin content usually increases later in their formation. This shows the edge of a mitral valve cusp, and the most prominent feature is an amorphous deeply eosinophilic mass (a vegetation) which consists mostly of fibrin (double arrow) and is very tightly adherent to the surface of the cusp (thin arrow). The base of the vegetation (centre of field) is being phagocytosed by macrophages (small lymphocytes are also present) and the boundary between the cusp and the vegetation is ill-defined. The cusp is thicker than normal and more fibrous, and in it there are macrophages (with pleomorphic nuclei), fibroblasts, lymphocytes, plasma cells and a small blood vessel (thick arrow). Organization of the vegetation produces collagenous fibrous tissue which deforms the mitral cusp and tends to render the valve incompetent and/or stenotic. HE ×235

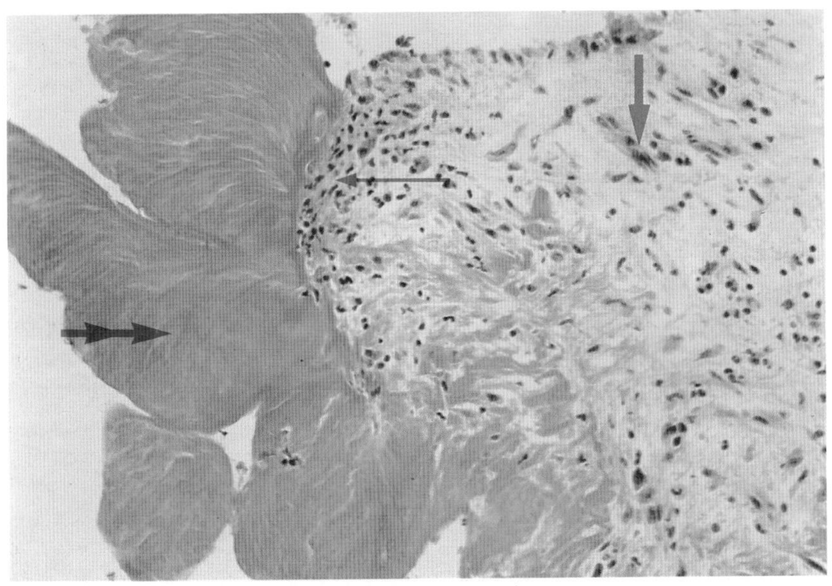

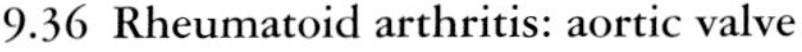

9.36 Rheumatoid arthritis: aortic valve

Necrosis of connective tissue is a frequent occurrence in rheumatoid arthritis and it is particularly common in the skin in the form of rheumatoid nodules. Rheumatoid nodules occasionally form in other tissues however, and this one was in the aortic valve of a man of 43. The valve was removed surgically and a prosthesis implanted. The shows part of a rheumatoid nodule (lower half of field). The centre of the nodule consists of amorphous necrotic eosinophilic material (double arrow) (much of it has disintegrated), enclosed by a wall of large elongated histiocytes (thin arrows) with ovoid vesicular nuclei, some with a coarsely granular pattern and others containing a nucleolus. The histiocytes are roughly aligned side-by-side (palisaded). Peripheral to the histiocytic zone there is a very cellular exudate (thick arrows) of moderately large macrophages with a round or ovoid vesicular nucleus (some containing a nucleolus) and (even more peripheral) small lymphocytes. The presence of the destructive necrotizing lesion illustrated here had rendered the aortic valve incompetent and led to its removal. HE ×360

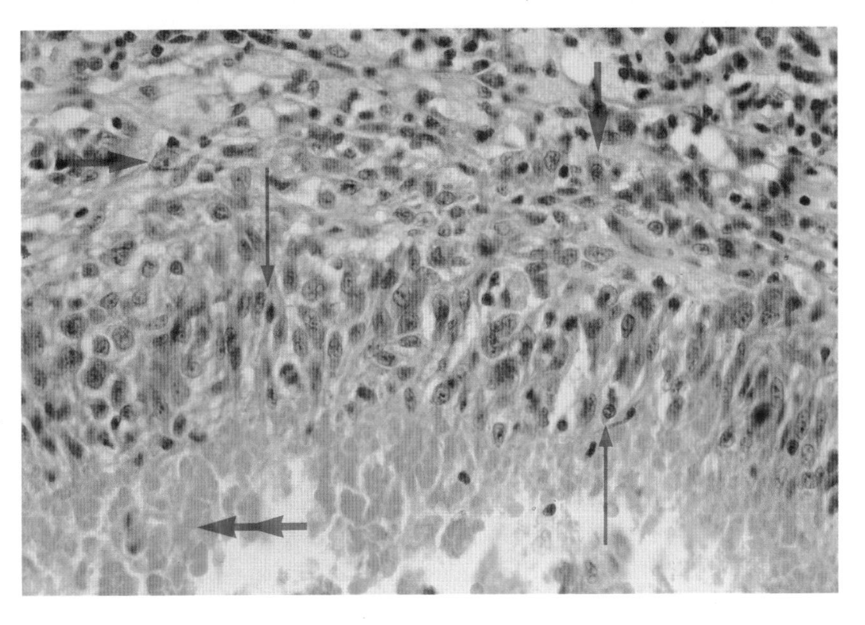

9.37 Infective endocarditis: aortic valve

In infective endocarditis, vegetations containing microorganisms form on the endocardium, generally on a valve cusp. It usually involves one or more heart valves but it may also occur in a patent ductus arteriosus. Unlike the small, firm closely-adherent sterile vegetations in acute rheumatism, the vegetations in infective endocarditis are often large and friable; and parts tend to break off and form emboli. Of the two forms, acute bacterial endocarditis progresses rapidly and is very destructive (if untreated), whereas subacute endocarditis progresses more slowly and is less destructive. In this case of subacute endocarditis, there is a large crumbling vegetation on an aortic cusp (heavily scarred by previous attacks of rheumatic endocarditis). The most superficial part of the vegetation (thick arrows) consists of eosinophilic platelets and fibrin, with a surface layer of mononuclear macrophages with ovoid basophilic nuclei (thin arrow). The inner (eosinophilic) platelet/fibrin layer encloses a purple granular mass of bacteria (*S. viridans*) (double arrow). The platelet/fibrin layer is protective and isolates the bacteria, which are thus able to grow freely. At the same time, the phagocytes are excluded from the bacteria, and antibiotics are correspondingly less able to overcome the infection. HE ×470

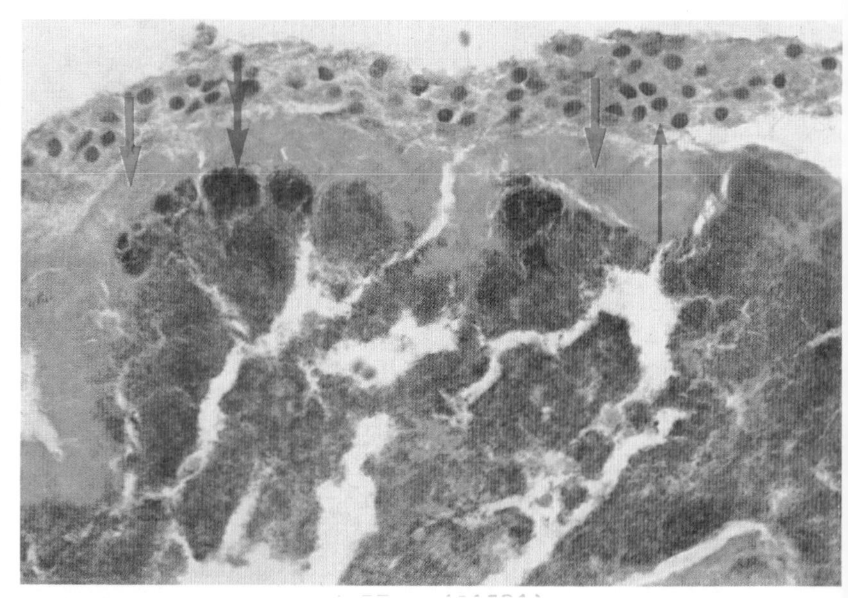

9.38 Infective endocarditis (Q fever): aortic valve

Q fever is a relatively mild Rickettsial disease. The causative organism is *Coxiella burneti* and the illness develops after inhalation of an aerosol from infected animals. It resembles typhus, with pneumonia and also granulomas in the liver and bone marrow. Very occasionally also chronic Q fever manifests chronic infective endocarditis. The organism colonizes the valves of the heart and produces a destructive form of endocarditis. The illness is similar to subacute bacterial endocarditis but the blood cultures are persistently negative for *Streptococcus viridans*. This shows a small part of a vegetation on an aortic cusp. The diagnostic feature is the presence of very large or extremely large macrophages (thick arrows), with their greatly swollen distended cytoplasm containing enormous numbers of basophilic *Coxiella burneti*. The huge number of microorganisms gives the macrophage cytoplasm a distinctive purple colour. The macrophages, some of which are breaking down, are surrounded by paler amorphous material (thin arrow), composed mainly of fused platelets, and they are accompanied by a small number of basophilic (blue-black) lymphocytes. HE ×200

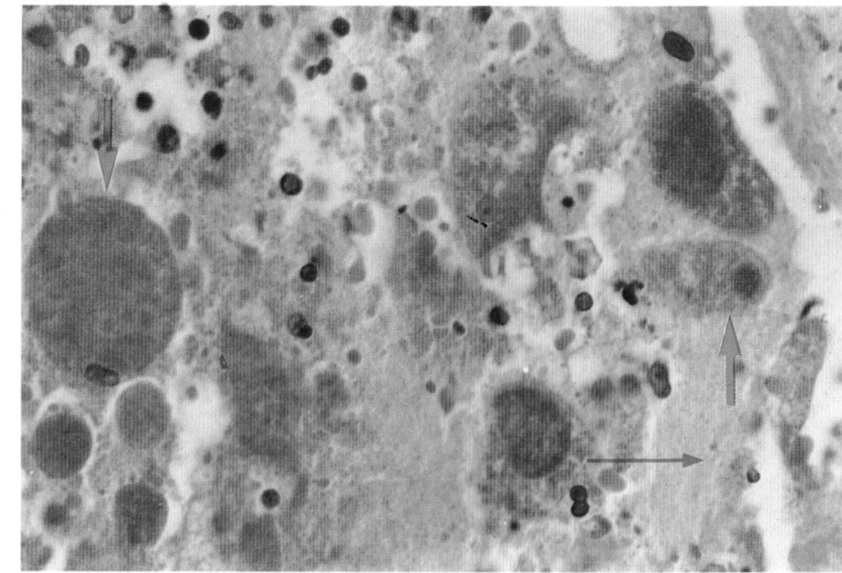

9.39 Myxoma: left atrium

A myxoma can arise in any chamber of the heart but the majority are located in the left atrium. An atrial myxoma tends to produce chronic left atrial hypertension, pulmonary hypertension and chronic venous congestion of the lungs, in the same way as mitral stenosis. Myxomas are generally spheroidal (up to 10cm dia) and gelatinous. Most are pedunculated. A woman of 63 was found to have mitral incompetence, and investigation revealed a 'tumour' within her left atrium. A soft mass (5 × 4 × 3cm) with a shiny blue capsule was removed surgically. Its cut surface had a variegated appearance, and histologically it is myxomatous, consisting of slender cords of spindle-shaped cells with elongated or oval basophilic nuclei and ill-defined vacuolated cytoplasm (thin arrow), surrounded by a large amount of pale amorphous matrix (thick arrow). There is also a dilated capillary blood vessel (double arrow) and (elsewhere in the mucoid mass) there is a well-developed network of capillaries and a considerable amount of fibrin. Special stains revealed large quantities of connective tissue mucin in the matrix. HE ×335

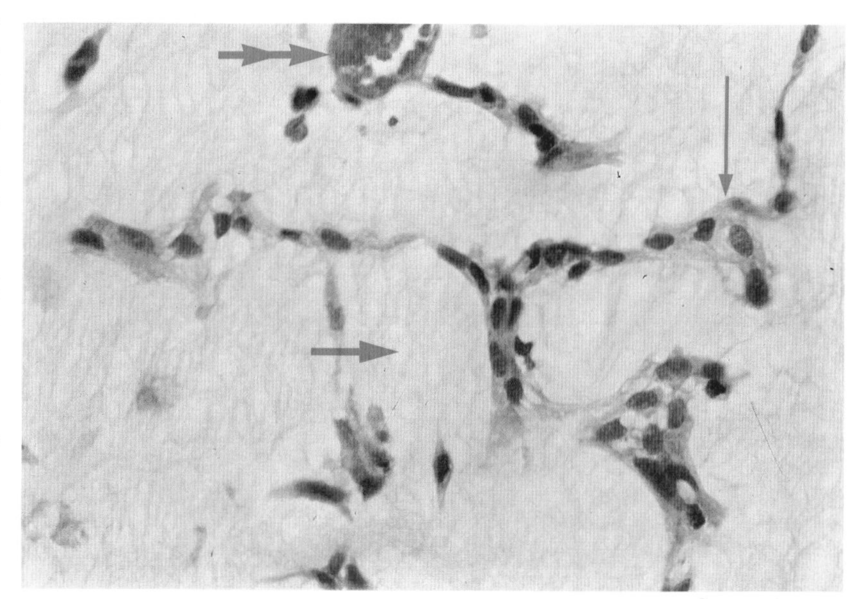

9.40 Chemodectoma: carotid body

Chemodectomas (sometimes incorrectly called non-chromaffin paragangliomas) are rare tumours of the chemoreceptor system. They include tumours of the carotid body, aorticopulmonary bodies and glomus jugulare. They do not produce any endocrine effect. Tumours of the carotid body are uncommon, but the incidence is considerably greater in those who live at high altitudes. It is a benign tumour, but a minority are locally invasive. A woman of 46 developed a firm swelling in the left side of the neck which slowly increased in size over a period of years. An ovoid mass, brownish in colour and measuring 3 × 2 × 1.5cm, was removed from the bifurcation of the right common carotid artery. The tumour was enclosed in a fibrous capsule. Histologically it consists of solid nests of polyhedral cells with eosinophilic cytoplasm (thin arrows) (and indistinct cells boundaries) and a slightly pleomorphic but generally round or ovoid nucleus, separated by strands of fibrous tissue (thick arrow). There is usually a rich sinusoidal blood supply but it is not evident in this case. There are no mitotic figures. HE ×150

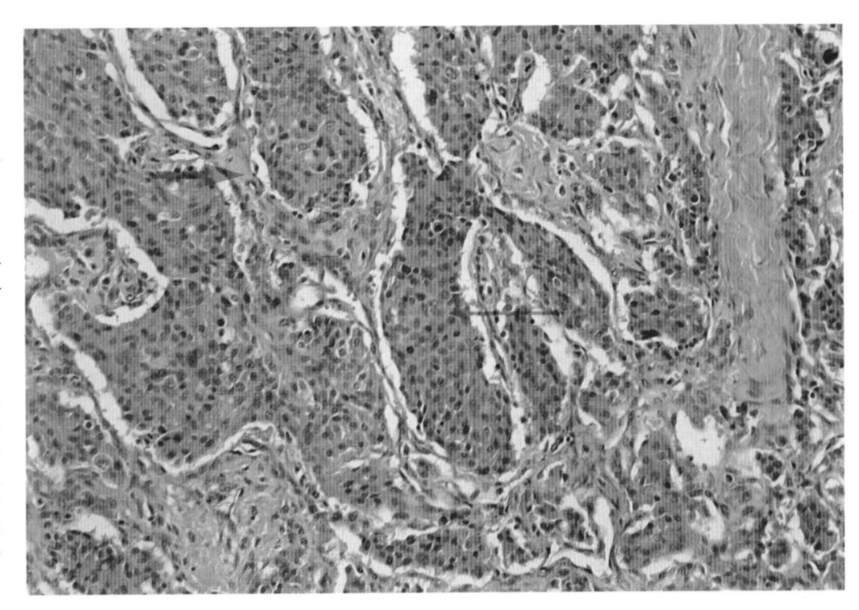

9.41 Chemodectoma: carotid body

The commonest site for chemodectomas is in the carotid body, and chemodectomas at other sites have the same general features. Carotid body tumours have a very characteristic stromal pattern, strongly reminiscent of the structure of the normal carotid body. The structural pattern is brought out particularly clearly by a reticulin stain for connective tissue fibres. The nuclei of the tumour cells are pale and 'vesicular' but visible (thick arrows). The cytoplasm of the tumour cells is even paler than the nuclei but just visible), and it is evident from these features that the tumour cells have formed 'nests' within a delicate 'capsule' of darkly-stained reticulin (thin arrows). There are many vascular sinusoids lying between the reticulin fibres in the stromal trabeculae, but these sinusoids are not readily detectable in either this reticulin-stained section or in HE sections. Reticulin stain ×360

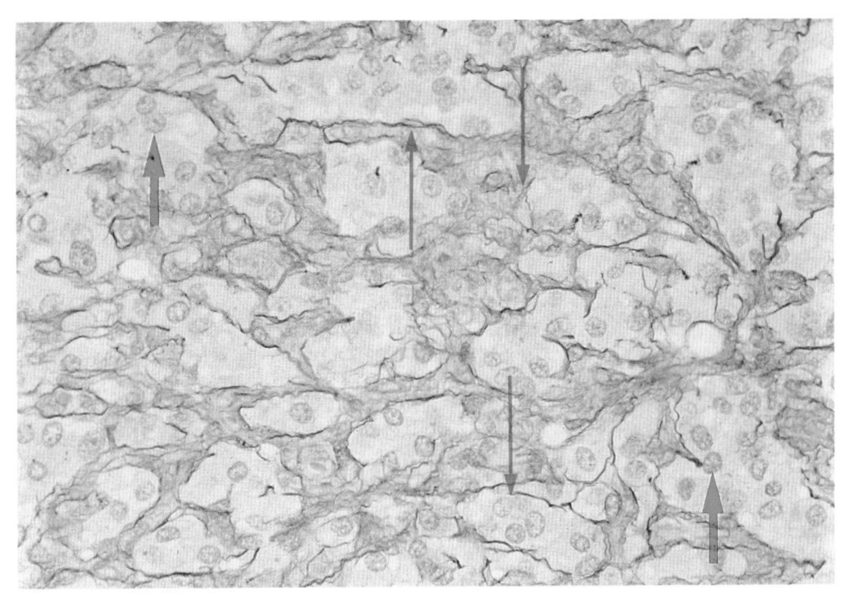

9.42 Hemangiosarcoma: skin

Hemangiosarcoma is a poorly differentiated malignant tumour of vascular endothelium which tends to be very aggressive and highly invasive. Hemangiosarcoma of the skin is usually restricted to the head and neck region of elderly people of either sex, and sometimes it arises in a lymphedematous limb of an elderly female 10 or more years after mastectomy. This lesion, in the skin of the forehead of a man of 59, was an irregular purplish-red slightly elevated lesion (4 × 3cm) with several small satellite nodules. It consists of closely packed blood vessels (thin arrow), many dilated and lined by plump elongated endothelial cells with spindle-shaped nuclei. Large pleomorphic spindle-shaped cells, which may be vasoformative, are dissecting between bundles of collagenous fibrous tissue. Some of their nuclei are extremely pleomorphic (double arrows) and there is also considerable mitotic activity. The walls of some of the blood vessels are attenuated, and there is much hemorrhage into the stroma. There are some hemosiderin-laden phagocytes (thick arrows). Also present is one normal large (clear) fat cell. HE ×360

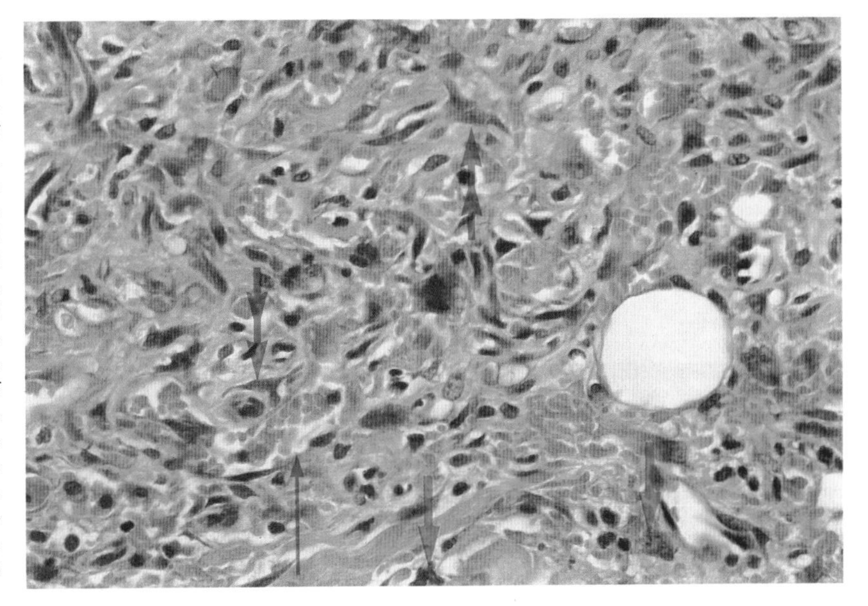

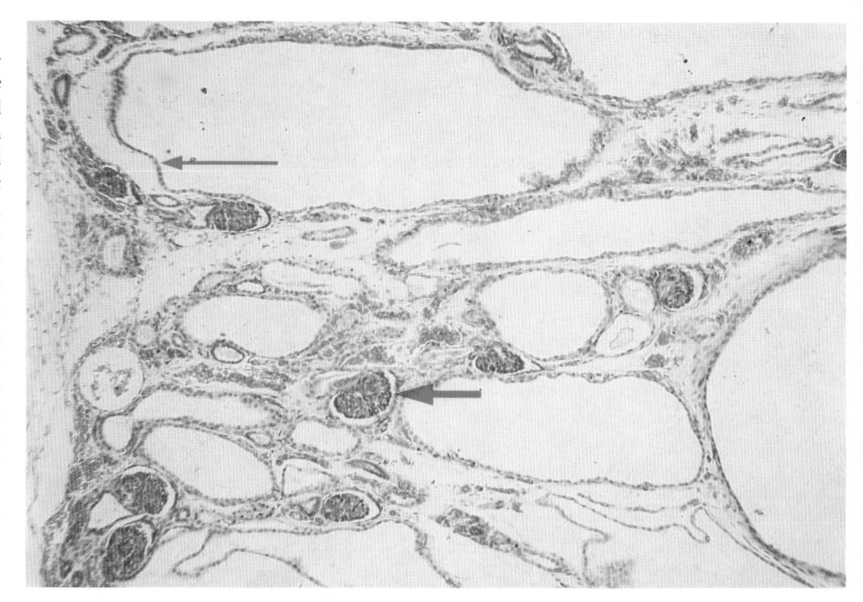

10.1 Adult polycystic disease: kidney

Adult polycystic disease is the commonest form of congenital cystic disease of the kidneys, it is also one of the most common dominantly inherited renal or nonrenal conditions (estimated prevalence of 1 in 1,000). It is an autosomal dominant. The gene responsible (designated PKD1) has been identified. Another gene for polycystic disease 2 (PKD2), a somewhat milder form of the disease, has recently been identified. The disease may be complicated by hypertension, hematuria and cardiac valve abnormalities, but the most important complication is the presence of berry aneurysms of the cerebral arteries. 10% of patients die of subarachnoid hemorrhage due to rupture of an aneurysm. But 77% of patients suffer terminal renal failure. The disease does not usually become clinically apparent until adult life. Both kidneys are usually greatly enlarged from the presence of large numbers of cysts, which may be several cm in dia. Weights of 4,500g for a single kidney have been recorded. This is the 'cortex' of a polycystic kidney, with the capsule on the left. No normal tubules are present, the bulk of the tissue consisting of cysts of various sizes and lined by flattened epithelium (thin arrow). Many glomeruli remain however between cysts, and despite being compressed by the cysts, look remarkably normal (thick arrow). HE ×55

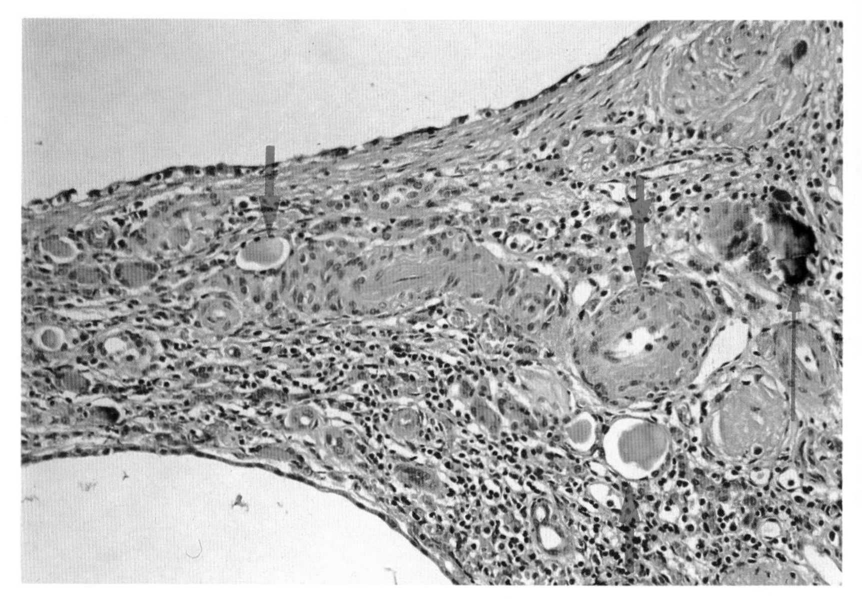

10.2 Adult polycystic disease: kidney

Part of the lower pole of a kidney removed surgically from a woman of 57. Parts of two cysts (top left and bottom left) and the interstitial tissues between them. The cysts are lined by flat attenuated cells. They, mostly, contain clear watery light yellow fluid frequently discoloured by old and recent hemorrhage. Their watery contents have been lost during processing of the tissue. Between the cysts are no apparent normal structures. It is surprising how these patients can survive the quite long time it must take for these destructive changes to develop. The interstitial tissue is infiltrated with lymphocytes, and a multinucleated giant cell is present, adjacent to a focus of calcification (thin arrow). Some tubules have survived (thick arrows), but they are small and atrophic and several contain dense eosinophilic material. The wall of the small artery (double arrow) is thickened and fibrosed and the lumen of the vessel is reduced, possibly due to hypertension. The mechanism which leads to the formation of the cysts is unknown. Cysts may be present also in the liver in about a third of the cases, but they are usually functionally insignificant. HE ×150

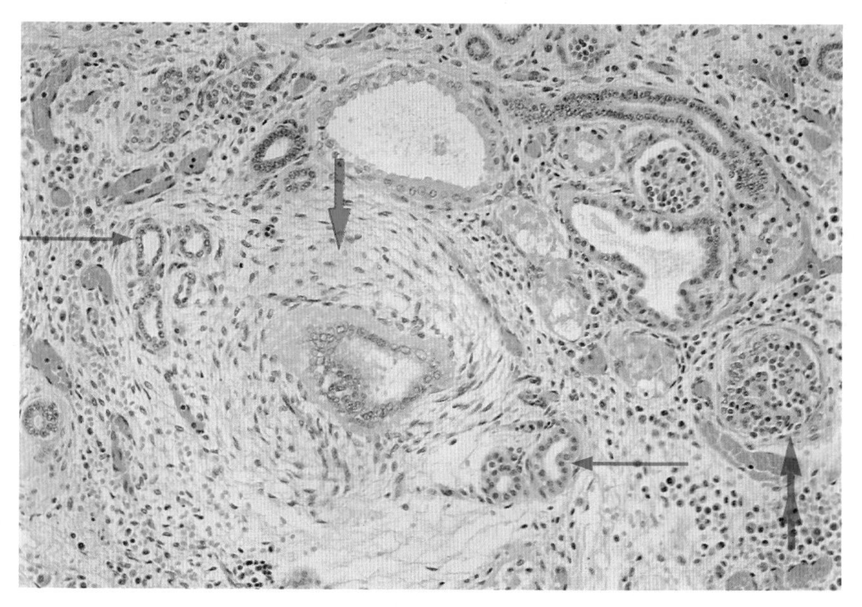

10.3 Renal dysplasia: kidney

In renal dysplasia structures are present in the kidney or region of the kidney which are represented in normal nephrogenesis. It may affect all or part of the kidney, or it may be present as foci scattered through the kidney . In the newborn, total renal dysplasia usually presents clinically as an abnormal abdominal mass. Histologically there are focally dilated ducts lined by cubical or columnar epithelium. These ducts may be surrounded by loose mesenchyme. There are smaller ductules lined by darkly staining epithelium. There may be cartilage in the interstitium. In this example the dysplastic tissue consists of immature ductules (thin arrows) surrounded by a cellular mesenchymal stroma (thick arrow). The ductules vary in size and are lined by a variety of types of epithelial cells; in most, the epithelial cells are cuboidal, with compact basophilic nuclei, and in others the cells have vesicular nuclei and eosinophilic cytoplasm. Two normal-looking glomeruli (double arrow) are present. Plasma cells and lymphocytes are present in small numbers in the stroma, and hemorrhage has occurred from the many small blood vessels. HE ×150

10.4 Acute pyelonephritis: kidney

Acute pyelonephritis is caused by bacterial infection which in most instances reaches the kidneys from the bladder. The common causative organism is *Escherichia coli*. The other important factor is lower urinary tract obstruction. In the male, prostatic obstruction is important. Acute pyelonephritis occurs in pregnancy. Dilatation of the ureters can be detected early in pregnancy. The dilatation is possibly hormonally induced, but more probably mechanical and caused by the enlarged uterus. The third important cause of obstruction is vesicoureteral reflux, i.e. leakage back from the bladder into the ureter. In severe cases, areas of suppuration are visible macroscopically, usually as elongated yellow streaks in the medulla. Destruction of tubules tends to be greater than damage to glomeruli. Here the epithelium of the convoluted tubules (thin arrows) is swollen and granular (severe cloudy swelling). In places, the lining cells are necrotic and contain large numbers of bacteria (staining deep blue). One tubule (thick arrow) is full of pus and has lost most of its epithelial lining. The interstitial tissues are infiltrated with polymorphs, lymphocytes and plasma cells. HE x200

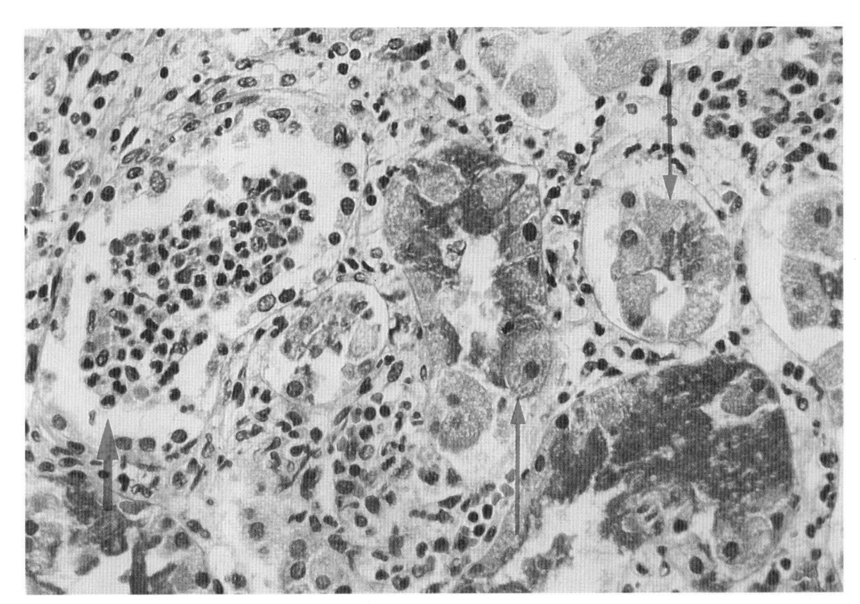

10.5 Papillary necrosis: kidney

If the inflammatory process is very intense (the patient not infrequently has diabetes mellitus with obstruction of the lower urinary tract), necrosis of renal papillae occurs. The tips of the papillae are particularly susceptible. The base of this papilla (left) is still viable and several tubules retain their epithelial lining. The part of the papilla towards the tip however (centre and right) is necrotic (thin arrow), and the collecting tubules (thick arrows) are full of necrotic cellular debris and bacteria and are disintegrating. The absence of a leukocytic and vascular response at the junction of the living and necrotic tissues is noteworthy. A more chronic form of papillary necrosis is associated with overconsumption of analgesic drugs. First described in Switzerland and Australia, where it accounted for 20% of the cases requiring haemodialysis, this peculiar geographical distribution was almost certainly due to the cases being missed in other countries. The first analgesic implicated was phenacetin. Subsequently there has been controversy over whether other analgesics such as aspirin might be involved, hence the name analgesic nephropathy.

HE × 95

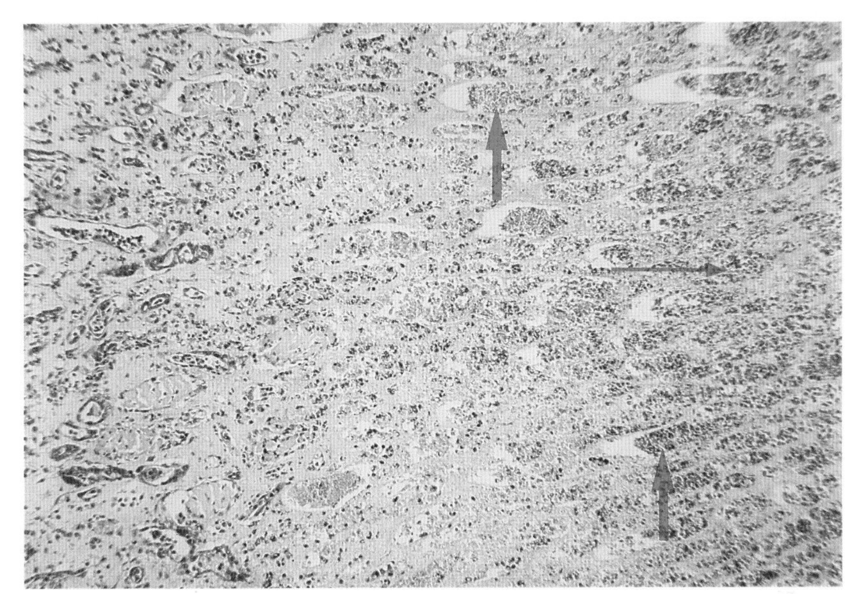

10.6 Chronic pyelonephritis: kidney

Chronic pyelonephritis sometimes develops after recurrent attacks of acute pyelonephritis; many cases have no history of preceding acute attacks. The kidneys are reduced in size, often asymmetrically, and scarred, with fibrous thickening of the pelvis. The scars are localised with adjacent areas of near-normal kidney and affect the full thickness of the cortex. The capsular surface is depressed in the scarred area. The associated medullary pyramid is often shrunken and distorted. This association of a distorted medullary pyramid with a depressed cortical scar distinguishes pyelonephritic scars from scars due to previous infarction, in which the medullary pyramids are intact. These gross findings are often important, establishing a diagnosis of chronic pyelonephritis. This is cortex of an advanced case. The glomeruli are nearly all completely fibrosed and avascular. There is atrophy of most of the tubules which, apart from a few very small tubules, have practically no lumen. The result is crowding of the hyalinised glomeruli (thick arrow). The remaining tubules are dilated and contain densely eosinophilic ('colloid') casts (thin arrows). The interstitial tissue is heavily infiltrated with lymphocytes and plasma cells. HE ×65

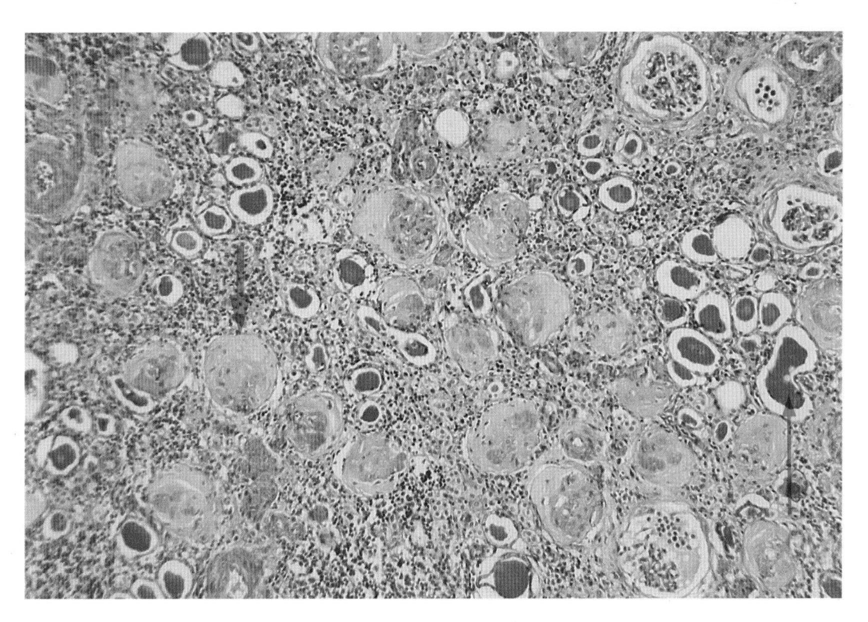

10.7 Infarct: kidney

The branches of the renal artery are end-arteries. Occlusion of one from embolism or thrombosis results in infarction. Sources of emboli are the left atrium in mitral stenosis, the left ventricle in myocardial infarction or atheromatous plaques of the aorta. Thrombosis may result from vascular disease of the intrarenal arteries, such as atheroma or from acute arteritis as in polyarteritis nodosa. This is the edge of a recent infarct. The cells lining the tubules (left) are necrotic (thick arrow): there is no nuclear staining and the cytoplasm is deeply eosinophilic. The tissues in the right half of the field are probably viable, though the left half of the glomerulus appears necrotic (thin arrow). The capillaries of the boundary zone (centre) are greatly distended and the stroma is edematous, with separation of the tubules. After a few days, macrophages, polymorph leukocytes and fibroblasts appear in the boundary zone and organization of the dead tissue results in the formation of a depressed subcapsular scar. This scarring is usually confined to the cortex, sparing the medullary pyramids a feature that is helpful in distinguishing between healed infarcts and pyelonephritic scars (**10.6**). HE ×135

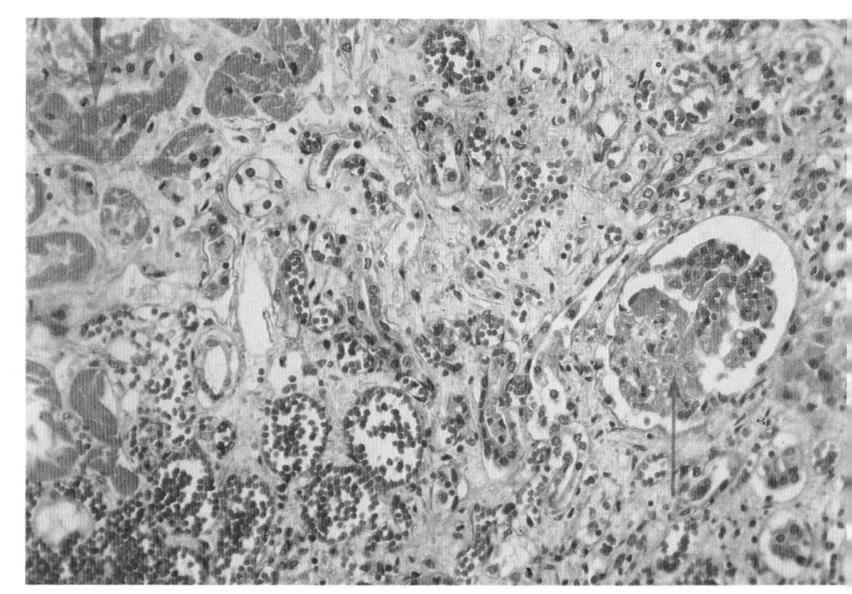

10.8 Acute tubular necrosis: kidney

Necrosis of the epithelium of the renal tubules, particularly of the proximal convoluted tubules, may be widespread throughout the kidney, causing anuria or severe oliguria and acute renal failure. The lesion is associated with shock following trauma and incompatible blood transfusion. A number of chemicals, i.e. mercury compounds, carbon tetrachloride and ethylene glycol, are also toxic to tubular epithelium. In the United Kingdom hemodialysis was first developed during the war to treat this form of renal failure in the victims of crush injuries as a temporary means supporting the patient until the tubules had regenerated, not as a long-term support as it is now used. The epithelium has considerable powers of regeneration, and in the acute phase of the recovery quite numerous mitotic figures may be seen. Renal function can recover, being heralded by profuse diuresis (the diuretic phase of the recovery). This patient died from renal failure seven days after an operation for relief of constrictive pericarditis. Most of the epithelium lining the collecting tubules has died and sloughed into the lumen (thick arrow). The surviving cells have made considerable attempts at repair and already the tubules are lined by flat elongated cells (thin arrows). HE ×200

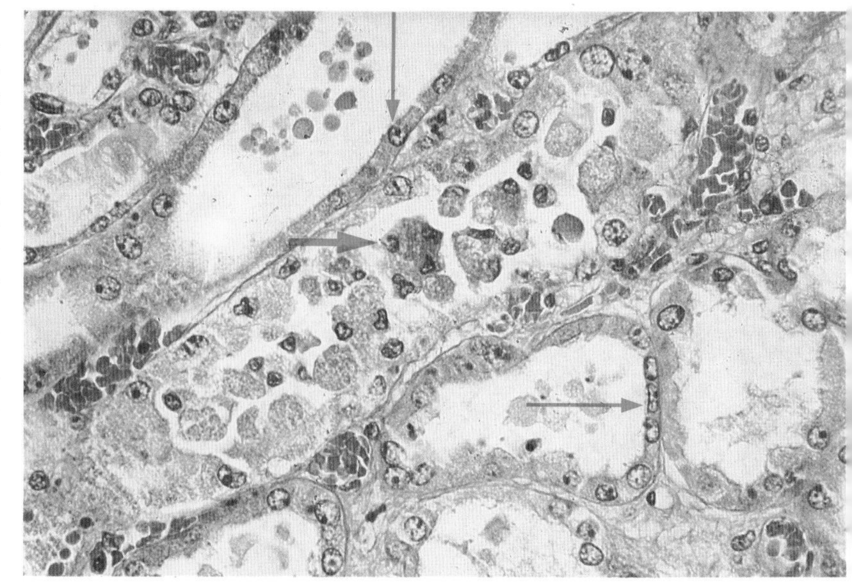

10.9 Hydropic change: kidney

All the cells lining the proximal convoluted tubules are pale and swollen due to hydropic change. This can be caused by the administration of osmotic diuretics, e.g. sucrose, intravenously. It is also seen in patients who have a low serum sodium from a variety of causes. In these circumstance there is a correlation between the degree of hyponatremia and the extent of the lesion. When the change is produced by the administration of osmotic diuretics such as sucrose, it results from swelling of the lysosomes forming numerous vacuoles within the cell. This change affects not only the cells of the kidney but many cells throughout the body. It is particularly strikingly seen in the parenchymal cells of the liver. In this case all the cells of the proximal convoluted tubules are pale and swollen (thick arrow). The glomerulus to the right is normal (thin arrow). The tubules can recovery rapidly and completely. HE ×150

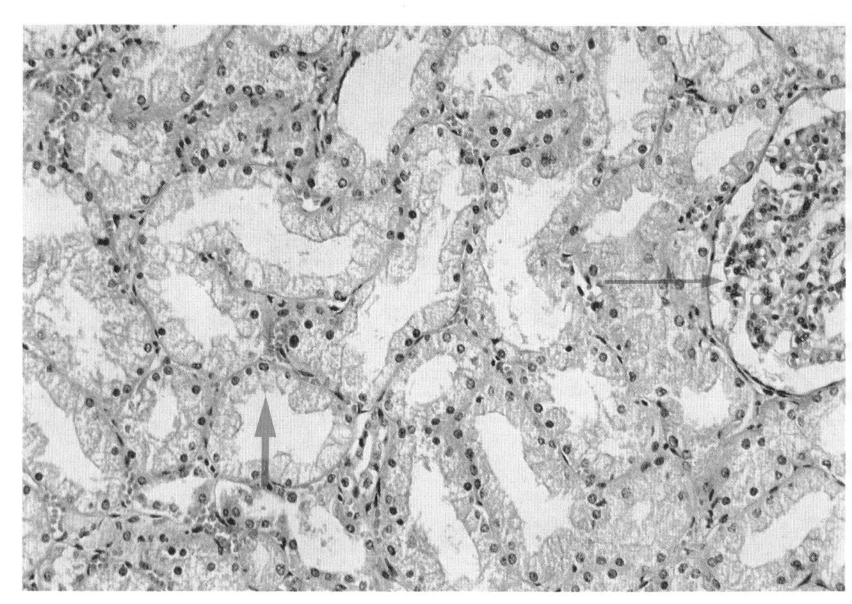

10.10 Fat embolism: kidney

When fatty tissues such as the marrow of a large bone are severely traumatized, particles of fat may enter the venous circulation. Most are filtered off by the capillaries of the lungs but some get through the lungs and form small emboli in the systemic circulation. This is the kidney of a young woman who died from multiple injuries, including fracture of a femur. The glomerular capillaries are distended with fat globules (arrow) and a small amount of fat is present in the subcapsular space. The gaps in some droplets were caused by fat dissolving in the stain (Sudan IV). In conventional paraffin sections the fat is completely dissolved during the preparation. The clear round spaces left can be seen distending the glomerular capillaries. Fat embolism of the kidneys and other organs happens not infrequently after severe injury without altering the clinical outcome, unless it produces lesions in a vital part of the central nervous system (4.6).

Sudan IV ×335

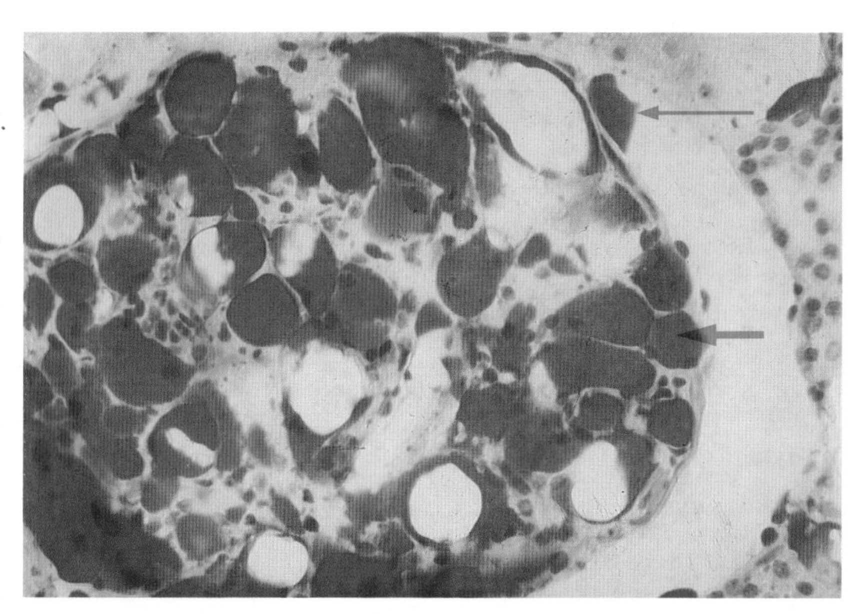

10.11 Diabetic glomerulosclerosis: kidney

Renal complications are important in diabetes mellitus resulting in renal failure. Severe vascular disease may result in much renal damage. This consists of atherosclerosis involving the larger vessels and hyalinization of the arterioles, which may be severe and widespread. Acute and chronic pyelonephritis may occur, sometimes accompanied by necrosis of the medullary pyramids (10.5). In this case the glomerular lesion of diabetes mellitus is illustrated. Lesions develop in the glomeruli of a significant proportion (up to 50%) of diabetic individuals, in the form of deposits of hyaline material in the mesangium of the lobules of the glomerulus. It may be deposited diffusely and more or less evenly throughout the glomerulus, or unevenly as one or more nodules. The two types of lesion are often present together, as in this case. There is diffuse infiltration of the glomerular tuft with eosinophilic material and also heavy focal deposition (thin arrow). The diffuse infiltrate appears to be in the basement membranes of the capillaries, and the capillary bed has been obliterated in places. In time this can lead to more or less complete hyalinization of many glomeruli. The afferent arteriole (thick arrow) shows hyaline change.

HE ×335

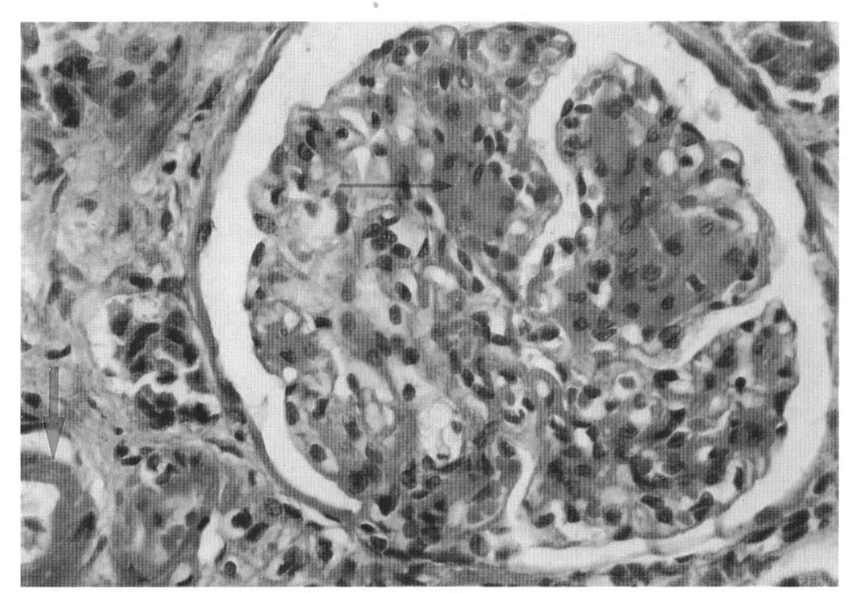

10.12 Diabetic glomerulosclerosis: kidney

This is the classical Kimmelstiel-Wilson lesion of diabetic glomerulosclerosis. The hyaline material has been deposited in round, practically acellular, nodules (thin arrows) in the glomerular tuft. The cuff of red cells around the larger of the two main nodules is a greatly dilated capillary blood vessel. There is also a considerable deposit of hyaline material thickening in Bowman's capsule. The arterioles, appearing as narrow ovals, to the left of the glomerulus also show quite marked, strongly eosinophil hyaline thickening (thick arrow). Diabetes mellitus is the only disease in which both the afferent and efferent glomerular arterioles show hyaline thickening. The Kimmelstiel-Wilson lesion occurs virtually only in diabetes. Claims to have located such nodules in non-diabetic are mostly unconvincing, because of the difficulty of rigorously excluding diabetes. The nodules are found very frequently in diabetic glomerulosclerosis, but the number of glomeruli showing the lesions may vary widely. Diabetic glomerulosclerosis may be confused histologically with renal amyloidosis (10.15) or lobular membranoproliferative glomerulonephritis (10.29). Amyloidosis can readily be excluded by Congo red staining, and in lobular glomerulonephritis virtually every glomerulus is affected.

HE x235

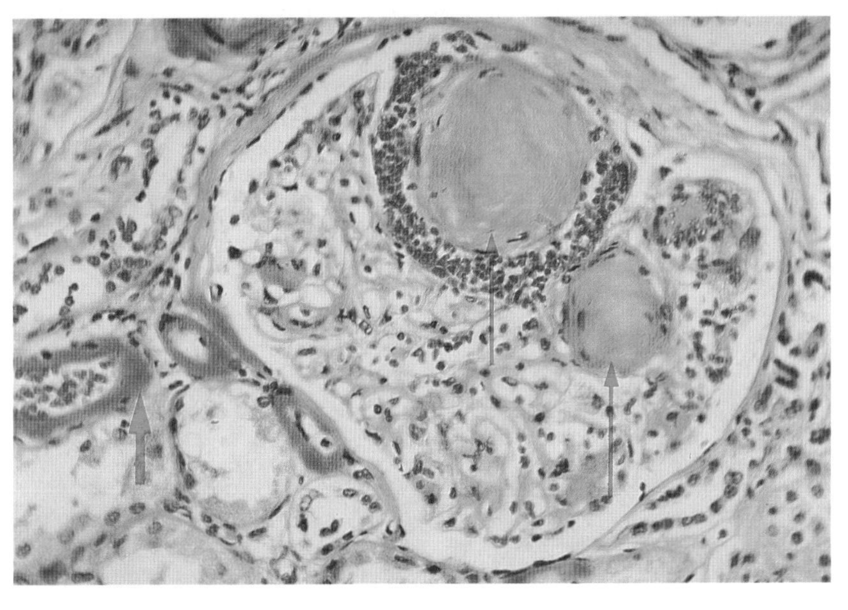

10.13 Cytomegalic inclusion disease: kidney

Up to 80% of adults have been reported as having antibodies to cytomegalovirus, and the infection is persistent. However in adults the virus rarely causes disease, except in immunosuppressed individuals. This may happen in immunosuppressed renal transplant recipients when the virus may affect numerous organs, such as the kidney, liver, spleen and lungs. The fetus is sometimes infected in utero with the cytomegalovirus, and if it happens early in pregnancy it may cause developmental abnormalities in the central nervous system, including mental retardation, but the infection may be quite localised. This is the kidney of a newborn infant, showing a renal tubule in longitudinal section. Most of the epithelial cells have been colonized by the virus and are greatly swollen, and in each there is a large round basophilic viral inclusion in the nucleus. In several cells there appears to be also a cytoplasmic inclusion (thin arrow). Similar changes are present in the adjacent tubule cut in cross-section (thick arrow). The interstitial tissues (top left) are heavily infiltrated with lymphocytes. HE ×360

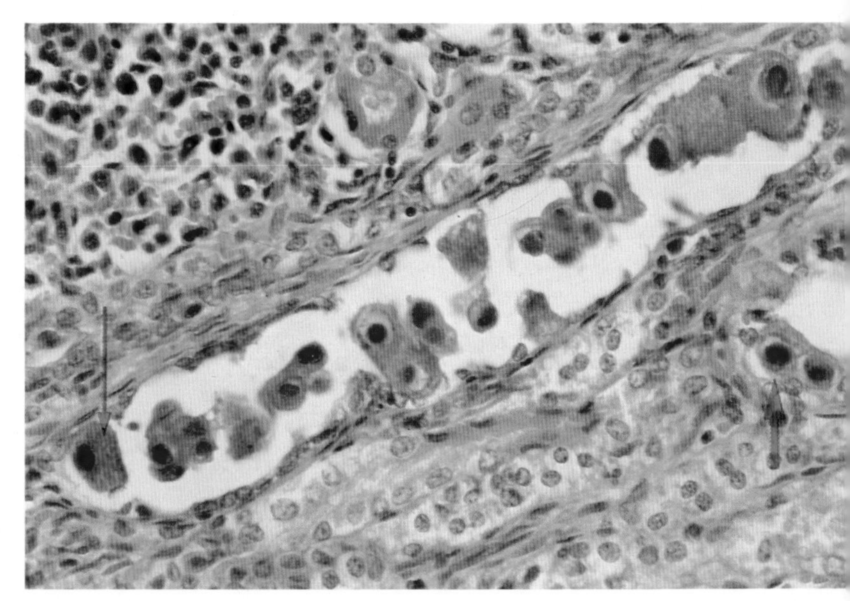

10.14 Metastatic calcification: kidney

Calcium salts may be deposited in living tissues when calcium metabolism is abnormal and the calcium level in the blood is raised (hypercalcemia). This process is metastatic calcification and should not be confused with dystrophic calcification, in which calcium salts are deposited in necrotic or dying tissue in the presence of a normal blood calcium level. Calcium may be deposited in the kidneys in sarcoidosis, when there is sometimes excessive intestinal absorption of calcium. There may be excessive mobilisation of calcium from the bones in widespread skeletal metastases or multiple myelomatosis. Renal deposition of calcium may result from overdosage with vitamin D. This patient had a parathyroid carcinoma and hyperparathyroidism, with a very high blood calcium level. He died eventually from renal failure. Parts of the glomerular tuft (left) are heavily calcified and deeply basophilic (thin arrow). The epithelium lining the convoluted tubules (right) is greatly swollen, with pale-staining hydropic cytoplasm (thick arrow). . HE ×200

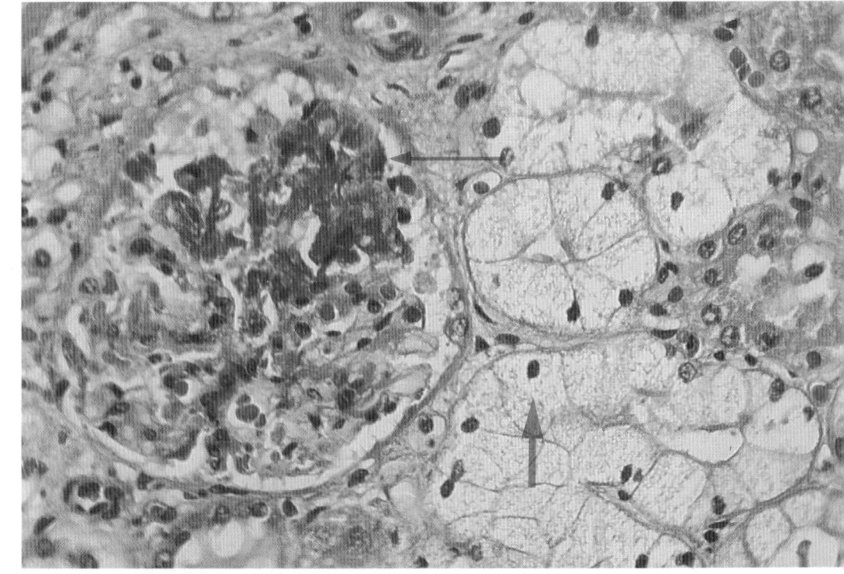

10.15 Amyloidosis: kidney

Amyloid is translucent hyaline material deposited extracellularly in various organs in chronic inflammatory disease, such as pulmonary tuberculosis. It also occurs in some non-inflammatory conditions. All the amyloid fibrils have the same basic protein structure, the ß-pleated sheet (as in silk), probably accounting for its persistence in the tissues. The amyloidogenic protein is different in the different forms of amyloid. In chronic inflammation it is amyloid protein A, derived from serum amyloid A (SAA), in multiple myelomatosis it is derived from the light chains of immunoglobulin, and in some endocrine glands and tumours it is derived from the polypeptide hormone. It always contain another protein component, serum amyloid P component (SAP). In amyloidosis associated with chronic inflammatory conditions there is atrophy and loss of parenchymal cells. In the kidneys it usually produces a nephrotic syndrome. In this case the patient had had pulmonary tuberculosis for many years and amyloid was present in many organs. This shows one glomerulus and the associated tubules. The tubules (thin arrow) are relatively unaffected, but the glomerular tuft is enlarged and the basement membrane of the capillaries infiltrated by eosinophilic amyloid (thick arrow). Where the infiltrate is greatest, the lumen of the vessels is obliterated, and in severe lesions many nephrons are rendered functionless. HE ×250

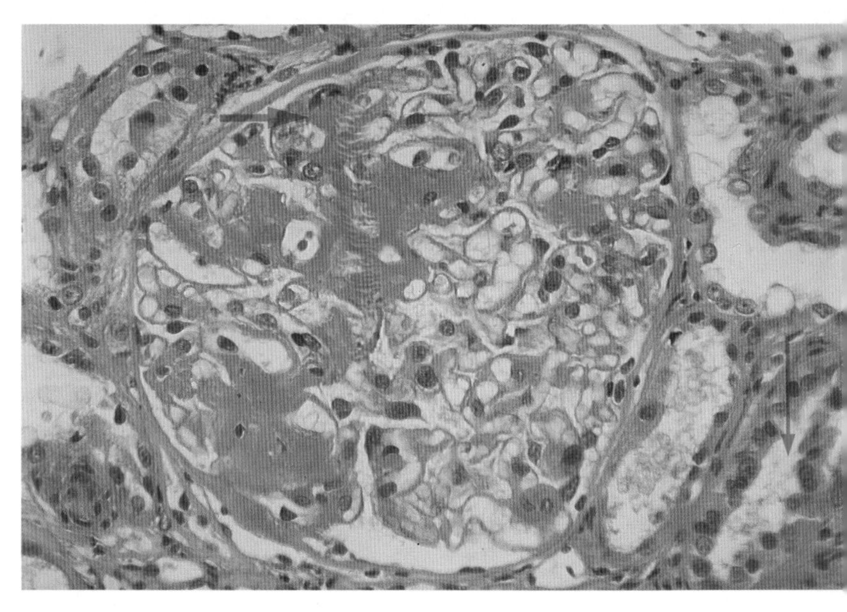

10.16 Amyloidosis: kidney

In this case the amyloid has infiltrated the basement membrane of the collecting tubules (thin arrow) and the loop of Henle (thick arrow). The convoluted tubule (double arrow) is free from deposits but its epithelial cells are swollen and their cytoplasm is granular as a result of the proteinuria produced by the disease. The amyloid deposits are eosinophilic, and so in the glomerulus might be mistaken for diabetic glomerulosclerosis (**10.11**), but amyloid stained with Congo red shows a striking range of colours in polarised light, varying from lemon yellow to lime green to orange on rotating the analyser. In renal amyloidosis the intrarenal veins have an increased tendency to thrombose and the main veins may be involved secondarily. Thrombosis of the renal veins may occur in other forms of the nephrotic syndrome, so it is now accepted the thrombosis is the result of the nephrotic syndrome; a consequence of the gross changes in the plasma proteins, although the precise change responsible is uncertain HE ×335

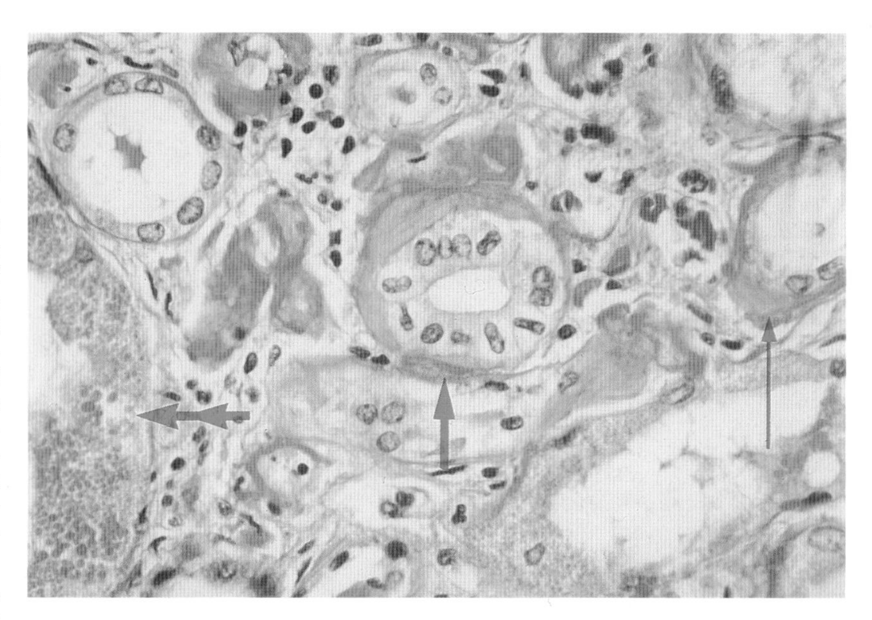

10.17 Myelomatosis: kidney

Myelomatosis is a neoplastic overgrowth of cells of the plasma cell series, usually confined to the hemopoietic bone marrow (ribs, sternum, skull). It diffusedly affects the bone marrow and may also give rise to localised tumours. The malignant plasma cells are derived from a single cell; they are a single clone. The immunoglobulin molecule they produce consists of only one type of light chain, either lambda or kappa (monoclonal gammopathy). The excess of light chains is readily excreted in the urine as its molecular weight is in the range of 20,000 to 40,000, compared with, for example serum albumen, molecular weight, 69,000. The excretion of this "myeloma protein" (so-called Bence-Jones protein) was detected in the mid-nineteenth century by its distinctive reaction to heating the urine. The protein first precipitates, but then redissolves on further heating. In this kidney there is deeply eosinophilic material, precipitated immunoglobulin light chains, filling the lumen of two collecting tubules and effectively blocking them (thick arrows). These casts are dense and they are pressing on and causing atrophy and destruction of the epithelial cells lining the two tubules. The cells of another tubule (thin arrows) are also degenerate. The interstitial tissue appears edematous. HE ×335

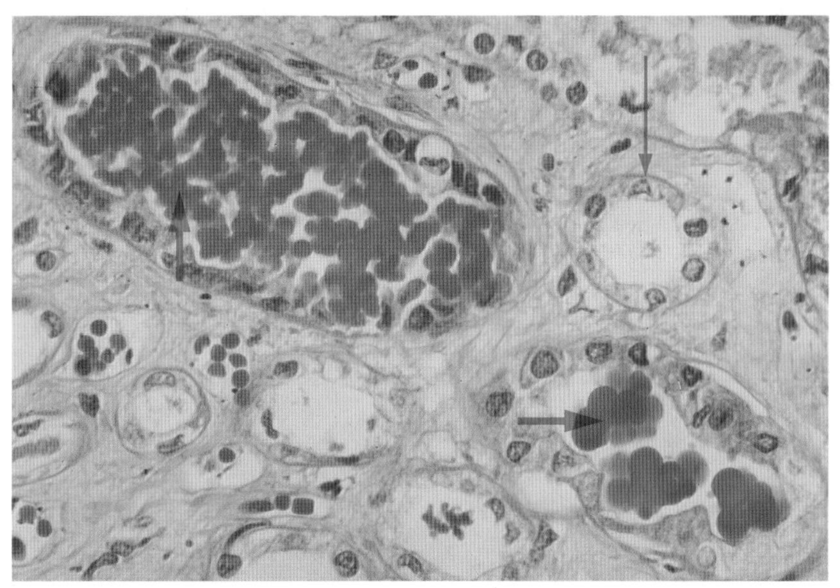

10.18 Myelomatosis: kidney

This is a biopsy specimen of kidney from a man of 59. The lumen of most of the collecting tubules is blocked by dense hyaline casts of precipitated light chains. The casts have caused atrophy and loss of the epithelial cells in many places, with disruption of the walls of the tubules (thin arrows). The protein casts in multiple myelomatosis are very unusual, if not unique, in that they are often surrounded by an intratubular cellular reaction. In this case macrophages and multinucleated foreign-body giant cells (thick arrows) surround the exposed parts of the casts. The myeloma protein may have other effects on the kidney. Intracellular hyaline protein droplets may be present in the cells of the proximal convoluted tubules; more rarely crystals of protein may be found in these cells. The interstitial tissues are edematous and infiltrated by lymphocytes and plasma cells. Elsewhere many glomeruli were globally sclerosed. Tubular destruction can occur on a wide scale in myelomatosis and lead to renal failure. Hypercalcemia is often also present, and producing nephrocalcinosis. HE ×235

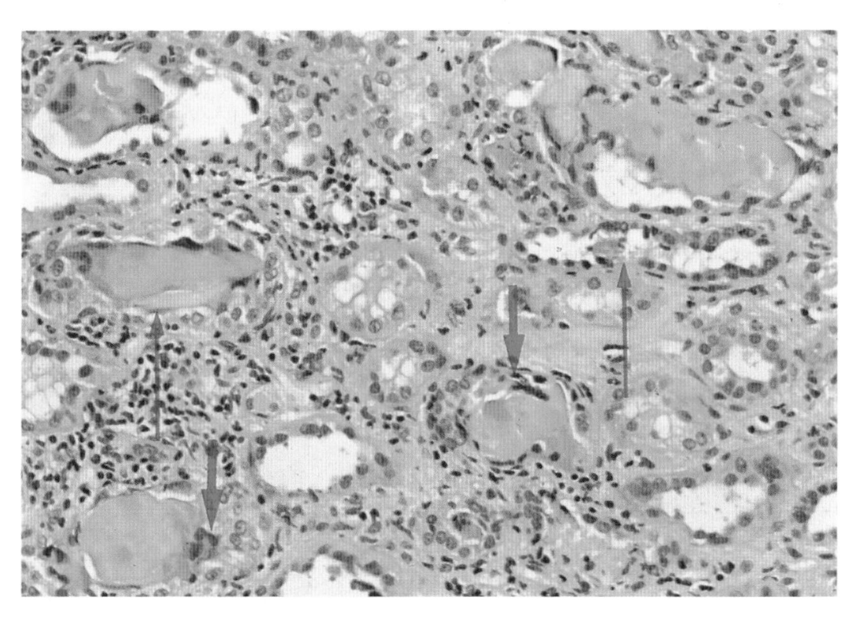

10.19 Minimal change glomerulonephritis: kidney

Minimal change glomerulonephritis occurs most often in young children (1-4 years), but can also occur in adults. It usually presents with a nephrotic syndrome, i.e. heavy proteinuria, low serum albumen and generalised edema. The proteinuria is selective, consisting almost entirely of serum albumen and smaller serum proteins. Most patients recover completely; the remissions being induced by steroid therapy. There is no impairment of renal function. This glomerulus has been stained by the periodic acid-Schiff (PAS) method. There is no cellular proliferation in the glomerulus and no thickening of the basement membrane, the amount of purplish-red material at the centre of the glomerular lobules being within the normal range of variation. The walls of the capillaries therefore show no thickening (arrow). Electron microscopy showed that the foot processes of the epithelial cells were fused, forming a continuous layer of epithelial cell cytoplasm over basement membrane. PAS ×375

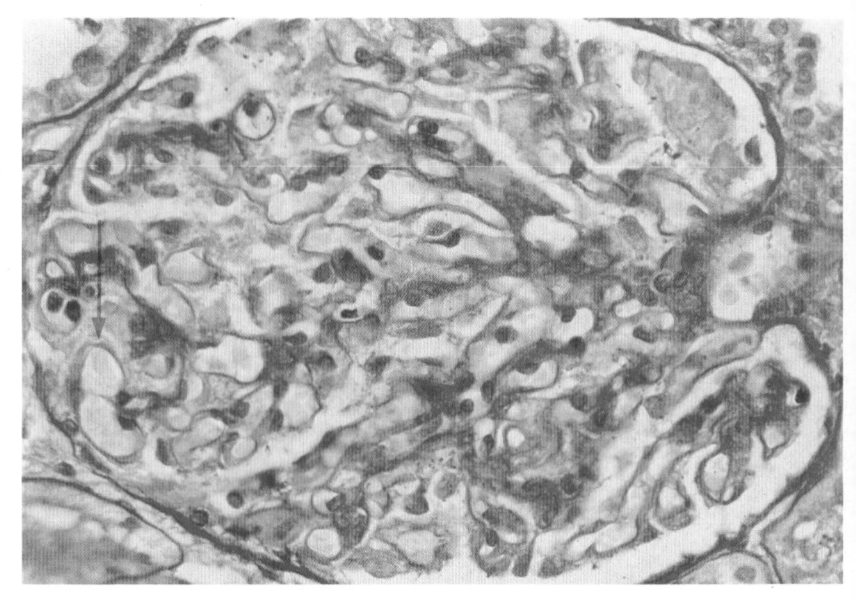

10.20 Membranous nephropathy: kidney

Patients with membranous nephropathy generally present with the nephrotic syndrome. The long term prognosis is much less favourable than in minimal change glomerulonephritis. The non-selective proteinuria is quite heavy. The characteristic lesion is a diffuse thickening of the basement membrane, as shown in this glomerulus stained by the PAS method (arrow). The change is diffuse, affecting all capillaries in the glomerulus equally, and all the glomeruli in both kidneys. There is no proliferation of endothelial cells or of mesangial cells, and no infiltration of the mesangium by leukocytes. Granular deposits of IgG along the basement membrane are found in virtually all cases. Similar deposits of the complement component C3 are also very common. A small minority of cases occur sufficiently frequently in association with a variety of conditions to provide some support an immunological mechanism. These include hepatitis B, a variety of carcinomas, and treatment with number of substances, including gold and penicillamine. In these cases the glomerular changes have been observed to resolve after the stopping of the penicillamine or after removal of the carcinoma. PAS ×375

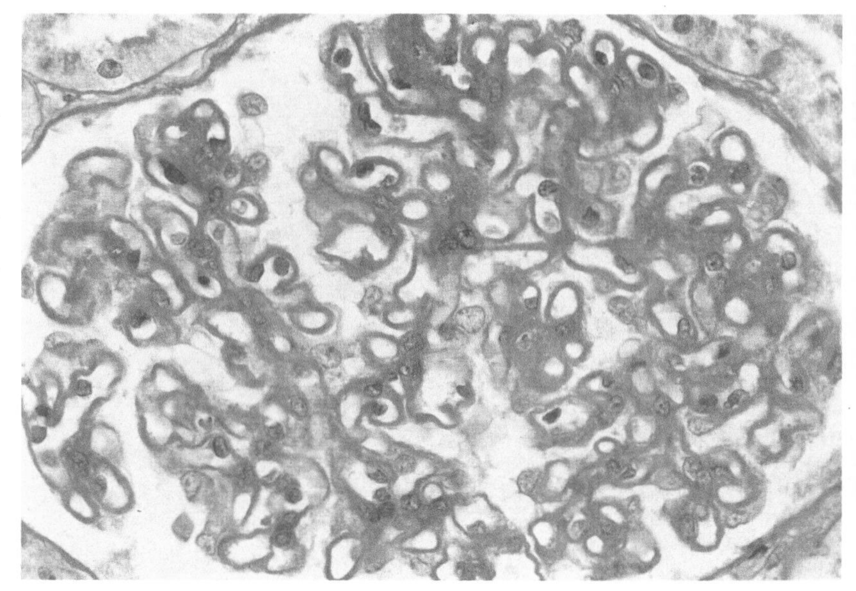

10.21 Membranous nephropathy: kidney

It is occasionally difficult to distinguish between membranous nephropathy and membranoproliferative glomerulonephritis and also between early membranous nephropathy and minimal change glomerulonephritis. The use of thin (1 m) sections stained by the periodic acid-methenamine silver method is very helpful. In this preparation, several capillaries show changes typical of membranous glomerulonephritis: instead of being a smooth black line, the glomerular basement membrane now consists of an inner continuous black line with stumpy black "bristles" projecting from its outer surface (arrow). These little " bristles" overlie one another in thicker sections and so can not be resolved. In early cases of membranous nephropathy the "bristles" are few in number and small. As the disease progresses the "bristles" become larger and more numerous, covering the whole of the outer surface of the glomerular basement membrane. In the late stages of the disease the ends of the "bristles" become linked up to one another to produce the appearance of the links of a chain.

Periodic acid-methenamine silver ×1200

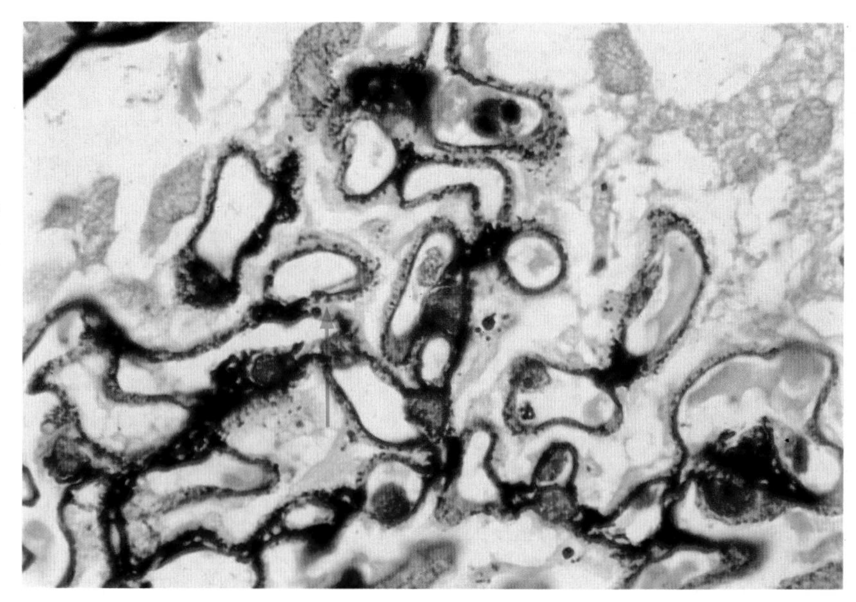

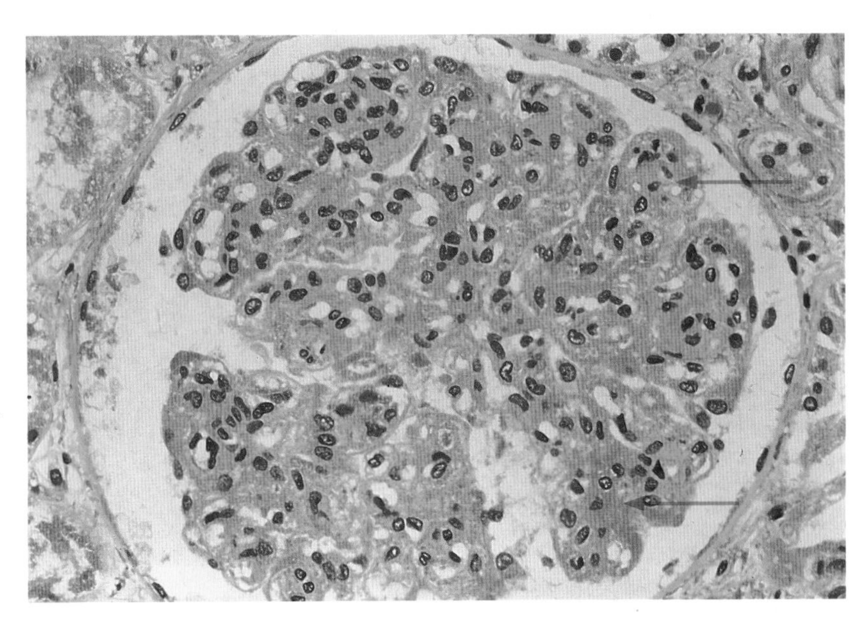

10.22 Membranoproliferative glomerulonephritis: kidney

Membranoproliferative glomerulonephritis may present with malaise, pyrexia, hematuria and edema or, more commonly, with the nephrotic syndrome. The proteinuria is non-selective. The prognosis is generally poor, but a small minority do recover. The glomeruli are enlarged and show a diffuse proliferative change, with increase in the numbers and size of the endothelial and mesangial cells. The mesangial changes are particularly marked and, in this case, have produced diffuse eosinophilic sclerosis of the glomerulus. The lobular structure of the glomerulus is more obvious than normal (arrows), and this has lead to the name lobular glomerulonephritis being applied to these cases. No definite etiology for membranoproliferative glomerulonephritis has been demonstrated, but a significant number of cases have a raised titre of antibodies to streptococcal antigens. However a role for streptococcal infection has not been confirmed. A reduced serum complement is commonly found, as is also a granular deposition of the C3 component of complement along the basement membrane, but a convincing immunological mechanism for this disease has not been demonstrated. HE ×335

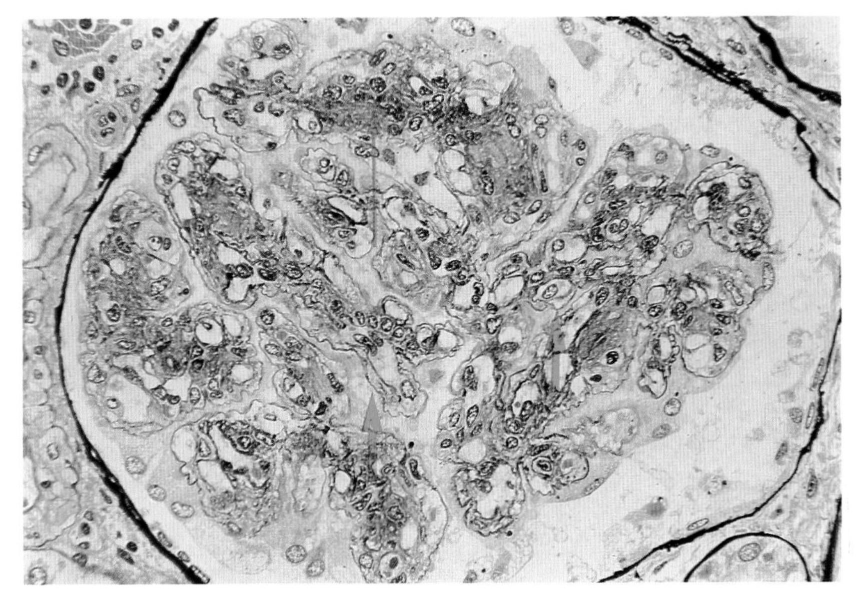

10.23 Membranoproliferative glomerulonephritis: kidney

Thin (1 m) sections and the periodic acid-methenamine silver method make it possible to see the structural changes in the glomeruli in membranoproliferative glomerulonephritis more clearly. Membranoproliferative glomerulonephritis can readily be distinguished from membranous nephropathy by the absence of " bristles" on the outer surface of the glomerular basement membrane. The characteristic changes of membranoproliferative glomerulonephritis are also more easily seen. There is an increase in the endothelial cells. There is also glomerulosclerosis in the form of fine black-staining fibres (thin arrow). In some areas the glomerular basement membrane, particularly in the peripheral capillaries, is a double line (thick arrows) as a result of new fibres being laid down within the existing basement membrane. The inner line of black fibres are mesangial fibres formed by the extension of mesangial cell cytoplasm which lies between the two lines of black fibre.

Periodic acid-methenamine silver ×450

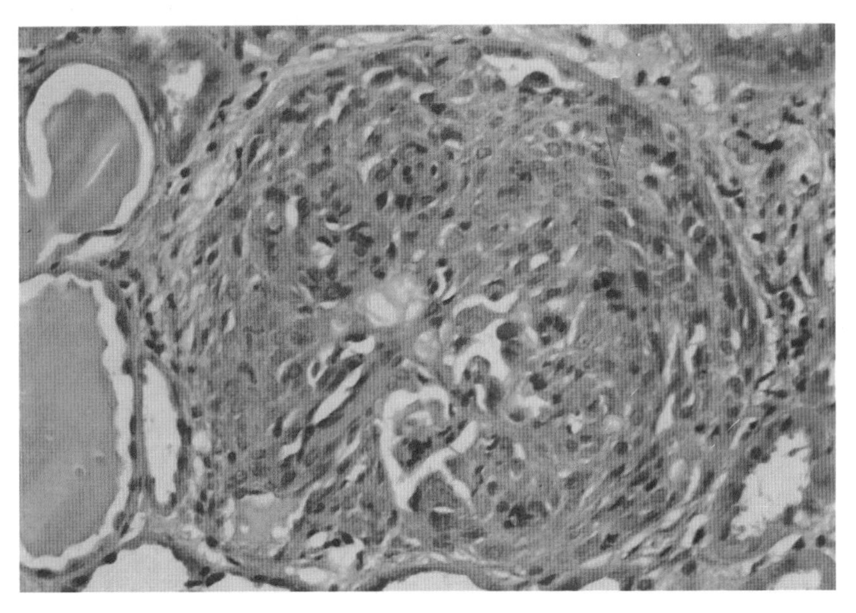

10.24 Goodpasture's syndrome: kidney

Goodpasture's syndrome affects mainly the lungs and kidneys. There is extensive intra-alveolar hemorrhage. The glomerular changes vary with the course of the disease. In early cases there is acute focal glomerulonephritis, with hematuria and proteinuria. Later, rapidly progressive glomerulonephritis may develop. The prognosis is very poor. Uniquely, an autoantibody is present in the serum which reacts specifically with the basement membrane of the glomerular capillaries and of the pulmonary capillaries. The antibody can be demonstrated immunohistologically. It can also be detected in the serum. That it is important is evidenced by the finding that the disease recurs in renal transplants if the antiglomerular antibody persists in the serum. This shows a severely affected glomerulus. It is shrunken and atrophic (thick arrow) and surrounded by, and closely adherent to, a large epithelial crescent which fills Bowman's space. A considerable number of pyknotic and probably necrotic nuclei are also present in the glomerulus. There is eosinophilic proteinaceous material in the adjacent tubules. The tubules are lined by atrophic epithelium, probably as a result of secondary ischemic damage. HE ×310

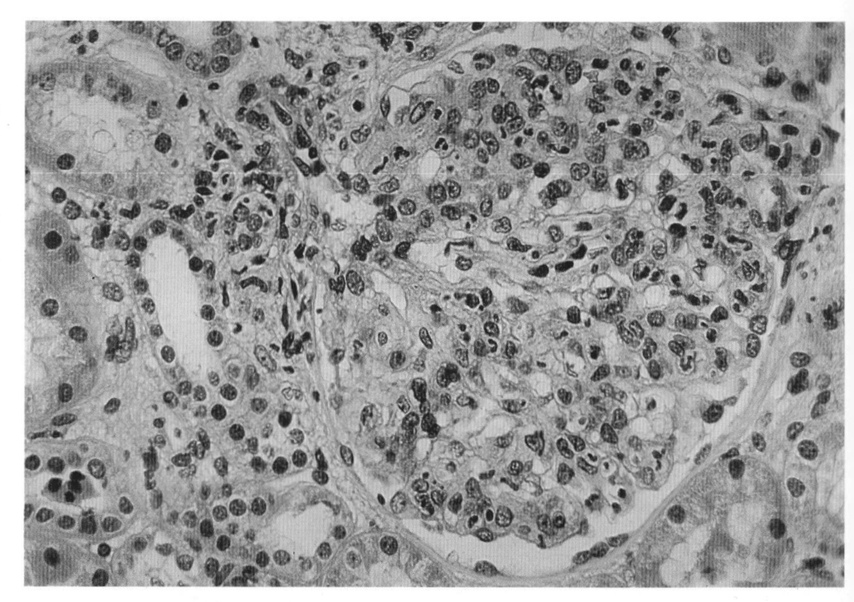

10.25 Proliferative glomerulonephritis: kidney

This form of nephritis develops 1-4 weeks after an infection with ß-hemolytic streptococci (Group A), often in the throat. The relation to streptococcal infection would suggest an immunological mechanism, but there is no convincing evidence for this. However, a very interesting relationship between the type of infecting streptococcus and the development of glomerulonephritis has been demonstrated. These nephritogenic streptococcal types include type 12 and type 49. There is malaise, fever and edema. Hematuria is also a feature. Children and young adults generally recover completely in a week or two, but a minority of adults develop rapidly progressive glomerulonephritis, or the condition persists in a clinically silent form. The glomerular tuft shows marked increase in cellularity, as a result of proliferation of endothelial cells and infiltration with polymorph leukocytes. Immunohistological studies show a granular deposition of IgG and the C3 component of complement in the glomeruli. The increased number of swollen endothelial cells has blocked the lumen of many capillaries, and the swollen tuft has almost obliterated Bowman's space. The interstitial tissues (left) are edematous, causing separation of the tubules. HE ×335

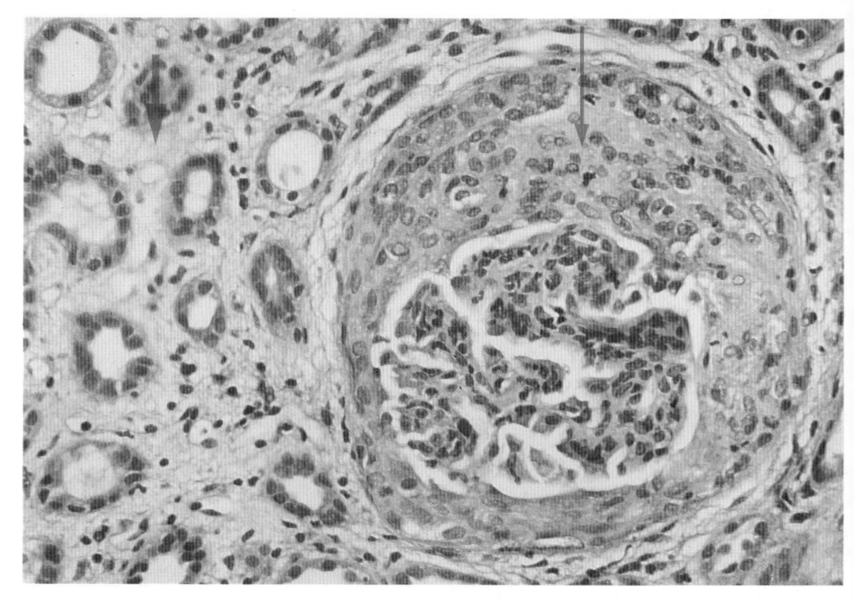

10.26 Proliferative glomerulonephritis: kidney

This patient had an attack of acute diffuse proliferative glomerulonephritis which did not clear up. There is a large cellular crescent (thin arrow) which fills Bowman's space (extracapillary glomerulitis). Crescent formation is associated with previous severe damage to the glomerulus, and the glomerulus is shrunken. The tubules (left) are widely separated from one another by edematous interstitial tissue (thick arrow). The normal epithelium of the tubules is replaced by a low simple epithelium, possibly as a result of regeneration following previous tubular damage. There is good evidence from immunohistological studies that the stimulus to the formation of the crescent is deposited fibrin. Previously it was almost universally accepted that the cells forming the crescent were glomerular epithelial cells, although there was controversy as to whether they were visceral or parietal epithelial cells, or possibly both. More recently the suggestion has been made that they are in fact infiltrating macrophages. HE ×270

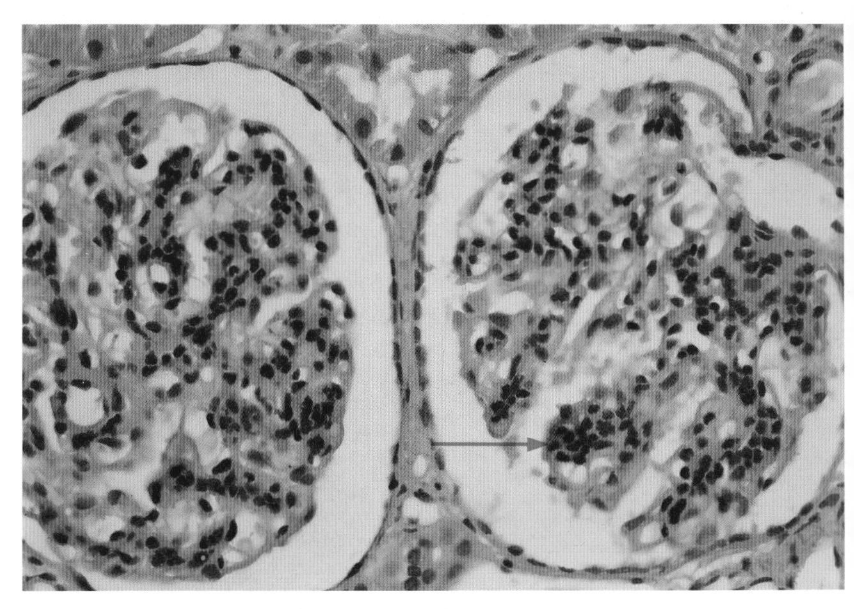

10.27 Proliferative glomerulonephritis: kidney

A boy of 16 had an attack of acute diffuse proliferative glomerulonephritis (post-streptococcal). This biopsy specimen was taken 12 weeks later because of persistent proteinuria. There is fairly pronounced proliferation of mesangial cells throughout both glomerular tufts without much increase of mesangial matrix. The endothelial and epithelial cells and the capillary basement membranes appear normal. Increased numbers of cells in the mesangium may persist for many weeks after an attack of acute proliferative glomerulonephritis, and they may provide retrospective confirmation of the diagnosis. The lobular pattern of the glomeruli and the mesangial proliferation (arrow) in this case are therefore not unexpected. It is generally held, clinically, that the prognosis for recovery in post-streptococcal glomerulonephritis is very good. However biopsy studies have shown that even in cases with no clinical evidence of disease and no urinary abnormalities, there may still be an increase in endothelial cells in the glomeruli. HE ×360

10.28 Proliferative glomerulonephritis: kidney

This is the same case as shown in 10.27. The changes in the glomerulus are seen more clearly in this thin (1μm) section stained by the periodic acid-methenamine silver method than in ordinary HE sections. The lobules of the glomerulus are clearly demonstrated. There is no abnormality of the endothelial or epithelial cells or of the peripheral capillary basement membranes; and Bowman's capsule is not thickened. In all the lobules however the mesangium is more membrane prominent than normal, from increase of nuclei (arrow). At higher magnification a double basement was detectable in several capillary loops. The changes in the basement membrane did not allow a firm diagnosis of early membranocapillary glomerulonephritis.

Periodic acid-methenamine silver ×440

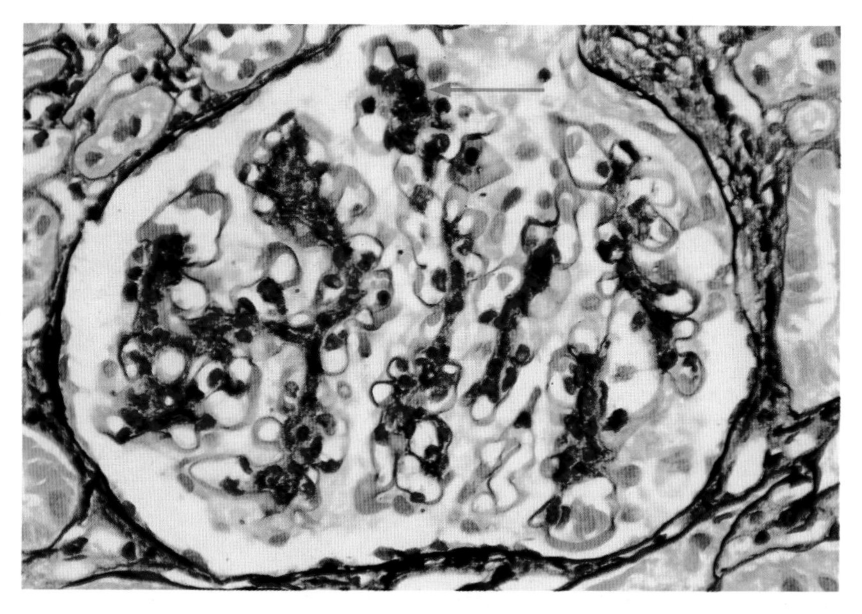

10.29 Lobular membranoproliferative glomerulonephritis: kidney

Lobularglomerulonephritis is a form of membranoproliferative (or mesangioproliferative) glomerulonephritis which is characterized by accentuated lobulation of the glomerular tuft with solidification of the centrilobular or mesangial region. The lobules assume a club shape (thick arrows), and all glomeruli are affected. The changes are demonstrated particularly effectively in thin (1 μm) resin-embedded sections stained by the periodic acid methenamine silver method, and in this example the increased size and argyrophilia of the mesangium are very obvious (thin arrow). This morphological variant of membranoproliferative glomerulonephritis was originally considered to be a separate entity, and in HE-stained sections was sometimes confused with diabetic glomerulopathy or with amyloidosis; but with the method used in staining this section the nature of the changes can be seen much more clearly and its relation to classical membranoproliferative glomerulonephritis is apparent. Periodic acid-methenamine silver ×440

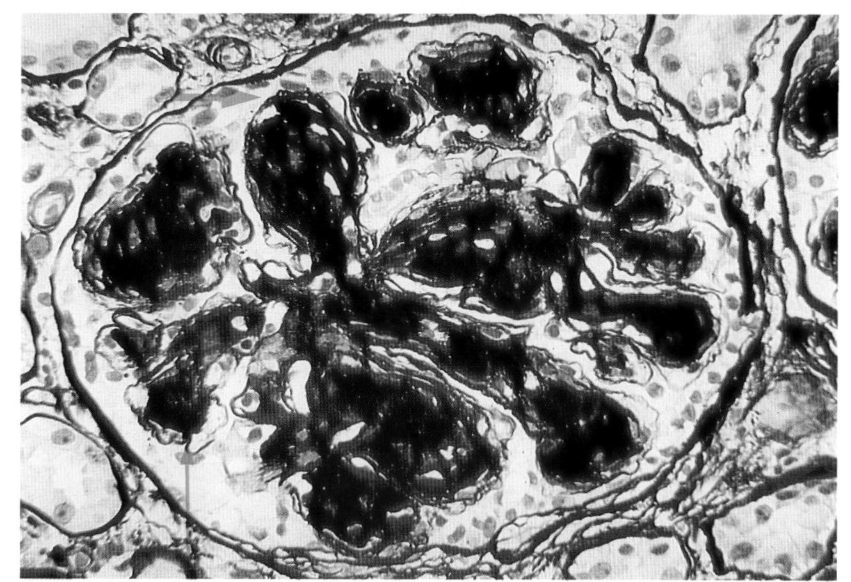

10.30 Chronic glomerulonephritis: kidney

Chronic glomerulonephritis is the end-stage of various forms of glomerulonephritis. The patient is uremic, hypertensive and in chronic renal failure. The glomerular tuft is sclerosed and many of its capillaries are obliterated (thin arrow). There are extensive adhesions between the tuft and Bowman's capsule, and Bowman's space is reduced to several narrow slits lined by proliferated enlarged epithelial cells. There is marked periglomerular (thick arrow) and interstitial fibrosis. The tubules on the left (double arrow) are so damaged that it is not possible to identify them with certainty, but they are probably grossly altered proximal convoluted tubules. Changes similar to these were present throughout both kidneys, involving all the glomeruli. The glomerulosclerosis, the loss of tubules, and the interstitial fibrosis may progress to such an extent that it is impossible to diagnose the original disease. This happens frequently nowadays when patients in complete renal failure are kept alive by hemodialysis. The cause of the slowly progressive destruction of the kidney over many years after the damage produced by the original disease is uncertain. One theory is that the reduced number of nephrons left by the initial disease have to cope with the same volume of glomerular filtrate and so are subject to hyperfiltration that slowly damages them. It is also thought that the persistent hypertension may be a factor HE ×335

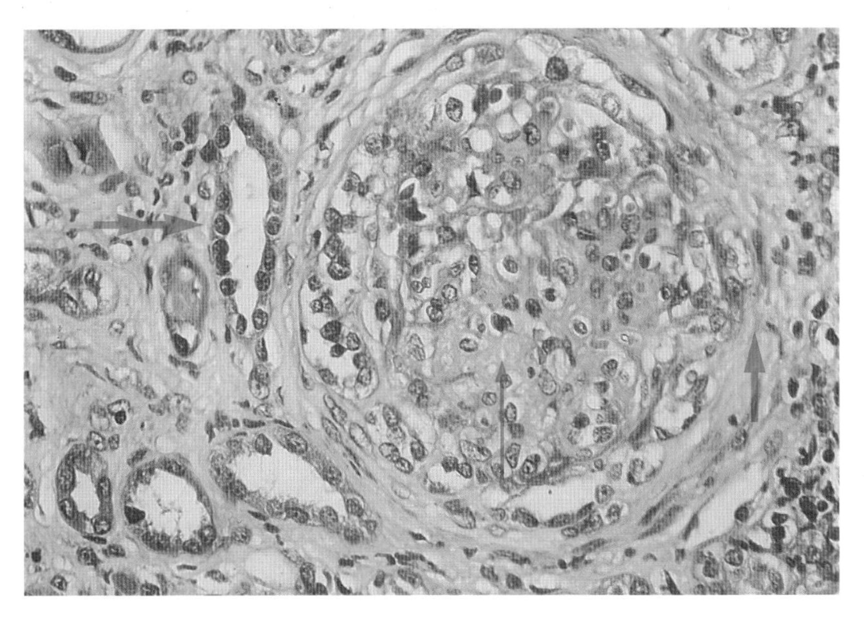

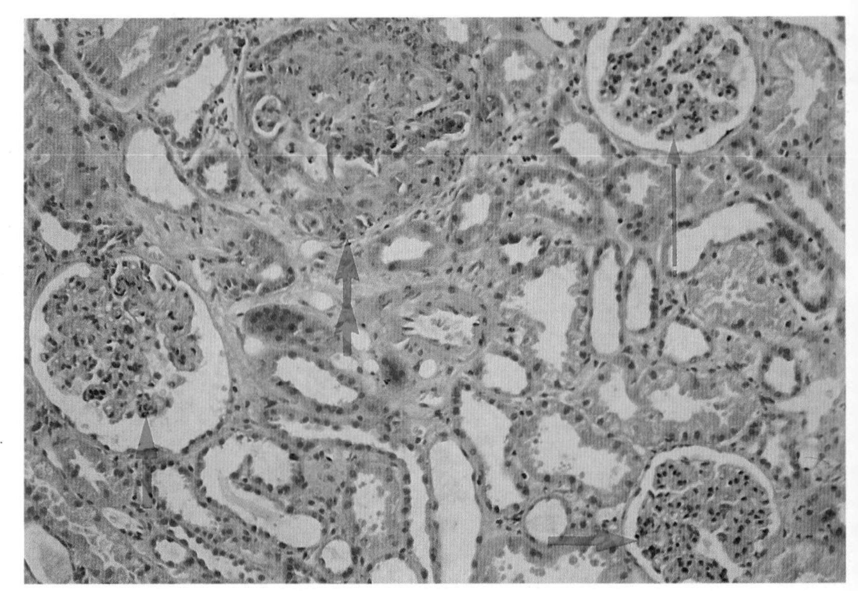

10.31 Focal (segmental) glomerulonephritis: kidney

In focal glomerulonephritis the lesions are confined to a part of each glomerulus, and it is said that only some glomeruli have lesions. This is difficult to prove for, as may be seen in this figure, only a relatively small part of the glomerulus is affected. Many sections through the glomerulus would miss the lesion. There is a strong association with certain diseases, including subacute bacterial endocarditis, systemic lupus erythematosus, Goodpasture's syndrome, Henoch-Schönlein purpura and polyarteritis nodosa. The changes were interpreted as being due to very small emboli, and so the name focal embolic nephritis was applied to it. This is now considered to be mistaken and the name has been discarded. It is generally thought that there is an underlying immunological cause. The presenting sign is usually hematuria. A woman of 64 with rapidly progressive renal failure, hematuria and sinusitis was suspected of having Wegener's syndrome. One glomerulus (thin arrow) appears normal but foci of necrosis and disruption of the capillary loops are present in two others (thick arrows). The fourth glomerulus (double arrow) is severely (globally) damaged; and there is an accumulation of cells in Bowman's space. The tubules are lined by a low simple epithelium.

HE ×150

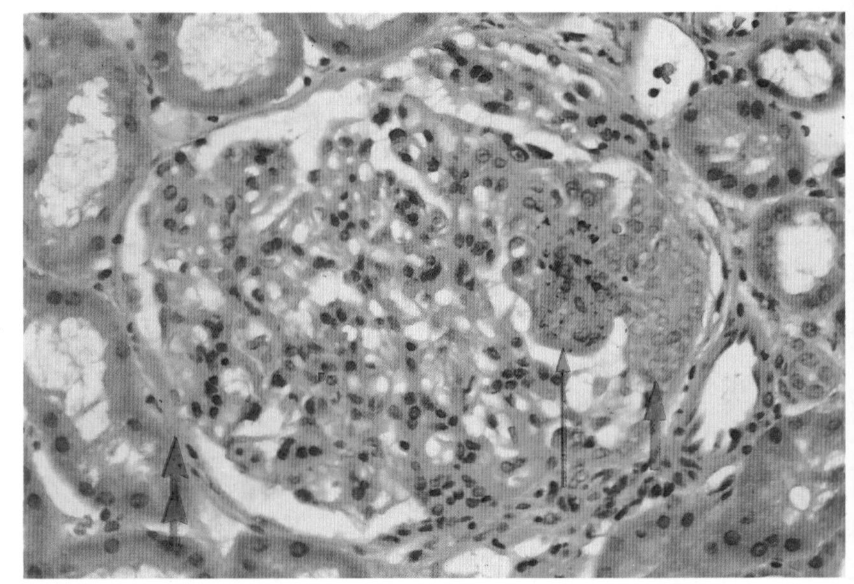

10.32 Focal (segmental) glomerulonephritis: kidney

This shows one glomerulus at higher magnification. Most of one lobule (thin arrow) is necrotic and disrupted, containing many nuclear fragments. It is adherent to a small epithelial crescent on Bowman's capsule (thick arrow). Several other foci in the tuft show similar but less severe changes, and one is adherent to Bowman's capsule (double arrow). The remainder of the tuft appears fairly normal, apart from some increase in cells in the mesangium. The tubules show no significant lesion. The lesion in this glomerulus has the appearance of a recent active lesion. Frequently in this disease glomerular lesions of different ages may be seen, some active and cellular as here, and other showing varying decrees of sclerosis.

HE ×290

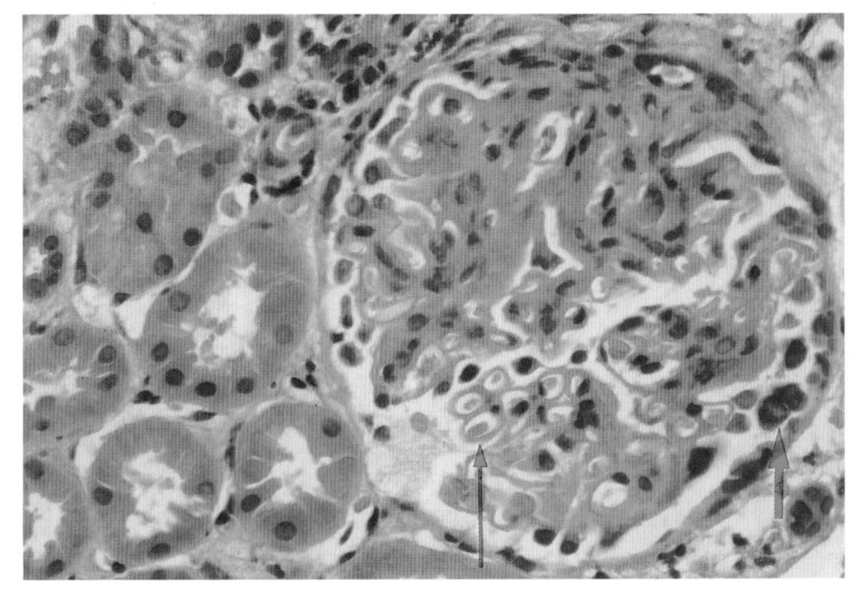

10.33 Systemic lupus erythematosus: kidney

Renal lesions are very common in systemic lupus erythematosus. A considerable majority of affected individuals will show some clinical signs of renal disease (nephrotic syndrome, proteinuria, etc.) and many die from renal failure. The glomerular lesions take various forms. These include focal glomerulonephritis, membranoproliferative glomerulonephritis, and membranous nephropathy. In this case the glomerular tuft is excessively lobulated. In one half of the glomerulus the pink hyaline thickening of the mesangium is so marked that the capillary lumens are almost obliterated. In another area the walls of the capillaries are infiltrated to a varying extent with a homogeneous eosinophilic material which gives many of them a "wire-loop" appearance (thin arrow). This characteristic feature is produced by a thick immune deposit, including immunoglobulins, on the inner surface of the glomerular basement membrane. Another characteristic feature of system lupus erythematosus is the presence of hematoxyphil bodies. There are several here in Bowman's space (thick arrow). The tubules (left) appear normal.

HE ×440

10.34 Arteriolosclerosis and glomerulosclerosis: kidney

The characteristic lesion in benign essential hypertension is hyaline thickening of the arterioles by the deposition of an eosinophilic amorphous material beneath the endothelium and in the media. This affects virtually all arterioles, but in contrast to the arteriolar hyalinization seen in diabetic nephropathy, the efferent glomerular arterioles are not involved. This glomerulus is globally sclerosed, with greatly reduced cellularity (thin arrow). It is adherent to Bowman's capsule at several points (double arrow). The arteriole (thick arrow) has a thick hyalinized wall and a much-reduced lumen, from the deposition of eosinophilic amorphous material beneath the endothelium and in the media. The narrowing of the lumen of the arteriole reduces the flow of blood to the glomerulus and the resulting ischemia leads to glomerulosclerosis. As the arterioles are diffusely involved, the ischemic damage is also diffuse, resulting in small subcapsular areas of ischemic damage, producing a fine granularity. HE ×470

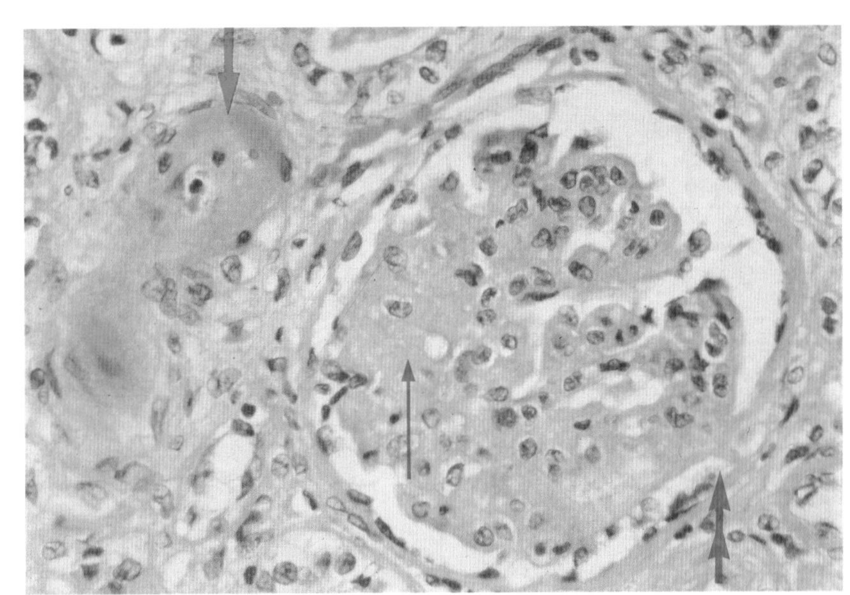

10.35 Malignant hypertension: kidney

Malignant hypertension, i.e. a diastolic blood pressure of more than 130 mm Hg accompanied by retinopathy and papilledema, causes a characteristic lesion in the afferent glomerular arterioles consisting of fibrinoid necrosis of the walls of arterioles which commonly extends into the glomeruli. In the arcuate and interlobular arteries there is marked intimal thickening with concentric layers of loose cellular fibrous tissue. The prognosis is poor. The afferent arteriole and the adjacent part of the glomerular tuft are necrotic (thick arrow). The necrotic tissue resembles fibrin in its strongly eosinophilic staining reaction and the term fibrinoid necrosis is used. Immunohistological studies show that the material in the arteriolar wall consists of fibrinogen with an admixture of other plasma proteins. The rest of the tuft is shrunken, lobulated and slightly fibrosed (thin arrow). The epithelial cells lining Bowman's capsule are prominent. There is a dense protein cast in the tubule (double arrow). The capillary blood vessels are very congested. HE ×400

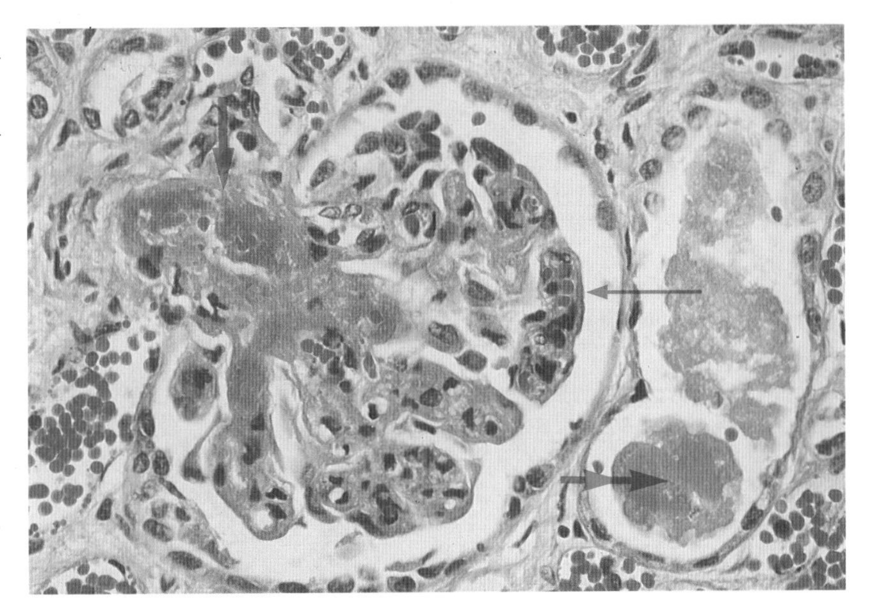

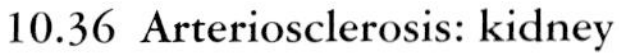

10.36 Arteriosclerosis: kidney

Arteriosclerosis is a diffuse change which affects all coats of the artery. In the kidney the changes are markedly accentuated, if not initiated, by benign essential hypertension. In the early stages there is hypertrophy of the muscular media, but later there may be some fibrosis of the media. There are marked intimal changes with considerable fibrous thickening and newly formed elastic fibres. The elastic fibres form new incomplete elastic laminae internal to the original elastic lamina (reduplication of the elastic lamina). This artery, from a person who was hypertensive, is an arcuate artery; that is, an artery that runs in an arc between the cortex and medulla of the kidney. The media is hypertrophied, with an increase in the number of smooth muscle cells (thick arrows). As in the normal state, the muscle fibres are arranged circularly, as is evident from the pattern of their nuclei. The intima is also very thick and fibrous (thin arrow) and the lumen consequently much narrowed. The elastic lamina and the intimal elastic fibres cannot be clearly seen in this preparation, but there is some suggestion of increased elastic fibres internal to the elastic lamina in the lower left quadrant. HE ×175

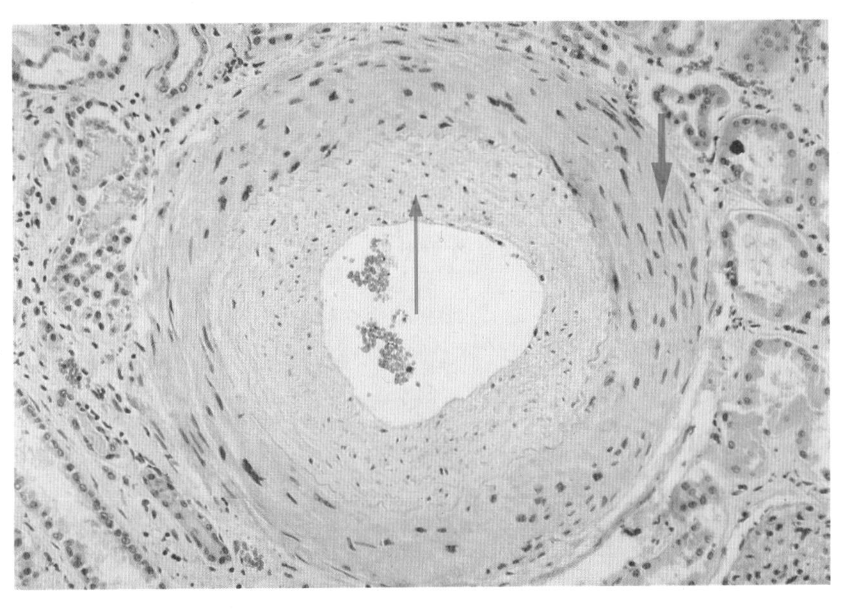

10.37 Rejection: renal allograft

A transplanted kidney induces an immunological reaction in the host. The histological appearances consequent upon this are complex, variable and alter with time. There is immunological damage to the blood vessels as well as the renal parenchyma so that the histological appearances are complicated by the presence of ischemic as well as immunological damage The transplanted kidney induces a cellular and humoral response. Cellular rejection develops during the first few weeks after transplantation and is generally controllable by immunosuppressive drug therapy. However, acute rejection may occur at almost any time after transplantation. This kidney, transplanted 7 months previously into a 13-year-old girl, shows a severe cellular rejection reaction. The glomerulus (centre) is shrunken (thin arrow) and the endothelial cells are swollen. There is severe tubular damage, with replacement of the epithelium by flattened cells. Many of the epithelial cells are vacuolated and some appear necrotic. The interstitial tissues are edematous, with wide separation of the tubules (double arrow). In the interstitial tissues there are small hemorrhages and an infiltrate of chronic inflammatory cells which tends to concentrate around the tubules (thick arrow) HE ×150

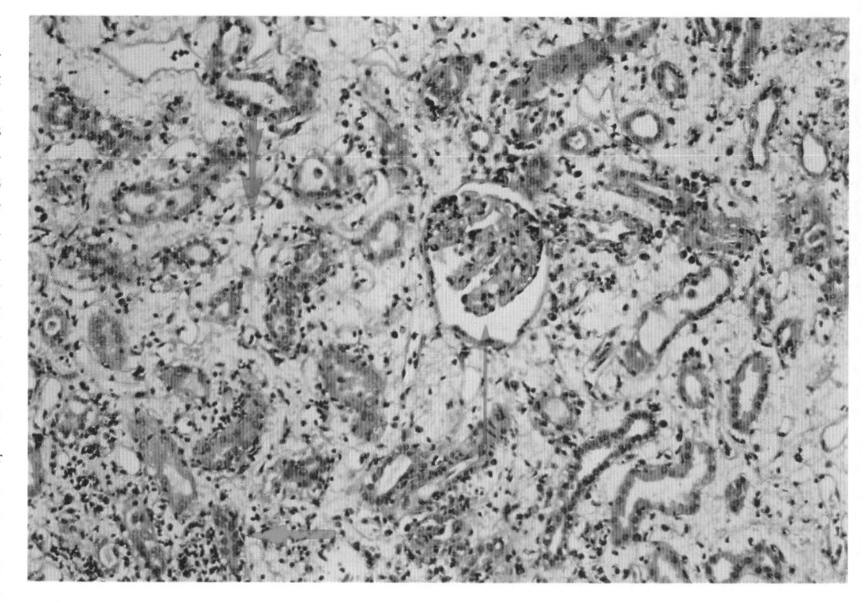

10.38 Acute vascular and cellular rejection: renal allograft

This renal allograft of 14 days' duration in a man of 34 was removed from the recipient because of a severe vascular and cellular rejection reaction. It was swollen (265g) and its surface was mottled and hemorrhagic. This shows the collecting tubules in longitudinal section. There is extensive necrosis of their epithelium (thin arrow) and several tubules contain eosinophilic fluid or blood (thick arrow). There is also extensive hemorrhage into the interstitial tissues (double arrow). The arteries also showed severe rejection damage (**10.39**) and some arterioles were necrotic. The glomeruli were hypercellular.

HE ×235

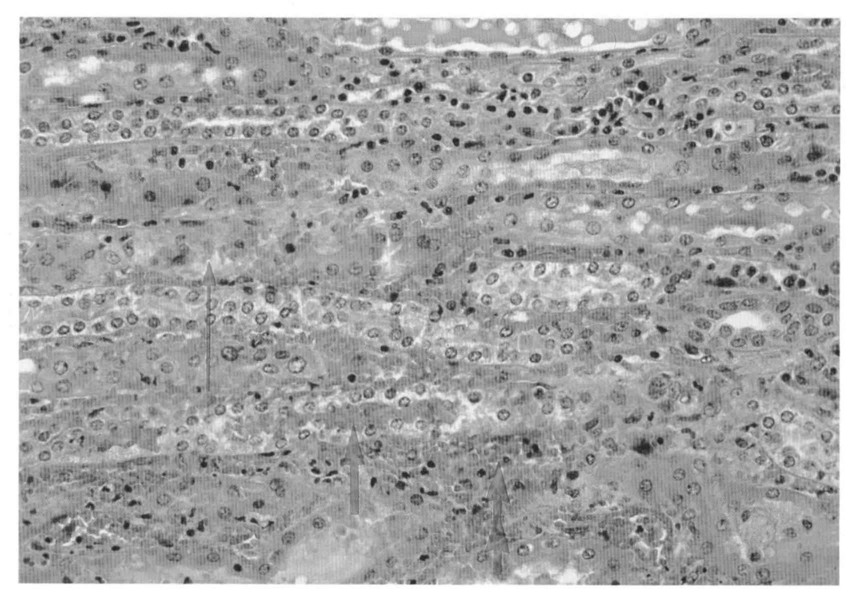

10.39 Acute vascular and cellular rejection: renal allograft

This is the same kidney as that shown in **10.38**. Immunological induced vascular damage is an important cause of loss of all sorts of grafts, liver and heart as well as kidney. The changes seen in the arteries are complex and vary with time. Initially there is swelling of the endothelial cells and an infiltrate of inflammatory cells. There then may be marked intimal thickening with clear foamy cells that almost occlude the lumen. Finally the intimal thickening may become organised (**10.42**). This is a small muscular artery in cross-section. The media appears normal apart from the presence of a few lymphocytes. The intima however is greatly thickened by proliferated and swollen endothelial cells and an infiltrate of mononuclear inflammatory cells (arrow). The lumen is so small that the vessel is probably non-functional. Its adventitia and the interstitial tissues of the kidney are packed with an infiltrate of small lymphocytes, plasma cells and histiocytes. HE ×360

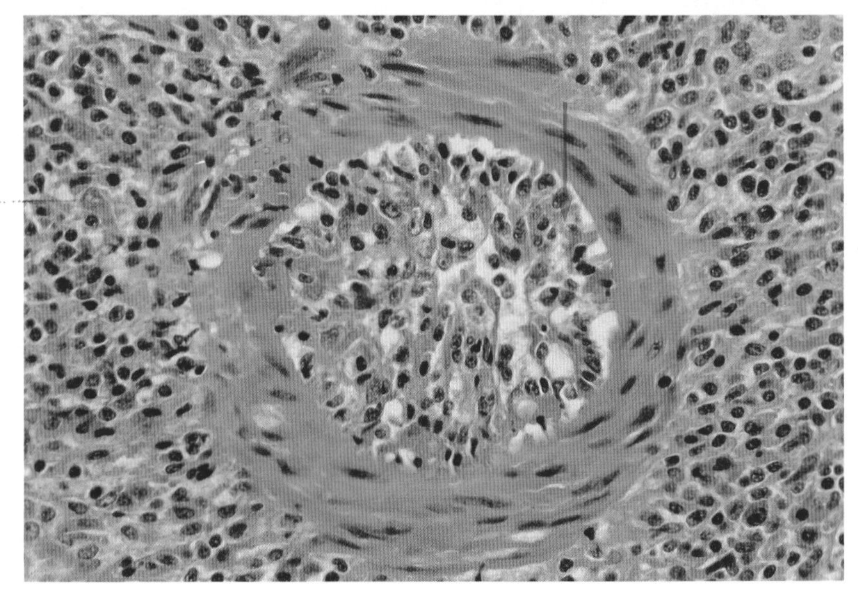

10.40 Severe chronic vascular rejection: renal allograft

In chronic rejection of a renal allograft, vascular lesions predominate and may cause renal failure through ischemia. Once the arterial changes have become severe and organised the damage is irreversible and the kidney is inevitably lost. The arterial damage may be accompanied by venous thrombosis. This case illustrates the complexity of the changes in late grafts. This is an allograft of 19 months' duration in a man of 53. The most marked change is the loss of tubules; and many of those remaining (e.g. bottom left) are small and lined by very atrophic epithelium. The interstitial tissue is considerably expanded, severely fibrosed and heavily infiltrated by chronic inflammatory cells (thin arrow). One glomerulus is atrophic (thick arrow). There is some epithelial and mesangial proliferation in the others but they are fairly well preserved. The loss of tubules which has resulted in a crowding together of the glomeruli is predominantly due to ischemia. The heavy interstitial infiltrate with lymphocytes is more difficult to interpret, but is probably an immunological response. HE ×150

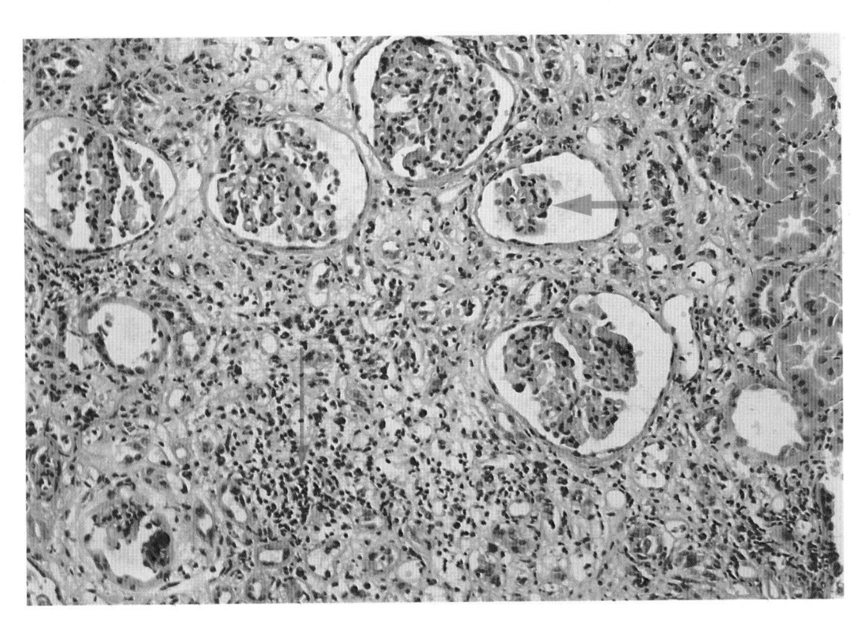

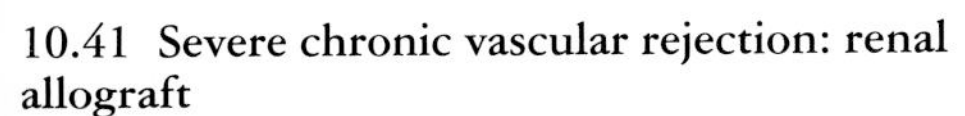

10.41 Severe chronic vascular rejection: renal allograft

This is the same kidney as that shown in 10.40. The two glomeruli show predominantly ischemic change. There is thickening of the basement membrane of Bowman's capsule (thin arrow). There is also some mesangial and extracapillary cell proliferation. The glomerular basement membrane shows ischemic corrugation. There is severe loss of tubules and those surviving are very atrophic (thick arrows). An infiltrate of inflammatory cells is present in the interstitial tissues. HE ×360

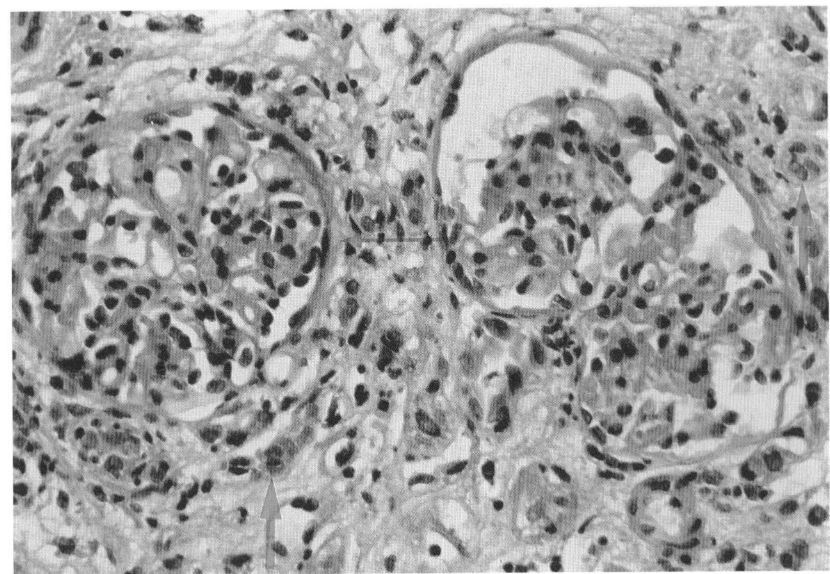

10.42 Chronic vascular rejection: renal allograft

This is a biopsy specimen from a renal allograft of approximately 3 months' duration in a boy of 15. It shows the final stages of the organisation of the intimal thickening in the small arteries. At this stage the intimal thickening is clearly irreversible. The previously cellular intimal thickening of the small arteries has become organised. There is a very thick layer of edematous poorly vascular fibrous tissue (double arrow). Around the much reduced lumen is a layer of circumferentially arranged smooth muscle (thin arrows) closely resembling the intact original muscular media of the arteries. Elastic laminae may be formed in such muscular layers, increasing the resemblance to rudimentary arterial walls. With these arterial changes it can be readily understood that much of the damage to the renal parenchyma, i.e. marked loss of tubules, interstitial fibrous and the glomerular damage results from chronic ischemia consequent upon the vascular damage. HE ×235

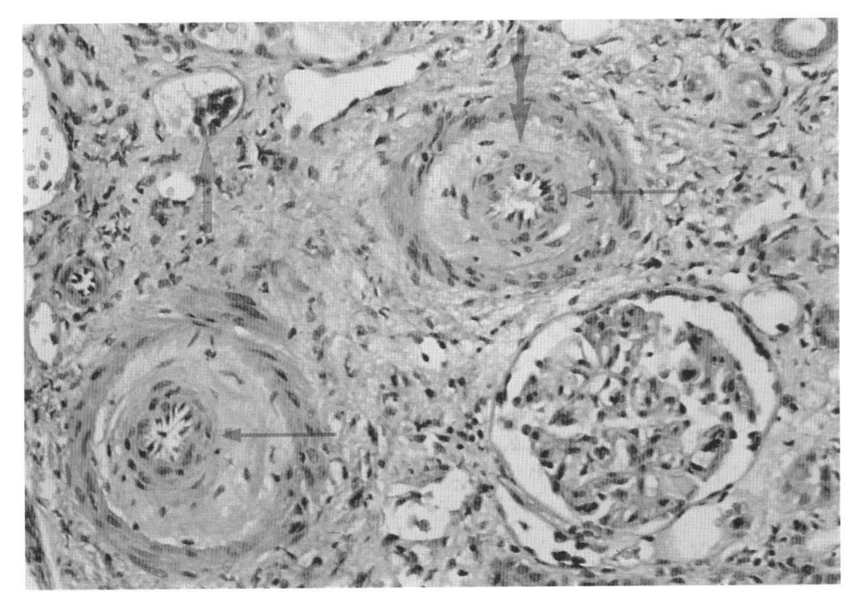

10.43 Adenoma: kidney

Adenomas of the kidney are located most usually in the subcapsular cortex. Most commonly they are quite small, only a few mm in dia and as they are generally regarded as insignificant their incidence is underestimated, but they are said to be present in about 4% of all kidneys examined at autopsy. They are generally thought to be more common in scarred contracted kidneys. They are yellowish nodules which appear encapsulated. Because of their yellow colour they are sometimes confused at autopsy with rests of adrenal tissue in or beneath the renal capsule. Such rests do occur but are much less common. The tumour (left) has a branching papillary structure, consisting of delicate cords of connective tissue covered with a single layer of cuboidal epithelial cells (thin arrow). The epithelial cells have small round nuclei which show no pleomorphism or mitotic activity. There are many pyknotic nuclei, some belonging to necrotic desquamated epithelial cells. The cytoplasm of the epithelial cells is weakly eosinophilic and in many cells it is vacuolated (the vacuoles contain lipid). There is no capsule and the tumour is bounded (right) by normal tubules lined by large epithelial cells. The wall of the arteriole is hyalinized (thick arrow). HE ×150

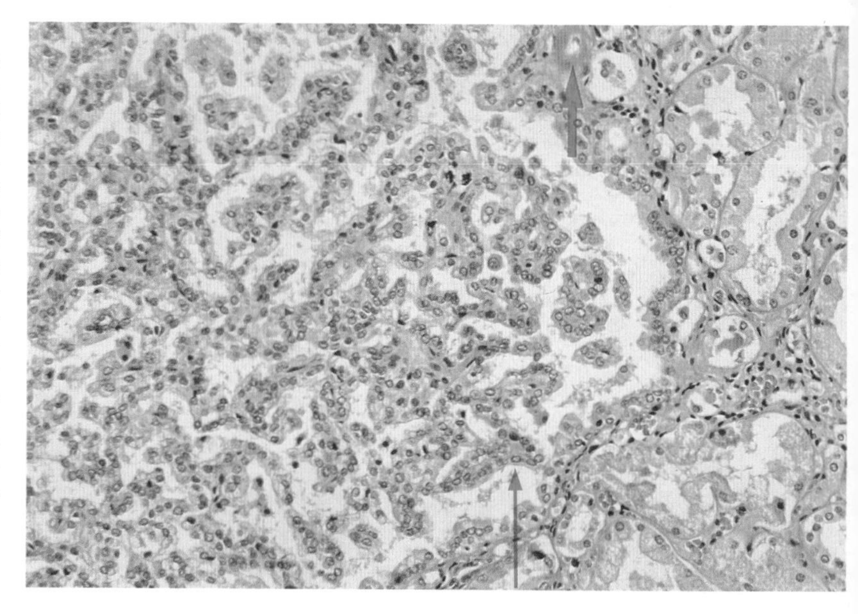

10.44 Adenoma: kidney

This shows the boundary between the tumour and the normal kidney (left) at higher magnification. There is no fibrous capsule between the tumour and the kidney. The epithelial cells covering the finger-like processes are well-differentiated, with round or ovoid vesicular nuclei which show no pleomorphism or mitotic activity. Their cytoplasm is granular and vacuolated (thick arrow). The histological appearances of an adenoma are such that it may be impossible to distinguish certainly between an adenoma and a small primary renal adenocarcinoma but lesions less than 2.5cm dia can generally be regarded as adenomas since they almost never metastasize. The wall of the arteriole is hyalinized (thin arrow). HE ×335

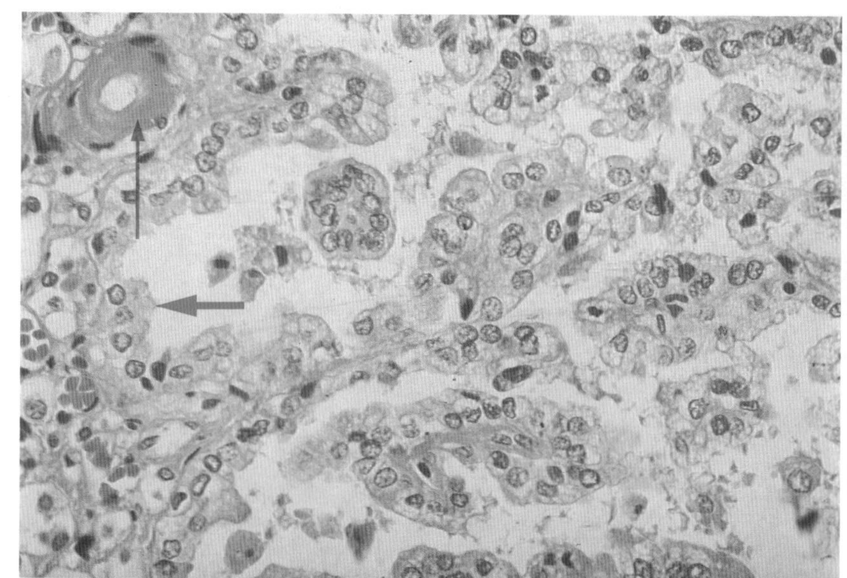

10.45 Wilms' tumour: kidney

Wilms' tumour (embryoma or nephroblastoma) is uncommon, but of the malignant tumours of infants and young children, it is the commonest. It occurs most frequently in the first three years of life, being occasionally found in the neonate or the fetus. It may form a large fleshy mass. It invades blood vessels and tends to metastasize to the lungs and elsewhere. It arises from embryonic nephrogenic tissue, though neural elements may be present. This tumour (3.5 × 3.5 × 3.0cm), in a girl of 3, was yellow and seemed to be encapsulated. It contains the two elements usually present: rudimentary glomerular ('glomeruloid') structures (thick arrows), and a loose immature spindle-cell stroma (thin arrow). The epithelial cells of the glomeruloid structures have ovoid deeply basophilic nuclei, and several mitotic figures are present. Tubules and muscular elements are often also present. The fibrous capsule was incomplete. Recent chromosomal studies have shown a loss of a gene designated WT-1, located on chromosome 11, which is a growth regulating gene.

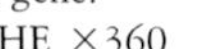

HE ×360

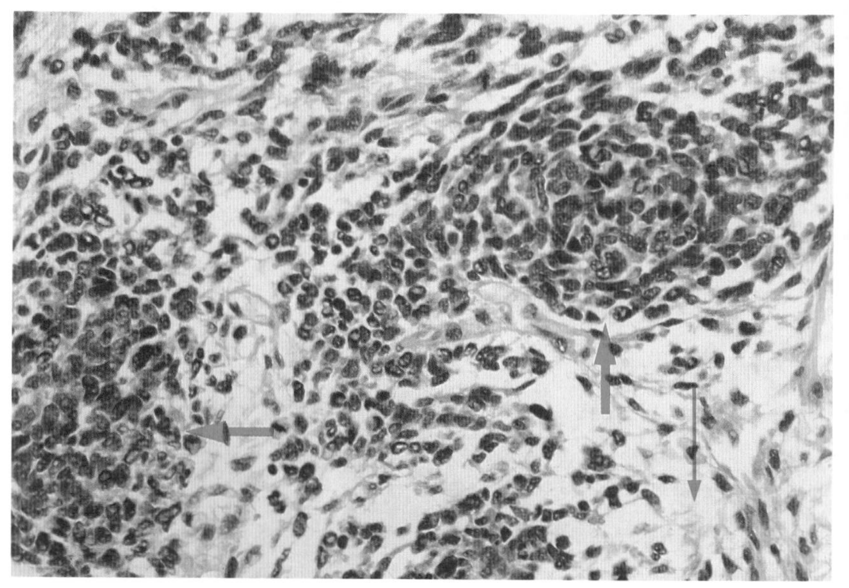

10.46 Carcinoma: kidney

Renal carcinoma occurs two to three time more frequently in men than women. There is an increased incidence in von Hippel-Lindau's disease, but as this is a rare genetic disorder it does not contribute significantly to the total number of cases. There is also an increased incidence in the extremely scarred shrunken kidneys of patients on chronic hemodialysis. The tumour originates from the renal tubular epithelium. Macroscopically it is often yellow, with extensive areas of necrosis and hemorrhage. Hematuria is frequently the presenting sign, but it may occur late in the history of the tumour so that the tumour may be quite large on presentation.. This tumour consists of large pale cells with abundant cytoplasm (thick arrows), foamy from the presence of lipid and glycogen. The nuclei are vesicular and fairly pleomorphic. They have a prominent nucleolus but there are no mitoses (they were present elsewhere in the tumour). The cytoplasmic lipid which gives the tumour its yellow colour may cause the cytoplasm to appear 'clear': clear cell carcinoma. The scanty stroma consists largely of thin-walled blood vessels (thin arrow) which tend to rupture and bleed (bottom left). HE ×135

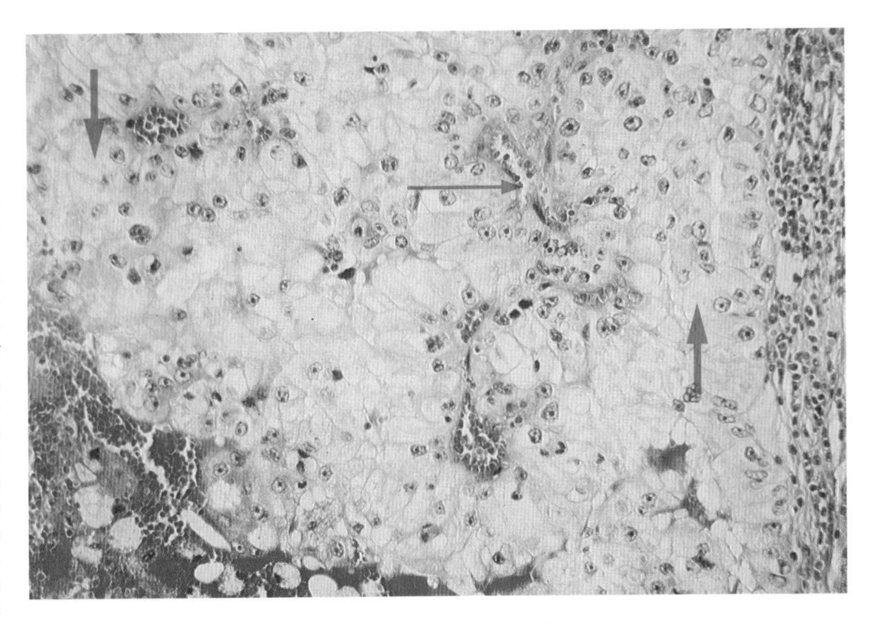

10.47 Carcinoma: kidney

The cells of renal carcinoma vary considerably in their morphology from 'clear' cells to 'solid' cells with eosinophilic cytoplasm; and not infrequently the various types are found within one tumour. The cells of this tumour are round and have eosinophilic cytoplasm (thin arrow). They are forming acini which contain pale granular secretion (thick arrow). Their nuclei are round and vesicular and fairly uniform in structure. There is no mitotic activity. The small deeply-staining nuclei are either lymphocytes or pyknotic nuclei of tumour cells. The stroma consists of thin-walled blood vessels. Cells with granular eosinophilic cytoplasm are termed oncocytes, and sometimes renal carcinomas of the type shown here are called oncocytomas. These tumours have a marked tendency to spread by the blood vessels. This may result from the numerous thin-walled blood vessels in the stroma. Not infrequently this spread may consist of a large mass of the tumour extending along the main renal vein, even reaching the inferior cava HE ×360

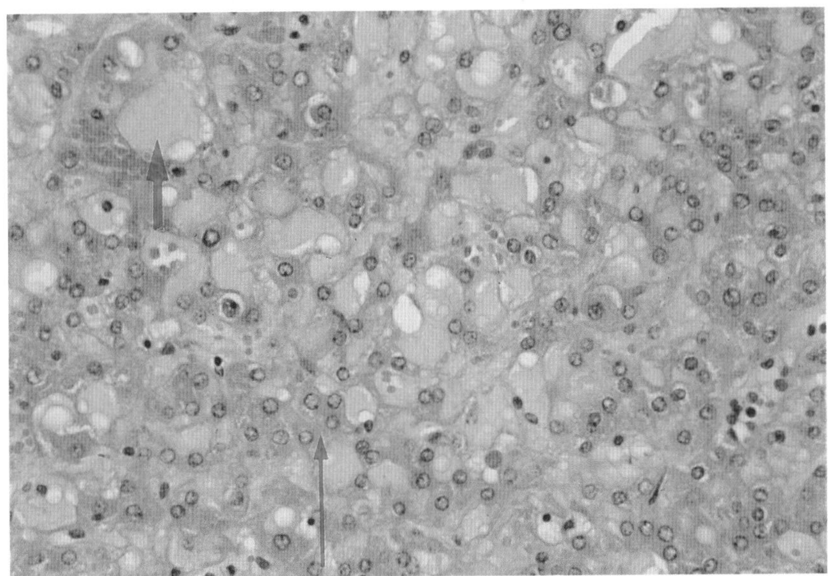

10.48 Transitional cell papilloma: renal pelvis

This tumour consisted of long delicate papilliform processes and this is the tip of one of them. It has a core of vascular connective tissue covered with a layer of fairly well-differentiated transitional epithelium (thin arrow). The cells show some loss of polarity and their nuclei are more pleomorphic than normal. The epithelial basement membrane however is intact. A mitotic figure (thick arrow) is present. As in the bladder, papillomatous tumours of transitional epithelium, however well-differentiated, are liable to recur and should be regarded not as benign papillomas but as well-differentiated papillary carcinomas (Grade I). As can be seen here there are quite numerous thin-walled blood vessels in the connective tissue core of the papillae just beneath the layer of tumour cells. Such delicate vessels are liable to bleed, and painless hematuria is often the presenting sign. In addition to the industrial carcinogens that induce transitional tumours of bladder, an increased incidence of transitional tumours of the renal pelvis has been observed in cases of analgesic abuse. These patients also suffer from papillary necrosis (10.5) but the tumours develop some years after the papillary necrosis.

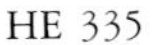
HE 335

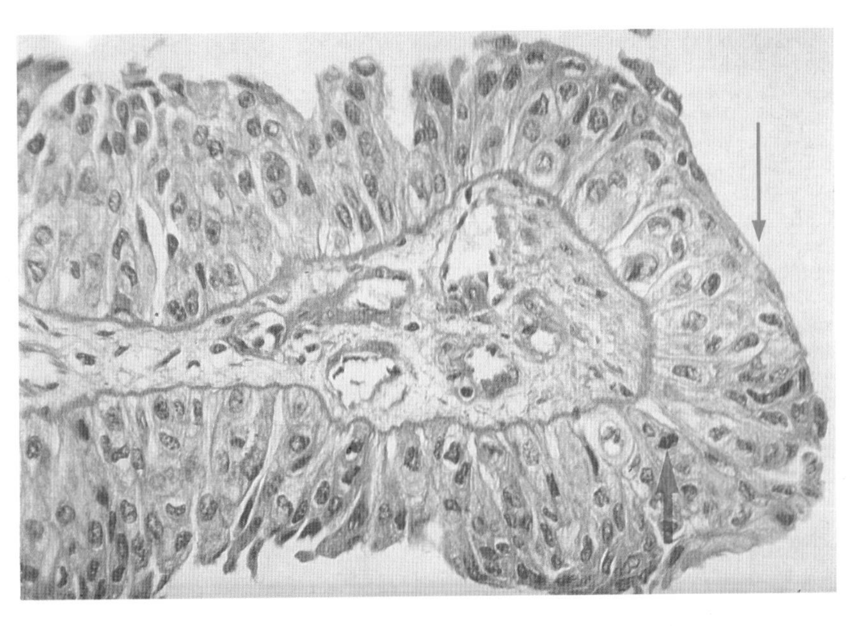

10.49 Chronic pyelitis: renal pelvis

In pyelitis the renal pelvis and calyces are inflamed. Infection spreads to them more readily from the bladder via the ureters when there is an obstruction to urinary outflow. Further spread to the renal parenchyma leads to pyelonephritis. The organism is commonly *Escherichia coli* but a mixed infection not infrequently establishes itself. The inflammatory reaction may be acute, with excretion of large numbers of polymorph leukocytes in the urine. In this case the lesion was chronic. The transitional epithelium of the renal pelvis (thin arrow) is on the left. It is intact and appears normal, apart from the presence within it of a few lymphocytes. The tissues beneath the epithelium are edematous and hyperemic and heavily infiltrated by chronic inflammatory cells, mostly plasma cells (thick arrow). HE ×135

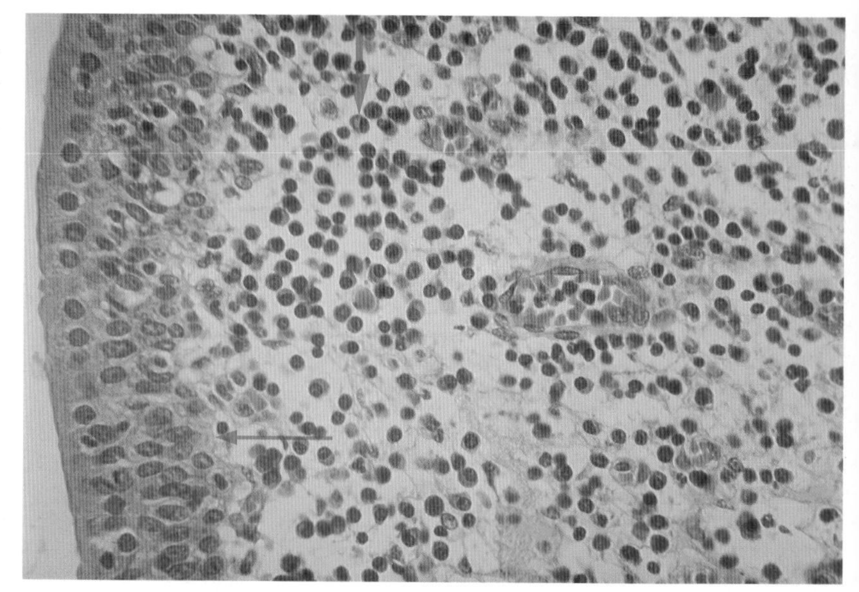

10.50 Idiopathic retroperitoneal fibrosis

Retroperitoneal fibrosis is a chronic inflammatory lesion of the para-aortic region which leads to the formation of dense fibrous tissue around the ureters. They are drawn medially and narrowed; and complete obliteration of the lumen may occur. There is an association with idiopathic fibrosing lesions in other sites (pseudotumour of the orbit, Riedel's thyroiditis, etc.) and an autoimmune basis for the disorder is suspected. In this example the ureter is on the left. The para-aortic tissues (double arrow) are heavily fibrosed and the dense fibrous tissue has spread into the muscular wall (thin arrow) of the ureter and into the submucosa. As a result there is marked narrowing of the lumen. There are two granulomas (thick arrows) in the muscle coat of the ureter. HE ×13

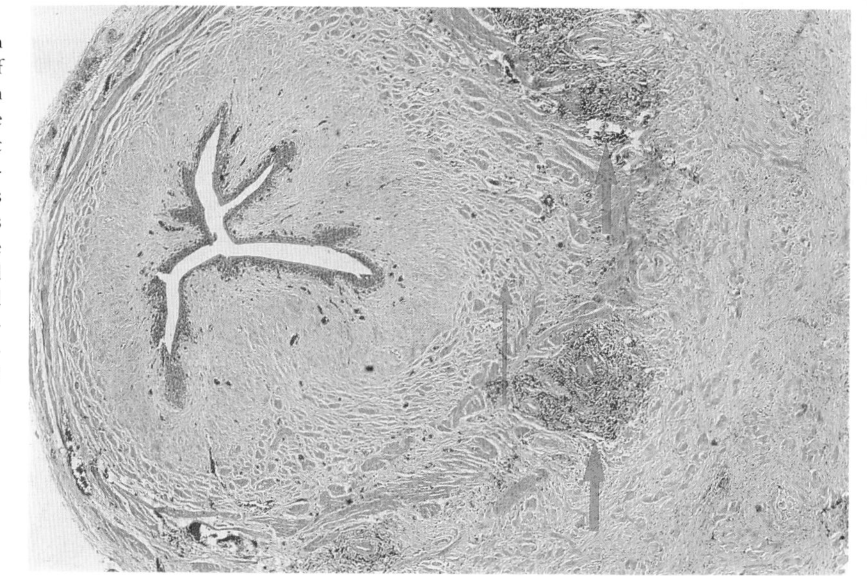

10.51 Chronic cystitis: bladder

Women are more liable to cystitis than men, although prostatic obstruction is a major predisposing factor in older men. A woman of 60 had repeated attacks of cystitis, and polypoid bladder mucosa was removed for diagnostic purposes. The transitional epithelium (left) is hyperplastic and thicker than normal (arrows). Slight nuclear pleomorphism is evident. There are no mitoses, however, and the polarity of the cells is preserved. The epithelium is infiltrated with polymorph leukocytes (bottom left) and occasional lymphocytes. The underlying lamina propria (centre and right) is edematous and hyperemic and infiltrated by chronic inflammatory cells, mostly plasma cells. The appearances are those of chronic cystitis, and the epithelial changes were presumed to be secondary to the persistent inflammatory reaction. HE ×235

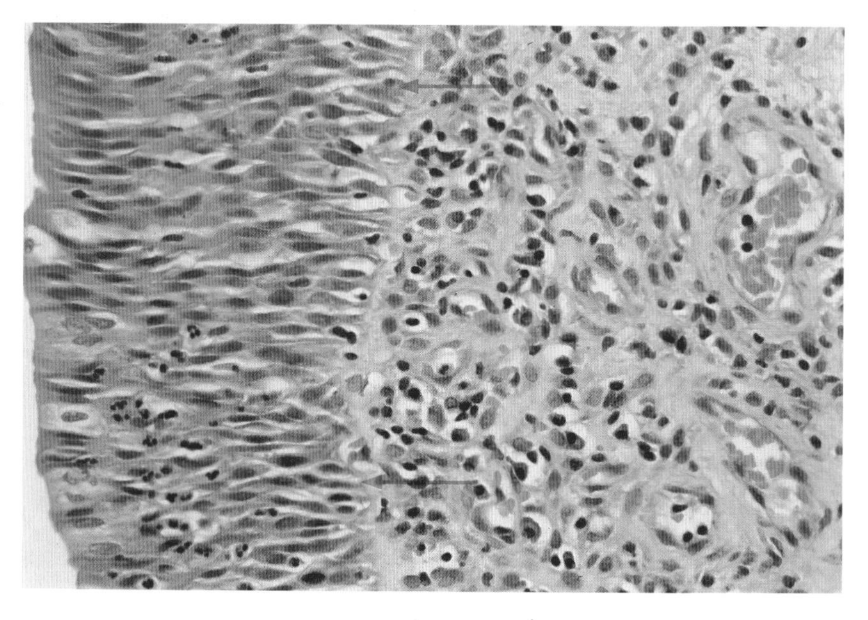

10.52 Pseudomembranous trigonitis: bladder

Sometimes in chronic cystitis the trigone of the bladder is particularly affected and the transitional epithelium there undergoes squamous metaplasia. Macroscopically, it loses the normal translucency of transitional epithelium and appears whitish and opaque. Histologically, it consists of a thick layer of well-differentiated squamous epithelium with elongated interpapillary processes. Many of the epithelial cells are vacuolated, and can be shown histochemically to contain glycogen. The resemblance therefore to vaginal epithelium is close, and the condition is sometimes called "vaginal metaplasia". The underlying submucosa is hyperemic but the number of chronic inflammatory cells is small. HE ×150

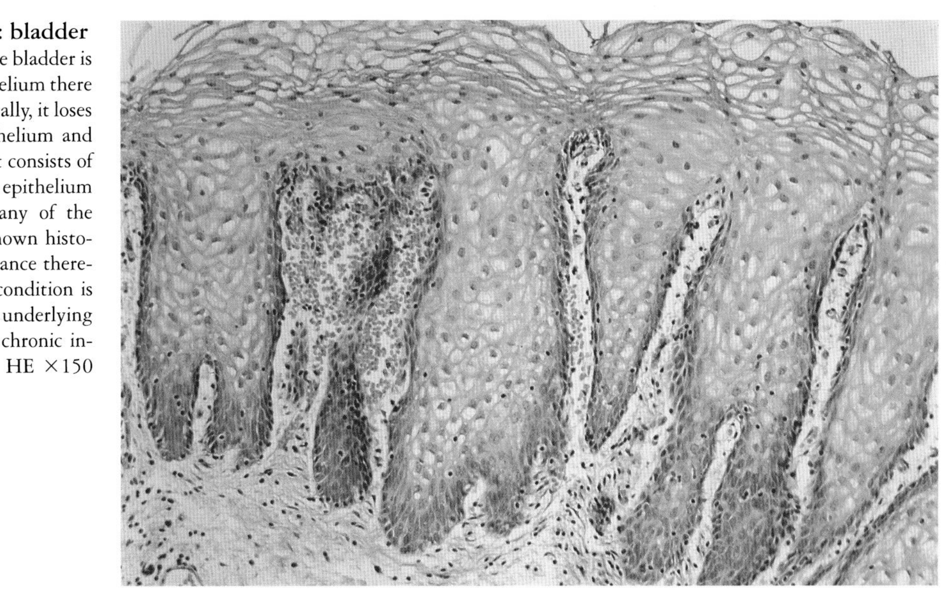

10.53 Ureteritis cystica: ureter

In a chronically inflamed bladder (cystitis) or ureter (ureteritis), the transitional epithelium may proliferate downwards into the lamina propria to form the cell-nests of von Brunn. Fluid collects in the centres of these cell-nests and with increase in the fluid they become cystic. This shows cell-nests of various sizes. The lumen of the bladder is on the left. Two large cell nests, filled with eosinophilic fluid and lined by flattened transitional epithelium (thin arrow), project into the lumen of the bladder. Smaller cell nests (thick arrows), also containing eosinophilic fluid, are being formed by epithelial downgrowths. HE ×120

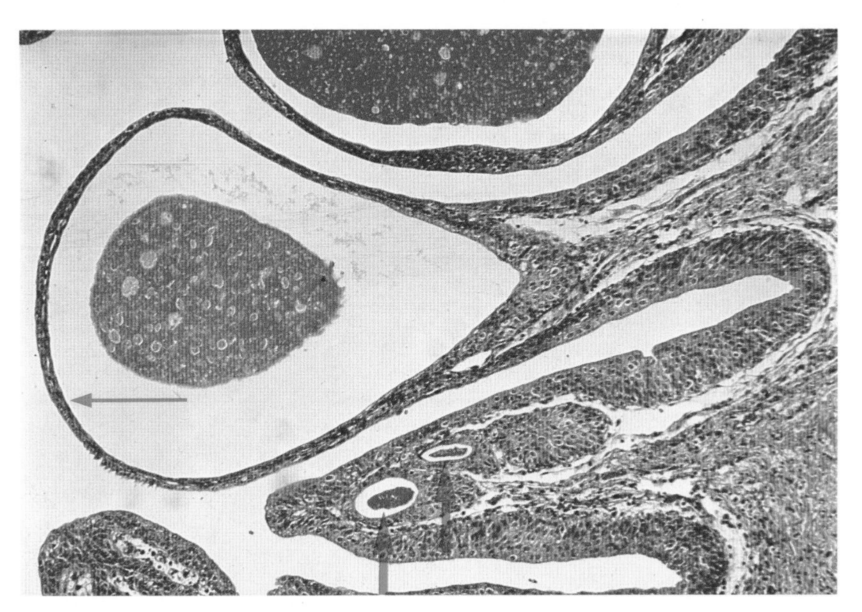

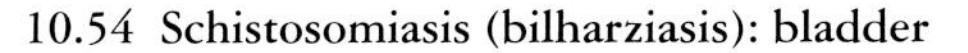

10.54 Schistosomiasis (bilharziasis): bladder

The parasitic worm Schistosoma haematobium tends to lodge in the veins of the bladder where the adult female deposits its ova in the adjacent venules. The ova (150 × 50 m), which are oval with a characteristic terminal spine escape into the bladder and leave the body in the urine, to start the next phase of the worm's life-cycle in fresh-water snails. They hatch in water to form free-swimming miracidia which infect the snails. They undergo further development in the snail, and the next phase of the infective cycle is initiated by the release from the snail of free-swimming cercaria, which can penetrate the skin of man and form the adult worms that come to rest in the veins of the bladder. In endemic areas such as Egypt and parts of East Africa, the incidence of infestation is very high, a majority of the population being affected. This disease is therefore responsible for a great burden of illness in these communities. A gravid adult female-worm (thick arrows) lies in the submucosal connective tissues of the bladder wall. There is an intense cellular infiltrate (of eosinophil leukocytes) around the worm and throughout the edematous submucosa. The transitional epithelium (top left) is hyperplastic, with downgrowths of finger-like processes (thin arrows) into the lamina propria. This hyperplasia sometimes proceeds to malignancy, and carcinoma of bladder is common in those countries in which schistosomiasis is endemic. HE ×55

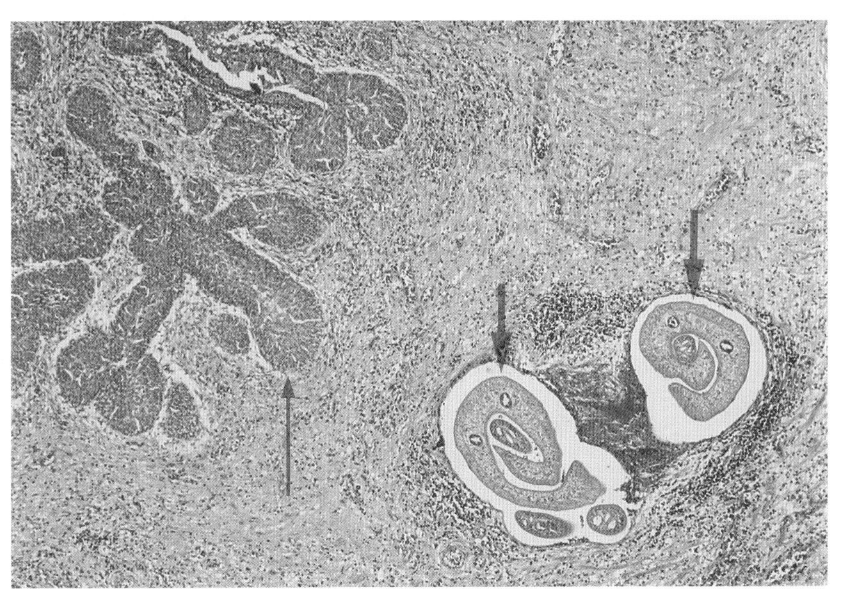

10.55 Transitional carcinoma: ureter

Transitional cell carcinomas vary widely in malignancy from Grade I, the best differentiated 'papilloma', to Grade IV, the most malignant. However even a well-differentiated 'papilloma' of transitional epithelium may recur locally and should be regarded as a low grade carcinoma. Bladder carcinomas tend to arise in the trigone region and usually present with hematuria. This neoplasm was an irregular friable mass (6 × 2.5 × 1.5cm), blocking the distal end of the left ureter in a man of 75, and the kidney was hydronephrotic. It is a papilliform lesion, consisting of short broad papillae. The papillae have a fibrovascular core (thick arrow), covered with transitional epithelium several times thicker than normal epithelium (thin arrow). The polarity of the epithelial cells is reasonably well preserved. HE ×150

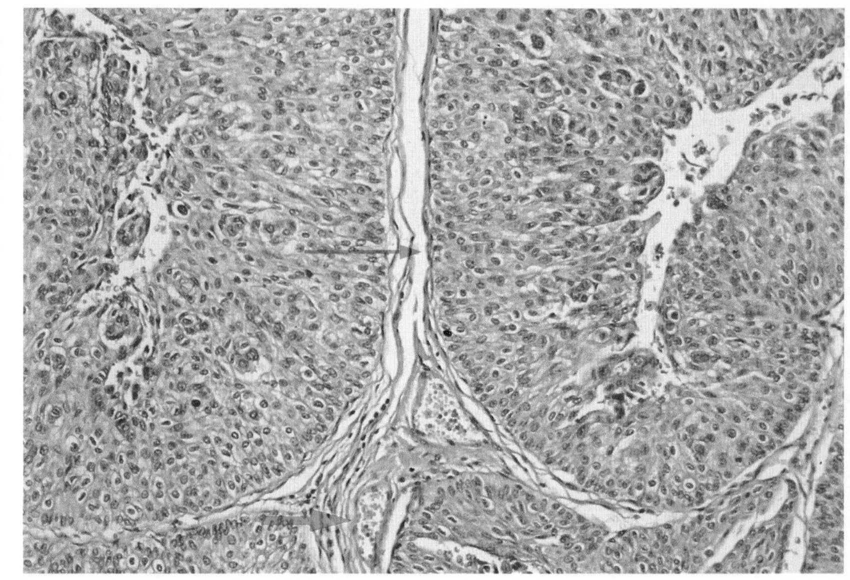

10.56 Transitional carcinoma: ureter

This shows the fibrous core (thin arrow) of a papilla and the basal layers of the covering epithelium. The epithelial cells show some loss of polarity. Their nuclei are large and vesicular and in each there is a prominent nucleolus. They are slightly pleomorphic and one mitotic figure is present (thick arrow). This tumour was classified as a fairly well-differentiated transitional cell carcinoma of ureter (Grade II). This carcinoma is important in the development of our knowledge of carcinogenic substances. It was the second carcinoma to be shown to have a chemical cause, the first being carcinoma of the scrotum in boy chimney sweeps, described by Percival Pott in England in 1775. In 1895 Rehn described an increased incidence of carcinoma of the lower urinary tract in workers in the aniline dye industry in Germany. It was subsequently shown that the carcinogenic substance involved is ß-naphthylamine. In recent years it has been shown that workers in the rubber industry and in the electric cable industry also have a increased incidence of this carcinoma. Benzidine has also been shown to be a causative chemical. HE × 360

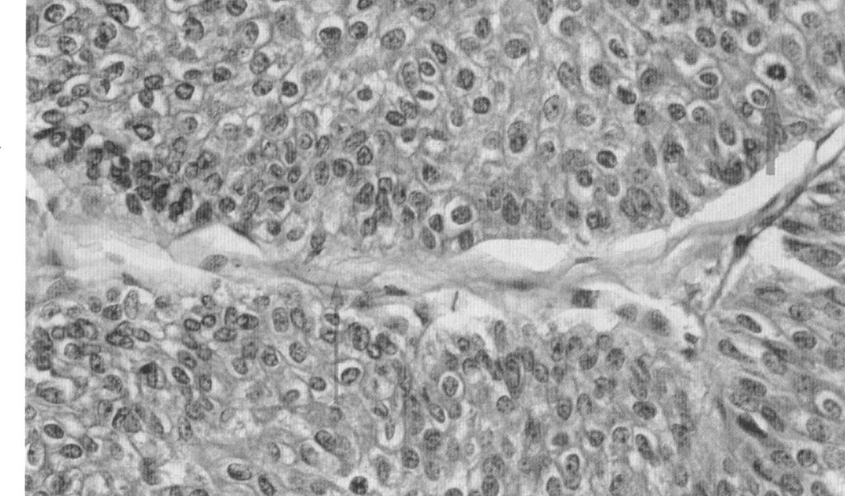

10.57 Squamous cell carcinoma: bladder

Squamous cell carcinoma of bladder arises from transitional epithelium that has undergone metaplasia to squamous epithelium as a result of chronic 'irritation', e.g. from calculi present in the bladder. This lesion in a man of 87 contained areas of both transitional cell carcinoma and squamous cell carcinoma. This area consists of cords of fairly well-differentiated squamous cells which form keratin (thin arrow). The more 'basal' cells towards the surfaces of the cords are pleomorphic, and mitotic activity is evident (thick arrow). The stroma is fibrous and infiltrated with chronic inflammatory cells. The squamous cell carcinoma component but not the transitional cell part was invading the muscle coat of the bladder and was also present in perineural lymphatics, indicating its more aggressive nature. HE ×235

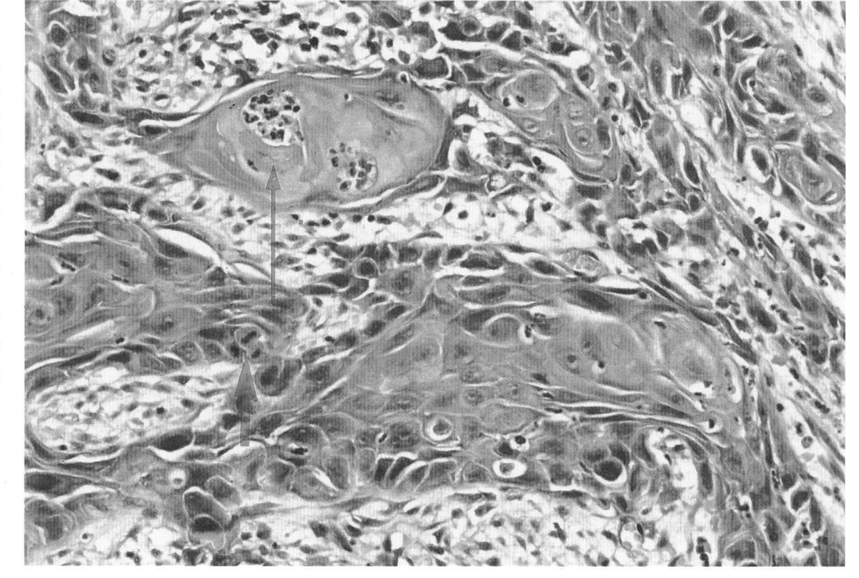

10.58 Inverted papilloma: bladder

Inverted papilloma of bladder is sometimes confused with transitional cell carcinoma or papilloma but it is a separate entity. It is a benign lesion and its structure is not papilliferous. Instead it is generally a smooth-surfaced mass, formed by the neoplastic epithelium growing beneath the epithelial lining of the bladder. This lesion was in a man of 69. It consists of cords of basophilic epithelial cells (double arrow) lying in a pale-staining loose connective tissue (thin arrow). The epithelial cells are well-differentiated and there is no nuclear pleomorphism. The cells on the outsides of the cords are columnar and similar to the basal layer of transitional epithelium. Small cystic spaces containing secretion are present within the epithelium (thick arrow). The blood vessels in the connective tissue are dilated and there are small numbers of lymphocytes. HE ×150

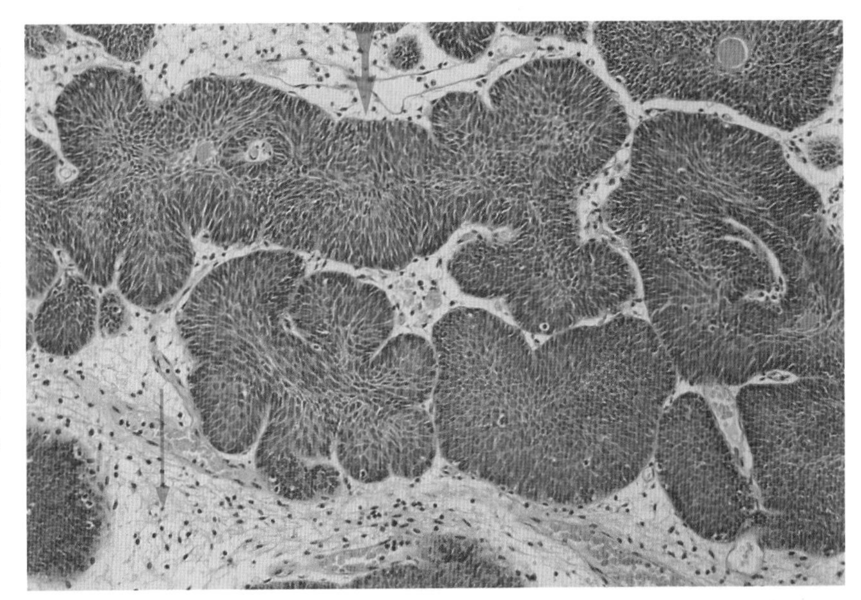

10.59 Inverted papilloma: bladder

At higher magnification the tumour epithelium is seen to be well-differentiated, resembling a double layer of normal transitional epithelium. The epithelial cells at the periphery of the cords of epithelial cells, i.e. the 'basal' layers, are columnar and palisaded, and similar to the basal layer in normal transitional epithelium. They rest on a well-formed basement membrane (thin arrow). The stroma is very loose connective tissue, and occasional lymphocytes are present in it, along with a thin-walled blood vessel (double arrow). There is a small cystic space containing eosinophilic secretion (thick arrow). Inverted papilloma is generally located in the region of the trigone or bladder neck, and it presents with either hematuria or obstruction of the urethra. There is a close association with chronic cystitis. HE ×360

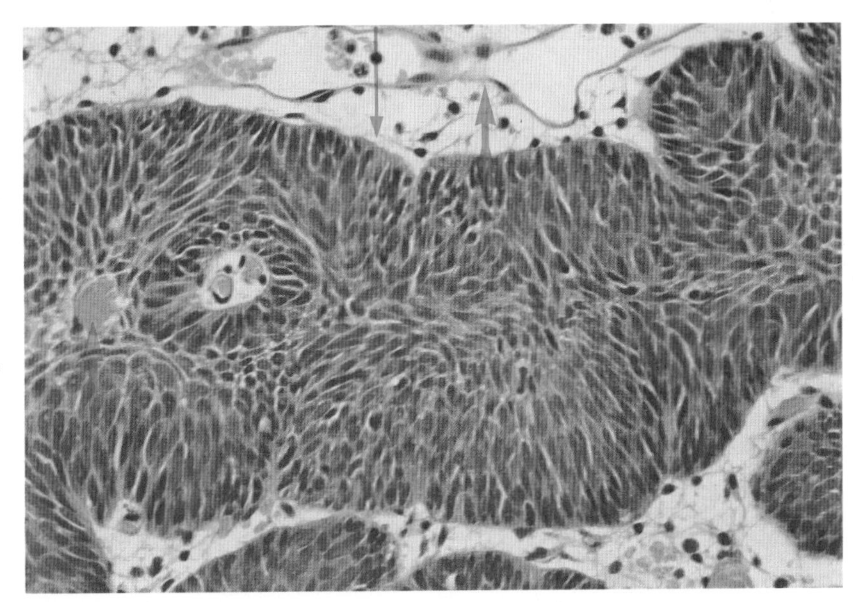

10.60 Pheochromocytoma: bladder

Pheochromocytoma occasionally arises from sympathetic paraganglia in sites other than the adrenal. This tumour arose in the bladder, a rare occurrence. The tumour cells form cords separated by connective tissue stroma. Their nuclei are large and round and the nucleoli small. Nuclear pleomorphism is moderate. The brown colour of the cytoplasm (arrow) was produced by the reaction of the catecholamines in it with the dichromate in the tissue fixative (Orth's solution) - the chromaffin reaction. The stroma is vascular but the blood vessels are inconspicuous. A small proportion of pheochromocytomas are genetically determined and then they occur in association with medullary carcinoma of thyroid, and parathyroid adenoma or hyperplasia. This is one form of the multiple endocrine neoplasia syndrome, designated MEN2A; and when it occurs with submucosal neuromas and a Marfan's habitus, it is designated MEN2B. HE ×360

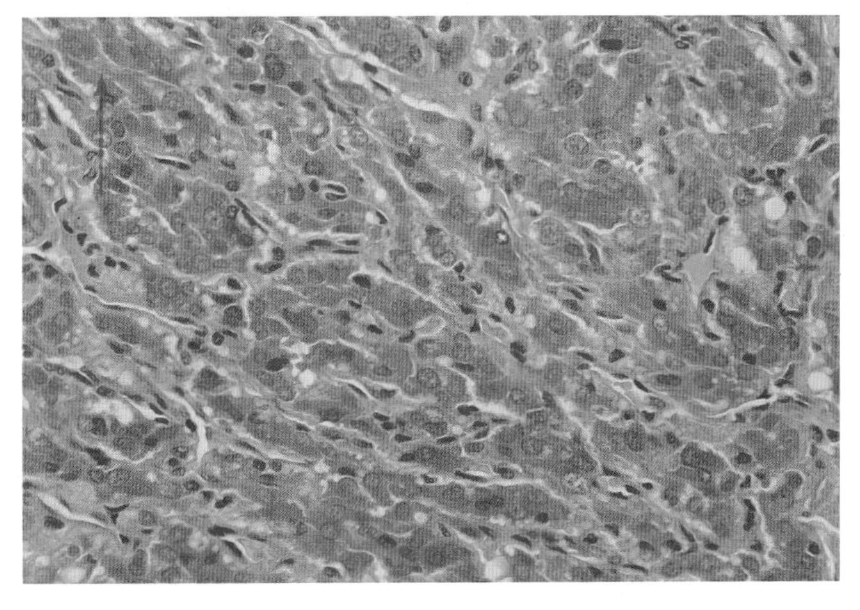

11.1 Congenital hepatic fibrosis: liver

Congenital hepatic fibrosis is regarded as a form of cystic disease of the liver, and occurs in infants, adolescents or young adults. The disease is familial and sometimes accompanied by cystic disease of the kidneys. In this case the patient was aged 15, his liver was enlarged and fibrotic and he had portal hypertension. Septa of dense fibrous tissue extended throughout the liver, enclosing islands of essentially normal parenchyma and numerous small bile ducts. In this field there is one such broad fibrous septum within which, characteristically, there is a large number of small mature bile ducts and a smaller number of large dilated (cystic) ducts (thick arrow). The cystic ducts, usually not more than 3cm dia, are lined by a single layer of uniformly cuboidal epithelial cells and contain plugs of brown dense inspissated bile (thin arrow). A small nodule of liver cells (double arrow) is also present within the fibrous tissue. The kidneys were polycystic, a condition known to be present in about a third of the patients with adult cystic disease. HE 55

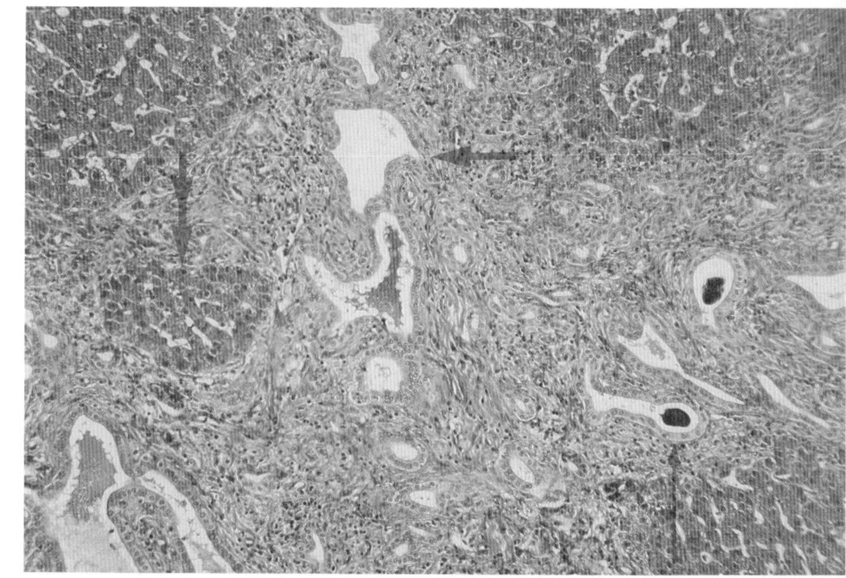

11.2 Dubin-Johnson syndrome: liver

The Dubin-Johnson syndrome (hereditary hyperbilirubinemia) is an uncommon benign condition which does not interfere with life or longevity. The disease is inherited as an autosomal recessive trait with a high frequency of consanguinity of parents. The condition is characterized by a chronic or intermittent non-hemolytic type of jaundice, resulting from the partial failure of the hepatocytes to secrete normally-conjugated bilirubin into the bile canaliculi. Conjugated bilirubin is therefore released into the bloodstream. The other constituents of the bile are unaffected. The patient is mildly jaundiced but the intensity of the jaundice fluctuates intermittently. In the liver cells, as shown here, large coarse granules of a brown melanin-like pigment (arrow) accumulate within lysosomes, in amounts sufficient to turn the liver black. The architecture of the liver is however undisturbed.

HE ×360

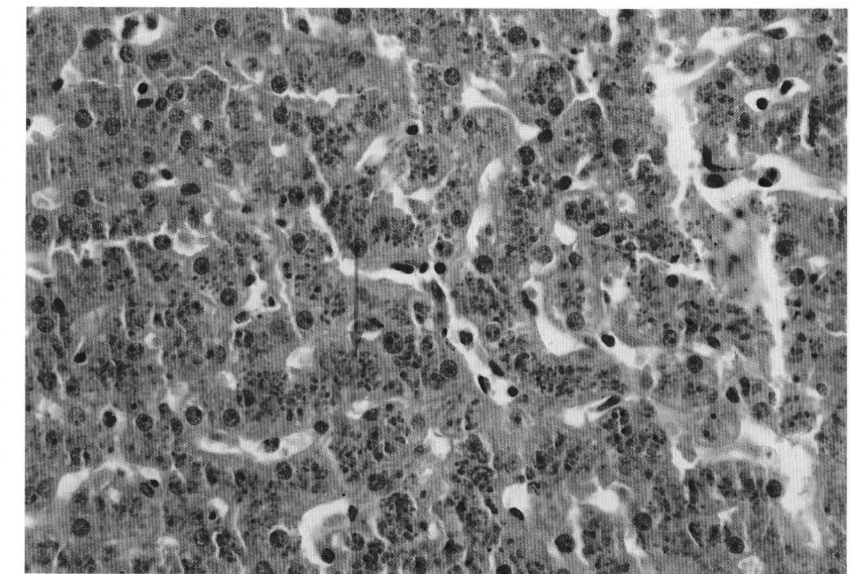

11.3 Alpha-1-antitrypsin deficiency: liver

Alpha-1-antitrypsin is formed in the liver and circulates in the blood. Its normal function is to inhibit the action of trypsin in the blood. Individuals with very little alpha-1-antitrypsin deficiency in their plasma often develop pulmonary disease, usually emphysema (usually panacinar) and sometimes chronic pancreatitis; and globules of abnormal antitrypsin are retained within the endoplasmic reticulum of the hepatocytes. The abnormal antitrypsin is well-demonstrated in the liver, as round bodies, by the periodic acid-Schiff (PAS) method. This shows two lobules of liver, separated by a portal tract within which there is a small bile duct (thin arrow). Large numbers of small round bodies, stained a deep purplish-red, are present within the hepatocytes (thick arrow). The staining reaction of the bodies is unaffected by pretreatment of the section with diastase. Most of the hepatocytes are vacuolated, showing severe fatty change. There is marked increase of fibrous tissue in this portal tract, and in severe cases macronodular cirrhosis develops. PAS ×360

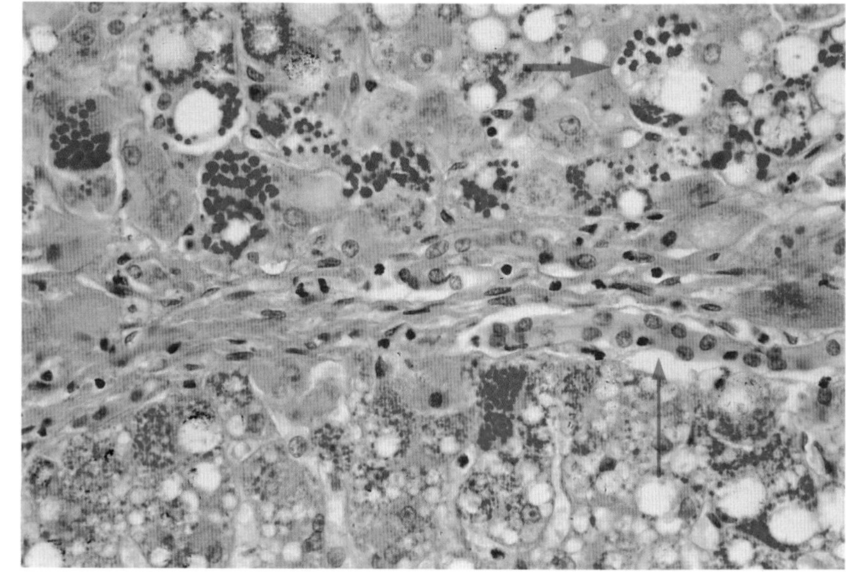

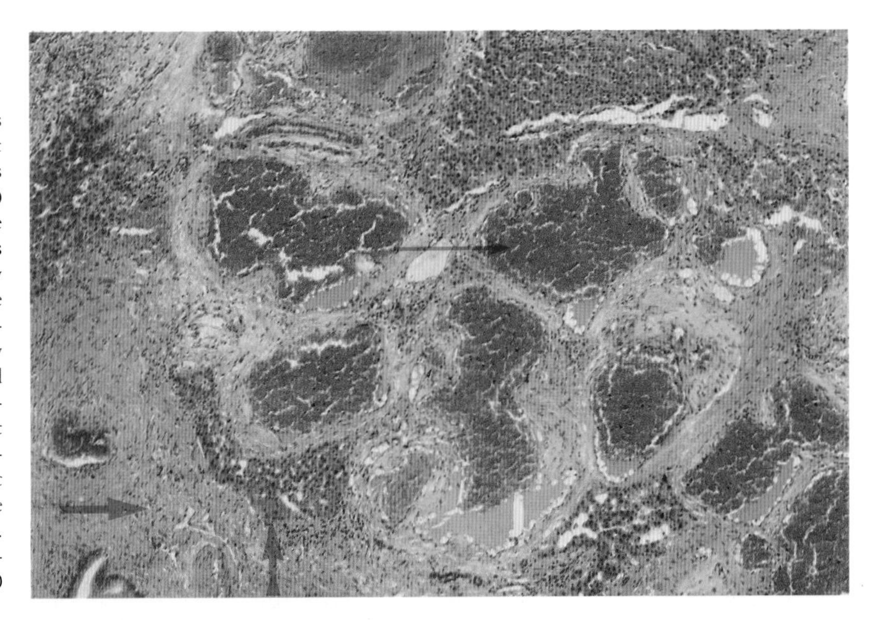

11.4 Hereditary hemorrhagic telangiectasia (Osler-Weber-Rendu syndrome:) Osler's disease): liver

Osler's disease (hereditary hemorrhagic telangiectasia) is a genetic disorder, transmitted as an autosomal dominant trait of high penetrance. The lesions are in skin, mucous membranes & viscera (particularly the nose and bowel) and they take the form of superficial punctate purple spots, a few mm in diameter. They consist of collections of small thin-walled capillaries and venules, which may cause problems of bleeding. In the liver the lesions are sometimes regarded as discrete hemangiomas. This example consists of thin-walled vascular channels, lined by a single layer of endothelial cells and filled with blood (thin arrow). The vascular channels, some of them enormously dilated, are located in the vicinity of a portal tract and surrounded by an irregular sheet of eosinophilic fibromuscular tissue (thick arrow) and islands of atrophic hepatocytes (double arrow). The lesions may be extensive and fibrosis may develop, to produce a form of cirrhosis. Recurrent bleeding may also occur, and increase in frequency & severity with age. HE ×60

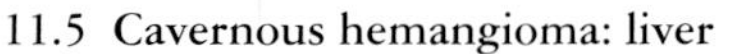

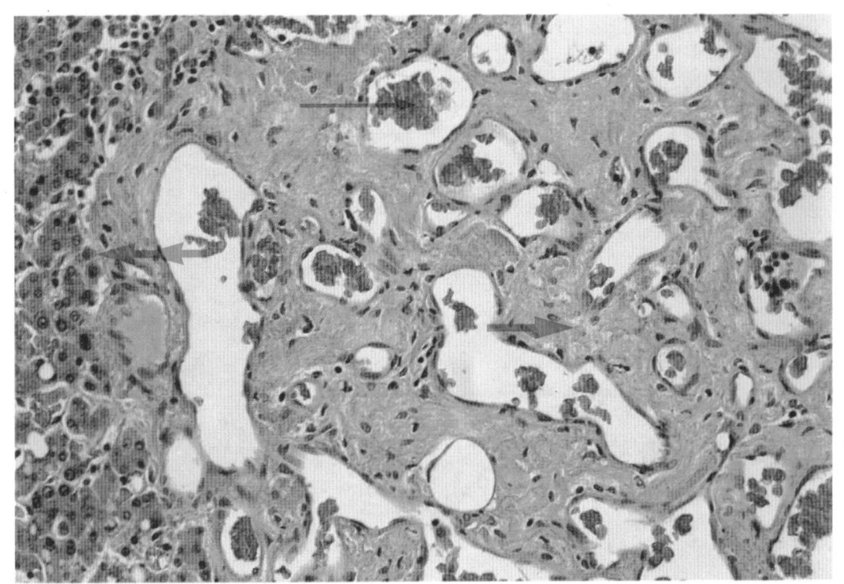

11.5 Cavernous hemangioma: liver

Most hemangiomas of liver are cavernous, and cavernous hemangioma of liver is generally single and rarely a large number. It is probably hamartomatous rather than neoplastic in nature, and it is a not uncommon incidental finding during post-mortem examinations. It appears as a spongy dark purplish-red nodule (usually less than 2cm dia), sharply demarcated from the surrounding hepatic tissue and sometimes wedge-shaped. It is generally located under the liver capsule and projects only slightly above the surface of the liver. This hemangioma of liver is composed of large thick-walled vascular channels (thin arrow), lined by normal very flat endothelial cells and supported by thick septa of eosinophilic fibrous tissue (thick arrow). Some normal liver cells are visible at the left margin (double arrow). A hemangioma of liver rarely bleeds into the peritoneal cavity or produce symptoms, and it is usually of little or no clinical significance.
HE ×235

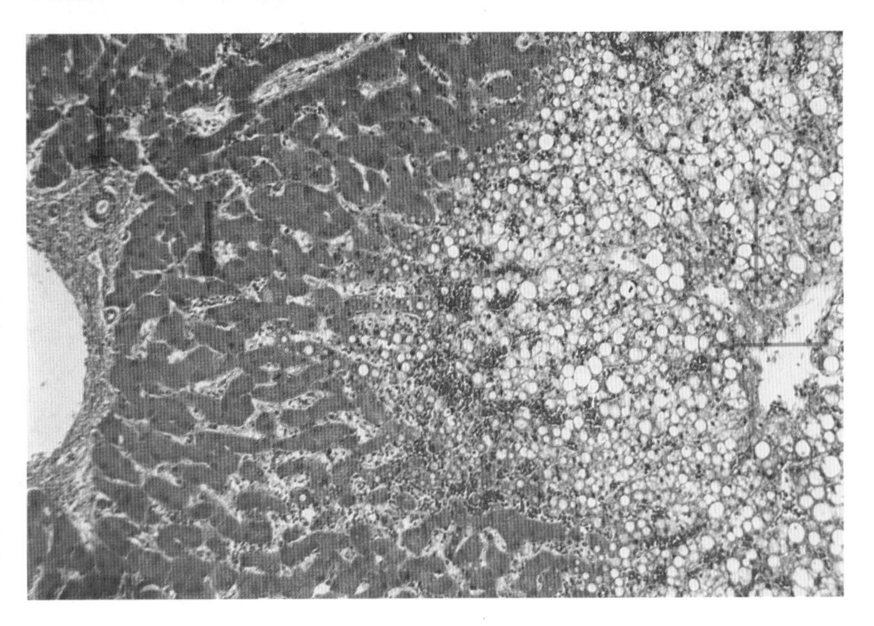

11.6 Chronic venous congestion and fatty change: liver

In chronic heart failure, when the right side of the heart fails to maintain its output, the inferior vena cava and hepatic veins become congested, and the continued effects of compression by dilated sinusoids and hypoxia lead to loss of liver cells. When venous congestion is prolonged, perivenular loss of hepatocytes may be extensive, and perivenular fibrosis may occur. In this case, the hepatocytes on the left are relatively large and normal in appearance, and adjoining them there is a portal tract containing a small bile duct and a dilated branch of the portal vein (double arrow). The sinusoids in the mid-zonal and centrilobular regions are very congested however (thick arrow). The centrilobular zone shows severe fatty change (thin arrows) and many hepatocytes are atrophic. In more severe cases, many hepatocytes disappear. Macroscopically, the contrast between the brown colour of the peripheral parts of the lobules and the yellow colour of the fatty central zones produces the 'nutmeg' pattern characteristic of chronic venous congestion. Fibrous tissue appears to increase and cardiac cirrhosis results. HE ×55

11.7 Budd-Chiari syndrome: liver

The Budd-Chiari syndrome is caused by narrowing or obstruction of the superior vena cava or of the main hepatic vein. Thrombosis is the most common cause, but its etiology is often unknown. If the obstruction occurs suddenly, the liver becomes intensely engorged, swollen, purple and acutely painful. The hepatic sinusoids are dilated, there is perivenular congestion and considerable hemorrhage, and severe ascites develops. Atrophy of the hepatocytes commonly occurs in the centres of the lobules. Slowly-developing obstruction produces less acute clinical signs and symptoms, and the patient may live for months or years. In this example, the sinusoids in the centre of the lobule are distended and full of blood, and most of the hepatocytes in that area have undergone necrosis and disappeared, apart from a number of swollen degenerate bile-stained cells. In the less affected mid-zonal region, the hepatocytes are moderately atrophic (thin arrow) but at the periphery of the lobule they look comparatively normal (thick arrow). HE ×150

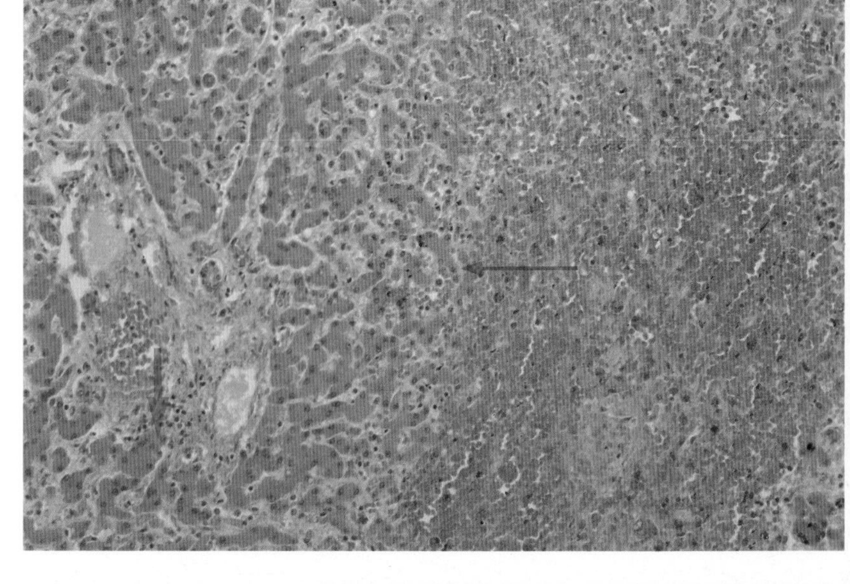

11.8 Peliosis hepatis: liver

Peliosis hepatis is an uncommon condition in which angiomatoid lesions develop throughout the liver. The lesions are associated with wasting disease such as advanced tuberculosis or malignancy, and with the consumption of anabolic and contraceptive steroids. Macroscopically they take the form of a few (or sometimes many) bluish dots a few mm or so across in the parenchyma. Histologically, the 'dots' consist of several large round blood-filled 'spaces' (thin arrow) which vaguely resemble dilated sinusoids. The spaces, which are obviously compressing the adjacent parenchymal cells, are well-defined but do not appear to have a distinct wall. The spaces have no obvious connection with the hepatic sinusoids, which are not distended, but very occasionally some of them do have a sinusoidal lining. Hemosiderin-laden phagocytes are present in the adjacent liver (thick arrow). The blood in the spaces is usually fluid but it may thrombose. Organization of thrombus in a space produces a stellate scar. HE ×60

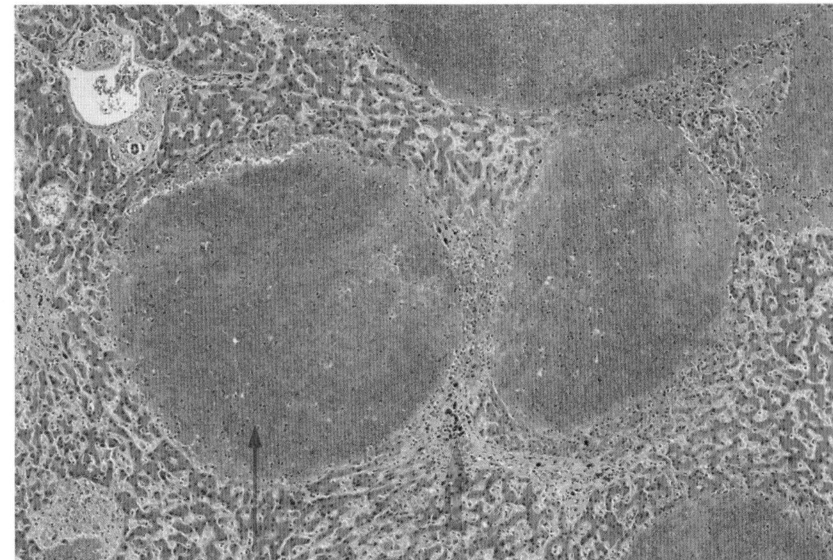

11.9 Nodular regenerative hyperplasia: liver

The etiology of nodular regenerative hyperplasia (nodular transformation of the liver) is uncertain but the condition may be an incidental finding or associated with various other conditions, including rheumatoid arthritis, chronic circulatory impairment and long-sustained drug therapy. There are no symptoms as a rule but, rarely, portal hypertension or hepatic failure may develop. Throughout the liver there are very large numbers of small hyperplastic round nodules (1-5mm dia) of regenerating hepatocytes but no fibrous septa. The nodules are paler than normal liver parenchyma. The nodules compress and largely replace the hepatic parenchyma, and the condition can simulate micronodular cirrhosis fairly closely. Two nodules are shown here (thin arrows), and between them there are cords of liver cells which look relatively normal, apart from the fact that the sinusoids are much wider than usual (thick arrow). There is little or no fibrosis in or around the nodules. HE ×60

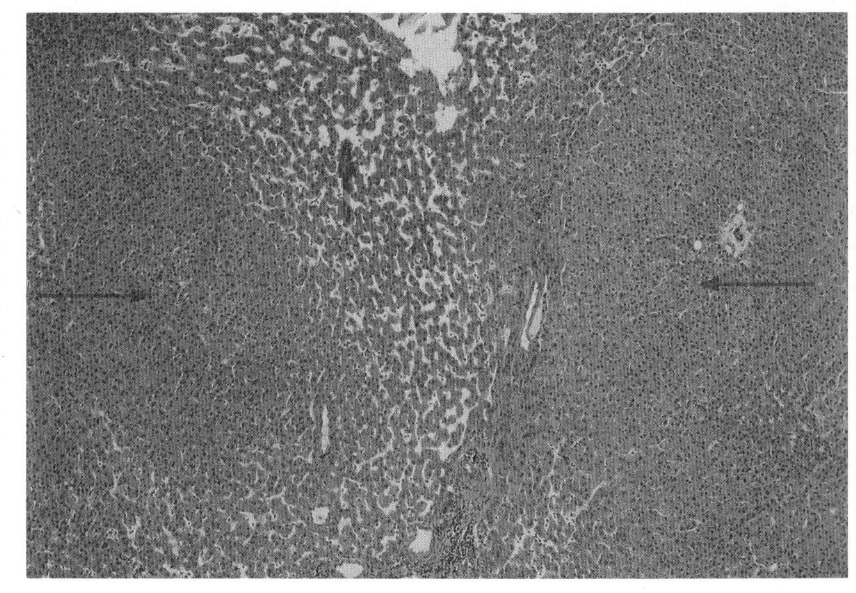

11.10 Amyloid: liver

Amyloid is a fibrillar material which is laid down in the tissues, usually extracellularly. It is associated with chronic inflammatory diseases such as rheumatoid arthritis and certain neoplastic conditions. In the liver, amyloid is occasionally laid down in considerable amounts, usually in the walls of the sinusoids (in the spaces of Disse, small spaces between the sinusoids and the hepatocytes). The amyloid compresses and destroys large numbers of hepatocytes, but liver function may still be well preserved In this case the patient had suffered from severe rheumatoid arthritis for many years. The amyloid takes the form of bands of dense strongly eosinophilic amorphous material (thin arrows) which separate the hepatocytes from the lumen of sinusoids (thick arrow). The hepatocytes apposed to and occasionally completely surrounded by the bands of amyloid are atrophic, presumably from pressure atrophy and ischemia. Many hepatocytes appear normal however. HE ×335

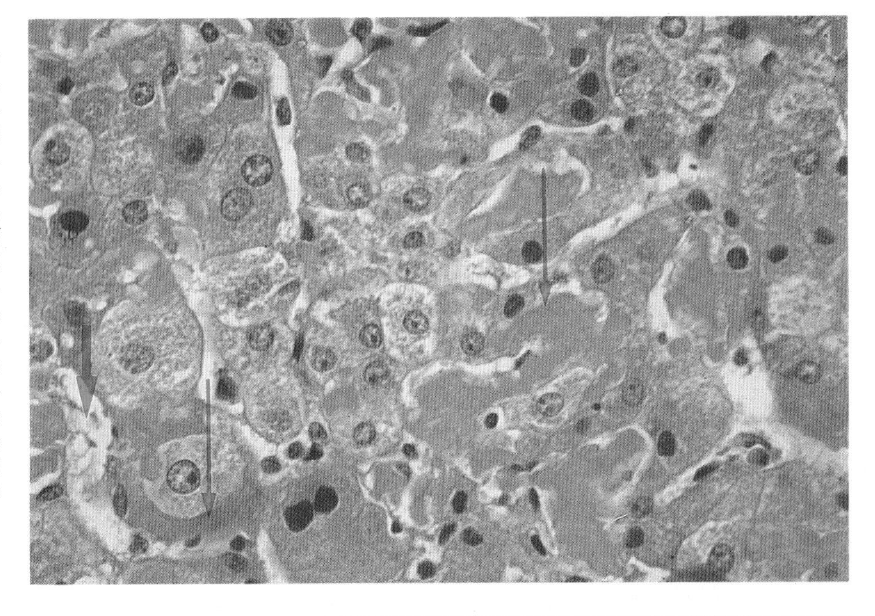

11.11 Alcoholic hepatitis: liver

Individuals vary considerably in their susceptibility to the toxic effects of alcohol, and alcoholic hepatitis develops in only about one-third of chronic alcoholics. The liver always undergoes fatty change and patchy hepatocellular necrosis. Cellular necrosis is most marked around the terminal hepatic veins but it may be widespread. The dying cells tend to shrink and become hyalinized or ballooned. The condition may progress to cirrhosis. This specimen was a wedge biopsy of liver removed at laparotomy from a man of 57 who was a known chronic alcoholic. There is ballooning degeneration of hepatocytes in the centrilobular region around the branch of the hepatic vein (thick arrow), and also panlobular fatty change in the middle of the lobule (thin arrow). The hepatocytes at the periphery of the lobule, around the portal tract (double arrow), are much less affected. It should be noted that ballooned hepatocytes have abundant pale cream-coloured cytoplasm and a central nucleus, whereas the fatty cells have much larger cytoplasmic vacuoles and a nucleus that is located at the periphery of the cell or not visible. There is no evidence of cholestasis. HE ×60

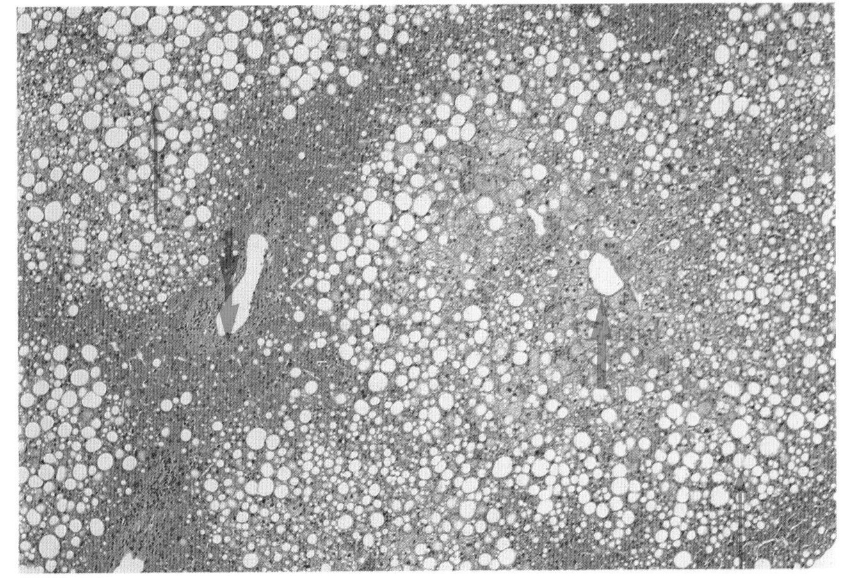

11.12 Alcoholic hepatitis: liver

Cholestasis is not usually pronounced in alcoholic hepatitis, being severe only occasionally. This is a close-up view (at higher magnification) of 11.11. The hepatocytes are swollen, and in them there are numerous fat-containing vacuoles of widely varying size, many small and some very large (the vacuoles are empty, the fat having dissolved in reagents). Some hepatocytes have small pyknotic nuclei and are probably necrotic. Irregular masses of amorphous deeply eosinophilic alcoholic hyaline (composed of filaments of cytokeratin) are present in several cells (arrow). A very mild infiltrate of polymorph leukocytes is also present. There is no evidence of cholestasis. Sometimes the cytoplasmic envelope around the larger droplets of fat ruptures and the droplets coalesce to form a large extracellular fat cyst which undergoes phagocytosis. Fibrosis usually follows. A stain for reticulin however showed no increase in reticulin fibres in this liver. There was also no increase in stainable iron. HE ×360

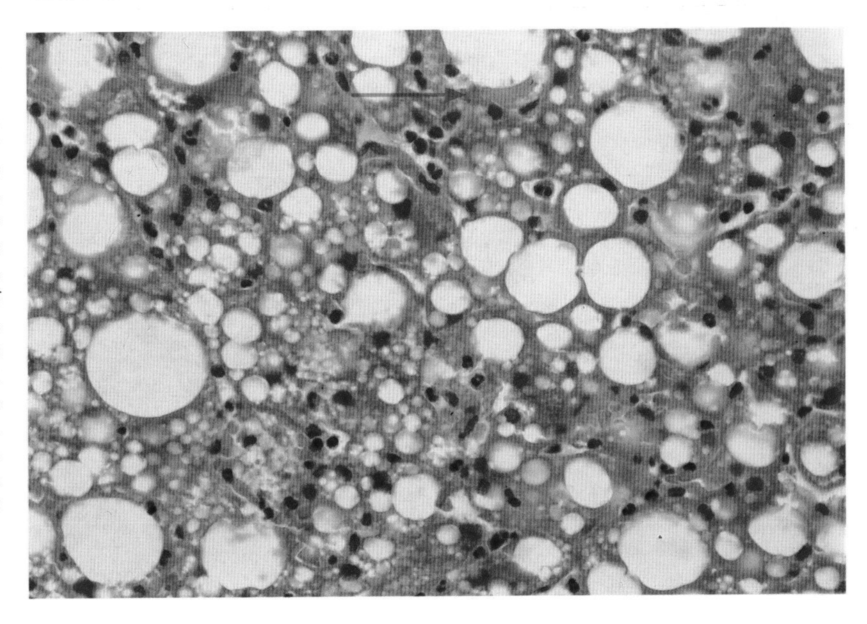

11.13 Gumma: liver

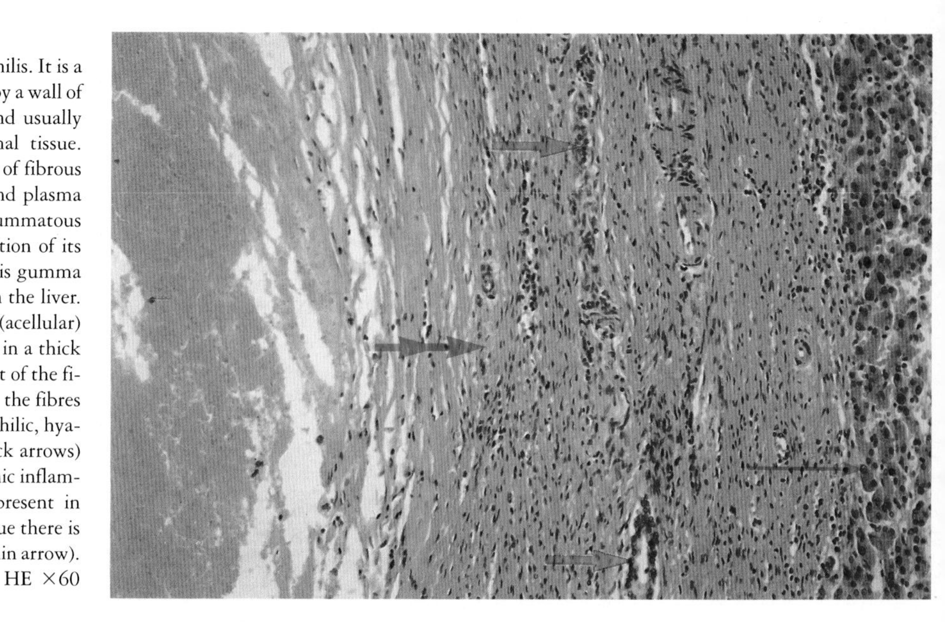

A gumma is a lesion of the tertiary stage of syphilis. It is a granuloma with a necrotic centre, surrounded by a wall of macrophages. Necrosis is usually extensive and usually accompanied with destruction of parenchymal tissue. The gumma is generally enclosed in a capsule of fibrous tissue, in which there are also lymphocytes and plasma cells. Subsequently much scar tissue forms. Gummatous scarring of the liver may cause marked distortion of its structure (hepar lobatum). Macroscopically, this gumma is a yellowish mass (approximately 5cm dia) in the liver. Histologically most of it consists of amorphous (acellular) deeply eosinophilic necrotic material, enclosed in a thick layer of densely collagenous fibrous tissue. Most of the fibrous tissue is very cellular (double arrow), but the fibres closest to the necrotic material are very eosinophilic, hyaline and acellular. Several small bile ducts (thick arrows) are trapped within the fibrous tissue, and chronic inflammatory cells (mainly plasma cells) are also present in moderate numbers. External to the fibrous tissue there is a sheet of compressed and atrophic liver cells (thin arrow). HE ×60

11.14 Visceral leishmaniasis: liver

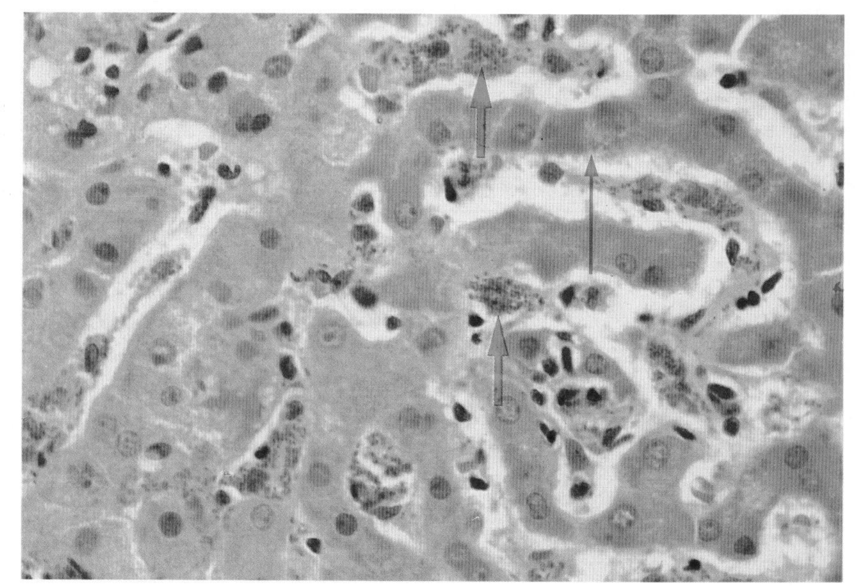

The three kinds of leishmaniasis are visceral, cutaneous and mucocutaneous, and different species of sandfly are involved in the different forms of the disease. Visceral leishmaniasis (kala-azar) is caused by the protozoon *Leishmania donovani,* which is 4-5μm dia and contains nuclei (1-2μm dia). The parasite is transmitted by the bite of the sandfly *Phlebotomus papatasii* which, as it feeds, regurgitates the motile promastigotes that are proliferating in its gut into the wound, entering macrophages in which they divide and then escape into the blood. In a person with visceral leishmaniasis, the affected organs (spleen, liver, kidneys etc) are swollen from the presence of large numbers of macrophages full of Leishmann-Donovan bodies. The fine structure of the *L. donovani* is not well demonstrated by histological sections, a smear stained by Giemsa or Leishman's stain being much more effective. In this liver, the cords of hepatocytes appear atrophic (thin arrow) (some fixation shrinkage has occurred), whereas the phagocytic Kupffer cells lining the sinusoids are swollen, their cytoplasm containing large numbers of the protozoon, the nuclei of which appear as very small blue dots (thick arrows). HE ×575

11.15 Cryptococcosis: liver

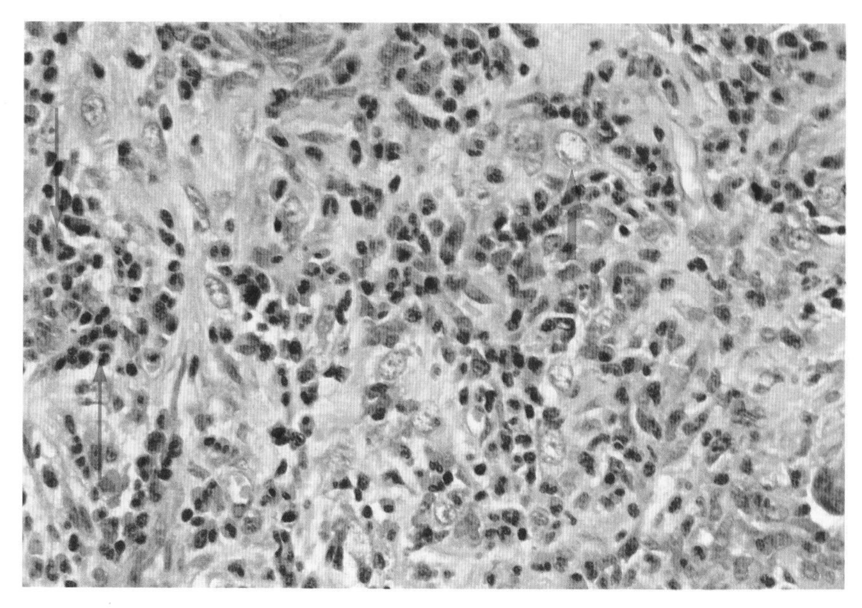

The fungus *Cryptococcus neoformans (Torula histolytica)* is ubiquitous in the environment around the world, particularly in places contaminated by pigeon droppings. In tissue, the microorganism grows as a round oval or elliptical yeast-like fungus 5-20μm dia, and it has a thick mucinous capsule, usually thicker than the diameter of the fungus, which is difficult to stain. It evokes a chronic inflammatory reaction which is usually granulomatous, but is sometimes non-specific and may be very slight. A woman of 31 was found at laparotomy to have many small white nodules in her liver, and a portion of liver was removed for diagnostic purposes. Histologically, each nodule consists of necrotic liver surrounded by an inflammatory cellular infiltrate. The inflammatory response is generally slight. The cells are epithelioid-type macrophages, multinucleated giant cells and large numbers of eosinophil polymorphs (thin arrows). The nuclei of the giant cells are large pale and vesicular (thick arrow). No microorganisms are visible. HE ×360

11.16 Cryptococcosis: liver

Cryptococci are saprophytic fungi which are difficult to detect in sections stained with hematoxylin and eosin, since they are enclosed in a mucinous capsule which surrounds the organism. The capsule generally appears as a clear halo, but the periodic acid-Schiff method for mucin stains the capsule and so demonstrates clusters of the microorganism effectively. In this section of the lesion shown in 11.15, in a background of purplish-red acellular tissue and a few small cells, there are two very large (giant) multinucleated cells with large uniform pale vesicular ovoid nuclei (thin arrows), arranged around the periphery of the abundant purplish-red cytoplasm (double arrow). Within large clear vacuoles in the cytoplasm of the giant cells there are round capsules (containing the proliferating cryptococci) which appear as bright purple-red PAS+ve (mucinous) circles (thick arrows).

PAS ×740

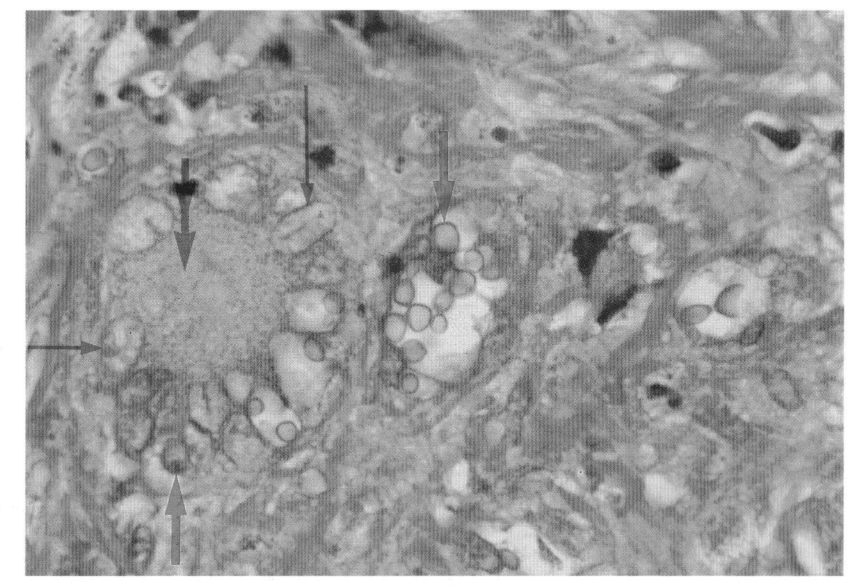

11.17 Cryptococcosis: liver

The range of inflammatory responses which *Cryptococcus neoformans*, may induce is broad, varying from very little inflammation to a granulomatous reaction. The microorganism is not contagious but it may produce severe disease in an individual with a markedly defective immune system. Sometimes there is no evident host response. The periodic acid-Schiff (PAS) method for demonstrating mucin is effective, but an even more effective method for detecting microorganisms, such as fungi which have a mucinous capsule, is the Grocott method, which reveals the mucinous capsule by depositing silver within it. The silver appears black and, in this section of the lesion shown in 11.15, clusters and single forms of the microorganism stand out as densely black ovoid shapes (arrows), in a sheet of uniformly blue-stained tissue.

Grocott silver method ×360

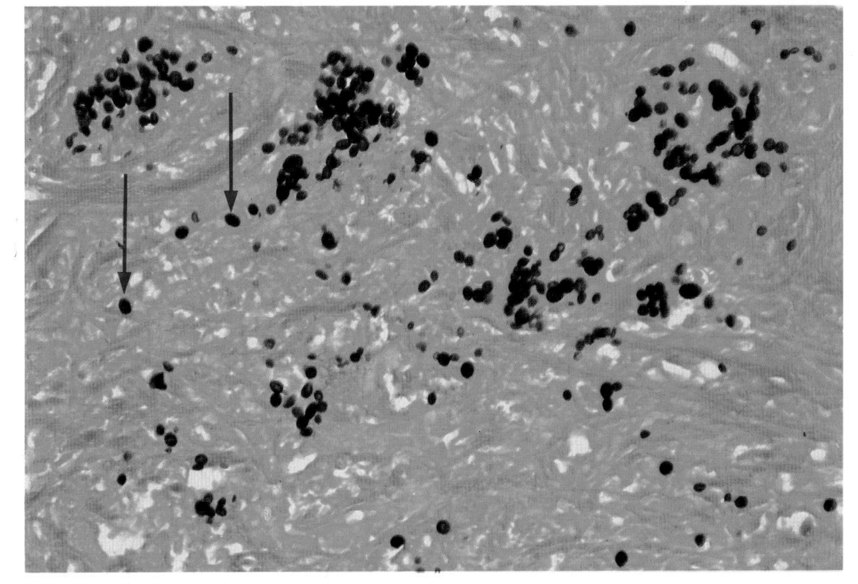

11.18 Schistosomiasis (Bilharziasis): liver

The liver is always involved in Schistosomiasis. *Schistosoma mansoni* and *Schistosoma japonicum* are flukes which inhabit the branches of the portal vein. Man acquires Schistosomiasis by drinking or bathing in water which contains free-swimming cercariae. *S. mansoni* and *S. japonicum* lay their ova in the portal vein, and the ova are then washed into the liver via the portal vein. There they excite an inflammatory reaction which is initially acute but becomes granulomatous. In the centre of this field there is a degenerate ovum (thin arrow), enclosed in a layer of phagocytes (thick arrows) and a wall consisting of concentric layers of cellular collagenous fibrous tissue (double arrow) in which there numerous fibroblasts and fibrocytes. The architecture of the surrounding liver is markedly disturbed, and many of the hepatocytes vary in size and have pleomorphic nuclei. Other hepatocytes are atrophic, and there are a few inflammatory cells. Schistosomiasis does not lead to cirrhosis but may cause extensive fibrosis of the liver (pipe-stem fibrosis) and portal hypertension.

HE ×360

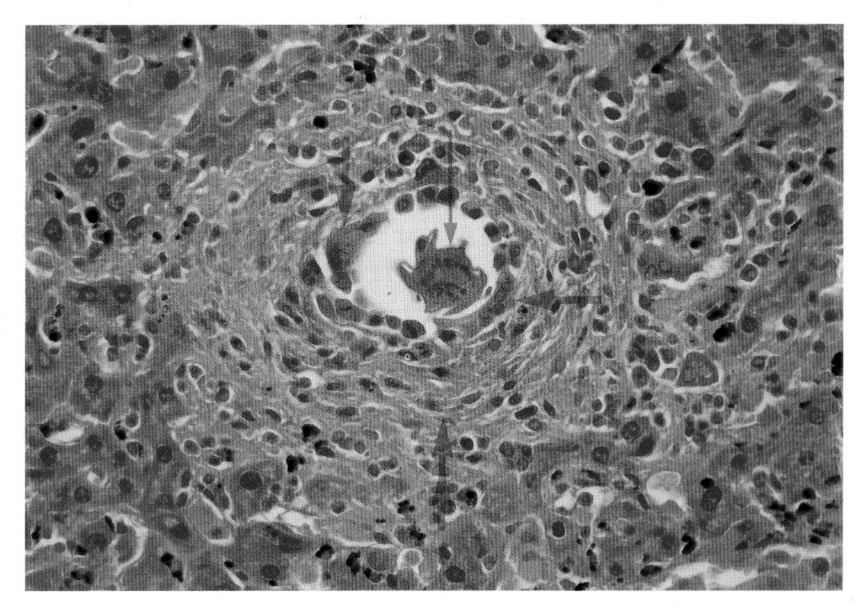

11.19 Viral hepatitis: liver

There are several common types of viral hepatitis, including hepatitis A (HAV), hepatitis B (HBV), hepatitis C (HCV), non-A non-B hepatitis and hepatitis D. It is not possible to distinguish between them histologically. In acute viral hepatitis there is diffuse inflammation of the liver and widespread necrosis of parenchymal cells, hepatitis B, hepatitis C and hepatitis D being more severe than hepatitis A and more likely to progress to chronic hepatitis. This patient died several weeks after the onset of hepatitis B, a disease which is more severe than hepatitis A and can occur in any age group. The hepatic cell plates have been destroyed (lobular disarray), and there is very marked disarray and extensive destruction of hepatocytes. The surviving hepatocytes are pleomorphic and form clusters of various sizes (double arrow, many hepatocytes being atrophic. There is an infiltrate of lymphocytes and plasma cells (thin arrow) which is widespread but most intense in the portal tracts (triaditis). Occasional bile capillaries are blocked by bile (thick arrows), evidence of severe cholestasis, but many small bile ducts have survived in the portal tracts. HE ×150

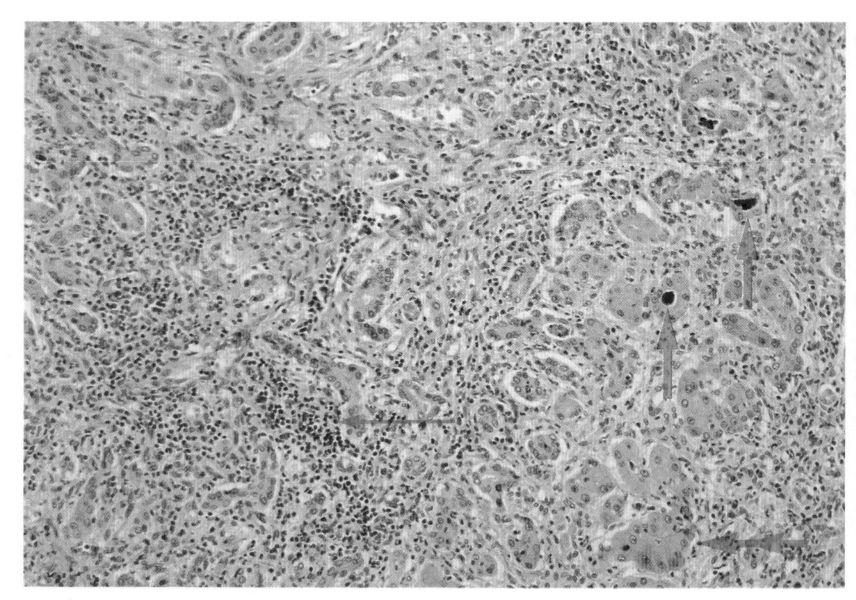

11.20 Viral hepatitis: liver

In viral hepatitis, severity of infection varies considerably, from a mild pyrexial illness without jaundice to a fulminant hepatic lesion with diffuse necrosis and hepatic failure. This is a less severe illness than that shown in **11.19** and it is at a later stage of its development. The numerous eosinophilic hepatocytes that remain viable are very swollen, each cell having a large amount of weakly eosinophilic hydropic mottled cytoplasm (ballooning degeneration) (thick arrow). In some of the distended cells there are also irregularly-shaped vacuoles of various sizes (mostly small, some possibly artefactual). In each of the two portal tracts, which are considerably expanded, there is an infiltrate of small deeply basophilic chronic inflammatory cells (mostly lymphocytes and plasma cells) which is dense and concentrated to a large extent in the portal tracts (thin arrow). Several degenerate hepatocytes in the form of acidophil bodies are also evident. HE ×150

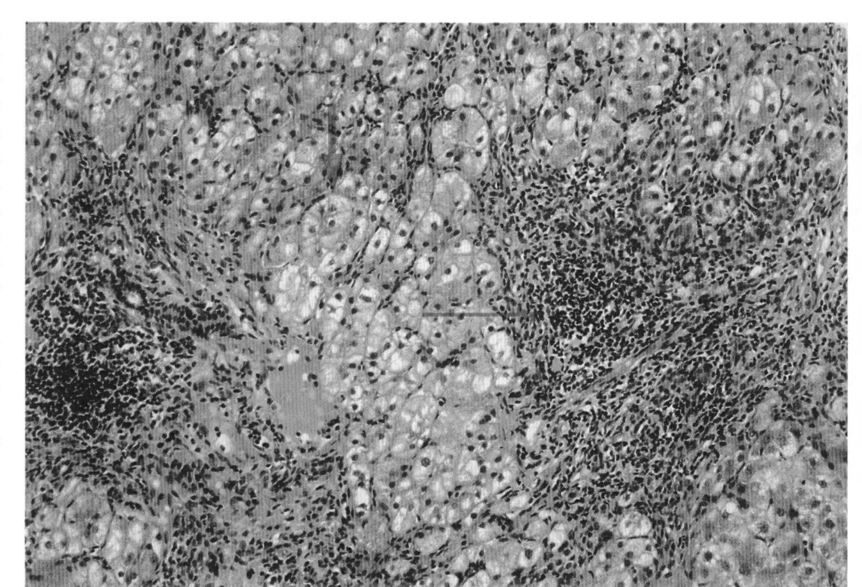

11.21 Viral hepatitis: liver

Most infections with type A virus (HAV) are mild, as are some of those with hepatitis B virus or others with non-A non-B viruses. HAV also rarely causes chronic hepatitis. This is a case of hepatitis A. In HE sections of the liver there was little evidence of hepatocyte damage and only a moderate infiltrate of inflammatory cells in the connective tissue. A silver stain for fine connective tissue fibres (reticulin) has been used to demonstrate the delicate reticulin network and lobular structure of the liver; and it reveals broad bands of dark-staining fibres (thin arrow) linking several portal tracts. The degree of bridging fibrosis visible in this field, some of which is probably attributable to condensation of the stroma following destruction of liver cells, is probably reversible. It may however be a precursor of cirrhosis. There is no increase of fibres around the central veins (thick arrows). Reticulin stain ×55

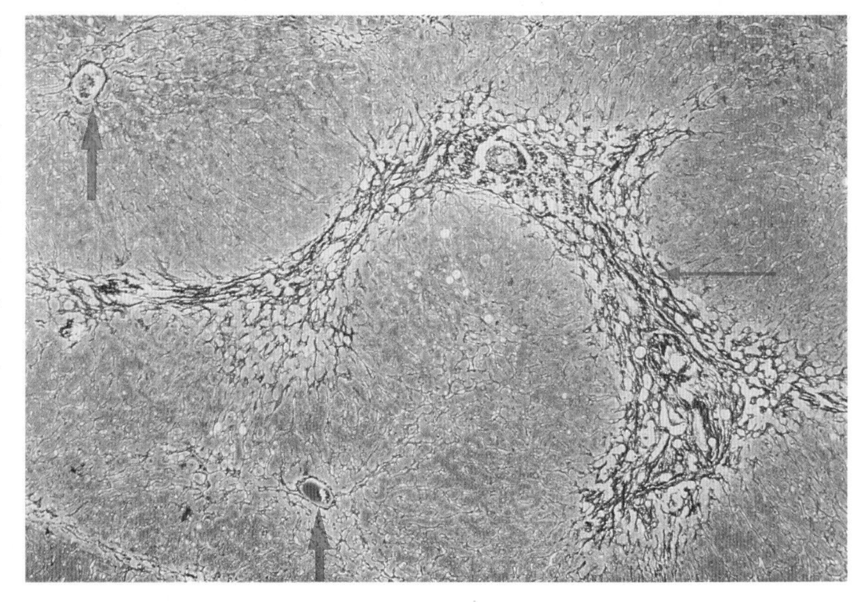

11.22 Subacute viral hepatitis: liver

The hepatitis B virus is not cytopathic, and the damage to the liver is probably caused by an immunological attack on the infected hepatocytes. In this field, from a fatal case of hepatitis B, there is extensive destruction of hepatocytes with resultant condensation of fibrous stroma (centre and bottom). There is a moderate infiltrate of chronic inflammatory cells in the connective tissue. The surviving hepatocytes have been regenerating and are still doing so, thereby leading to the formation of single forms and small irregular clusters of hepatocytes at the bottom of the field, and also much larger well-defined rounded nodules of hyperplastic hepatocytes (double arrows), surrounded by fibrous tissue, with much eosinophilic cytoplasm and vesicular nuclei. However there is evidence of biliary stasis in one of the nodules, as demonstrated by dense dark brown plugs of bile in the canaliculi (thin arrows). A small bile duct (thick arrow) is also visible.
HE ×150

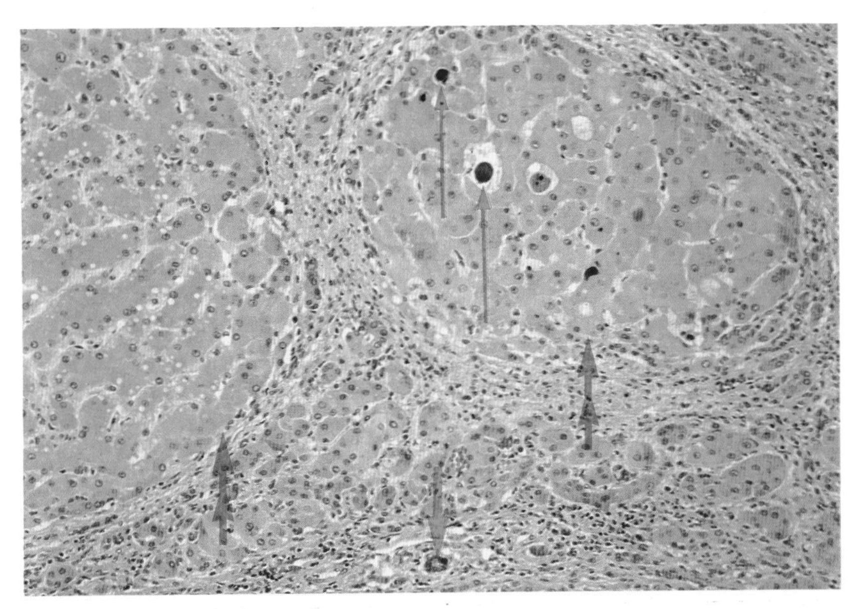

11.23 Chronic active hepatitis: liver

Some patients (3-5%) with acute B-viral hepatitis progress to chronic active hepatitis. Others present with chronic active hepatitis without a history of an acute phase. The milder form of the disease is confined to the portal triads and the parenchyma around them. Bridging necrosis is typical of the more severe form. The severity of injury to a liver may vary, with an exudate only of lymphocytes in some triads, and severe triaditis with destruction of surrounding parenchyma in other regions. This patient had had acute hepatitis. The portal tract is enlarged and heavily infiltrated with small basophilic chronic inflammatory cells (thick arrow) which have eroded the limiting plate of hepatocytes and extended irregularly into the lobule, accompanied by necrosis of individual hepatocytes (piecemeal necrosis). Most of the hepatocytes are swollen and hydropic (ballooning degeneration) (thin arrows), but some individual cells are shrunken and necrotic (acidophil bodies). Connective tissue stains demonstrated an increase of fibrous tissue in the portal tract.
HE ×150

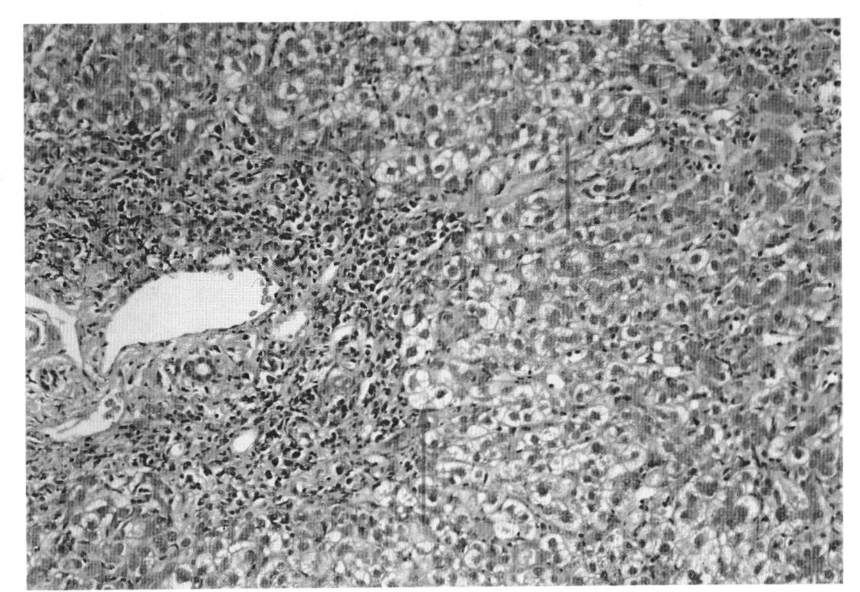

11.24 Chronic active hepatitis: liver

Idiopathic chronic active hepatitis may lead to cirrhosis. This field is from the same case as that shown in 11.23. The hepatocytes in the centre and left parts of the field are very swollen and hydropic (severe ballooning degeneration) (double arrow), with only wisps of cytoplasm around the nucleus (hepatocytes more distant from the portal tracts than these swollen hepatocytes are generally normal, although isolated foci of necrosis, as in acute viral hepatitis, may develop). Also present among the ballooned hepatocytes there is a bile canaliculus plugged with bile (thick arrow). Adjacent to the hepatocytes there is a portal tract with a small bile duct lined with cuboidal epithelial cells (thin arrow) and an increased amount of fibrous tissue, as well as fibroblastic activity. The number of chronic inflammatory cells in this part of the portal tract is comparatively small. The latter features are suggestive of progression to cirrhosis and a poorer prognosis.
HE ×360

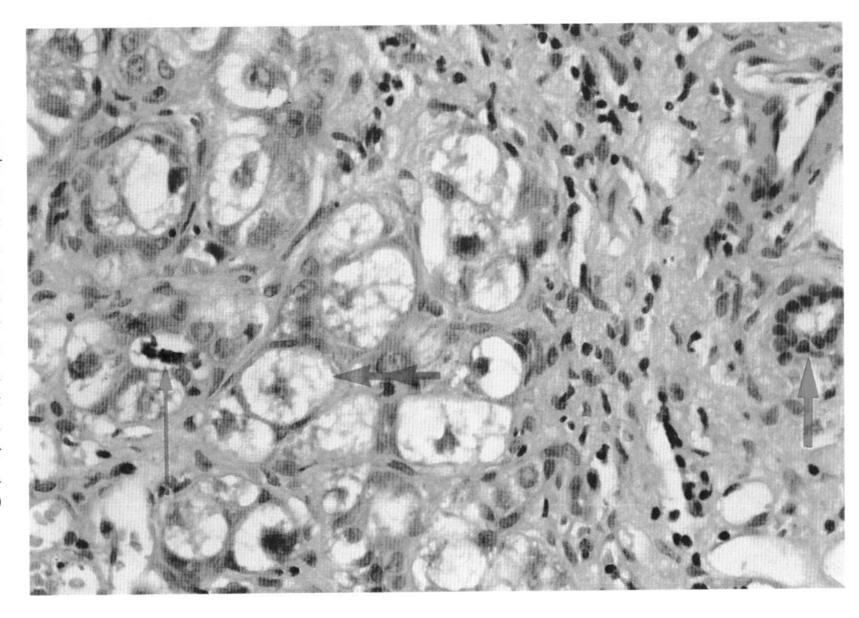

11.25 HBsAg in viral hepatitis: liver

Hepatitis B is most often diagnosed by demonstrating the surface antigen of the virus (HBsAg) in the plasma. In this case, the patient suffered from chronic hepatitis, and the portal tract is infiltrated by chronic inflammatory cells (thin arrow). By means of the indirect immunoperoxidase method, this histological section of liver has been reacted with an antibody to the surface antigen of the B virus; and in the cytoplasm of most of the slender brownish-yellow hepatocytes there is a fairly large well-defined dark brown round or ovoid mass (thick arrow) which represents the surface antigen of hepatitis B virus (HBsAg). Electron microscopy confirms that cells giving this reaction contain HBsAg in the smooth endoplasmic reticulum of the cell. In HE sections, cytoplasm containing HBsAg in high concentrations has a ground glass appearance. HBsAG also stains with orcein. In some countries a significant minority of the population are carriers of HBsAg.

Indirect immunoperoxidase method for HBsAg ×235

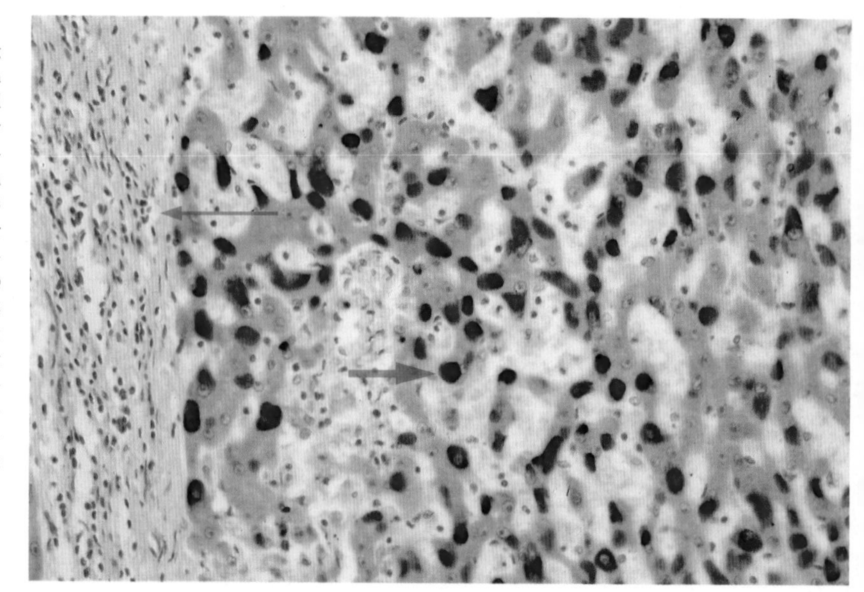

11.26 Macronodular cirrhosis (early): liver

In macronodular cirrhosis, septa of collagenous fibrous tissue join portal tracts to portal tracts and portal tracts to terminal hepatic veins. The general pattern however is more irregular than in micronodular cirrhosis, some of the portal tracts and hepatic veins remaining intact. In this field, there are two fairly large hyperplastic nodules of hepatocytes (regenerative nodules) (double arrows). Between the two nodules there is a septum of mature fibrous tissue (thick arrow), infiltrated by comparatively few lymphocytes, which extends to the nodules from a portal tract (top right), in which there is a very dilated thin-walled blood vessel. The junction between the fibrous septum and the regenerating nodules is well-defined. Within the nodules the cords of hepatocytes are very irregular, and some of the hepatocytes are large, containing two or more nuclei (thin arrow) in which there are prominent nucleoli (multinucleated hepatocytes are evidence of regeneration). The cytoplasm of some of the hepatocytes contains large droplets of fat droplets, and some of the other hepatocytes show ballooning degeneration. A reticulin stain demonstrated that the hepatocyte plates are two or more cells thick. HE ×235

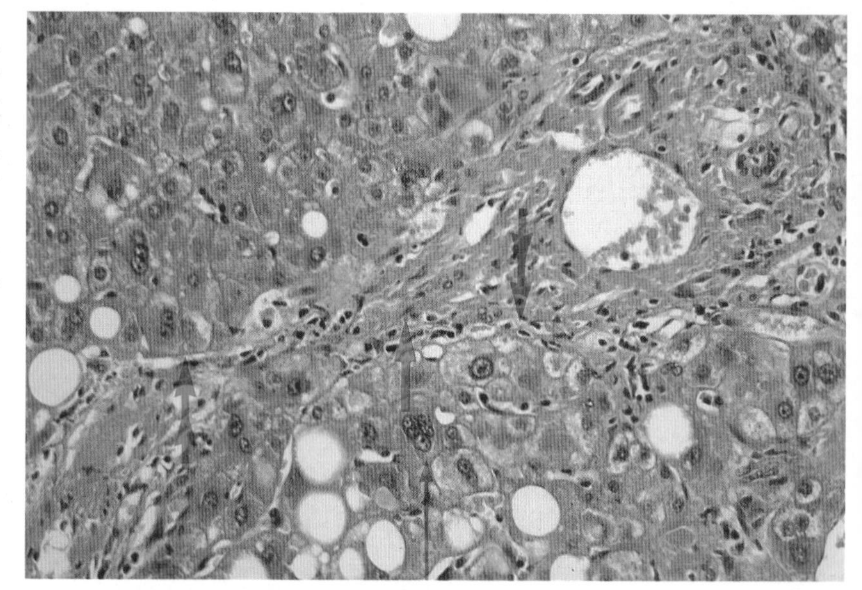

11.27 Ischemia of cirrhotic nodules: liver

Anastomoses may form between (hypertensive) portal veins and systemic veins, the best-known being the esophageal varices that develop in the proximal part of the stomach and the distal end of the esophagus. The varices in the esophagus are readily torn by minor trauma, and since the blood supply to the nodules of regenerating hepatocytes is often precarious, hemorrhage from the varices may produce severe ischemia and necrosis in a cirrhotic liver. When the ischemia is less pronounced, the hepatocytes undergo fatty change instead of necrosis. In the centre in this nodule, most of the hepatocytes contain round clear (fat-filled) vacuoles of various sizes, whereas the hepatocytes at the periphery of the nodule are affected only slightly or not at all. In contrast to the focal fatty change in this ischemic nodule, in alcoholic fatty cirrhosis fatty change would occur diffusely throughout the whole of the nodule.

HE ×150

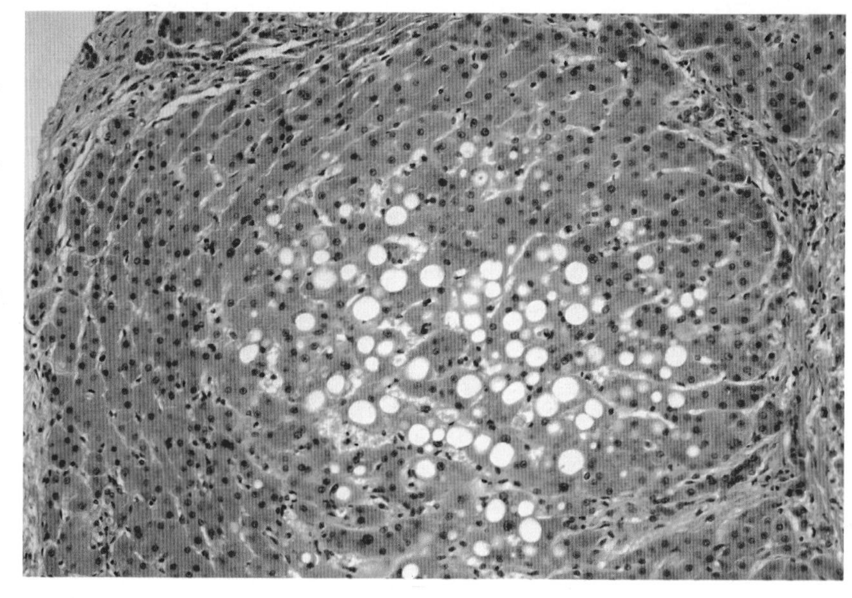

11.28 Cryptogenic cirrhosis: liver

Not infrequently cirrhosis develops without any obvious cause, and it is therefore termed cryptogenic cirrhosis. The cirrhosis pattern is generally macronodular. Development of cirrhosis may be halted but there is no obvious cure for it. It has been suggested therefore that chronic non-A non-B viral infection or an episode of subclinical hepatitis might be responsible. This is a section of the liver, stained for reticulin, from a man who had had portal hypertension for many years before dying of liver failure. The cause of his liver disease was not known. Several large pale sharply-defined nodules of parenchymal cells are present (double arrow), separated by broad bands of closely packed darkly-staining reticulin fibres (thick arrow). The weakly stained or unstained elongated clefts in the sheets of reticulin are vascular channels. There is also a well-developed reticulin framework throughout the nodules of hepatocytes, and in places it is evident, from their width, that the cords of hepatocytes are two cells thick (thin arrows).

Reticulin stain ×60

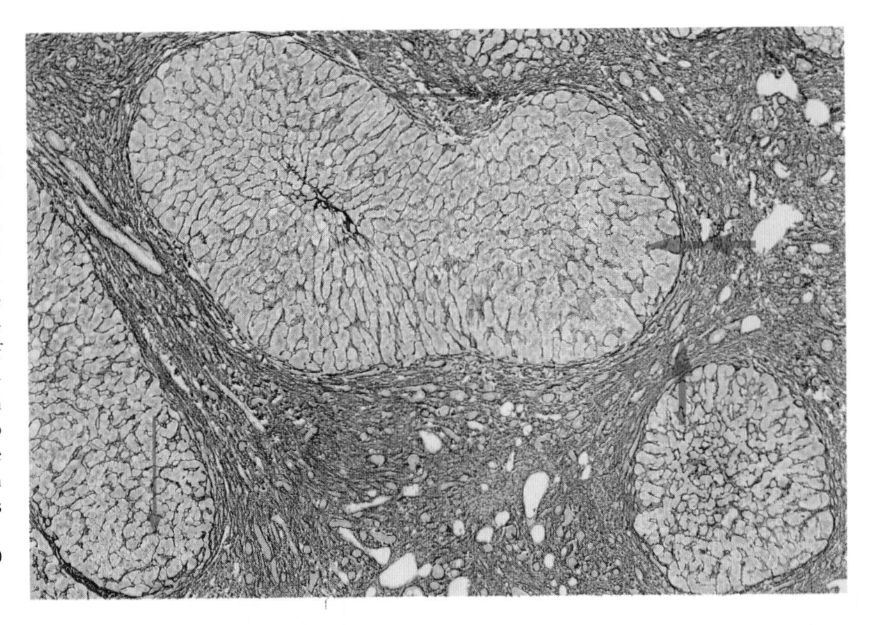

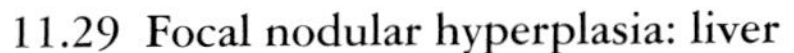

11.29 Focal nodular hyperplasia: liver

During laparotomy for resection of a carcinoma of colon, a woman of 48 was found to have a whitish lesion 4mm dia in her liver. The lesion was resected, and it was found to consist of ill-defined nodules of hepatocytes. In this field the nodules are separated by the bands of delicate connective tissue in which there are bile ductules and a fairly intense infiltrate of small basophilic lymphocytes. The hepatocytes within the nodules are arranged haphazardly, and in the centre of one of the nodules they are accompanied by a collection of lymphocytes (arrow). The hepatocytes are relatively small, each having a round compact solid-looking central nucleus and moderate amount of weakly staining or vacuolated cytoplasm. At the periphery of the lesion there was no fibrous capsule, and the nodules merged with normal-looking liver. Focal nodular hyperplasia may be mistaken for cirrhosis, but it is a localized lesion, probably of a hamartomatous nature. It is liable to bleed.

HE ×150

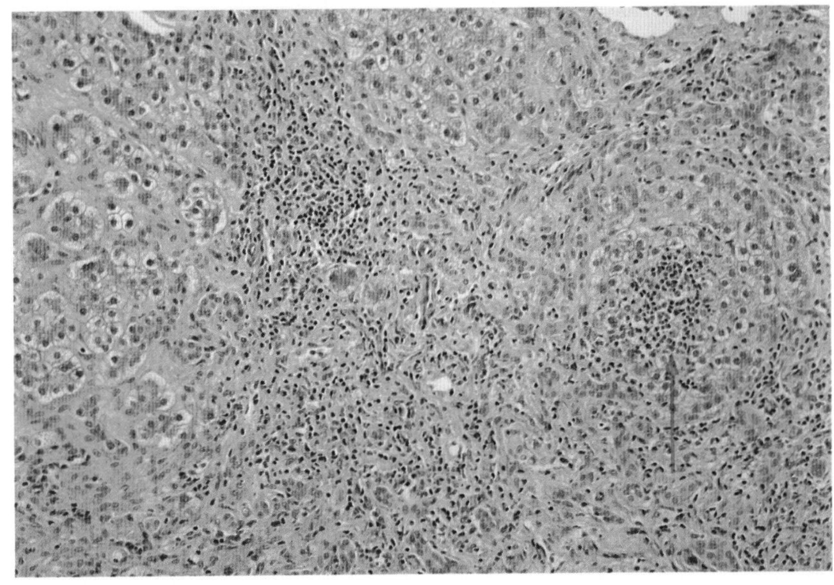

11.30 Primary hemochromatosis: liver

In primary (idiopathic) hemochromatosis, an inborn error of metabolism (inherited as an autosomal recessive character) leads to excessive absorption of iron from the gut. Much of the iron is stored as hemosiderin in the liver, in hepatocytes and bile duct epithelium. Hepatocytes are destroyed, and fibrosis develops which eventually leads to cirrhosis, generally micronodular in type. A large majority of cases are men. This section has been stained by Perls' method, which colours the iron blue or blue-black (the Prussian blue reaction), and in this field there are three discrete nodules of regenerating eosinophilic hepatocytes, separated by broad bands of dense fibrous tissue (double arrow). Nearly all the hepatocytes contain well-defined round black masses of iron (thin arrow), in high concentration in their cytoplasm, but the Kupffer cells in the sinusoids contain comparatively little. In the broad bands of fibrous tissue there is a considerable amount of black iron in collections of phagocytes, and much less in the epithelial cells lining the small bile ducts (thick arrow).

Perls' method ×55

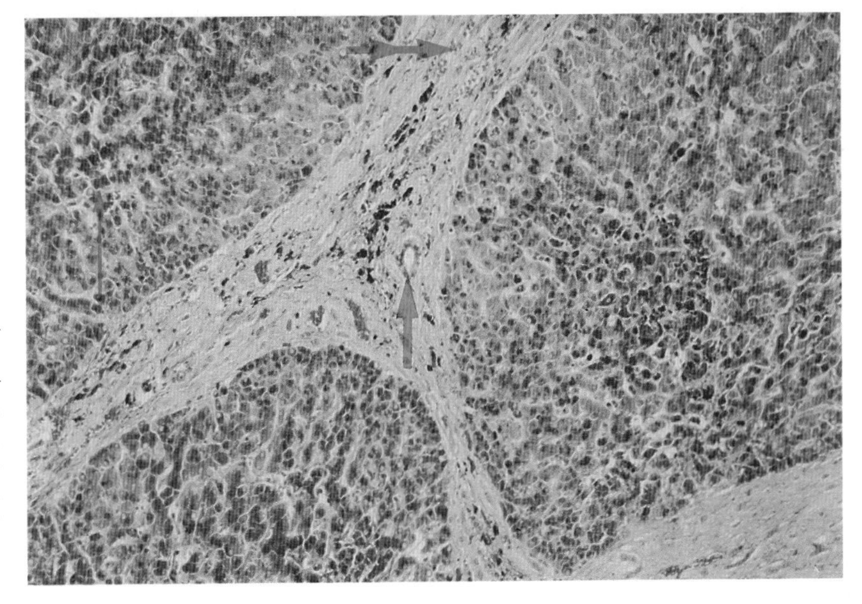

11.31 Drug-induced intrahepatic cholestasis: liver

This is a central vein (double arrow) in part of a hepatic lobule. There are also many distended bile canaliculi, each containing a plug of very dark brown inspissated bile (thin arrow). This appearance is characteristic of very marked centrilobular cholestasis. The hepatocytes appear comparatively normal, with round or ovoid vesicular nuclei and (in many) a prominent nucleolus (thick arrow). There is a notable lack of inflammatory cell infiltrate, and no evidence of necrosis or hepatitis was detected elsewhere. The fact that the cholestasis is centrilobular is very typical of the jaundice induced by anabolic steroids and oral contraceptives. In this case, a woman of 52, the cause was thought to be chlorpromazine, even though there was (unusually) no evidence of necrosis of liver cells or of a cellular inflammatory infiltrate in the portal tracts. The condition usually resolves completely when the hormone or drug is stopped. HE ×360

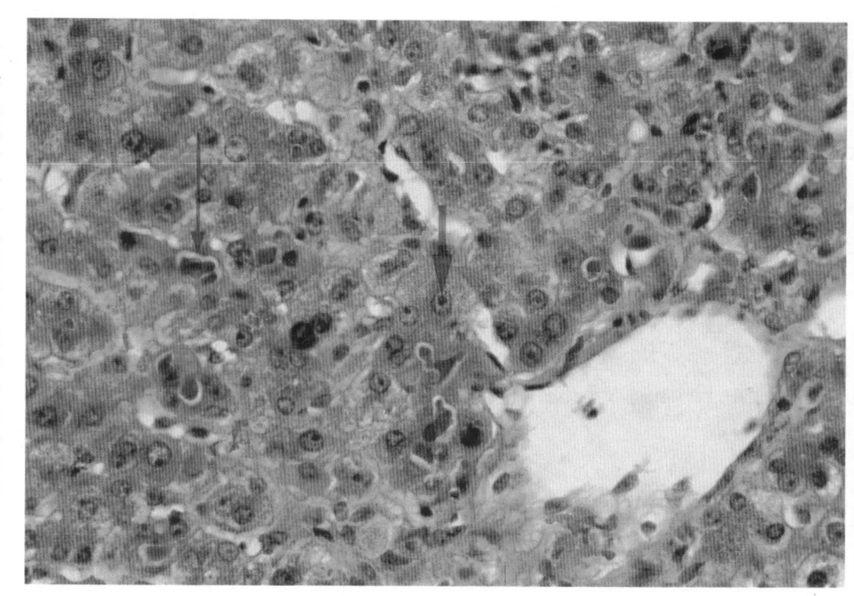

11.32 Biliary atresia: liver

In biliary atresia, the extrahepatic ducts fail to develop normally, and sometimes the whole extrahepatic biliary system becomes atretic. Biliary atresia is not a single entity, since a number of different conditions, including viral infections of the liver and cholangitis, are capable of damaging the extrahepatic and intrahepatic bile ducts; and a similar lesion occurs in association with various chromosomal defects. Atretic bile ducts may be reduced to fibrous cords without a lumen, and occasionally, in children, the intrahepatic ducts in the fibrous tissue gradually disappear. This section is from the liver of a child who had long-standing cholestatic jaundice, and the most important feature is the presence of large amounts of fibrous tissue (thin arrow) in the vicinity of the portal tracts. No interlobular bile ducts are visible in the fibrous tissue however and very few inflammatory cells are present. Just within or very close to the margin of the sheet of comparatively normal-looking hepatocytes, alongside the abundant fibrous tissue, there are distended canaliculi containing brownish-black inspissated plugs of bile (thick arrows). HE ×60

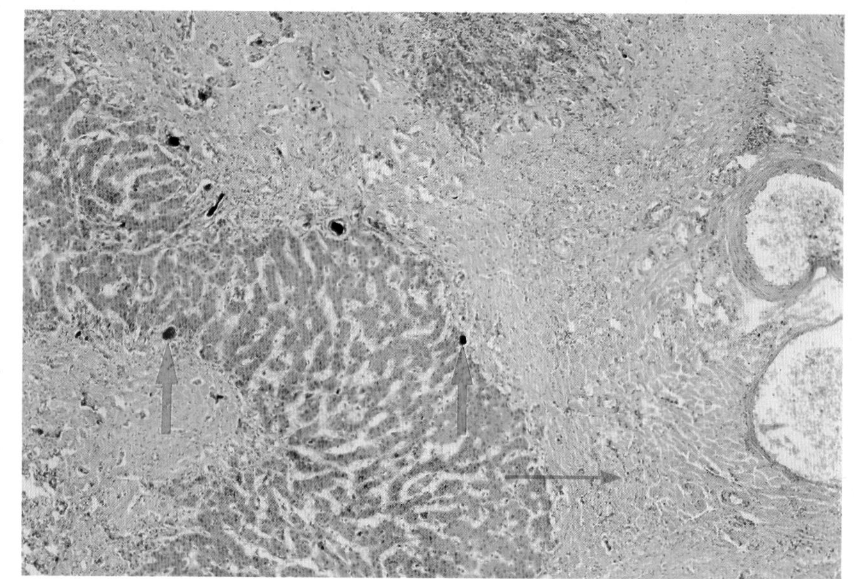

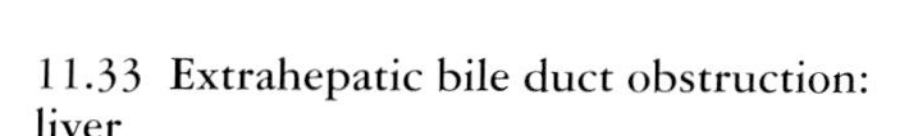

11.33 Extrahepatic bile duct obstruction: liver

Benign stricture of the common bile duct or of another extrahepatic duct is very often caused by surgical injury or other type of trauma. In extrahepatic bile duct obstruction there is often evidence of cholangitis and portal inflammation. Secondary infection, usually low-grade, tends to occur. When the extrahepatic ducts are involved, they become progressively thickened, fibrotic and stenosed. In the centre of this field, there is a portal tract which is wider than normal and in which there is a greatly dilated interlobular bile duct filled with inspissated fragments of dark brown bile (double arrow). The duct is surrounded by concentric layers of collagenous connective tissue. The single layer of epithelial cells lining the duct is flattened and deficient in places. The number of inflammatory cells in the connective tissue is fairly small, but at one point where there is loss of the limiting plate, they are fairly numerous (thin arrow). Proliferation of small ducts is evident (thick arrows). HE ×75

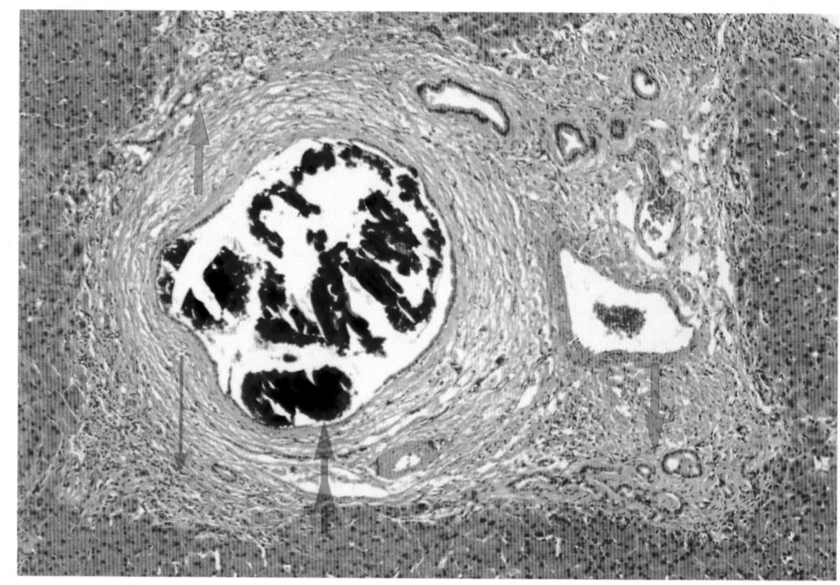

11.34 Extrahepatic bile duct obstruction: liver

After several days or a few weeks of extrahepatic biliary obstruction, the portal tracts are edematous and lose their typical angular shape, becoming rounded. The most notable feature then is marked proliferation of the small bile ducts at the margin of the portal tracts. This patient had long-standing obstruction of the common bile duct, and this field is filled with a 'trilobed' section of liver (resembling a jigsaw 'piece') which looks fully viable. Characteristically the centrilobular zones (thin arrow) are unaffected. However, chronic cholangiohepatitis has led to the formation of a considerable amount of edematous fibrous tissue in the portal tracts, which are consequently enlarged and round and within which there are many proliferating bile ductules (thick arrow). Most of the proliferating ductules are adjacent to the periphery of the hepatic lobules which are themselves delineated by the enlarged portal tracts. The widened portal tracts tend to coalesce and produce secondary biliary cirrhosis of a monolobular type. HE ×60

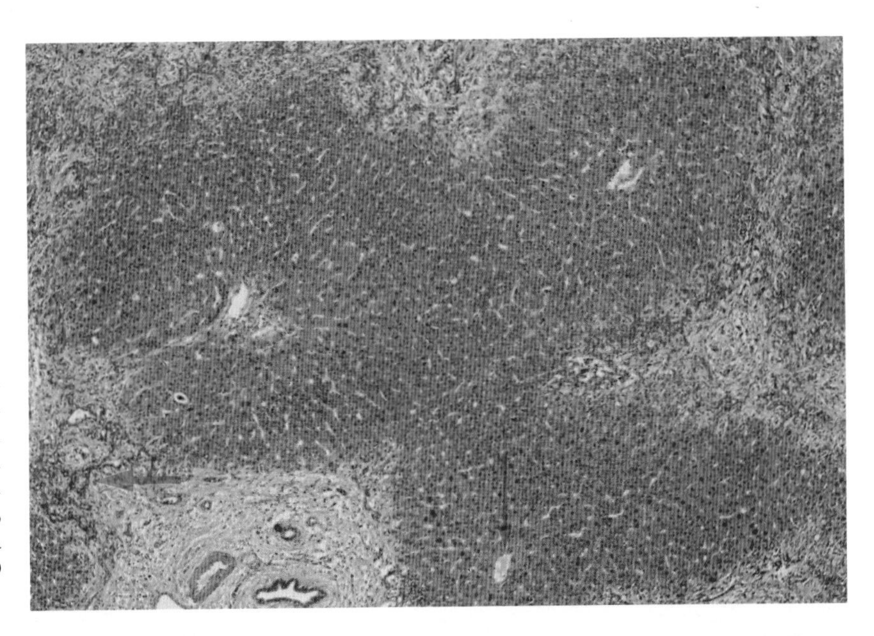

11.35 Extrahepatic bile duct obstruction: liver

This is the same lesion (secondary biliary cirrhosis) as that illustrated in 11.34. The deeply eosinophilic centrilobular zone of liver parenchyma (centre and left), in which there is a dilated central vein (thick arrow), is unaffected. The hepatocytes appear fully viable, but there is some pleomorphism of the nuclei. The periphery of the hepatic lobule is fairly well delineated and adjacent to a greatly widened portal tract (a small part of another hepatic lobule is just visible at the left margin of the field). The portal tract consists mainly of pale edematous cellular connective tissue, and at its margin and within it there is a complex network of proliferating small irregularly shaped basophilic bile ductules (thin arrow) lined by a single layer of pleomorphic epithelial cells. A modest population of chronic inflammatory cells is also present in the tract. Sometimes the proliferating ductules form spurs which extend out from the portal tracts and join the tracts together. HE ×150

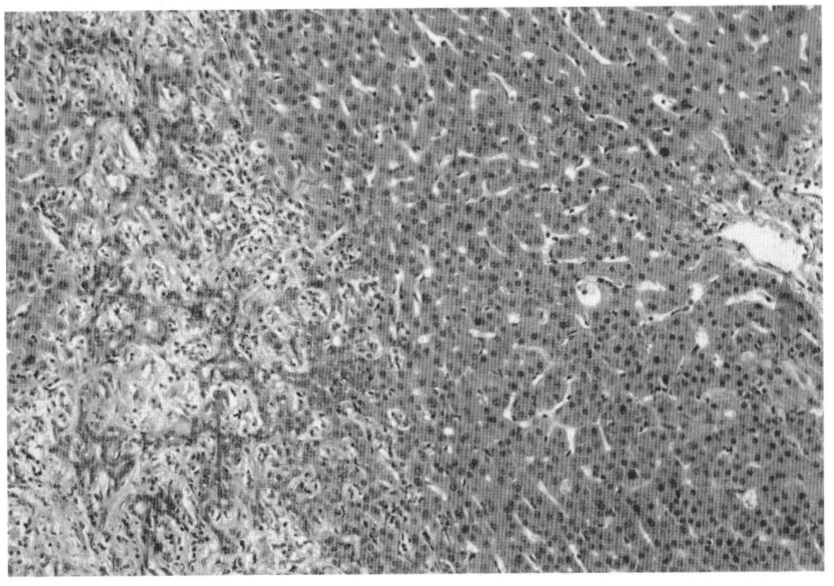

11.36 Extrahepatic bile duct obstruction: liver

If extrahepatic biliary obstruction is prolonged, bile accumulates in the hepatocytes and bile plugs in the canaliculi. Occasionally a large duct ruptures and produces a granulomatous reaction. Single hepatocytes or small groups of hepatocytes undergo feathery degeneration and are greatly swollen. Subsequently they become necrotic and lyse. In this case, there is a sheet of swollen eosinophilic hepatocytes (thin arrow) with fairly normal-looking vesicular nuclei and a few atrophic hepatocytes (left of centre) with pyknotic nuclei. Among the hepatocytes there are scattered bile canaliculi (thick arrows), plugged with dark brown bile. On the left there is a deeply eosinophilic sheet (with a greenish tint) of necrotic hepatocytes into which extravasated bile has seeped, forming a so-called bile lake or bile infarct (double arrow). The cytoplasm of macrophages and some atrophic hepatocytes adjacent to the bile lake also contain bile. Bile lakes, like bile infarcts, are usually located near portal tracts. They tend to be found in large duct obstruction, but they may be found also in primary biliary cirrhosis and alcoholic cirrhosis. HE ×360

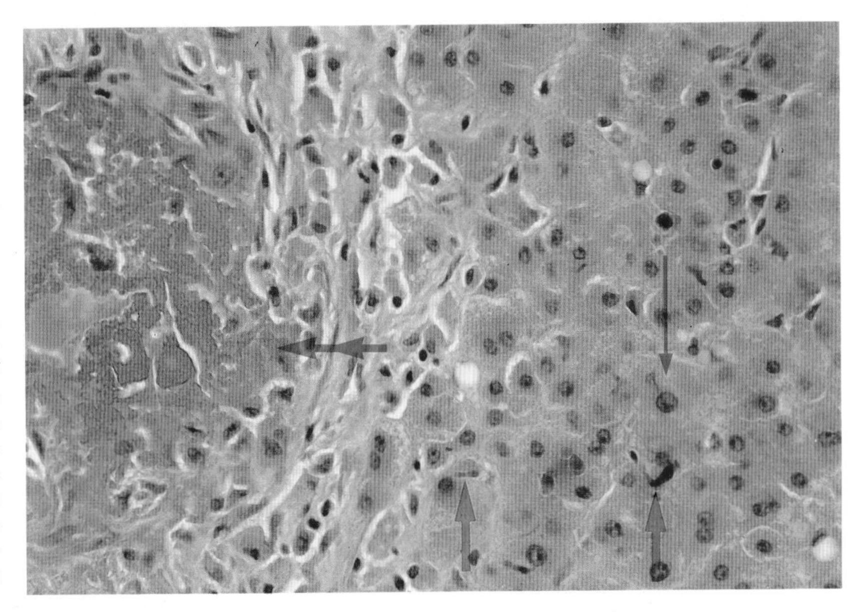

11.37 Primary biliary cirrhosis: liver

Primary biliary cirrhosis is probably immunologically mediated, and the patient's serum generally contains an anti-mitochondrial antibody. The disease, also called chronic non-suppurative destructive cholangitis, causes progressive destruction of the bile ducts in the portal tracts of the liver. Cirrhosis develops patchily early in the disease and diffusely only later in the disease. An inflammatory process, consisting mainly of lymphocytes, causes degeneration of the epithelium of the smaller (interlobular and septal) intrahepatic bile ducts (50μm or less in diameter). Necrosis of hepatocytes occurs later. Sometimes macrophages, plasma cells and polymorph leukocytes also accumulate, to form granulomas. The inflammatory infiltrate varies in intensity from one tract to another. In this case, large numbers of small deeply basophil lymphocytes (thin arrow) and far fewer large pale macrophages have accumulated around the bile ducts, filling and enlarging the affected triads of the portal tracts. Small bile ducts and ductules are absent, and there is neither cholestasis nor significant damage to the liver parenchyma, apart from a few acidophil necrotic hepatocytes (thick arrows). Piecemeal necrosis is occurring in the most severely affected tract.

HE ×60

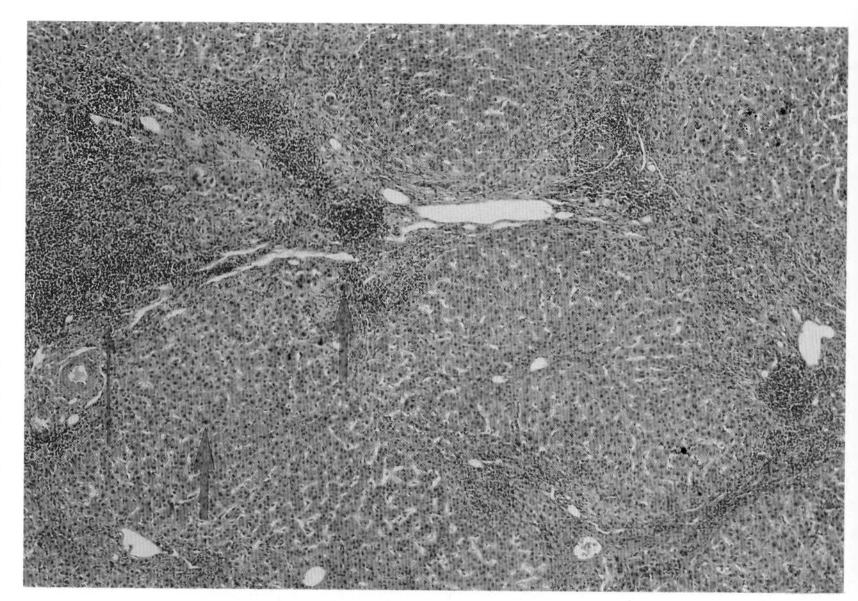

11.38 Primary biliary cirrhosis: liver

The lesions produced by primary biliary cirrhosis suggest an immunological attack against the epithelium of the intrahepatic bile ducts, and possibly of other types of secretory duct. This field, from the same case as in **11.37** at higher magnification, contains only one portal tract, in the centre of which there is a compact rounded group of swollen strongly eosinophilic cells (thick arrows), each with abundant cytoplasm and a relatively large pale ovoid or kidney-shaped vesicular nucleus. In the centre of the group there is a lumen-like space in which there are several smaller cells with less cytoplasm but similar nuclei. Many small basophilic lymphocytes (thin arrow) (but relatively few plasma cells) surround and also invade the group of swollen cells. It has been suggested that the group is a damaged interlobar duct (in cross-section), lined by single layer of epithelial cells, but on closer inspection it seems much more likely to be an unusually compact epithelioid granuloma, composed of large eosinophilic histiocytes. In the top right corner of the field there is ballooning degeneration of some hepatocytes and some erosion of the adjacent limiting plate. HE ×360

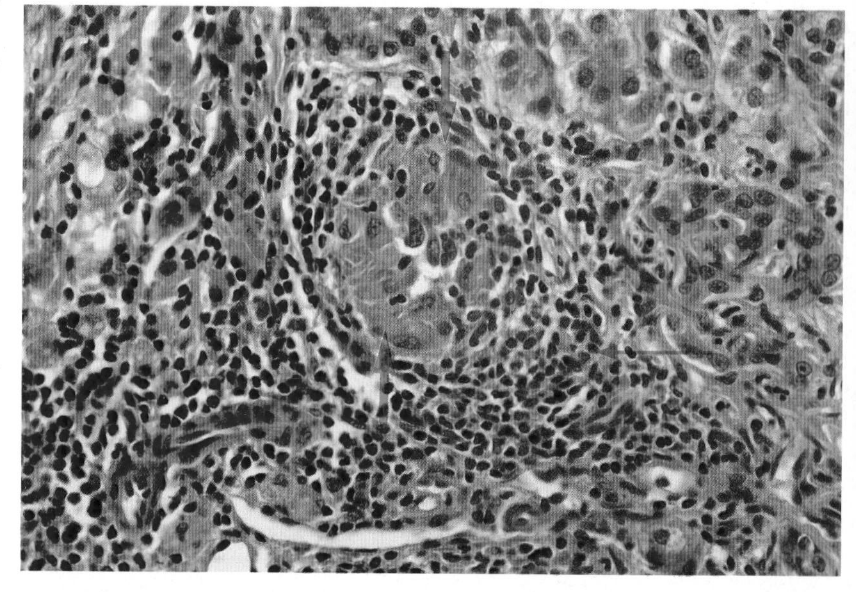

11.39 Primary biliary cirrhosis: liver

In primary biliary cirrhosis, the distribution of the duct lesions is irregular, and the large intrahepatic and extrahepatic ducts are unaffected. The exudate in the portal tracts consists initially of lymphocytes, but later there are numerous macrophages and plasma cells. Frequently also the macrophages aggregate around the ducts and form a granuloma, and there is a round granuloma of the same type in the left half of this field, the portal tract apparently having developed in relation to a damaged bile duct. The granuloma is composed mainly of closely packed large pleomorphic epithelioid macrophages (thin arrow) with deeply eosinophilic cytoplasm and large vesicular nuclei, in some of which there is a prominent nucleolus (giant forms are also occasionally present, but not in this granuloma). None of the macrophages in the granuloma is necrotic. There are fairly numerous small basophilic lymphocytes and occasional plasma cells in the portal tract, and some lymphocytes have infiltrated the granuloma. The large swollen hepatocytes adjoining the portal tract have undergone ballooning degeneration and piecemeal necrosis (thick arrow). HE ×360

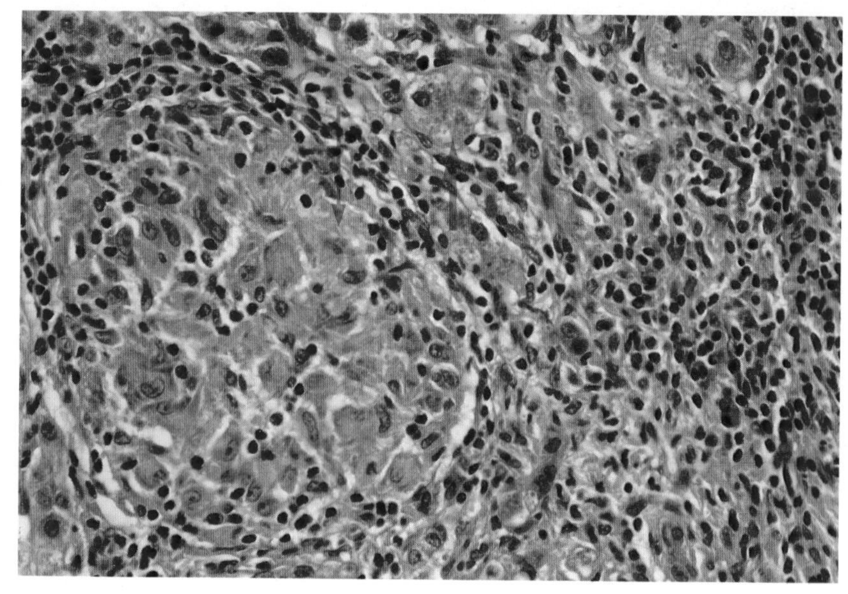

11.40 Primary biliary cirrhosis: liver

Primary biliary cirrhosis can usually be distinguished from extrahepatic bile duct obstruction by the absence of bile ducts and the presence of a more intense infiltrate of lymphocytes in the portal tracts. As primary biliary cirrhosis progresses to a later stage of the disease, as illustrated by this field, the portal tracts are markedly enlarged and within them there are large network of small basophilic ductules (thin arrow), proliferating at the margins of the tracts and accompanied by loose connective tissues. A considerable population of small lymphocytes and plasma cells is also present in the expanded irregularly-shaped tracts. Previously, segments of the bile ducts have been destroyed and obliterated by the exudate of lymphocytes and other inflammatory cells, and consequently no bile ducts now remain in the portal tracts. The limiting plate of the hepatocytes (top right) has also been eroded, as exhibited by the piecemeal necrosis of some hepatocytes (thick arrow). HE ×235

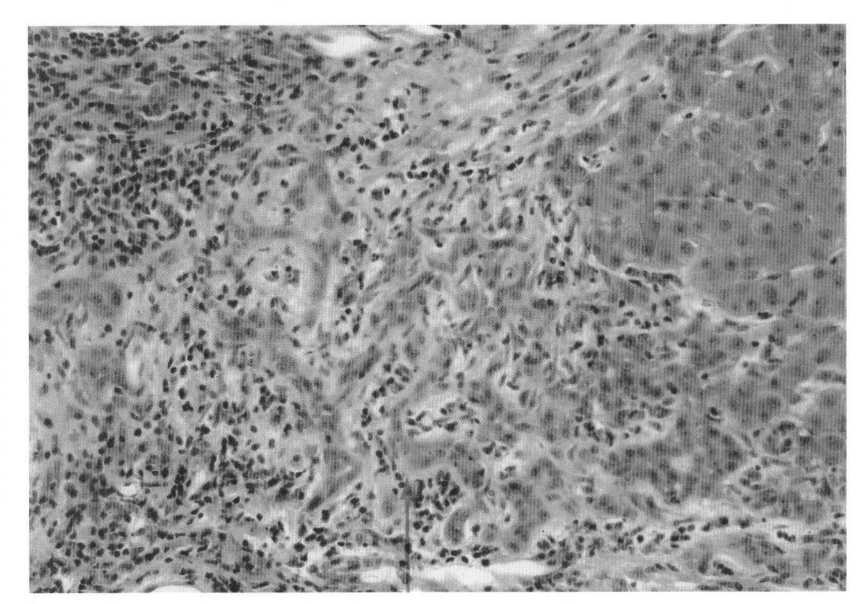

11.41 Primary biliary cirrhosis: liver

Primary biliary cirrhosis may persist for a period which may vary from months to many years, death resulting from liver failure or from the complications of portal hypertension. This is a more advanced stage of the disease than that in **11.40**, and in this field fibrosis has progressed to the formation of portal-portal fibrous septa (thin arrow). The fibrous septa have joined up adjacent portal tracts, splitting and encircling the lobules but leaving the centrilobular regions unaffected (thick arrow), thereby producing a pattern of monolobular fibrosis similar to that seen in extrahepatic bile duct obstruction. There is patchy lymphocytic infiltration of the portal tracts, but proliferation of bile ductules is not a feature. Persistent loss and nodular regeneration of hepatocytes complete the final stage of cirrhosis. The cirrhotic liver is usually micronodular in type. HE ×60

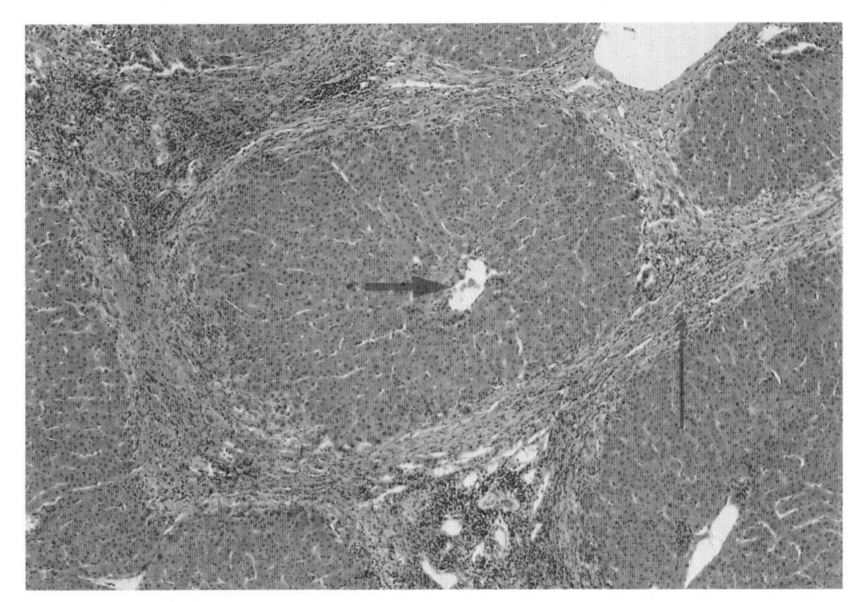

11.42 Ulcerative colitis: liver

Lesions are not infrequently seen in the liver in patients with chronic inflammatory bowel disease, but they are usually mild and cause no dysfunction. In this case, a man aged 60, with severe long-standing ulcerative colitis affecting the whole colon and rectum but now inactive, developed sclerosing cholangitis which caused fibrosis and narrowing of the common bile duct. There is severe cholestasis and there is also marked increase in fibrous tissue within the liver. In this field, the fibrous tissue surrounding the small interlobular bile ducts in the portal tracts is fairly heavily infiltrated with lymphocytes (thin arrow). These lymphocytes are also extending into the adjacent nodule of hepatic parenchyma and eroding its periphery. There is considerable disorder in the arrangement of the hepatocytes, which also vary greatly in size. A considerable proportion of the hepatocytes show ballooning degeneration (thick arrow) and some hepatocytes have two or more nuclei. Some of the hepatocytes are stained with bile, and numerous canaliculi are distended with large plugs of brownish-black bile (double arrow). The changes in the liver were diagnosed as secondary biliary cirrhosis. HE ×150

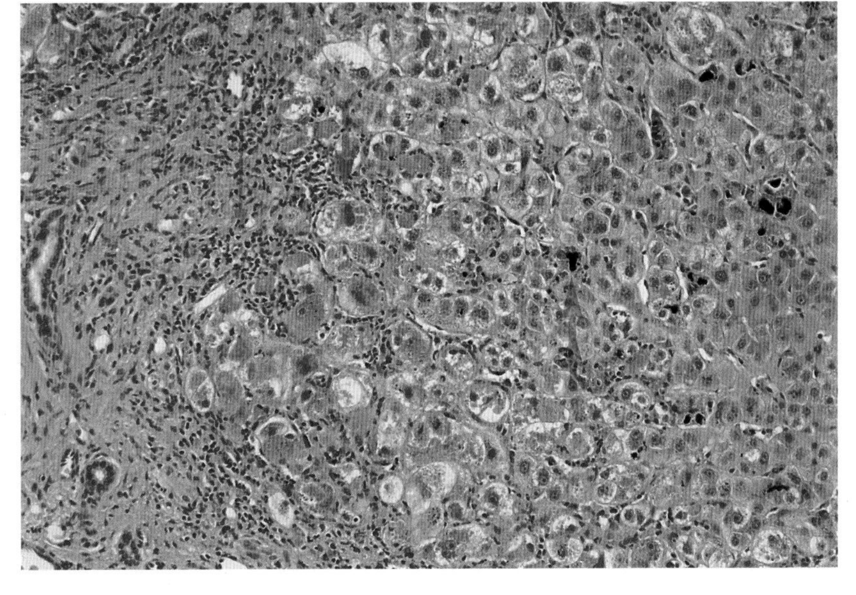

11.43 Liver cell adenoma: liver

Liver cell adenoma (benign hepatoma) is very uncommon but it is increasing in incidence, probably because of the use of the oral contraceptive pill and sex hormone therapy. It is lighter in colour than the surrounding liver. It usually has a fibrous capsule it is generally incomplete, and tumour cells do not invade the adjacent parenchyma. The cells of the adenoma closely resemble normal hepatocytes but are slightly larger, and they form cord-like arrangements (two or three cells thick) around bile canaliculi (which can be detected). The neoplastic cells have a considerable amount of eosinophilic cytoplasm and very uniform round basophilic nuclei. There is little or no mitotic activity (none visible in this field). There are no bile ducts or portal tracts. A notable feature of the tumour is its vascularity, and there are two areas of necrosis and hemorrhage in it (arrows). A high percentage of the adenomas may rupture during pregnancy or post-partum period, resulting in serious intraperitoneal hemorrhage,

HE ×150

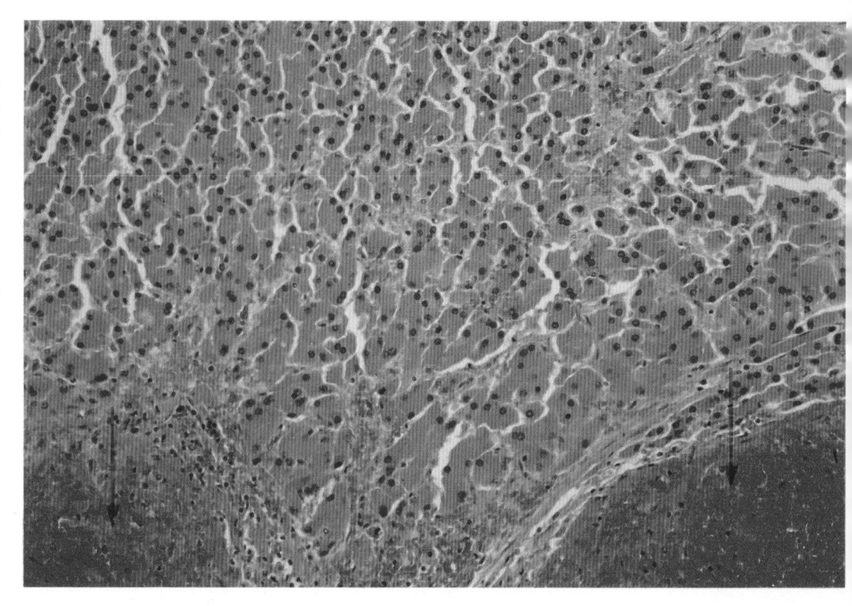

11.44 Hepatocellular carcinoma: liver

The incidence of hepatocellular carcinoma (hepatoma) varies markedly in different parts of the world, being relatively much more common in parts of Africa and Asia, hepatitis B virus playing a part in its etiology. The great majority of tumours arise in cirrhotic livers, and men are affected more often than women. Hepatocellular carcinomas often spread intrahepatically by the portal vein, but they also frequently metastasize to other organs and tissues. This lesion was in the cirrhotic liver of a man of 67. It consists of broad trabeculae (2-8 cells thick) of large polyhedral cells (malignant hepatocytes), closely apposed to the thin-walled capillary blood vessels (thin arrow). The neoplastic hepatocytes are markedly uniform in this field but including spindle-shaped or giant forms, have a large amount of eosinophilic granular multivacuolated cytoplasm and large round vesicular nuclei in which there is a very prominent central nucleolus (double arrows). Some acini, which are lined by malignant ductal-epithelial cells, contain bile-stained debris (thick arrows). Glycogen could be demonstrated in the cells but an orcein stain for HBsAg was negative. HE ×360

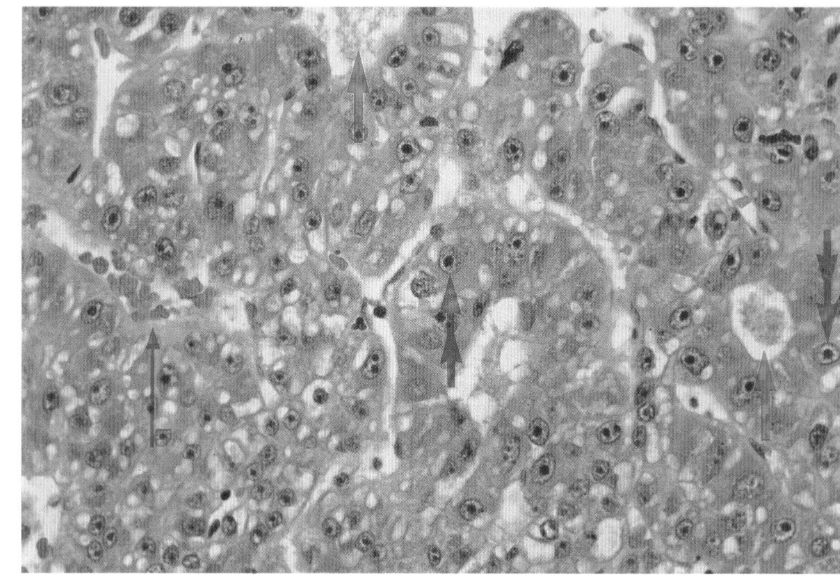

11.45 Hepatocellular carcinoma: liver

A hepatocellular carcinoma may be a single discrete mass or multicentric or diffusely infiltrative, and the tumour is often bile-stained. In contrast, this tumour, in a woman aged 41, weighed 6,120g and caused enormous enlargement of the liver. There was no evidence of cirrhosis. The tumour consisted of multiple rounded masses, several of which showed extensive necrosis and hemorrhage. Histologically there was a wide range of structure. Much of the tumour consisted of solid trabeculae (mostly several cells thick), but acinar formation was common. In this part of the tumour the neoplastic cells are arranged in irregular groups, aligned along thin-walled vascular channels (thick arrow). The neoplastic cells are large and pleomorphic, with much eosinophilic cytoplasm, in which there are numerous round clear vacuoles, mostly large (thin arrow). The vacuoles had contained fat (which dissolved in reagents) and it was also possible to demonstrate abundant glycogen in them. The tumour cells have uniform round nuclei, and the majority are vesicular in appearance and contain a nucleolus. The structural pattern of this tumour is reminiscent of renal carcinoma (hypernephroma).

HE ×360

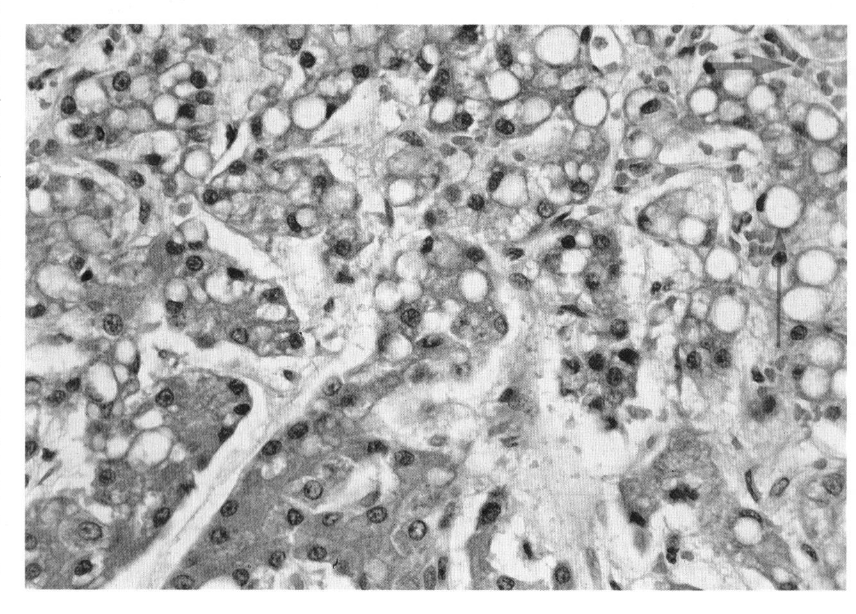

11.46 Hepatocellular carcinoma: liver

In some hepatocellular carcinomas there are well-differentiated acini. In this case, a woman of 72 with no history of ethanol abuse and no evidence of jaundice was admitted to hospital because of the recent onset of ascites and persistent diarrhea. She died 6 weeks later, and post-mortem examination revealed cirrhosis and a hepatocellular carcinoma. The tumour was bile-stained in places. It is a poorly-differentiated carcinoma, but the tissue in this area has a marked tendency to form acini. The acini are fairly large and regularly spaced and lined by cuboidal tumour cells (thick arrow). The neoplastic cells have relatively scanty cytoplasm, but their nuclei are large (some very large) markedly basophilic and pleomorphic. There are frequent mitoses elsewhere in the tumour but few in this field. In the lumen of several acini there are desquamated cells or cell debris. HBsAg was not detectable in the tumour cells. The tissue at the bottom consist of compressed and markedly atrophic trabeculae of non-neoplastic hepatocytes (thin arrow). HE ×235

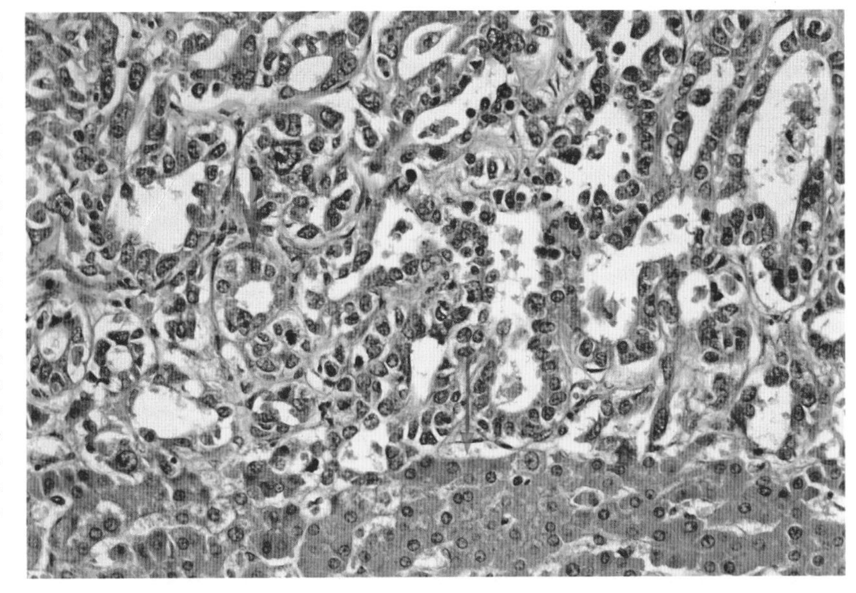

11.47 Cholangiocarcinoma: common bile duct

Cholangiocarcinoma most often arises in the porta hepatis at the junction of the right and left hepatic ducts. The presenting sign is usually jaundice. This tumour, however, was a small mass within the terminal portion of the common bile duct, near the ampulla of Vater. Typically it infiltrated the submucosa of the common bile duct and occluded and dilated the duct. It is a papilliferous adenocarcinoma, consisting of gland-like structures and acini of widely varying sizes, lined by deeply basophilic tall columnar or cuboidal malignant epithelial cells. Long finger-like papilliform processes, with a fibrovascular core and their surfaces covered with a single layer of columnar epithelial cells (thin arrow), project into the larger gland-like structures. There are also clusters of desquamated tumour cells and a considerable amount of cell debris in the lumen of the gland-like structures. Cholangiocarcinomas are generally sclerosing (desmoplastic) tumours and characteristically there is abundant fibrous stroma (thick arrow) between the gland-like structures of this tumour. The fibrous stroma is also heavily infiltrated with lymphocytes. HE ×120

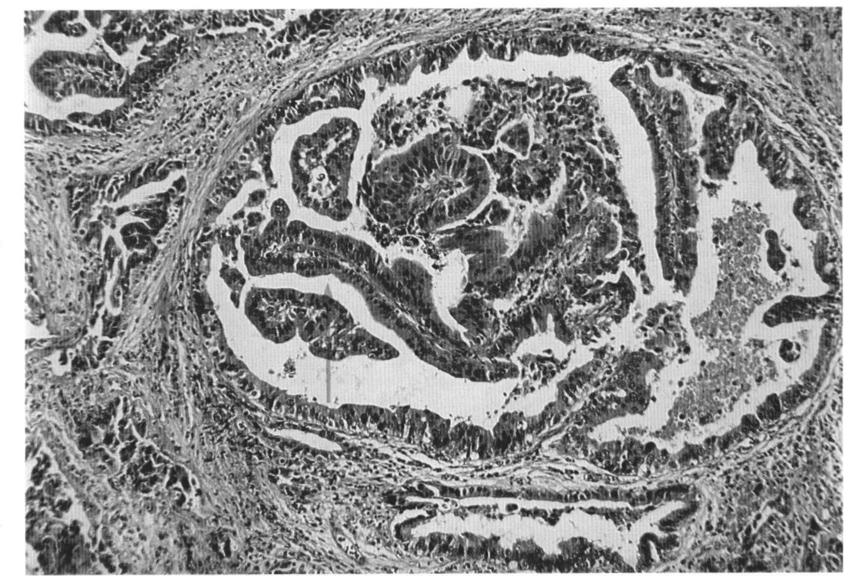

11.48 Secondary melanoma: liver

The liver is a common site for secondary tumours, usually carcinomas, the metastasizing cells being carried to the liver in the portal vein blood or by the hepatic artery. The metastases are usually multiple, often large, well-demarcated and tending to reproduce the microscopic structure of the primary tumour. Sometimes however the metastatic malignant cells infiltrate the liver diffusely, without forming large masses, and in this case the malignant cells are lying within the sinusoids. The malignant cells have a moderate amount of cytoplasm, and in their nuclei there is a prominent central nucleolus (thin arrows). The nucleoli of the malignant cells are also generally larger than the nucleoli in the hepatocyte nuclei (thick arrows). Nuclear pleomorphism is comparatively slight however in the malignant cells, and there are no mitotic figures in this field. The brown pigment (top right) in the cytoplasm of the hepatocytes is hemosiderin. A special stain did reveal small quantities of melanin within the tumour cells, confirming that the deposit was metastatic malignant melanoma. HE ×360

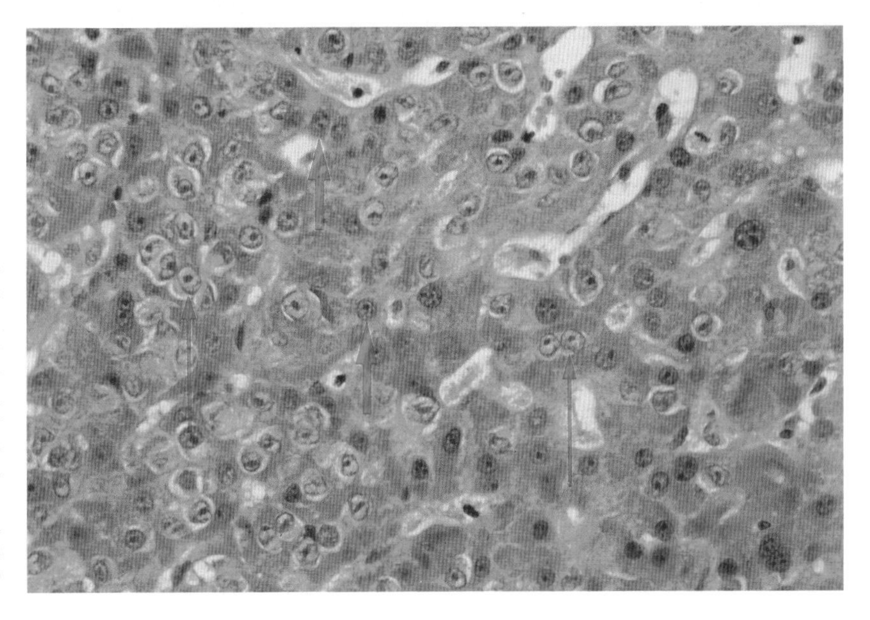

11.49 Cholesterolosis: gall bladder

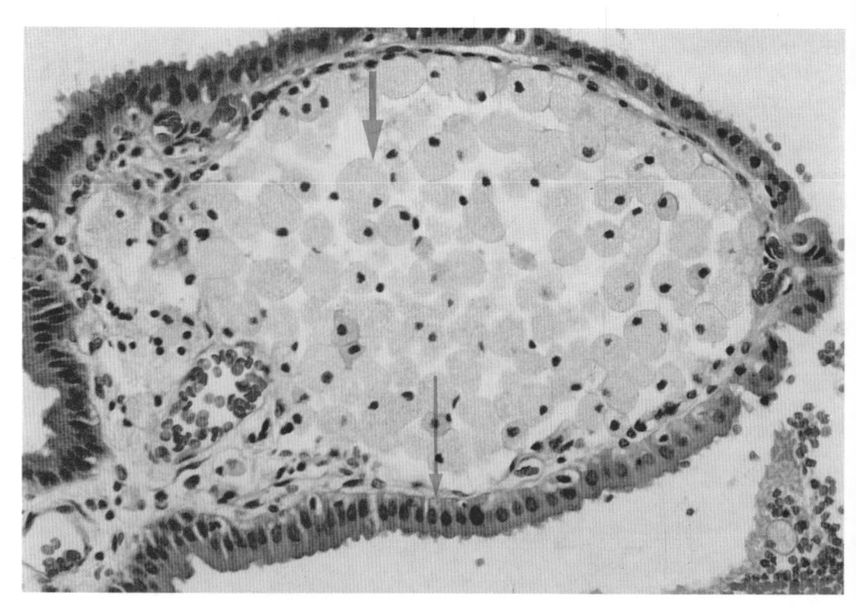

Cholesterolosis of the gall bladder precedes formation of gallstones, and gallstones are usually present in gall bladders showing cholesterolosis. Gall-bladders showing cholesterolosis have a thin wall and they usually function normally, producing no symptoms. The mucosa lining this gall bladder, from a man of 72, was yellow from the presence within it of small bright yellow flecks, scattered over the (usually bile-stained) folds of the mucosa. The flecks are usually less than 1mm dia but may become larger and polypoid. The flecks resemble the seeds of a strawberry — hence the term 'strawberry gall-bladder'. In this field there is one mucosal fold, in cross-section. The fold, its surface covered with cuboidal or low columnar epithelial cells, most of them 'hob-nail' type (thin arrow), is greatly swollen from the presence within it of many large round macrophages with abundant pale well-defined finely granular ('frosted-glass') cytoplasm (thick arrow). The frosted-glass appearance is caused by the presence of lipid (mostly cholesterol ester), and it is the lipid which gives the mucosal folds their (macroscopic) yellow colour. HE ×320

11.50 Chronic cholecystitis: gall bladder

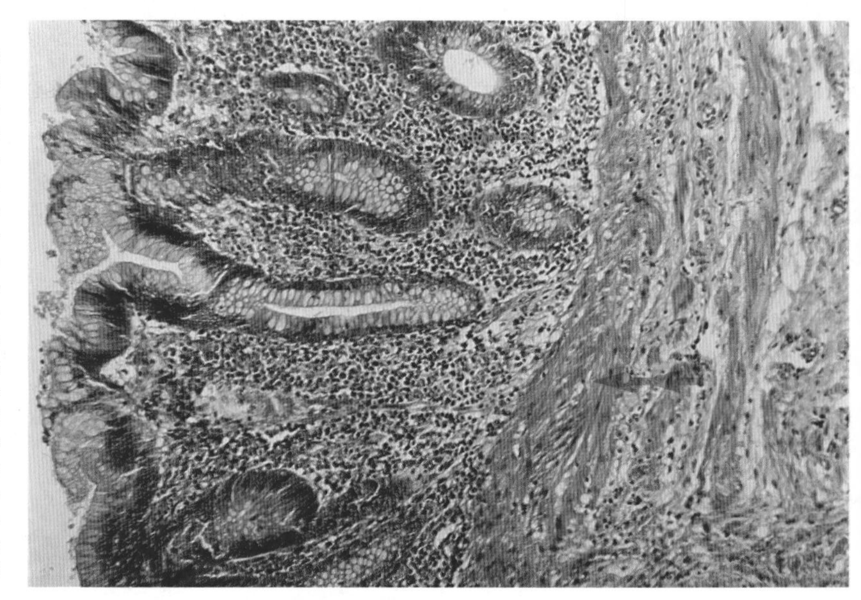

Almost all patients with chronic cholecystitis have cholelithiasis, and vice versa. In chronic cholecystitis, the wall of the gall bladder is generally thick, collagenous fibrous tissue being the most important component. The gall bladder may be of normal size or small, and in this patient it was small and shrunken, with a thick opaque fibrous wall. It also contained many 'mixed' (as usual) gallstones. The mucosa lining the gall bladder is chronically inflamed and thickened. The elongated mucosal glands are lined by a single layer of tall columnar epithelial cells (thin arrow), distended with pale mucin, with deeply basophilic nuclei at the cell base (oblique sectioning has given a mis-leading appearance of nuclear multilayering at the mucosal surface). The normal mucosal folds are lacking, and there is a dense infiltrate of closely packed inflammatory cells (thick arrow) (lymphocytes, plasma cells and eosinophil leukocytes) between the glands. The eosinophilic muscle coat (double arrow) is thick, from hypertrophy, and infiltrated by relatively few chronic inflammatory cells. Increase of fibrous tissue in the wall is fairly slight. HE ×120

11.51 Acute hemorrhagic pancreatitis: pancreas

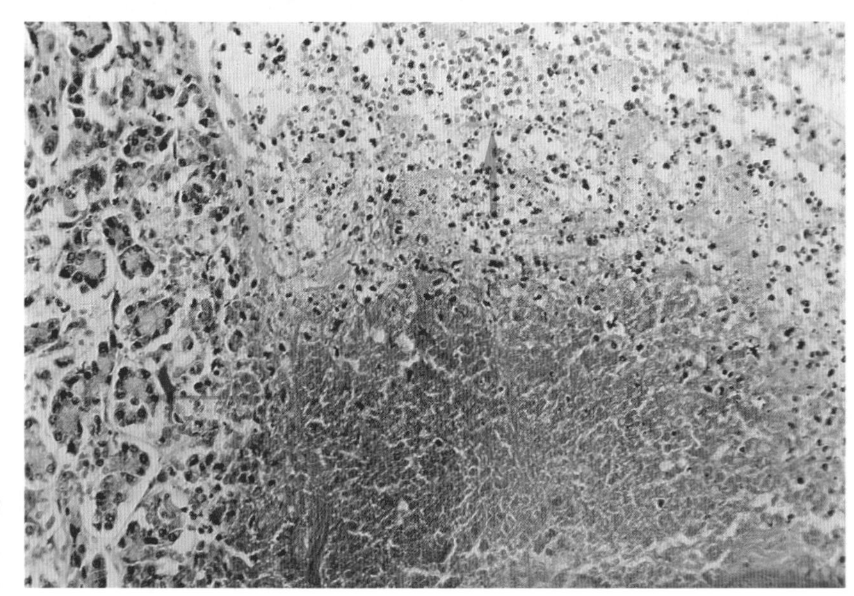

The etiology and pathogenesis of acute pancreatitis are still uncertain, but most cases are associated with disease of the biliary tract (generally gall stones), trauma or alcoholism. In the more severe forms of acute pancreatitis, the pancreas is inflamed and edematous, and foci of necrosis appear throughout the organ after a few days. In acute hemorrhagic pancreatitis, necrosis is even more extensive and accompanied by hemorrhage. There is also an intense infiltrate of neutrophil leukocytes. Pancreatic enzymes, particularly lipase and trypsin, are released in an active form into the pancreas itself and also into adjacent tissues such as the omentum, where they cause necrosis. In this case, the exocrine tissue of the pancreas (thin arrow) has been spared to limited extent, much of the adjacent tissue (centre and right) being completely necrotic and disintegrated, leaving only cell debris and numerous red cells (thick arrow). Most of the necrotic tissue is diffusely and intensely basophil (bluish-purple) (double arrow), following the rapid deposition of calcium in it, calcium having a high affinity for necrotic tissue. HE ×135

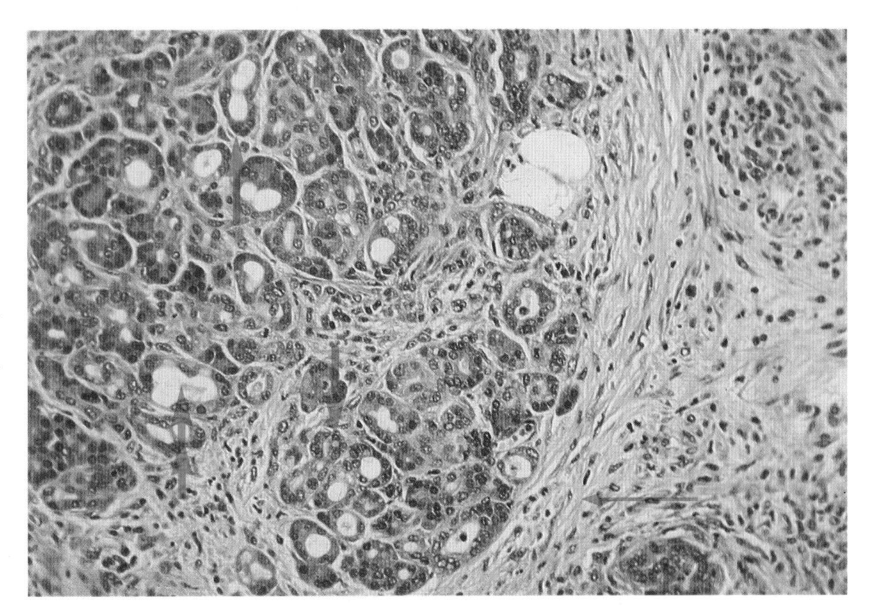

11.52 Chronic sclerosing pancreatitis: pancreas

In this form of chronic pancreatitis, which is associated with alcoholism, the pancreas becomes hard and nodular. It is sometimes larger than normal but is more often reduced in size. Histologically the most pronounced change is marked increase in collagenous fibrous tissue, in the form of bands of fibrous tissue (thin arrow) around and within the pancreatic lobules (interlobular and intralobular fibrosis). The fibrous tissue contains a fairly scant mixture of lymphocytes, plasma cells and polymorph leukocytes. The exocrine tissue is abnormal. The lumen of many of the glands is much increased (double arrow) and, instead of the normal columnar epithelial cells, most of the glands are lined with flat or cuboidal epithelial cells (thick arrow)s. The nuclei of the epithelial cells however (except for the smaller cells) are more or less uniformly round and pale and lack a nucleolus. There are no mitoses in this field. It may be difficult to differentiate chronic pancreatitis from carcinoma of the pancreas, but the comparatively normal appearance of the nuclei of the epithelial cells is very helpful in distinguishing chronic sclerosing pancreatitis from carcinoma. HE ×150

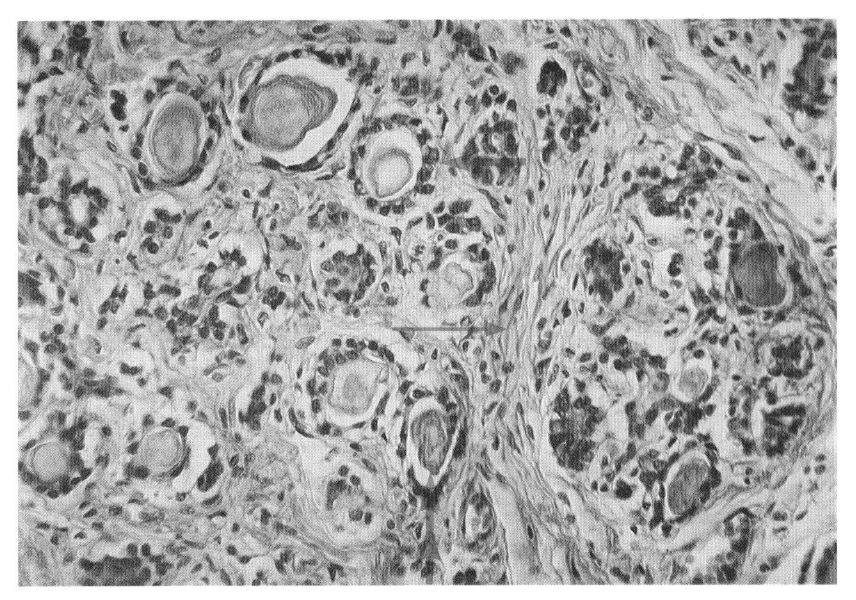

11.53 Cystic fibrosis: pancreas

Cystic fibrosis (also termed as mucoviscidosis or fibrocystic disease), common in white people but rare in black people, is inherited as an autosomal recessive character. The secretory activity of exocrine glands is abnormal in many organs, including pancreas, liver, alimentary tract, lungs and sweat glands. The pancreas looks normal at birth, but fibrosis of the pancreas increases steadily, and it becomes small, firm and gritty. Small cysts are also generally present. Loss of the exocrine secretion of the pancreas produces a malabsorption syndrome. This field contains one lobule of pancreas. Dense collagenous fibroblastic tissue (thin arrow) has formed around the lobule and between the individual ductules and acini that remain (interlobular and intralobular fibrosis). The ductules and acini are markedly atrophic, lined by a single layer of flat or low cuboidal cells (thick arrow) with very little cytoplasm and a small inert-looking round basophilic nucleus. The lumen of the larger exocrine structures is distended with dense eosinophilic laminated secretion (double arrow). Elsewhere a similar type of secretion filled the ducts.

HE ×160

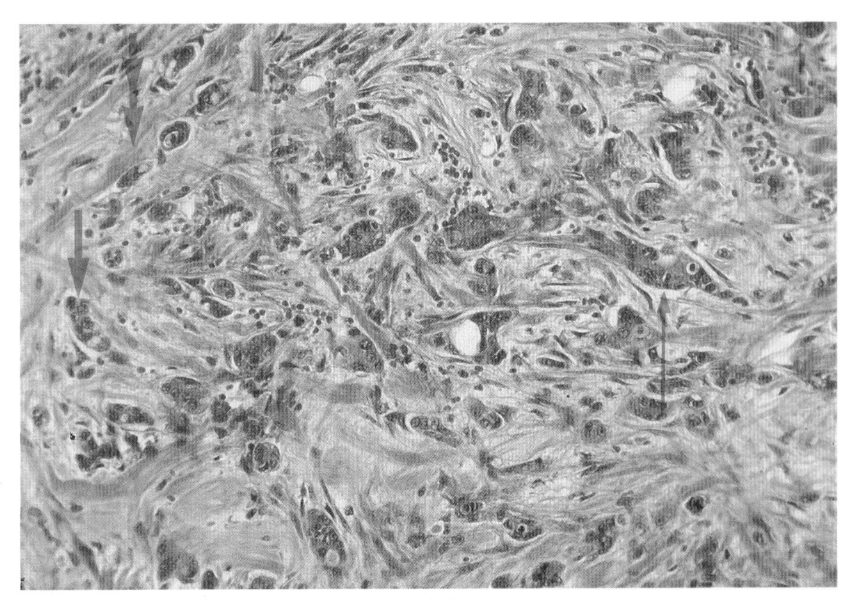

11.54 Carcinoma: pancreas

Carcinoma of pancreas is a not uncommon tumour which arises most frequently in the head of the pancreas and less often in the body of the organ. It rarely occurs in the tail of the pancreas however. The tumour usually obstructs the main ducts of the pancreas, and the pancreatic secretions fail to reach the duodenum. Malabsorption results. The common bile duct also is obstructed and jaundice develops. Carcinoma of pancreas (which is histologically an adenocarcinoma) is usually a scirrhous type of tumour. In this example of pancreatic carcinoma, the growth pattern of the tumour is markedly disordered. The tumour consists of single forms and small groups of pleomorphic malignant epithelial cells (thick arrow), as well as cords and acinar structures of similar malignant epithelial cells with more eosinophilic cytoplasm (thin arrow) (the acini, though rudimentary, are reminiscent of the exocrine tissue of the pancreas). All of these single and multiple malignant cell forms are surrounded by a very abundant stromal background of connective tissue, in which there are broad bands of eosinophilic collagen (double arrow). HE ×135

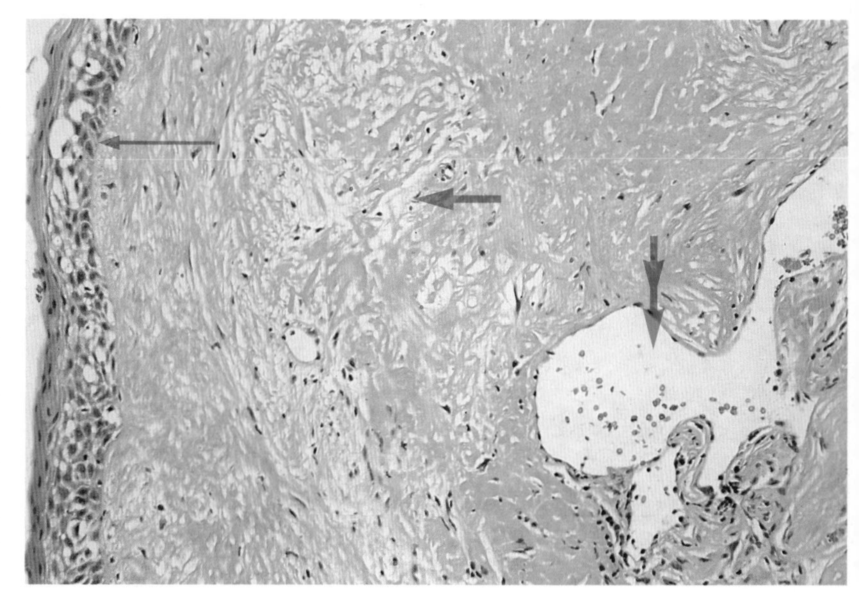

12.1 Laryngeal nodule: vocal cord

Laryngeal nodules (singer's or preacher's nodes) are common, arising in adults, more often than in men (30-50 years of age) than in women. They are probably the product of chronic 'irritation', with heavy smoking and singing the main predisposing factors. The nodule is usually single, and generally located on the anterior part of the true vocal cords or on the anterior commissure. Initially it is edematous but as the nodule ages, the small blood vessels in it become widely dilated. It is not neoplastic. This lesion was a smooth swelling (10 × 5mm) on the right vocal cord of a woman of 68. It consists typically of strongly eosinophilic but widely vacuolated connective tissue (thick arrow) in which there are thin-walled blood vessels, one greatly dilated (double arrow), and only a sparse population of slender elongated fibrocytes. The stratified squamous epithelium of the vocal cord is intact, with a layer of mildly dysplastic keratinized squamous epithelial cells (thin arrow). In the cytoplasm of the squamous epithelial cells there are one or more vacuoles. Some of the vacuoles, in the more superficial (non-keratinized) cells, are very large. HE ×150

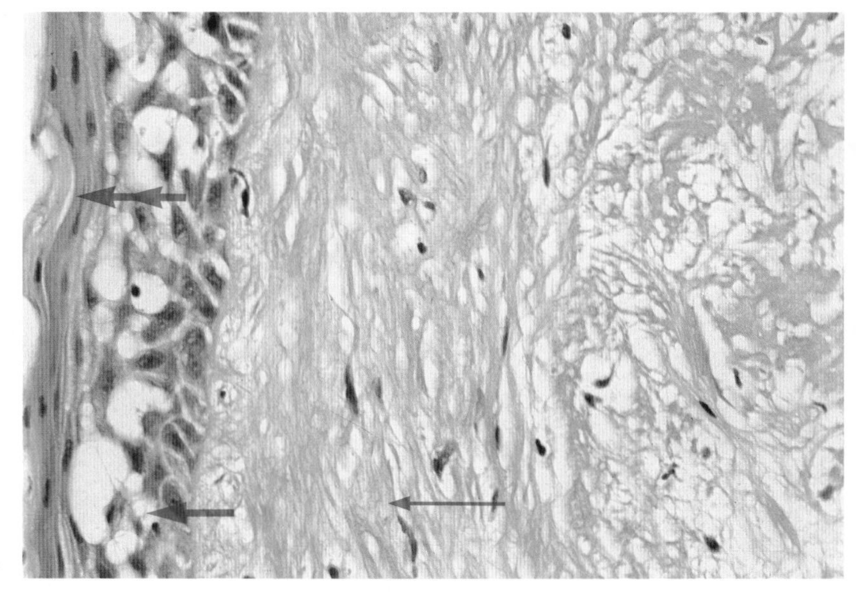

12.2 Laryngeal nodule: vocal cord

Hyperkeratosis sometimes develops on the (nodule-free) vocal cord, along the line where it comes into regular contact with the nodule on the other vocal cord. This is the same lesion as 12.1, at higher magnification. This shows the stroma of the nodule and the surface epithelium. The most superficial layer of stratified squamous epithelial cells on the surface of the vocal cord (double arrow) is keratinized, and beneath it the (non-keratinized) epithelial cells are extensively vacuolated (thick arrow) but showing only slight dysplasia of no neoplastic significance. The epithelial cells in the basal layer are only slightly edematous and vacuolated. The sub-epithelial stroma consists of a large quantity of eosinophilic amyloid-like connective tissue (thin arrow) and a sparse population of elongated slender fibrocytic cells. Although the eosinophilic connective tissue seems to be amyloid-rich, it is actually hyalinized poorly cellular collagenous fibrous tissue, with a fibrin content. The many elongated (clear) vacuoles in the stroma confirm the edematous nature of the nodule. In some nodules (elsewhere) the stroma is vascular and almost hemangiomatous, but in others it is more dense and fibrous (there are no vessels in this field). HE ×360

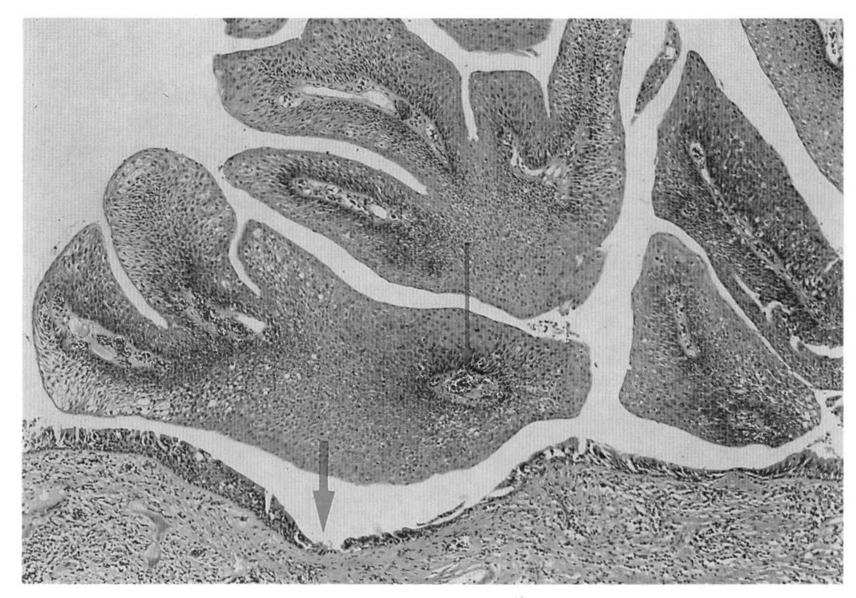

12.3 Juvenile papilloma: larynx

Juvenile papilloma is probably caused by a virus. It is often multiple (papillomatosis), and usually diagnosed in children ages 1 to 6 years. There are fewer episodes after 10 years of age but a majority have the disease well into adulthood. It is located on the true vocal cord, the anterior half more often than posterior, but it may also be on the false cord and in the subglottic region. It may grow to a considerable size and block the larynx. This lesion is a branching structure, composed of multiple papillary processes, each one consisting of a vascular core of connective tissue (thick arrow) and a thick layer of well-differentiated non-keratinized stratified squamous epithelial cells on its surface. There is also extensive perinuclear vacuolation of non-atypical keratinocytes, with only a thin rim of cytoplasm around the periphery of the cells. One part of the respiratory-type epithelium lining the larynx is atrophic (thin arrow), having been compressed by the tumour; and submucosa beneath it is infiltrated with chronic inflammatory cells. HE ×60

12.4 Juvenile papilloma: larynx

Papillomas of the larynx are probably unrelated to solitary squamous papilloma of larynx. In children papillomas tend to recur over a long period but remain well-differentiated. They seldom become malignant, and they sometimes disappear at puberty. Adult papillomas are usually single, whereas juvenile papillomas are often multiple (papillomatosis). Papillomatosis is a non-neoplastic reaction, almost certainly to a virus of papova group. This shows part of the papilloma in 12.5, at higher magnification. The maturation pattern of the stratified squamous epithelial cells is orderly, and the epithelial cells have a moderate amount of eosinophilic cytoplasm and uniform vesicular nuclei. However in the most superficial layers of the stratified squamous epithelium, there is perinuclear vacuolation of many of the epithelial cells (thick arrow). The nuclei in the basal layers of epithelial cells are large, ovoid and vesicular (thin arrow), but there is no dysplasia or loss of polarity. There is however some mitotic activity.
HE ×350

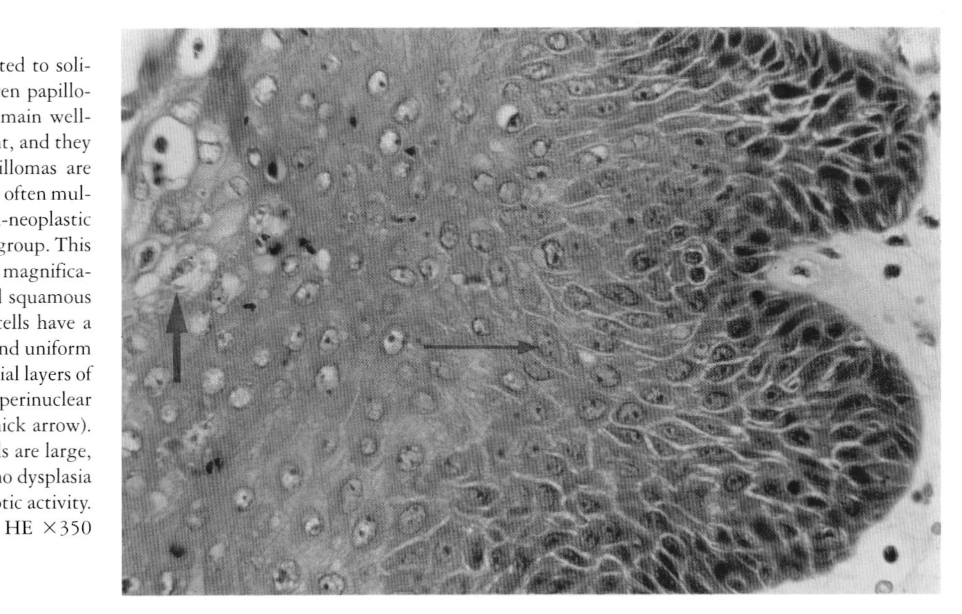

12.5 Squamous cell carcinoma (SCC): larynx

Squamous cell carcinoma of the larynx occurs most often in older men. It arises almost exclusively in smokers, & the risk is even greater in those who also abuse ethanol. Most are located in the vocal cords, but they may also be found above or below the cords or on the aryepiglottic folds. Almost all arise from the stratified squamous epithelium and they are usually well-differentiated. If the tumour is confined to the compartment of origin, the survival rate is around 90%.This lesion was an ulcerated mass 1cm dia on the left vocal cord of a man of 60 who had suffered for some months from progressive hoarseness and difficulty in swallowing. The eosinophilic squamous epithelium on the surface of the larynx is very attenuated but unbroken (double arrow), and beneath it there are small collections of dark-staining lymphocytes. The tumour in the underlying tissues, a squamous cell carcinoma, consists of sheets of pleomorphic (mostly spindle-shaped) keratinocytes (thin arrow). Within the sheets there are several round compact strongly eosinophilic foci of keratinization (thick arrows).
HE ×60

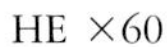

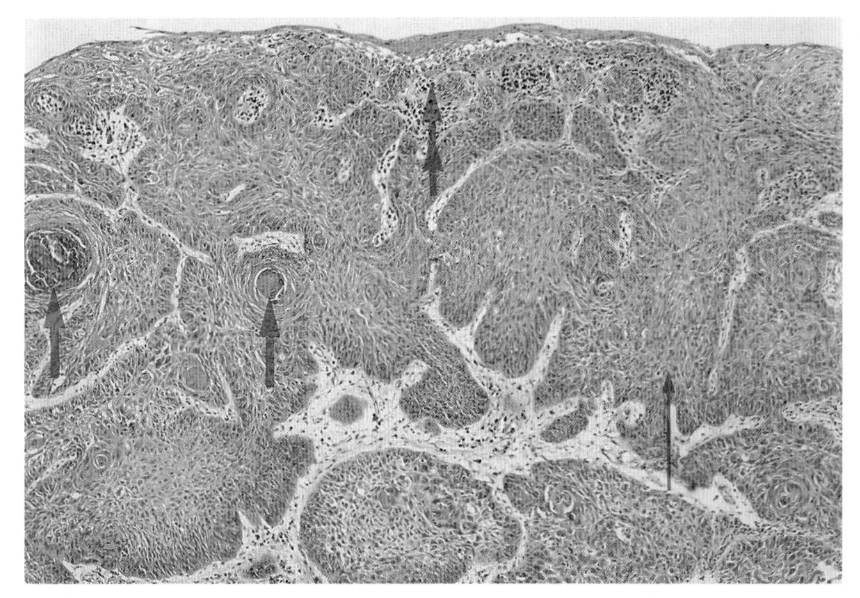

12.6 Squamous carcinoma: larynx

Carcinoma of the larynx tends to remain localized. It is locally destructive however, and ulceration may lead to infection and eventually to bronchopneumonia through inhalation of infected material. This is the same tumour as in 12.7, at higher magnification. The laryngeal surface epithelium (just visible at left margin) is extremely attenuated but not ulcerated. There is a small number of lymphocytes in the (non-neoplastic) stromal connective tissues near the surface of the tumour. The tumour consists of sheets of moderately well-differentiated squamous epithelial cells, each with abundant eosinophilic cytoplasm. Many of the tumour cells are elongated, and their nuclei are ovoid or spindle-shaped, vesicular and pleomorphic (double arrow). The neoplastic epithelial cells in the basal layer are generally large cuboidal or columnar and palisaded (thin arrow), and their nuclei are very pleomorphic. The number of mitotic figures is small however, and in general cellular dysplasia is moderate. There is one round mass of dense laminated keratin (thick arrow). HE ×150

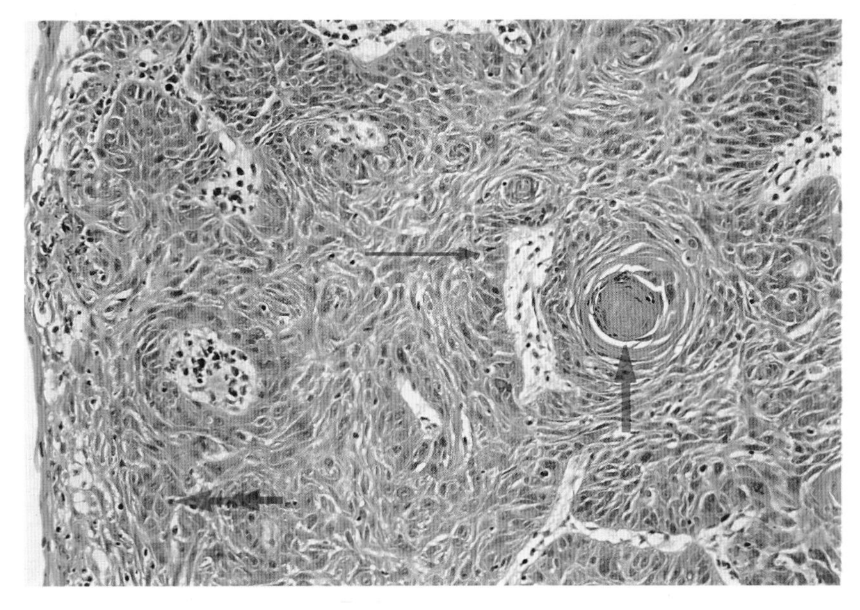

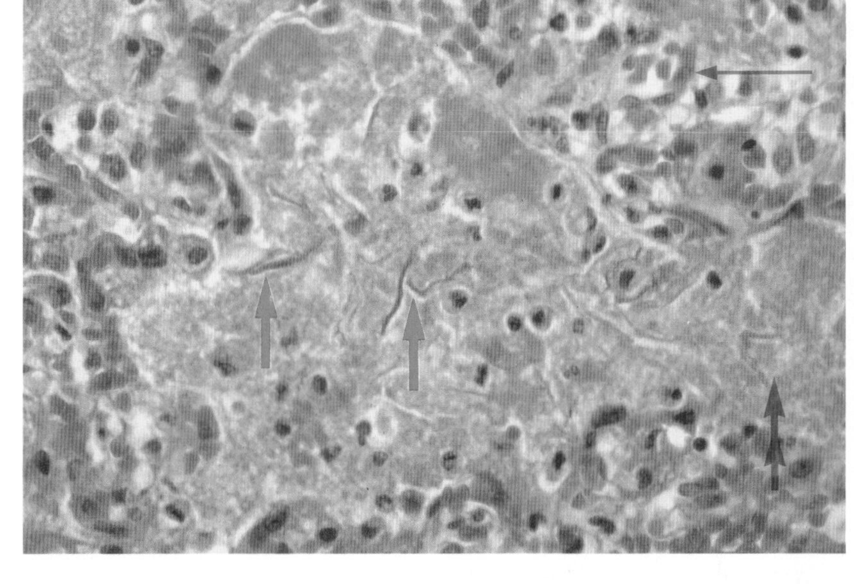

12.7 Aspiration of amniotic fluid: lung

When there has been some difficulty during childbirth, the fetus may draw excessive amounts of amniotic fluid into its lungs and subsequently fail to expel it completely. This is more liable to occur in premature infants with respiratory difficulties. This is the lung of a newborn infant. The air spaces are distended with dense granular material in which there are numerous slender elongated keratotic epithelial squames (thick arrows). Scattered throughout the granular material (double arrow), which consists mainly of coagulated protein, there are fairly numerous polymorph leukocytes and macrophages. The capillaries in the walls of the alveoli are intensely congested (thin arrow), which suggests the onset of pneumonia. The presence of mucus and lipid can also demonstrated in the alveoli by special stains. Rarely, during pregnancy or at delivery, a large amount of amniotic fluid may enter the maternal circulation and cause pulmonary edema and respiratory distress to develop in the mother (the process is termed amniotic embolism). The coagulation system may also be activated. HE ×200

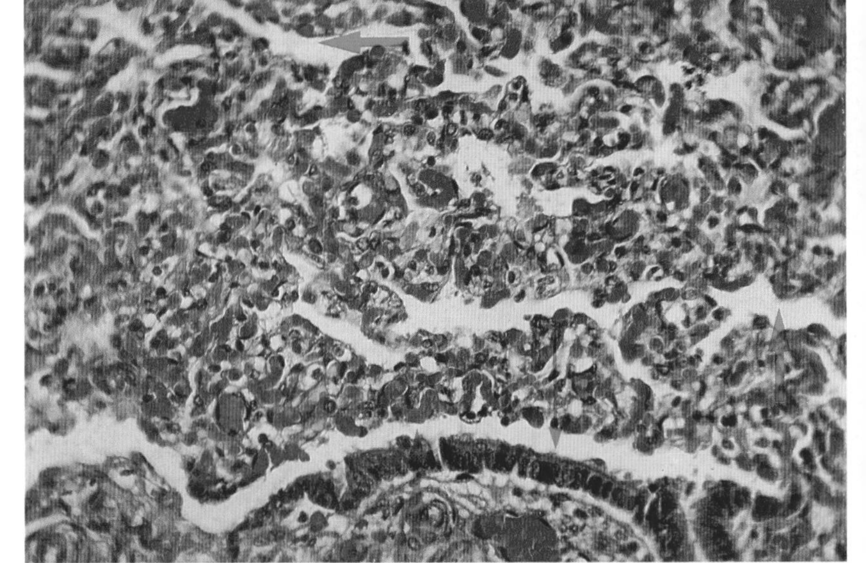

12.8 Atelectasis neonatorum: lung

Atelectasis means imperfect ineffectual stretching or expansion of part or all of a lung. The lungs of a stillborn child never expand. The lungs of a newborn infant do expand, but they may fail to expand fully, and this is an important cause of hypoxia and death. The condition is particularly common in infants born prematurely and in those suffering from birth trauma. This section of lung is from an infant who lived for only a few hours and whose lungs were small and rubbery. The structure of the infant's lung is markedly reminiscent of fetal lung. At the bottom of field there is a bronchiole, lined by a single layer of palisaded tall columnar epithelial cells (thin arrow) with ovoid deeply basophilic nuclei. Above the epithelial lining there are numerous slender empty clefts (thick arrows) which represent large numbers of closely packed unexpanded and virtually airless pulmonary alveoli. The capillaries in the walls of the alveoli are tortuous and prominent (double arrow), being packed with fused purplish-red erythrocytes. HE ×200

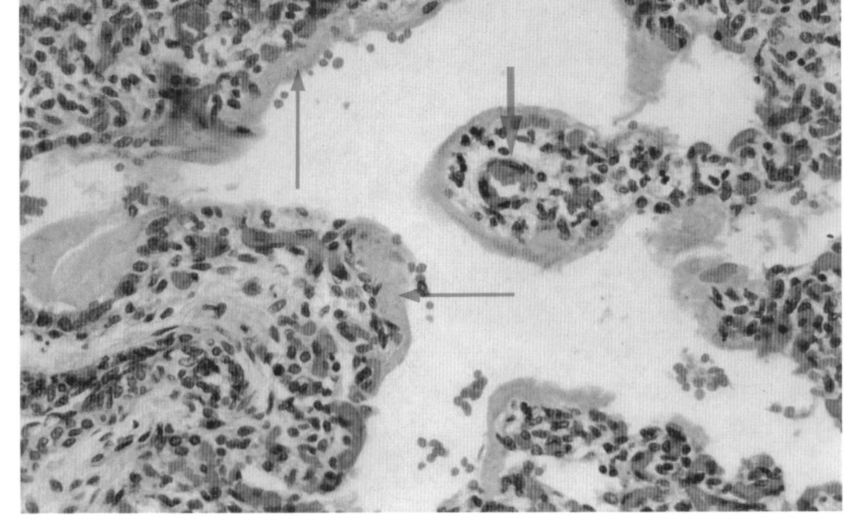

12.9 Respiratory distress syndrome (hyaline membrane disease): lung

Respiratory distress syndrome is particularly liable to affect premature infants. The child develops dyspnea and cyanosis, and its blood pressure falls. The cause is a deficiency of surfactant secretion by the type II cells in the pulmonary alveoli. The child's respiratory movements then fail to keep the alveoli fully expanded, with subsequent exudation of plasma proteins and particularly fibrin into the air spaces. The lungs are of normal size and weight but are fleshy and dull red, containing so little air that they sink in water. The bronchioles and alveolar ducts are widely dilated; and in this section from the lung of an infant the surface of the alveolar duct (part of a bronchiole is just visible on the left) is lined by a wide band of eosinophilic hyaline material (thin arrows) which probably consists of fibrin and debris from desquamated pulmonary and amniotic cells. The associated alveoli are collapsed and solid-looking, and the capillaries in their walls are extremely congested (thick arrow). There is also an infiltrate of inflammatory cells in the alveolar walls. HE ×280

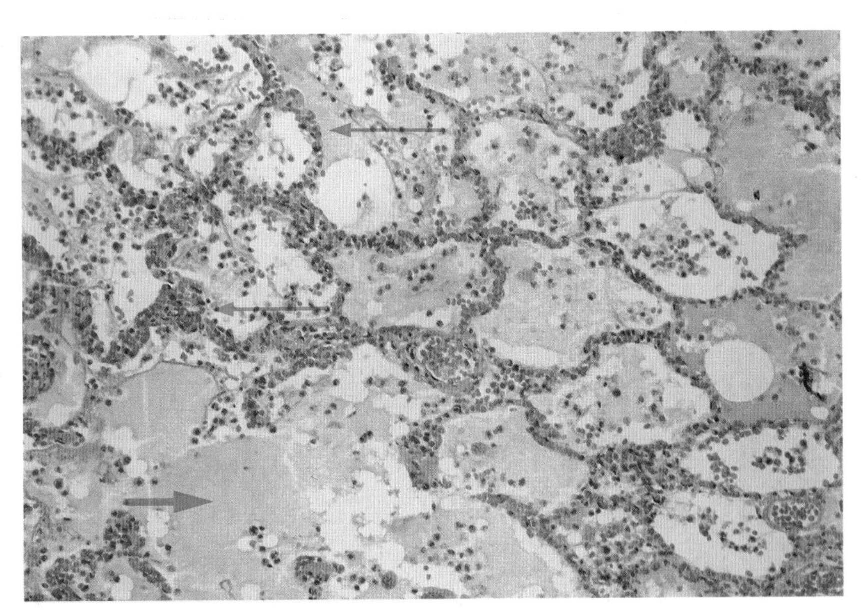

12.10 Congestion and edema: lung

Failure of the left ventricle causes the blood pressure to rise abruptly in the pulmonary veins, and passive congestion in these vessels makes the lungs heavy and edematous. In more severe cases, pulmonary hypertension develops and leads to failure of the right side of the heart. This patient died of acute left ventricular failure. The lungs were edematous and there was also frothy fluid in the air passages. In this field, the small veins in the lung are swollen, and the capillaries in the alveolar septa are markedly distended and tortuous (thin arrows). The pulmonary alveoli are full of amorphous eosinophilic fluid (thick arrow) which has leaked from the congested capillaries. A few eosinophilic strands (probably fibrin) are also present in the lumen of some of the alveoli. There are also fairly numerous leukocytes (predominantly polymorphs) within the alveoli and in the alveolar septa. The fluid in the lungs is a transudate, which is usually cell-free. The polymorph leukocytes in the fluid within the alveoli suggest therefore that bronchopneumonia was starting to develop. HE ×150

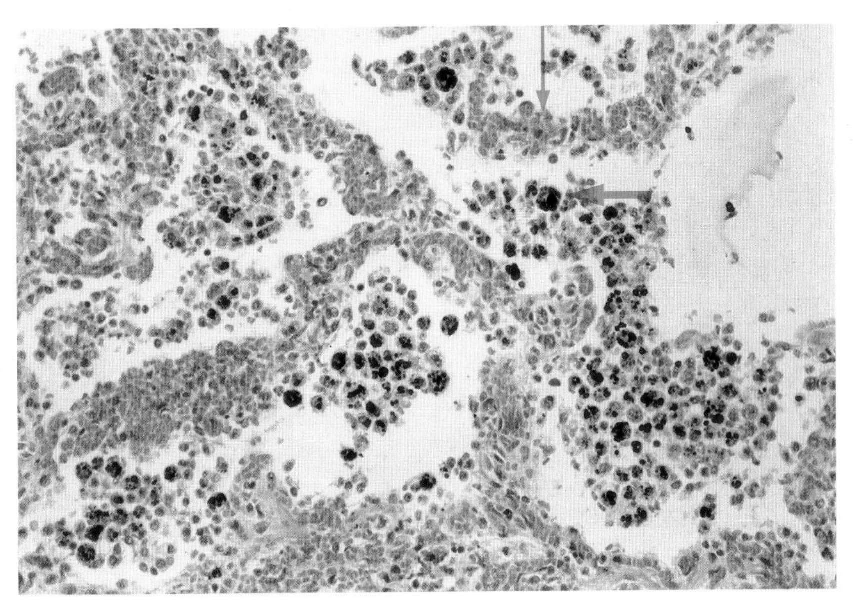

12.11 Chronic venous congestion: lung

The section of lung is from a person with mitral stenosis and long-standing pulmonary venous hypertension. The raised blood pressure has caused the pulmonary capillaries to become extremely swollen and tortuous (thin arrow) (the endothelium of the distended capillaries is usually damaged). Large numbers of erythrocytes have leaked readily from the capillaries into the lumen of the pulmonary alveoli, and a large population of macrophages has congregated in the alveoli and ingested the erythrocytes. Many of the macrophages are golden-brown and dark-brown cells (generally the largest) which contain a considerable amount of golden- or dark-brown granular pigment in their cytoplasm (thick arrow). The granules of pigment are hemosiderin, and it has come from the many extravasated erythrocytes ingested and digested by the macrophages (pulmonary hemosiderosis). Hemosiderin-laden macrophages also tend to congregate around the respiratory bronchioles, and they may release iron-containing salts which are deposited in the connective tissue fibres of the lung. When the amount of connective tissue increases in the lungs, the appropriate term is brown induration. HE ×235

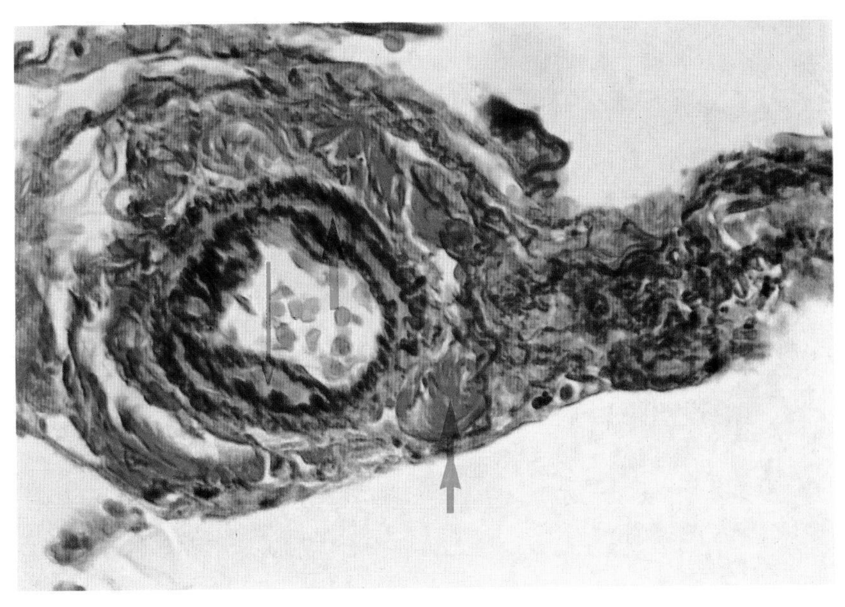

12.12 Pulmonary (arterial) hypertension: lung

Many diseases can cause pulmonary arterial hypertension and pulmonary vascular disease. Secondary pulmonary hypertension may produce hyperplasia of muscle in pulmonary arteries between 1000μm and 100μm dia, and also extend muscle fibres distally into arterioles which are less than 100μm dia and have little or no muscle in their walls. In this pulmonary arteriole (60μm dia), the wavy elastic fibres are coloured black, the dense collagen fibres are deep red (double arrow) and the muscle fibres are orange-yellow. There are areas of localized thickening of the intima (thin arrow), from the presence of longitudinally-orientated bands of smooth muscle fibres (cut in cross-section), and also of a well-developed hypertrophied muscular media (thick arrow) similar to that in systemic arterioles. The changes in this pulmonary arteriole are characteristically termed 'muscularization' of the terminal parts of the pulmonary vascular tree. This patient had very severe chronic bronchitis and emphysema, with consequent chronic hypoxia, and this led to increased resistance in the pulmonary vascular (arterial) system and to pulmonary hypertension. Elastic-van Gieson ×580

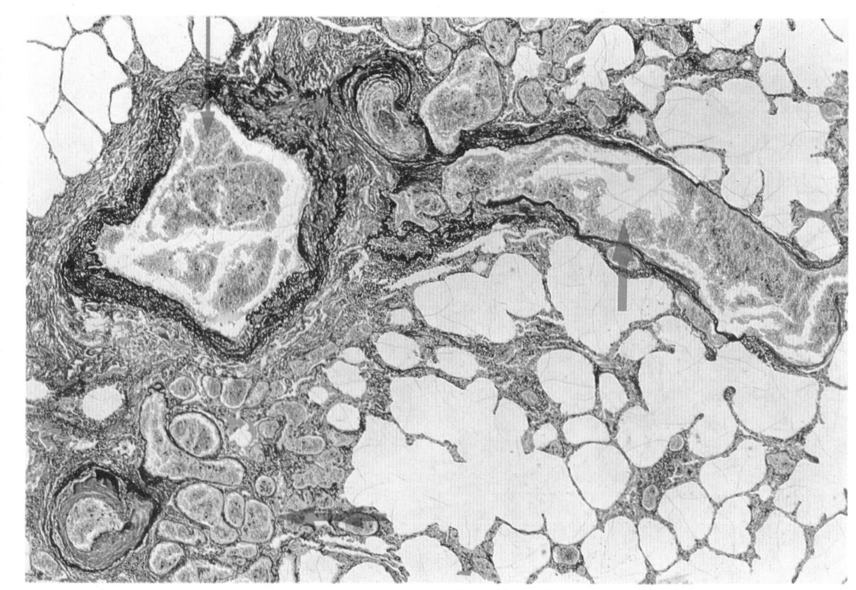

12.13 Pulmonary (arterial) hypertension: lung

If pulmonary hypertension is severe, and especially if it develops suddenly, a hypertrophied muscular artery may give rise to a thin-walled branch that divides into a maze of thin-walled sinusoids. The result is a plexiform lesion which drains into a capillary. This patient had a patent ductus arteriosus. The flow of blood from the aorta to the pulmonary artery had caused severe pulmonary hypertension which had been present for many years. The elastic tissue is stained black and the blood is orange-yellow. The branch of the pulmonary artery (thin arrow) has a thick hypertrophied media. Closely associated with this artery are numerous closely packed small abnormal thin-walled blood vessels with their lumens full of golden-yellow erythrocytes (top centre and bottom left). The thin-walled blood vessels are markedly dilated small branches of the pulmonary artery proximal to sites of occlusion of the artery, and they are arranged in a plexiform pattern (double arrow), thus giving rise to a so-called angiomatoid lesion. Adjoining the angiomatoid lesion there is a thin-walled blood vessel of very wide calibre, cut longitudinally (thick arrow). It resembles a vein but it is a greatly dilated arteriole.

Elastic-van Gieson ×70

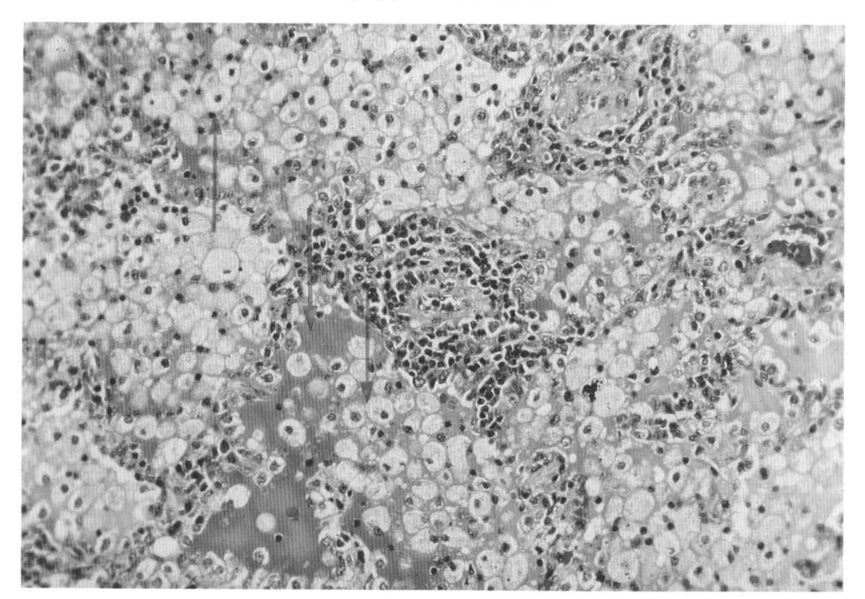

12.14 Obstruction of bronchus: lung

When a tumour obstructs a bronchus, the air trapped beyond the obstruction is absorbed and the related part of the lung collapses relatively slowly (when a bronchus is obstructed suddenly, the lung collapses much more quickly). In this case, the bronchus was obstructed by a primary carcinoma. The lung distal to the obstruction collapsed, and the bronchial secretions and desquamated cells were retained in the affected lung. Histologically, the alveoli are full of large round macrophages (arrows) with abundant pale foamy (lipid-laden) cytoplasm and relatively small round or ovoid strongly basophilic nuclei. The large foamy macrophages are accompanied by smaller numbers of plasma cells and lymphocytes. The alveoli contain varying amounts of deeply eosinophilic fluid exudate (thin arrow). Macroscopically, cut surface of the affected segment of lung is a definite yellow colour, from the presence of a considerable amount of lipid within the macrophages. This type of lesion is sometimes referred to as endogenous lipid pneumonia. Exogenous lipid pneumonia is caused by the inhalation of lipoid material.

HE ×160

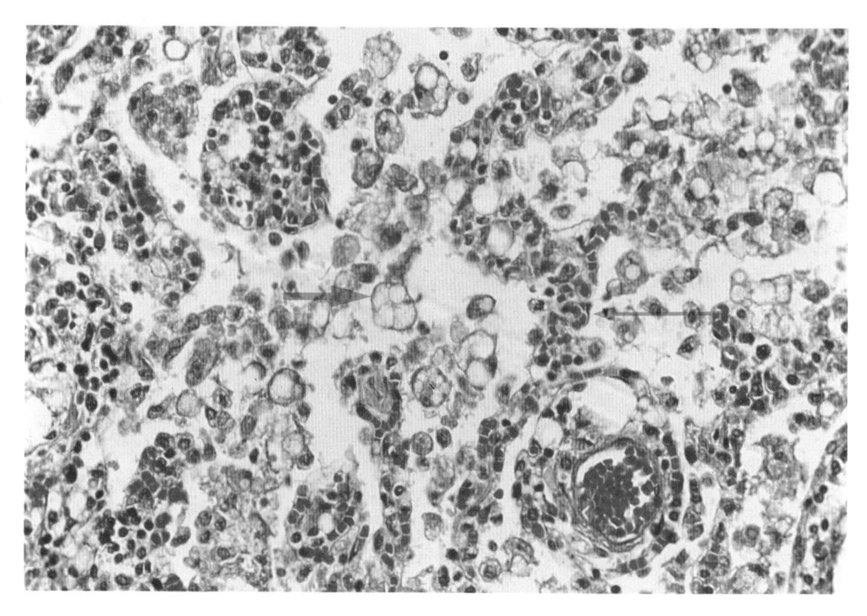

12.15 Lipid (aspiration) pneumonia: lung

Aspiration of irritant liquids causes injury to the lungs, and especially to the bronchi. Sometimes the inhaled liquid is lipid, and it may be aspirated from a variety of sources. The inhaled materials include drops or sprays used for nasal conditions, or mineral oil (liquid paraffin) taken as a laxative; or radio-opaque material used for bronchography (and which has remained in the lungs). The lipid tends to be irritant and it may produce a chronic inflammatory reaction which can lead to considerable fibrosis. In this case, a mass was detected in the patient's right lower lobe. Histologically, in the pulmonary alveoli there are large numbers of macrophages with a considerable amount of cytoplasm in which there are several large vacuoles containing pale material (thick arrow). The pulmonary tissues are hyperemic, with dilated tortuous capillaries (thin arrow) and a moderate infiltrate of polymorph leukocytes in the alveolar septa, evidence of a more acute inflammatory reaction. A specific stain confirmed that the material in the vacuoles in the macrophages is lipid, and that the patient had used nasal drops containing mineral oil.

HE ×200

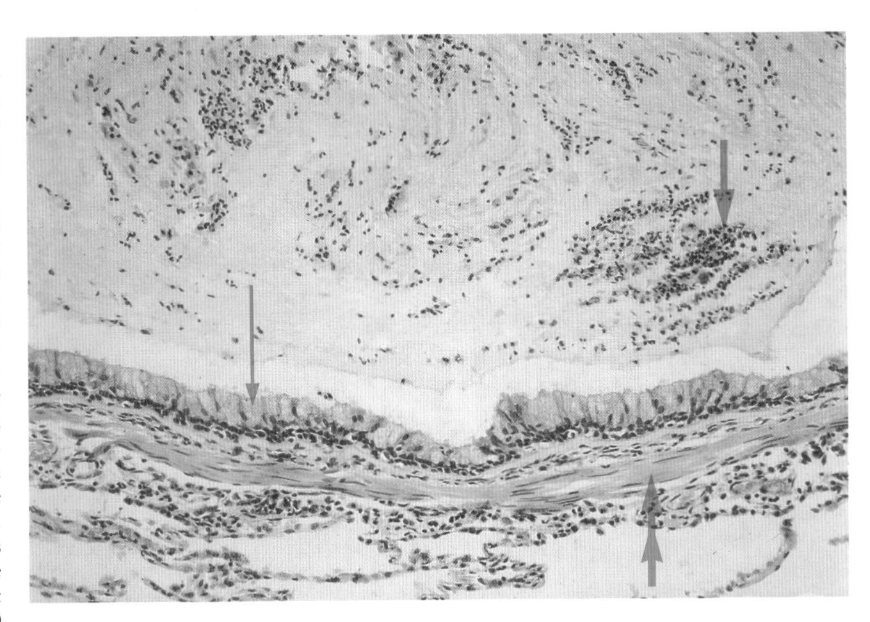

12.16 Asthma: lung

In asthma, the patients suffer repeated attacks of bronchospasm, usually of sudden onset. In an attack, there is onset of hypersecretion of thick tenacious mucus (and a serous component) into the narrow bronchi which tends to block the small air passages. A woman aged 27 years who had suffered from asthma for 4 years died in status asthmaticus. At postmortem examination the small bronchi and bronchioles were obstructed by plugs of viscid secretion and there was patchy collapse of both lungs. The right ventricle of the heart was neither hypertrophied nor dilated. The lumen of this small bronchus contains a pale bluish firm-looking exudate (with a well-defined boundary) in which there are many cells, mostly eosinophil leukocytes (thick arrow). The bronchus is lined by single layer of large palisaded epithelial cells, distended with of bluish mucus (thin arrow), on a relatively thick basement membrane. In the wall of the bronchus, there is also a much thicker band of hypertrophied eosinophilic smooth muscle cells (double arrow) beneath the basement membrane). There is also a moderate infiltrate of eosinophil leukocytes and lymphocytes on each side of the smooth muscle. The adjacent alveoli appear normal and emphysema was not present. HE ×150

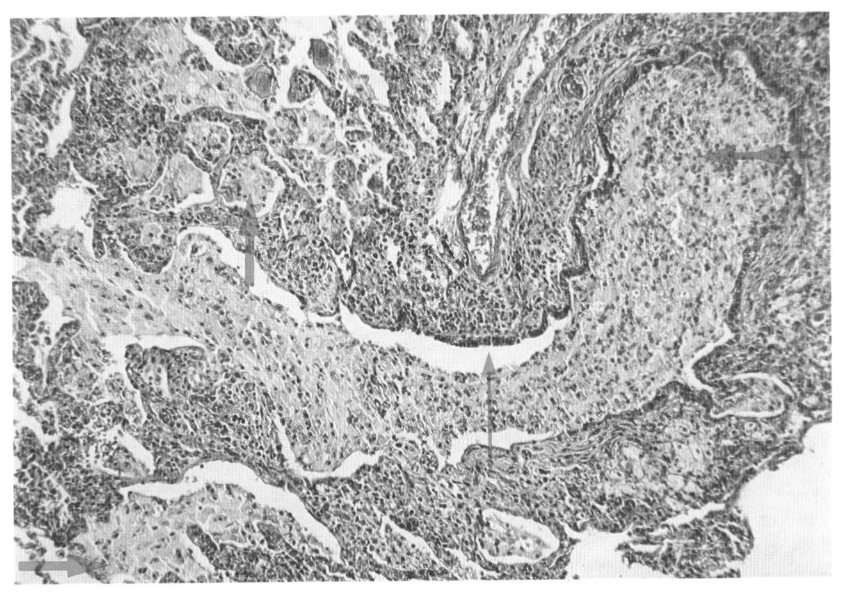

12.17 Fibrocystic disease (cystic fibrosis): lung

Fibrocystic disease (also termed cystic fibrosis or mucoviscidosis) is autosomal recessive (with good penetrance but variable expressivity) and consequently it affects cells throughout the body (heterozygous carriers are usually asymptomatic). The secretions of the exocrine glands, including those in bronchi, bowel, pancreas, sweat glands and reproductive organs, are abnormally viscid, and inspissated tenacious mucoid secretion blocks ducts and causes atrophy of acini. In the lungs, the secretion plugs bronchi and bronchioles, and saccular bronchiectasis tends to develop. Secondary infection and severe inflammation are liable to develop in mucus-filled bronchioles and lead to destruction and obliteration of the lumen by fibrous tissue (obliterative bronchiolitis). In this field there is a dilated bronchiole, the epithelial lining of which is intact and of normal structure (thin arrow). The lumen of the bronchiole is occupied by a solid-looking well-defined plug of basophilic (bluish) mucus (double arrow), and the associated alveoli are also full of similar bluish mucus (thick arrow). There are many inflammatory cells within the mucus and also in the walls of the alveoli. Many small blood vessels, mostly capillaries in the alveolar septa, are dilated. HE ×120

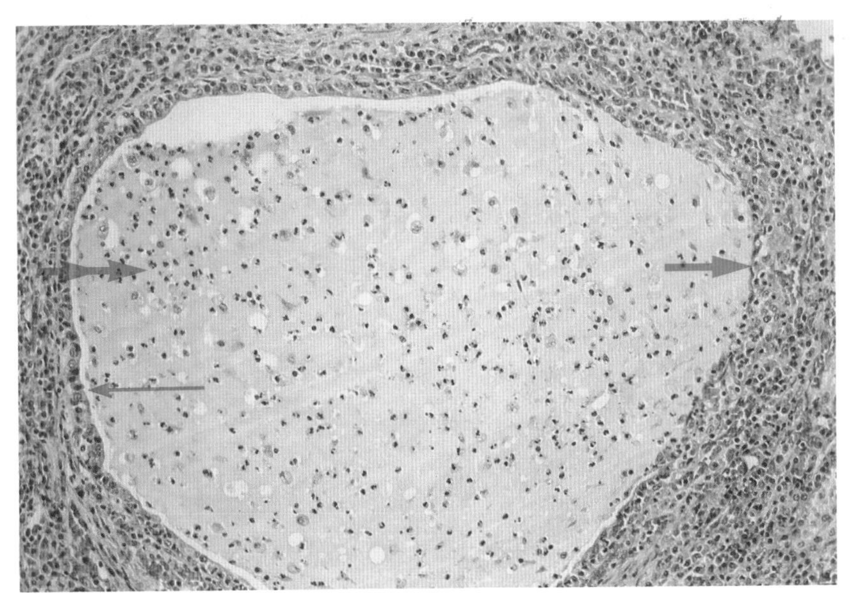

12.18 Fibrocystic disease (cystic fibrosis): lung

The lungs are severely damaged in most patients with fibrocystic disease who survive for a considerable time, and repeated attacks of pulmonary infection (notably *Pseudomonas aeruginosa*) usually follow. Chronic obstructive pneumonia develops, and the lungs become increasingly fibrotic. This is a small bronchus from another case, in cross-section. It is markedly ectatic, and the lumen is filled with well-defined plug of weakly eosinophilic mucoid secretion (double arrow) in which there are many polymorphs and large macrophages. The even distribution of cells throughout the mucus suggests that its consistence is firmer than that of normal mucus. The bronchus is incompletely lined by mucosal epithelium which consists of a slightly disorganized single layer of pleomorphic cuboidal cells (thin arrow) which do not appear to secrete mucin. The other part of the bronchial wall (thick arrow) is extensively ulcerated, having lost its epithelial lining. The wall of the bronchus and the tissues surrounding it are hyperemic and heavily infiltrated by polymorphs, lymphocytes and plasma cells. HE ×150

12.19 Bronchiectasis and emphysema: lung

Dilatation of bronchi is termed bronchiectasis, and it is caused by weakening of the bronchial walls. One of the most effective ways of studying bronchiectasis (and emphysema) is a thin (300μm thick) slice of the whole lung (a Gough-Wentworth section). In this thin slice, the lower lobe and part of the upper lobe are macroscopically visible. The changes in the structure of the lower lobe extend as far as the pleura, practically all the bronchi in the lower lobe being dilated (ectatic) (arrow) and in close proximity to each other. The ectatic bronchi were filled with greenish mucopus but it was lost during processing of the lung tissue. The walls of the bronchi are thin, and no cartilage is visible in them. There is no fibrosis around the ectatic bronchi, the lung surrounding them being generally normal. Several bronchi in the upper lobe are similarly affected. Much carbon is present in the centres of many lobules, and dilatation of the respiratory bronchioles has produced focal dust emphysema (coal worker's pneumoconiosis).

Whole lung section, unstained ×1

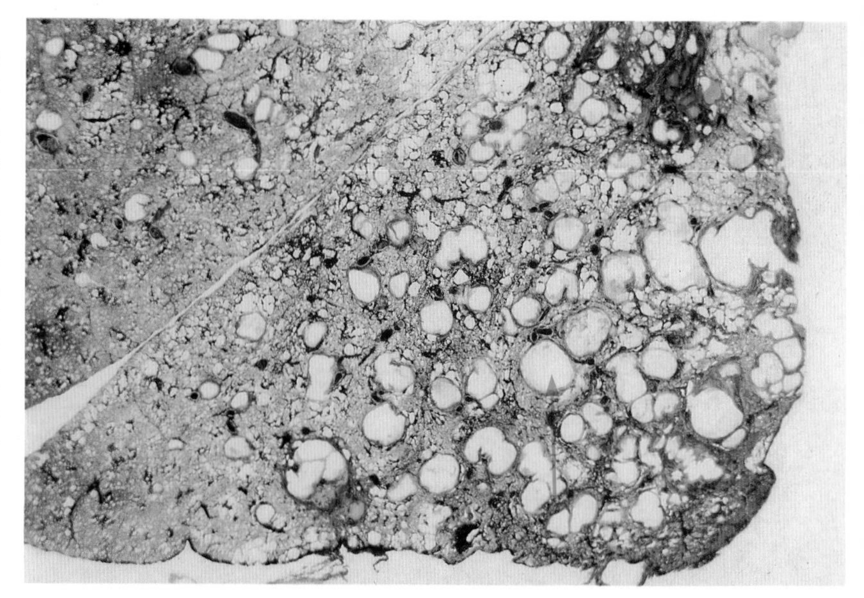

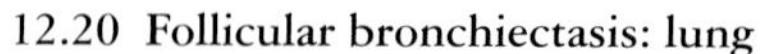

12.20 Follicular bronchiectasis: lung

Occasionally, in bronchiectasis, the bronchial wall is thickened by fibrosis, often accompanied by muscular hypertrophy and hyperplasia of mucous glands. Inflammatory changes are usually pronounced, and in many instances there is much lymphoid tissue (predominantly lymphocytes and plasma cells), sometimes including mature lymphoid follicles. When lymphoid follicles are a prominent feature, the term follicular bronchiectasis is sometimes applied. Sometimes foci of acute inflammation are superadded. This shows a terminal bronchiole (left and top). The lumen of the bronchiole is filled with numerous polymorph leukocytes and large macrophages with pale ovoid vesicular nuclei. The bronchiole is lined by single layer of uniform palisaded closely packed cuboidal and columnar epithelial cells (thin arrow) with ovoid vesicular nuclei. Adjacent to the bronchiole there is a large follicular structure, consisting entirely of mature lymphocytes (double arrow) with small round deeply basophil nuclei, but without a germinal centre. Penetrating the follicle there are several prominent venules with thick deeply eosinophilic hyalinized walls (thick arrow).

HE ×135

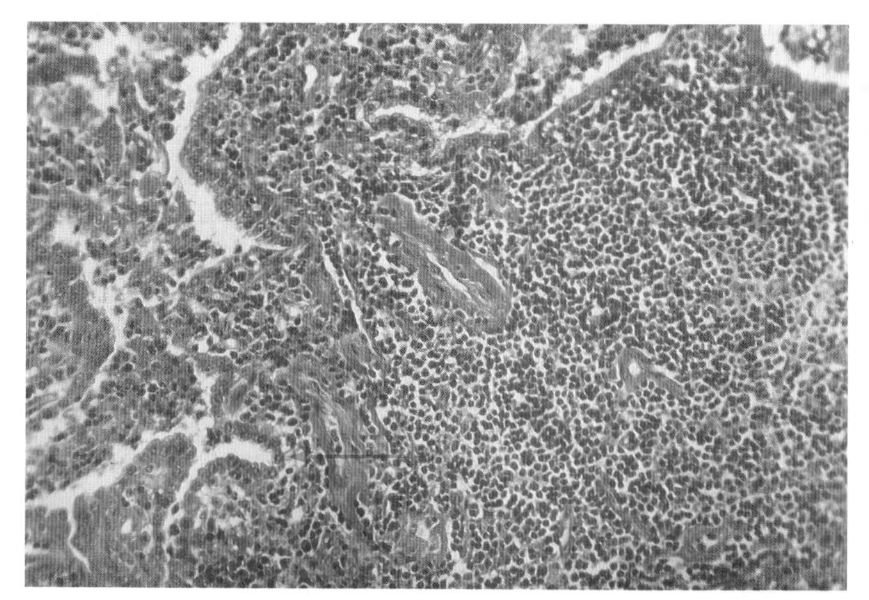

12.21 Centrilobular emphysema: lung

The term pulmonary emphysema is applied to air spaces which are increased in size and distal to the terminal bronchioles (respiratory bronchioles, alveolar ducts, atria or alveoli). Enlargement of air spaces is also accompanied by some destruction of tissue. In centrilobular emphysema, the abnormal air spaces are dilated respiratory bronchioles in the centres of the acini (also termed centriacinar emphysema). Carbonaceous dust is often present in town-dwellers, in the same site as the emphysematous lesion, but its presence is not invariable. This is a part (9 × 6cm) of a whole lung section prepared by the Gough-Wentworth technique. A linear deposit of carbonaceous dust is present beneath the pleura (just visible at the bottom margin). Large abnormal air spaces (up to 2cm dia) (double arrow) are present in the centres of almost all the lobules, and within the emphysematous spaces there are carbon-laden septa. The alveoli in the peripheral parts of the lobule (adjacent to the pleura) appear relatively normal (thin arrow), as do the branches of the pulmonary artery (thick arrows).

Whole lung section, unstained ×1.3

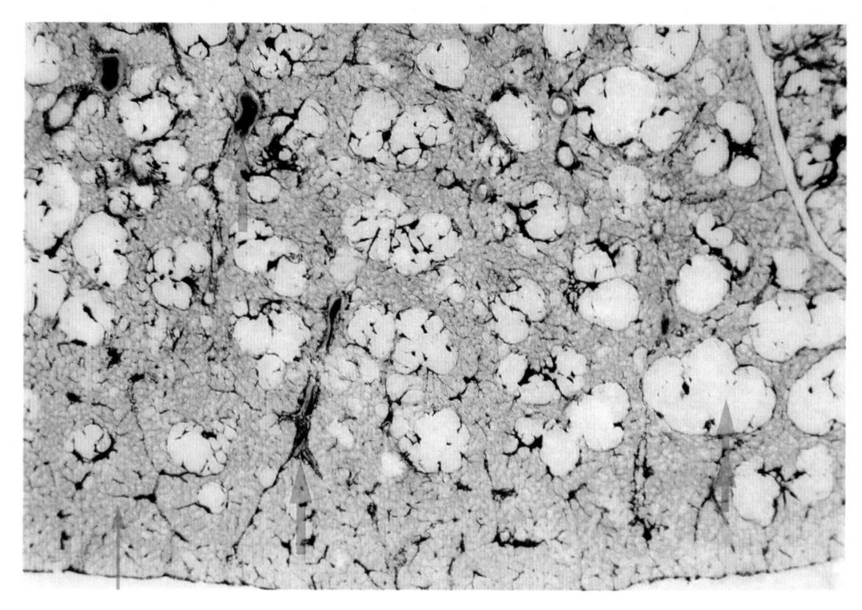

12.22 Panacinar emphysema: lung

Panacinar emphysema (sometimes termed panlobular) may be widespread or limited to a few lobules. It tends to be most severe in the lower and anterior parts of the lung. If it is severe and widespread, the lungs are enlarged (overinflated) and seemingly lack substance. Alveolar ducts and respiratory bronchioles are involved in the more severe forms of panacinar emphysema. The whole of each pulmonary acinus is disorganized, all the alveolar walls becoming increasingly attenuated and fenestrated, until some of them are lost and replaced by large thin-walled spaces. This is a part (9 × 6cm) of a whole lung section prepared by the Gough-Wentworth technique. Apart from the large blood vessels, the normal architecture of almost all the pulmonary acini has been damaged, so that the lung now consists entirely of thin-walled air spaces of variable size and shape (arrow). There is no evidence of inflammation or of fibrosis. The branches of the pulmonary artery appear normal.

Whole lung section, unstained ×1.3

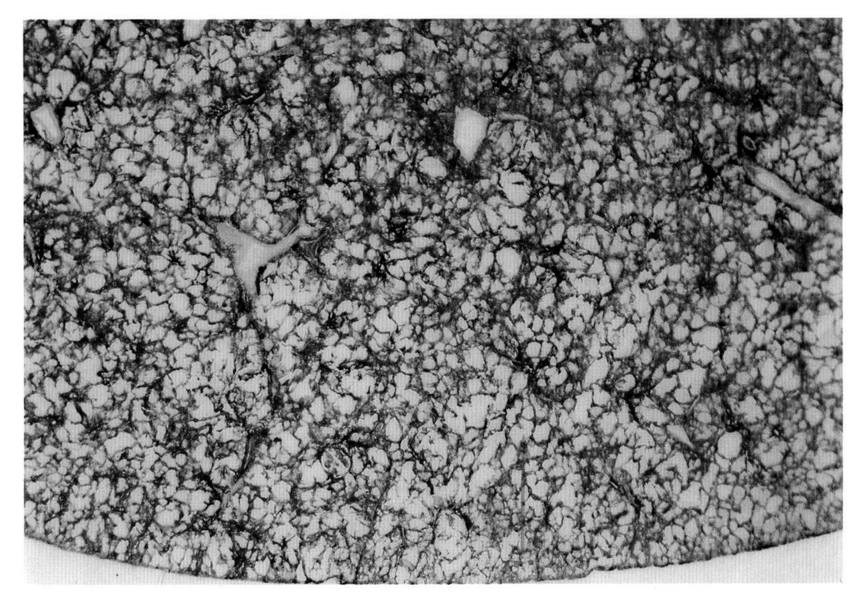

12.23 Panacinar emphysema: lung

In panacinar emphysema the emphysematous spaces are formed by the loss of alveolar walls and coalescence of adjacent alveoli. This is a stained histological section from paraffin-embedded tissue, whereas **12.25** is a thin slice of whole lung, fixed in formaldehyde and unstained. The pleura consists of a thin layer if fibrous tissue, and beneath it there are small deposits of carbonaceous (black) dust. The walls of nearly all the alveoli are remarkably atrophic and thin (double arrow), so much so that it is almost impossible to detect the presence of capillaries in the alveolar walls. Moreover, almost all the alveolar walls have broken down and merged to form spaces considerably larger than normal alveoli. In one such enlarged alveolus there are clusters of pigment-laden macrophages (thick arrow), and within the pleural tissues there are small deposits of carbonaceous dust (thin arrow).

HE ×110

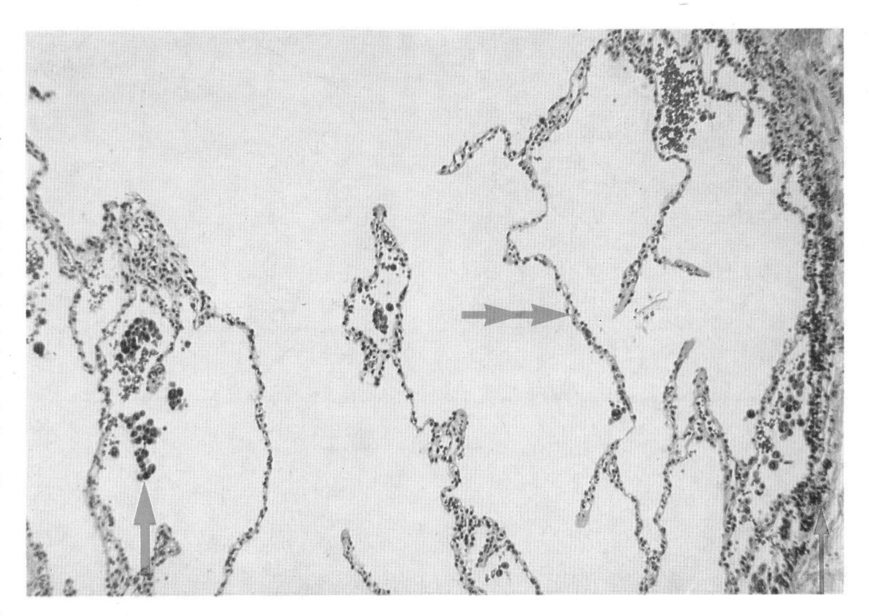

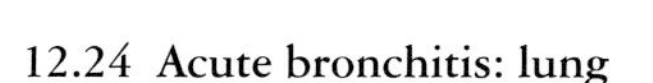

12.24 Acute bronchitis: lung

Acute bronchitis usually follows viral bronchitis, chronic bronchitis or asthma. Acute inflammation of the bronchi is probably initiated in most cases by viruses or mycoplasmas, with subsequent invasion by pyogenic bacteria such as *Haemophilus influenzae* or *Staphylococcus aureus*. The inflamed mucosa is red and congested and edematous, and the respiratory epithelium secretes increased quantities of mucus (catarrhal bronchitis). There is a sparse cellular exudate in the bronchial wall, usually of lymphocytes and plasma cells, but if there is secondary bacterial infection, inflammation becomes more intense, polymorphs appear in increasing numbers and the mucus becomes mucopurulent or even purulent. This is a very acute lesion. The lumen of the bronchus is full of pus-like secretion which consists mostly of closely packed basophilic neutrophil polymorphs, and it lined by tall columnar (ciliated respiratory-type) epithelial cells (double arrow). The mucosal epithelium, which has been infiltrated by polymorphs, is ulcerated at one point (thin arrow). Beneath the mucosa there are polymorphs and also a thin layer of eosinophilic fibrin (thick arrow). On the right, deeper in the submucosa, there are greatly dilated thin-walled blood vessels.

HE ×200

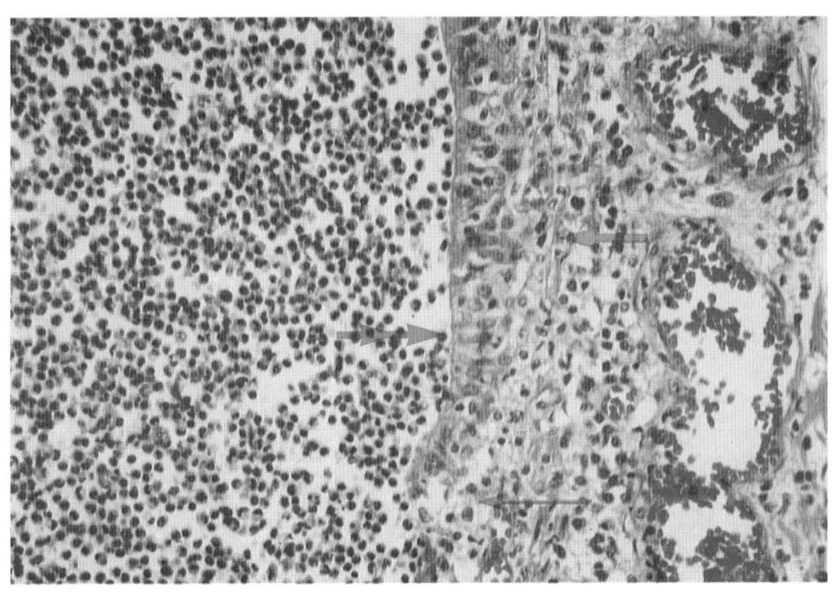

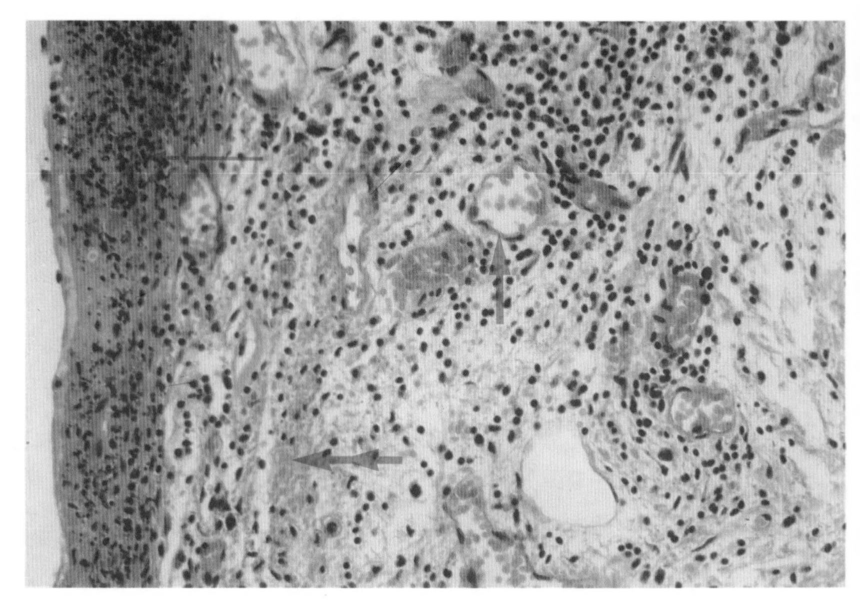

12.25 Influenzal bronchitis: lung

Influenzal bronchitis is an abrupt illness. The influenza virus attacks the respiratory epithelium, and the mucociliary defence mechanism of the respiratory tract is weakened. Secondary bacterial infection is liable to occur, and the mucosa of trachea and bronchi becomes fiery red and edematous. The cellular exudate is moderate however, consisting mainly of lymphocytes. There may be focal desquamation of the bronchial mucosa, and extensive necrosis may develop. Bronchopneumonia may follow with great rapidity and severity, particularly when *Staphylococcus aureus* is present. This shows the mucosa and submucosa of a small bronchus from a fatal case of viral bronchopneumonia. The lumen of the bronchus is just visible on the left, and its epithelial lining has been destroyed by the viral infection, to become just a layer of necrotic cells and cell debris (thin arrow). The submucosa is intensely hyperemic, with widely dilated small blood vessels (thick arrow) and a cellular infiltrate consisting almost entirely of numerous small basophilic lymphocytes. There are also eosinophilic strands of fibrin in the submucosa (double arrow), and among the strands there are red cells. In a less severe case, bacterial infection would tend to increase the number of polymorph leukocytes. HE ×235

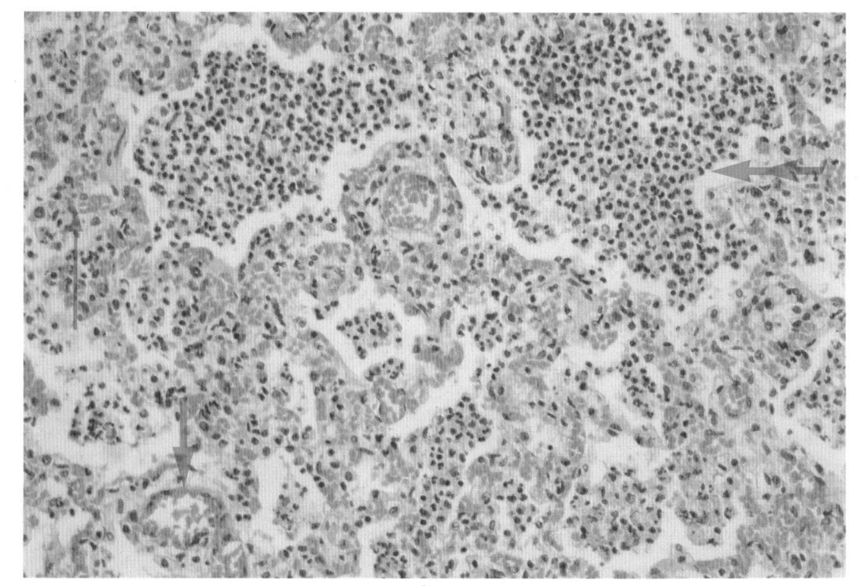

12.26 Bronchopneumonia: lung

In allergic alveolitis, the inflammatory reaction is centred on the walls of the alveoli, whereas in pneumonia the lung is acutely inflamed and the causative agent (usually a microorganism) is in the alveoli. In bronchopneumonia the microorganism colonizes the air passages and bronchioles and penetrates to the alveoli. It evokes an acute inflammatory reaction in the associated alveolar spaces, and the exudate which collects in the alveoli takes the form of numerous discrete solid foci (consolidation). In this histological section, the lung is notably hyperemic. The alveolar walls are thicker than normal (thin arrow), and the alveolar capillaries are greatly dilated and tortuous. The venules (thick arrow) also are dilated. Polymorphs are also present also in the walls of the alveoli. An exudate of polymorph leukocytes and more numerous red cells almost fills the alveoli, and the alveolar ducts are distended by a much larger and denser (pus-like) sheet of polymorph leukocytes (double arrow). The inflammatory exudate in the lung contains fibrin and bacteria, and these can be demonstrated by special stains. HE ×150

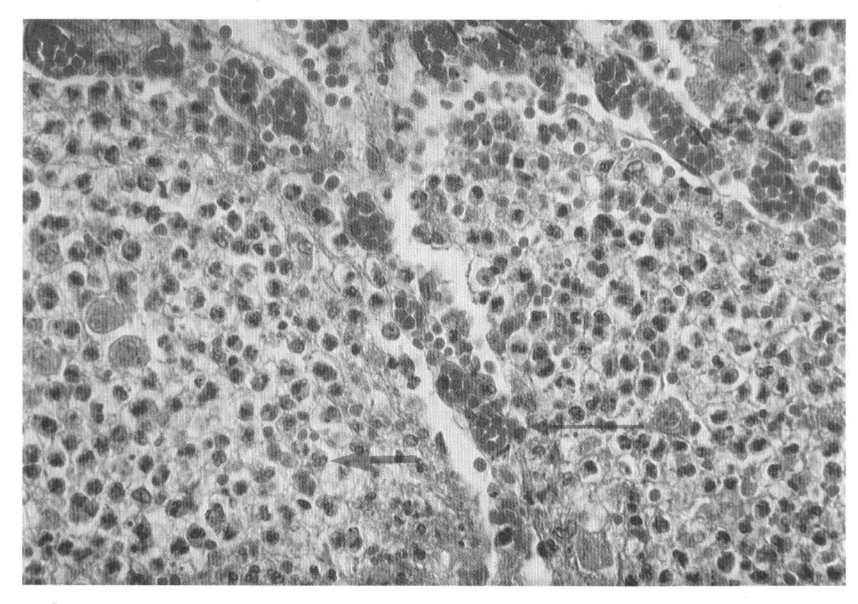

12.27 Lobar pneumonia: lung

As in bronchopneumonia, the route of infection in lobar pneumonia is via the bronchi and bronchioles, but within the lung the reaction is more acute, and a watery inflammatory exudate forms in the alveoli. The exudate spreads directly into the bronchioles and related alveoli. It then spills over into the adjacent lobules and through the lung tissue until it reaches the pleural surface. In this way the affected part of the lung undergoes rapid diffuse consolidation. The consolidated lung tissue is sharply confined to a whole lobe or more than one lobe. Macroscopically, the cut surface of this lobe of a lung appeared brownish-red and solid, typical of red hepatization. Histologically, this shows lobar pneumonia at a fairly early stage. The capillaries in the alveolar walls are greatly dilated (thin arrow), and the alveoli are completely filled with an inflammatory exudate (thick arrow) which contains large numbers of closely packed polymorph leukocytes, along with red cells, degenerate macrophages and fibrin. A Gram stain would reveal large numbers of microorganisms, usually *Streptococcus pneumoniae*. HE ×335

12.28 Lobar pneumonia: lung

Post mortem, the consolidated lobes were (macroscopically) not red and hyperemic, as in 12.30, but grey in this case. The cut surface was dry granular and grey, as a result of prolonged (4-8 days) consolidation (grey hepatization). Histologically, the alveolar walls are thin (thick arrow), and in many places the alveolar capillaries are largely collapsed and inconspicuous, perhaps as a result of compression of the walls by the large amount of inflammatory exudate (double arrow) which fills the alveoli (it is the reduction in the vascularity of the consolidated lung that makes it appear grey to the naked eye). In some of the alveolar spaces, the inflammatory exudate consists of a network of inspissated eosinophilic fibrin (thin arrow) (embedded in abundant pale amorphous material) and a moderate number of polymorph leukocytes (centre), many of them pyknotic dead and disintegrating. Likewise many red cells also are degenerating. Elsewhere however there are many more polymorph leukocytes and usually less fibrin in the alveoli. HE ×135

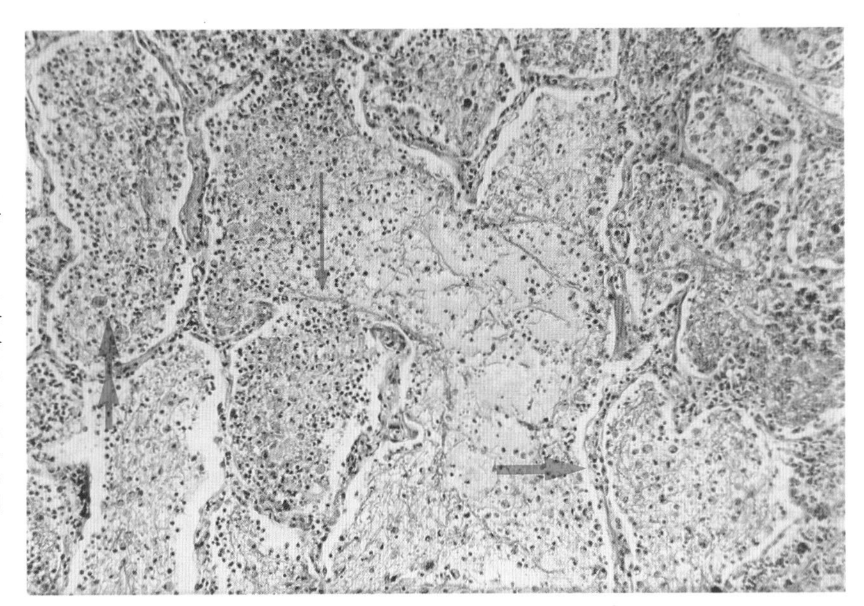

12.29 Fibrinous pleurisy: lung

In acute inflammatory conditions of the lung such as lobar pneumonia, an inflammatory exudate may form in the pleural cavity, with deposition of fibrin on the visceral pleura (fibrinous pleuritis). After the acute phase of the illness, fibrin on the pleural surface undergoes organization. Organization is already well advanced in this case. In the subpleural tissues beneath the undulating layer of eosinophilic elastic tissue of the pleura (bottom margin), there are small clusters of carbon-laden (black) macrophages (thick arrow). There are no serosal cells on the pleural surface, but above it there is a thick layer of granulation tissue and closely packed strand of eosinophilic fibrin (double arrow). The granulation tissue consists of large numbers of greatly dilated capillary-type blood vessels (thin arrow) and a relatively small number of macrophages and fibroblasts. Between the blood vessels there is abundant pale loose (edematous) connective tissue. Eventually this tissue digests the remaining fibrin and organizes (converts) the granulation tissue and loose connective tissue into fibrous tissue. HE ×235

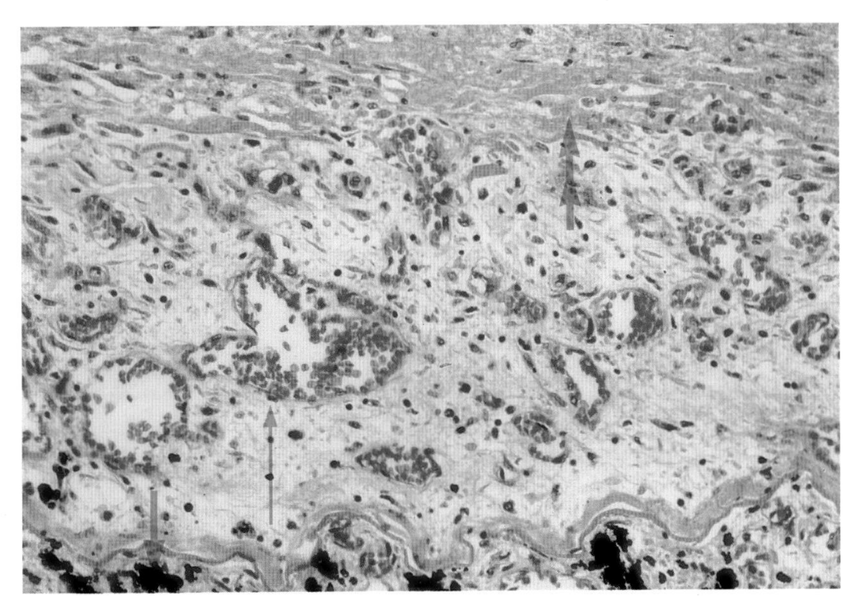

12.30 Fibrinous pleurisy: lung

The process of organization of the layer of fibrin on the surface of the visceral pleura has reached a more advanced stage than that shown in 12.32. Initially, after digestion and organization by macrophages and capillaries, all the fibrin on the surface of the pleura had been replaced by a thick layer of granulation tissue which, in turn, has now been converted into a large sheet of pale collagenous fibrous tissue (double arrows). The newly formed collagenous tissue is still fairly vascular, with numerous slender capillaries; and within the collagenous tissue there are large numbers of both elongated plump fibroblasts and smaller slender fibrocytes. Beneath the pleural surface there is a thin sheet of eosinophilic elastic tissue (thin arrow) and layer of subserosal connective tissue in which there are dilated capillaries (thick arrow). The end-result of this fibrinous 'pleuritis' might be a layer of dense fibrous tissue which, if sufficiently abundant, could greatly restrict the respiratory movements of the lung. HE ×134

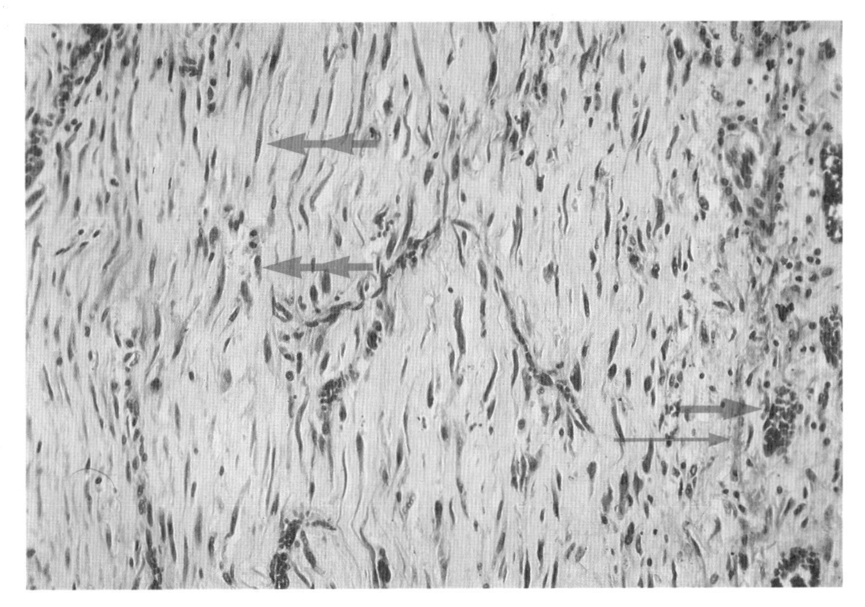

12.31 Pleural plaque: lung

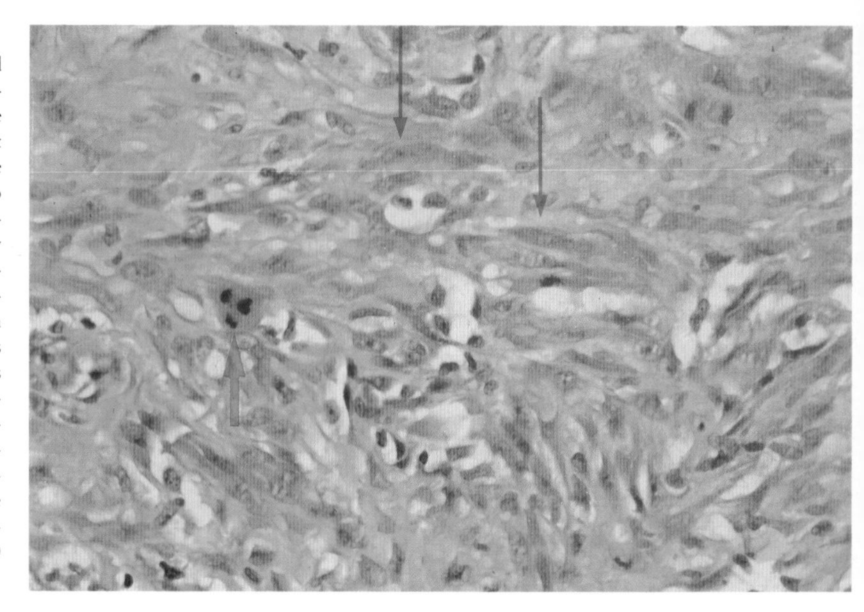

Pleural plaques are the most common lesion associated with asbestos, and in people exposed to asbestos, distinctive plaques form not infrequently on the pleural surface of the diaphragm and on the parietal pleura of the chest wall. No asbestos (ferruginous) bodies are found in these plaques as a rule. The plaques take many years to develop but do not become mesotheliomatous. They are also usually symptomless. They are well-defined, with a shiny smooth or knobbly ivory-coloured surface, and are usually bilateral. Cutting reveals a firm consistence, not unlike that of cartilage. This plaque is from a man of 41 with a history of occupational exposure to asbestos. It consists of interlacing bundles of large fibroblasts and fibrocytes (thin arrows), surrounded by eosinophilic collagenous fibrous tissue. The fibroblastic cells have ill-defined cytoplasm and large pale-staining ovoid vesicular or pleomorphic nuclei. An abnormal (tripolar) mitotic figure is visible (thick arrow). Elsewhere, other parts of the plaque were less cellular, with proportionately more hyaline fibrous tissue. HE ×360

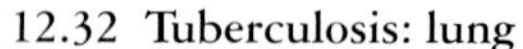

12.32 Tuberculosis: lung

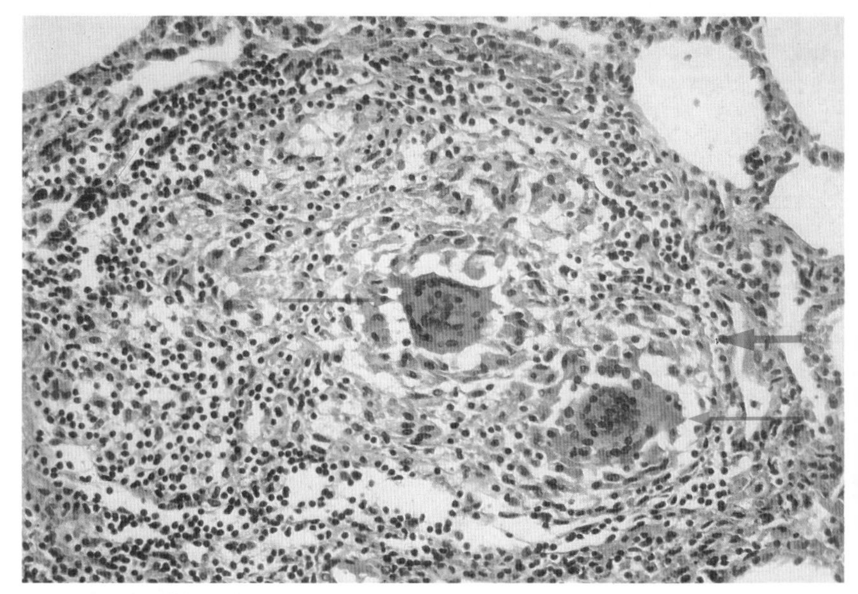

Tuberculosis is caused by *Mycobacterium tuberculosis,* and the route of infection is generally inhalation of droplets from other individuals with the disease. The tubercle bacillus evokes a mononuclear cell response in the tissues, although polymorphs sometimes appear initially. In this case, however, the infection has been blood-borne and has given rise, in the pulmonary tissues, to a fairly large miliary tubercle around which there are several normal alveolar spaces (top right). The paler macrophages in the tubercle have evolved into epithelioid cells with eosinophilic cytoplasm and adopted a follicular arrangement (thick arrow). In the centre of the tubercle there are two closely apposed groups of epithelioid histiocytes with heavily stained ovoid nuclei and poorly-defined cytoplasm (much of it disintegrating). Accompanying the epithelioid cells there are two giant multinucleated cells (thin arrows). At the periphery of the miliary tubercle there are a few plasma cells and numerous lymphocytes with minimal cytoplasm and a small round deeply basophilic nucleus. In a histological section stained by the Ziehl-Neelsen method, tubercle bacilli would be detectable. HE ×235

12.33 Tuberculous bronchopneumonia: lung

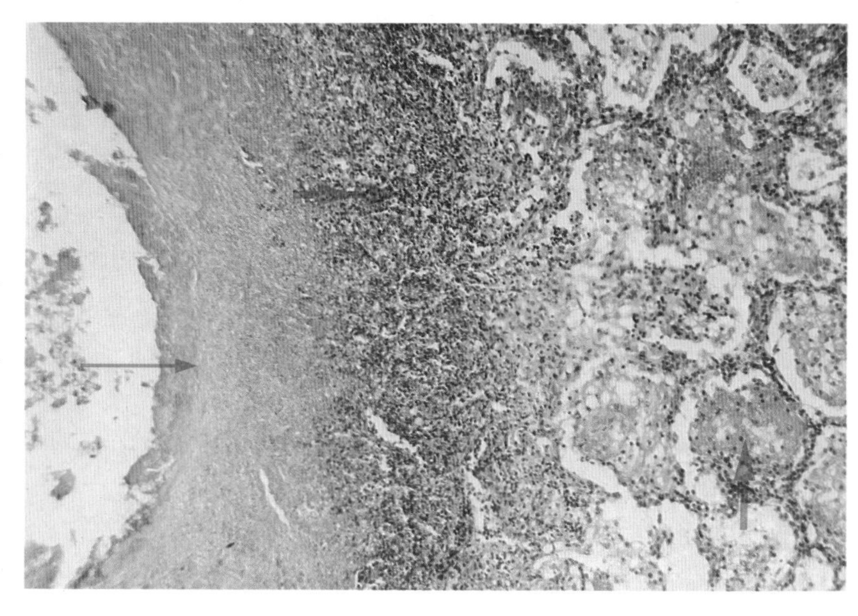

Large numbers of tubercle bacilli may be discharged into a bronchus, from a caseous lymph node or from a caseous focus in the lung, and inhaled. Tuberculous bronchopneumonia results. An inflammatory exudate, consisting of fibrin, edema fluid, large numbers of macrophages and a few other inflammatory cells fill the infected alveoli, and the lung undergoes consolidation. In this more advanced lesion, all the alveolar spaces are filled with abundant consolidated deeply eosinophilic exudate (thick arrow) in which only a relatively small number of viable macrophages have survived. The consolidated lung on the left has become necrotic (caseated), and the necrotic (caseous) tissue now consists of a solid mass of amorphous pink material (thin arrow). The centre of the mass has disintegrated and been coughed up, to form a cavity in which there are only a few fragments of necrotic material. A broad ring of densely packed blue-staining nuclear debris (double arrow) separates the caseous tissue from the macrophage-containing alveolar spaces on the right. A Ziehl-Neelsen stain would reveal large numbers of tubercle bacilli throughout the focus. HE ×70

12.34 Tuberculous pneumonia: lung

Foci of tuberculous pneumonia, consisting of pale crumbly (caseous) 'pus', tend to form at the margin of a lesion in the lung and then destroy more and more pulmonary parenchyma. Tuberculous lesions tend to undergo necrosis on a large scale, and the whole of a consolidated lung may become caseous. This field illustrates, at high magnification, a large pulmonary alveolar space which has undergone consolidation. The capillaries in the walls of the alveolar space are distended (in some parts of the vessels) by round or lobulated groups of red cells which appear to have fused together (thick arrow), to form thrombi. The large alveolar space is full of inflammatory exudate which consists of large numbers of cells of various types. Most of the cells are round macrophages with a considerable amount of cytoplasm and an ovoid or slightly pleomorphic nucleus. Small numbers of polymorph leukocytes are also present. Many of the cells in the exudate are degenerate however and some have completely disintegrated into fragments of cell debris.

HE ×335

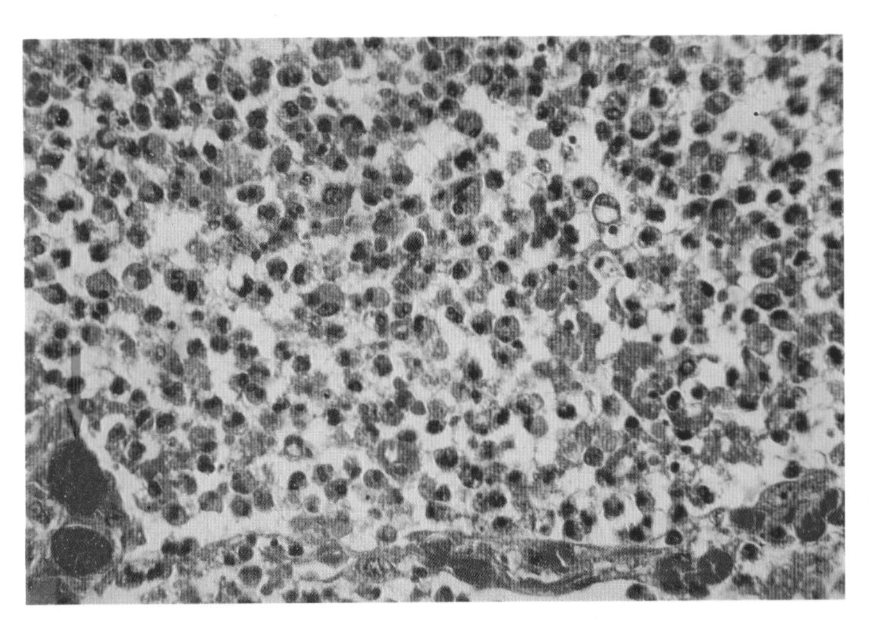

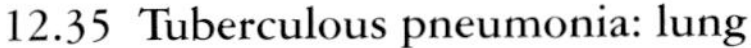

12.35 Tuberculous pneumonia: lung

This field is similar to the lesion in 12.37, but visible at higher magnification. Staining a histological section of a tuberculous lung with HE is of little or no value, since tubercle bacilli are very difficult to stain and not easily rendered visible by other stains, including an ordinary Gram stain. The Ziehl-Neelsen method however stains acid-fast bacilli successfully, by using three components, namely a powerful stain (carbol fuchsin), heat and a mordant. In this histological (paraffin) section, stained by Ziehl-Neelsen method, there is an alveolar space which is filled with a consolidated inflammatory exudate. The exudate consists, almost exclusively, of closely packed large macrophages. The macrophages have a considerable amount of ill-defined pinkish cytoplasm and ovoid or round pale blue vesicular nuclei (arrow). Very strikingly there are, in the cytoplasm, an enormous number of bright purple-red tubercle bacilli, stained a bright purple-red colour. Many of the bacilli are curved rods and they congregate in clumps. However there are also many single forms.

Ziehl-Neelsen ×580

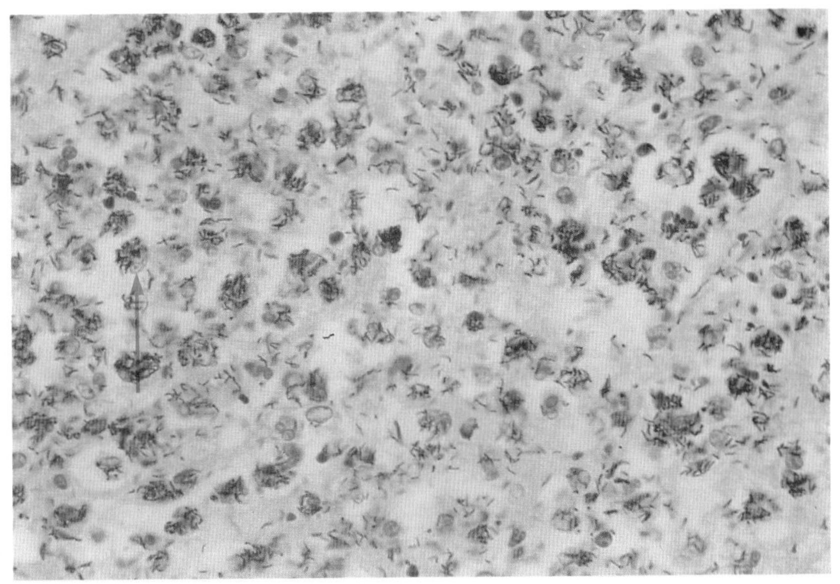

12.36 Nodular silicosis: lung

Nodular silicosis develops slowly in the lungs, mostly in the lungs of men. Small particles (0.5-5μm dia) of free silica (silicon dioxide) are inhaled into alveolar spaces in the lungs and are ingested there by alveolar macrophages. The silica particles in the alveolar macrophages are toxic and kill the macrophages which ingested them. The cycle of particle ingestion followed by macrophage necrosis is persistently repeated but fibroblasts are eventually activated, forming bundles of delicate collagen fibrils which envelop the particles in abundant dense fibrous tissue. Mature silicotic nodules are generally round and several mm in diameter, and their consistence is hard. In this case, there were many silicotic nodules scattered throughout both lungs, and in this histological section part of a nodule is shown. It is composed of dense hyalinized collagenous fibrous tissue which is virtually acellular and more or less avascular (thin arrow). There are accumulations of dark brown particles (thick arrow) (small fragments of non-fibrogenic coal dust) in the nodules, whereas the silica particles are colourless and invisible. The clear 'cracks' in the fibrous tissue were caused by shrinkage during processing.

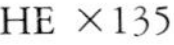

HE ×135

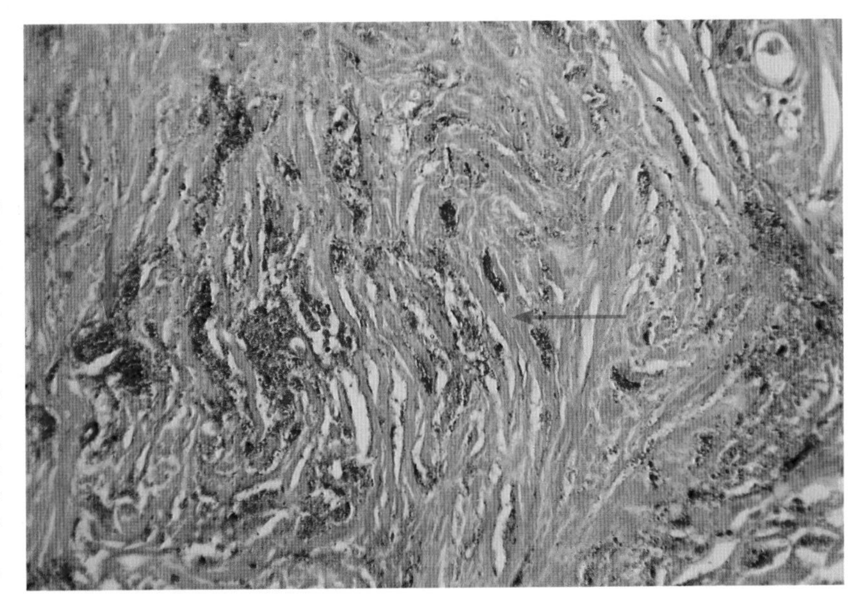

12.37 Asbestos (ferruginous) bodies: lung

Fibres of asbestos in the lung are too large to be phagocytosed but generally acquire a proteinaceous golden-yellow 'coat' which is impregnated with (iron-containing) hemosiderin and other minerals. Golden-yellow asbestos bodies (2-5μm dia and mostly about 100μm long) are unstained, but when stained for iron their colour is a brilliant blue. In this field there are several tight clusters of dark brown or golden-brown asbestos bodies (thin arrow) of very variable length in the bronchiole and alveolus. The coat of most of the bodies is beaded or highly segmented, and most have pointed or bulbous (knob-like) swellings, usually at the ends of the fibre. Eosinophilic vacuolated amorphous exudate (thick arrow) and macrophages with large vesicular nuclei are also present in the air spaces. There is also an unusual macrophage with a relatively enormous very pleomorphic pale granular nucleus (double arrow) With sensitive methods, asbestos bodies are detectable in the lungs of a large proportion of the population of many countries. Their significance is uncertain but their presence in the lung or in the sputum does not signify asbestosis. HE ×360

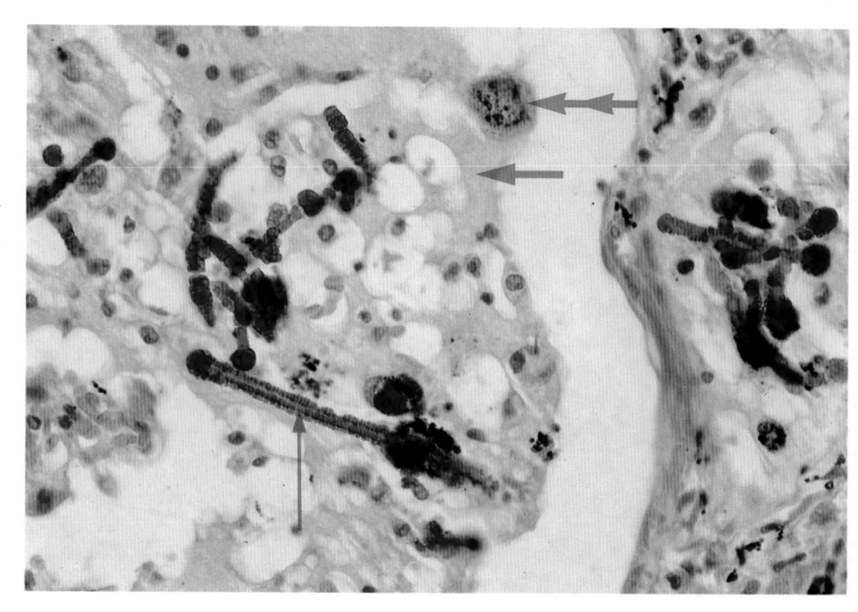

12.38 Alveolar proteinosis: lung

Alveolar proteinosis is a rare disease of the lungs, of unknown etiology, which can occur at any age. The symptoms are cough and shortness of breath, with loss of weight and increasing weakness. Usually both lungs are affected, often the lower lobes. About one-third of those with the condition die. Post-mortem there are areas of consolidation in the lungs. This shows one such area. The alveoli are greatly distended, from the presence of a large quantity of eosinophilic amorphous exudate (double arrow) in which there are many clefts which contained cholesterol crystals. The stretched alveolar walls are compressed and thin (thin arrow), apparently from compression by the exudate in the alveoli. The exudate consists mainly of cell debris. The alveolar capillaries and the epithelial cells lining the alveoli are inconspicuous. There is a very scant population of lymphocytes in the pulmonary tissues and no fibrosis. The eosinophilic exudate is rich in protein and lipid and probably comes from degenerate granular pneumocytes, some of which are visible (thick arrow). HE ×150

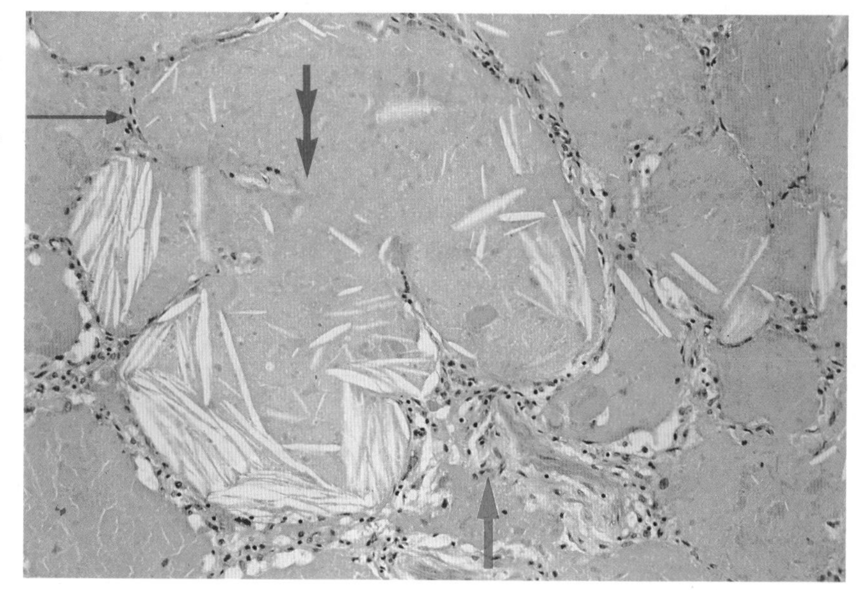

12.39 Alveolar proteinosis: lung

The abundant amorphous material which fills the alveoli contains protein, cholesterol and phospholipids (similar to surfactant). Most of the contents of the material probably comes from cell fragments, the sources being mainly macrophages and desquamated alveolar epithelial cells. Cell fragments are often also visible in the material. This is part of the lesion shown in 12.41, at higher magnification. The alveolar spaces are larger than normal and their walls are notably thickened and infiltrated with lymphocytes. The alveoli are distended with eosinophilic material (thin arrows) (the material also stains a bright purple-red colour with the PAS method) but the epithelial lining of the alveoli is indistinct or absent. Much of the material in the alveoli is homogeneous, but much of it is also finely granular (double arrow) and similar in texture to that of the cytoplasm of the large round pale cells (thick arrow) in the exudate. These large round cells are granular pneumocytes, with abundant granular cytoplasm, and many of them in the alveoli have small pyknotic nuclei, an appearance which suggests strongly that they are degenerate and disintegrating. HE ×235

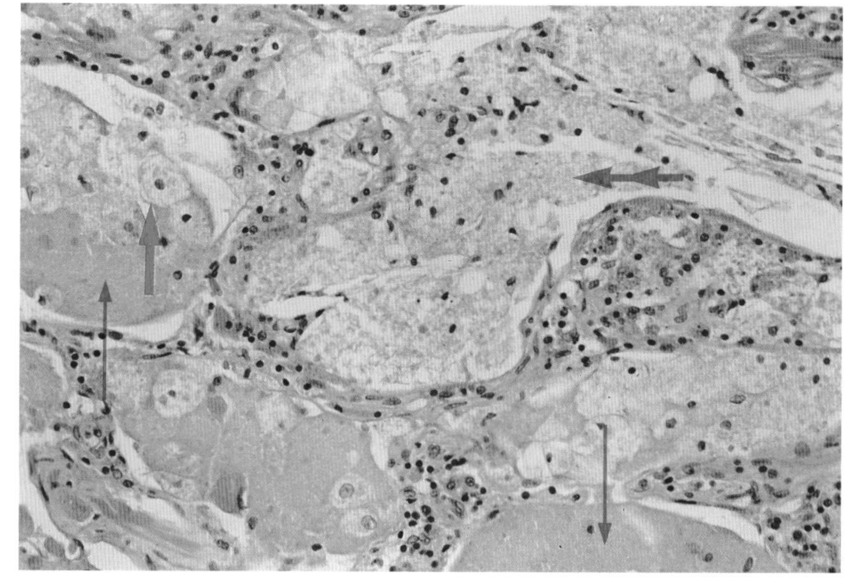

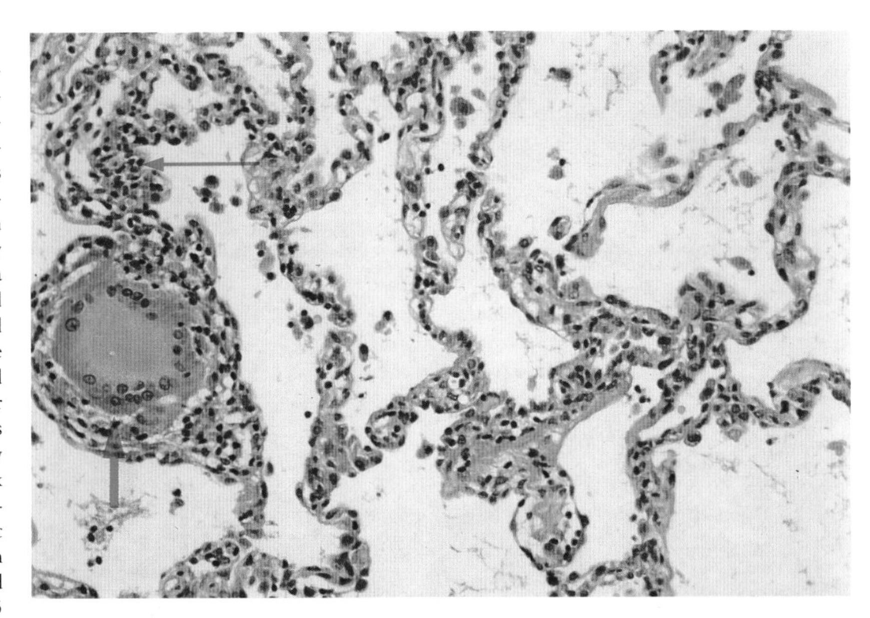

12.40 Extrinsic allergic alveolitis: lung

Inhaled organic dusts (inhaled antigen) can induce an Arthus (type III) reaction in the walls of the pulmonary alveoli, by reacting with circulating precipitating antibodies. The dust may be derived from moulds or bird droppings (bird-fancier's lung), and the clinical syndromes produced by this reaction are termed collectively as extrinsic allergic alveolitis and also linked individually with the patient's occupation (e.g., a response to mouldy hay in a farmer's lung). In this diagnostic specimen from a 36-year-old woman, the alveolar walls are thickened (thin arrow), from the presence of lymphocytes and plasma cells. The epithelial cells lining the alveoli are more prominent than normal, and a few desquamated cells lie within the alveoli. Also present in the alveolar wall is a large (giant) multinucleated cell of the Langhans type, with the many nuclei located around the periphery of the abundant strongly eosinophilic cytoplasm (thick arrow). Multinucleated giant cells are characteristic of extrinsic allergic alveolitis, in which an identifiable organic antigen has been inhaled. The source of the antigen in this case was a budgerigar and the illness was termed bird-fancier's lung. HE ×235

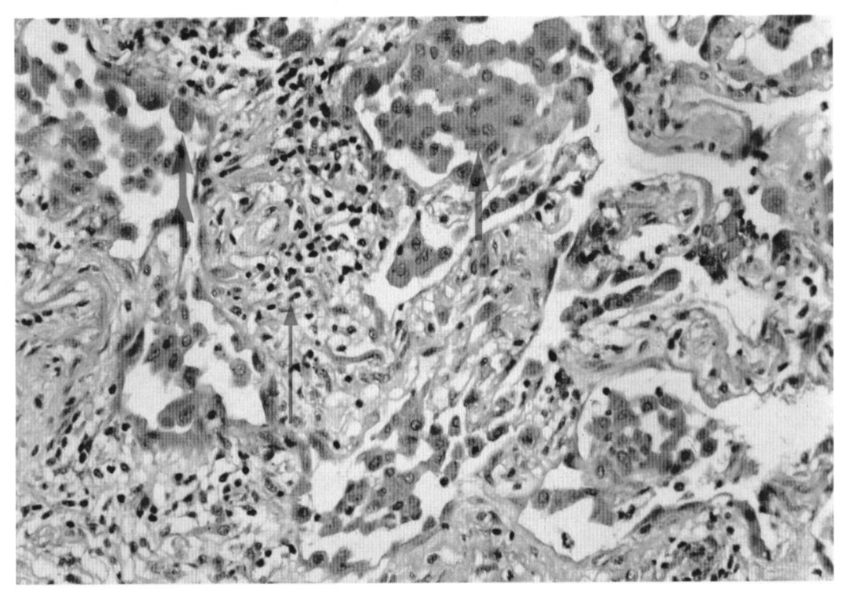

12.41 Cryptogenic (idiopathic) fibrosing alveolitis: lung

The cause of the lung damage in cryptogenic fibrosing alveolitis is unknown. An autoimmune mechanism may operate, serum autoantibodies occurring in some patients. A not infrequent association with connective tissue diseases, and inhalation of an external agent of an unknown nature may also play a part. The basic cause of the disease appears to be diffuse damage to the walls of the alveolar spaces, which then thicken. Macrophages and granular (Type II) pneumocytes also congregate in the alveolar spaces. In this diagnostic specimen from a man of 52, the air spaces vary in size and shape and their walls are very thick (thin arrow), consisting of eosinophilic fibrous connective tissue in which there are many small clear vacuoles. In the walls there are also groups of relatively small cells, mainly lymphocytes and plasma cells, with heavily stained round or ovoid nuclei. The air spaces are still recognizable as alveolar in form, containing clusters (varying markedly in size) of mononuclear cells with a considerable amount of deeply eosinophilic cytoplasm (thick arrow) and ovoid or round vesicular nuclei (and often nucleoli). The alveolar spaces are lined (partly) by prominent epithelial cells with fairly similar eosinophilic cytoplasm (double arrow). HE ×235

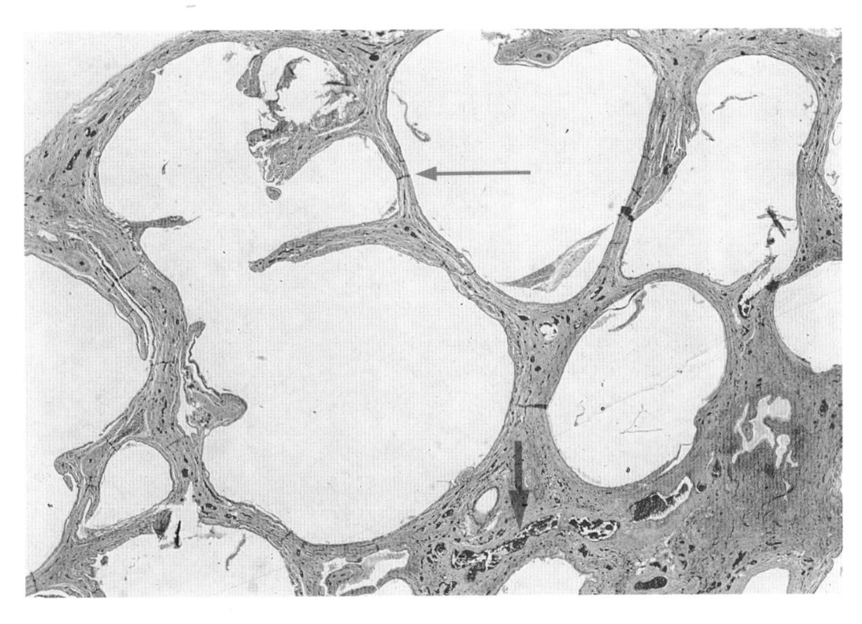

12.42 Honeycomb lung

As with extrinsic allergic alveolitis and cryptogenic (idiopathic) fibrosing alveolitis, fibrosis of the interstitial tissues of the lung may progress until large parts of the lungs are converted into small cystic spaces (1-2cm dia) with thick fibrous walls. The affected parts of the lung resemble a honeycomb and the condition is termed honeycomb lung. Honeycomb lung is associated with a variety of diseases, particularly the connective tissue group, and various drugs and toxic substances (including beryllium and cadmium). In this case the underlying disease was progressive systemic sclerosis. The normal structure of the patient's lungs has been replaced by large air-filled spaces with thick walls of collagenous fibrous tissue (thin arrow). There are also numerous thin-walled blood vessels, some dilated (thick arrow), in the fibrous tissue. High-power magnification shows air-filled spaces lined (incompletely) with cuboidal epithelium of the bronchiolar type and many lymphocytes and plasma cells in the fibrous tissue. HE ×8

12.43 Sarcoidosis: lung

Sarcoidosis is a granulomatous disease of unknown etiology, characterized by the formation in many tissues (mostly thoracic) of (macroscopically) small round whitish granules similar to miliary tubercles. Histologically the granules are spheroidal collections of macrophages. Each macrophage has one or more elongated or kidney-shaped vesicular nuclei, and its cytoplasm is characteristically strongly eosinophilic. The macrophages are therefore generally referred to as epithelioid cells. The epithelioid cells are usually closely packed, with cytoplasmic boundaries so poorly defined as to be indistinguishable. The follicles are located most often in lymphoid tissue, but the lungs are also involved fairly frequently. This is a diagnostic biopsy specimen from the lung of a woman of 30 suspected clinically of having asbestosis. The alveolar walls are thickened and infiltrated by lymphocytes and macrophages. Several round epithelioid follicles (thin arrows) are also present. There are very large (giant) multinucleated cells (Langhans-type) within the follicles, and one follicle is enclosed (at least partly) in fibrous tissue (thick arrow). There is no necrosis in the follicles. In several alveolar spaces there are a few macrophages. A minority of cases of sarcoidosis progress to honeycomb lung. HE ×150

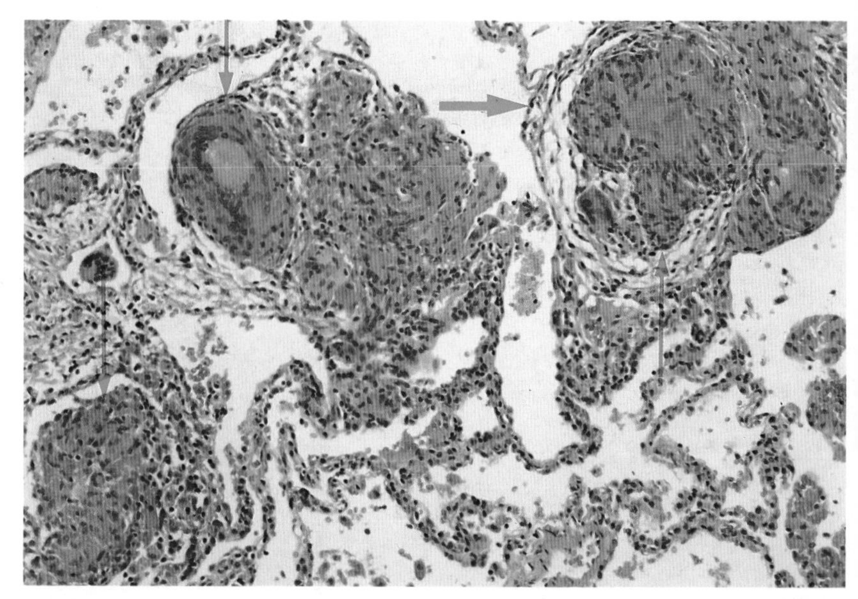

12.44 Wegener's granulomatosis: lung

In Wegener's granulomatosis the basic lesion is a necrotizing vasculitis with granulomatous inflammation (including giant cells), usually in the nose or in the maxillary sinuses. Similar lesions often arise in the lungs and kidneys however, and polyarthritis or polyneuritis occasionally develops. Sometimes, in the dermis and subcutis, not only are small vessels involved but so also are medium-sized vessels. In the lungs, the affected tissues are consolidated and reddish-grey, but necrosis is often extensive and accompanied by cavitation. In this field there is a sheet of cellular granulomatous tissue (double arrow) which consists of closely packed macrophages, lymphocytes, plasma cells and connective tissue cells and fibres. Also present, at the periphery of the granulomatous tissue, are occasional giant cells of the Langhans type (thin arrow). This central tissue is still viable and it has replaced lung tissue. On both sides of the viable tissue there are sheets of deeply eosinophilic solid tissues which are necrotic and composed of lung and granulomatous tissue. Small amounts of carbon dust (thick arrow) are visible in the necrotic tissue. HE ×55

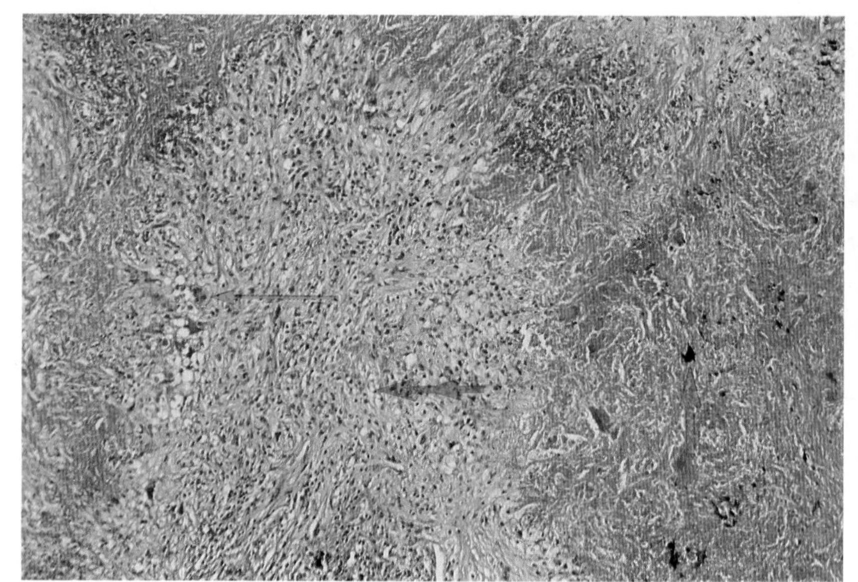

12.45 Kaolin pneumoconiosis: lung

Kaolin (china clay) is silicate of aluminium, and inhaled particles are not fibrogenic. The dust is not harmless however, and kaolin pneumoconiosis occasionally occurs if exposure to the dust is very severe. The patient in this case was a china clay worker who had been heavily exposed to kaolin dust over many years. At post-mortem examination, both lungs had a distinctly nodular texture. The visceral pleura is a thin sheet of cellular connective tissue (double arrow), and above the alveolar spaces are lined by a single layer of uniform prominent cuboidal epithelial cells with ovoid vesicular nuclei (thick arrow) and their lumen distended with sheets of closely packed large macrophages (thin arrow) with abundant pink cytoplasm and uniform ovoid or round vesicular nuclei (the 'cracks' between the clusters of macrophages are probably artefactual). Kaolin dust is practically colourless but at higher magnification the cytoplasm of the macrophages was seen to be full of dust particles (which give the cytoplasm a brownish tint). The macrophages show no sign of degeneration and there is no evidence of fibrosis. HE ×360

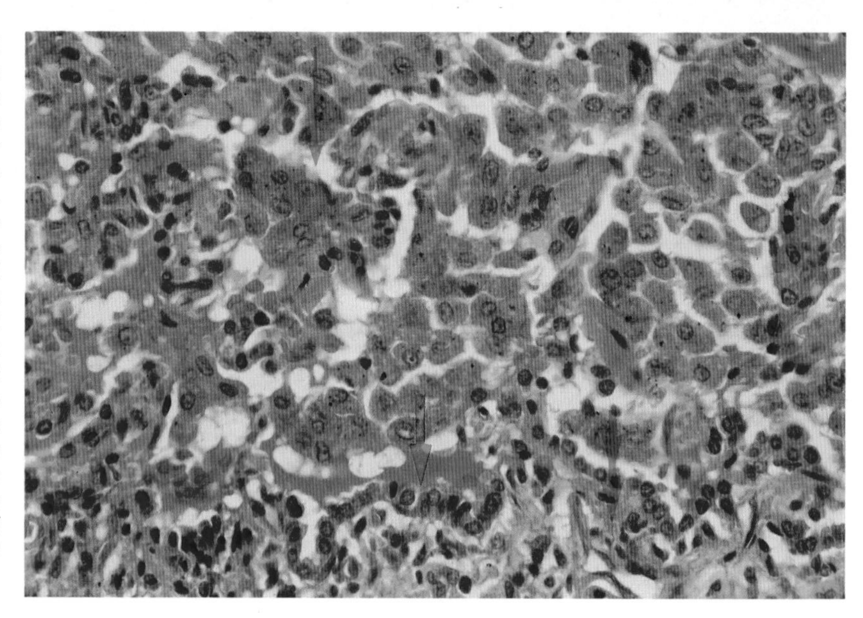

12.46 Hydatid disease (Echinococciasis granulosus): lung

Hydatid disease is caused by the tapeworm *Echinococcus granulosus*. The adult worm is only 3-5mm long and has only a few segments. It is a common parasite of dogs, and it can occur anywhere in the world. Hydatid disease is produced in another animal when it acts as intermediate host, as a result of swallowing ova from a dog's feces. Hydatid cyst forms a slowly growing space-occupying mass up to 20cm dia. It is multilocular, containing many daughter cysts. The cuticular layer of the cyst wall, which is on the left of this field (the lumen and the innermost germinative layer are out of the picture), consists of a sheet of pale acellular laminated chitinous material (thick arrow) (densely-stained in parts) which is being digested by a small population of macrophages. The cuticular layer is enclosed by the adventitial layer (centre and right) of dense collagenous fibrous tissue (thin arrow), which is infiltrated by large numbers of eosinophil leukocytes (double arrow). HE ×120

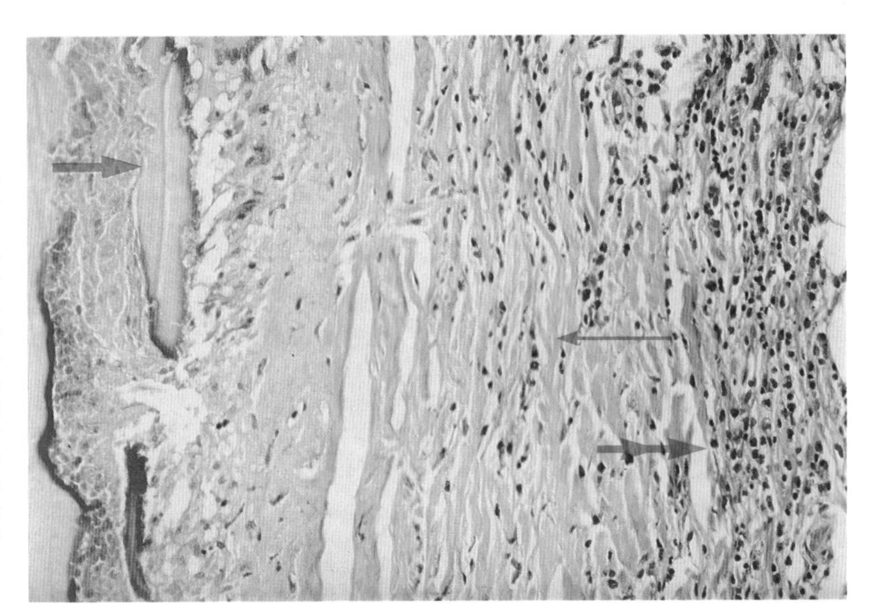

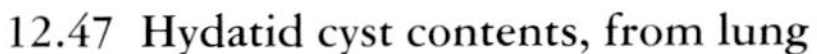

12.47 Hydatid cyst contents, from lung

Tapeworm (*Echinococcus granulosus*) from a hydatid cyst in the lung. This wet preparation exhibits the head of a new worm, with a crown of 30-50 invaginated hooklets (arrow).

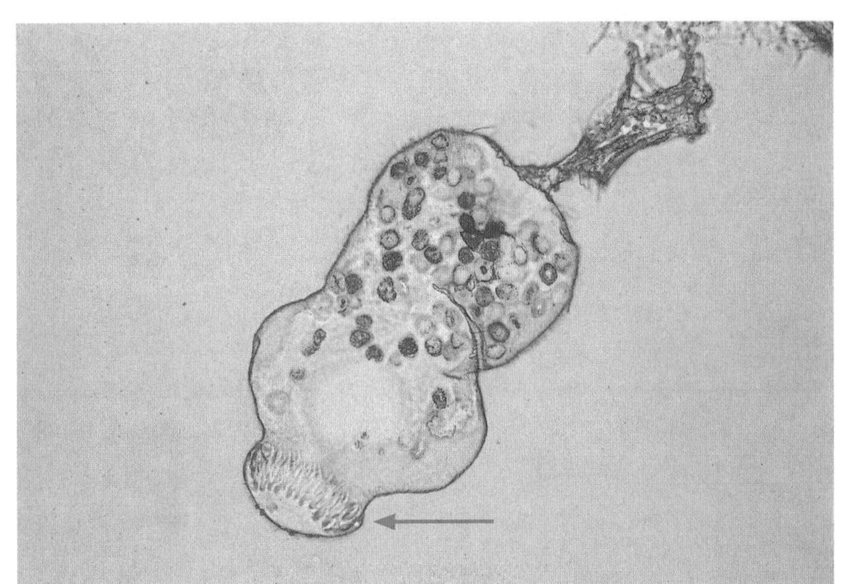

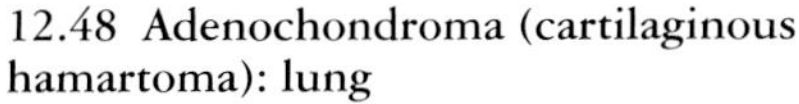

12.48 Adenochondroma (cartilaginous hamartoma): lung

Adenochondroma of lung is uncommon, not present in infants and usually occurring in adults. It is a firm, discrete (sharply defined) benign tumour-like lesion, generally loculated, at the periphery of a lung. Very occasionally however it takes the form of a polypoid intrabronchial mass (2-5cm dia). It is often found by chance, e.g. on X-ray of the chest. Its cut surface is firm, with glistening bluish-white nodules of cartilage and small foci of calcification. The lesion grows slowly but does not invade the surrounding tissues or metastasize, and does no harm. The major component of this tissue consists of well-differentiated plates of eosinophilic cartilage, evenly populated by large (mostly stellate-shaped) chondrocytes (thin arrows) with very basophilic nuclei in clear (vacuolated) lacunae. The cartilaginous plates are partly surrounded by fibrous connective tissue (thick arrow), and the chondrocytes within the plates are fully mature, exhibiting no pleomorphism of nuclei or mitotic activity. The adjacent loose connective tissue is infiltrated by large numbers of small lymphocytes (double arrow) with round deeply basophilic nuclei. It is also intersected by extremely elongated cleft-like spaces which are lined by a single layer of flattened or cuboidal epithelial cells rather than by respiratory-type cells. There is also some cell debris in the lumen of the clefts. The precise nature of adenochondroma of lung is uncertain but it is probably primarily a hamartomatous overgrowth of the connective tissue elements of the wall of a bronchus with secondary involvement of bronchial epithelium. HE ×150

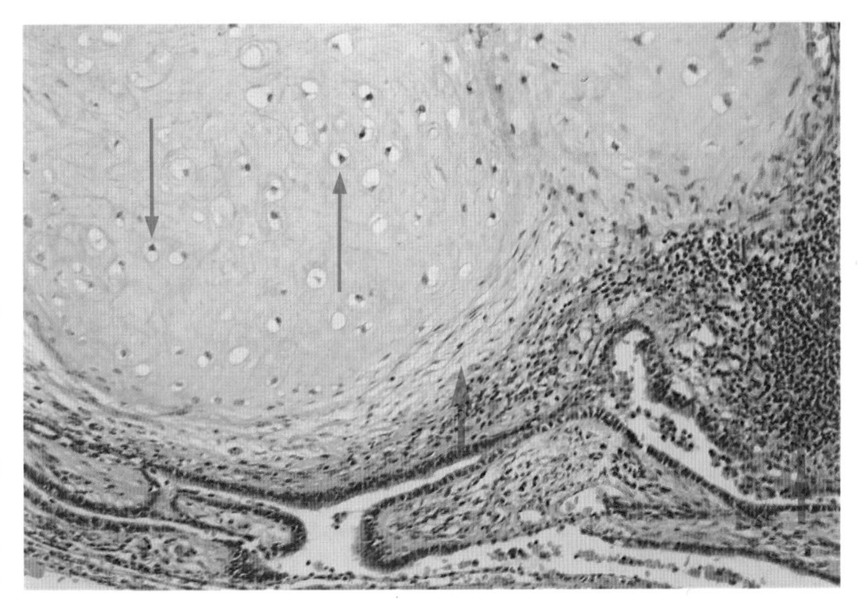

12.49 Carcinoid: bronchus

Carcinoid originates from Kulchitzky-type cells and tends to form a vascular nodule or polypoid mass in a central bronchus or a small bronchus or bronchiole at the periphery of the lung. The tumour may cause chronic cough or hemoptysis, or obstruct a bronchus and collapse part of the lung. The tumour is slow-growing and locally invasive. The prognosis is usually good but less so in atypical carcinoids. In this tumour, the neoplastic cells are uniform in size and shape and arranged in closely packed cords (double arrow). They have a moderate amount of eosinophilic cytoplasm and regular round or ovoid vesicular nuclei which contain one or more small nucleoli. No mitoses are present. Although hyalinized elsewhere in the tumour, the stroma is sparse, pale and rich in connective tissue mucin (thin arrow). The small blood vessels are narrowed and inconspicuous (thick arrow). Bronchial carcinoid cells are argyrophil-positive but argentaffin-negative, and electron microscopy reveals neurosecretory granules in the cytoplasm. HE x360

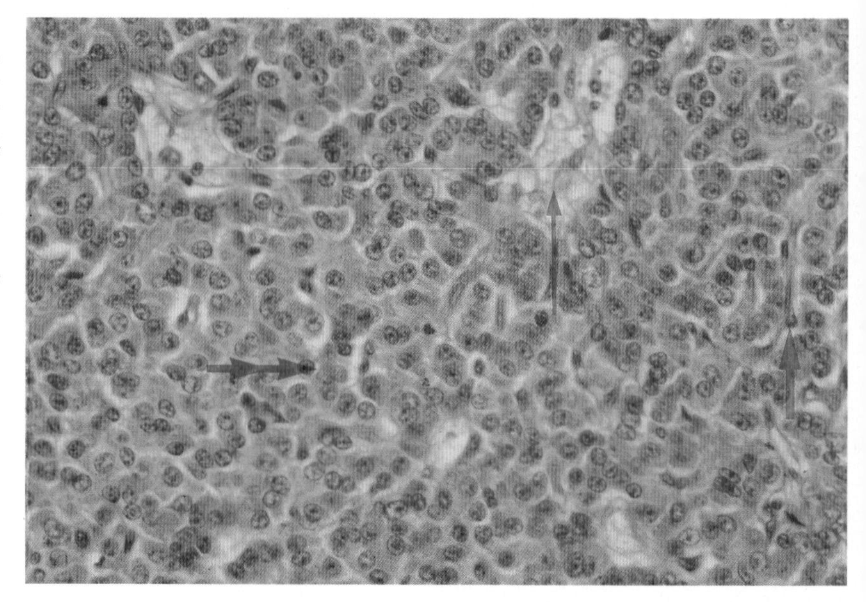

12.50 Carcinoma, small cell anaplastic: bronchus

Small cell anaplastic carcinoma of bronchus is closely linked with cigarette smoking, and it arises from Kulchitsky cells. Neurosecretory granules can be demonstrated in the cytoplasm by a positive argyrophil reaction. It is a highly malignant tumour, spreading rapidly to nodes (hilar, mediastinal) and to other organs via the blood. The bronchial epithelium, on a thick eosinophilic basement membrane, consists of a single layer of cuboidal or low columnar epithelial cells (double arrows). It is intact, but atrophic and stretched over the tumour. The tumour is a diffuse sheet of small cells (slightly larger than lymphocytes) of uniform shape and size, with a negligible amount of cytoplasm and a small ovoid deeply basophilic nucleus. There are numerous mitoses (thin arrow), and pyknotic nuclei and nuclear fragments are fairly numerous. An area of necrosis consists of shrunken cells with pyknotic nuclei (thick arrow). HE ×235

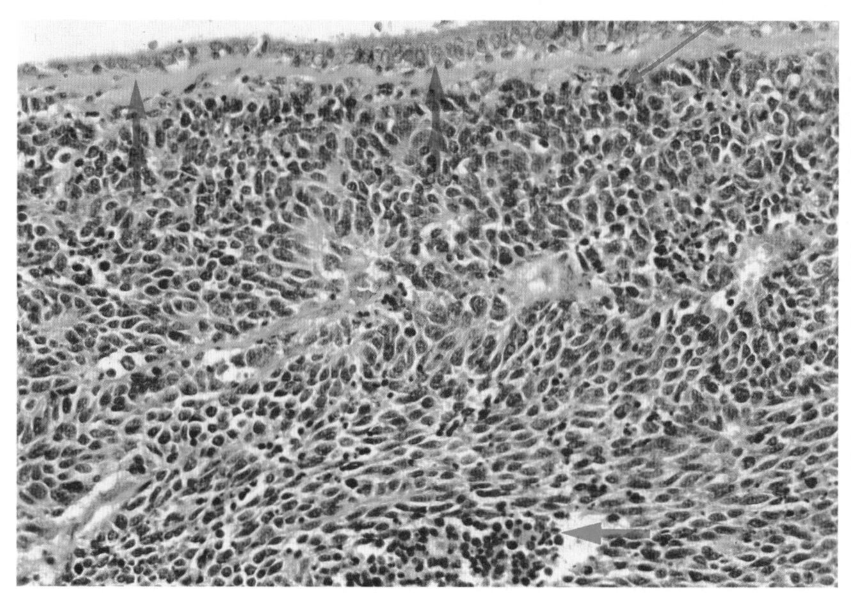

12.51 Carcinoma, large non-small-cell: bronchus

Large cell (non-small-cell) carcinoma) consists of well-formed anaplastic malignant epithelial cells. It has a strong association with smoking, grows rapidly and has a poor prognosis. Tumours of this type show no evidence of squamous, glandular or small-cell differentiation, but they may be poorly differentiated variants of adenocarcinoma, squamous cell carcinoma or combined adeno- and squamous carcinoma. This is a biopsy of bronchial mucosa several cm from a primary carcinoma of bronchus. The lumen of the bronchus (top margin) is lined by a sheet of ciliated respiratory epithelium (thin arrow), beneath which there are a prominent basement membrane and the muscularis mucosae. At the bottom of the field there is a slender sheet of pale blue hyaline cartilage (double arrow). Between the cartilage and the muscularis mucosae there is a dilated lymphatic channel (thick arrow), cut longitudinally, more or less full of compact groups of large malignant cells with abundant cytoplasm, pleomorphic nuclei and prominent nucleoli. There is lymphocytic infiltration in the vicinity of the lymphatic channel. Permeation of lymphatic channels and embolic spread to the lymph nodes are well-recognized modes of spread of highly malignant tumours, and the tumour cells in this channel are probably part of a finger-like extension of the primary tumour along it. HE ×235

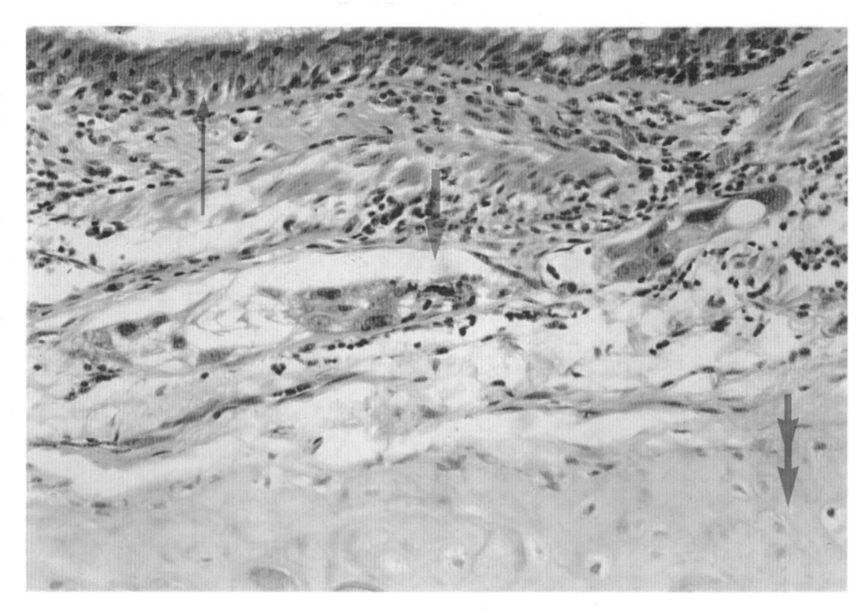

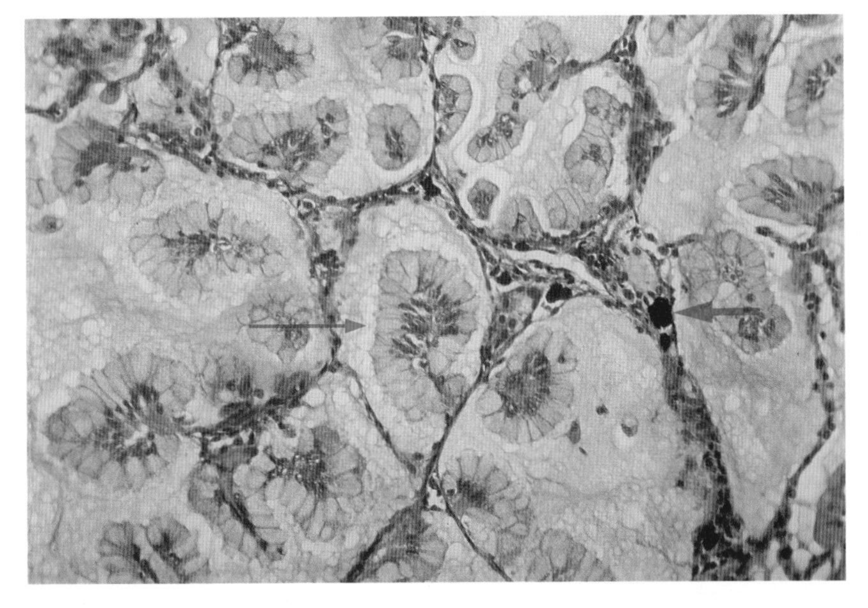

12.52 Bronchioloalveolar carcinoma: lung

Bronchioloalveolar (non-small-cell) carcinoma) arises in the periphery of the lung distal to bronchial epithelium. Possible cells of origin are Type II (granular) pneumocytes, Clara cells or metaplastic bronchiolar cells. The existing air spaces serve as stroma, and in this case the tumour cells use the alveolar walls. The tumour is composed of palisaded mucin-secreting columnar cells (thin arrow), shaped like tall goblets with ovoid or elongated nuclei. They line the alveolar walls and form papillary growths which protrude into the lumen. None of the neoplastic cells shows mitotic activity. The alveolar walls are thin but apparently intact, and the alveolar spaces are distended with secreted mucin. A few small round black deposits of carbonaceous dust (thick arrow) are also present in the alveolar walls. Secondary adenocarcinoma can produce a similar lesion in the lungs, and a diagnosis of alveolar carcinoma is valid only after the presence of a primary carcinoma in another organ such as the alimentary tract has been excluded. This is generally possible only by postmortem examination. HE ×135

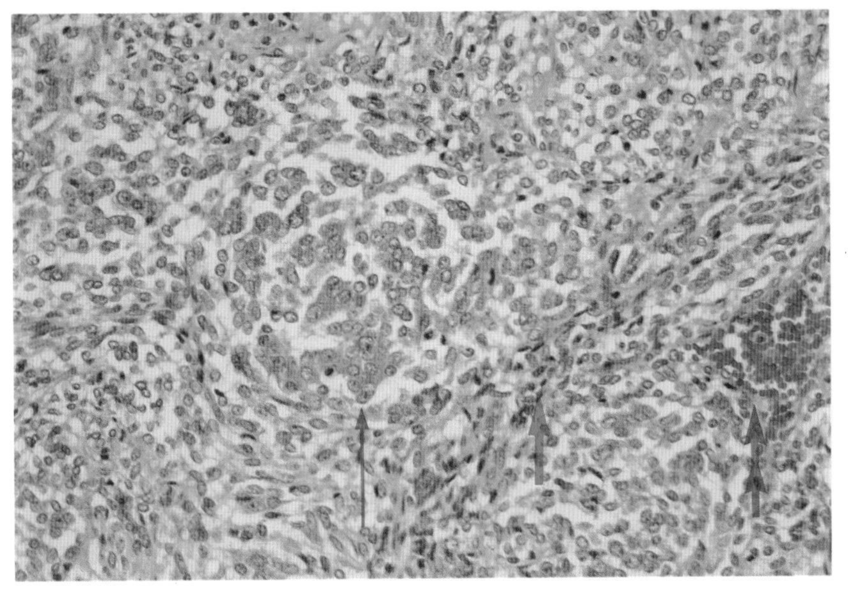

12.53 Pulmonary blastoma: lung

Pulmonary blastoma is a rare lesion, usually a large fairly well defined mass, located peripherally, which may present with hemoptysis but is sometimes detected on routine X-ray examination of the chest. It is biphasic and probably best regarded as a 'mixed' tumour, and this firm well-circumscribed lobulated lesion is composed of elongated basophilic mesenchymal cells and loosely packed epithelial cells. The large numbers of epithelial cells are arranged in clusters, the largest just left of centre (thin arrow). The epithelial cells are regular in size and shape and have a small or moderate amount of ill-defined cytoplasm. Their nuclei are pale, round or ovoid, and vesicular. A nucleolus is visible in some nuclei, but no mitotic activity is evident and there is no necrosis. The epithelial elements are traversed by strands of mesenchymal tissue, which consist of elongated spindle-shaped basophilic connective tissue cells (thick arrow) and thin-walled blood vessels, some greatly dilated (double arrow). HE ×235

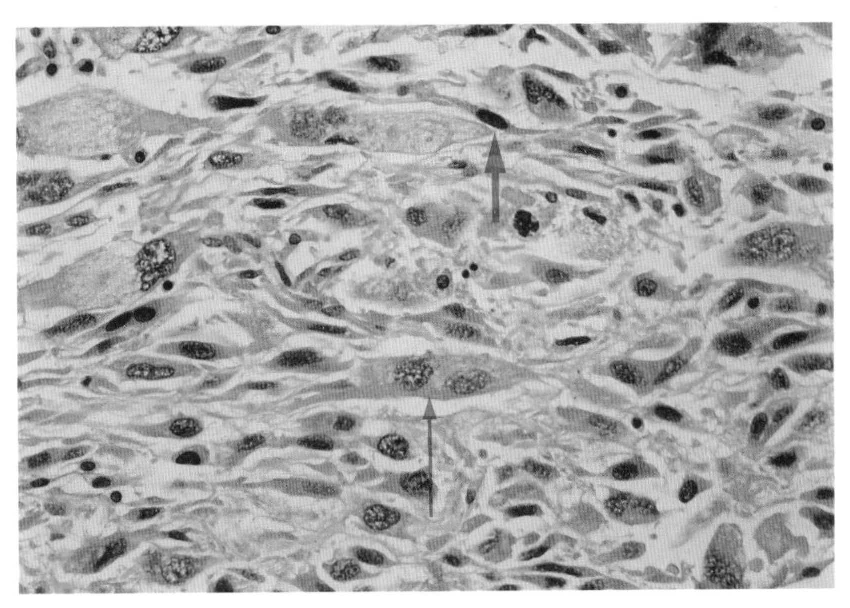

12.54 Secondary sarcoma: lung

The capillary bed of the lungs forms an effective filter, and malignant cells in the bloodstream are frequently retained. The lungs are therefore a common site for metastatic tumour which takes the form of multiple discrete masses or occasionally of a solitary metastasis. This metastasis was a hemorrhagic necrotic mass (4 × 4 × 3cm) in the right lower lobe of a man of 76. It appeared to be solitary and was removed surgically. It is a sarcoma, composed of malignant cells of widely varying size and shape, from small slender forms (thick arrow) with minimal cytoplasm to large or elongated cells with considerable amounts of strongly eosinophilic cytoplasm (thin arrow). With few exceptions, the neoplastic cells have one or more pleomorphic vesicular nuclei with coarsely granular chromatin and no prominent nucleoli. The most prominent cells however are elongated or enormous strap-like cells with equally large quantities of cytoplasm. The appearance and texture of the cytoplasm (focally pale and granular) suggest that the cells are rhabdomyosarcomatous but cross-striations could not be demonstrated and the expected diagnosis was not confirmed. The site of the primary was unknown. HE ×360

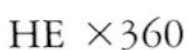

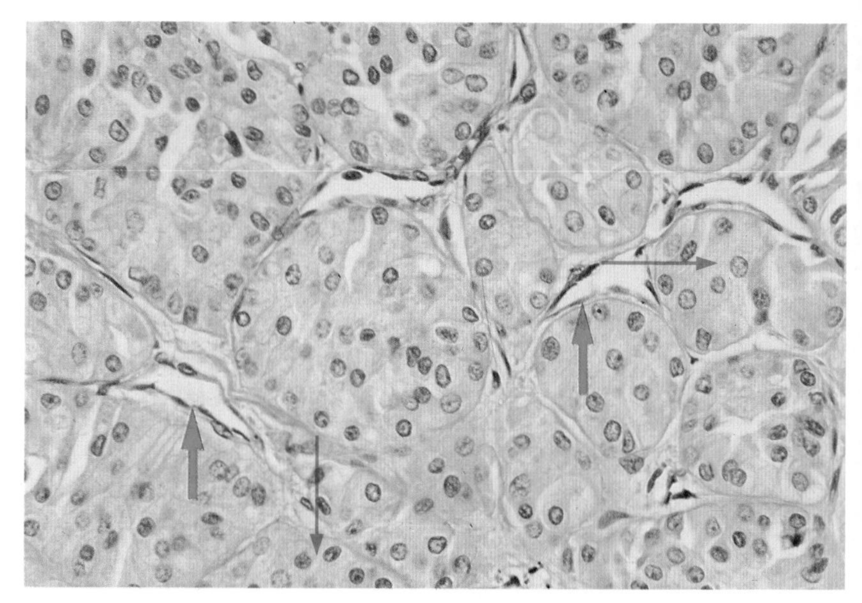

12.55 Secondary carcinoma: lung

A 'shadow' was found on X-ray examination in the upper lobe of the right lung of a man of 51. The lobe was excised surgically and found to contain a firm pale mass 3cm dia, close to the main bronchus. It consists of cords of large neoplastic cells, separated by a delicate stroma which consists almost wholly of thin-walled blood vessels lined by flat endothelial cells (thick arrows). The tumour cells have abundant pale (weakly eosinophilic) granular cytoplasm (thin arrows). Their nuclei show very little pleomorphism and are round or ovoid and vesicular. There is no mitotic activity. Despite its well-differentiated appearance, the tumour had infiltrated the adjacent lung deeply. The appearance of the cells and the sinusoidal structure of the stroma suggested that it was almost certainly a metastasis from a primary renal carcinoma. Although apparently encapsulated, primary renal carcinoma invades the kidney and perirenal tissues. It also invades the renal veins very readily, lining them or filling them with tumour. It also has a marked tendency to remain in direct continuity with the tumour mass in the kidney. HE ×360

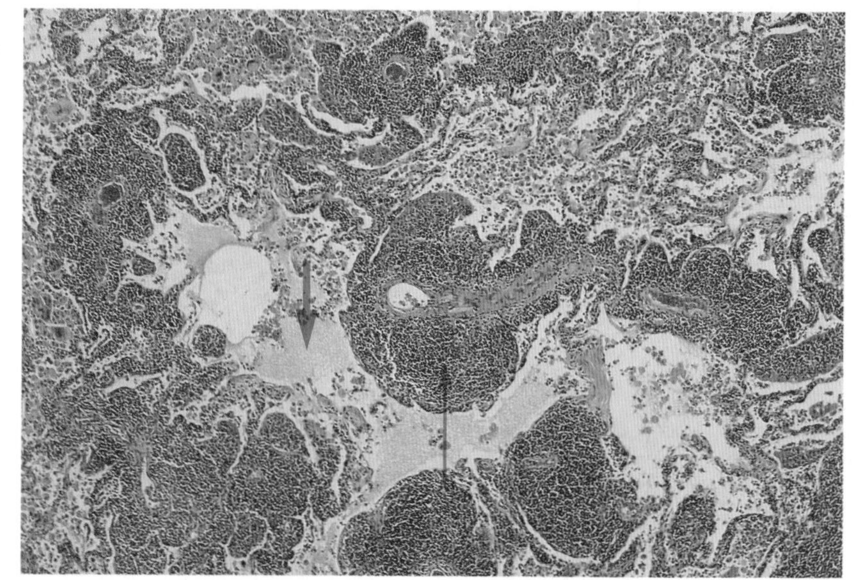

12.56 Lymphocytic lymphoma: lung

In the lung, lymphocytic lymphoma may take the form of a soft well-defined mass or of small pale nodules with a moderately defined edge, scattered throughout the lung. It may also consolidate part or all of a lobe of the lung. This is a lobectomy specimen from a man of 42 with an undiagnosed lesion in the left lower lobe. The lesion took the form of a soft creamy-white wedge-shaped mass which had its apex at the main bronchus and extended 5cm to the pleura, where it was 8cm dia. Multiple fine white nodules were also detected in the surrounding lung. Histologically, the interstitial tissues of the lung are diffusely and heavily infiltrated with small lymphocytes which have almost no cytoplasm and a single small round deeply basophilic nucleus. The lymphocytic infiltrate is greatest in the walls of the bronchioles and the larger blood vessels (thin arrow), but it also extends deeply into the alveolar walls. No germinal centres are present in the groups of lymphocytes. There are large numbers of eosinophilic macrophages and desquamated epithelial cells, as well as a considerable amount of eosinophilic fluid (thick arrow), in most of the air spaces, including bronchioles and alveoli. HE ×60

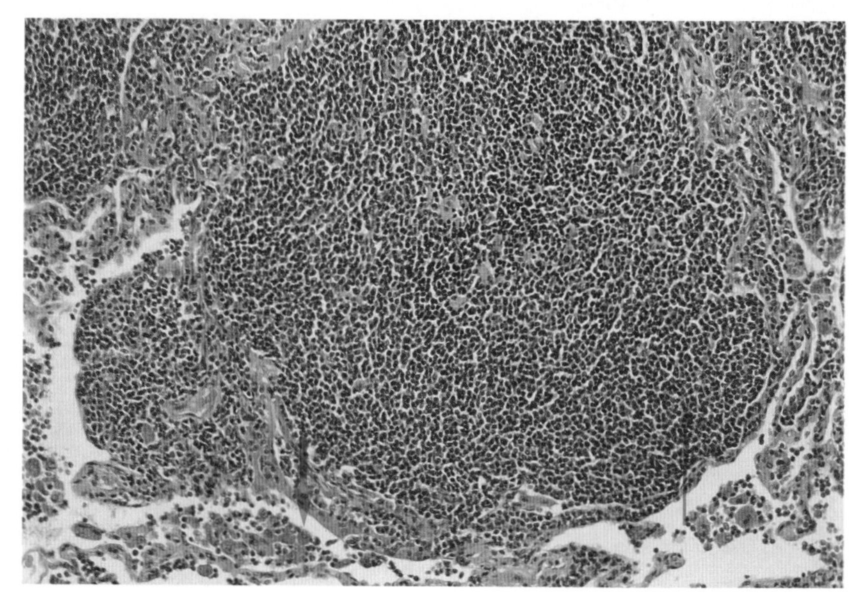

12.57 Lymphocytic lymphoma: lung

Primary lymphomas of lung are mainly B cell lymphomas, often of follicle centre cell origin. This is the same lesion as in 12.59, at higher magnification. In this field, there is a dense infiltrate, throughout the interstitial tissues of the lung, of densely packed uniformly round lymphomatous lymphocytes. The neoplastic lymphocytes are arranged in smaller collections and larger groups (thin arrow) in the interstitial tissues, each lymphocyte having a small round extremely basophilic nucleus and only a barely detectable moderately defined rim of cytoplasm. There is no visible pleomorphism among the lymphomatous lymphocytes, and they closely resemble mature small lymphocytes. There are also very few histiocytes in the sheets of lymphocytes but in the collapsed alveolar spaces there is, in addition to fairly numerous neoplastic lymphocytes, a very considerable number of hemosiderin-containing alveolar-type macrophages and desquamated eosinophilic epithelial cells (thick arrow). The tumour was diagnosed as a low-grade lymphocytic lymphoma, a type of neoplasm which may almost completely replace the lung tissue. HE ×150

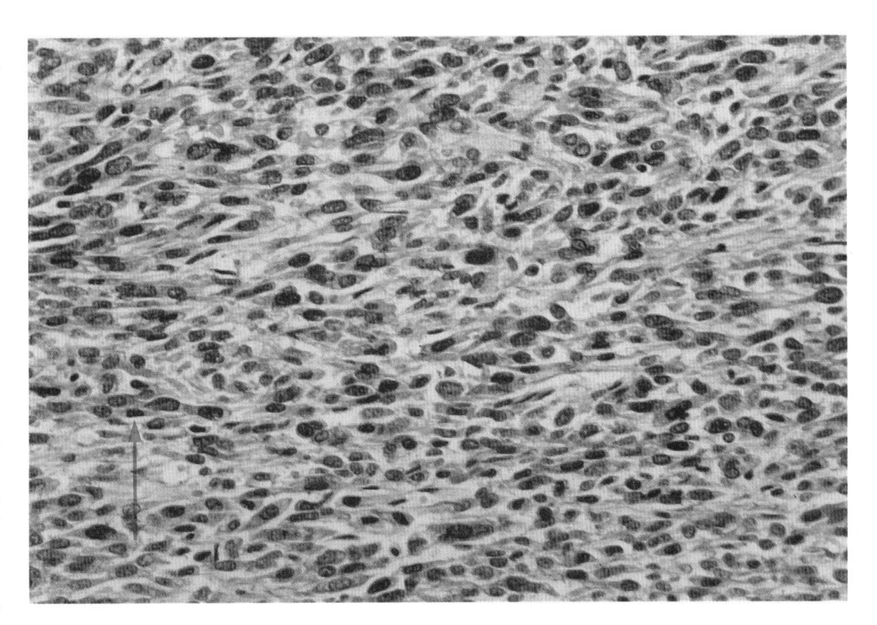

12.58 Mesothelioma: pleura

Mesothelioma is an increasingly common neoplasm of pleura and peritoneum, in the over-50 age group, strongly related to asbestos exposure. Exposure to the dust may be comparatively slight, and many years may elapse between exposure and development of the tumour. The tumour forms a continuous layer over the pleural surfaces, encasing the lung and obliterating the pleural cavity. It does not as a rule penetrate deeply into lung tissue. This tumour has a sarcomatous structure, consisting of sheets of closely packed elongated cells resembling fibroblasts or smooth muscle cells, with ovoid (mostly blunt- or round-ended) basophilic nuclei and a moderate amount of fairly well defined eosinophilic cytoplasm (arrow). There is considerable nuclear pleomorphism, but no mitoses are visible in this field. Nor are any connective tissue fibrils evident. There is however a network of small capillaries, containing a few red cells and lined by small very slender elongated endothelial cells. At higher magnification small vacuoles were detectable in the cytoplasm of some of the malignant (mesothelial) cells. HE ×235

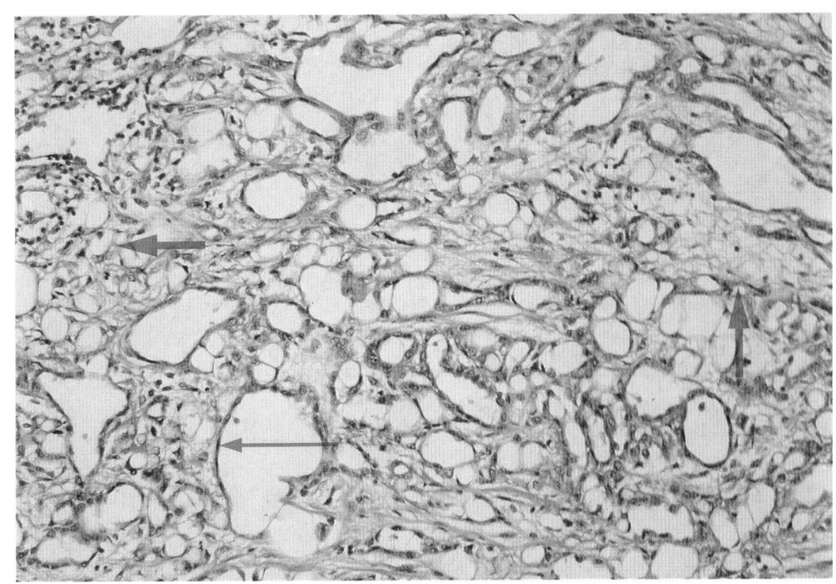

12.59 Mesothelioma: pleura

Histologically, mesotheliomas are biphasic and (generally) consist of a sarcomatoid spindle cell component and epithelial elements that form tubular and papillary structures. Mesotheliomas which form pseudoacini are termed epithelial mesotheliomas, and the malignant cells in this mesothelioma consist almost entirely of tubular and gland-like spaces (also termed pseudoacini) which vary in size and shape from single (individual) cells to clusters of cells (thick arrows), each cell containing a vacuole, and tubular structures. Also present are large and extremely large pseudoacini. Only a minority of the pseudoacini are lined by cuboidal cells, most of them being lined by flat attenuated malignant cells (thin arrow) which look more like endothelial or mesothelial cells than epithelial cells. No mitoses are evident among the neoplastic cells. Between the tubules and pseudoacini there is a large amount of weakly eosinophilic stroma-like tissue, in which there are only a small number of eosinophilic fibres and a sparse population of small pale fibroblast- and fibrocyte-like cells. All the spaces in the tumour are empty ('clear'), apart from a few strands of eosinophilic secretion in the lumen, and it must be assumed that (before the tissue was processed) the spaces were full of connective tissue mucin.

HE ×150

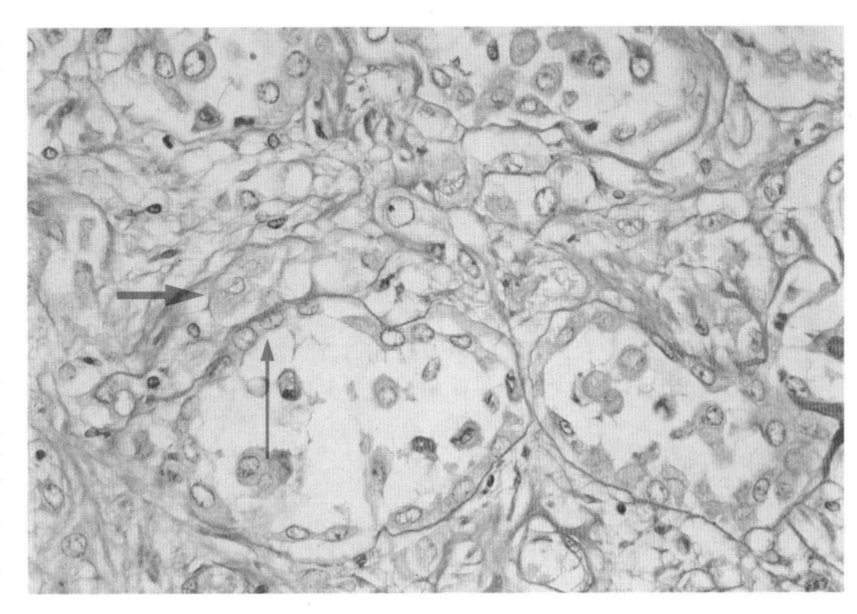

12.60 Mesothelioma: pleura

The structure of this tissue is more or less identical with that in **12.62**, but stained with the PAS method instead of HE. The most notable feature is the presence of spaces of various size and shape, from large pseudoacini (gland-like spaces) lined by flat or low cuboidal cells (thin arrow) to small cytoplasmic vacuoles in single cells (thick arrow) in the 'stroma' between the pseudoacini. The periodic acid-Schiff (PAS) method reacts positively with the numerous delicate (reticulin) fibrils between the tumour cells, which form a kind of basement membrane to the tubules, but there is no purplish-red (PAS-positive) epithelial mucin. The vacuoles within the individual neoplastic cells are unstained (hyaluronic acid being PAS-negative) and there is no PAS-positive secretion within the tubules (the strongly-staining material is cell debris). The absence of Schiff-positive epithelial mucin helps therefore to exclude adenocarcinoma. Mesothelial cells secrete hyaluronic acid, and a positive result with appropriate stains for connective tissue mucin (rich in hyaluronic acid) facilitates the diagnosis of mesothelioma. The nuclear structure of the malignant cells is incidentally well demonstrated by the PAS method.

PAS ×360

13.1 Gaucher's disease: spleen

Patients with the adult form of Gaucher's disease have a deficiency of glucocerebroside-ß-glucosidase in the lysosomes in their macrophages of the mononuclear phagocyte system. Large amounts of glucocerebroside (from the breakdown of erythrocytes) are stored in many tissues, the spleen being greatly increased in size by the presence within the distended sinusoids of large distinctive Gaucher cells (macrophages with abundant cytoplasm). The massive infiltrate of Gaucher cells causes the lymphoid elements, including the Malpighian bodies, to undergo atrophy. This spleen weighed more than 5kg. Most of the cells are Gaucher cells with a single round vesicular nucleus of moderate size (thin arrow), generally eccentric. A few Gaucher cells are binucleated. The cytoplasm is eosinophilic (thick arrow) and often has a striated pattern, produced by the presence in it of fine wavy kerasin fibrils which lie parallel to the long axis of the cell. The pattern is not present in this field however. A small number of lymphocytes is visible (double arrow).

HE ×360

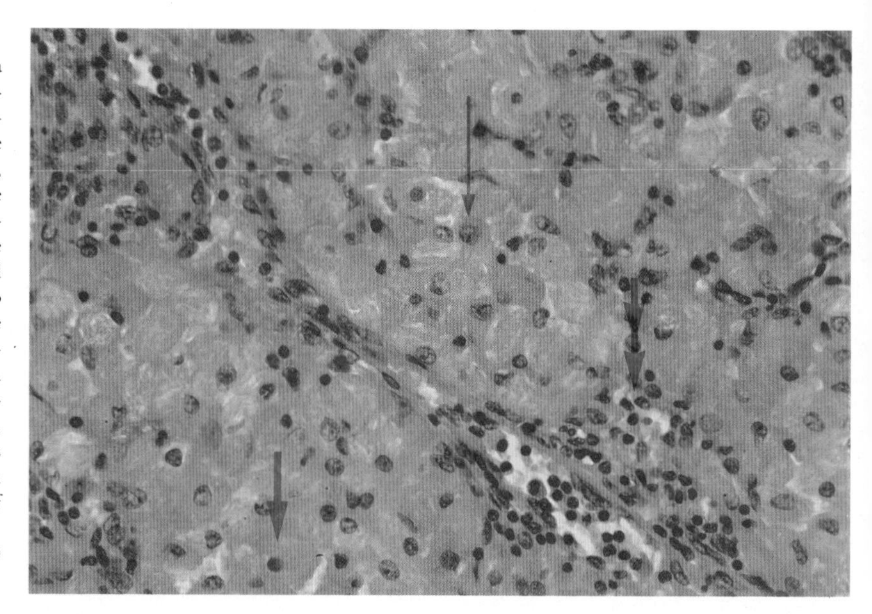

13.2 Portal hypertension: spleen

In portal hypertension, the spleen, from various causes such as cirrhosis, schistosomiasis etc, is intensely congested and generally considerably enlarged (weighing up to 1.5kg) (congestive splenomegaly). The changes in the spleen are more marked than in systemic venous congestion. In this case the capsule of the organ was thickened and adherent to the neighbouring tissues, and the cut surface of the spleen was firm and 'meaty' in appearance. Histologically the Malpighian bodies underwent atrophy and caused some periarterial fibrosis, and in this field the venous sinuses (the red pulp) are markedly dilated and lined by prominent endothelial cells (thin arrow). The walls of the sinusoids are thickened, having become more fibrous than normal (thick arrow), the increase of fibrous tissue being more obvious with stains for reticulin. Periarteriolar hemorrhages may also occur and become converted into brown or yellow pigmented fibrous nodules (so-called siderotic nodules or Gamna-Gandy bodies).

HE ×235

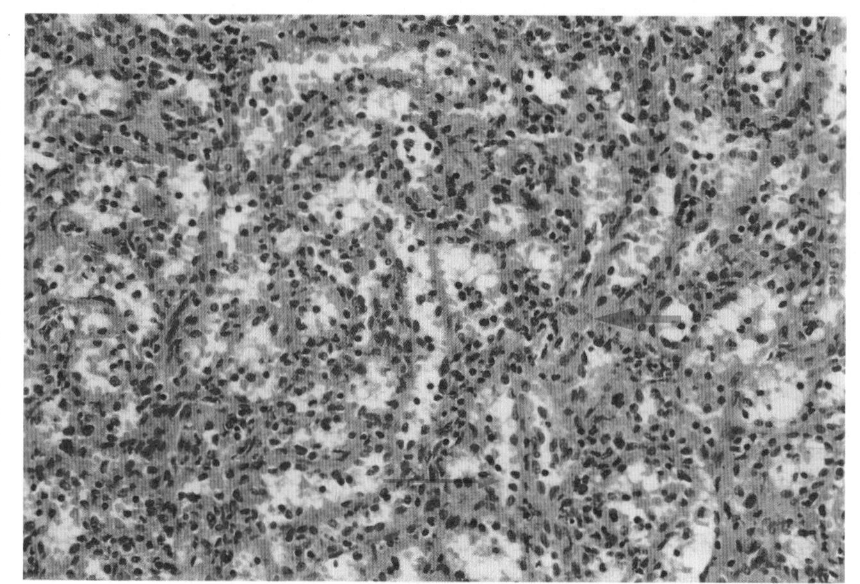

13.3 Siderotic nodules (Gamna-Gandy bodies): spleen

When the blood pressure increases markedly in the portal vein, the spleen enlarges markedly (congestive splenomegaly) and hemorrhage from the congested vessels within the spleen tend to occur repeatedly. When the extravasated blood is organized, it gives rise to focal fibrotic lesions rich in hemosiderin (siderotic nodules or Gamna-Gandy bodies). These range up to 3 or 4mm dia and macroscopically appear as brown spots ('tobacco' nodules) on the cut surface of the spleen. In this field, recent hemorrhage is clearly evident, mostly around the left side of nodule (thin arrow). The nodule consists mainly of dense collagenous fibrous tissue, which is heavily impregnated with iron and calcium salts (thick arrow). The numerous crystals of iron encrusted on the degenerated connective tissue fibres are deeply basophilic (bluish-black). Deposits of hemosiderin were also present in the fibrous trabeculae throughout the spleen.

HE ×55

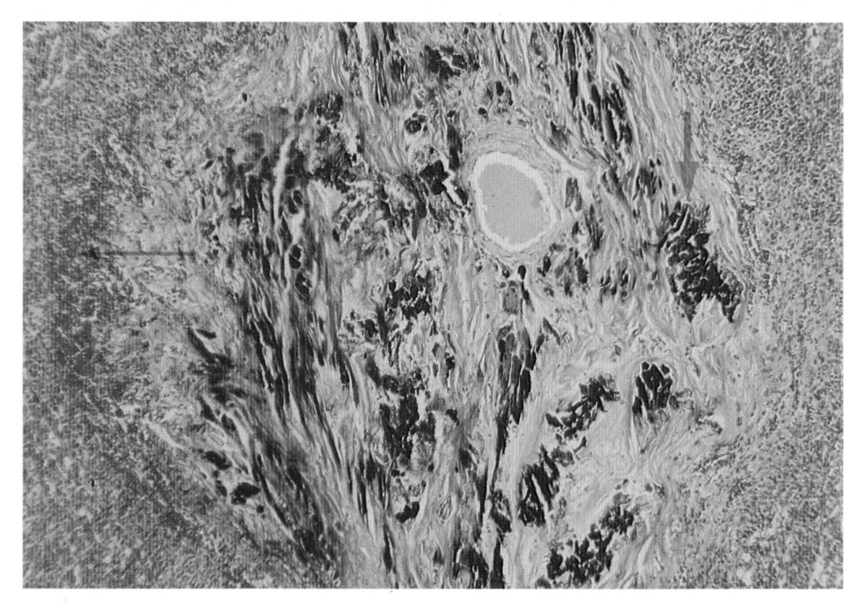

13.4 Systemic lupus erythematosus: spleen

Systemic lupus erythematosus (SLE) is a classical example of a non-organ-specific autoimmune disease of unknown etiology which ranges from mild to fulminating and affects mainly middle-aged women. There are, typically, many autoimmune phenomena, including hypergammaglobulinemia, and environmental factors which predispose to the development of SLE include drugs and sex hormones. Vascular lesions are prominent in the disease, and there is often widespread and progressive degeneration of the connective tissues. The skin is a frequently-involved organ, with the classical malar rash which occurs in about one third of patients. In this case of SLE, one manifestation is a marked increase in fibrous tissue around two penicillary arteries, with closely packed concentric lamellae of collagen fibres (thin arrows) surrounding fragmented elastic laminae and deposits of eosinophilic material (thick arrow) in the wall of the vessels: this appearance is termed 'onion-skinning'. Sometimes this change is so pronounced as to amount to fibrinoid necrosis. HE ×135

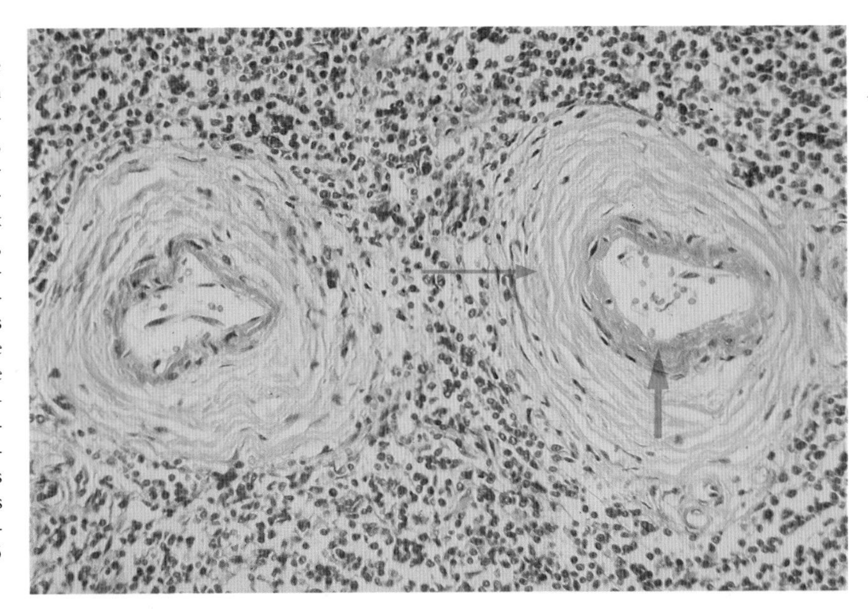

13.5 Myelofibrosis: spleen

In myelofibrosis, as a result of increased fibroblast activity there is a progressive increase in reticulin and collagen fibres in the hemopoietic bone marrow, replacing it with fibrous tissue. Consequently extramedullary hemopoiesis frequently occurs, mainly in liver and spleen. The disease, not being monoclonal but apparently reactive rather than part of a neoplastic process, was at an advanced stage in this case. The spleen weighed 820g and was dark brownish-red in colour; and histologically the normal lymphoid elements (the Malpighian bodies) were very small and atrophic. The spleen, as shown in this field, consists very largely of moderately large immature cells of the granulocyte and erythrocyte series. Cells of the granulocyte series have a pale cytoplasm and a vesicular nucleus, in many of which there is a prominent central nucleolus. A few of the cells have a bigger more pleomorphic basophilic nucleus. Some of the cells in the erythrocyte series are relatively small, with a small round deeply basophilic nucleus. HE ×135

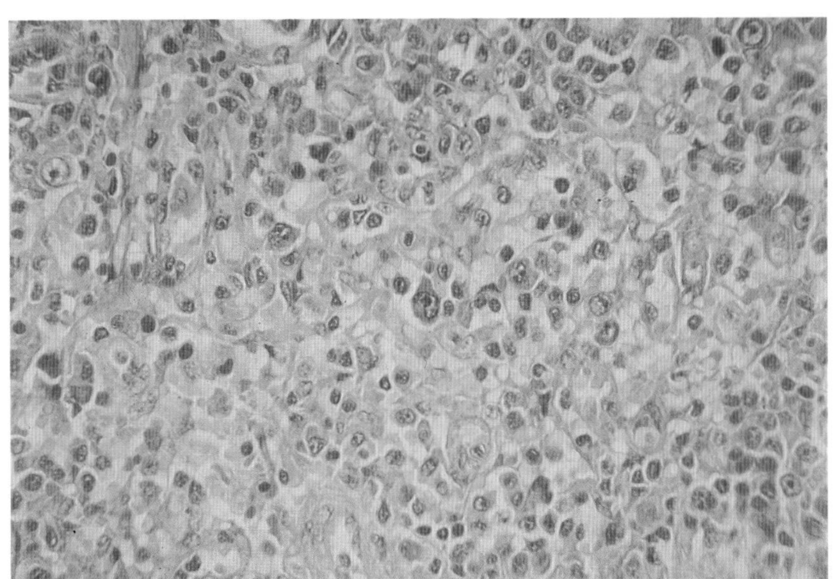

13.6 Secondary carcinoma: spleen

In contrast to the bone marrow and lymph nodes, the spleen, macroscopically at least, is for unknown reasons a rare site for metastatic tumour deposits. In this case the patient had a primary carcinoma of bronchus, and it had metastasized to the spleen, infiltrating it extensively. Nearly all the splenic sinusoids are filled with closely packed malignant cells (thin arrows), which confirms that the tumour cells have formed cords which permeate the sinusoids. The neoplastic cells are undifferentiated malignant cells of moderate size. Each of them has a basophilic pleomorphic hyperchromatic nucleus and only a small amount of cytoplasm. The Malpighian body on the left, consisting of small lymphocytes and a central small penicillary artery (thick arrow), is slightly atrophic but otherwise normal. The penicillary artery has undergone marked hyaline change in its wall and also narrowing of the lumen, a not infrequent finding in elderly individuals. HE ×150

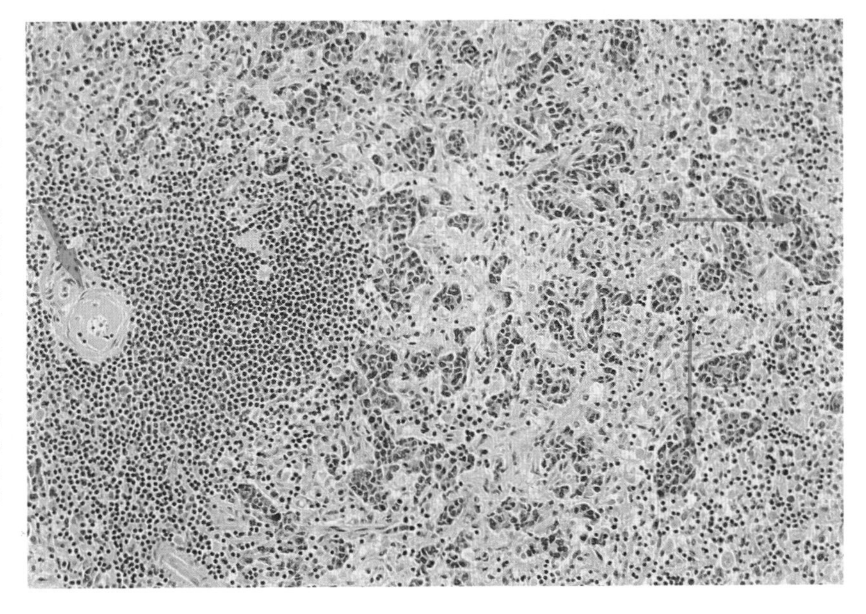

13.7 T cell lymphoma: pleural fluid

Classes of lymphocytes cannot be differentiated on morphological grounds. B cells have immunoglobulin on their surface, but T cells do not. However T cells can be identified by the presence of CD3 antigen on its surface. The presence of a 'dot' of acid phosphatase on the cell membrane is another useful marker for T lymphocytes. This patient, who had a lymphoma, developed a pleural exudate which was aspirated. This is a smear of the cells in the fluid, and the cells have been stained blue (methylene blue). The nuclei are round and vary moderately in size (the larger paler nuclei also present in the smear are from mesothelial cells). The lymphocytes have little cytoplasm, but in a high proportion of them there is a 'dot' of acid phosphatase on the surface which, when suitably reacted, developed an orange yellow colour (thick arrow). This result confirmed that the patient had a T-lymphoblastic lymphoma with involvement of the pleural cavity.

Acid phosphatase-methylene blue x850

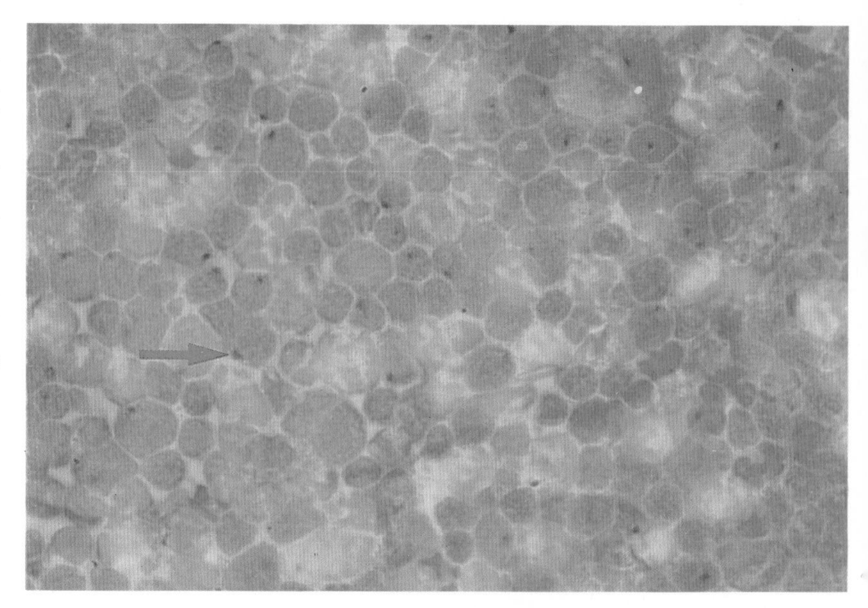

13.8 Atrophy: thymus

The thymus normally increases in size during childhood, reaching its maximum size (30-40g) around puberty, most cell-mediated immunity being effected by long-lived T cells. The population of cortical thymocytes decreases and the thymus weighs about 15g in adult life. Severe secondary atrophy occurs in prolonged protein malnutrition and immunosuppression by drugs and chronic viral infections (especially HIV-1). The architecture of the medullary epithelium is relatively spared, but the epithelial component gradually atrophies. In this case a mixed lymphocytic and epithelial thymoma was resected surgically from a woman aged 57. Within it there are nodules of atrophic thymic tissue and a considerable amount of fatty tissue. In the centre of each nodule there is a Hassal's corpuscle (thick arrows), a cluster of large strongly eosinophilic squamous epithelial cells, surrounded by a broad cuff or cluster of small thymocytes with deeply basophilic nuclei. Cortex and medulla can be distinguished, the closely packed outermost cells (cortex) staining more deeply (thin arrow) than the more loosely-packed and slightly more eosinophilic cells (medulla) (double arrow) nearer the Hassal's corpuscles. HE x60

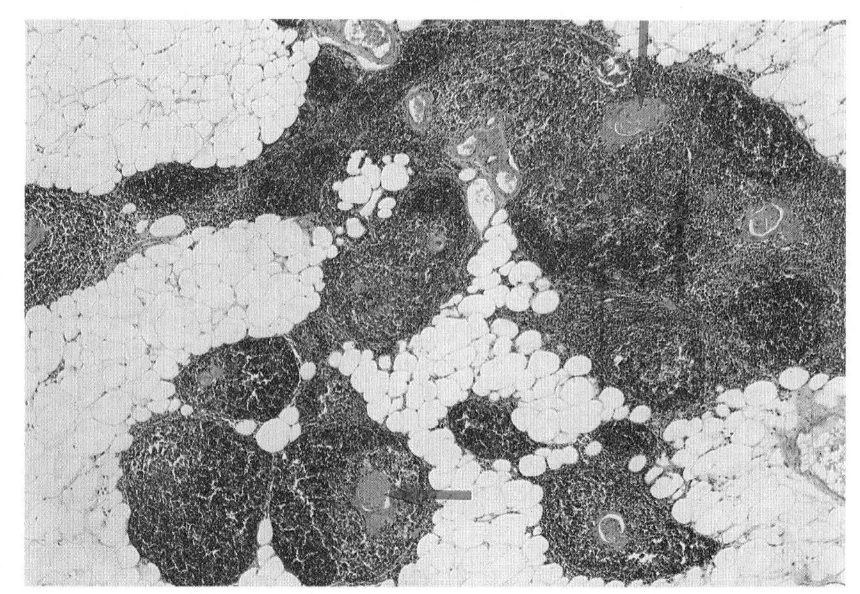

13.9 Atrophy: thymus

The thymus is a primary lymphoid organ, composed of lymphocytes and epithelial cells, but its functions are almost wholly independent of antigen and it plays no part in the induction of the immune response to specific antigens. An intact thymus is necessary for the normal development and function of T cells, a role which it performs almost exclusively during fetal life or in the early neonatal period. When there is persistent loss of thymocytes from the thymus, the thymus's lobular architecture may progressively collapse and fibrosis may result. This is part of an atrophic thymus, the thymic tissue (at higher magnification) is seen to consist of parts of several Hassal's corpuscles, each surrounded by lymphocyte-type cells (thin arrow) of the adjacent medulla. The Hassal's corpuscles are composed of closely packed large squamous epithelial cells with abundant deeply eosinophilic cytoplasm and large pale vesicular nuclei (double arrow). The centres of the two larger corpuscles contain keratinized cell debris (thick arrows). The cells of the medulla are almost exclusively lymphocyte-type cells with sparse cytoplasm and deeply basophilic round nuclei (thymocytes), but few epithelial cells are evident. HE ×360

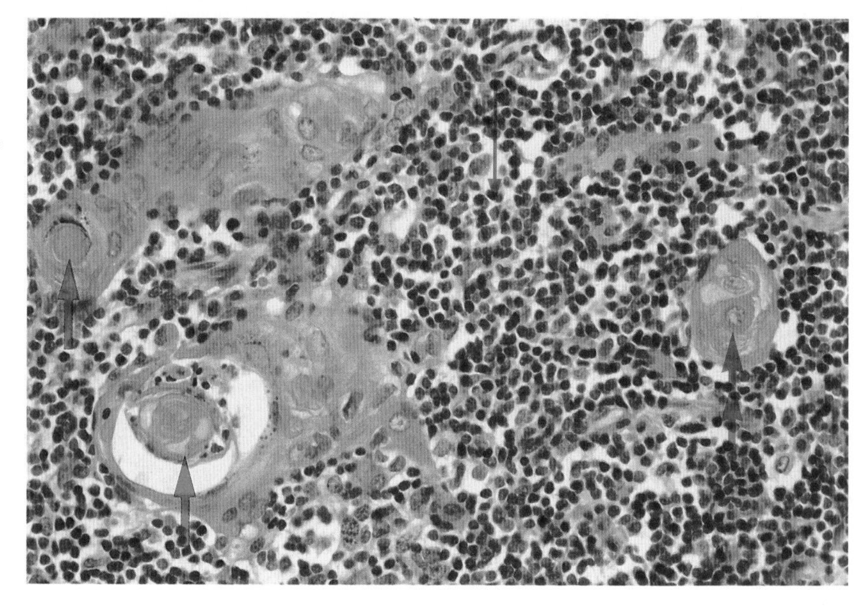

13.10 Myasthenia gravis: thymus

Human thymoma is a thymic epithelial cell tumour which often contains a large number of immature T cells and is frequently associated with autoimmune diseases. Lymphoid follicles with germinal centres develop in the thymus in patients with autoimmune disease, especially myasthenia gravis, and a thymoma is present in 10-20% of cases of this disease. Antibodies to acetylcholine receptors, on the motor end-plates of striated muscle, can be demonstrated in the serum. They block the action of acetylcholine and thereby produce muscle weakness. Thymectomy is generally beneficial in the early stages but has little effect later in the disease. In this case, a thymoma is present. It was apparently benign and it is encapsulated, with a fibrous capsule (thin arrow). The tumour is of mixed type, consisting of a network of very large pale-staining epithelial cells (thick arrows), with much weakly eosinophilic cytoplasm and very large vesicular nuclei, in most of which a prominent nucleolus is visible, and small lymphocytes (double arrow) with deeply basophilic nuclei and little cytoplasm, lying in the interstices of the network of epithelial cells. HE ×360

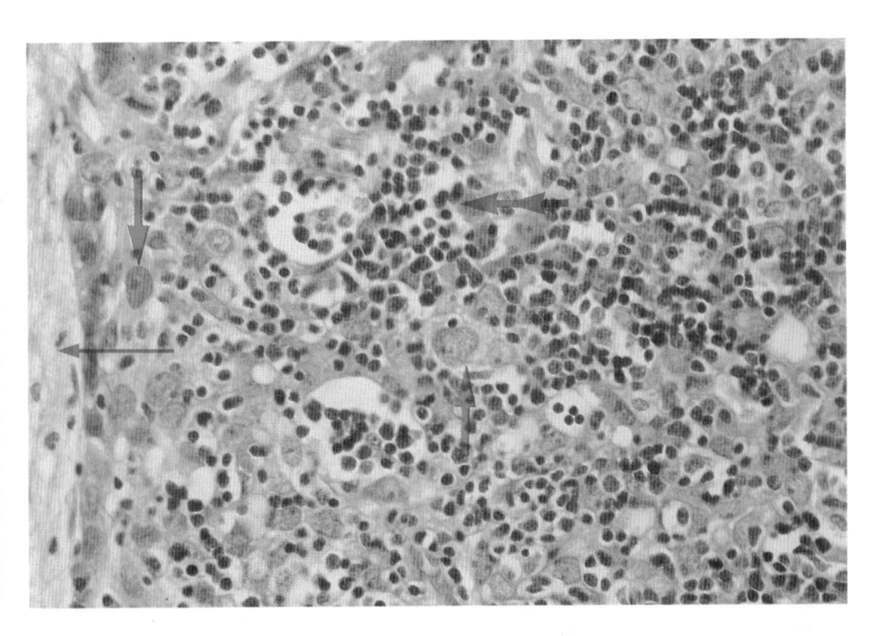

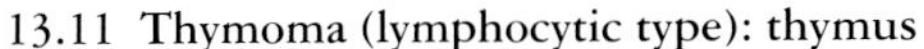

13.11 Thymoma (lymphocytic type): thymus

Thymomas are relatively rare, and diverse both in morphology and in behaviour. The average of the patient is about fifty, and the incidence is the same for men and women. Most thymomas are benign, do not produce symptoms and are discovered incidentally. They may however cause pressure symptoms or very occasionally myasthenia gravis. Other systemic manifestations such as systemic lupus erythematosus or red cell aplasia may also occur. The majority of thymomas are of mixed composition, containing both epithelial and lymphocytic elements, but may be predominantly epithelial or predominantly lymphocytic. Lymphocyte/medullary type thymomas have a much better prognosis than the epithelial/cortical type tumours. This lesion is predominantly lymphocytic, consisting of nodules of closely packed small deeply basophilic lymphocytic cells (thin arrow), among which there are occasional larger paler cells. Broad dense bands of connective tissue (thick arrows) separate the cellular nodules. The presence of fibrous bands is a common feature of thymoma, as is a thick fibrous capsule.
HE ×60

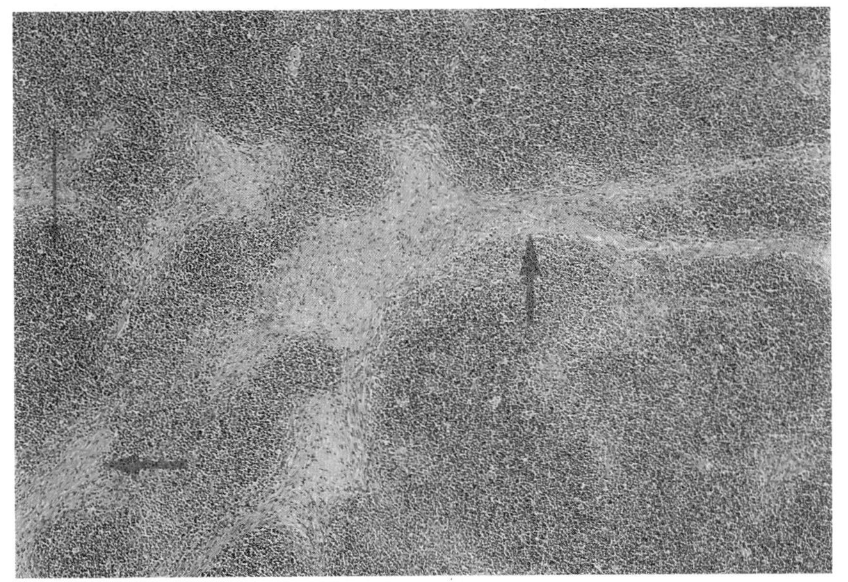

13.12 Thymoma (lymphocytic type): thymus

As a rule, thymomas consist of closely packed neoplastic spindle-shaped or round epithelial cells (which may show squamous differentiation) and normal (non-neoplastic) cortical and medullary lymphocytes, the open vesicular nuclei of the epithelial cells contrasting with the small solid lymphocyte nuclei. The sheets of epithelial cell usually have a palisaded border. This is the same thymoma as in 13.11, at higher magnification. Occasional large cells with a vesicular nucleus and pale-staining cytoplasm (thick arrows) are scattered throughout the tumour, but the tumour consists largely of small cells, each with a compact round basophilic nucleus and a small amount of eosinophilic cytoplasm (thymocytes). These cells have a marked tendency to form long slender cords, with one cell behind the other in 'Indian file' (thin arrows). An Indian file pattern of infiltration is a notable feature of T-lymphoblastic lymphomas. No mitoses are evident among these cells.
HE ×360

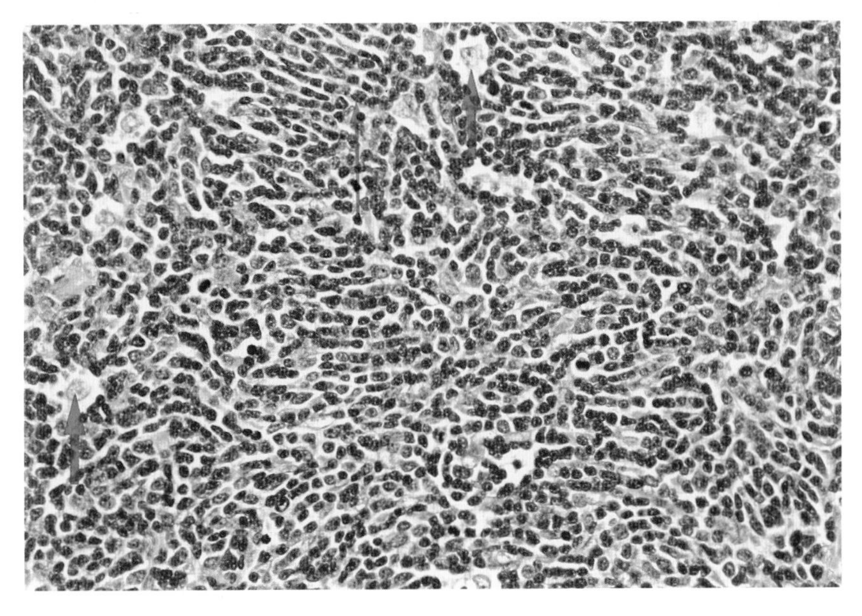

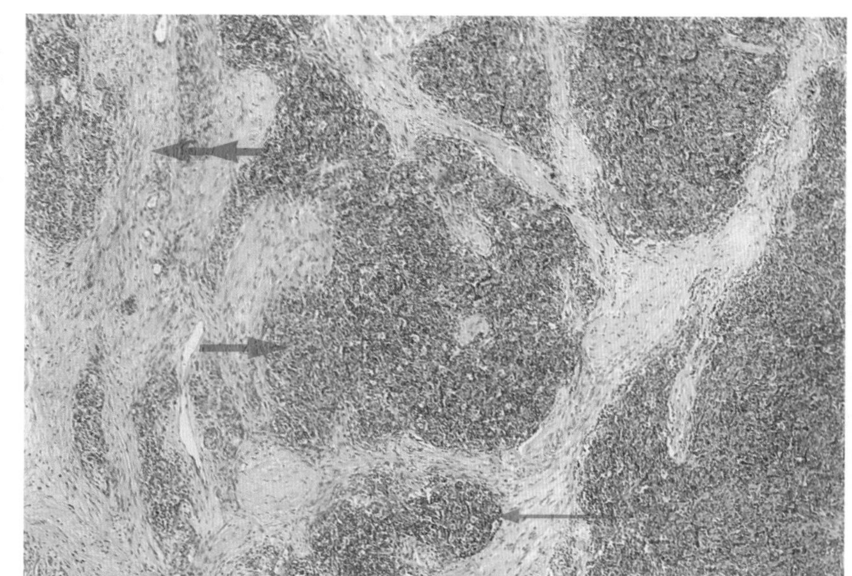

13.13 Thymoma (mixed type): thymus

Of low grade malignancy, thymomas invade locally (sometimes to pleura or pericardium) but seldom metastasize. Many take the form of a firm well-circumscribed mass (up to 20cm dia) with a thick fibrous capsule, but some are more invasive and less well-defined, encasing adjacent organs. It is usually intersected by broad dense trabeculae of collagenous connective tissue which, on section, give it a 'lobulated' appearance. The patient in this case had a mixed type of thymoma, containing both epithelial and lymphocytic elements. A systemic manifestation was also present in the form of hypercalcemia. The hypercalcemia was relieved by thymectomy. This thymoma has a structure similar to that of the lymphocytic-type lesion shown in **13.11**, consisting of deeply basophilic cellular nodules of various sizes (thin arrow), separated by broad bands of eosinophilic collagenous fibrous tissue (double arrow). The staining of the cellular nodules however is not as uniform as in the lymphocytic type, a large population of paler-staining epithelial cells (thick arrow) being present alongside darkly-staining lymphocytes. HE ×60

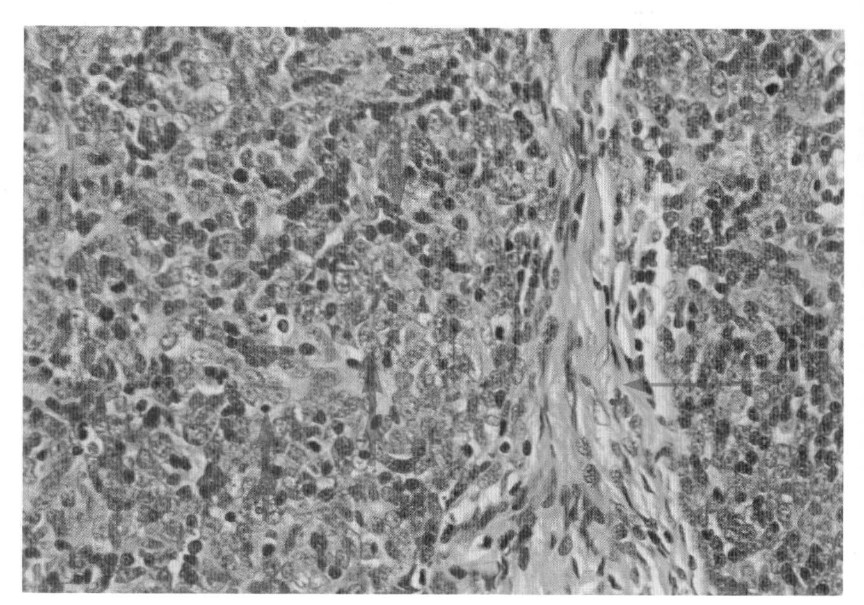

13.14 Thymoma (mixed type): thymus

Thymomas tend typically to be surrounded by a thick capsule of dense collagenous fibrous tissue and also frequently intersected by dense trabeculae of similar tissue which thereby gives the mass a lobulated or nodular structure. Histologically, the neoplastic cells may be spindle-shaped or round cells which may show squamous differentiation, and in most cases they are interspersed with normal cortical or medullary thymocytes. The structure of this thymoma is also typical, showing, at high magnification, two sheets of tumour cells separated by a broad band of dense collagenous tissue (thin arrow). Most of the cells are closely packed fairly large pale-staining neoplastic epithelial cells (double arrows) with vesicular nuclei, many containing a nucleolus, and a relatively small amount of cytoplasm. The epithelial cells are accompanied by a much smaller population of small deeply basophilic lymphocytes (thick arrow). The open vesicular structure of the nuclei of the epithelial cells contrasts with the solid virtually pyknotic appearance of the nuclei of the lymphocytic cells. HE ×360

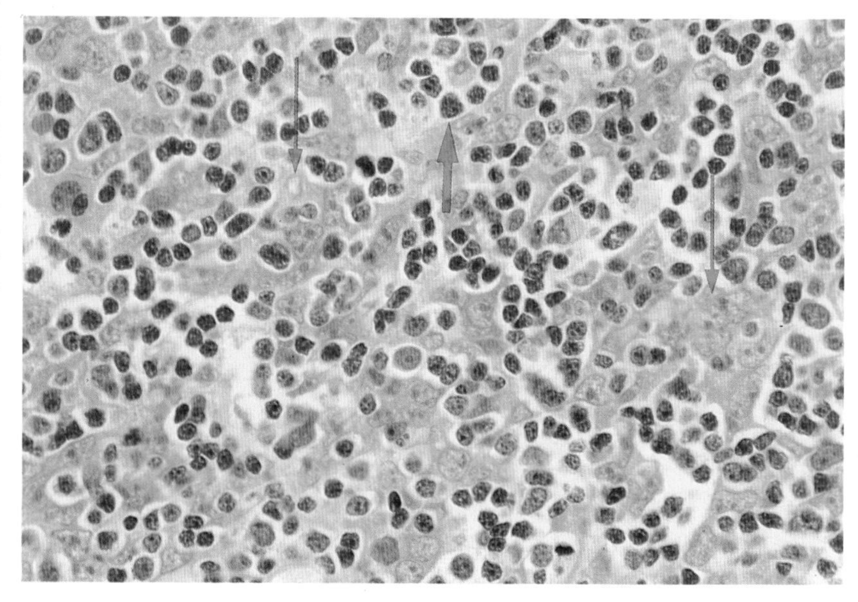

13.15 Secondary deposit of thymoma: marrow

Malignant thymoma is a rare type of neoplasm, and metastasis of a thymoma to bone marrow is extremely rare. A man of 37 had a thymoma removed surgically. It proved to be a malignant mixed type of thymoma. Nine months later a trephine specimen of bone marrow was taken from his iliac crest. This shows that the normal fat cells and almost all the hemopoietic cells have been largely replaced by a mixture of large pale-staining epithelial cells and small lymphocytic cells with small basophilic nuclei, the general appearance being similar to that of a mixed type of thymoma. The epithelial cells are arranged as cords of very irregular shape and they have a considerable amount of moderately eosinophilic cytoplasm (thin arrows). Their nuclei are large pale pleomorphic and vesicular and contain one or more prominent nucleoli. The association between the lymphocytes and the epithelial cells is close.

Moderate numbers of other mononuclear cells, very probably hemopoietic, with moderately-sized round or ovoid nuclei (thick arrow) which contain basophilic granules of chromatin and often a prominent nucleolus. HE ×580

13.16 Secondary carcinoma: marrow

Hemopoietic marrow is frequently the site of metastasis of malignant tumours. This specimen of bone marrow is from the iliac crest of a man of 62, and a very eosinophilic trabecula of normal lamellar bone is visible on the left side of this field. All the hemopoietic tissue has been replaced by a vascular moderately cellular connective tissue in which a number of compact well-defined nodules of tumour cells are growing (thick arrow). Alongside these nodules there are two eosinophilic trabeculae of new (woven) bone which contain spindle-shaped osteocytes (double arrow) and have a more or less complete layer of prominent plump osteoblasts on their surfaces (thin arrows). The new bone which has replaced the hemopoietic marrow (osteosclerosis) has been induced by the malignant (carcinomatous) cells. The site of the primary tumour was not known clinically but the presence of cytoplasmic granules, which were argyrophilic (but not argentaffin), suggested an endocrine-cell origin. Unlike this example, most deposits of metastatic tumour are osteolytic. HE ×235

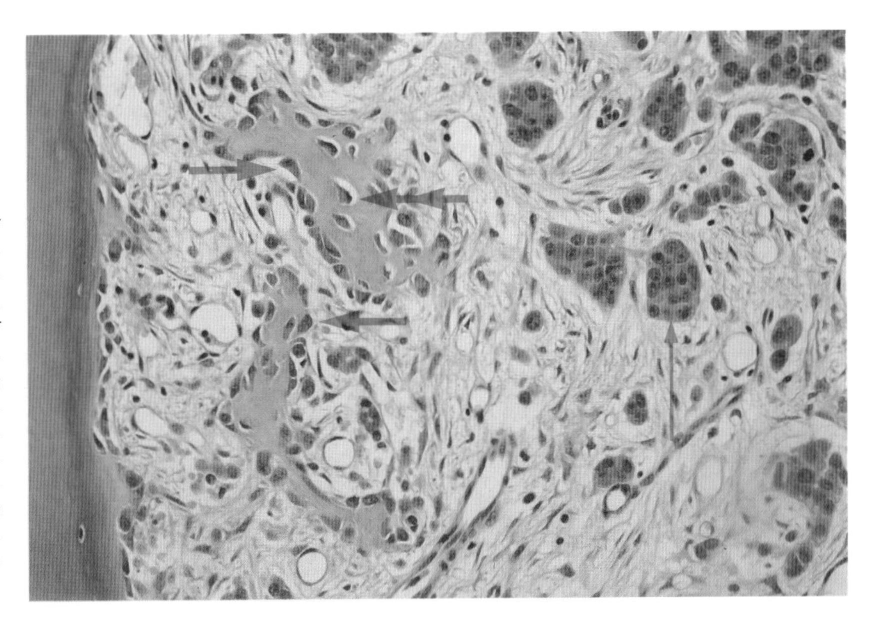

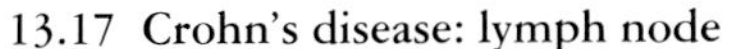

13.17 Crohn's disease: lymph node

The main symptoms in Crohn's disease are those of obstruction, and even the esophagus may be constricted and obstructed, especially at the lower end. Fistulae often develop between lesions in the intestine and structures adjacent to them, and perianal fistulae are especially troublesome. This is a lymph node from the mesentery of a woman of 61 who had the terminal ileum and part of the ascending colon removed surgically for Crohn's disease. The capsule of the node is on the left. The node shows marked reactive changes. The sinuses, including the subcapsular sinus (thin arrows), are dilated and contain a large population of very pale-staining histiocytes. The lymphoid follicles underlying the subcapsular (peripheral) sinus are large, and have germinal centres (double arrow). The adjacent paracortical zone is well-developed and very vascular, with many prominent high endothelial venules (thick arrows). At higher magnification numerous small granulomas consisting of epithelioid cells and small multinucleated giant cells were evident. HE ×60

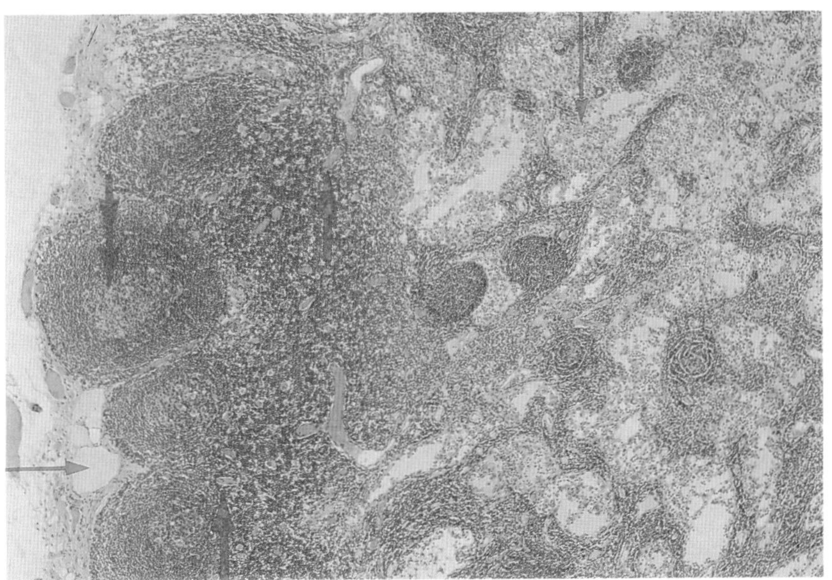

13.18 Intestinal lipodystrophy (Whipple's disease): lymph node

Intestinal lipodystrophy is a rare multisystem disorder which is associated with disturbance of fat metabolism and malabsorption of fat in the small intestine. It is marked by diarrhea with fatty stools and deposition of fat in intestinal lymphatic tissue. Other organs may be involved. The mucosa of the small intestine, and notably the villi, are diffusely infiltrated with large histiocytes, and neutral fat also enters the mesenteric lymph nodes. Electron microscopy shows bacilliform bodies in the cytoplasm of the distended histiocytes, and treatment with antibiotics usually control the bacteria. In this field there is a node with a fibrous capsule (thin arrow) and a subcapsular sinus, the lumen of which is dilated and full of droplets (thick arrow) of neutral fat, lost (unstained) through tissue processing. The droplets of fat may lie "free" in the sinus but the presence of small dark nuclei in close association with the fat droplets suggest that at least some of the fat may be inside histiocytes. The cortical tissue is composed mostly of small lymphocytes, but unstained droplets of fat are also present (e.g. bottom right corner) along with strands of eosinophilic amorphous material (double arrow). HE ×235

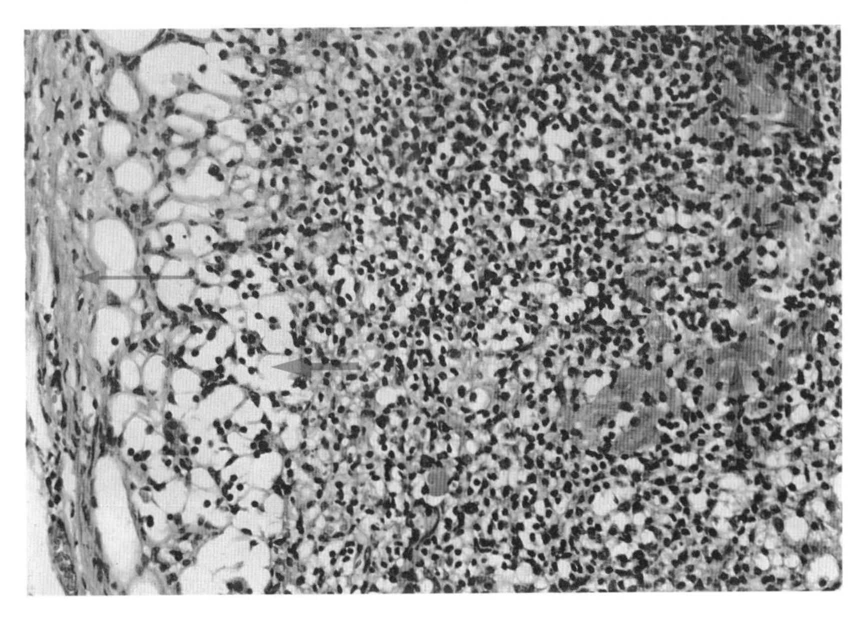

13.19 Sinus histiocytosis (reactive sinus hyperplasia): lymph node

In sinus histiocytosis there is marked proliferation, and increase in number, of the histiocytic cells normally present in the sinus network, which includes the peripheral sinus. The histiocytic response in the sinuses occurs in many chronic inflammatory and reactive states. It is also frequently prominent in the axillary nodes (without metastases) draining a breast which is the site of a primary adenocarcinoma. Affected nodes may also show the various changes that occur in an immune response. Two medullary lymphatic sinuses are shown. They are greatly distended, and their lumens are filled with large numbers of large eosinophilic histiocyte-like cells (thin arrows). Many of these are part of the network of 'fixed' histiocytes in the sinuses. The small deeply basophilic cells accompanying the histiocytes in the sinuses are lymphocytes. Fibromuscular septa (thick arrows), which divide each sinus into twin channels, can be seen. The medullary lymphoid tissue (double arrow) consists of small lymphocytes, plasma cells and histiocytes. HE ×150

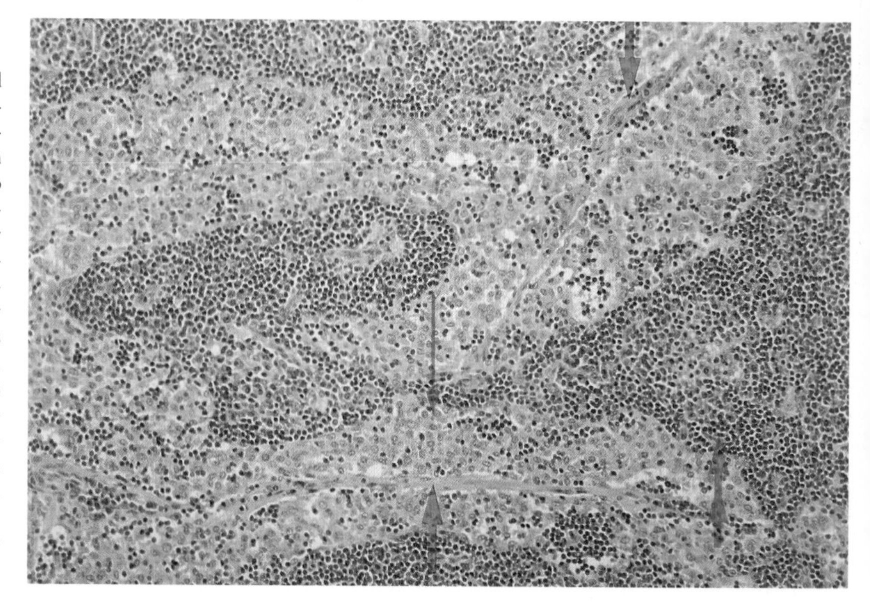

13.20 Sinus histiocytosis (reactive sinus hyperplasia): lymph node

This shows, in more detail, a lymphatic sinus in the medulla of the same lymph node as in 13.19. The fibromuscular septum (thick arrow) is clearly visible in the centre of the sinus, and the channel on each side of the septum is filled with large well-differentiated histiocyte-like cells (thin arrow) and a small number of basophilic lymphocytes. The histiocytes have abundant eosinophilic cytoplasm and each has a large round or ovoid pale vesicular nucleus, sometimes containing a nucleolus. Most of the cells in the medullary lymphoid tissue are closely packed lymphocytes (double arrow) with a round heavily stained nucleus, but a small number of histiocytes (with a large vesicular nucleus) and plasma cells are also evident among them. The significance of sinus histiocytosis in lymph nodes is uncertain but the same pattern is sometimes seen in lymph nodes in which there is continued destruction of cells. HE ×360

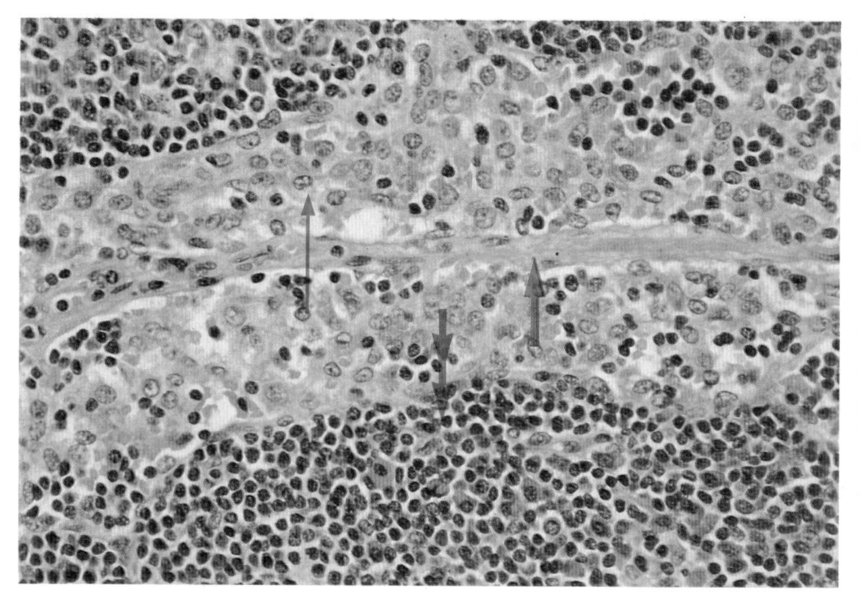

13.21 Sinus hyperplasia with massive lymphadenopathy (Rosai-Dorfman syndrome): lymph node

This syndrome is a painless cervical lymphadenopathy, often bilateral. There is no specific therapy and the disease is protracted. Complete recovery generally takes place however in most patients. There is massive enlargement of lymph nodes (mainly in the neck) s accompanied by fever, leukocytosis and hypergammaglobulinemia. Characteristically the capsule of the node is thick and fibrous, and the architecture of the node is altered by very pronounced dilatation of the lymphatic sinuses. This sinus (filling most of field) is very dilated and full of eosinophilic lymph (thin arrow) and a mixture of lymphocytes and histiocytes. Some of the histiocytes are round, with a pale vesicular nucleus and a relatively enormous amount of well-defined cytoplasm (thick arrows). In the cytoplasm there is a large number of phagocytosed small lymphocytes. Very large cells with this appearance are a diagnostic feature of this syndrome. The intersinusoidal tissue (above and below the sinus) consists of dark-staining small lymphocytes. HE ×360

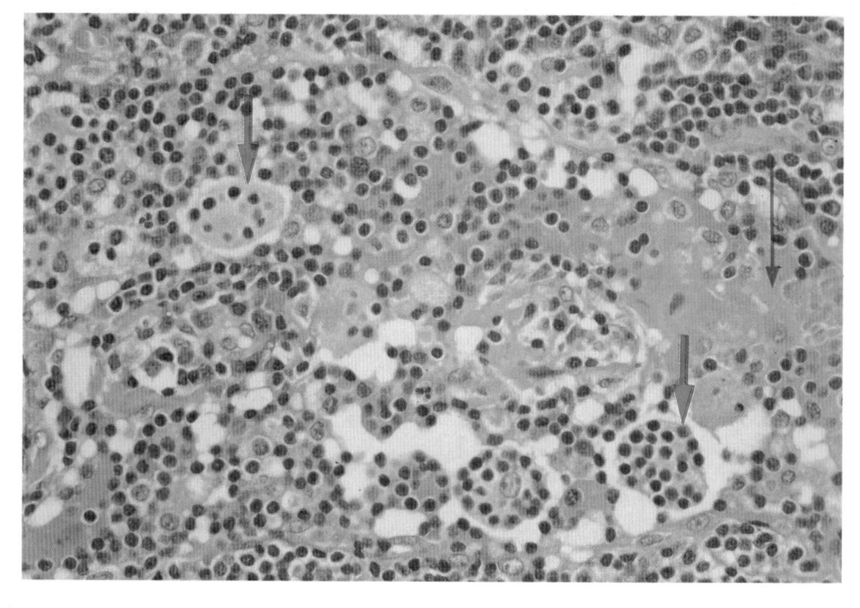

13.22 Lymph node: porta hepatis

Although the liver has no lymphatic system, lipid and bile pigment sometimes drain to the lymph nodes in the porta hepatis and produce a reaction in the lymphatic sinuses. This is a very dilated lymphatic sinus (occupying most of the field), and within it there are numerous round "droplets" of lipid (neutral fat, which dissolves in reagents), most of them apparently occupying vacuoles in the cytoplasm of the macrophages. The macrophages have large pale vesicular nuclei (thin arrows) in which there is generally a prominent nucleolus. Also present are three very large (giant) multinucleated phagocytes which contain (vacuolated) lipid droplets of various sizes (thick arrow). The cytoplasm of these giant cells is remarkably eosinophilic, and in one of the giant cells there is a cluster of deeply purple nuclei (thick arrow). The lymphoid tissue adjacent to the sinus (bottom right) consists of lymphocytes and histiocytes. Bile pigment is not evident in these tissues but it is sometimes present, along with the lipid within phagocytes. HE ×360

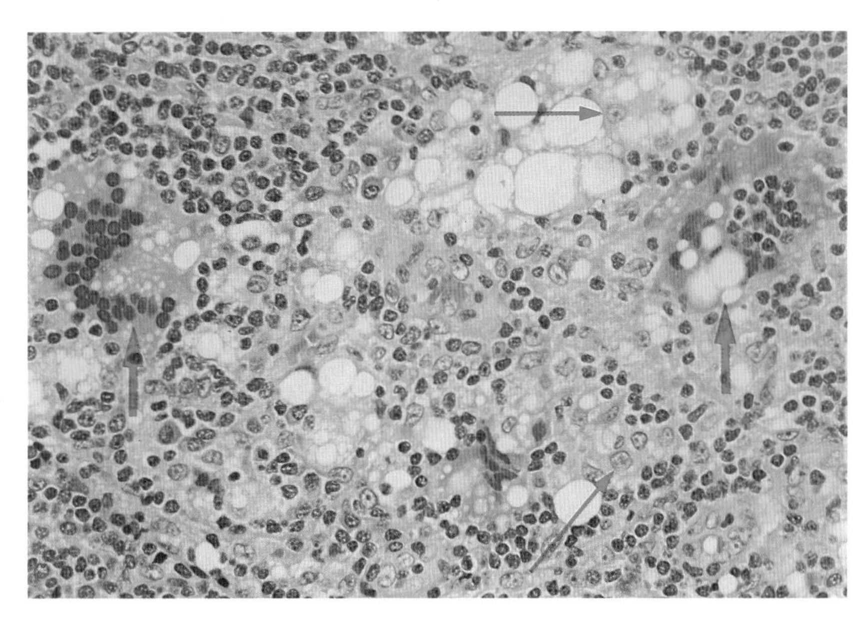

13.23 Lymph node: secondary (mucoid) carcinoma:

Lymph drains into the peripheral sinus of lymph nodes at the capsule, and malignant cells carried to the node in the lymph tend therefore to be found within the peripheral sinus, at least initially. A large mucoid adenocarcinoma was resected from the sigmoid colon of a man aged 76. This is a lymph node in the mesentery. Beneath the fibrous capsule of the node (thin arrow), the peripheral sinus has been infiltrated by large numbers of large pale round malignant cells, distending the sinus and invading the underlying lymphoid tissue. Each cell contains a large droplet of very weakly stained mucin which has pushed the relatively small nucleus to one side. All the malignant cells have a characteristic signet-ring appearance (thick arrow). There is no visible mitotic activity. There is some evidence that mucoid carcinomas metastasize less readily than other forms but it is not conclusive. HE ×150

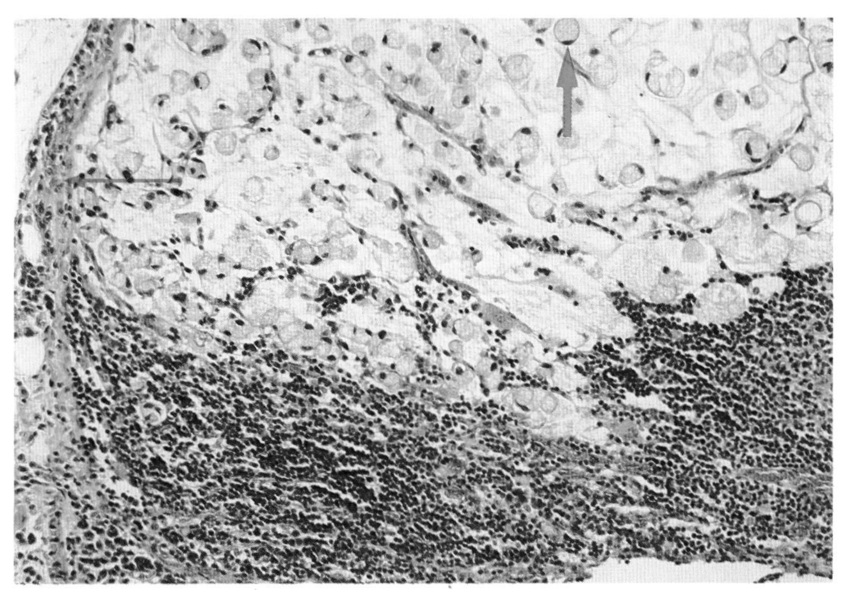

13.24 Lymph node: carcinoma:

Lymph node showing infiltration through the sinuses by metastatic malignant epithelial cells. This is demonstrated by means of immunostaining for broad-spectrum cytokeratins. Small carcinoma cells such as these could easily be missed on conventional staining.

Malignant epithelial tumours (carcinomas) contain cytokeratin molecules. Immunostaining, using antibodies to keratins (broad-spectrum cytokeratins) demonstrates keratin intermediate filaments in epithelial cells, including carcinomas.

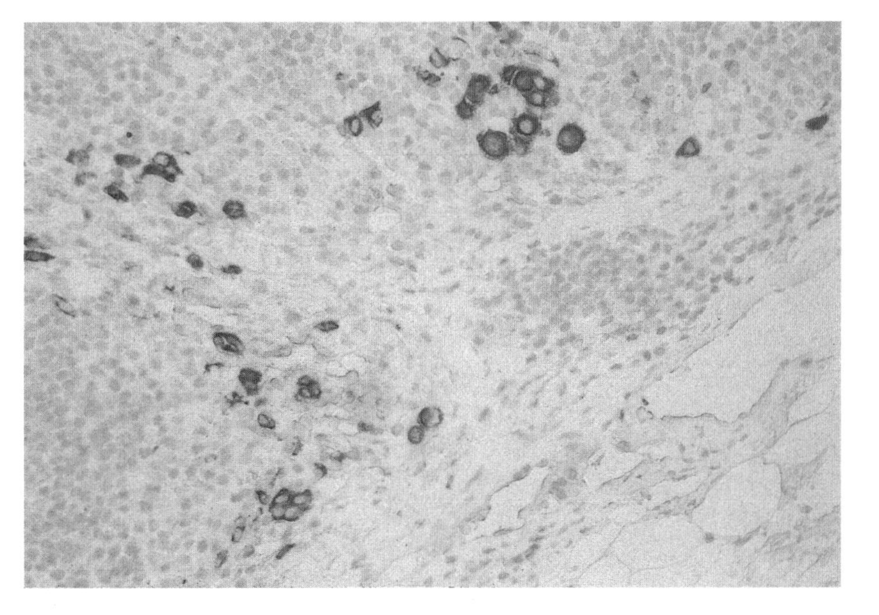

13.25 Dermatopathic lymphadenopathy: lymph node

In certain skin diseases, particularly chronic dermatitis and mycosis fungoides, the lymph nodes draining the affected area of skin enlarge. Histological examination of this node shows reactive hyperplasia. The fibrous capsule of the node is at the left margin. The architecture of the node is preserved and the principal change is in the paracortical zone. The paracortex is greatly enlarged (thin arrows), consisting of lymphocytes and large numbers of large pale-staining mononuclear histiocytes. Many of them are of macrophage type, and some of them are laden with melanin. The small blood vessels lined by plump endothelial cells are high endothelial venules (thick arrows). The lymphoid follicles in the cortex of the node are also enlarged and part of one follicle is visible. The follicle has a broad corona of small lymphocytes and a large germinal centre (double arrow) in which there is mitotic activity. HE ×150

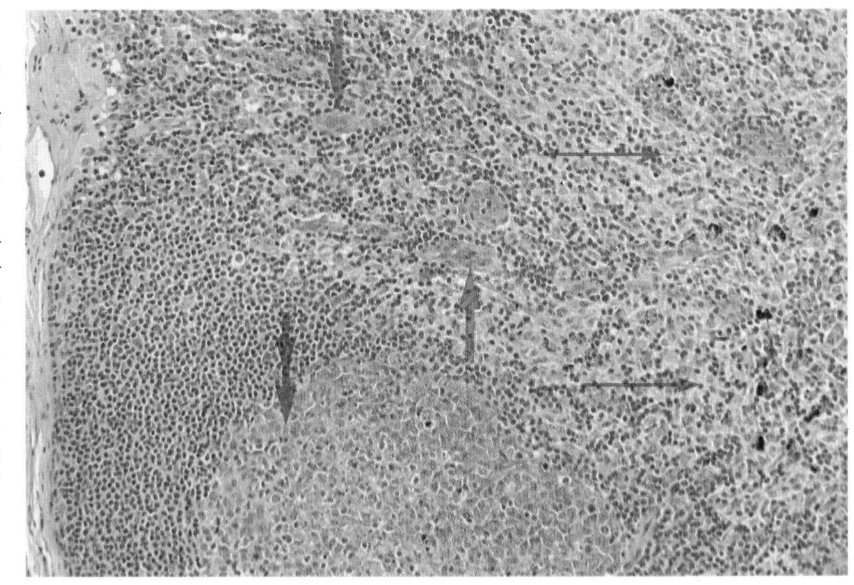

13.26 Dermatopathic lymphadenopathy: lymph node

This shows, at higher magnification, part of the paracortical tissue of the lymph node in 13.25. Some of the histiocytes in this tissue have been shown to be Langerhans cells and interdigitating reticulum cells. The small cells with darkly-staining nuclei (right) are readily identifiable cells. They are lymphocytes (mainly T cells). The blood vessels (thick arrows) lined by tall plump endothelial cells are post-capillary venules (HEV). The predominant cells however are histiocytes, large cells, each with a vesicular nucleus (thin arrows), a central nucleolus (often) and abundant weakly eosinophilic cytoplasm. Many of the cells are macrophages, containing melanin pigment in amounts which vary from a few granules to dense deposits of coarse granules which fill and distend the cell (double arrow). A frozen section stained for lipid would demonstrate the presence also of lipid within these macrophages. The melanin pigment and cell-wall lipid in the macrophages have been released by the breakdown of epidermal cells in the inflamed skin.

HE ×360

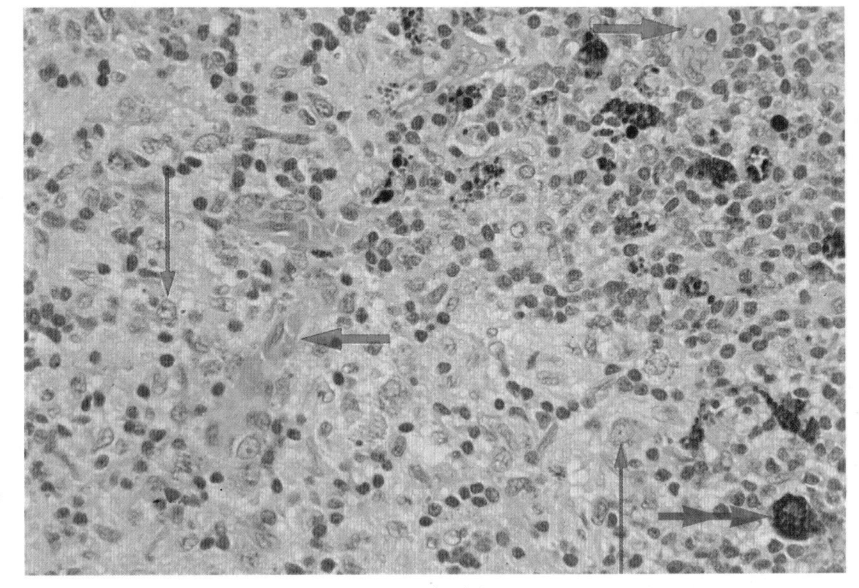

13.27 Histiocytosis X (Langerhans' cell histiocytosis)

A lymph node from a child with Histiocytosis X. Many eosinophils are seen in the centre of the picture, and round the edges here are large pale atypical histiocytes (Langerhans cells).

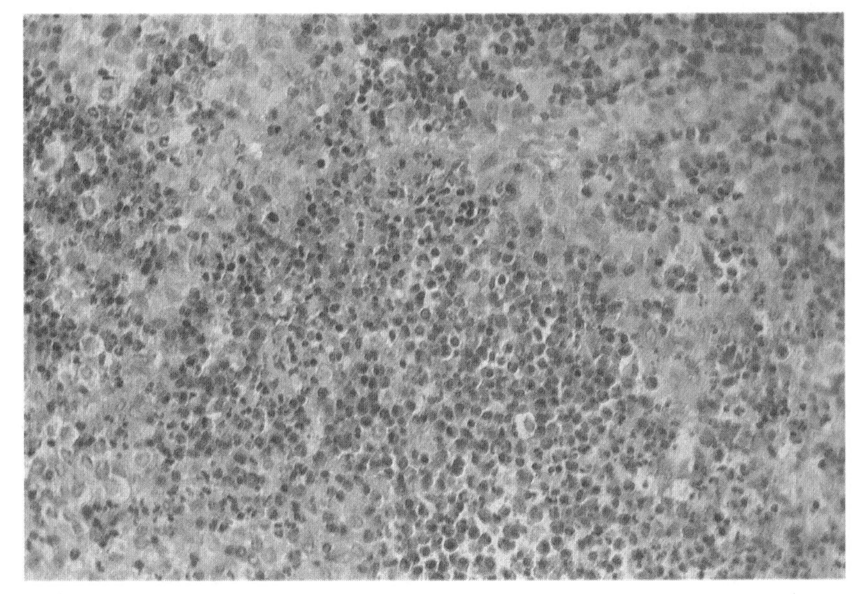

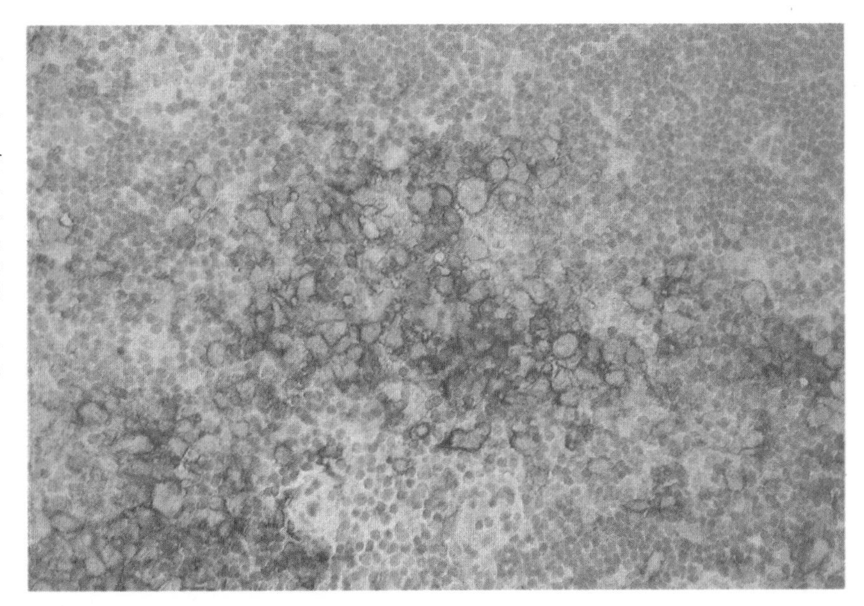

13.28 Histiocytosis X

The same lymph node as in 13.27, with a reaction for CD1a. This is specific for the cells of Histiocytosis × (H.X.) and can be seen in the atypical histiocytes (Langerhans cells).
Histiocytosis × is a granuloma-like lesion, consisting of pale-staining proliferating Langerhans cells and often numerous eosinophils. Langerhans cells are antigen-presenting dendritic cells (APC) with CD1 antigen on their surface. In the cytoplasm of the Langerhans cells there are very characteristic Birbeck granules, very small and shaped like a tennis racket.
A localized form of histiocytosis × (eosinophil granuloma) may develop at any age or site but is commonest in children and young adults.

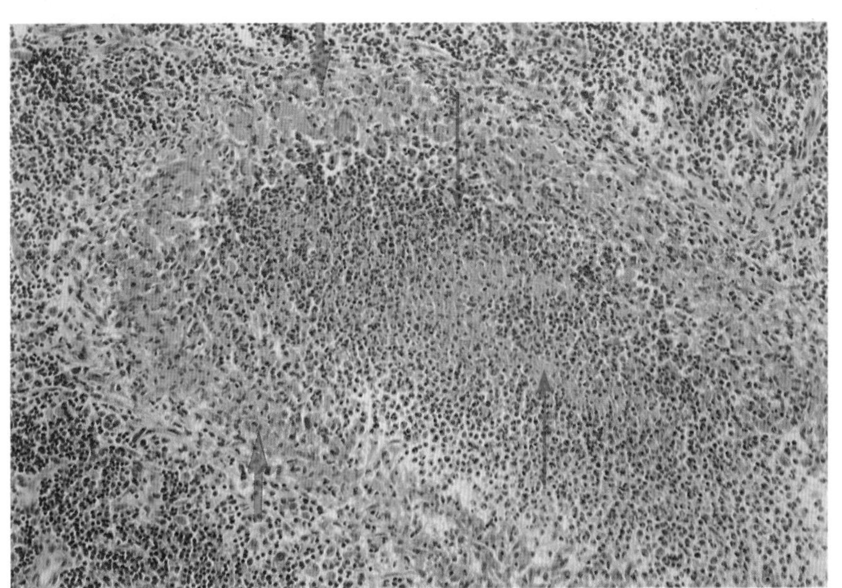

13.29 Cat-scratch disease: lymph node

Some cats carry an infectious agent which, when inoculated by a scratch from the claws of the cat, causes a systemic illness of a benign self-limiting nature. A papule forms in the skin and the regional nodes become inflamed and enlarged. A characteristic granulomatous reaction develops in the node, and abscesses, which tend to be serpiginous or stellate in outline, often form. A woman of 25 developed a tender swelling on the left side of her neck. Part of it (1 × 0.6 × 0.6cm) was removed surgically for diagnostic purposes. Histologically, several 'abscesses' had formed in the node but no normal architecture remained. In this field there is one abscess, the pus-like contents in the centre consisting of large numbers of polymorph leukocytes and necrotic cells (thin arrows). The contents of the abscess are surrounded by a fairly thick band of markedly eosinophilic histiocytes (thick arrows). The tissue outside this band of histiocytes is the lymphoid tissue of the node. HE ×150

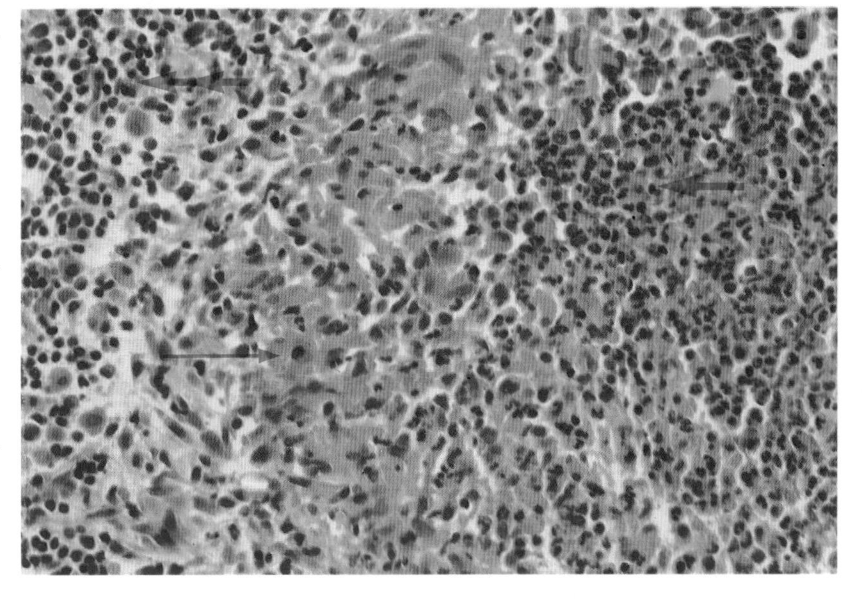

13.30 Cat-scratch disease: lymph node

The granulomatous inflammation characteristic of cat-scratch disease tends to develop in the cortex of the node and then extend to the perinodal tissue and to the medullary part of the node. This field shows part of the abscess at higher magnification. The contents of the abscess (right) are suppurative or pus-like material, consisting mostly of polymorph leukocytes (thick arrow), many of the necrotic. Adjacent to the polymorphs there is a central band of large mononuclear histiocytes with ovoid vesicular nuclei and a considerable amount of deeply eosinophilic cytoplasm (thin arrow). The histiocytes have formed a 'capsule' round the polymorphs and are showing a tendency to palisade. The cells external to this histiocytic capsule are the small lymphocytes (double arrow) of the surrounding lymphoid tissue. It has been suggested that the agent causing cat-scratch disease belongs to the psittacosis-lymphogranuloma group of microorganisms but there is some uncertainty about its origin. HE ×360

13.31 Toxoplasmosis: lymph node

Toxoplasmosis is a not uncommon systemic infection by the protozoon *Toxoplasma gondii*. Only very rarely can the parasite be demonstrated. Cats are probably the definitive host. Any tissue may be affected, the trophozoites proliferating within cells and destroying them. Lymphoid tissue is often involved, particularly in the cervical region, the nodes becoming enlarged. The architecture of the node is not destroyed, and the most striking feature, shown here, is the presence of clusters of large eosinophilic mononuclear histiocytes (thin arrow), with numerous clear vacuoles of various sizes (mostly small) in the cytoplasm of most of them. Their nuclei are large, weakly basophilic, and many contain a nucleolus. These are epithelioid-type histiocytes, and when they increase greatly in number they may encroach on the lymphoid follicles of the node. The small blood vessels are high endothelial venules and deeply eosinophilic (thick arrow). The small round deeply basophilic cells (double arrow) are the remaining lymphocytes of the lymphoid tissue. An occasional Langhans cell may be present. Necrosis is usually absent. HE ×235

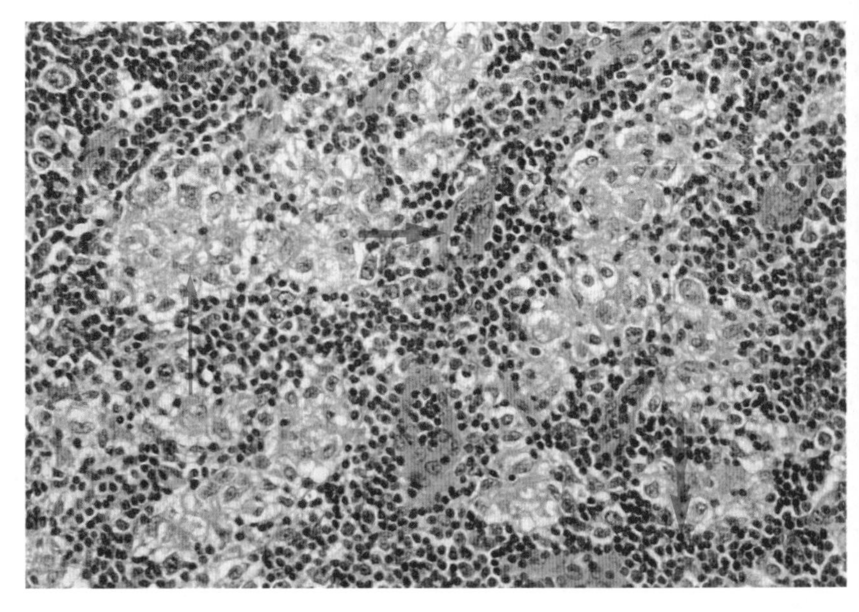

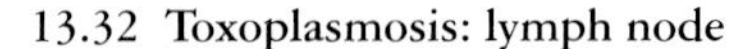

13.32 Toxoplasmosis: lymph node

Section of the node with immunohistochemical staining for *Toxoplasma gondii*, giving a brown staining of the organisms. These would not be apparent on conventional HE staining. The distribution of the protozoon *Toxoplasma gondii* is world-wide. It is usually asymptomatic but a small minority develop one of a group of syndromes, including acute acquired toxoplasmosis and congenital toxoplasmosis. The disease may mimic lymphoma, with enlargement of lymph nodes, usually in posterior cervical nodes. Toxoplasmosis may also affect the myocardium of neonates.

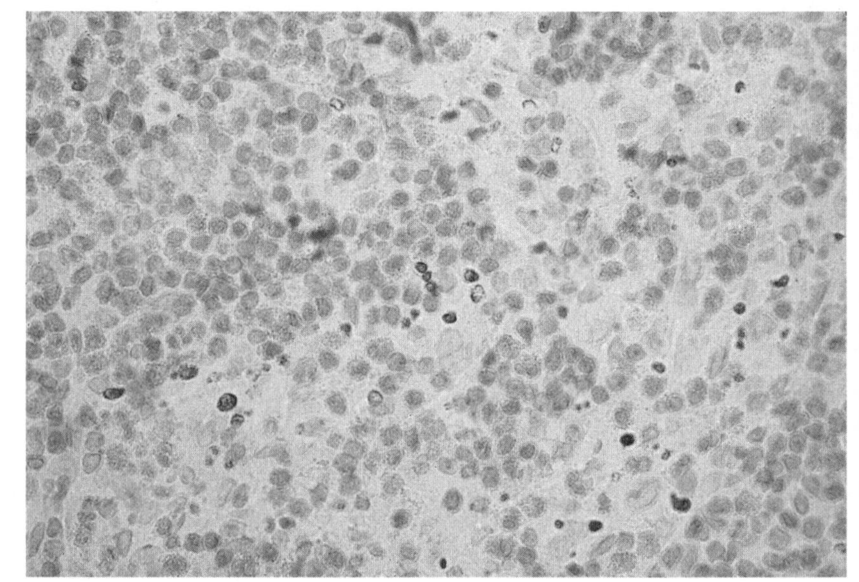

13.33 Sarcoidosis: lymph node

Sarcoidosis is a granulomatous inflammatory disease which affects many tissues, including lymphoid tissue. This is a cervical lymph node, which measured 3.5 × 1.5 × 0.5cm, from a woman of 51 with severe sarcoidosis. Part of the capsule of the node is just visible (double arrow). It is thick and fibrous. There are numerous round eosinophilic (sarcoid) follicles (thin arrow), consisting of epithelioid histiocytes, scattered throughout the blue-staining lymphoid tissue beneath the capsule. The follicles vary in size from very large collections of epithelioid histiocytes, several mm in diameter, to similar but smaller clusters. Some follicles are grouped closely together. The normal architecture of the node has been largely destroyed, but some normal lymphoid tissue survives beneath the capsule and between the follicles. Early fibrosis can just be detected at the periphery of several follicles. There is no necrosis within the follicles, but some contain laminated black (calcified) Schaumann bodies (thick arrows). HE ×60

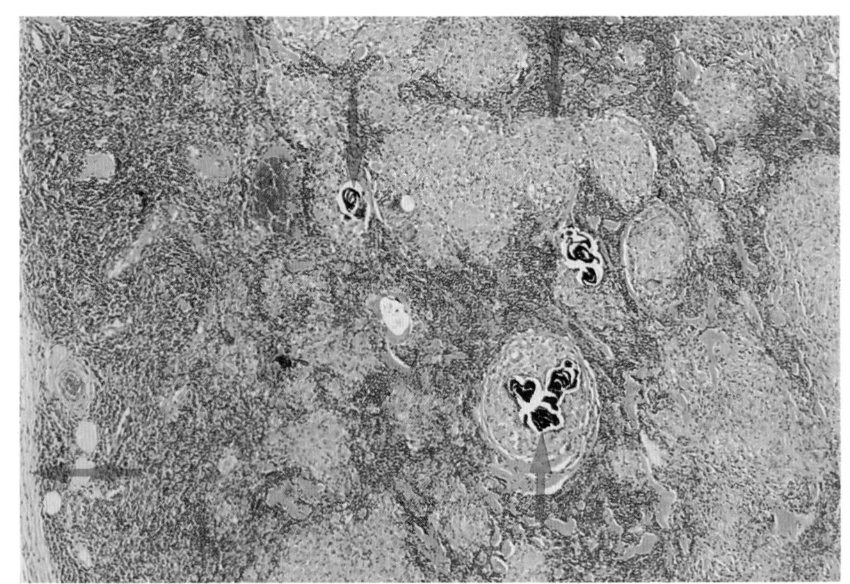

13.34 Infectious mononucleosis (glandular fever): lymph node

Infectious mononucleosis is caused by the Epstein-Barr (EB) virus, which grows mainly in B cells and seriously damages the B-cell areas of lymph nodes. There is also a striking paracortical T-cell reaction and marked proliferation of immunoblasts. It is a systemic illness, but the lymph nodes and particularly the cervical lymph nodes are swollen and tender. The architecture of this node has been characteristically obscured by the presence of numerous large lymphoid blast cells (thick arrows). Each of these cells, which predominate, have a large vesicular nucleus in which there are one or more prominent or very prominent nucleoli. The blast cells have a moderate amount of cytoplasm, with well-defined margins. These cells are considered to be T-immunoblasts, and they are accompanied by moderate numbers of other cells of the lymphocyte series, notably small lymphocytes with a small round densely basophilic nucleus. The general histological features in this field are very suggestive of a malignant lymphoma. Atypical lymphoid cells could also be demonstrated in smears of the peripheral blood.

HE ×360

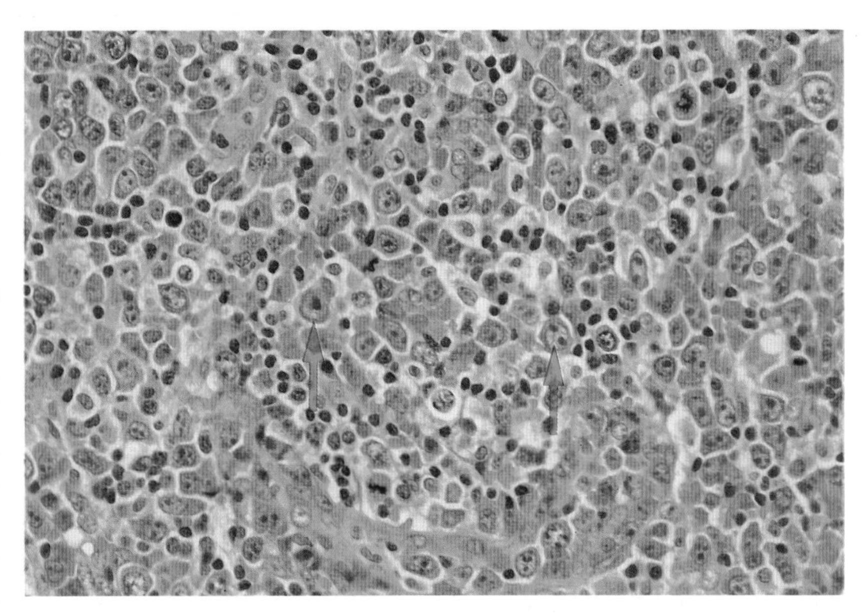

13.35 Hodgkin's disease: nodular sclerosis

Much the most common presenting feature of Hodgkin's disease is enlargement of lymph nodes in the neck or mediastinum, and it rarely occurs in an extranodal site. Eventually however there may be local spread to adjacent lymph nodes and organs. The disease differs from other lymphomas in that histologically it is not monomorphic but involves, generally, a variety of different cell types, including histiocytes, lymphocytes, plasma cells and eosinophil leukocytes, as well as a characteristic and diagnostic type of large cell with two or more nuclei, the Reed-Sternberg cell. This is the nodular sclerosis form of Hodgkin's disease, the most common type, characterized by the presence of cellular nodules of lymphomatous tissue, surrounded by broad bands of birefringent collagen (thin arrow). The central lymphoid nodule (thick arrow) consists of lymphocytes and a small number of eosinophilic histiocytes, as does the part of the larger cellular nodule on the right. A moderate number of lymphocytes are scattered throughout the dense collagenous tissue.

HE ×65

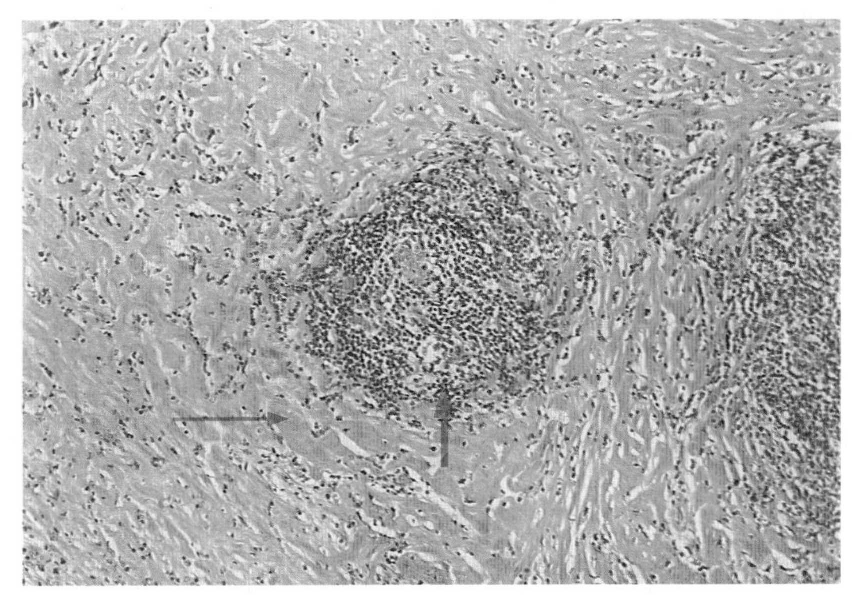

13.36 Hodgkin's disease - Reed-Sternberg cells

This is Hodgkin's disease immunostained for CD30 illustrating the positive reaction of Hodgkin/Reed-Sternberg cells. This marker is characteristic of these cells and is used regularly in diagnosis. The diagnosis of Hodgkin's lymphoma is still based on histological features, and finding classical RS cells in the tissues is essential for diagnosis. There are relatively few RS cells in lymphocyte-predominant Hodgkin's lymphoma, and the presence of large polypoid variants of the RS cell with lobulated nuclei (popcorn cells) is characteristic.

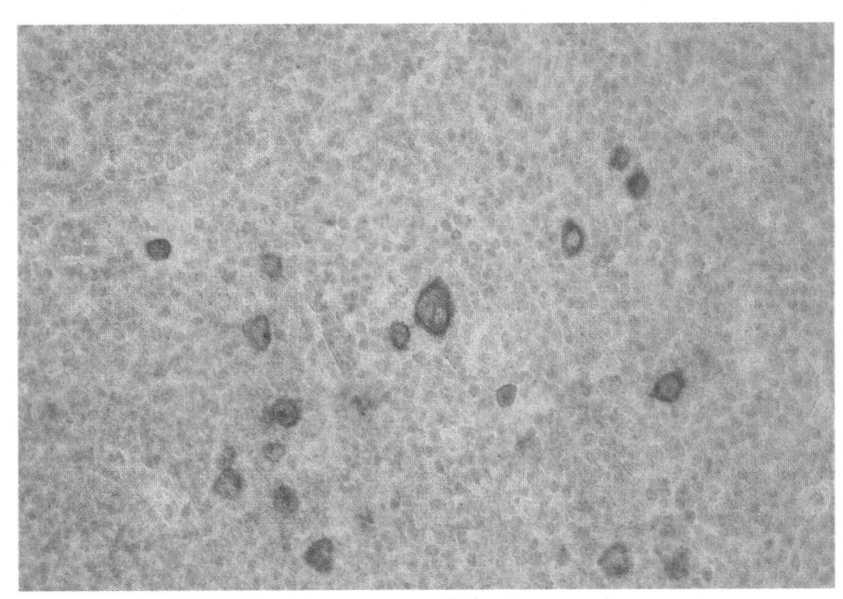

13.37 Hodgkin's disease: mixed cellularity

This is the mixed cellularity form of Hodgkin's disease, and the tissue consists of several different types of cell. On the right side of the field there is a large area of necrosis, staining deep red (double arrow), and about two-thirds of the tissue (centre and left) is viable. Necrosis is often a striking feature of Hodgkin's disease and was widespread in this lymph node. The most prominent type of cell in the sheet of viable tissue is the pleomorphic mononuclear histiocyte, with its large vesicular nucleus (thin arrows). It is the most numerous type of cell. Another form of histiocyte is the Reed-Sternberg (RS) cell, a relatively small multinucleated giant cell (thick arrow) containing several pleomorphic basophilic vesicular nuclei and prominent nucleoli. The small cells with the deeply-staining nuclei are lymphocytes, and a moderate number of polymorph leukocytes with eosinophilic cytoplasm are also present. A tangled network of reticulin fibres usually spreads throughout the Hodgkin's tissue. HE ×335

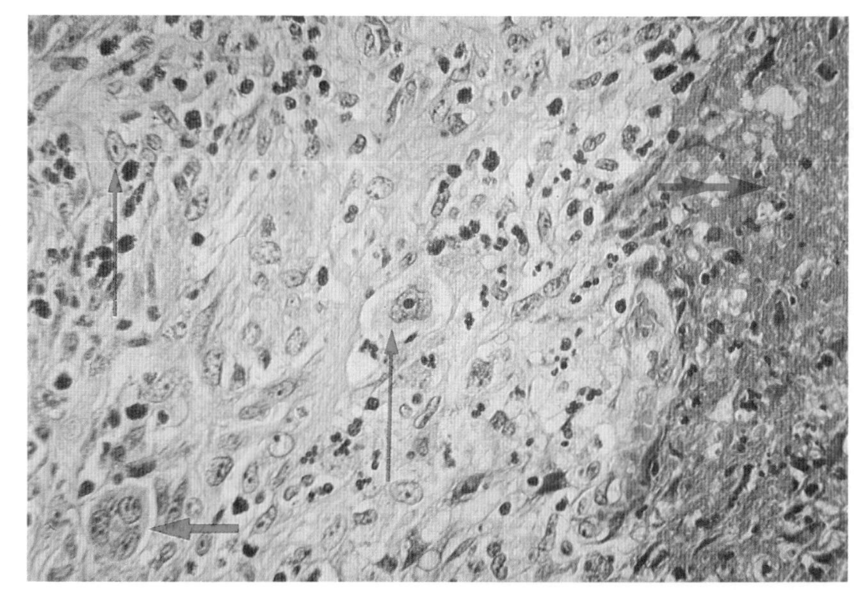

13.38 Hodgkin's disease: lymphocyte predominance

The lymphocyte predominance type of Hodgkin's disease is found mostly in young adult males. Lymphocytes make up the bulk of the tissue and the number of classic Reed-Sternberg (abnormal histiocytes) is relatively small, most of the neoplastic cells being L & H cells with multilobated or convoluted nuclei ('popcorn' cells). In this field there are many small lymphocytes with compact basophilic nuclei (thick arrow), several normal-sized histiocytes with vesicular nuclei (e.g. in top right corner of field (double arrow) and two relatively enormous histiocytes of classical Reed-Sternberg (RS) form. Each RS cell is binucleated, containing two very large nuclei, apposed to each other in a 'mirror-image' pattern (thin arrows). The nuclei in both RS cells are pale and vesicular and in each nucleus there is a prominent or very prominent heavily red-stained and pleomorphic central nucleolus. The origin of Reed-Sternberg cells is uncertain, but their presence is a very important, indeed essential, factor in the histological diagnosis of Hodgkin's disease. HE ×950

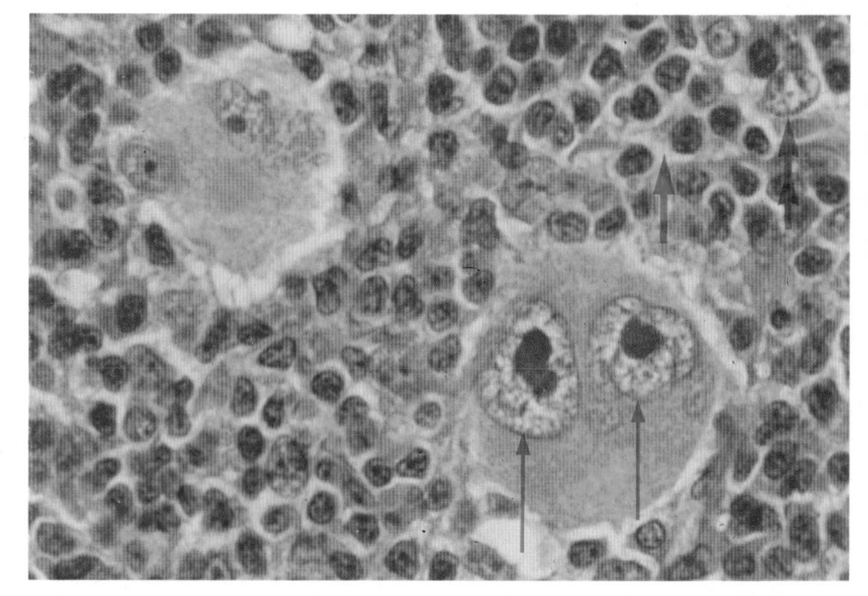

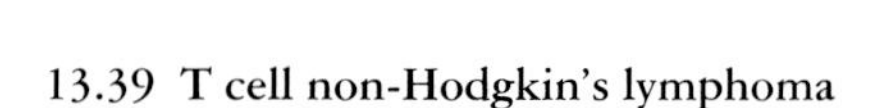

13.39 T cell non-Hodgkin's lymphoma

The interfollicular areas are expanded by lymphoma cells, which are surprisingly regular in sizes and shapes (the grading and assessment of T cell lymphomas is notoriously difficult). T cell lymphomas are less common than B cell lymphomas and a well-developed follicular pattern is seen only in the B cell type.

13.40 Anaplastic high grade lymphoma

This lymphoma is called "Ki1 lymphoma" for historical reasons because it was initially recognised by its reaction with an antibody to CD30, called Ki1. We can now identify this tumour, which is usually of T-cell phenotype by means of its labelling with antibodies such as BerH2, which reacts with conventional sections.

It is a lymphoblastic (convoluted T cell) lymphoma, with diffuse proliferation of primitive cells, composed of large pleomorphic cells which lack distinctive features but include many binucleated giant forms and grossly abnormal mitoses.. The cells express activation antigens, notably CD30. In lymph nodes the neoplastic cells form focal expanding aggregates or involve the sinusoids. Children and young adults tend to be affected.

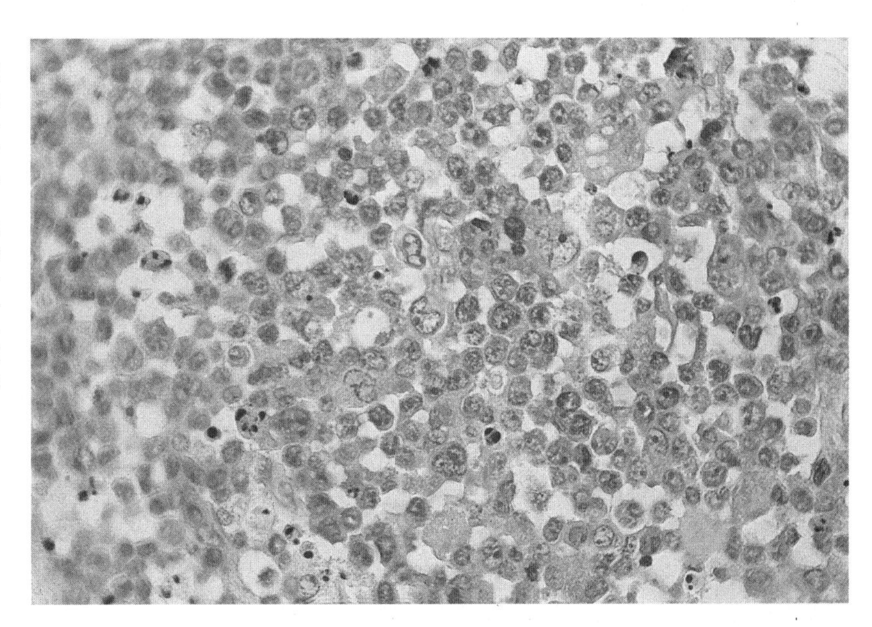

13.41 Angioimmunoblastic lymphadenopathy

Individuals with angioimmunoblastic lymphadenopathy (AIL) are adult and often elderly. The illness usually presents with generalized lymphadenopathy. In addition to the enlarged lymph nodes, the patients generally have skin rash, fever, hemolytic anemia and a polyclonal hypergammaglobulinemia. The condition may be mistaken for malignant lymphoma but differs in its rapid onset and fluctuant course. In this node, a few atrophic follicles remain but the architecture of the lymph node has otherwise been completely destroyed by the formation of new tissue which consists of very numerous proliferating small blood vessels, between which there is a cellular infiltrate of small lymphocytes, large immunoblasts with a prominent central nucleolus (thick arrows), plasma cells and eosinophil leukocytes. The small blood vessels are lined by plump endothelial cells (thin arrows) with a large pale vesicular nucleus and resemble high endothelial venules. The small lymphocytes are neoplastic T cells, usually CD4+, and often have clear cytoplasm. The multinucleated giant cells which are sometimes present tend to be mistaken for Hodgkin's cells. HE ×360

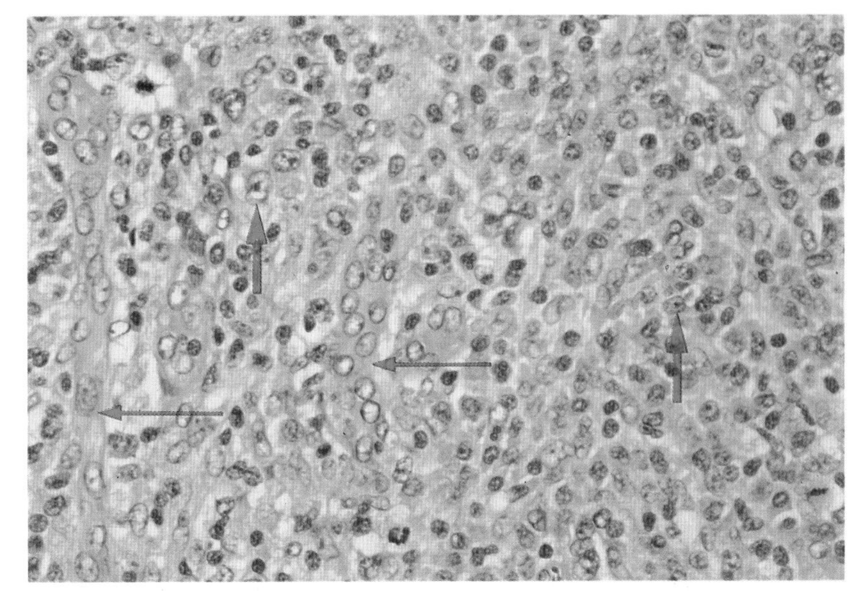

13.42 Angioimmunoblastic lymphadenopathy

The large numbers of arborizing small blood vessels in the lymph nodes in angioblastic lymphadenopathy (AIL) form an important diagnostic feature but they are relatively difficult to detect fully in ordinary HE sections. To facilitate and confirm the diagnosis, the silver method for reticulin has been applied to a histological section of part of a lymph node. The silver method stains the basement membranes of the blood vessels dark grey or black, thereby revealing the membranes very clearly as reticulin fibres. Consequently, with the tissue architecture made much more obvious, the network of small thick-walled branching (arborizing) blood vessels (like post-capillary venules) is demonstrated much more vividly than staining with HE. Significantly the fact that no lymphoid follicles can be seen in this silver preparation is in agreement with the knowledge that lymphoid follicles are usually absent from lymph nodes in AIL.

Silver method for reticulin ×150

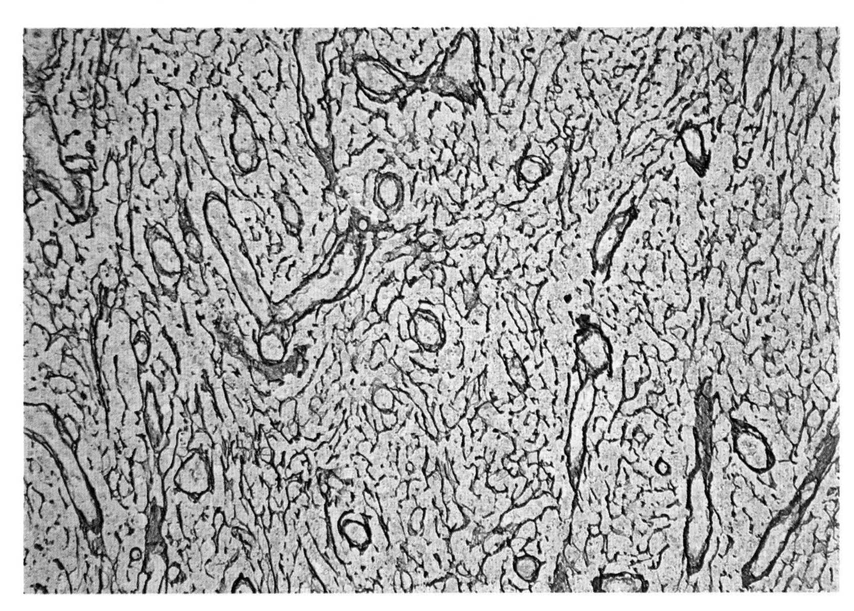

13.43 Angiofollicular lymph node hyperplasia

The cause of angiofollicular lymph node hyperplasia (AFLNH) is obscure. The lesion, usually in young adults, is benign and generally a large encapsulated mass of abnormal lymphoid tissue, in which there are comparatively few sinusoids but large numbers of follicular structures. The abnormal lymphoid tissue is located most often in the mediastinum or neck and usually an incidental finding, e.g. when the thorax is X-rayed. The tissue consists of compact lymphoid follicles with well-defined boundaries. There is interfollicular tissue on the left and a lymphoid follicle on the right. Running into the centre of the follicle and occupying part of it is a hyalinized blood vessel with a thick hyaline wall (thick arrow). The vessel ends in a small germinal centre of pale-staining histiocytic cells. Peripheral to germinal centre there is a mantle of lymphocytes, arranged in tight concentric circles (thin arrow) and forming an 'onion-skin' pattern. The interfollicular tissue consists of an extensive network of small blood vessels with an eosinophilic hyalinized wall and a small lumen (double arrow). Between the vessels there are many small lymphocytes, some in clusters, and occasionally macrophages. In plasma cell type of of AFLNH, the interfollicular tissue is massively infiltrated by plasma cells, and the patient may have systemic symptoms, including fever and loss of weight. HE ×150

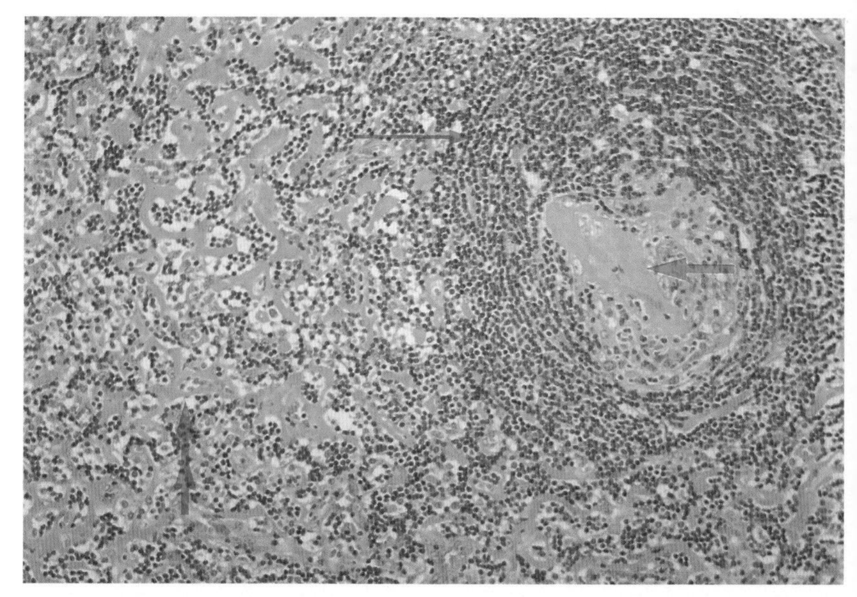

13.44 Angiofollicular lymph node hyperplasia

This is the same interfollicular tissue as that in 13.43, at higher magnification. In consists of small vessels, part of the complex network of vessels in the interfollicular tissue, separated by a large population of small lymphocytes, each with a compact strongly basophilic nucleus and very little cytoplasm (and shown to be T cells); and occasional macrophages (in some lesions, numerous plasma cells and eosinophil leukocytes mingle with the lymphocytes). The vessels have the structure of high endothelial venules, being lined by large cuboidal endothelial cells (thick arrows) with a large round vesicular nucleus and often a central nucleolus. In this area the walls of the vessels are only slightly hyalinized but the walls of the small vessels elsewhere (not in this field) are heavily infiltrated by strongly eosinophil hyaline material, a striking feature of the hyaline vascular form of AFLNH. HE x360

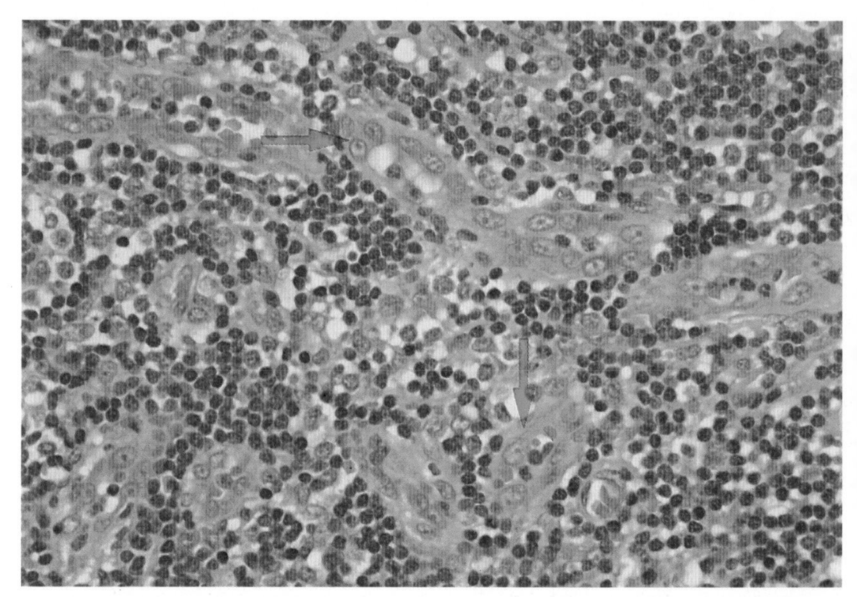

13.45 Lymphocytic lymphoma (diffuse): lymph node

Well-differentiated lymphocytic lymphoma may be considered as the counterpart, in the tissues, of chronic lymphocytic leukemia. In this lymph node the normal architecture has been replaced by a diffuse sheet infiltrate of closely packed small round cells, fairly uniform in size and shape. They resemble mature small lymphocytes, most of them having a thin rim of cytoplasm and a small round deeply basophilic nucleus. None of the nuclei is indented. There is also no evidence of follicle formation. Among the predominant smaller lymphocytes there is also a small number of slightly larger lymphocyte-type cells with a vesicular nucleus. In a few of these vesicular nuclei there appears to be a nucleolus but this is unlikely. Scattered among the lymphocyte-type cells there are reactive histiocytes (thin arrows), much larger than the lymphocyte-type cells. Each of the histiocytes has a much larger paler vesicular nucleus, in which there is a prominent nucleolus. Also present in these tissues there are scant high endothelial venules, lined by plump endothelial cells (HEVs) (thick arrows). HE ×150

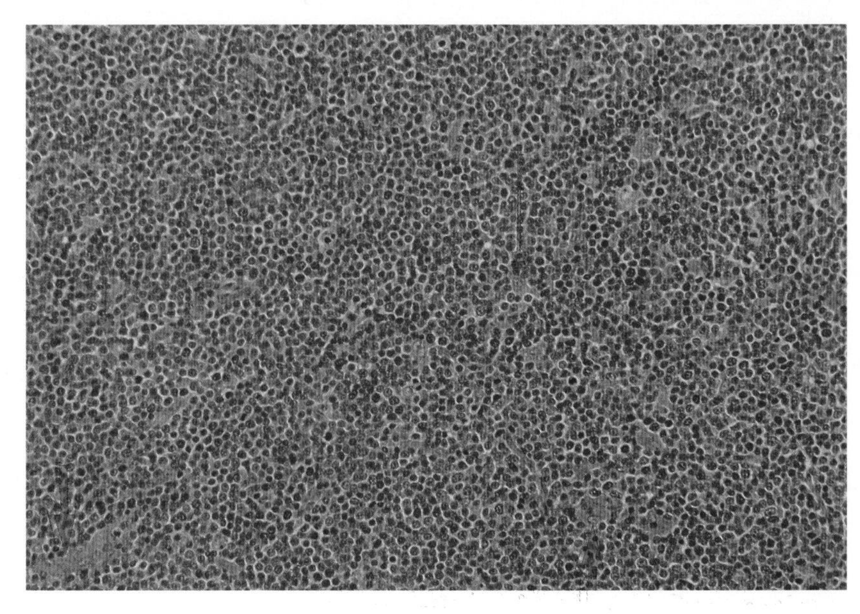

13.46 Lymphocytic lymphoma (diffuse): lymph node

This is the lymphoma shown in 13.45, at higher magnification. The tissue consists almost entirely of a diffuse infiltrate of closely packed small round B lymphocytes, resembling mature lymphocytes and showing no plasmacytic differentiation. Variable numbers of prolymphocytes and lymphoblasts also tend to be present. The cells in this field have a thin rim of cytoplasm and round or ovoid strongly basophilic nuclei which vary only moderately in size and pleomorphism (thin arrows). There is no folding or indentation of the nuclei. The nuclear chromatin is generally coarsely granular, and very occasionally there appears to be a central nucleolus in the nucleus. However this may be just a solitary granule of chromatin. The reactive histiocytes are invariably larger than the lymphocyte-type cells, but some of the histiocytes are comparatively very large, with abundant well-defined eosinophilic cytoplasm and a large pale vesicular pleomorphic nucleus in which there is a prominent nucleolus (thick arrows). HE ×360

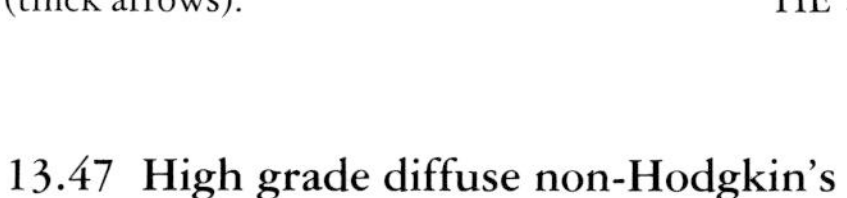

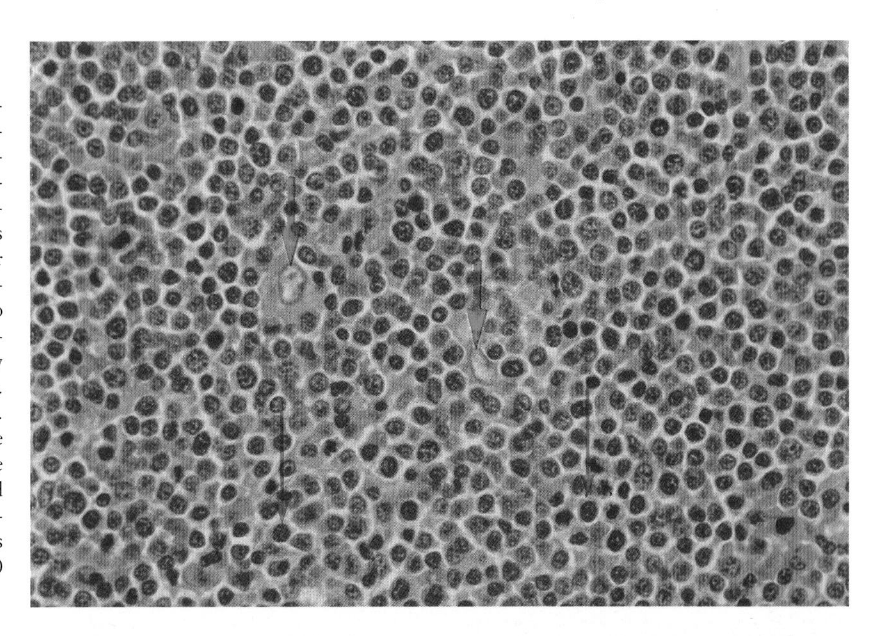

13.47 High grade diffuse non-Hodgkin's lymphoma

High grade diffuse non-Hodgkin's (NHL) lymphoma, stained with HE. The cells are large and have pale rounded nuclei with, usually, a large single nucleolus (thin arrow). Mitoses are frequent (thick arrow). This is a large non-cleaved lymphoma (FCC), follicular in approximately 10% of cases. Behaviour is aggressive, with rapid dissemination. The cell surface is typically monoclonal Ig: IgM or IgG. Other markers include bcl-2.

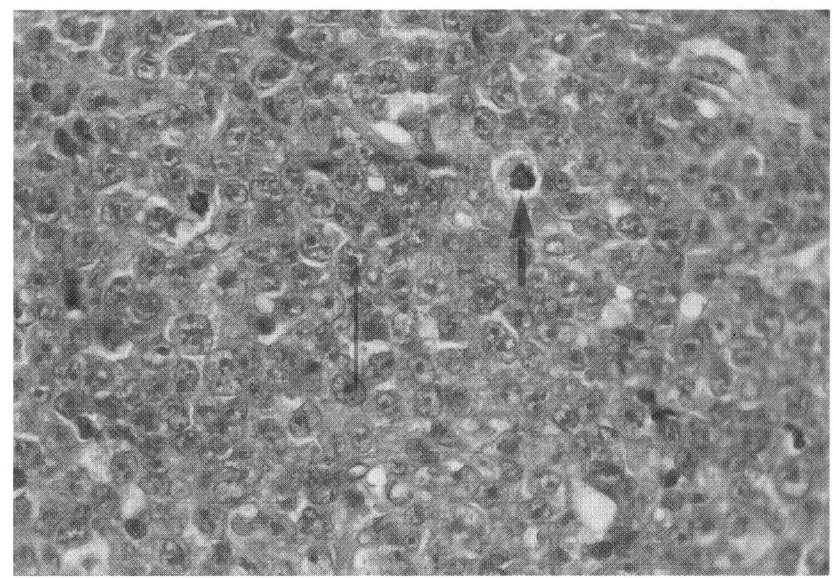

13.48 High grade diffuse non-Hodgkin's lymphoma

Same tumour as 13.47, immunostained for CD79a, which is a highly restricted B-cell antigen. This is clearly positive and proves the B-cell origin of the tumour.

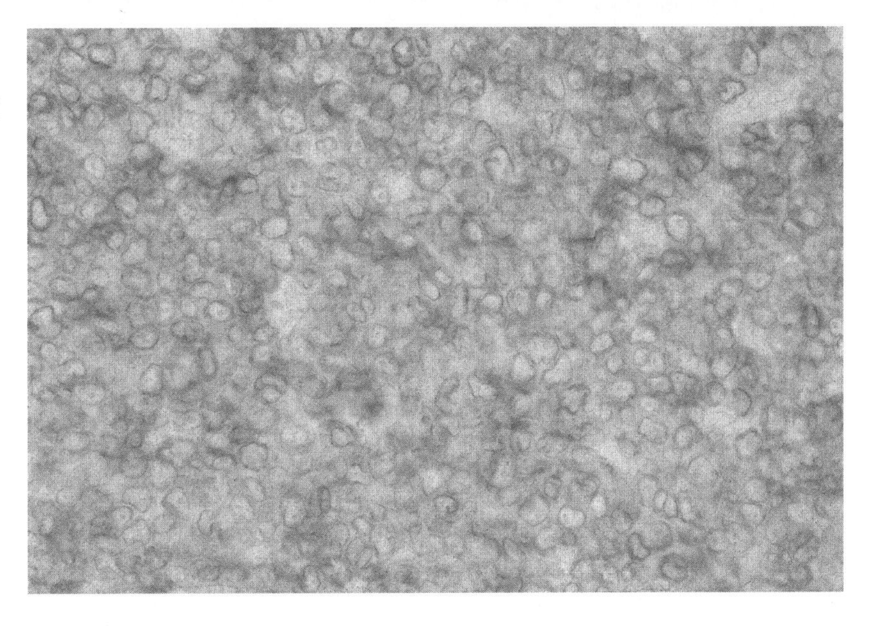

13.49 Lymphocytic lymphoma: marrow

The bone marrow is, rarely, the site of origin of a primary lymphoma. In many instances, however, it is involved secondarily in the form of either a diffuse infiltrate or as focal deposits. Biopsy of the bone marrow is very useful in staging the disease and in determining treatment. Focal or diffuse involvement of the marrow does not, however, reflect the lymph node pattern (follicular or diffuse) of a lymphoma. This is a section of a biopsy of iliac crest. In this field, the normal hemopoietic marrow has been replaced by a uniform population of small lymphocyte-type cells which are closely apposed to a trabecula of dense lamellar bone (thick arrow). A plump capillary vessel (thin arrow) traverses the sheet of cells. The cells are neoplastic, each with a small very heavily stained slightly pleomorphic nucleus and very little cytoplasm. In a few of the cells there is mitotic activity, but from the changes in the lymph nodes, the lesion was classified as a low-grade lymphocytic lymphoma of diffuse type. HE ×360

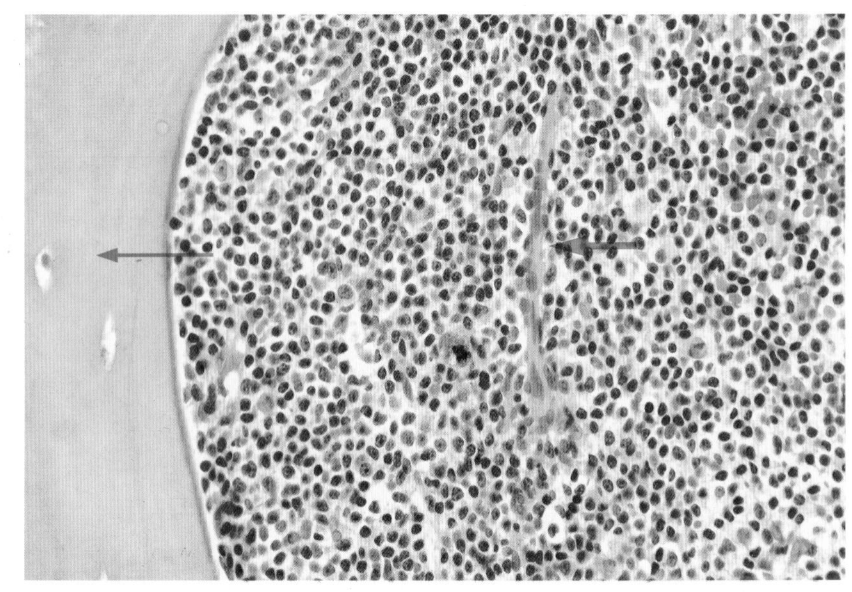

13.50 Lymphocytic leukemia: marrow

In chronic lymphocytic leukemia, the number of lymphocytes in the peripheral blood is increased, often very markedly. In about 95% of the cases the leukemia cells are of B cell origin and in about 5% of cases they are of T-cell lineage. There is often some enlargement of lymph nodes and spleen, and the bone marrow is not infrequently involved. Involvement of the bone marrow may be focal or diffuse, and in this trephine specimen of marrow from the iliac crest of a woman of 57, there is a diffuse uniform population of neoplastic lymphocytes which has infiltrated and almost completely replaced the hemopoietic elements, apart from the megakaryocytes. The neoplastic lymphocytes are small mature-looking cells with a small round very basophilic nucleus and minimal cytoplasm. In addition to the population of small neoplastic lymphocytes, there is a number of non-neoplastic megakaryocytes in the centre and lower left part of the field. They are very large (giant) cells, and each contains a very large and very pleomorphic nucleus in its abundant eosinophilic cytoplasm (arrow). HE ×360

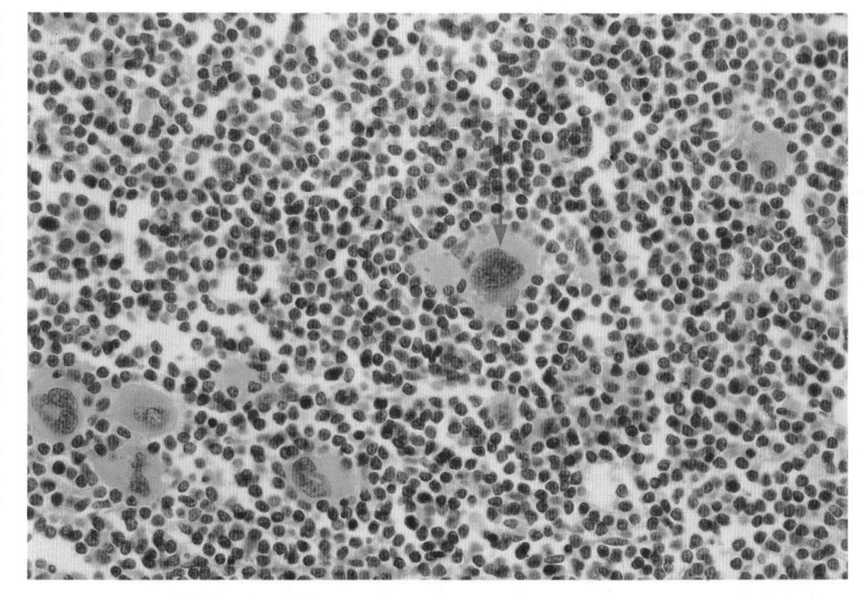

13.51 Follicular (centroblastic/centrocytic) lymphoma: lymph node

Lymphomas other than Hodgkin's lymphomas arise from lymphocytes (B cells or T cells) or from histiocytes (histiocytic lymphomas, malignant histiocytosis). All lymphomas are malignant. Follicular lymphoma (centroblastic/centrocytic), one of the commonest forms of low-grade non-Hodgkin's lymphoma (NHL), generally occurring in adults and arising from B cells. The growth pattern of centroblastic/centrocytic lymphomas may be follicular, follicular and diffuse, or diffuse (that is, lacking a follicular pattern). Follicular lymphomas have a better prognosis than diffuse lymphomas. In this lymph node the lymphomatous tissue consists of a fairly uniform population of centrocytes and centroblasts, with nuclei noticeably less basophil than the nuclei of lymphocytes. The neoplastic cells are arranged in round or ovoid poorly-defined 'follicles' (thin arrow) with indistinct boundaries, and are separated by connective tissue (thick arrow) with a large reticulin content and numerous small blood vessels (HEV). The 'follicles' do not have a corona of lymphocytes or a clearly defined germinal centre.
HE ×60

13.52 Follicular (centroblastic/centrocytic) lymphoma: lymph node

This is the same lymphoma as in 13.51 above. It consists largely of centroblasts and centrocytes, with centrocytes predominant. The centroblasts (thin arrows) are larger than the centrocytes and they have more cytoplasm with a well-defined cell boundary and a large round nucleus which usually contains several prominent nucleoli, located close to the nuclear membrane. The centrocytes (thick arrows) are more numerous and smaller than the centroblasts, and many of them are comparable in size to small lymphocytes. The centrocytic nuclei are less basophilic than those of small lymphocytes however and many of then are 'deformed' (kidney-shaped), the 'deformity' being caused by 'notching' of the nucleus or indentation of nuclear membrane. In the nuclei of some centrocytes there is a small central nucleolus. Follicular centre cell lymphomas tend to become diffuse, with centroblasts then much more numerous than the centrocytes.

HE ×360

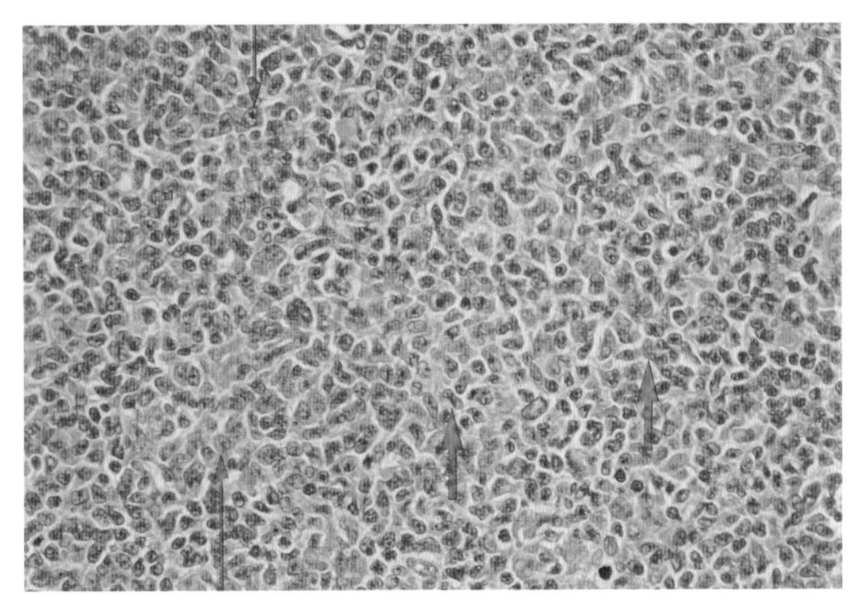

13.53 "Reactive" and malignant follicles: lymph node

Section of lymph node immunohistochemically stained for the protein product of the oncogene Bcl-2. On the top left is a malignant follicle (thick arrow) with Bcl-2 (brown) expression centrally. Adjacent to it is a benign follicle (thin arrow) with staining for the protein at the periphery ('mantle zone'). Bcl-2 is known to suppress apoptosis and can be used to differentiate between malignant and benign lymphoid follicles.

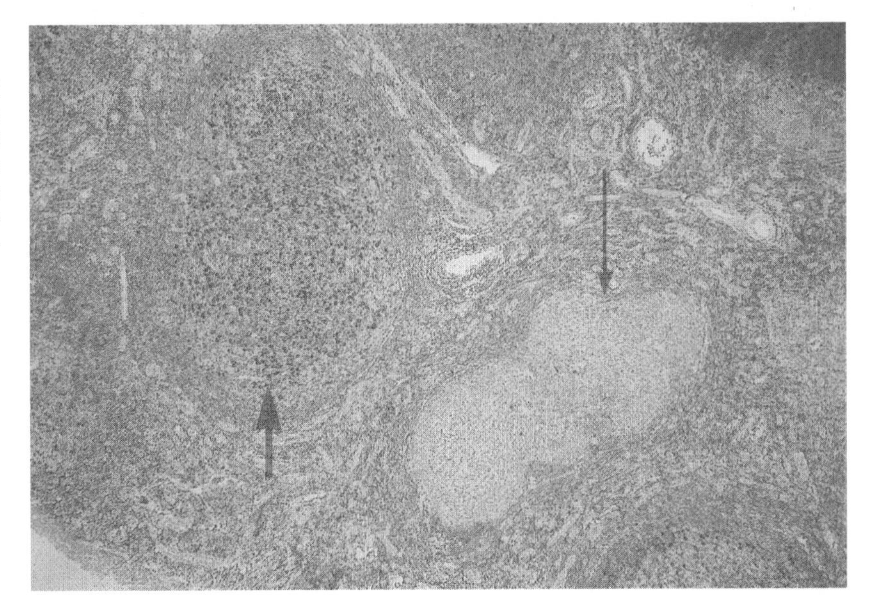

13.54 High grade diffuse (centroblastic) lymphoma (with immunoblastic transformation): lymph node

Lymphomas of centroblastic type may arise *de novo* or from a follicular centroblastic/centrocytic lymphoma, and they have a relatively poor prognosis. Immunoblasts are often present in small numbers in centroblastic lymphomas but in parts of this node they predominate. The cells on the right side of the field are mostly small lymphocytes with deeply basophilic small round nuclei (double arrow), and in the remainder of the field there are numerous large immunoblasts with strikingly pale round or ovoid vesicular nuclei (thin arrows). Characteristically the chromatin tends to concentrate at the nuclear membrane, and in most of the nuclei there is a single large prominent central nucleolus (thick arrows). In a few nuclei there are several nucleoli. The cytoplasm, which is abundant and has a well-defined boundary, tends to stain blue from the presence of many ribosomes, and immunoglobulin can usually be demonstrated in the cytoplasm.

HE ×360

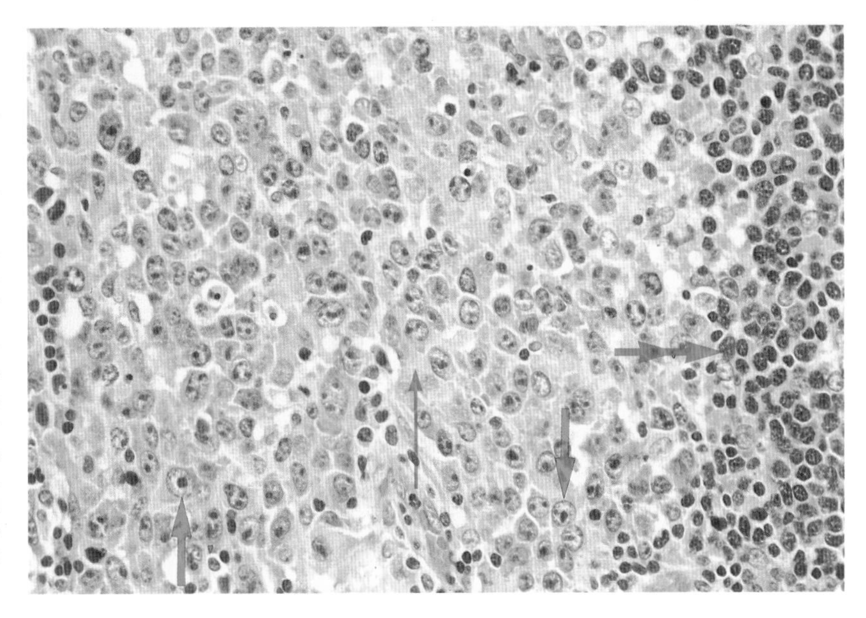

13.55 Lymphoblastic lymphoma: lymph node

Lymphoblastic lymphoma occurs at all ages but most often in children and adolescents. Many individuals later develop lymphoblastic leukemia. It is easier to study the detailed structure of lymphoma cells in thin (0.5-1.0μm thick) plastic sections than in thicker sections embedded in other materials such as paraffin wax. This is a 1μm plastic section of a high grade lymphoma of lymphoblastic type, in a lymph node. The normal population of cells in the node has been replaced by a monomorphic infiltrate of cells (lymphoblasts), each lymphoblast having a round or ovoid nucleus (a minority of lymphoblast nuclei are convoluted) in which the chromatin is evenly dispersed. In some of the nuclei there are one or more (two to five) small but clearly visible nucleoli (thin arrow). Cytoplasm is fairly scanty and not well-defined. There is considerable mitotic activity (thick arrows). The blood vessel (bottom centre) is a high endothelial venule (double arrow), lined by large plump endothelial cells, each with a pale vesicular nucleus. HE ×320

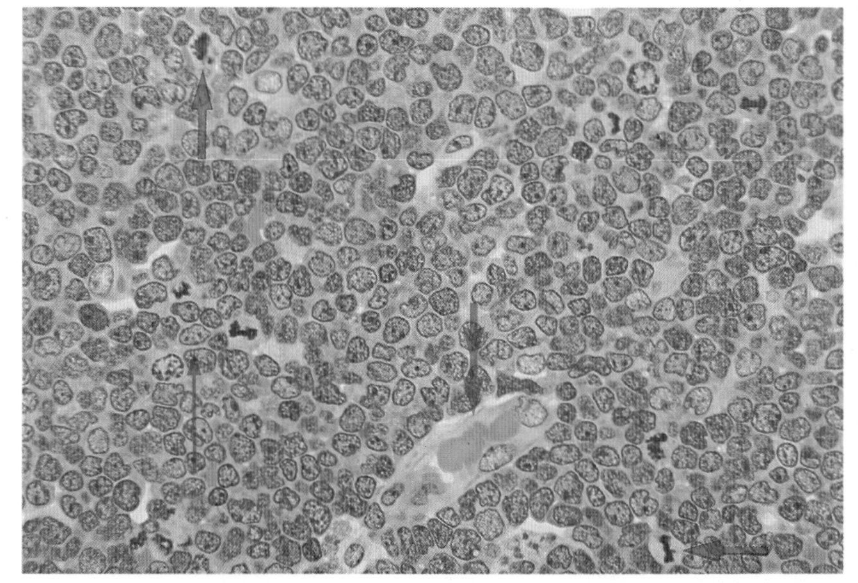

13.56 High grade diffuse non-Hodgkin's lymphoma (B cell)

This is a diffusely expansive lymphoma with large nucleolate nuclei (thin arrow) and many mitoses (thick arrow) and apoptotic bodies. The lymphoma proved to be of B-cell origin, having been stained for the antigenic markers CD20 and CD79a which are restricted to B cells.

This is an immunoblastic sarcoma (B cell), a large non-cleaved FCC but with nuclei more deeply basophilic. It is often plasmacytoid, with the nucleoli often central and large (prominent). margination of the chromatin gives a "vesicular" appearance.

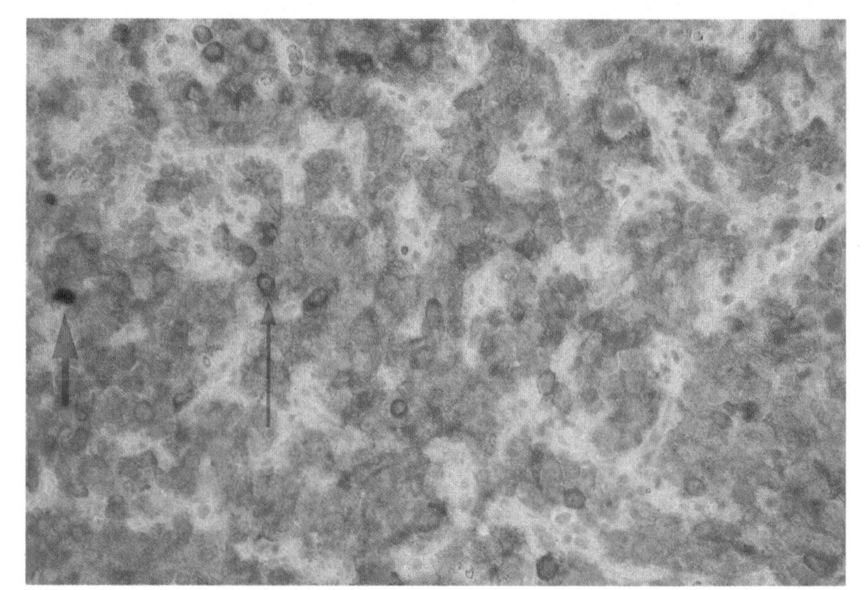

13.57 Lymphoblastic lymphoma: marrow

Lymphoblastic lymphoma is a high grade lymphoma which arises from the precursors of B cells or T cells. Lymphoblastic lymphoma of T-cell type occurs at all ages but most arise in first two decades. Lymphoblastic lymphoma is highly infiltrative, the cells tending to infiltrate in Indian-file, displacing the cells of the tissue but leaving the underlying structure intact. Many of the nuclei are round or oval with very distinctive chromatin, finely textured and evenly dispersed (thin arrows). A considerable proportion of lymphoblast nuclei are convoluted, i.e. they have a deep cleft or fold (double arrow), an appearance suggestive but not conclusive evidence of a T cell origin. Cell marker studies confirmed the T cell nature of this lesion. The cytoplasm is fairly scanty and ill-defined. Typically also, there are numerous mitotic figures (thick arrows). Scattered throughout the lesion are many reactive macrophages with a large amount pale more-or-less clear cytoplasm, thereby producing a 'starry-sky' appearance. HE ×360

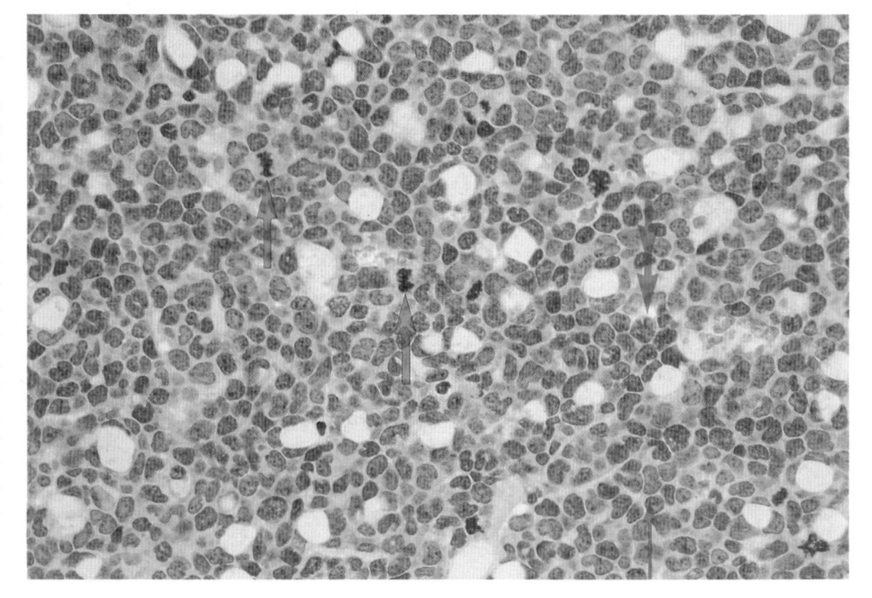

13.58 Lymphoblastic lymphoma (Burkitt's): omentum

Most cases of Burkitt's lymphoma arise in children and, at least in Africa, many organs and tissues including the jaws are involved. Lymph node involvement is often comparatively insignificant. This deposit of tumour in the omentum consists of sheets of closely packed uniform medium-sized blast cells with large round or oval nuclei, each containing three or four small basophilic nucleoli which tend to be located near the nuclear membrane (thin arrows). There are numerous pyknotic fragments of necrotic nuclei. The amount of cytoplasm in the lymphoblasts is small and strongly basophil, and intensely pyroninophil. Several large non-neoplastic macrophages are present (thick arrows) and within their abundant cytoplasm there are remnants of ingested cells, including many nuclear fragments. These (tingible-body) macrophages are a feature of lymphoblastic lymphoma and, being distributed throughout the lesion, consequently responsible for the 'starry-sky' appearance.

HE ×580

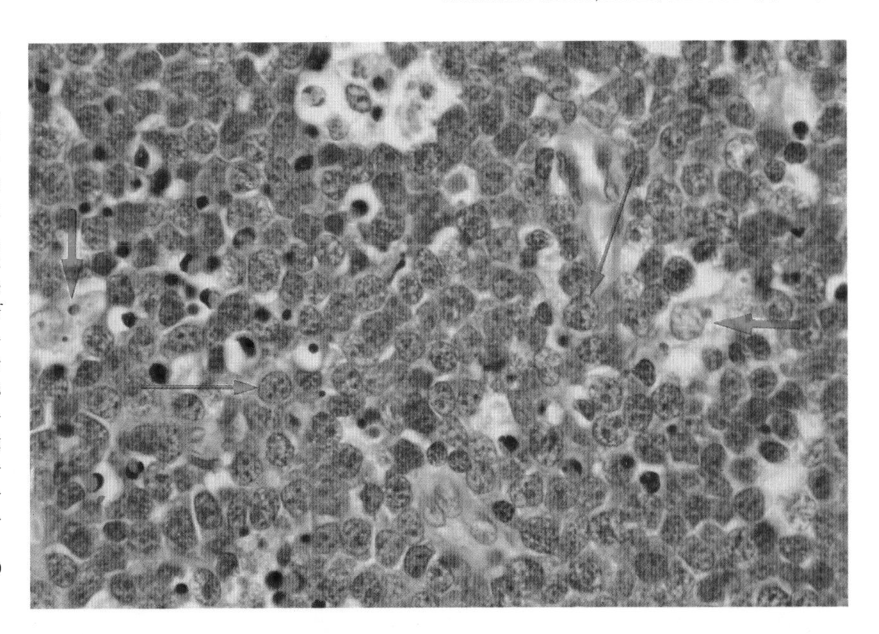

13.59 Lymphoplasmacytic lymphoma: lymph node

Lymphoplasmacytic lymphoma may present as a tumour, as chronic lymphoid leukemia, or as hyperviscosity syndrome. It is a tumour of B lymphocytes which shows differentiation towards plasma cells. The condition occurs most often in older people, and a paraprotein secreted by the tumour cells is usually present in the blood and urine. Histologically, the architecture of this node is effaced and diffusely infiltrated by small B-lymphocytes and lymphoplasmacytic cells of varying grades of maturity. The lymphoplasmacytic cells are slightly larger than lymphocytes and many show evidence of plasma cell differentiation. Their nuclei are ovoid or round and more vesicular than in lymphocytes. Occasionally there are intranuclear Ig protrusions (from cytoplasm). There is also hyaline thickening of blood vessels. This section has been treated with specific antibody against IgM, and many neoplastic cells (with round nuclei and a 'clock-face' pattern of chromatin resembling that of mature plasma cells) contain IgM (thin arrow). Other cells with the same nuclear structure (thick arrow), and less-well-differentiated cells with large pale nuclei, have not reacted for IgM.

Indirect immunoperoxidase method for IgM ×850

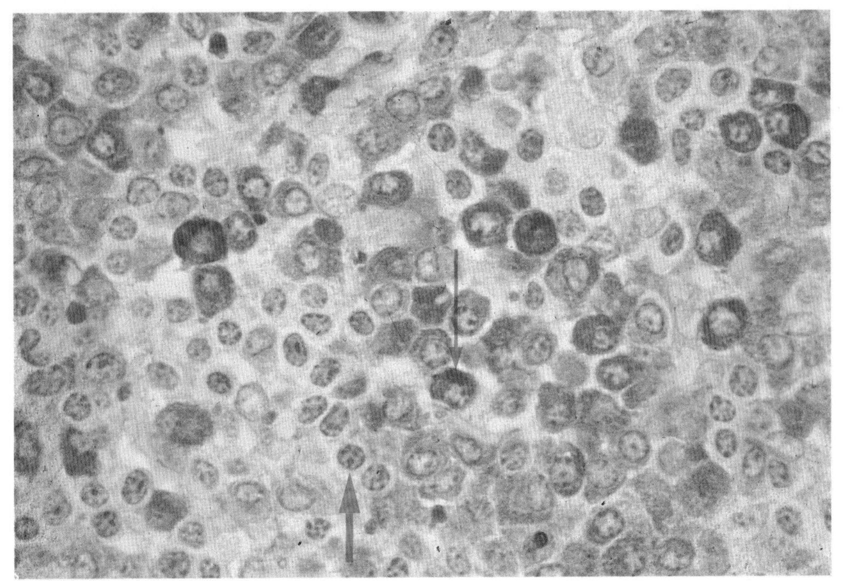

13.60 Multiple myeloma: marrow

Multiple myeloma is a malignant neoplasm of plasma cells which occurs in elderly patients. Their mean age is 60 years. The malignant cells usually arise in the hemopoietic bone marrow (vertebrae, skull, ribs, ends of long bones) and may spread to other sites. In the marrow they form nodules of soft red tissue which are osteolytic, destroying the bone lamellae and making visible, by the use of X-rays, characteristic 'punched-out' defects in the bone. Bone destruction may be very extensive. In this field, the hemopoietic tissue has been replaced by round or ovoid heavily stained neoplastic plasma cells which vary in their degree of differentiation. Most of them appear mature, with a clock-face nuclear chromatin pattern and abundant cytoplasm. The nucleus is typically located at one pole of the cell. The cytoplasm is well-defined and it has a purplish colour (arrow) produced by the large content of ribosomes. The ribosomes synthesize abnormal immunoglobulins (myeloma proteins) and a monoclonal protein is usually demonstrable in the serum &/or urine. HE ×335

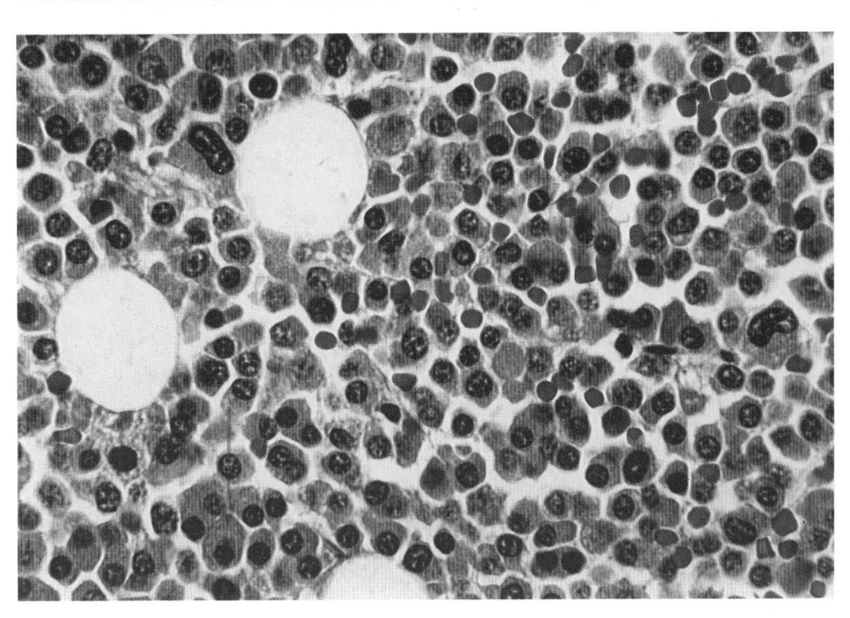

13.61 Extramedullary (solitary) plasmacytoma

Sometimes a single collection of plasma cells forms in the bone and occasionally in other (extramedullary) sites such as the lung and upper respiratory tract. The collection appears to be a solitary deposit and morphologically it resembles the lesions seen in multiple myeloma. Excision apparently effects a cure but multiple myeloma often develops subsequently in about two-thirds of the patients. Many of the neoplastic cells are recognizable as mature plasma cells, with polar location of the nucleus, a pale-staining halo adjacent to the nucleus (thin arrows), and a typical clock-face chromatin pattern in some of the nuclei. The more primitive cells (plasmablasts) have a large round or ovoid nucleus with a prominent nucleolus and relatively less cytoplasm (thick arrows). No mitoses are evident, a common feature of myelomatous deposits. To distinguish a plasmacytoma from a granuloma which contains an unusually large number of plasma cells, it may be necessary to determine whether the cells have a monoclonal origin. HE ×580

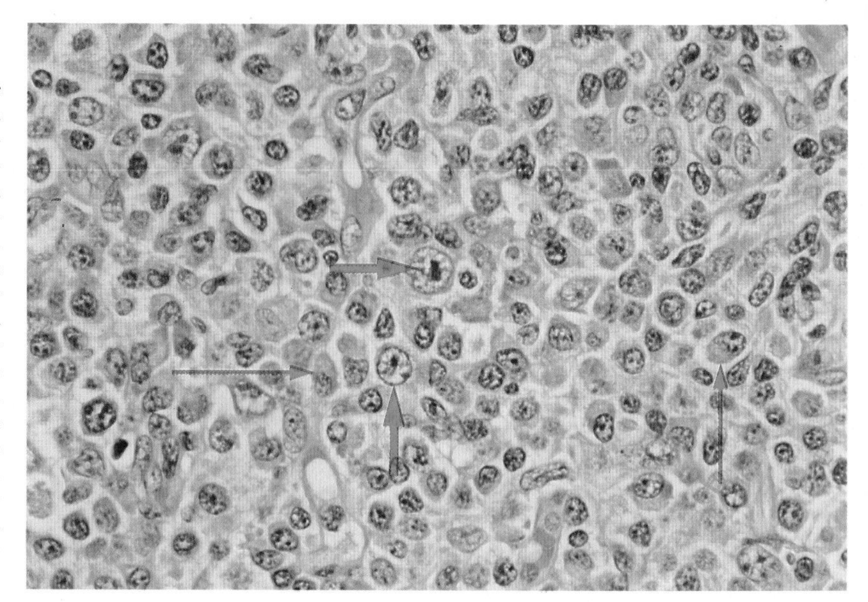

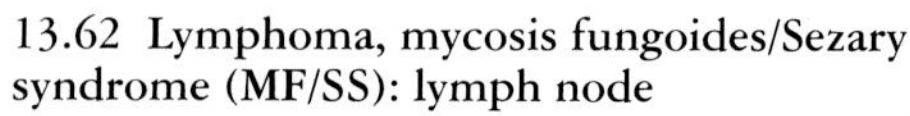

13.62 Lymphoma, mycosis fungoides/Sezary syndrome (MF/SS): lymph node

Sézary's syndrome produces skin lesions similar to those in mycosis fungoides with involvement of the lymph nodes, but there is in Sézary's syndrome also a leukemic blood picture. The cell of origin is the mature peripheral T cell, and Sézary cells have a distinctive morphology, particularly in smears of the peripheral blood. Affected lymph nodes are moderately enlarged and often rubbery. The paracortex of this node is infiltrated by large intermediate-size Sézary-type cells (resembling Lutzner cells) with their highly-convoluted (cerebriform) nuclei (double arrow), as well as small lymphocytes. The nuclear structure of the Sézary cells is reminiscent of that of centrocytes. The Sezary-cell nuclei are large pale vesicular and very convoluted, but the nuclear indentations are much more marked than in centrocytes. Several mitotic figures are present (thin arrows), and typically the Sézary cells are accompanied by large interdigitating reticulum cells with relatively abundant cytoplasm and a pale-staining nucleus (thick arrows). There are also prominent HEVs. HE ×580

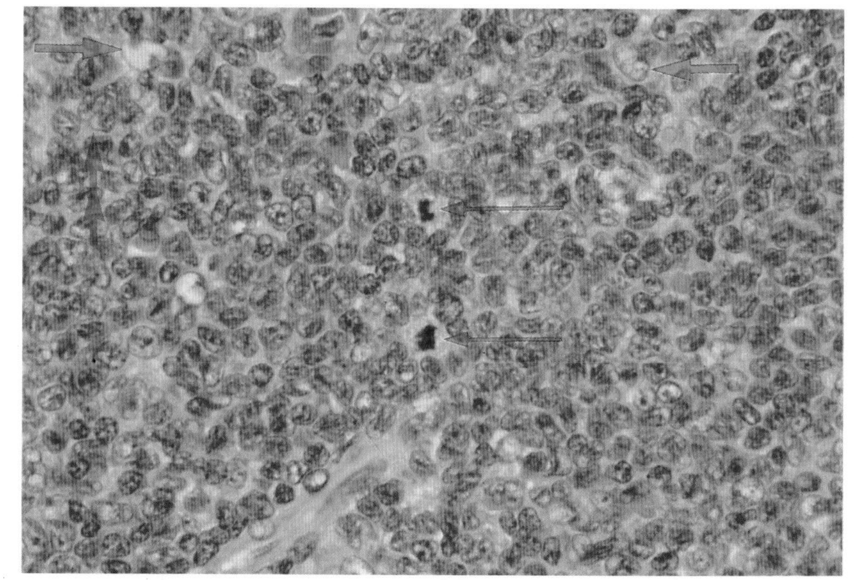

13.63 Chronic myeloid leukemia: marrow

Chronic myeloid leukemia affects mainly the middle-aged and elderly, and the number of leukocytes in the peripheral blood is often very large (300×10^9/l or more), most of them mature polymorphs. A more acute phase often develops eventually, with increase in the less mature forms. The liver and spleen are usually greatly enlarged. The normal red hemopoietic marrow is replaced by soft pale pink tissue which may appear almost pus-like. This tissue fills the medullary cavity and the bone trabeculae may be resorbed. The smear from this tissue consists of erythrocytes and cells of the granulocyte series. The cells of the granulocyte series including large promyelocytes with few cytoplasmic granules and large round or slightly indented nuclei (some containing multiple large nucleoli), myelocytes with round or ovoid nuclei and finely granular cytoplasm (thick arrows) (with one cell full of deeply basophil granules), metamyelocytes with indented nuclei (double arrow) and smaller neutrophil leukocytes with greatly lobulated nuclei (thin arrow).

Leishman's stain ×1200

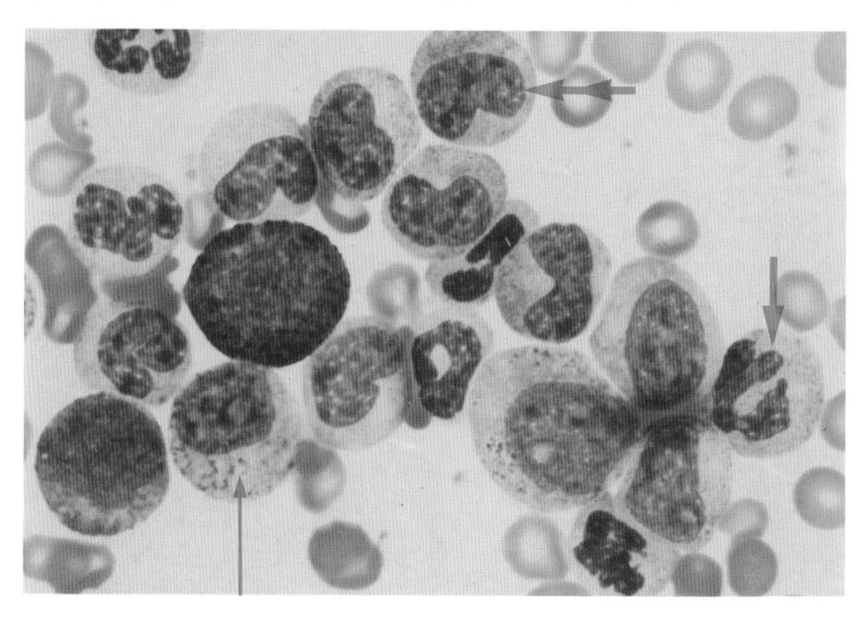

13.64 Chronic myeloid leukemia: spleen

The large size (3kg or more) of the spleen in chronic myeloid leukemia is frequently a source of considerable discomfort to the patient. The organ is firm, the cut surface pale and mottled, and pale infarcts are often present. There are also dilated congested blood vessels, in a sparsely cellular fibrous stroma. Organization of blood repeatedly extravasated from the congested splenic blood vessels tends to lead to the formation of deeply basophilic fibrous (siderotic) nodules (Gamna-Gandy bodies). The increase in size of the spleen is largely caused by the heavy diffuse infiltrate of immature myeloid cells in the red pulp of spleen, but extramedullary hemopoiesis is usually evident, in the form of non-leukemic erythroid cells and megakaryocytes. In this field, most of the myeloid cells are immature myelocytes with a large pleomorphic basophilic nucleus and a moderate amount of eosinophilic cytoplasm with well-defined boundaries (arrow). The other cells include normal erythroid precursors.

HE ×360

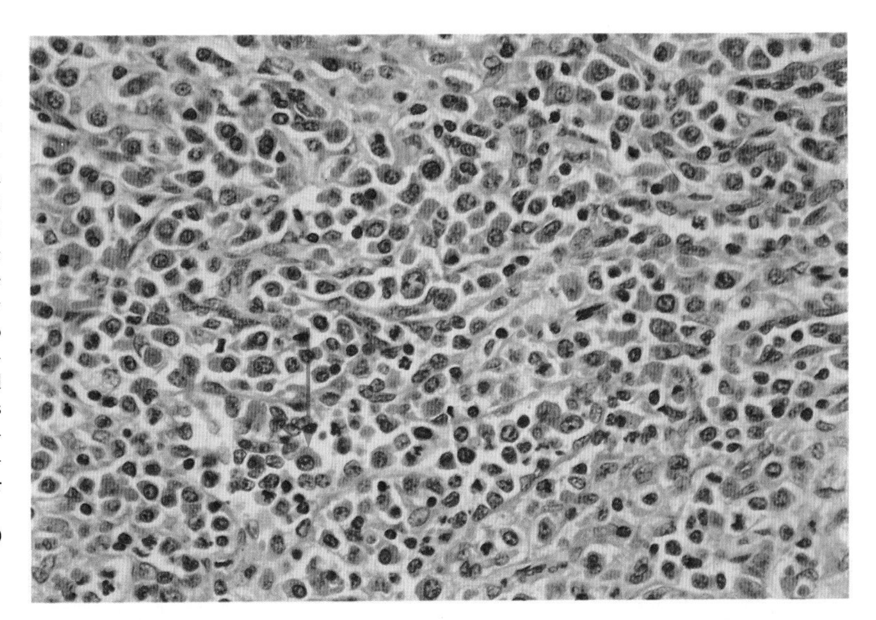

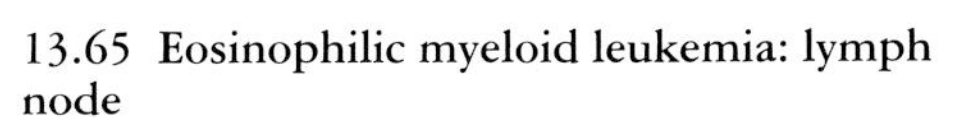

13.65 Eosinophilic myeloid leukemia: lymph node

In most cases of chronic myeloid leukemia, most of the cells in the peripheral blood are neutrophil leukocytes. Occasionally however eosinophil leukocytes are the dominant cell. Generalized lymphadenopathy may develop. and in the lymph nodes there is a diffuse infiltrate of leukemic eosinophil leukocytes in intrasinusoidal and paracortical tissues The presence of abundant eosinophilic granules in the leukocyte cytoplasm is evidence that the cells are mature and the leukemia is chronic. Also included usually are varying numbers of less mature leukemic cells, including myeloblasts (with large round or almost round vesicular nuclei), myelocytes (with smaller kidney-shaped nuclei) and metamyelocytes (with bilobed nuclei). In this lymph node from a man of 54 with eosinophilic leukemia, there is a dense infiltrate of round eosinophilic leukocytes, with abundant red-stained cytoplasm and an ovoid fairly inconspicuous nucleus (arrow). Less mature forms, with larger nuclei and paler cytoplasm, are also present. A trephine specimen of marrow showed that much of the hemopoietic tissue had been replaced by the same type of cellular infiltrate.

HE ×360

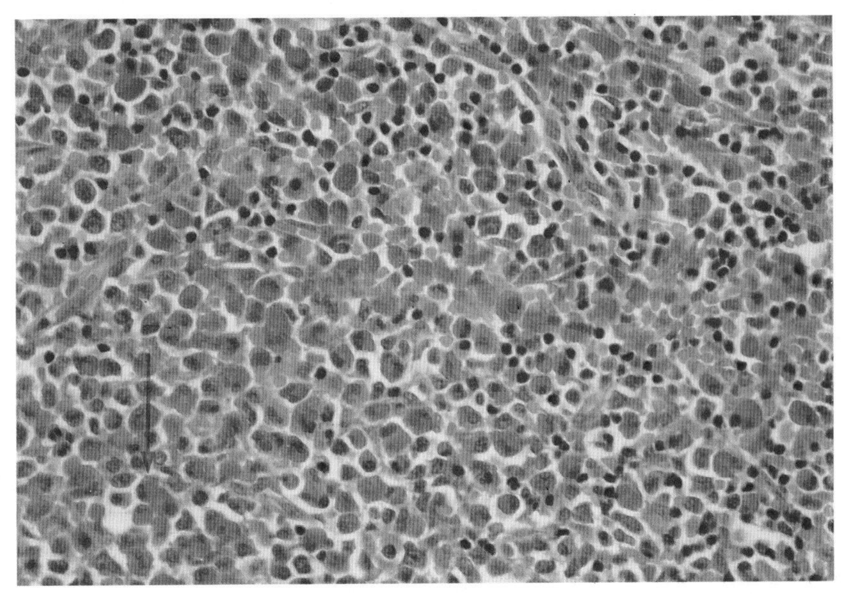

13.66 Acute myeloblastic leukemia: marrow

In acute leukemia the marrow is generally hypercellular from the presence of a diffuse infiltrate of leukemic cells (hypercellular pattern) which reduces and displaces normal hemopoietic elements. Sometimes however the pattern of the infiltrate, generally in the elderly, is hypocellular and the marrow predominantly fatty. The main clinical features are caused by failure of hemopoiesis with anemia, hemorrhage (from thrombocytopenia) and infection. In this field, the infiltrate consists of a compact sheet of closely packed uniform leukemic myeloblasts (thick arrows), large cells with a moderate amount of cytoplasm, a large round or oval nucleus (occasionally pyknotic) and small inconspicuous nucleoli. The myeloblasts have displaced the normal hemopoietic cells, including megakaryocytes. However the trabecula of bone is dense lamellar bone (thin arrow) and it shows no evidence of resorption.

HE ×120

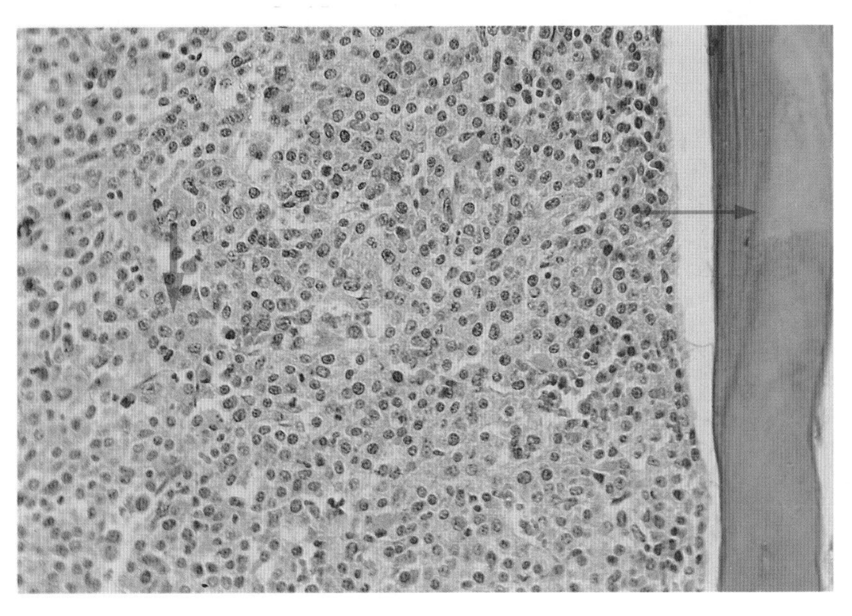

13.67 Monocytic leukemia: marrow

Monocytic leukemia originates in the marrow. It is a form of myeloid leukemia in which malignant monocytes are numerous in the blood, together with malignant granulocytes. It is uncommon. The morphology of the malignant cells is more uniform and infiltration of the bone marrow is usually more diffuse than in malignant histiocytosis. The leukemia is usually acute or subacute. Gingival hypertrophy is characteristic of acute monocytic leukemia. Monocytic leukemia infiltrates are relatively non-destructive. This is a trephine specimen of marrow from a woman of 55 who had acute leukemia of monocytic type. A bone trabecula is visible on the left. Closely applied to it and filling the medullary cavity is a solid sheet of large leukemic monocytoid cells, larger than leukemic myeloblasts, with fairly abundant cytoplasm and ovoid or indented vesicular nuclei (thin arrow). Several mitotic figures are present (thick arrows). There is a marked increase in reticulin in the marrow. Almost all the cells were shown to have lysozyme and cathepsin B in their cytoplasm. HE ×470

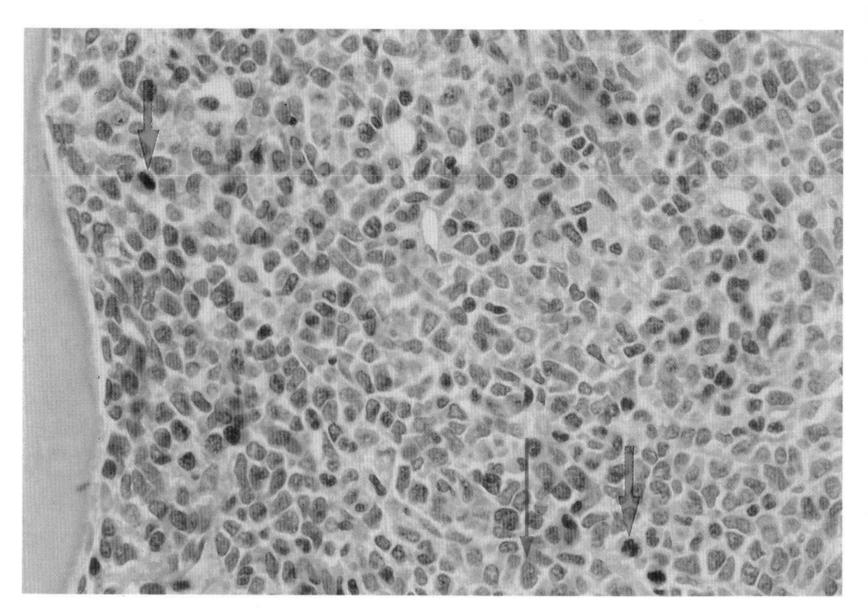

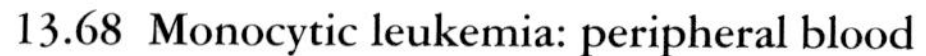

13.68 Monocytic leukemia: peripheral blood

Acute monocytic leukemia is type 5 in the French-American classification of acute myeloid leukemia. The total white cell count is not very high as a rule in monocytic leukemia, and most of the cells are monoblasts or monocytes. patients with acute monocytic leukemia have enlarged lymph nodes, leukemic infiltration of the gums and lesions in the skin, more often than in patients with other types of myeloid leukemia. On average the leukocyte count is $40\text{x}10^9$/litre in patients with acute monocytic leukemia (such a count is two to three times greater than the counts in acute myelomonocytic leukemia and acute myeloblastic leukemia). This is a smear of the peripheral blood, showing six characteristic malignant monocytes in the blood. As usual they are large cells, with a considerable amount of pale very finely granular cytoplasm (thick arrow) and a large irregular 'folded' nucleus (thin arrow). The cytoplasmic borders are irregular.

Leishman's stain ×1150

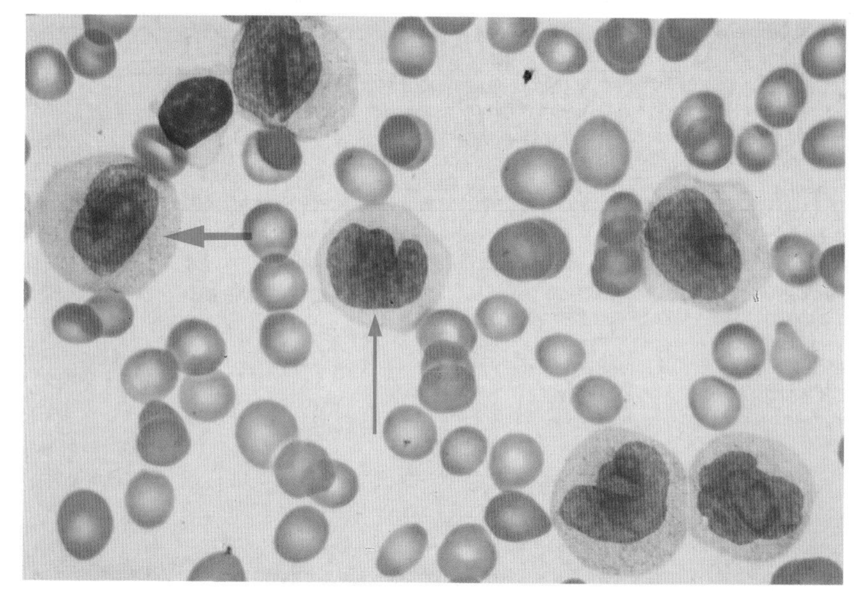

13.69 Histiocytic lymphoma: skin

The monocyte/macrophage system encompasses a wide range of cells of differing structure and function, and the term may cover a heterogeneous group of conditions. Moreover, non-neoplastic histiocytes are often present in large numbers in malignant lymphomas of lymphocytic origin. Histiocytic lymphomas have a greater tendency than other types of lymphoma to be located in tissues other than lymph nodes, such as the skin, alimentary system and skeleton, and this thin (1μm) resin-embedded section is from tissue taken from a purple cutaneous nodule. In this field there is a polymorphous infiltrate of large mature (possibly erythrophagocytic) histiocytes (thin arrows). They have a large amount of cytoplasm but their boundaries are ill-defined. Their nuclei are vesicular and pleomorphic, and many of them are elongated and some indented. Each nucleus possesses one or more prominent nucleoli (thick arrows).

HE ×360

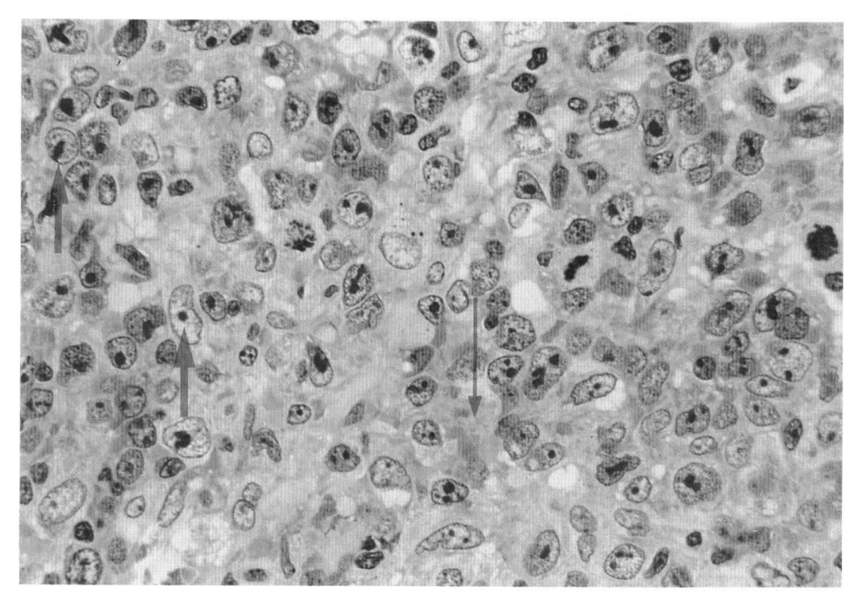

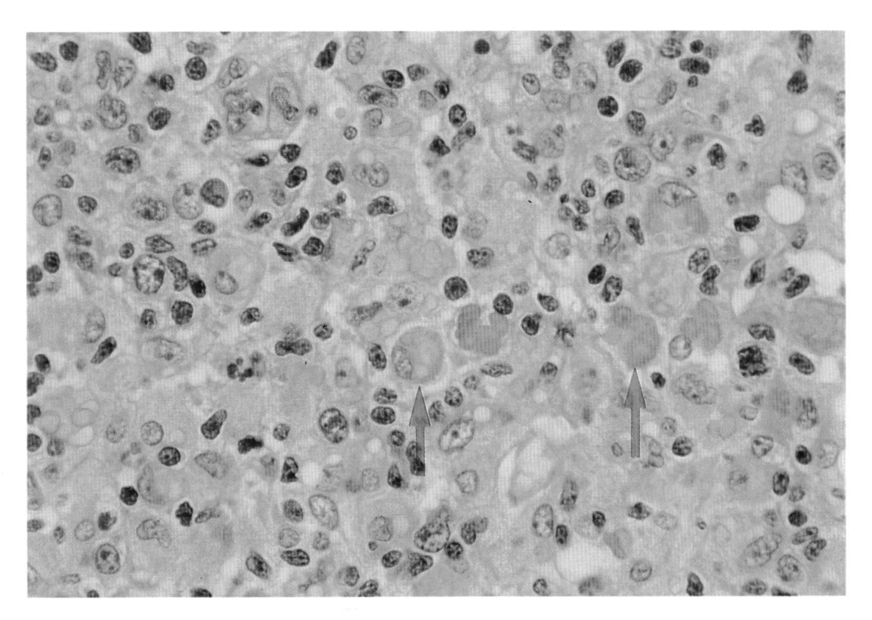

13.70 Malignant histiocytosis: lymph node

Malignant histiocytosis is a malignant and rapidly fatal lesion of the histiocytes of the bone marrow which usually spreads to lymph nodes, spleen and liver. It occurs at all ages and is commoner in males. In lymph nodes, as here, the malignant histiocytes are usually located, at least initially, within the lymphatic sinusoids. They frequently but not invariably phagocytose erythrocytes. In this field, there is a number of large atypical histiocytes with abundant cytoplasm, very pleomorphic pale vesicular nuclei and occasionally a prominent nucleolus. Some of the large histiocytes have a considerable amount of well defined eosinophilic cytoplasm in which there are many erythrocytes (thick arrow). The erythrocytes are being broken down, and many are pale and 'ghost-like'. At high magnification, remnants of erythrocytes could be detected in a high proportion of the other less-visible histiocytes.

Many conditions, classified as malignant histiocytosis, would now be better classified as T-cell non-Hodgkin's lymphoma. HE ×580

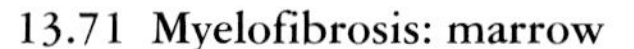

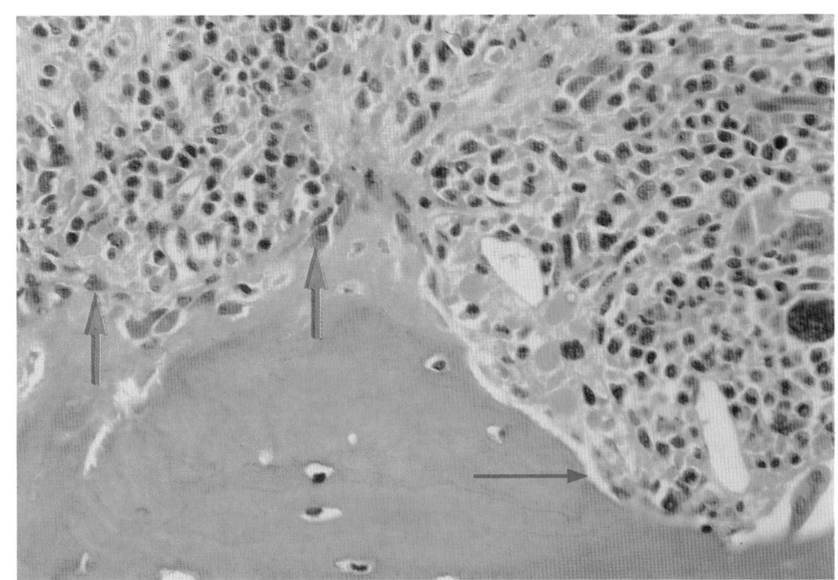

13.71 Myelofibrosis: marrow

Myelofibrosis develops in the older age group (over 50 years of age). It is probably reactive to an underlyng myeloproliferative disorder lesion, with increasing fibroblast activity in the hemopoietic marrow leading to the formation of a considerable amount of reticulin and collagen. Myelofibrosis may not be a primary disorder however, since chronic granulocytic leukemia (CGL) and polycythemia rubra vera also may transform to a myelofibrotic state. This is the marrow from a woman of 81. Histologically it was hypocellular, with hypercellular foci. This is one of the cellular areas. The cells are precursors of the granulocytic and erythrocytic series, and megakaryocytes are also present. Megakaryocytes were numerous elsewhere and many were structurally abnormal. There is however evidence of fibrosis, a stain for reticulin showing a very marked increase in reticulin throughout the marrow (myelofibrosis). The bone trabecula has been eroded at one point (thin arrow) and osteoblasts (thick arrows) are laying down osteoid and new bone. HE ×360

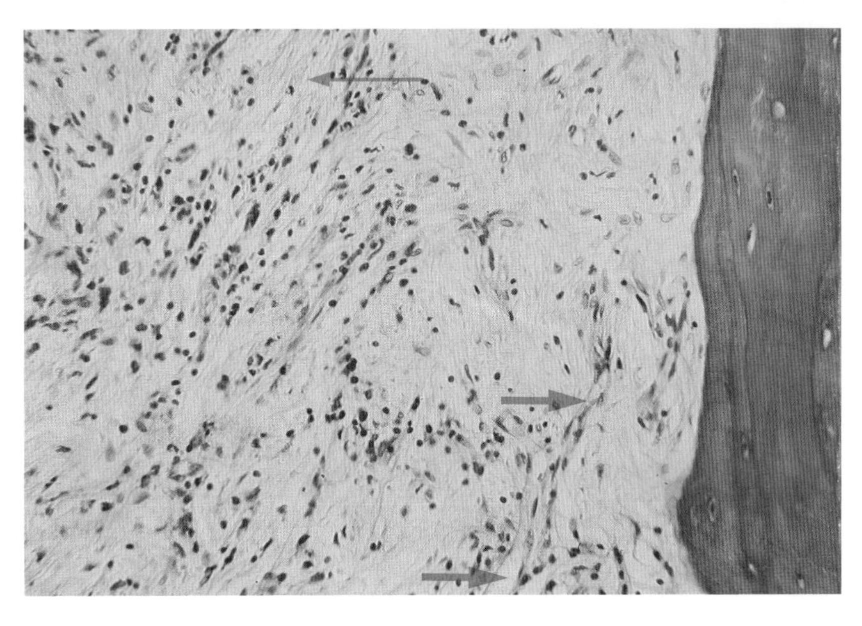

13.72 Myelofibrosis: marrow

In this field, the myeloproliferative lesion has now progressed to a late stage, the normal cellular hemopoietic tissue having been largely replaced by fibrous tissue. It is a fairly uniform sheet of pale fibrous tissue (thin arrow), scattered throughout which there is a scant population of cells of various types and sizes. In it there are also several dilated small blood vessels (thick arrows). At higher magnification, most of the cells can be identified as elongated fibroblasts, small round lymphocytes and larger plasma cells. No megakaryocytes can be detected. Formation of new bone trabeculae is sometimes a marked feature, and the term osteosclerosis is then applied. There was no increase in bone in this case however, the deeply eosinophilic bone trabecula at the right margin of the field being part of the normal spongy bone of the medullary cavity. The fibrosed state of the marrow usually leads to very active extramedullary hemopoiesis in the enlarged liver and spleen, the spleen in this case weighing 3kg. HE ×120

14.1 Epidermal cyst: skin

Epidermal cysts are situated in the dermis or subcutaneous tissue. They grow slowly to reach at most 5cm dia and elevate the overlying skin. They appear spontaneously as a rule, but may arise from epidermis transplanted into the deeper layers of the skin by trauma. This cyst (left) is filled with deeply eosinophilic laminated keratinous horny material and it is lined with true epidermis (stratified squamous epithelium) which, although stretched and thinned, has recognizable squamous, granular and keratinocyte layers (thin arrow). The wall of the cyst consists of a thick layer of collagenous fibrous tissue (double arrow). The sweat gland (thick arrow) outside the wall is a skin appendage and not related to the cyst. Epidermoid cysts are similar to epidermal cysts, benign, lined with stratified squamous epithelium and filled with keratin. They however are derived from embryonic remnants and usually located along the cerebrospinal axis, at sites such as the cerebellopontine angle, the surprasellar region and the lumbar region of the spinal cord (with spina bifida present). HE ×335

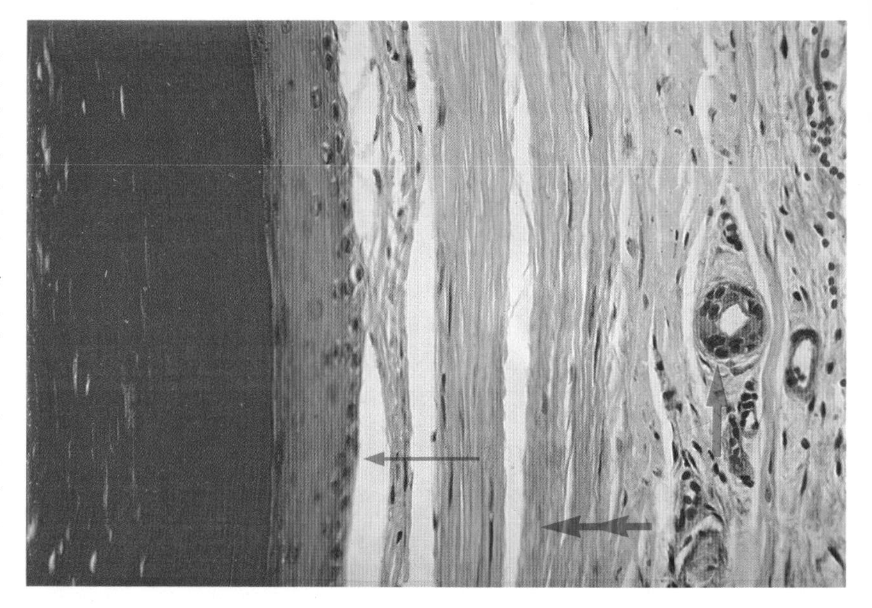

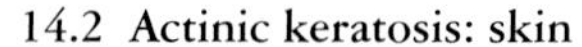

14.2 Actinic keratosis: skin

Actinic keratosis is a pre-malignant lesion which represents the effect on the skin of the ultraviolet component of sunlight. It occurs most frequently in fair-skinned people who have been exposed to sunlight, and particularly in countries such as Australia or southern USA. The lesions are present mainly in the skins of older individuals, but in tropical countries they may be found in older age groups. Actinic keratoses take the form of rough erythematous or brownish papules and are generally small or very small. Histologically there is dysplasia of the epidermis and degeneration of the dermal collagen (deeply eosinophilic 'elastosis'). In this lesion, there is pronounced hyperkeratosis and parakeratosis, with alternating columns of hyperkeratotic (thin arrow) and parakeratotic cells (thick arrows) on the surface. The granular layer of the epidermis is present in the hyperkeratotic area, but in the parakeratotic area it is absent, and the cells of the keratinocytic and basal layers show some dysplasia. There is an infiltrate of chronic inflammatory cell in the papillary dermis. HE ×190

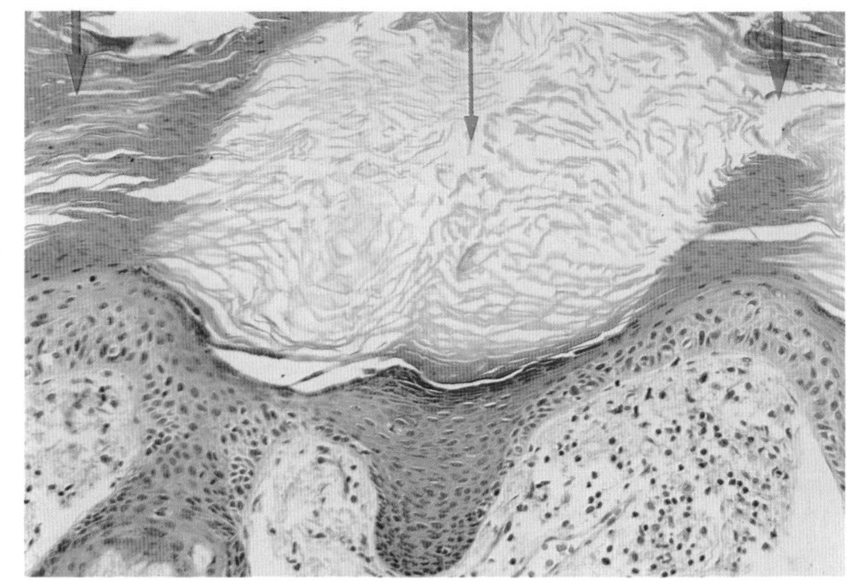

14.3 Radiodermatitis: skin

The total dose of ionizing radiation to the skin determines the severity of damage. After a few weeks of heavy exposure, the skin becomes erythematous and swollen, and cells desquamate from the epidermis (acute radiodermatitis). A therapeutic dose produces an almost immediate acute reaction and very different effects later; and after a long period, even fairly small doses may produce effects. In contrast, chronic radiodermatitis, which may persist for years, is characterized by atrophy of the epidermis, atypia of the epithelial cells, dermal fibrosis and development of telangiectasias and hyalinization of vessels. This patient had received therapeutic X-irradiation to the arm 6 months previously. The epidermis is hyperplastic and the surface markedly hyperkeratotic (double arrow), and the rete ridges are narrow, elongated and irregular (thick arrow). The normal dermis and its appendages have been destroyed and replaced by fibrous connective tissue in which there are many widely dilated blood and lymphatic vessels (telangiectasis). There is a scant population of chronic inflammatory cells and fibroblasts in the upper dermis (thin arrow) but the deeper collagenous tissue is practically acellular. HE ×120

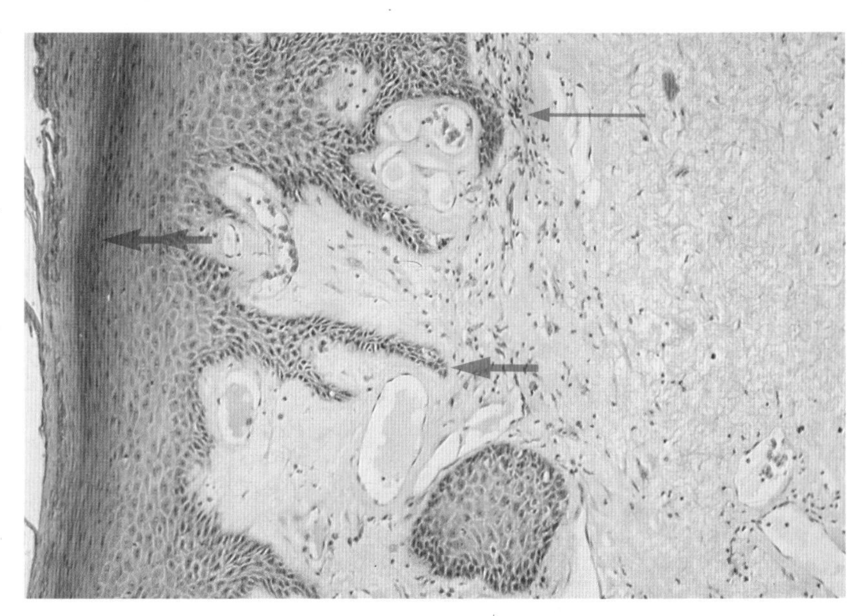

14.4 Pilonidal (piliferous) cyst

A pilonidal (piliferous) cyst is a sacrococcygeal dermoid cyst or sinus which contains hairs or fragments of hair and opens at a post-anal dimple in the sacral region. The hairs can drive fragments of epidermis through the epidermis into the dermis and subcutaneous tissues, where they may form epidermoid (inclusion) cysts. This is probably also the mechanism which leads to the formation of a pilonidal sinus. Sometimes lesions of this type occur in hairdressers and in individuals who habitually clip the hair of dogs. This is a section of the wall of such a sinus. The sinus is lined by a sheet of epidermis, of varying thickness, and the lumen is filled with many hairs (cut in cross-section) (thick arrow) and cell debris (double arrow). The wall of the sinus consists of a layer of vascular and highly cellular connective (thin arrow), infiltrated by chronic inflammatory cells. Elsewhere the sheet of epithelial cells lining the sinus has broken; and the hairs, desquamated cells and bacteria in the sinus have excited an acute inflammatory reaction in the surrounding tissues. HE ×150

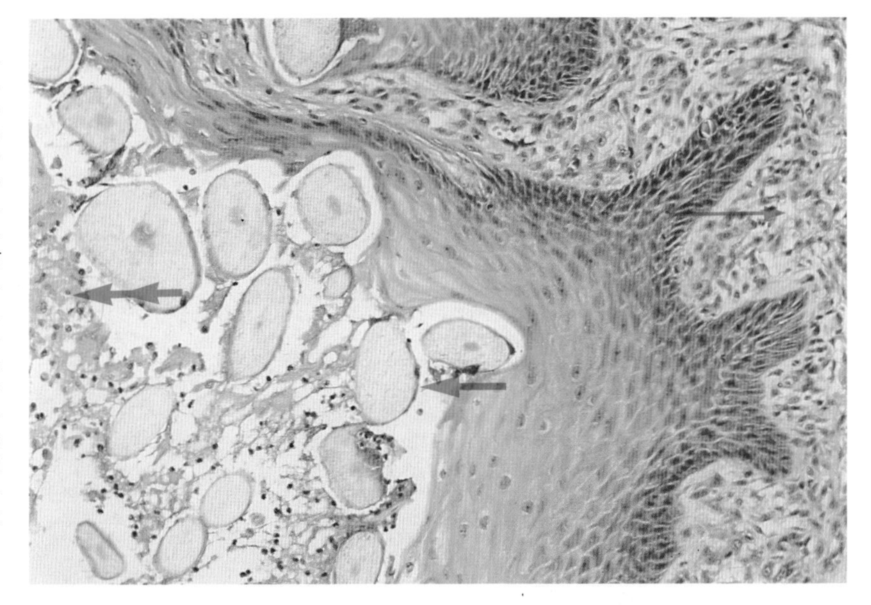

14.5 Keloid: skin

When a focus of dermal connective tissue becomes overactive and produces excessive amounts of collagen in a healing wound, it leads to the formation of abnormal nodular masses of collagen at the sites where skin is injured. The lesion is a keloid, an irregularly contracted skin nodule. Some individuals are prone to keloid formation, and attempts to remove a keloid not infrequently induce recurrence. This keloid is in a healed wound of skin. It consists of a sheet very large eosinophilic hyalinized collagenous fibres (thin arrow). The collagenous fibres are much broader than normal collagen fibres, and the margins of the fibres are irregular and ill-defined, appearing to merge with the cellular tissue between the fibres. The cellular tissue between the collagenous fibres consists of numerous unusually large fibroblasts (thick arrows) with elongated hyperchromatic spindle-shaped nuclei. In comparison with normal fibroblasts, the fibroblasts in the keloid are typically greatly hypertrophied, and most of them are also markedly elongated. Some tend to be irregular in shape however or even stellate. HE ×150

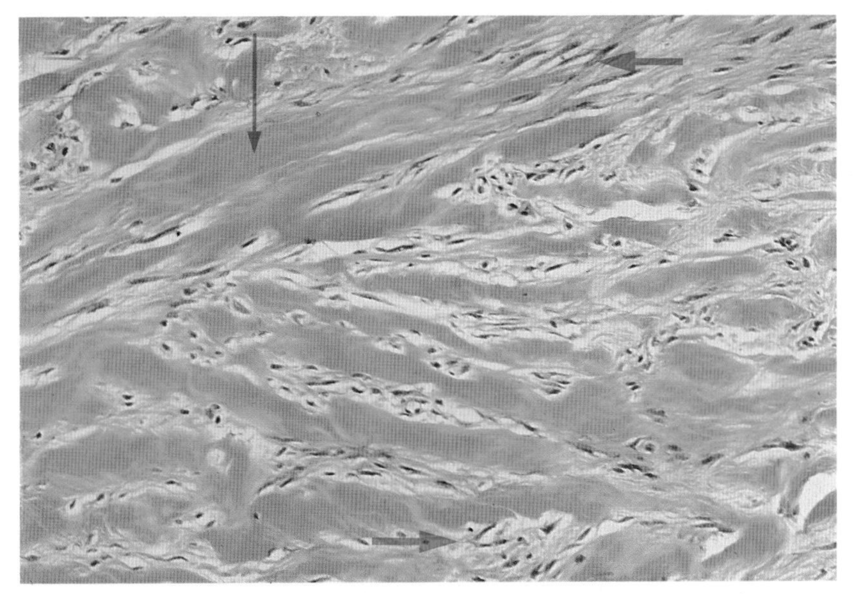

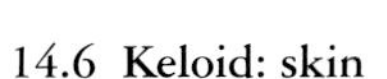

14.6 Keloid: skin

Keloids often arise in minor wounds of skin, and when a keloid is excised for cosmetic reasons, an even larger amount of new keloid may form. Keloid formation tends to occur more frequently in blacks and exhibits a familial tendency. However there is no recognizable single-gene inheritance pattern. The etiology of keloid formation is not known. This is part of the same keloid as in 14.5. It is composed of large fibroblasts (arrow), several times the length of a normal fibroblast and surrounded by very broad bands of eosinophilic collagenous connective tissue fibres. The fibroblasts also have remarkably large vesicular nuclei with rounded (blunt) ends, and in most of the nuclei there are one or more fairly prominent nucleoli. The nuclear chromatin is pale and very finely granular. Whereas the cellularity of ordinary scars grows less in time, a keloid usually retains its population of fibroblasts and they often become triangular in shape. HE ×360

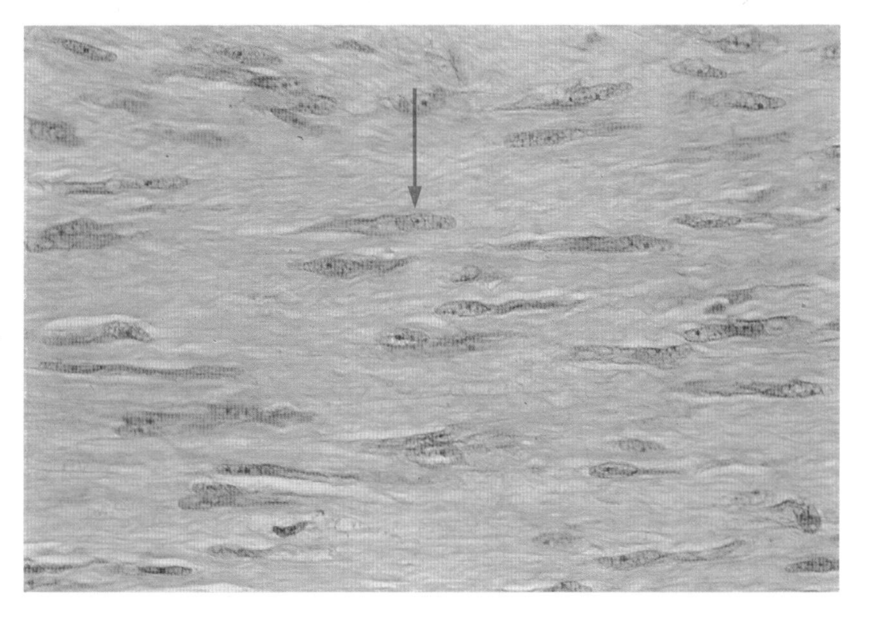

14.7 Secondary syphilis: skin

Syphilis is caused by *Treponema pallidum* The skin is often involved in secondary syphilis and occasionally in the tertiary form. In the secondary stage, a large range of skin rashes may develop, the plaque called *Condyloma latum* representing a specific skin lesion of secondary syphilis occurring in the anogenital region as a large moist papule. The histological changes in the skin are equally variable, and although plasma cells tend to be numerous and obliterative endarteritis is present, the appearances are not specific for syphilis. This is a biopsy specimen of skin from the right upper arm of man of 50 who was suspected clinically of having secondary syphilis. The epidermis is hyperkeratotic (thin arrow), but otherwise the structure of the epidermis and the upper dermis shows little change. The deeper dermis and subcutaneous tissues however are heavily infiltrated with chronic inflammatory cells (double arrows). The cellular infiltrate is concentrated around the blood vessels and the skin appendages. The walls of the small vessels are thickened (thick arrows). HE ×80

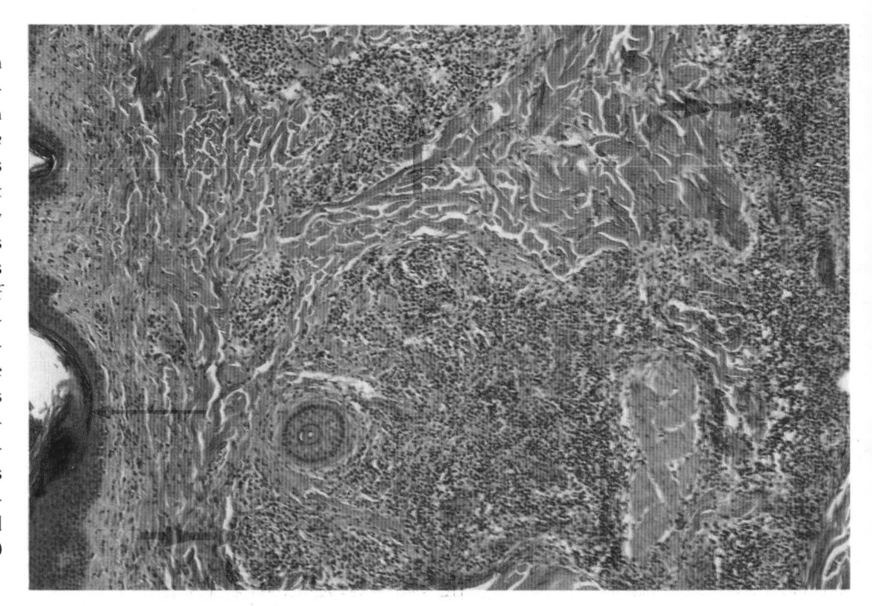

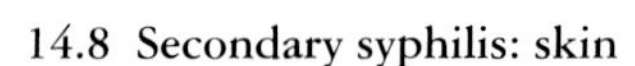

14.8 Secondary syphilis: skin

The skin is nearly always involved in secondary syphilis, with lesions such as pink macules and red papules, and mucosal lesions (mucous patches or 'snail tracks') around orifices such as the mouth, vulva etc. frequently develop. In almost patients some of the lymph nodes throughout the body are enlarged, and involvement of hair follicles often causes patchy loss of hair. The serous exudate from the broad moist flat *Condylomata lata* plaques in the anogenital region contains large numbers of treponemes and is highly infectious. This histological section however is part of same cutaneous lesion as in 14.7, at higher magnification. It shows an area of the fibrous connective tissue (double arrow) in the deeper dermis which is infiltrated with large numbers of chronic inflammatory cells of various types. Many of the cells are plasma cells (thin arrow), but there are also a considerable number of lymphocytes (thick arrow), fewer histiocytes and occasional neutrophils. HE ×360

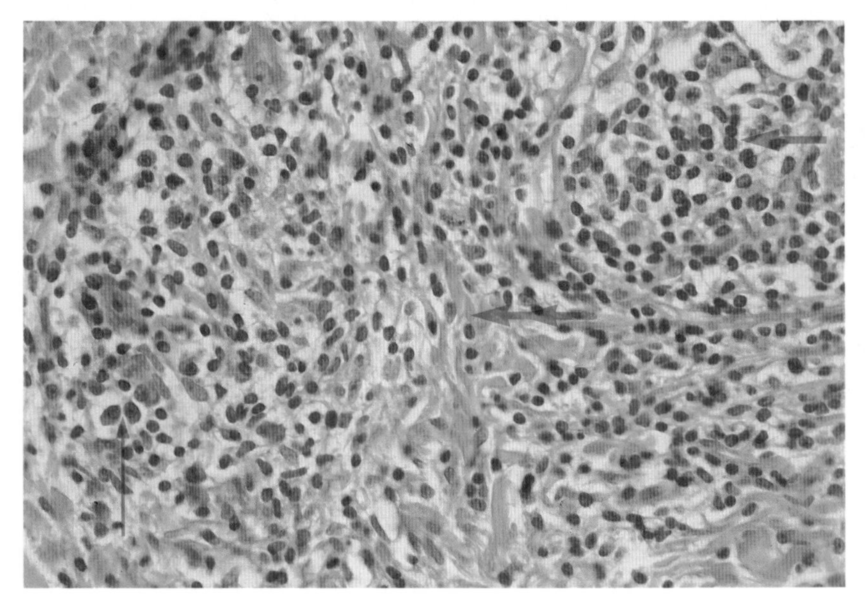

14.9 Tertiary syphilis: skin

The diseases that begin in the latent phase of tertiary syphilis affect a wide range of organs and tissues, such as the cardiovascular system, the eyes, the nervous system or other sites. Cardiovascular syphilis causes arteritis in small muscular arteries, and damage to the media of the aorta causes ectasia of the proximal part of the vessel. Neurosyphilis includes meningovascular syphilis, tabes dorsalis and general paresis of the insane. The disease in this case is affecting the skin and it is a late-stage tertiary lesion. Histologically, the epidermis is hyperplastic and its surface is covered with a thick layer of eosinophilic keratin (thin arrow). The most striking feature of the cutaneous lesion however is the very marked fibrosis of the dermis and adjoining subcutaneous tissue, along with considerable loss of the skin appendages. The dermal connective tissue is fibrous but also vascular (thick arrow) and fairly cellular, with sparse lymphocytes (double arrow) distributed throughout it. There is no infiltrate however of chronic inflammatory cells similar to that in secondary-stage skin lesions. HE ×120

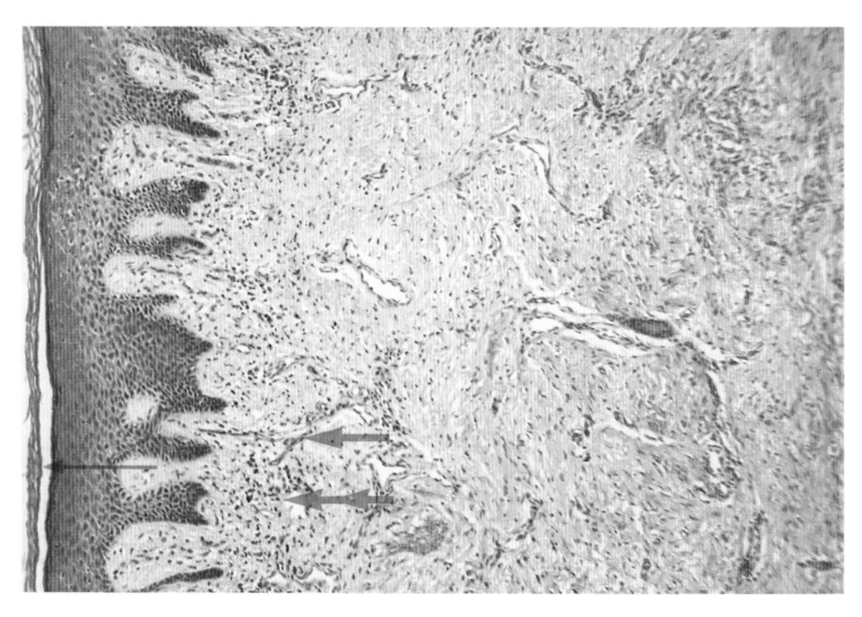

14.10 Sarcoidosis (Kveim test): skin

Sarcoidosis is a systemic disease characterized by the presence of noninfectious epithelioid cell granulomas in many tissues, especially lung, liver, lymph nodes and skin. Histologically the sarcoid granulomas look similar to the granulomas in tuberculosis but they do not undergo caseous necrosis in the same way as tuberculous granulomas do. Sarcoid granulomas often contain calcified (Schaumann) bodies but they are not specific for sarcoidosis. In the Kveim test for sarcoidosis, a sterilized suspension of sarcoid tissue is injected intradermally; and after 6-12 weeks the site of inoculation is excised and examined histologically. This is a positive result in a woman of 37, with two follicular granulomas in the dermis. The granulomas are composed of epithelioid cells (thin arrow), Langhans-type multinucleated giant cells (thick arrows) and small lymphocytes. The overlying epidermis is stretched but intact. It is essential that the material for the test be injected into the dermis and not into the fat of the subcutaneous tissues. Otherwise a granulomatous response to necrotic fat may give a false positive result. HE ×360

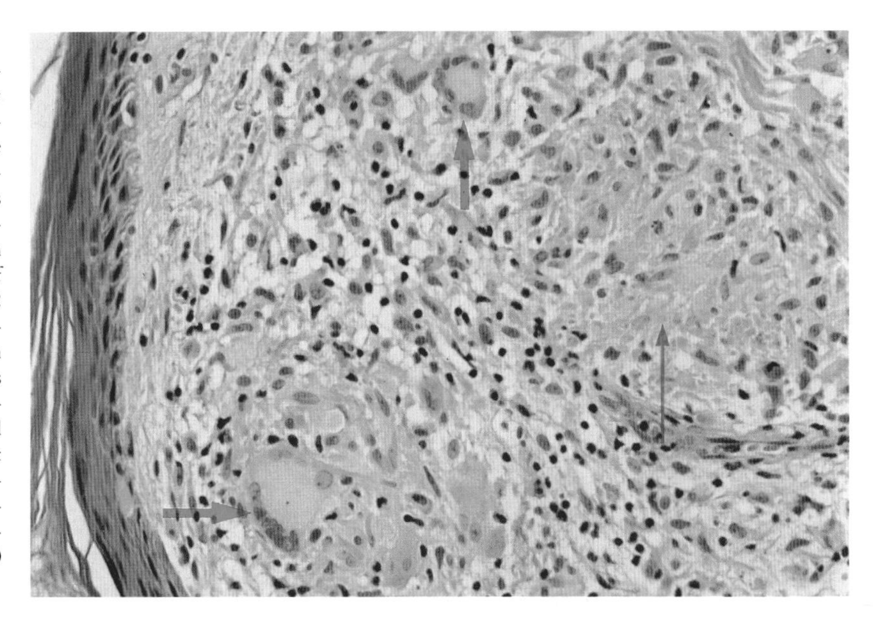

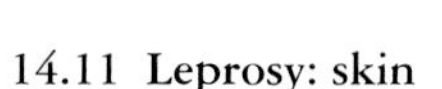

14.11 Leprosy: skin

Leprosy is a common disease in tropical countries. It is caused by *Mycobacterium leprae*, an acid-fast bacillus that has not been grown on artificial media. The behaviour of leprosy depends on the immunological reactivity of the host to the leprosy bacillus. When the host has a low level of cellular immunity, nodular lesions containing very large numbers of bacteria form in many tissues (lepromatous leprosy). When resistance is high, a follicular granulomatous reaction takes place, confined to the skin and peripheral nerves (tuberculoid leprosy). Some individuals have manifestations of both types of reaction. This is an example of lepromatous leprosy in the skin. The dermis is packed with large macrophages (thin arrows) with pale ovoid vesicular nuclei, finely granular chromatin and sometimes a prominent nucleolus. The macrophages have a considerable amount of fairly basophilic cytoplasm which is both granular and vacuolated, and in some of the vacuoles there are small dark-staining round bodies (thick arrows). These bodies are aggregates of lepra bacilli. Small lymphocytes are present and also several polymorphs. There is no necrosis or fibrosis. HE ×360

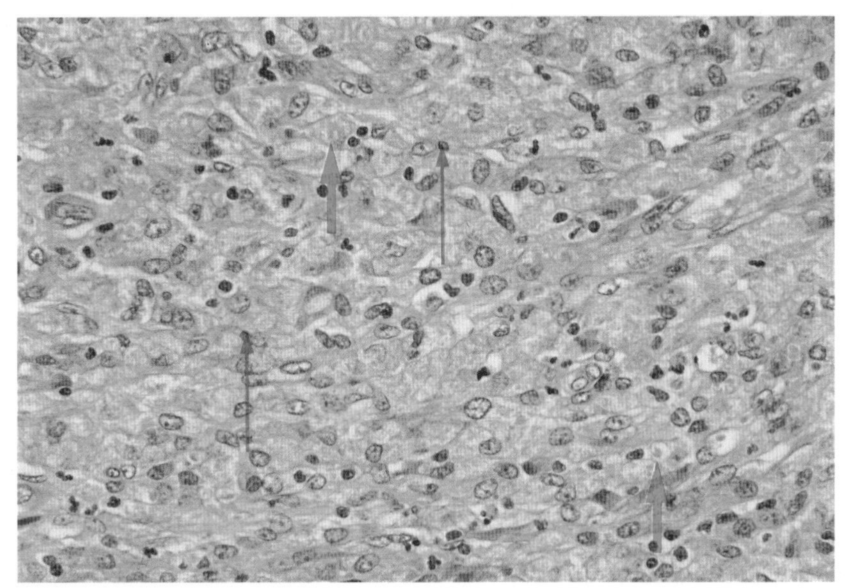

14.12 Lepromatous leprosy: skin

Lepromatous leprosy is a serious disease that causes extensive destruction of tissue, disfiguring the fingers, nose and ears. The bacillus also spreads widely by the bloodstream, and there are often lesions in the skin, eye, upper respiratory tract and testis. In the absence of an effective T cell response, the leprosy bacillus multiplies unchecked in skin macrophages, to form large foamy lepra cells. This lesion includes a small nerve and part of a larger nerve in the subcutaneous tissues, separated by a wavy band of dense fibrous tissue (double arrow). Both nerves are very swollen from the presence of large numbers of foamy macrophages (thin arrows) with heavily vacuolated cytoplasm. These cells are laden with lepra bacilli and they have no tendency to form granulomas. Clumps of bacilli are visible in some vacuoles (thick arrow), and acid-fast staining would effectively reveal very large numbers of leprosy bacilli in the cytoplasm of the macrophages. Superficial nerves are often extensively involved in this way, but anaesthesia and paralysis are often late features of lepromatous leprosy, unlike tuberculoid leprosy where they are usually early manifestations. HE ×235

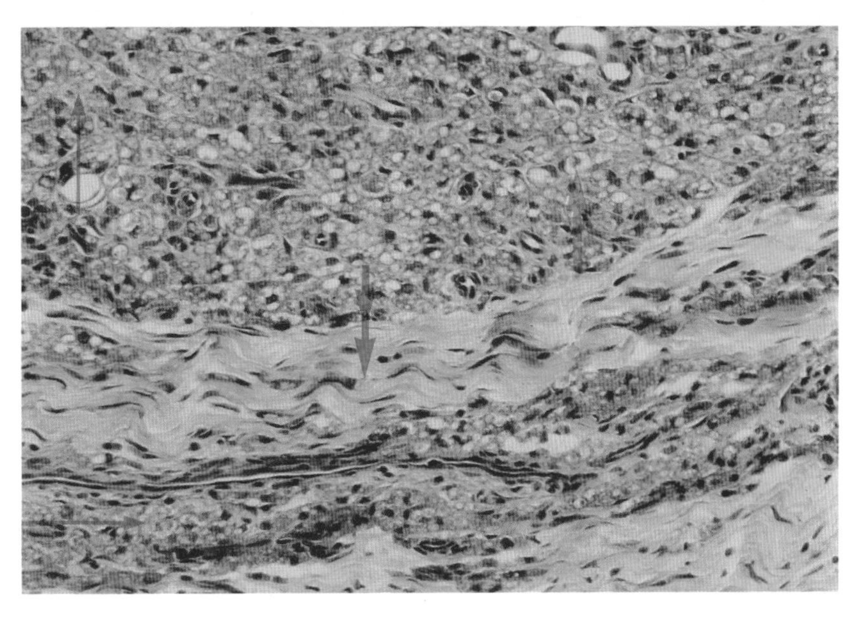

14.13 Onchocerciasis: skin

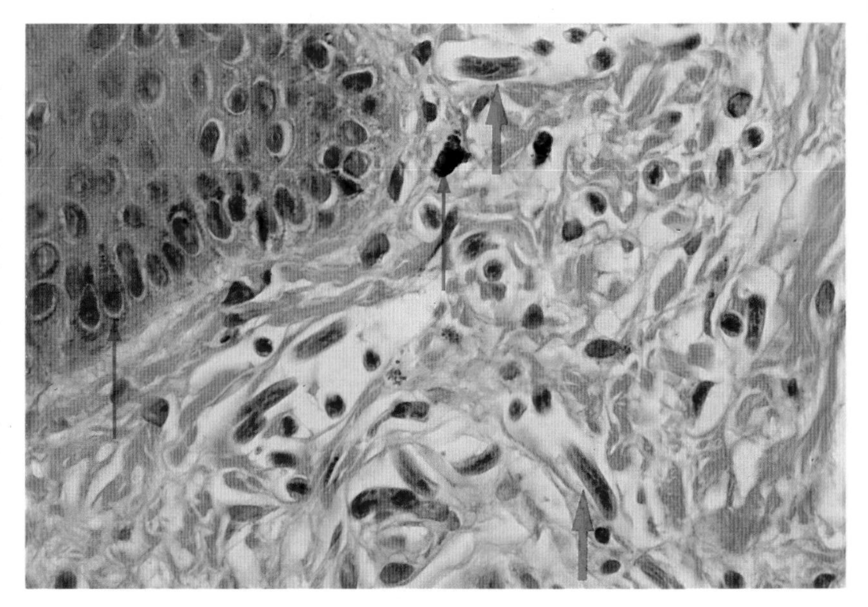

In Onchocerciasis (see 3.58), also called river blindness, microfilariae migrate into the adjacent dermis from the subcutaneous nodules (onchocercomas) which contain the adult worms (*Onchocerca volvulus*). This is the skin adjacent to a subcutaneous nodule. The normal-looking epidermis has been sectioned obliquely, and the epithelial cells of the basal layer contain granules of dark brown pigment (melanin) (thin arrows). There are also scattered melanin-laden macrophages in the dermis. Present in the dermis are numerous elongated very slender microfilariae (thick arrows), sectioned obliquely into short lengths (in the preparation of the histological section only a few microns thick). The microfilariae are within dilated channels, which are almost certainly dermal lymphatics. There is also evidence of edema in the dermis, and it has separated the eosinophilic collagenous fibres. Migration of the microfilariae irritates the skin, but initially they excite little reaction. However, as they die, they attract first neutrophils, then eosinophils, lymphocytes, plasma cells and macrophages. The epidermis becomes thickened and then atrophic. HE ×580

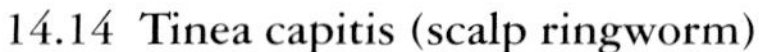

14.14 Tinea capitis (scalp ringworm)

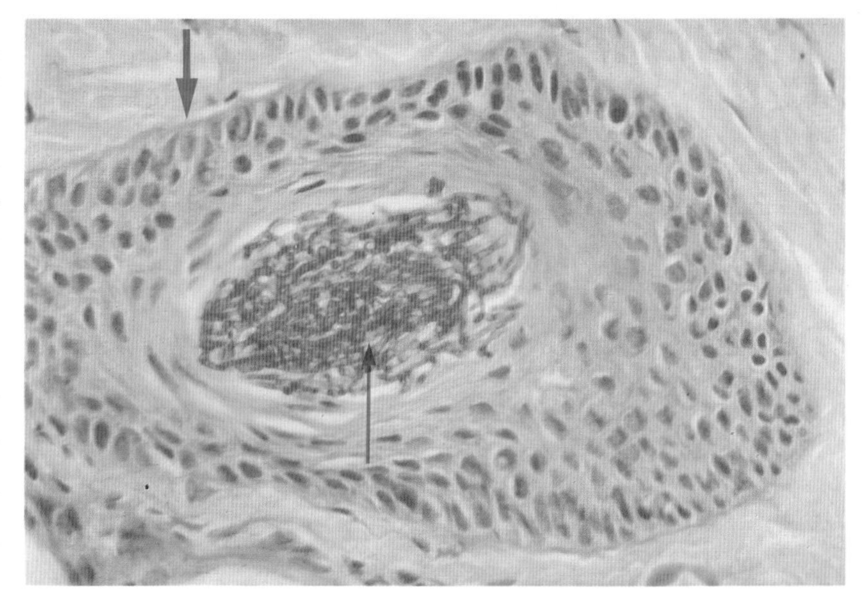

Ringworm of the scalp (*Tinea capitis*) is an infection of the hairs of the scalp, eyebrows or eyelashes with one of the two species of the fungus, Microsporum or Trichophyton. In the tropics, the fungus *Microsporon audouini* is often identified. The disease is commonest in children. A papule forms around an infected hair, and in a few days it becomes pale and scaly. The fungus invades the shafts of the hairs down to the zone of keratin formation, above the hair bulb, but does not invade the living cells of the hair bulb. The hairs become dull, the diseased hair shafts are fragile, and they break off close to the skin. The infected keratin remains in the follicle. The lesion enlarges as the fungus extends radially in the keratin, infecting new hairs. Plucking the hairs does not therefore effect a cure. This is a histological section of a hair follicle, surrounded by thin basement membrane (thick arrow) stained a weak purplish-red colour by the periodic acid-Schiff (PAS) method. In the centre of the follicle, the keratin of the hair shaft has been destroyed and replaced by a tangled mass of purplish-red (strongly PAS-positive) filamentous hyphae (thin arrow). PAS ×335

14.15 Molluscum contagiosum: skin

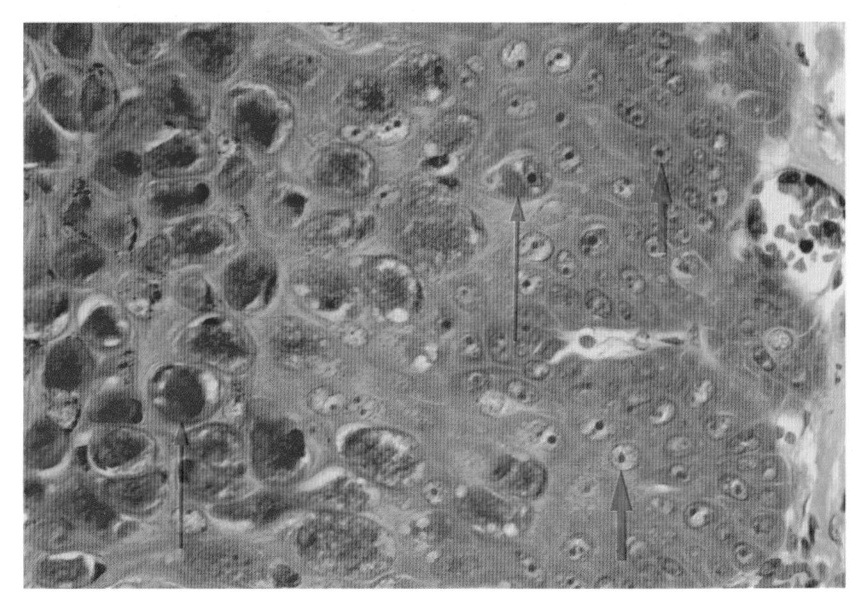

Molluscum contagiosum is caused by a virus of the poxvirus group. The lesions that form in the skin consist of small discrete dome-shaped nodules, each with an umbilicated centre. They eventually heal spontaneously, after several months. This histological section is from a nodule on the forehead of a woman aged 52. It is a flask-shaped lesion, and this shows part of the wall of the 'flask', in contact with the dermal connective tissue at the right margin. The lumen of the 'flask' is just out sight on the left. The wall of the flask-shaped lesion is a sheet of epithelial cells in the thickened epidermis. In the cytoplasm of each of the more superficial keratinocytes (left half), there is a very large round eosinophilic homogeneous inclusion (thin arrows). The nuclei in the infected cells are flat and pushed to one side of the cell by the inclusion. The inclusions are aggregates of elementary bodies of the virus, but the very much smaller round eosinophilic bodies (thick arrows) in the nuclei of the keratinocytes deeper in the epidermis and in the basal epithelial cells are nucleoli and not viral inclusions. HE ×360

14.16 Varicella (chickenpox): skin

Chickenpox is a common infection in childhood. After an attack in childhood, the varicella virus (also called varicella-zoster virus) may remain dormant in dorsal ganglia for as long as forty years after the initial illness and then become manifest in zoster (shingles). The virus enters via the respiratory tract and disseminates after an incubation period of 13-17 days. The varicella virus localizes mainly in the skin, where it produces vesicles (blisters). Histologically, the nuclei of the keratinocytes to become hyperchromatic and the cytoplasm to swell (balloon degeneration). Cells affected in this way eventually die but the cell walls tend to remain, to become a latticework within the vesicle that forms in the epidermis (reticular degeneration). This is the margin of an intraepidermal vesicle, part of which is visible on the right (thin arrow). The keratinocytes adjacent to the vesicle are swollen. Their cytoplasm is very edematous and pale-staining (thick arrow) (balloon degeneration), and in several cells large vacuoles have formed. The nuclei of the affected keratinocytes are also enlarged and some are hyperchromatic. HE ×480

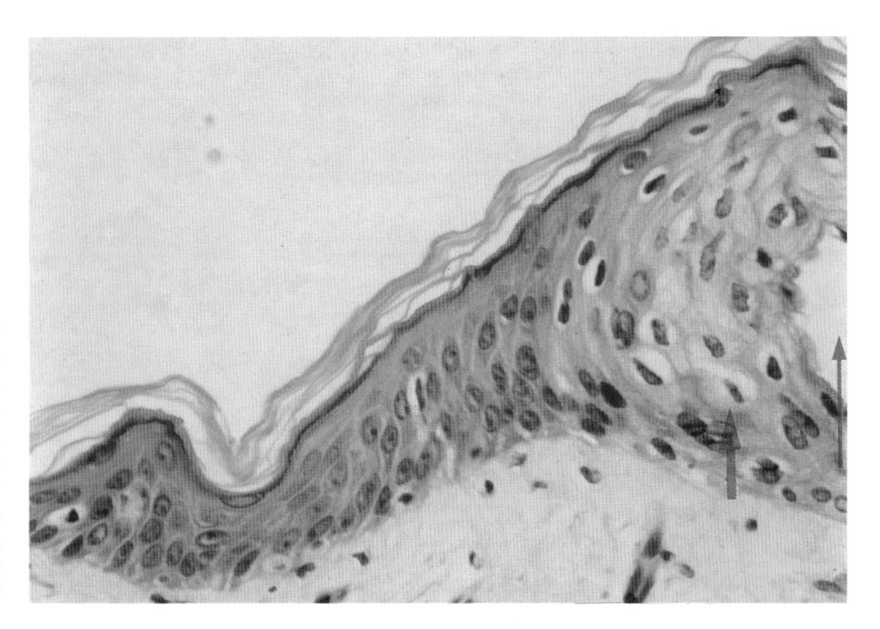

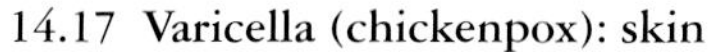

14.17 Varicella (chickenpox): skin

Chickenpox is highly contagious, the virus probably being carried, on droplets or dust, from the patient to a new host. The rash in chickenpox begins in the first day of pyrexia and progresses rapidly to form vesicles throughout the body. It is usually a mild self-limiting disease, but for three or four days successive crops of tense thin-walled vesicles continue to appear. Subsequent complications may include corneal lesions (impairing vision), pneumonia, encephalitis and especially disseminated disease (in immunodeficient individuals). This is part of the same lesion as in **14.16**. It shows the top of a fully-formed vesicle within the epidermis. The keratinized surface is still intact (double arrow), and part of the lumen is visible at the bottom margin. Practically all the keratinocytes are rounded-up and swollen (balloon cells), those lying within the lumen of the vesicle (thin arrow) showing the most severe changes. The nuclei in most of the cells are pleomorphic and hyperchromatic (thick arrows). Changes similar to those shown here are also liable to occur in herpes simplex and herpes zoster.

HE ×830

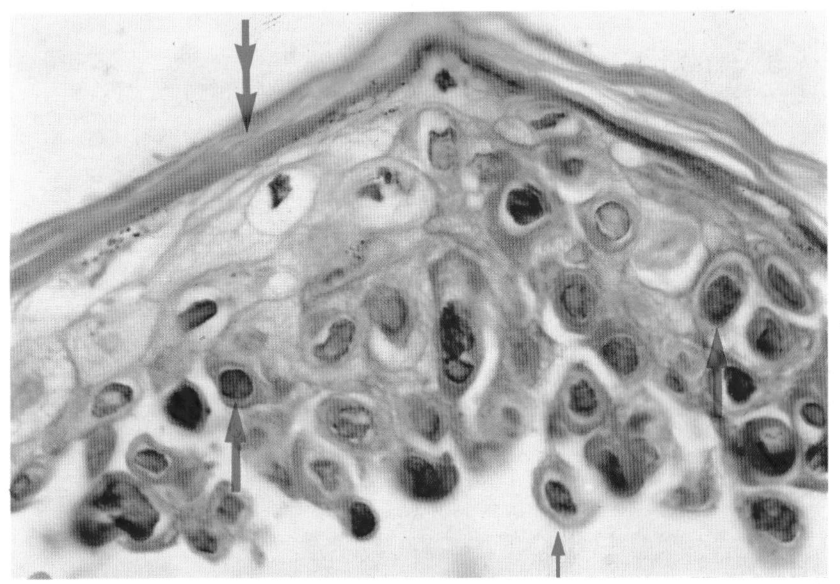

14.18 Herpes zoster (Shingles): skin

Herpes zoster (shingles) is caused by same (varicella-zoster) virus as in chickenpox. The strain of virus is different, but the tissue reactions are very similar in both diseases. The virus reaches sensory ganglia during an attack of chickenpox and after remaining dormant for long periods, becomes active in individuals over 50 years of age to initiate herpes zoster. This shows the base of an intraepidermal vesicle in herpes zoster. All the remaining cells of the epidermis are degenerate, and most of the cells have no nucleus or shrunken pyknotic nuclei and eosinophilic cytoplasm. Many rounded balloon cells are present, some in the lumen (thin arrows). Degenerate cells and cell debris form a network (double arrow) in the lumen, the cell walls of necrotic keratinocytes tending to adhere to each other, to form strands traversing the vesicle (reticular degeneration). The small blood vessels in the underlying dermis are dilated (thick arrow) and there is infiltration of the dermis by polymorph leukocytes (bottom left). HE ×320

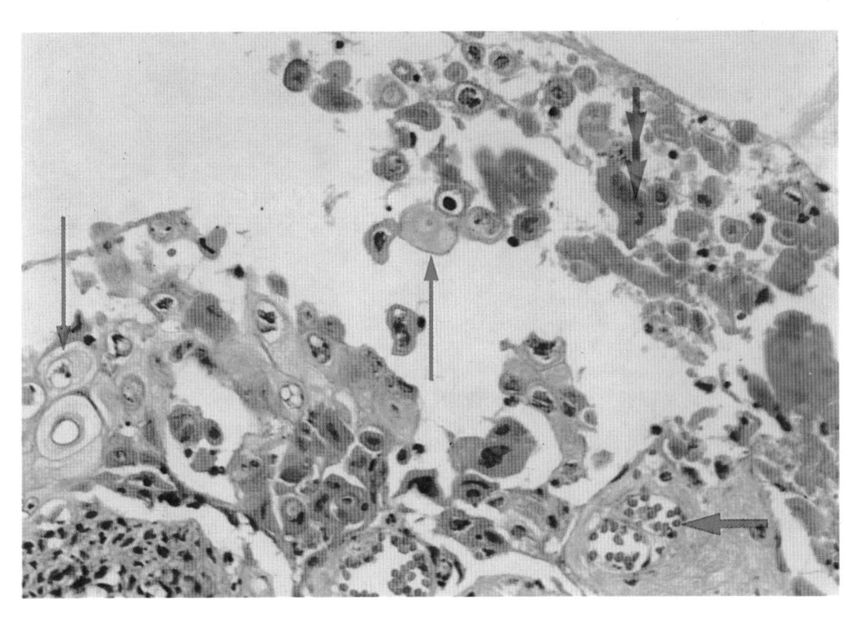

14.19 Allergic dermatitis (Eczema): skin

A large number of allergens produce dermatitis (eczema), by acting directly on the skin or via the blood stream (following ingestion). In many cases there are multiple allergens, and in other instances the allergen is obscure. The histological features tend to be the same irrespective of the cause. Acute dermatitis is involved with type I and type III hypersensitivity, whereas type IV hypersensitivity is responsible for chronic contact dermatitis. Initially the skin becomes red (erythema) and then vesicles tend to form. The vesicles may rupture, and the serous exudate forms crusts over the lesions. If the etiological factor persists, the lesions will tend to become chronic. Histologically the main features are edema within the epidermis (spongiosis), with separation and disintegration of clumps of epithelial cells to form vesicles. In this lesion, the edema has led to separation of the keratinocytes, and a vesicle (thick arrow) has formed high in the epidermis. The dermal papillae are swollen and edematous and their blood vessels dilated (thin arrow). The rete ridges are elongated (double arrow). There is an infiltrate of small lymphocytes in both the dermis and epidermis.

HE ×235

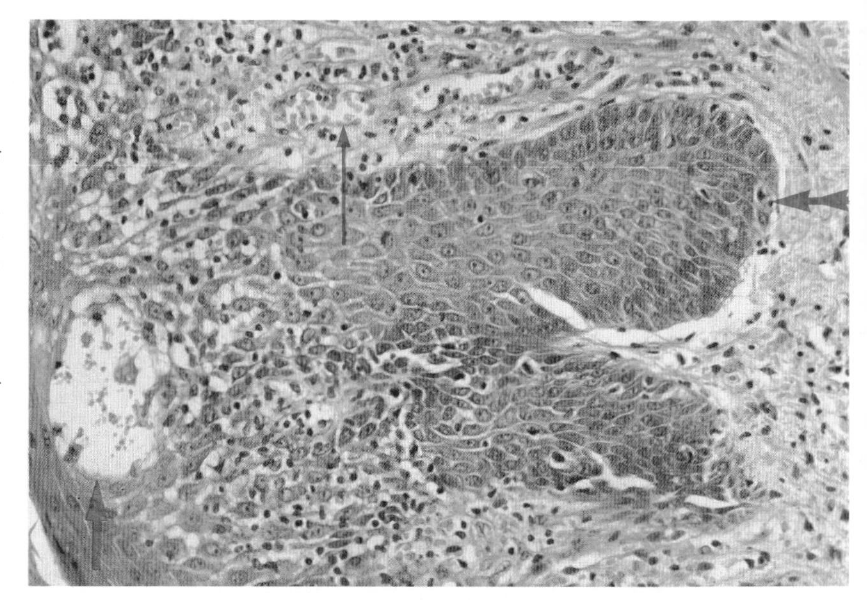

14.20 Lichen planus: skin

In lichen planus, crops of lilac-coloured itching papules and plaques form on the skin, oral mucosa and external genitalia. Women are affected more than men, and most of those affected are within the 30-60 age range. Decreased proliferation of epithelial cells leads to their prolonged retention in the epidermis increased amounts of keratinization. The decrease in cell turnover is probably caused by degeneration of the basal germinative layer. In this lesion, there is hyperkeratosis, the normal basket-weave keratin being replaced by dense laminated keratin (double arrow); the keratinocyte layer is prominent (it often shows more marked focal thickening); and the rete ridges are narrowed and pointed (thin arrows), caused by their being stretched over broadened dermal papillae. This gives the lower border of the epidermis a saw-toothed appearance. The basal layer of the epidermis is intact. Sometimes it is destroyed. There is a fairly intense infiltrate of lymphocytes and histiocytes (thick arrow) in the upper dermis which goes right up to the epidermis but is sharply limited to the papillary and subpapillary layer of the dermis. HE ×190

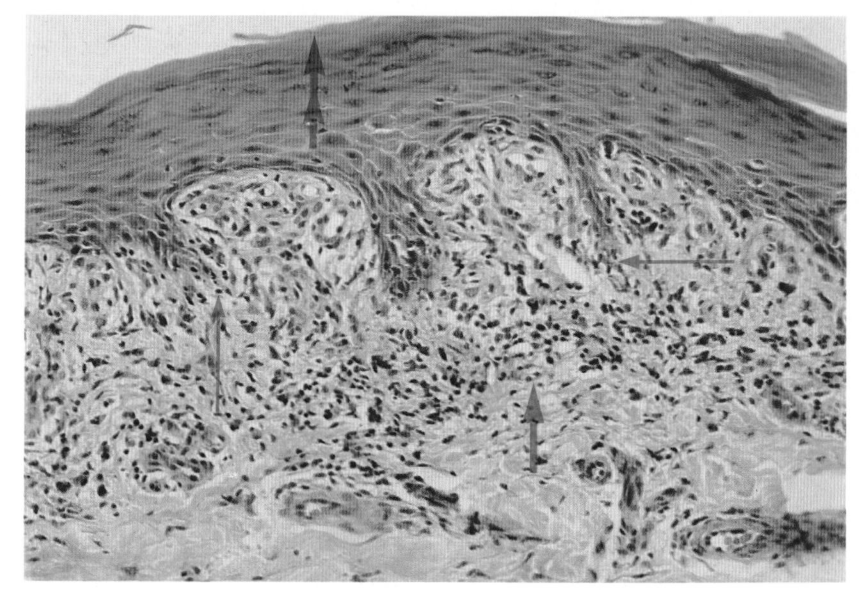

14.21 Urticaria pigmentosa: skin

Urticaria pigmentosa is a type of cutaneous mastocytosis which occurs in infants (infantile form) or in adults. All over the skin of the patient's body there are multiple red-brown macules and papules, from the presence of an excessive number of mast cells in the skin. In infants, the upper dermis may be packed with mast cells, but when the condition starts in adult life, as in this case, the number of mast cells is much smaller and they tend to be located around the blood vessels in the dermis. This is a section of the mid-dermis. The smooth muscle fibres (thin arrows) belong to the arrectores pilorum muscle; and the large round cells with eosinophilic cytoplasm and a small eccentric ovoid hyperchromatic nucleus are mast cells (thick arrows), congregated around the small vessels. The granules in the cytoplasm of the mast cells are not visible in HE sections but are well demonstrated by methylene blue or toluidine blue, particularly when the tissues have been fixed in non-aqueous solutions. The prognosis is good, and few patients develop systemic disease. HE ×200

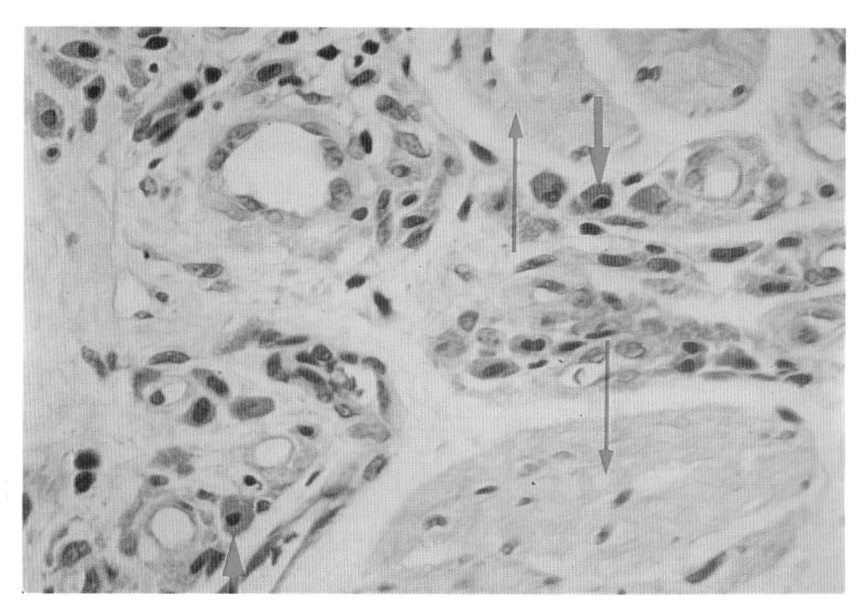

14.22 Lichen simplex chronicus (lichenification): vulva

Lichen simplex chronicus is a form of chronic eczema, in which there is thick scaling erythematous patches in the skin. The skin of the vulva may undergo lichenification as a reaction to chronic irritation of pruritic skin. The changes are fully reversible however. In this case, there is pronounced hyperplasia, of a selective nature, of the stratified squamous epithelium. Only the rete ridges are affected and not the surface layer of epithelium. As a result, the rete ridges are greatly elongated (thin arrow) and the dermal papillae are correspondingly very elongated (thick arrow). Keratin formation on the surface of the epidermis is disorganized, taking the form of a thick layer of deeply eosinophilic keratin and keratinized cells which retain their (very pale) nuclei (parakeratosis). In the dermis (right) the connective tissue is very vascular, with numerous dilated thin-walled capillary-type blood vessels; and in the dermis there is also an infiltrate of chronic inflammatory cells. HE ×135

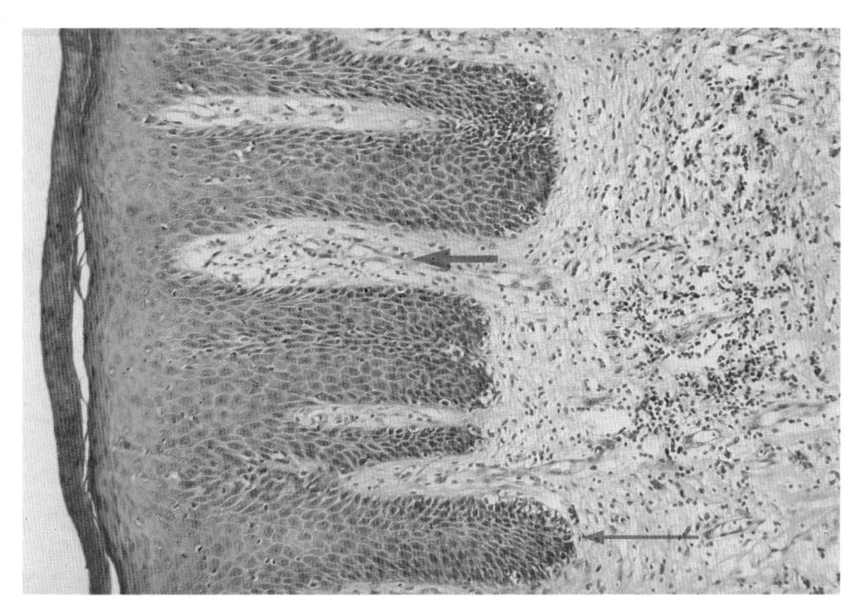

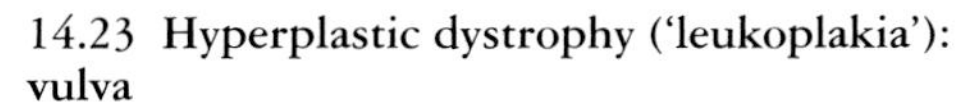

14.23 Hyperplastic dystrophy ('leukoplakia'): vulva

Hyperplastic dystrophy is a common lesion, occurring mainly in post-menopausal women. It appears clinically as leukoplakia. Histologically, in some lesions the epithelial cells mature normally, but in others cytological dysplasia occurs. Epithelial dysplasia may be sufficiently great as to suggest carcinoma-in-situ but malignant change seems to develop only rarely. In this case, the squamous epithelium of the vulva is thickened and hyperplastic. On the surface of the epidermis there is a very thick layer of keratin (thin arrow) (hyperkeratosis), and the deeply-staining stratum granulosum is equally prominent. The keratinocyte layer also is hyperplastic and thicker than normal (acanthosis) (thick arrow), and the keratinocytes show some loss of polarity. The rete ridges are irregular in shape and elongated (double arrow) (at higher magnification, there is increased mitotic activity in the keratinocytic and basal cell layers of the epidermis). The papillary processes of the dermis are also irregular in shape, and the connective tissues in the upper dermis are heavily infiltrated with chronic inflammatory cells (mostly lymphocytes). HE ×135

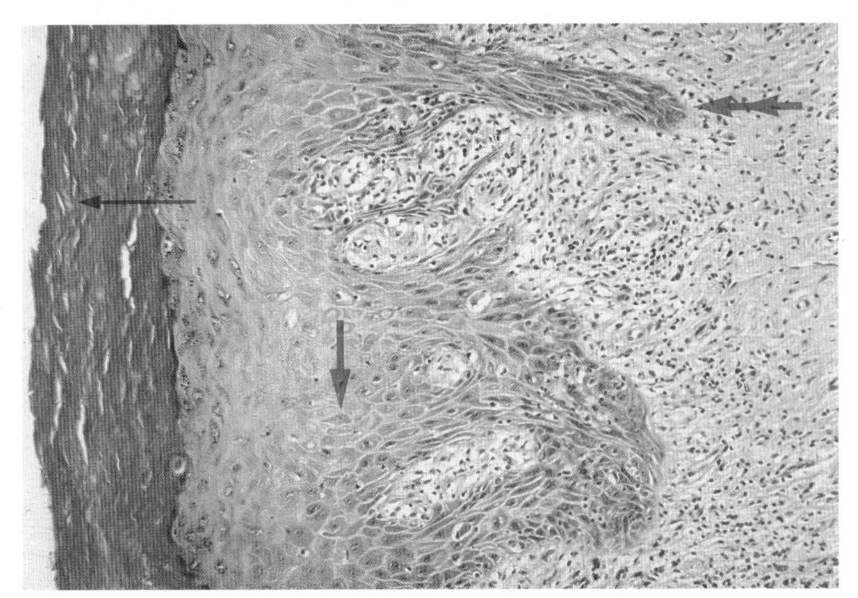

14.24 Lichen sclerosis (kraurosis): vulva

Lichen sclerosis is a chronic progressive disease which usually occurs in post-menopausal women. Its etiology is not known but it is not a premalignant type of lesion. Scaly and pruritic white plaques on the vulvar skin are characteristic features, but they may affect the skin of any part of the body. Sclerosis, shrinkage and atrophy of the epidermal and dermal components of the skin give it a parchment-like appearance. Histologically, the keratin (thin arrow) on the surface of the stratified squamous epithelium is moderately increased. The squamous epithelium however is flat and atrophic but intact (thick arrow), and the rete ridges have almost completely disappeared. An equally noteworthy change is the presence, beneath the epidermis, of a broad band of hyalinized collagenous tissue (double arrow) and complete absence of the dermal papillae. The hyalinized collagenous tissue is moderately edematous, with occasional small vacuoles in each of which there is a small lymphocyte-like cell with a round basophilic nucleus. A sharply-defined band of chronic inflammatory cells (centre of field) separates the collagenous superficial dermis from the deeper dermis (right). HE ×135

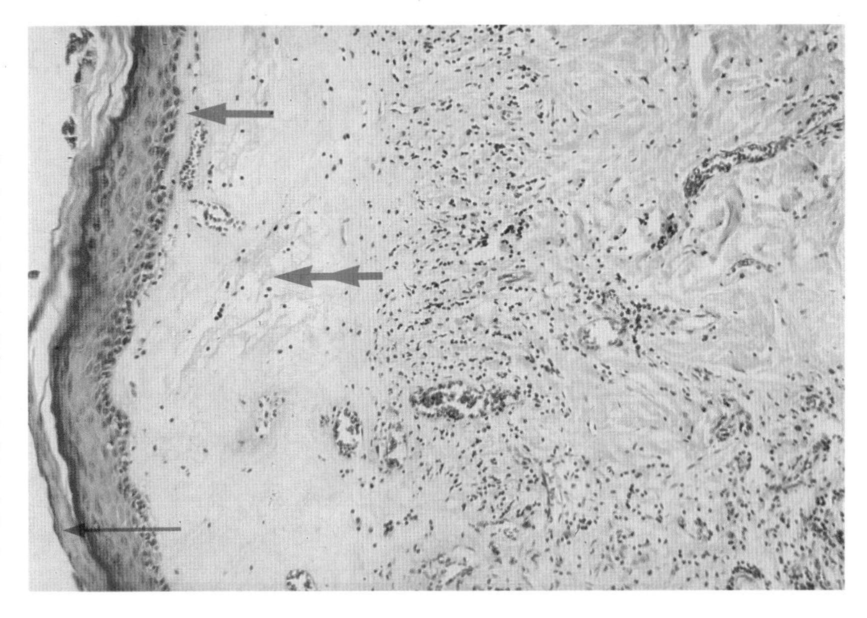

14.25 Pemphigus vulgaris: skin

Pemphigus vulgaris is a chronic severe and potentially fatal disease of individuals in the 40-60 are group. It is characterized by the formation of bullae (large blisters) in the skin and oral mucosa. The bullae are large and flaccid, and appear to rise on otherwise normal skin. They rupture readily, to leave raw tender areas which steadily enlarge. IgG autoantibodies in the serum react against the intercellular attachment sites of epidermal keratinocytes and allow the keratinocytes to lose cohesion (acantholysis). Consequently, intraepidermal (suprabasal) vesicles form between the keratinocytes and fill with serous fluid in which there are rounded-up acantholytic cells. In this case, an intraepidermal bulla is starting to form in the skin. The bulla (thin arrow) has formed suprabasally, and the keratinocytes are separating from the basal epithelial cells. The single layer of basal epithelial cells, attached to the basement membrane and separated from each other ('a row of tombstones'), will eventually form the floor of the bulla. Round acantholytic epithelial cells have formed and are detaching (thick arrows), to lie free in the lumen of the bulla. Small numbers of lymphocytes are present in the dermis. HE ×360

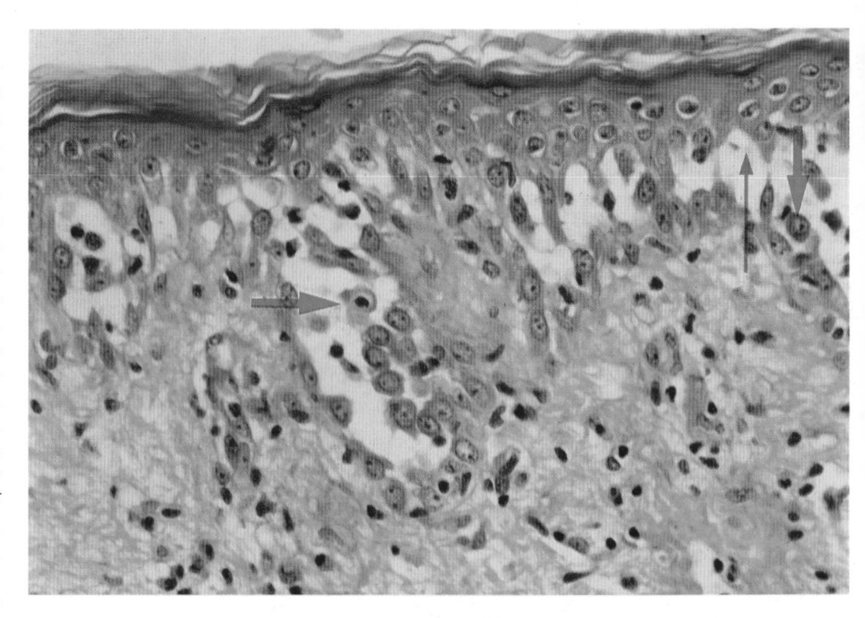

14.26 Dermatitis herpetiformis: skin

Dermatitis herpetiformis is a disease of adults, mostly 20-40 years of age, and it has a chronic course with spontaneous remissions and relapses. It is associated with gluten-induced enteropathy (celiac disease) but the dermatitis does not improve with a gluten-free diet. Macroscopically it is characterized by the formation of small clusters of intensely itchy erythematous vesicles or bullae, which tend to form in certain sites, such as the scapular and sacral areas or in the region of the elbows. Histologically, in this example, the papillary dermis (bottom) is edematous and vacuolated, and there are collections of eosinophil leukocytes in the papillae ('eosinophil abscesses') (thin arrows). The eosinophils in these are degenerate and disintegrating, and only a few have the characteristic eosinophilic cytoplasm. The cellular infiltrate is accompanied by eosinophilic material which is composed of serous exudate and debris from the eosinophils. Occasional eosinophils are present in the epidermis and also a small 'eosinophil abscess' (thick arrow) which is probably an extension of an abscess in a papilla. HE ×235

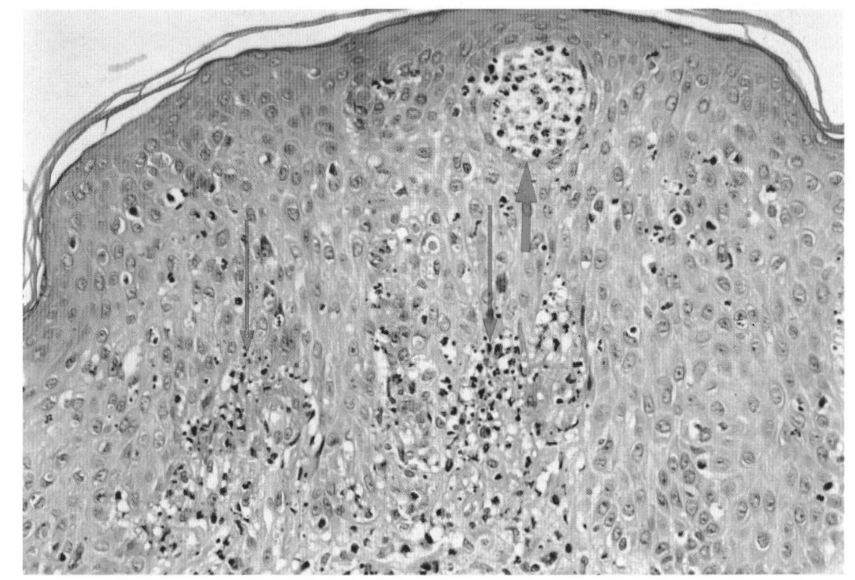

14.27 Dermatitis herpetiformis: skin

Dermatitis herpetiformis is associated with granular deposits of IgA at the dermoepidermal junction, especially at the tips of dermal papillae, and this is where vesicles tend to form and gradually coalesce. This is part of the same lesion in 14.26, showing the epidermis on the left and several papillae in the dermis (right and top). In the dermal papillae there are small 'abscesses' (thin arrows) which contain large numbers of eosinophil leukocytes, degenerate polymorphs and eosinophilic debris. Although the cytoplasm of the degenerate polymorphs stains weakly, examination at higher magnification confirms that many are eosinophil leukocytes which have shed most of their granules. The eosinophilic debris contains fibrin, and probably also collagen and debris from the degenerate eosinophils. Similar eosinophilic fibrillary material is present deeper in the dermis (thick arrows). The dermis is edematous and infiltrated with polymorphs and macrophages. The elongated interpapillary ridges of the epidermis eventually become detached, and the papillary microabscesses increase in size, to form a sub-epidermal vesicle. HE ×360

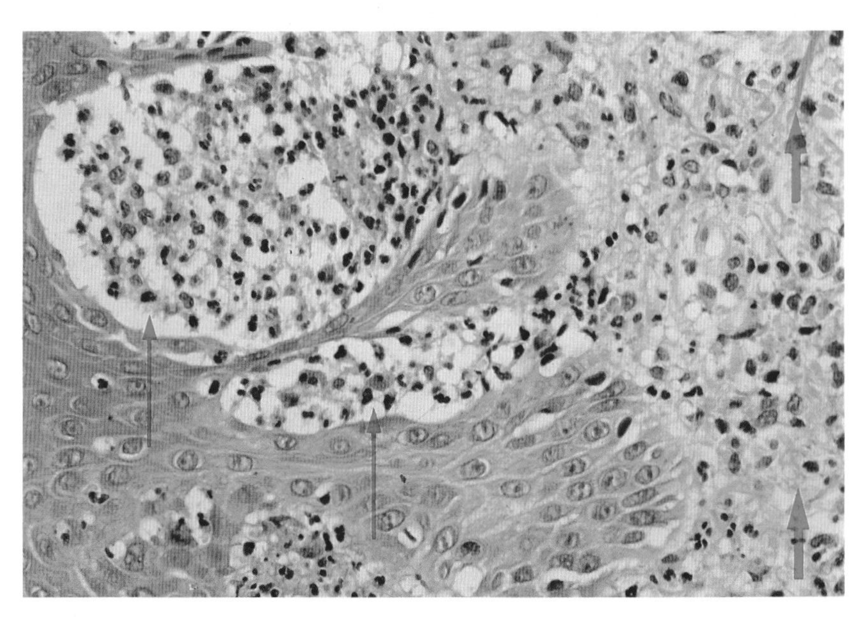

14.28 Pretibial myxedema: skin

In hypothyroidism of adults, increased amounts of mucopolysaccharides are deposited in the connective tissues. The changes in the interstitial tissues are termed myxoid degeneration (myxedema). Consequently the skin swells and develops a diffuse non-pitting dough-like texture. Remarkably, nodules (circumscribed patches) sometimes form in the skin over the tibia in individuals who are myxedematous or have untreated thyrotoxicosis. The nodules are the result of large localized accumulations of hydrophilic connective tissue mucin in the pretibial skin, and they almost never form in the absence of Graves' disease. The only symptom they produce is itching. In this section of pretibial skin, the epidermis is hyperkeratotic (thin arrow) and the dermal connective tissues are extremely pale and edematous (thick arrow), with few fibres and numerous large clear spaces. The large spaces separate the main components of the dermis (blood vessels, cells and connective tissue fibres) widely, and although seemingly empty, they are fully occupied with mucins (mucopolysaccharides) which do not stain with HE.

HE ×70

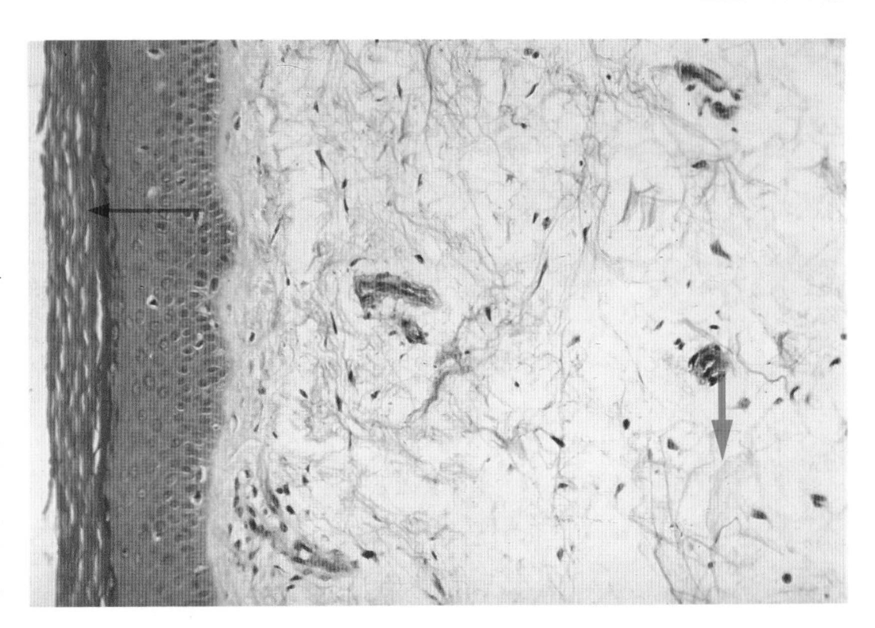

14.29 Pretibial myxedema: skin

Patients with myxedema are almost always hoarse, because their (edematous) vocal cords are swollen. Likewise, the interstitial tissues between the muscle fibres of the heart may be edematous and cause the heart to swell and perhaps eventually to fail. Connective tissue mucins (mucopolysaccharides) generally remain unstained in HE sections. They are also sensitive to the type of tissue fixative used, but in well-fixed tissues the colloidal iron technique displays the mucins effectively, colouring the connective tissue mucins blue, sometimes deeply. This is part of the same pretibial skin lesion as in 14.28. The histological section has been reacted with the colloidal iron technique. The epidermis (top margin) is brownish-yellow, the sparse collagenous fibres scattered throughout the dermis are brownish-black, and the dermis and subcutaneous tissues are a deep blue colour from the presence of greatly increased amounts of connective tissue mucin. Prior treatment of the section with hyaluronidase removed almost all the material giving the reaction, confirming that most of it was hyaluronic acid, the most hydrophilic type of connective tissue mucin.

Colloidal iron ×80

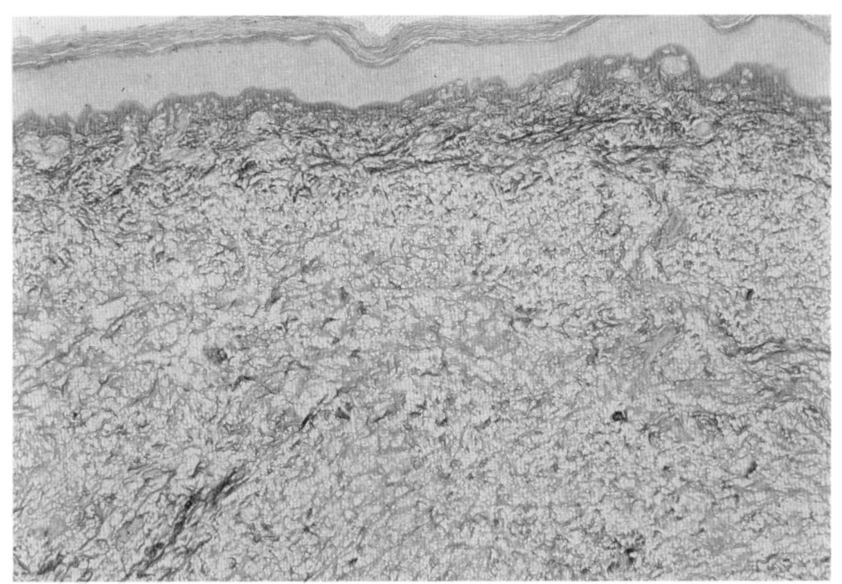

14.30 Lupus erythematosus (chronic discoid): skin

Lupus erythematosus is a connective tissue disease which takes two main forms. One is acute systemic lupus erythematosus (SLE), a progressive and often severe condition in which many tissues and organs are involved. The other is chronic (discoid) lupus erythematosus (CDLE), with lesions which dominate the skin and sometimes the mucous membranes, without systemic disease. Women are affected ten times more often than men, and the age of onset is generally between 20 and 40 years. This is a section of the skin below the eye of a man of 33 with chronic discoid lupus. The epidermis is thin, with a very atrophic stratum spinosum. There is hyperkeratosis which extends down into the pilosebaceous follicles (follicular plugging) (thin arrows). The basal layer of the epidermis shows liquefaction degeneration (thick arrows). The dermis is edematous and hyalinized, and within it there are deposits of eosinophilic fibrin. Beneath the damaged dermis there is a very intense infiltrate of chronic inflammatory cells (double arrow), mainly lymphocytes and tending to concentrate around blood vessels and pilosebaceous follicles. HE ×60

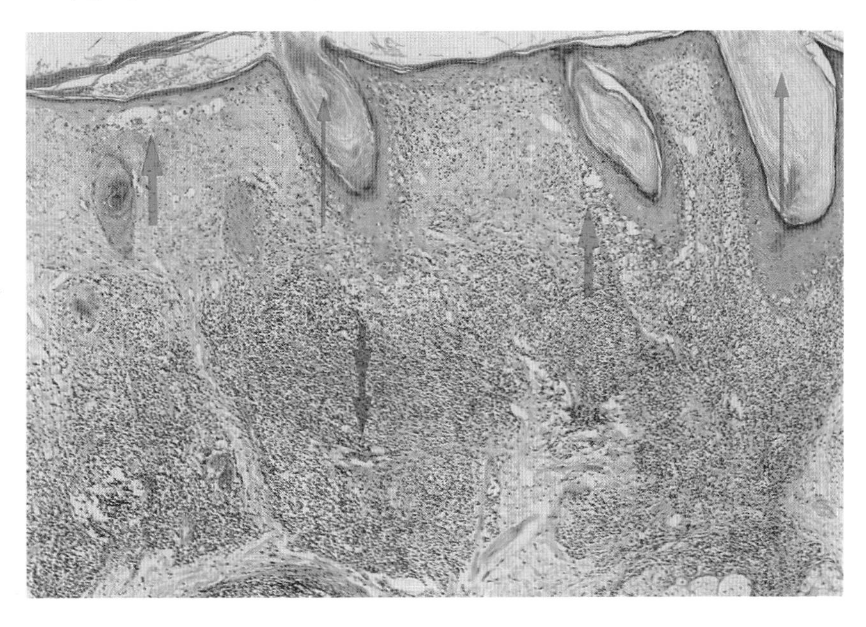

14.31 Lupus erythematosus (chronic discoid): skin

The cause of lupus erythematosus is not known, but there is little doubt that the pathological effects are mediated by an abnormal immune (probably autoimmune) response, associated with the presence of a range of antibodies and immune complexes in the plasma. This is part of the same lesion as in **14.30**. On the surface of the skin there is thick layer of keratin (hyperkeratosis), and the wide orifice of the large pilosebaceous follicle (thin arrow) which opens on to the surface of the epidermis is plugged with dense deeply eosinophilic keratin. The epidermis is atrophic, from change which particularly affects the keratinocyte layer (stratum spinosum). The whole basal layer of the epidermis has undergone liquefaction degeneration, but in some parts it is more severe and the basal layer has been completely destroyed (thick arrows). The connective tissue of the dermis is amorphous, weakly eosinophilic and apparently completely hyalinized. In some areas hemorrhage has occurred from the thin-walled blood vessels. Eosinophilic fibrin is also present. The pilosebaceous follicles are surrounded by an intense infiltrate of lymphocytes and plasma cells (double arrow).

HE ×150

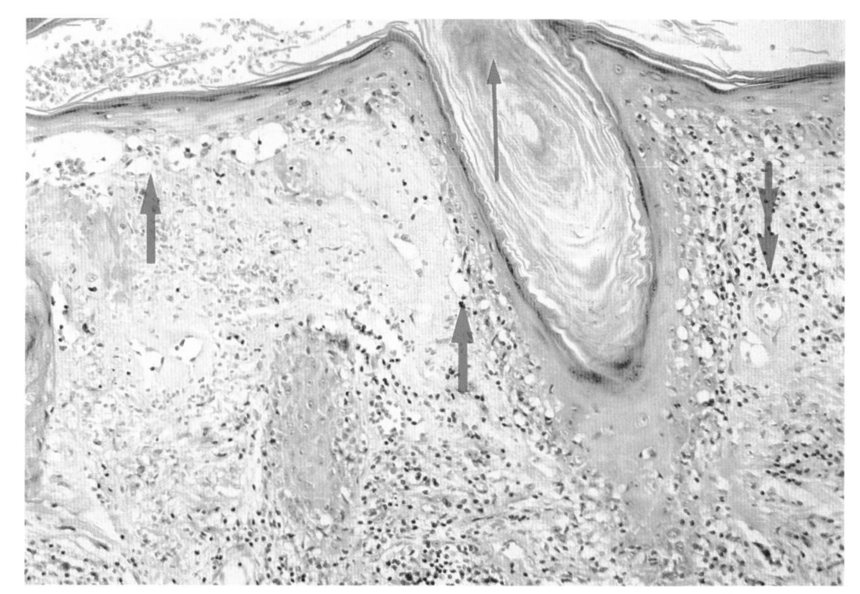

14.32 Rheumatoid arthritis: skin

Rheumatoid arthritis is a chronic disease and the exact cause of it is unknown. In the course of the disease, tender rheumatoid nodules form in the skin, and the number of nodules is considerably greater in the more severe forms of disease. Rheumatoid nodules are granulomas (1-2 cm dia) and they also form in tissues other than the skin. The granulomas consist of connective tissue with a relatively large central area of fibrinous necrosis. They are located in the subcutaneous tissues, generally in sites over bone and in the vicinity of joints, particularly the wrist and elbow joints. This shows part of a rheumatoid nodule. The strongly eosinophilic necrotic centre of the nodule consists of collagenous tissue which has undergone fibrinoid necrosis (thin arrow). The necrotic centre, in which there are some cells with pyknotic nuclei, is surrounded by a broad row of elongated histiocytes and fibroblasts, arranged in parallel with one another (palisading) (thick arrows). The necrotic material in the centre of the nodule is resistant to phagocytosis, and the nodules themselves are very persistent. HE ×235

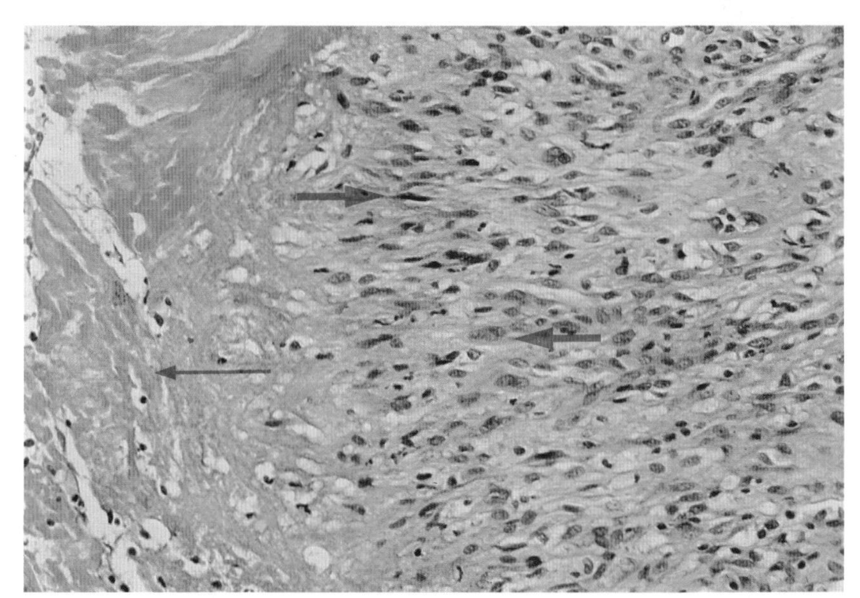

14.33 Progressive systemic sclerosis: skin

Progressive systemic sclerosis, previously called scleroderma, is an uncommon connective tissue disease, probably an autoimmune disorder closely related to systemic lupus erythematosus (SLE). The disease is characterized by vasculitis identical to that in SLE and affecting small vessels, and by widespread formation of collagenous tissue. There are lesions in many organs and tissues but the mechanism underlying the excessive fibrosis is unknown. The skin shrinks and becomes stiff, and the taut skin restricts movement, particularly of joints. The main clinical symptoms of this patient, a man of 60 with scleroderma, were caused by lesions in the esophagus and skin. The epidermis is extremely hyperkeratotic (double arrow), and the sweat ducts and glands in the subcutaneous tissues (thick arrows) are normal. The connective tissue of the dermis is homogeneous, swollen and poorly cellular (hyalinized) (thin arrow). However, since the distance from the sweat glands to the epidermis is only half the normal distance, the change in the dermis is not necessarily caused by fibroblastic proliferation and fibrous tissue formation but probably produced by marked atrophy of the dermis. HE ×80

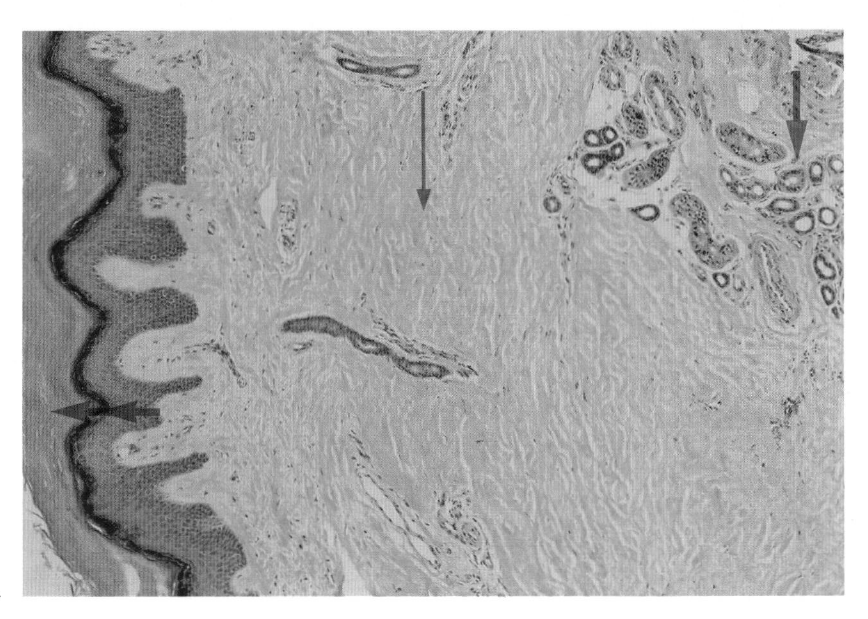

14.34 Verruca vulgaris (common wart): skin

Verruca vulgaris, the common wart, is caused by a papillomavirus, and papillomaviruses also cause verruca plantaris and condyloma acuminatum. Histologically, the wart is as squamous papilloma with variable keratinization and conspicuous keratohyaline granules. The virus is transmitted from one site to another, and from one person to another, by direct contact, and it may occur anywhere in the skin. Viral inclusions can be demonstrated in the nuclei of the cells by special techniques, but they are not visible in HE preparations. However in this active virus wart, as the epithelial cells moved outwards from the stratum spinosum (bottom) to form the granular layer, damage by the virus, caused many of them to become vacuolated; and instead of forming normal keratohyaline granules they develop deeply eosinophilic bodies (thick arrows) within their cytoplasm. These 'inclusions' are probably tangled masses of tonofilaments. The very thick deeply eosinophilic layer of keratin on the surface of the epidermis is nucleated (parakeratosis), the nuclei of the epithelial cells which produced by the keratin being damaged and weakly basophilic (thin arrow).

HE ×270

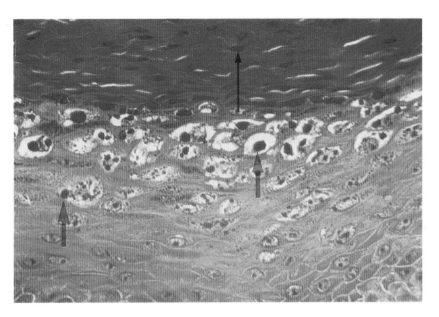

14.35 Keratoacanthoma (molluscum sebaceum): skin

Keratoacanthoma (molluscum sebaceum) is a benign tumour-like lesion of unknown etiology. It is usually a feature of middle age, most often present on the face or upper extremities. It grows comparatively rapidly, reaching its maximum size in a few weeks and followed by a static phase. It projects above the surface of the skin as a cup-shaped mass and undergoes keratinization in the centre. It then involutes, the whole cycle taking not more than one year to final scar formation. This shows a fully-formed lesion in cross-section. It is cup- or crater-shaped, the crater in the centre being full of keratin (double arrow) and strands of proliferating epithelium. The 'wall' of the crater is composed of a thick layer of hyperplastic epithelium which is invading the dermis (thin arrows). The epidermis and the skin appendages on both sides of the lesion seem to have been 'pulled up'. There is an infiltrate of chronic inflammatory cells in the dermis around the margins of the lesion. It is patchy but intense in some areas (thick arrow).

HE ×9

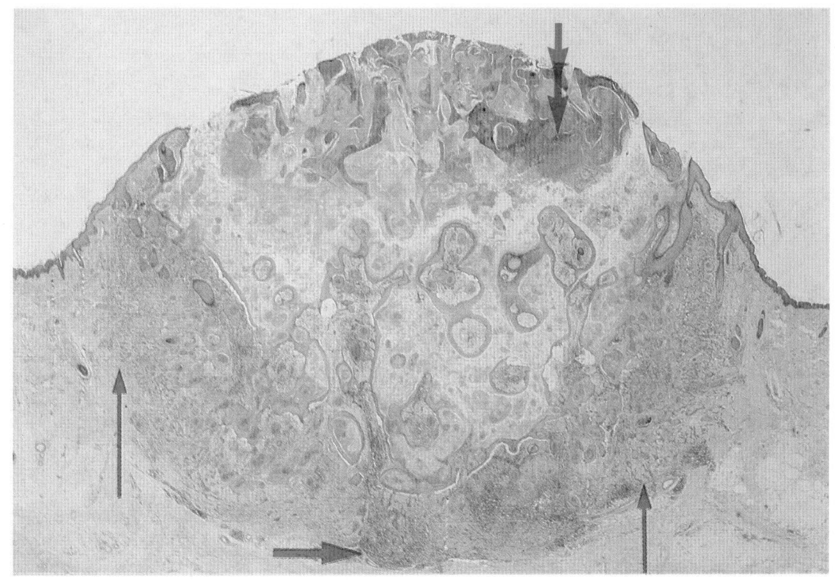

14.36 Keratoacanthoma (molluscum sebaceum): skin

The early growth phase of keratoacanthomas is much faster than that of its malignant counterpart, squamous cell carcinoma. Moreover, although the lesion seems to be invasive, its base is smooth and does not penetrate beyond the level of the hair follicles. Nevertheless it sometimes difficult to distinguish a keratoacanthoma, which consists of squamous epithelial cells (often showing mild atypia), dyskeratosis and mitotic activity, from a true squamous carcinoma. The squamous epithelial cells of the keratoacanthoma are invading the dermis; and the invading cells, which are arranged in slender cords and clusters ('cell nests') with central keratin formation (thick arrow), have hyperchromatic pleomorphic nuclei which are mitotically active. There is a heavy infiltrate of chronic inflammatory cells around the tumour margin. The histological appearances in this area are not distinguishable from those of the squamous carcinoma in **14.50**. Later in the evolution of the keratoacanthoma however, inflammatory cells invade the epithelial strands, involution follows, and a keratin plug fills the crater.

HE ×150

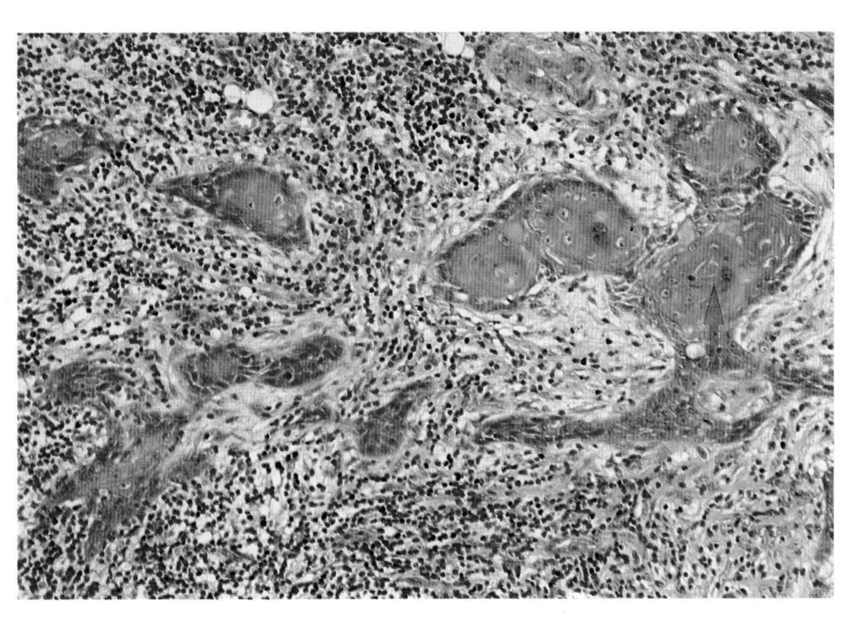

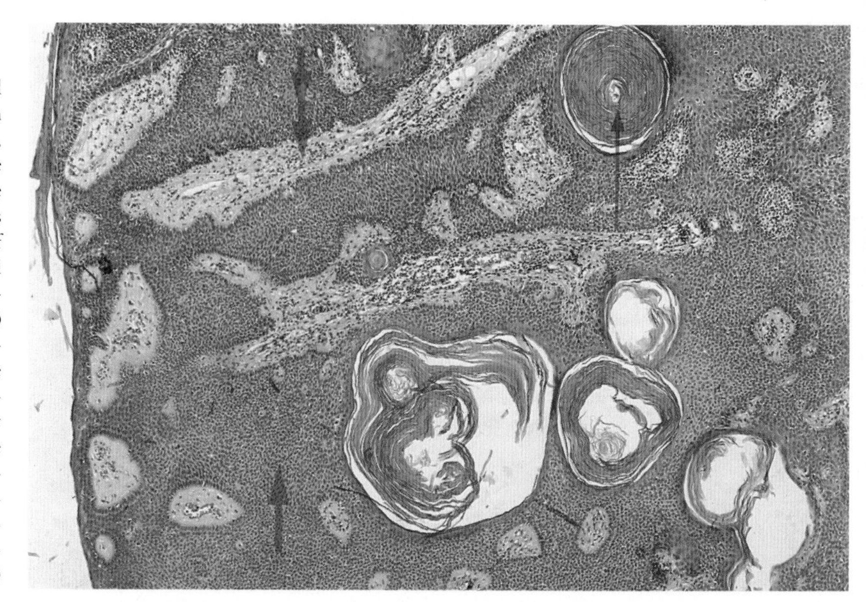

14.37 Seborrheic keratosis (seborrheic wart): skin

Seborrheic keratosis (also called seborrheic wart or basal cell papilloma) is a very common benign tumour which arises from the epidermis. A typical lesion is flat, soft, sharply demarcated and raised above the surface of the skin. It is often heavily pigmented and brown, and liable to be mistaken for malignant melanoma. However it is probably not a true neoplasm, and consists of a sheet of proliferating epithelial cells and numerous keratin-filled cysts (horn cysts). This is the solid type of papilloma, consisting of a mass of dark-staining cells (thick arrow) within which there are small round cysts full of eosinophilic laminated keratin (horn cysts) (thin arrow). The cysts are scattered throughout the tumour, and the keratin in them is characteristically in concentric layers. They probably arise in pilosebaceous follicles and can often be seen to open on to the surface. The surface is usually hyperkeratotic but the keratin has been lost during processing of the tissues. There is an infiltrate of chronic inflammatory cells in the connective tissue stroma (double arrow). HE ×60

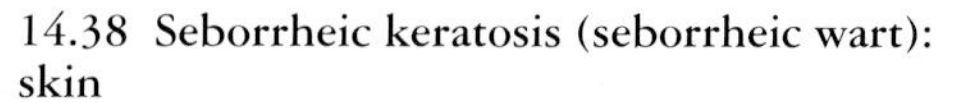

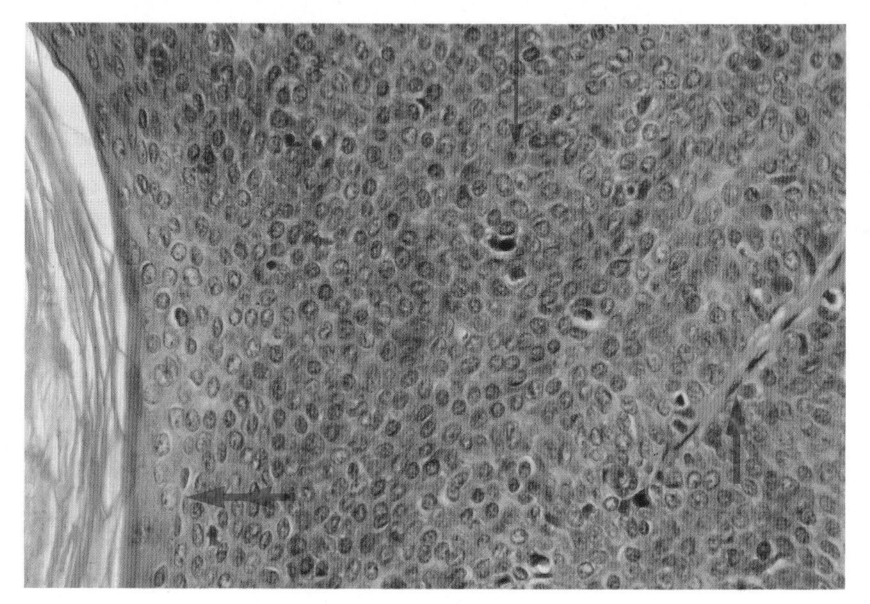

14.38 Seborrheic keratosis (seborrheic wart): skin

Seborrheic keratosis (seborrheic wart) is a sharply demarcated lesion usually elevated (along with its base) above the surrounding skin and apparently stuck to it. It rarely develops before the age of 40 or 50 years, and the number of lesions increases with age. The lesions are usually less than 1cm dia but are occasionally much larger. This shows part of the same lesion as in 14.37, at higher magnification. In the seborrheic keratosis (seborrheic wart) there is a keratin-filled horn cyst on the left and, on the right, a sheet of small closely packed 'basal' epithelial cells (thin arrow), intersected by a small stromal blood vessel (thick arrow). All the 'basal' epithelial cells have an ovoid vesicular nucleus and granules of brown pigment (melanin) in their cytoplasm. The layer of stratified squamous epithelial cells lining the horn cyst is extremely attenuated (double arrow), and the transition from the 'basal' cells of the tumour to the mass of eosinophilic laminated keratin in the horn cyst is abrupt, the boundary consisting of only a barely detectable very thin stratum granulosum. HE ×360

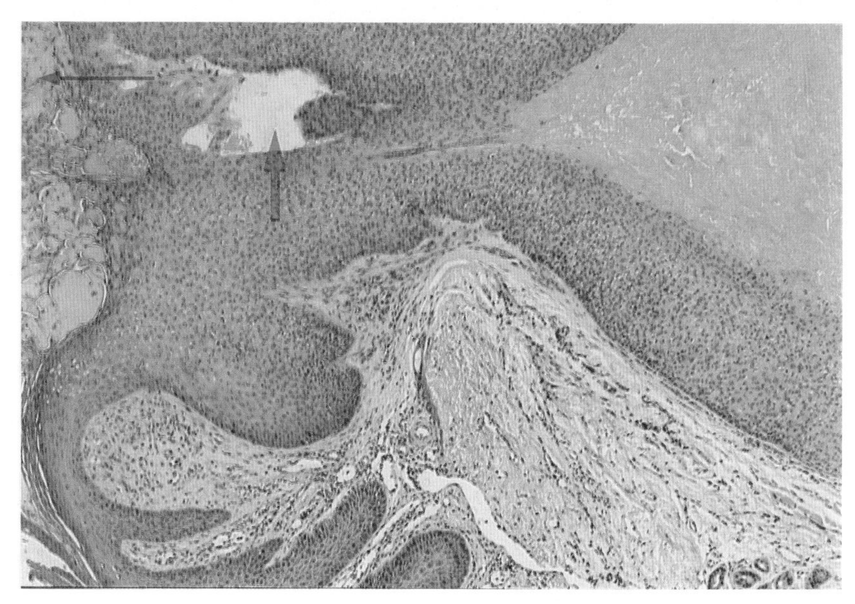

14.39 Eccrine poroma: skin

Eccrine poroma arises within the epidermis from the intraepidermal sweat duct and grows downwards into the dermis. It is a benign painless nodule, occurring most often on the palms and soles of the feet, mainly of individuals between 40 and 60 years of age. This lesion was a raised white hard nodule, 2mm dia, in the upper lip of a woman of 58. Histologically, the tumour is composed of a uniform population of round or cuboidal epithelial cells with a central ovoid nucleus . They are smaller than the squamous 'prickle' cells of the epidermis and sharply demarcated from them, but at higher magnification they are connected by intercellular bridges (desmosomes). The cells resemble the cells which form the outer layer of the intraepithelial part of the eccrine ducts. They do not keratinize except at the surface and are not mitotically active. They have formed a large cystic (flask-shaped) structure (top right), full of keratinous cell debris. The 'neck' of the flask-shaped structure (thick arrow) is blocked by desquamated neoplastic cells and keratin which have formed a 'plug' (thin arrow). HE ×60

14.40 Syringoma (sweat gland adenoma): skin

Syringoma (sweat gland adenoma) is a benign tumour which arises from the duct of an eccrine gland, though an origin from apocrine glands is possible. It usually takes the form of multiple nodules on the neck and face of young adolescents and young adults, many of them girls. This is atypical lesion. It consists of numerous small ducts in the dermis, widely separated by collagenous stroma and lined by a double layer of flattened eccrine ductal epithelial cells. Closer to the epidermis there are several small cystic structures (thick arrows) lined by stratified squamous epithelium and filled with laminated material which is pale and almost colourless but is purplish-red when reacted with the periodic acid-Schiff (PAS) method. If one of the cystic keratin-containing ducts ruptures, a foreign body reaction to keratin develops in the dermis. Some of the cystic structures have characteristic comma-shaped extensions (centre). There are also several solid strands of epithelial cells, similar to the cells lining the ducts. HE ×80

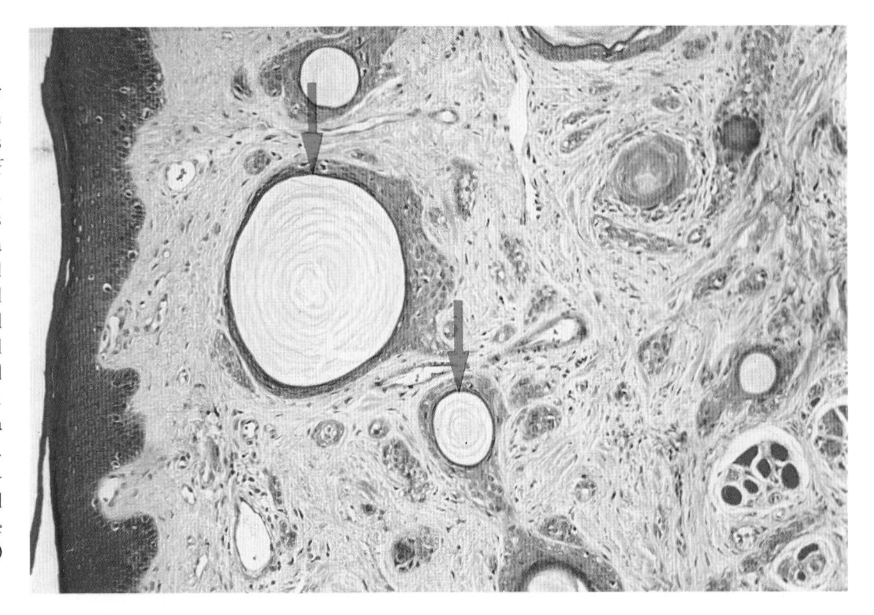

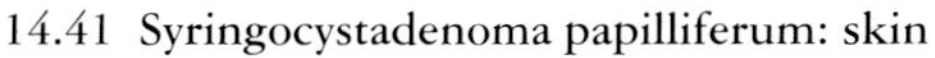

14.41 Syringocystadenoma papilliferum: skin

Syringocystadenoma papilliferum is a common benign hamartomatous lesion, most often located in the face or scalp. It probably arises from the ductal portion of an apocrine gland. The epidermis over the lesion is thick and often forms 'warty' folds. One or more cystic spaces extend downwards from the epidermis, the superficial part of the cyst being lined with keratinized epidermis and the lower part lined with a double layer of epithelial cells and filled with large papillary infoldings. This example of syringocystadenoma papilliferum is superficially situated and it opens on to the surface of the epidermis. Stratified squamous epithelium (thin arrow) has spread down from the surface epidermis, to form a cystic cavity, the wall of which (right) is partly lined by stratified squamous epithelium and a thick irregular epithelial layer (thick arrow). The cystic cavity is filled with eosinophilic material, into which papillary structures (double arrows) project. Each of the papillary processes is covered with a double layer of epithelial cells and has a fibrovascular core in which there are numerous chronic inflammatory cells. HE ×60

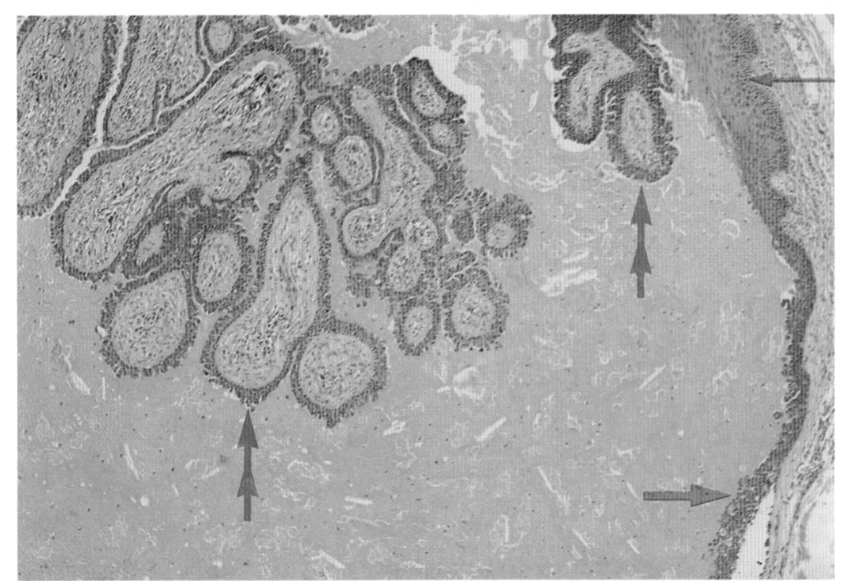

14.42 Syringocystadenoma papilliferum: skin

The origin of syringocystadenoma papilliferum is debatable. Some tumours apparently exhibit signs of apocrine differentiation in the neoplastic cells, but others show eccrine differentiation. This is part of the same lesion as in 14.41, at higher magnification. It consists of the tips of two of the papilliferous processes which are projecting into a large cystic space full of amorphous material. The core of each papillary process has a central core of vascular fibrous tissue in which there is a moderate infiltrate of plasma cells and lymphocytes. The surface of the process is covered with a double layer of epithelial cells. The inner layer, in contact with the fibrous core, consists of small flat epithelial cells with small very basophilic (almost pyknotic) nuclei (thin arrow), and the epithelial cells of the outer layer are mainly tall and columnar (thick arrow), with abundant eosinophilic cytoplasm and pleomorphic but mostly ovoid nuclei. A few of the epithelial cells are vacuolated and several appear to be desquamating into the cyst. The material in the lumen is also eosinophilic and amorphous, and unstained fragments of debris float in it (double arrow). HE ×235

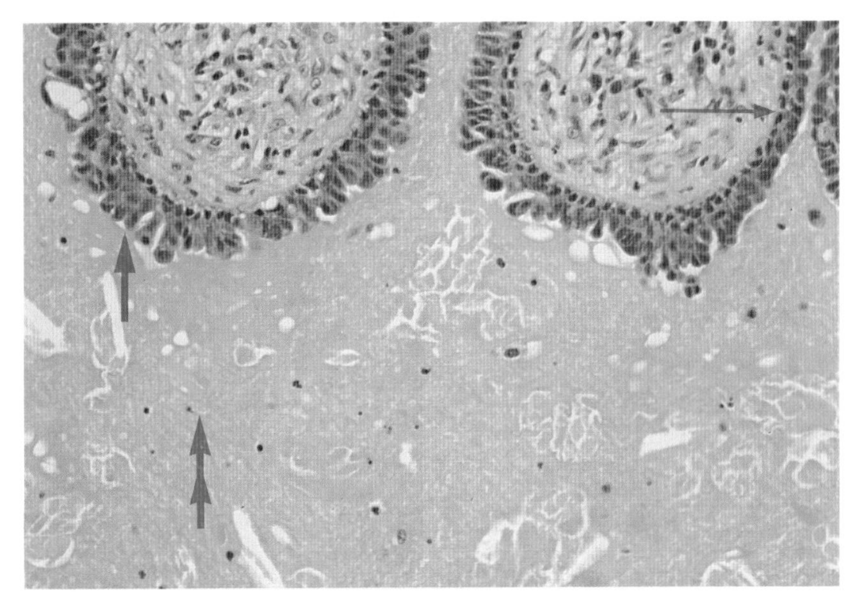

14.43 Cylindroma: scalp

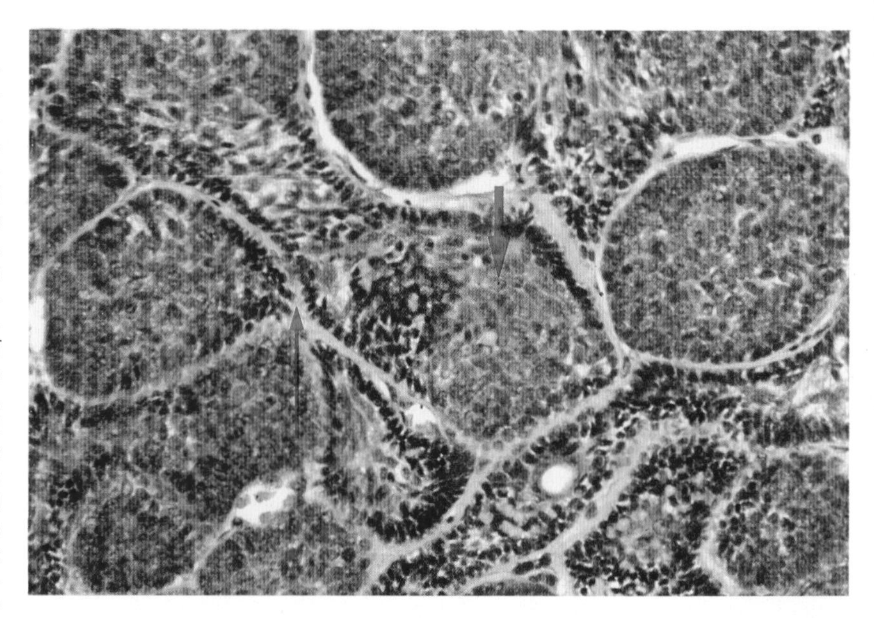

Cylindroma (also called turban tumour) is a benign tumour of apocrine gland origin. The solitary form of the lesion arises in adults and forms a single smooth dome-shaped mass (0.5-5cm), generally on the scalp or face. Multiple cylindromatosis, on the other hand, is a condition inherited as an autosomal dominant character; and lesions resembling the solitary type of tumour begin to appear in adult life and become increasingly numerous. They may grow to a large size and cover the entire scalp: hence the origin of the term turban tumour. This cylindroma is composed of thick intertwining cords ('cylinders') of epithelial cells, surrounded by thin bands of eosinophilic stroma (thin arrow). The stroma tends to be homogeneous and closely resemble basement membrane. The stroma is also accompanied by dilated small blood vessels. The tumour cells in the centres of the cords are closely packed and polyhedral, with scanty cytoplasm and large vesicular nuclei some of which contain a central nucleolus (thick arrow). The layer of epithelial cells at the periphery of the cords have elongated deeply basophilic ovoid nuclei which are palisaded and rest on the eosinophilic stroma. HE ×310

14.44 Cylindroma: scalp

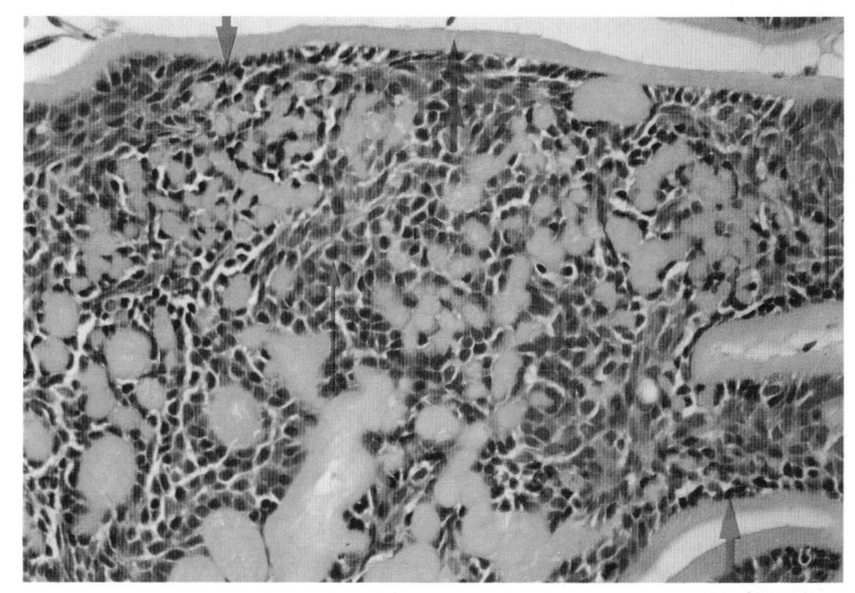

This cylindroma consists of two lobulated masses which arose in the scalp of a woman aged 66. The cut surface of each mass was brown and homogeneous, and the two tumours are histologically identical, each tumour consisting of narrow cords and small sheets of epithelial cells. This is one of the two tumours. The neoplastic epithelial cells in the centre of the cords have minimal cytoplasm and ovoid or round very hyperchromatic nuclei (thin arrow), and at the periphery of the cords there is single layer of closely packed small cells with even smaller deeply staining nuclei (thick arrows). These small cells are in contact with and tend to form a palisade upon the broad bands of strongly eosinophilic hyaline material which resembles basement membrane (double arrow). Apart from the much greater amount of the basement membrane material which surrounds and permeates the columns and sheets of epithelial cells in this tumour, its structure is essentially the same as that of the tumour in 14.43 HE ×360

14.45 Basal cell carcinoma: skin

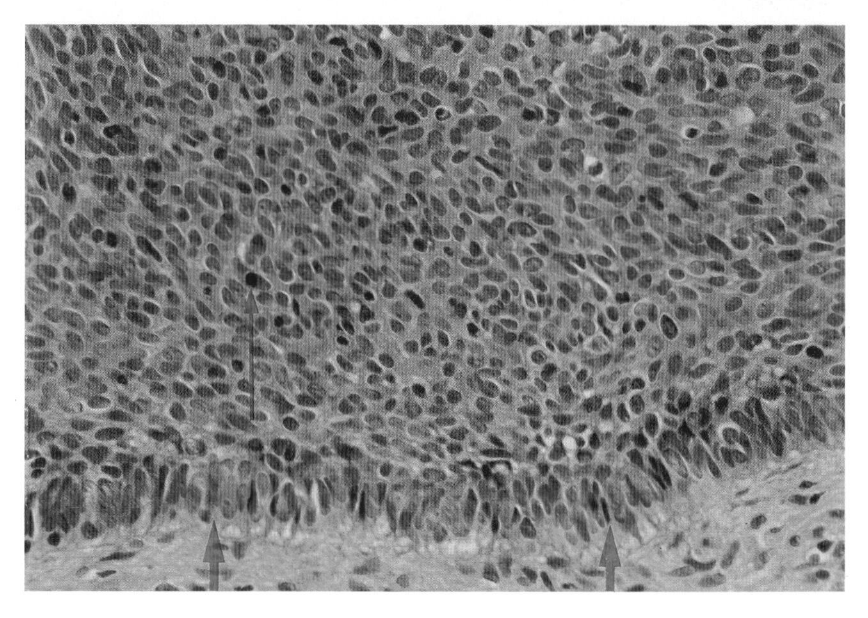

Basal cell carcinoma (also called rodent ulcer) is a common tumour of the skin. It usually affects skin, mainly of the face, that has been exposed to the sun, and fair-skinned individuals over 40 years of age are particularly susceptible. Basal cell carcinoma initially takes the form of a waxy papule with small telangiectatic vessels on its surface, necrosis in the centre produces a punched-out ulcer with rolled edges. It is malignant and locally invasive, but it grows slowly and almost never metastasizes. The skin covering this basal carcinoma is out of the picture at the top. The tumour consists of a sheet of basophilic uniform neoplastic cells which are invading the dermis (bottom margin). The cells are closely packed and polyhedral, with round or ovoid basophilic nuclei and a moderate amount of eosinophilic cytoplasm. The cell boundaries are indistinct (no intercellular bridges are detectable at higher magnification). Several mitoses are present (thin arrow). The cells at the periphery of the sheet of tumour cells are tall columnar cells with basal cytoplasmic vacuoles (thick arrows), with elongated nuclei which are aligned in parallel with each other (palisading of nuclei). HE ×360

14.46 Basal cell carcinoma: skin

Basal cell carcinomas arise from the basal layer of the epidermis. The neoplastic cells resemble basal cells, and tend usually to form a palisade (single layer of cells) at the periphery of the groups of tumour cells. Basal cell carcinomas are locally aggressive and may invade the tissues deeply, to involve bone and muscle, but they hardly ever metastasize. However they are sometimes pigmented (containing melanin) and may be mistaken for malignant melanoma.

This tumour was a pigmented smooth nodule in a man of 60, and (histologically) the tumour cells in this lesion have formed long slender cords and clusters of epithelial cells with basophilic ovoid nuclei and very little cytoplasm. The cells at the periphery of the cords however show palisading similar to that in the more 'solid' form of basal cell carcinoma shown in 14.42. There is considerable mitotic activity (thick arrow). In the centre of one group of tumour cells there is a collection of deep brown melanin-impregnated debris (thin arrow). Melanocytes can be detected by special stains in most basal cell carcinomas, and melanin is also present in about a quarter of all lesions. The amount of melanin is however is rarely large. HE ×235

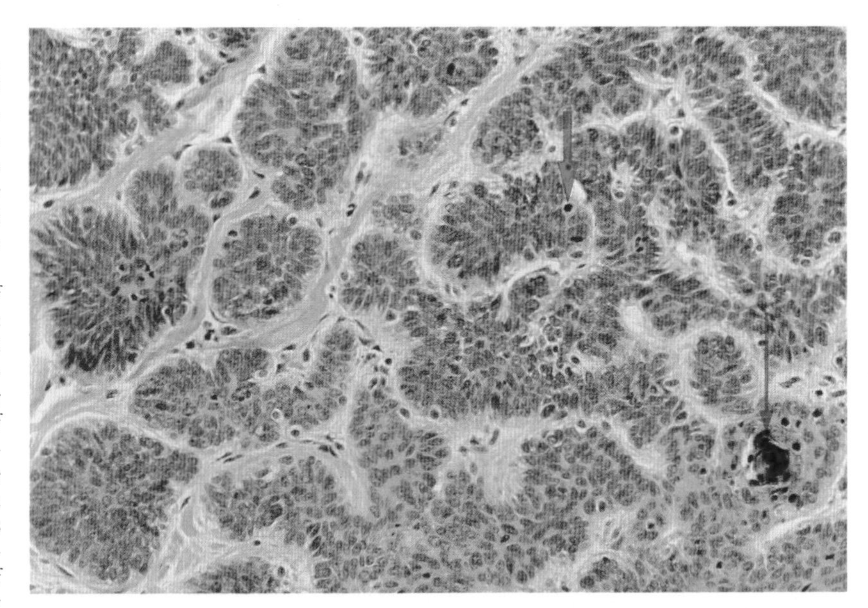

14.47 Fibroepithelioma: skin

Fibroepithelioma is an uncommon lesion, an uncommon distinctive variant of basal cell carcinoma. It is generally located on the skin of the back, where it forms one or more pedunculated or erythematous nodules. A pedunculated papilloma (2.5 × 2 × 1cm) was removed from the buttock of a man aged 57 years. Histologically it consists largely of long or very long anastomosing cords of tumour cells resembling those in other basal cell carcinomas. Most of the cords are slender but others are fairly thick (thin arrows), and they are in continuity with the surface epidermis (which is out of the picture at the top). Small groups of cells (thick arrow), looking like buds on a tree, project from the strands of neoplastic cells, and between the epithelial strands there is abundant fine loose connective tissue stroma. The neoplastic cells have also formed a very broad and well-demarcated invasive front of the closely packed tumour cells (bottom margin). Fibroepithelioma can change into an invasive basal cell carcinoma. It does not originate in the basal cells of the epidermis but probably from the keratinocytes of the intraepithelial portion of the pilosebaceous follicles and sweat duct. HE ×60

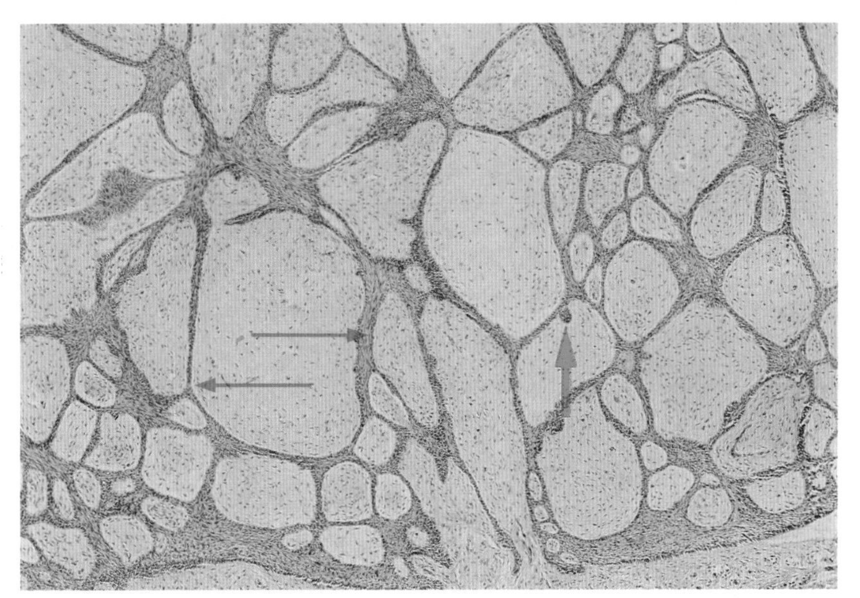

14.48 Pilomatricoma: skin

Pilomatricoma, often called calcifying epithelioma of Malherbe, is a benign tumour usually located on the face or scalp. It is the most common type of pilar tumours, and is derived from the hair root (the matrix). It can arise at any age and occurs predominantly but not exclusively in children and young adults. It forms a single firm well-defined nodule, deep in the dermis and enclosed within a pseudocapsule of fibrous tissue. This lesion is unusual however, in being situated on the front of the chest wall of a woman of 54. It is an ovoid yellowish nodule, about 1cm dia, in the dermis, and (histologically) it consists of a sheet of markedly uniform population of small epithelial cells (double arrow) with ovoid deeply-basophilic nuclei and very little cytoplasm, and also another population of larger and much paler cells with weakly eosinophilic cytoplasm (thin arrow). Within the sheet of neoplastic cells there is a central cystic area (thick arrow), full of amorphous keratin and cell debris. There is no evidence of mitotic activity in the sheet of small epithelial cells. HE ×200

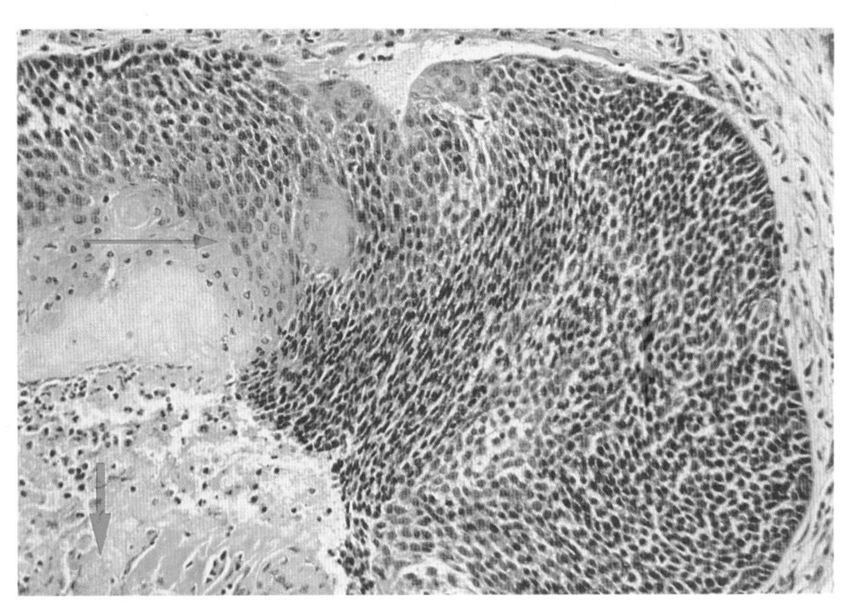

14.49 Pilomatricoma: skin

The transition between the two types of cells in pilomatricoma is sometimes sudden or sometimes gradual. Occasionally also, 'pearls' of keratin form in the sheets of small (dark) epithelial cells with basophilic nuclei. There are no keratohyaline granules however. This is a cystic lesion, from the upper eyelid of a man aged 26. The lumen of the cyst is out of the picture at the top, but in the upper half of the picture the cyst is lined by a sheet of 'shadow' ('ghost' cells), large eosinophilic cells which are necrotic and the nuclei of which are unstained (thick arrow). These eosinophilic cells are the produce of the deep layer of fully viable 'basal' cells with scant cytoplasm and deeply basophilic nuclei (thin arrows) which enlarge and keratinize abruptly, thereby constituting the actively-growing component of the tumour. This method of abrupt keratinization closely resembles the manner in which the cortex of the hair keratinizes without a granular layer. HE ×470

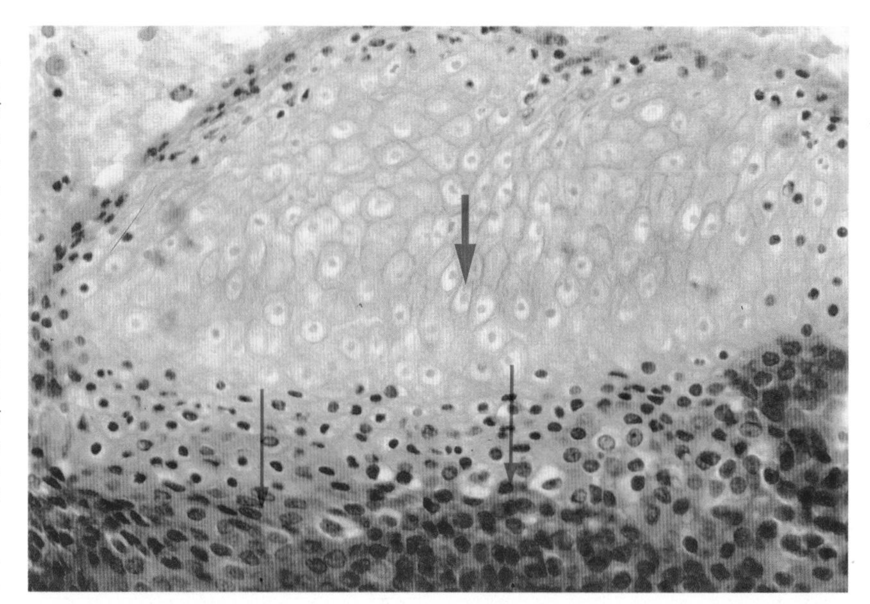

14.50 Squamous carcinoma: skin

Squamous carcinoma (also termed squamous epithelioma) is a very common lesion, especially in the sun-exposed skin of elderly fair-skinned individuals. It arises from the stratified squamous epithelium of skin and mucous membranes, and also from areas of squamous metaplasia in other types of epithelium. It is a malignant locally aggressive tumour but it rarely metastasizes. The incidence of metastasis is much higher however in chronic ulcers, scars of burns and infected sinuses. Squamous carcinoma arises from keratinocytes and makes keratin in amounts roughly proportional to the degree of differentiation. In this case, the malignant squamous epithelial cells have formed long strongly eosinophilic strands. In the centres of these strands there are relatively few tumour cells with eosinophilic cytoplasm, but also in several of the strands there are foci of laminated sheets of deeply eosinophilic keratinized epithelial cells (thick arrows). These foci are 'cell nests' or 'epithelial pearls'. Around the periphery of the strands there are larger cells with eosinophilic cytoplasm and large hyperchromatic pleomorphic nuclei, among which there is considerable mitotic activity (thin arrows). The stroma consists of loose connective tissue and a fairly dense infiltrate of lymphocytes and plasma cells. HE ×235

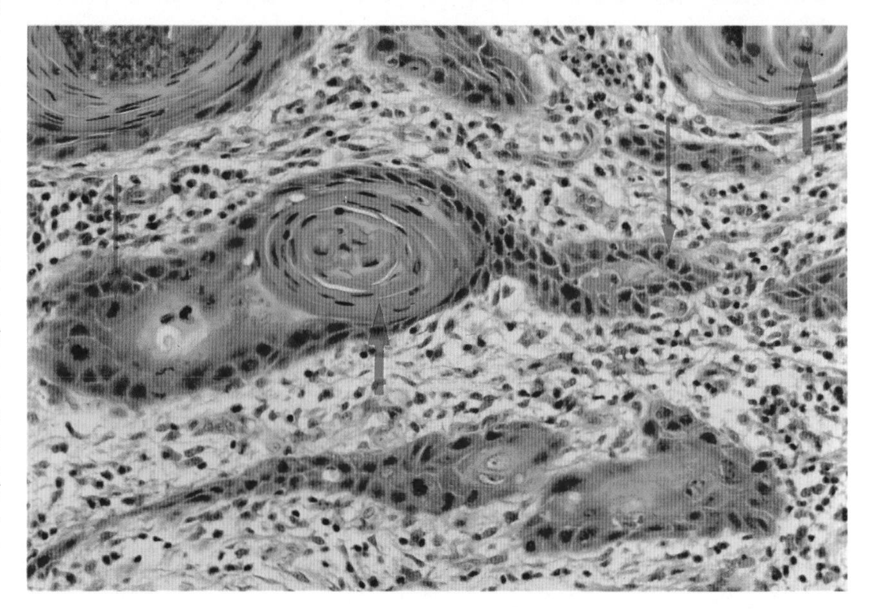

14.51 Melanocytic nevus (benign pigmented nevus): skin

Melanocytic nevi are formed by proliferation and maturation of the melanocytes of the epidermis. They develop from clusters of melanocyte precursor cells (nevus cells) which are arrested during the terminal phase of their migration from the neural crest to the epidermis, where they form melanocytes. Nevi develop in childhood but persist into adult life and are benign. Melanocytes are dendritic but appear as round cells with 'clear' cytoplasm, generally in the basal layer of the epidermis. This was a raised nodule 0.5cm dia on the face of a woman of 46. Histologically, it is a mature intradermal nevus. Melanocytes (thin arrow) in the basal layer of the epidermis show no proliferative (junctional) activity, whereas the dermis is occupied by packets (nests) of mature nevus cells, separated by strands of fibrous tissue (double arrow). The nevus cells exhibit some nuclear pleomorphism, but most of them have an ovoid basophilic nucleus and eosinophilic cytoplasm with ill-defined cell boundaries. Some of the nevus cells are multinucleated (thick arrow). There is no mitotic activity and no melanin pigment is visible. HE ×235

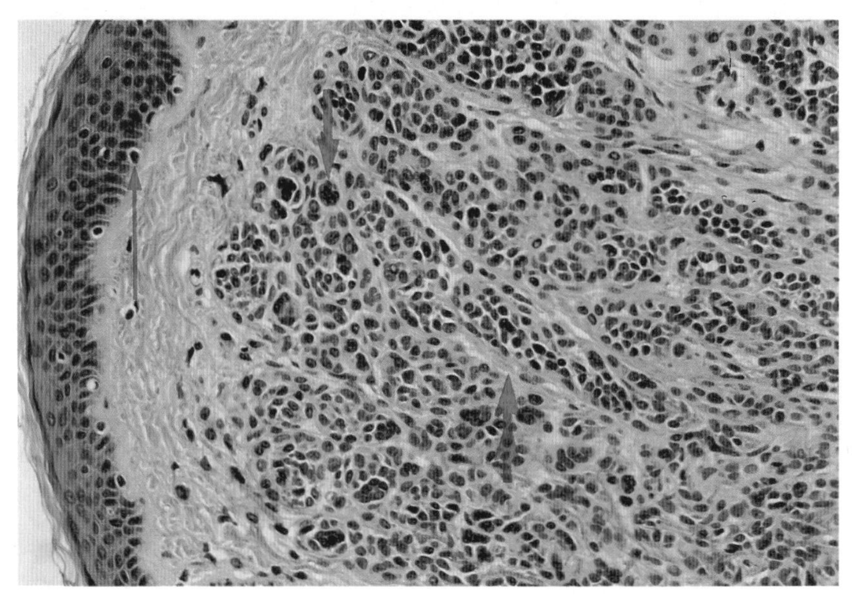

14.52 Juvenile melanoma: skin

In young individuals, compound nevi may show marked cellular atypia and pleomorphism, with proliferation of melanocytes in the junctional zone. Most juvenile melanomas are compound nevi and liable to be mistaken for a malignant melanoma. It is also recognized that juvenile melanomas are not confined to children, and a considerable proportion of them are found in older people. Despite its name however, juvenile melanoma, this type of nevus is benign, with no implication of malignant behaviour. Juvenile melanomas are flesh-coloured hairless nodules which are vascular and often look pink. Histologically they usually consist of large cells, some of which are spindle-shaped and the others epithelioid in appearance. In this nevus, there is active junctional activity, with nests of large melanocytes (thin arrows) in the epidermis and also in the immediately adjacent dermis (thick arrows). The melanocytes in these nests are mostly round and epithelioid, and their nuclei are fairly uniform. The cells in the epidermis (left) adjacent to the nevus cells contain melanin, and the dark brown (heavily pigmented) cells in the dermis are macrophages laden with melanin (double arrow).

HE ×360

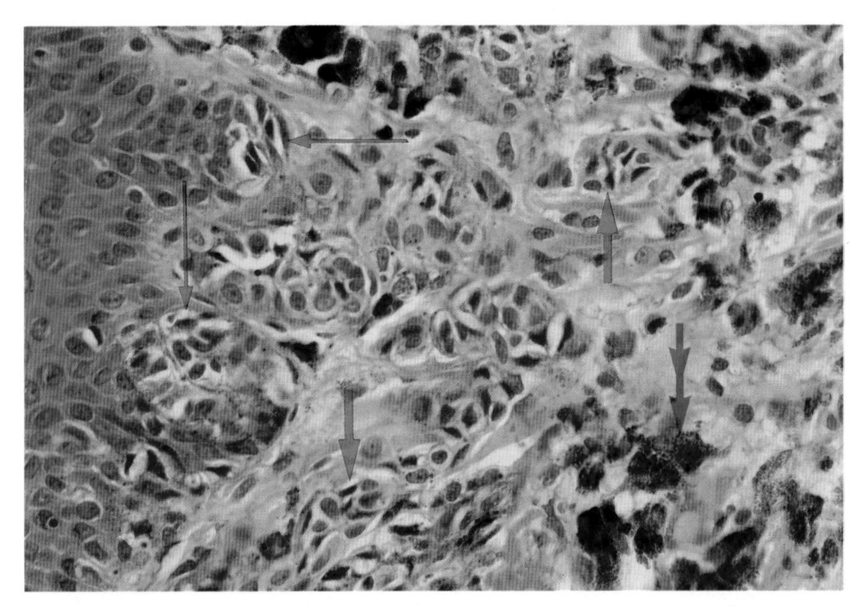

14.53 Juvenile melanoma: skin

When a juvenile melanoma arises in an older persons, it is sometimes difficult to differentiate it from malignant melanoma. Pseudoepitheliomatous hyperplasia is present in the epidermis in a minority of juvenile melanomas and the rete ridge (thin arrow) is elongated. The clusters of neoplastic nevus cells in the dermis are a mixture of epithelioid cells and elongated spindle-shaped cells (double arrow). The nevus cells are remarkably large, characteristically much larger than the keratinocytes of the epidermis, and they have a considerable amount of very well-defined eosinophilic cytoplasm. Their nuclei are large pleomorphic pale and vesicular, and contain one or more prominent nucleoli. Some are the nevus cells are very large and multinucleated. Although there is often considerable mitotic activity in a juvenile melanoma, there are no mitotic activity in this part of the nevus. There are however many small thin-walled but greatly dilated blood vessels (thick arrows), which is a diagnostically helpful feature in most juvenile melanomas. Small lymphocytes are also scattered throughout the dermal connective tissues.

HE ×235

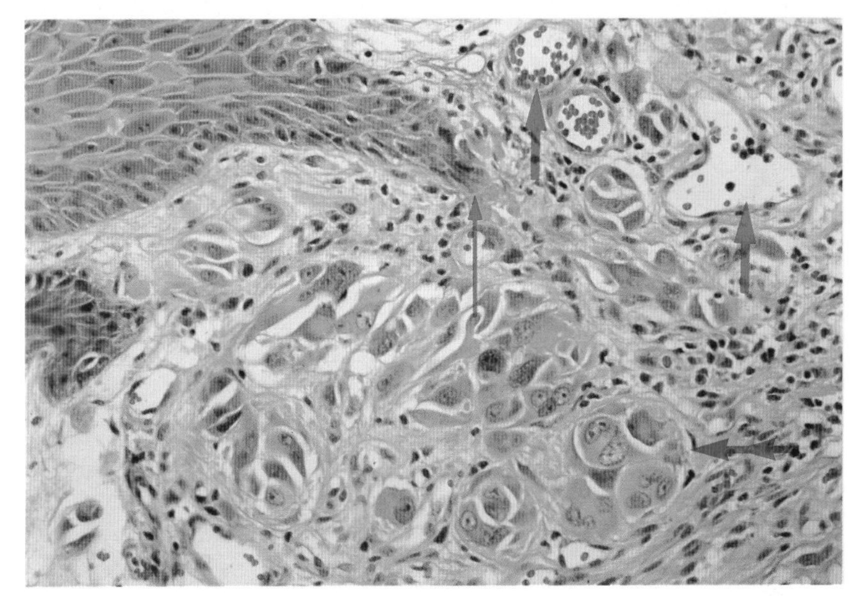

14.54 Intradermal nevus: skin

In most intradermal nevi, the nevus cells form small clumps in the dermis, and these are often arranged in rows at right angles to the epidermis. The nevus cells are cuboidal, with a uniformly round nucleus. Many intradermal nevi 'mature' and eventually involute, with progressive fibrosis until the lesion is replaced by a fibrous nodule which contains only a few nevus cells or structures resembling Meissner corpuscles. In this case, the epidermis (thin arrow) is attenuated, and the underlying dermis is occupied by the most superficial part of an intradermal nevus which has undergone a considerable degree of involution. The nevus cells have round or ovoid vesicular nuclei, containing pale finely granular chromatin. In some of the nuclei there is a central nucleolus. The cell cytoplasm, with fairly well-defined margins, is homogeneous and slightly hyalinized (thick arrows), which gives it a 'glassy' appearance. Several nevus cells contain melanin, and melanin-laden macrophages are also present. There is also a striking increase in fibrous tissue in the nevus, with eosinophilic connective tissue running between and around the individual nevus cells. A reticulin stain would show a well-developed network of delicate reticulin fibres.

HE ×400

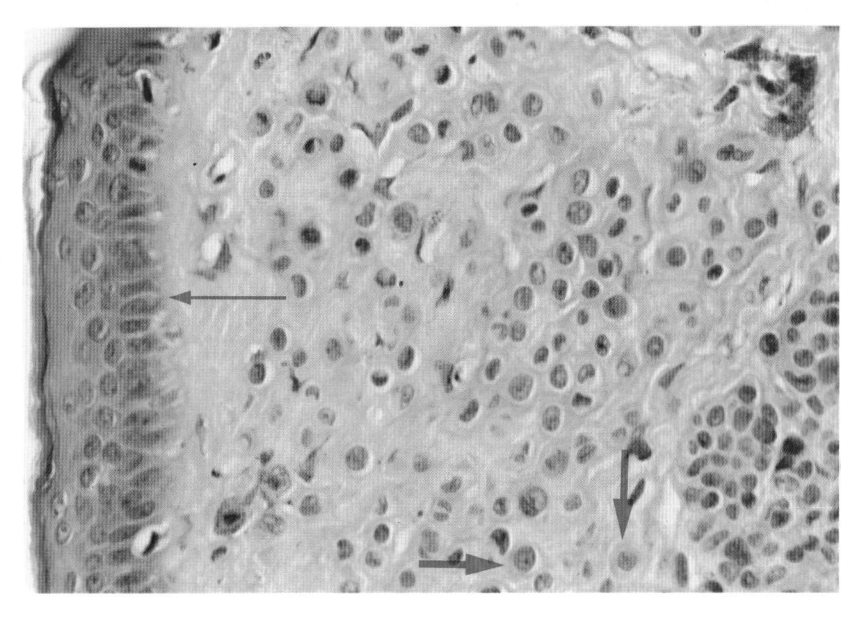

14.55 Blue nevus: skin

During development of the fetus, melanoblasts emigrating from the neuroectoderm to the epidermis may be retained in the dermis, where they mature to form blue nevi. In the sacral region, these cells form the Mongolian 'blue spots' present in some individuals at birth, but they may also form bluish nodules elsewhere. A blue nevus usually develops during childhood, and it is generally a solitary lesion. It is a small firm well-circumscribed bluish-black nodule, as a rule less than 1cm dia, and it is almost always benign. It consists of bundles of melanocytes, usually lying parallel to the epidermis and between bands of fibrous tissue in the dermis. Occasionally the nevus extends into the subcutaneous fat, and merges laterally with the dermis, without a clear margin between the two. In this lesion, the nevus cells, deep in the dermis, are mainly large spindle-shaped melanocytes with very long branching dendritic cytoplasmic processes (thin arrow) which contain melanin granules. The melanocytes are accompanied by similar numbers of large round or ovoid macrophages (melanophages) (thick arrow) with brown or dark brown cytoplasm which is heavily laden with ingested melanin produced by the nevus cells. HE ×335

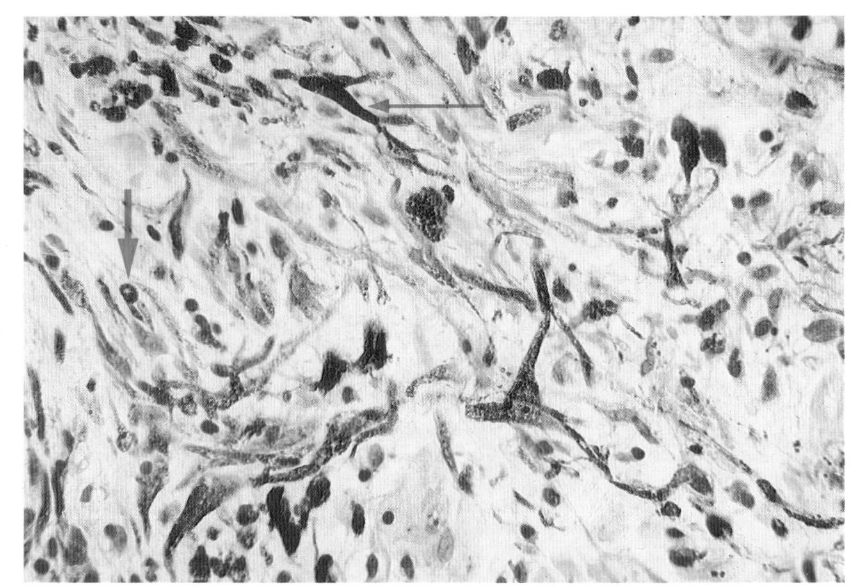

14.56 Lentigo maligna (Hutchinson's Freckle): skin

Lentigo maligna is a type of malignant melanoma in situ which occurs mainly in the skin of elderly individuals who have been heavily exposed to sunlight. It starts as a small unevenly pigmented macule which becomes progressively larger, sometimes extending to cover a large area. Histologically, lentigo maligna is characterized by a marked increase in the number of melanocytes in the basal layer of the epidermis. The lesion tends to remain in situ for long periods (10-15 years), but eventually one or more nodules of malignant melanoma may develop within it and then proceed to invade the dermis. In this case, the basal layer of the epidermis and that of the pilosebaceous follicle (top) have been replaced by a row, several cells thick, of large atypical melanocytes with pleomorphic hyperchromatic nuclei (double arrow). These melanocytes have not invaded the dermis however and the epidermal basement membrane is intact. Deep brown pigment-laden macrophages (melanophages) are present in the adjacent dermis (thin arrows). The collagenous fibrous tissue in the dermis (thick arrows) is basophilic and fragmented ('elastotic degeneration'), another effect of ultraviolet light.
HE ×235

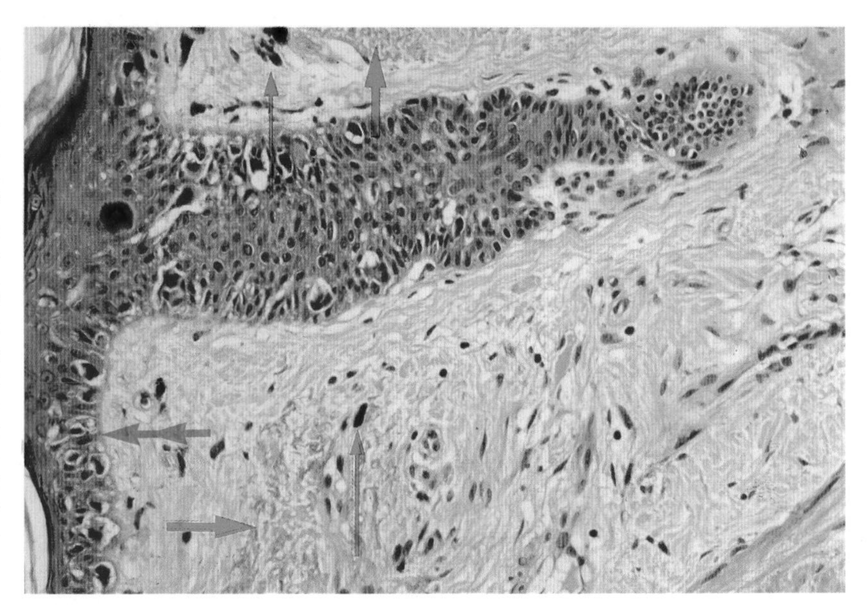

14.57 Lentigo maligna (Hutchinson's Freckle): skin

This is part of the same lesion as in 14.56. It is a particularly active area of junctional activity in the epidermis. On the surface of the epidermis, just visible at the left margin, there is a layer of keratin and trapped brown (melanin) granules (double arrow). Deep in the epidermis, large 'nests' (packets) of melanocytes with ovoid nuclei and abundant cytoplasm (greatly vacuolated and 'clear') (thin arrows) have formed and extended down to the dermis. The melanocyte 'nests' have also pushed upwards towards the surface of the epidermis. The packets of melanocytes are also expanding and stretching the basement membrane of the epidermis downwards, but it is still almost certainly intact (thick arrow), with no evident invasion of the dermis. There are numerous brown melanin granules within many of the melanocytes, but the elongated macrophages contain much greater amounts of the pigment. Most of the macrophages are located in the dermis, but there are also several within the epidermis. Not all cases of lentigo maligna go on to malignant melanoma. HE ×360

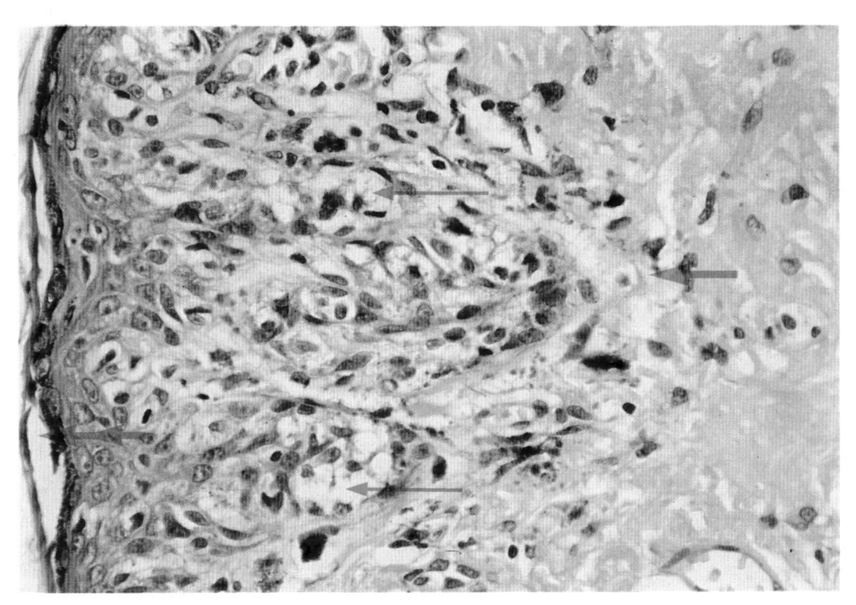

14.58 Malignant melanoma: skin

Malignant melanoma, generally a raised pigmented nodule on the skin, is a highly malignant type of tumour, growing rapidly and tending to bleed and ulcerate. This lesion arose in the nail-bed of the index finger of a woman of 63. Occasional pigment-laden cells are present in the stratum corneum (left margin), and there is pronounced junctional activity along basal layers of the epidermis and rete ridges, forming 'nests' (double arrow) full of abnormal melanocytes with hyperchromatic pleomorphic nuclei. Melanocytes have also migrated from the epidermis into the dermis and formed a large sheet of closely packed tumour cells (thin arrow), mostly elongated and with spindle-shaped nuclei. Many macrophages (melanophages), heavily laden with dark brown pigment, are present, particularly in the deeper aspects of the tumour (thick arrows). This tumour was diagnosed as a superficial spreading type of melanoma, with early dermal invasion (to a depth of 0.7mm). HE x150

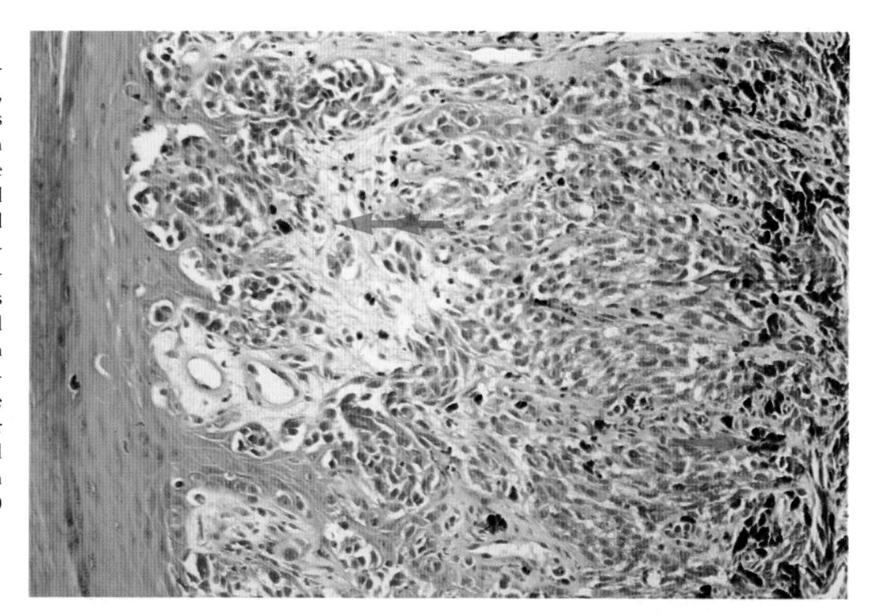

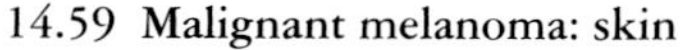

14.59 Malignant melanoma: skin

The neoplastic cells in malignant melanomas are generally markedly atypical and pleomorphic, with large hyperchromatic nuclei and a prominent nucleolus. Mitotic activity is increased. Melanin is usually present in the abundant cytoplasm, but absent in amelanotic melanomas. The two main types of tumour cell consist of malignant melanoma: spindle-shaped cells and epithelioid cells. The latter are large and round or polygonal with abundant deeply eosinophilic cytoplasm. Both types of tumour cell are often present in the same lesion. In this example, the epithelioid cells form fairly large clusters (thin arrows). Their cytoplasm is pinkish-brown, from the presence of very numerous fine melanin granules. The spindle cells are relatively few (thick arrows) and lie between the clusters of epithelioid cells. They have much less cytoplasm than the epithelioid cells and contain less melanin. The stroma (double arrow) is inconspicuous, but within it there are many pigment-laden macrophages (melanophages). No mitotic figures are present in this field but there were many elsewhere. HE x335

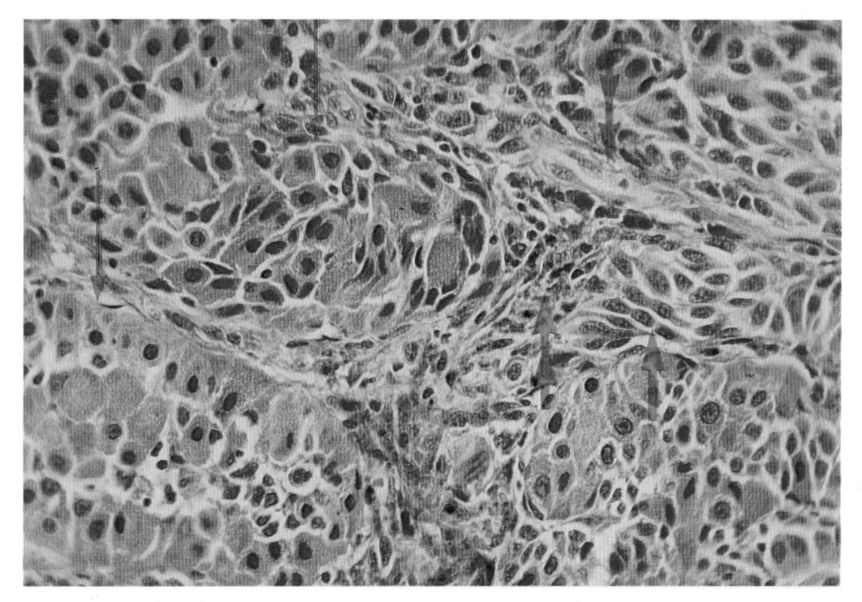

14.60 Malignant melanoma: skin

Malignant melanomas may arise in an existing benign pigmented nevus (junctional or compound but not intradermal) or arise de novo. Tumours in light-exposed skin which has been heavily exposed to sunlight tend to be flat (superficial malignant melanoma) with a better prognosis than tumours which tend to be nodular (nodular malignant melanoma). Nodular malignant melanomas tend to metastasize early, via the lymphatics and bloodstream, and useful signs of malignant change are the melanocytes with nuclei larger than keratinocyte nuclei. Upward penetration of the epidermis by abnormal melanocytes as far as the stratum granulosum is another lelptul indicator. In this example there is active proliferation of melanocytes (all melanin-containing) within the epidermis, and they have formed clusters (thin arrow), varying in size from a significant number deep in the epidermis, to single cells (thick arrow) which are being shed through the upper layers of the epidermis and into the keratin. The melanocytes in the relatively large clusters are mostly elongated and spindle-shaped, whereas those near the surface of the epidermis are round or ovoid. A large amount of near-black melanin (double arrow) is trapped in the thick layer of deeply eosinophilic keratin on the surface of the epidermis. HE ×335

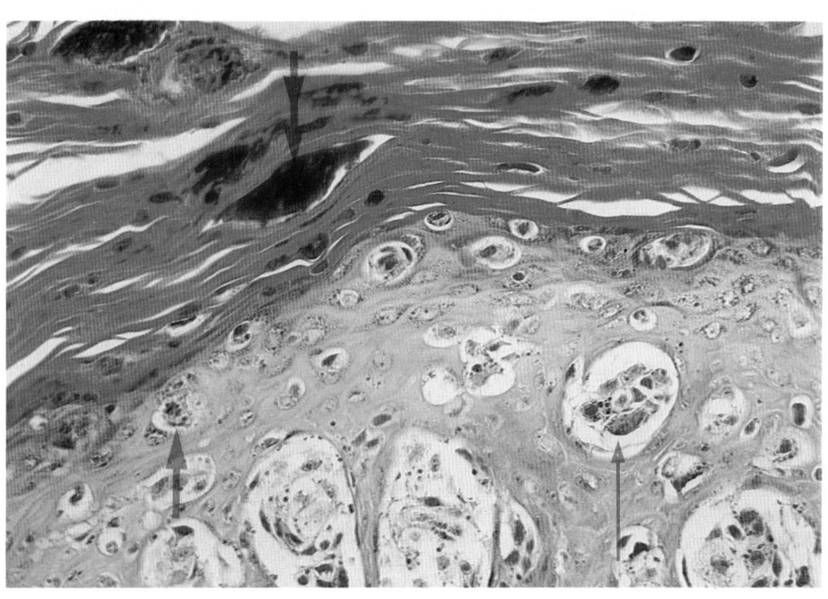

14.61 Malignant melanoma: conjunctiva

Malignant melanoma of the conjunctiva is rare, and may arise *de novo* or in a preexistent melanocytic nevus or a lentigo (acquired melanocytic hyperplasia). It generally takes the form of a nodule that may or may not be pigmented. Local excision of the more superficial lesions gives a good prognosis, but deeper invasion often leads to spread of the tumour via lymphatics and blood vessels. A man of 29 developed a small lesion at the limbus of the eye which was resected. Histologically, the tumour has an 'alveolar' pattern, consisting of groups of closely packed neoplastic cells (double arrow) separated by delicate strands of stromal connective tissue (thin arrows). The tumour cells are elongated, with scant cytoplasm and relatively large deeply basophilic hyperchromatic spindle-shaped nuclei. There is considerable mitotic activity (thick arrow) among the nuclei. There is no melanin, and only very small amounts could be detected elsewhere in the tumour. Dilated thin-walled blood vessels are present. The conjunctiva (top) is intact but was ulcerated over other parts of the tumour. There is a history of previous injury to the eye. HE ×350

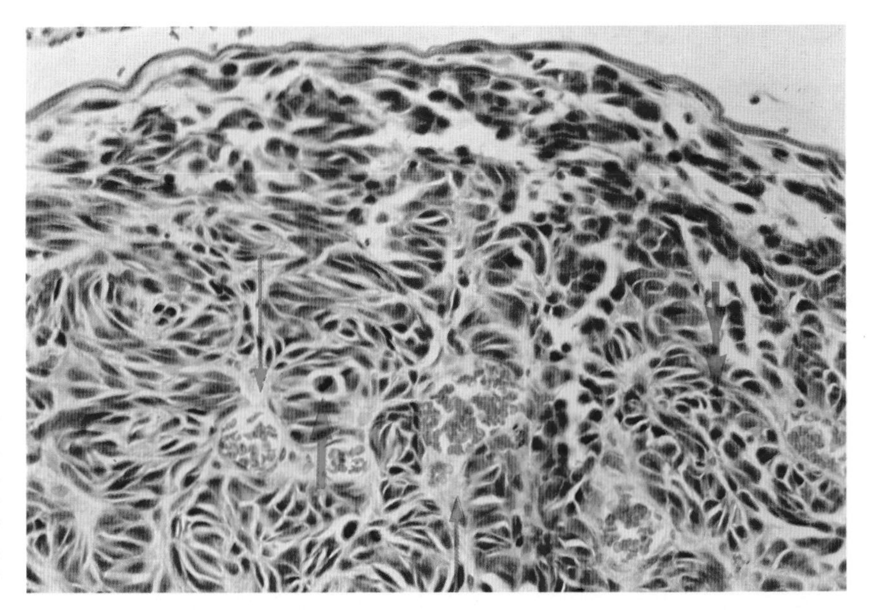

14.62 Gouty tophus: skin

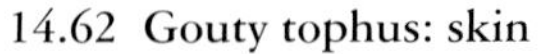

In gout, abnormal uric acid metabolism causes the level of uric acid in the plasma to rise (hyperuricemia), and consequently deposits of sodium urate crystals form in many sites, including the skin around joints. Deposition of microcrystals of sodium urate in the synovial membranes of joints causes acute gouty arthritis, whereas large masses of sodium urate crystals, large enough to produce a nodule (tophus), collect in the subcutaneous tissues and evoke chronic inflammation but not acute inflammation. This lesion is a gouty tophus, situated at the elbow (over the olecranon) of a man of 68. The tophus consists of clusters of pale or weakly eosinophilic urate crystals (thick arrows), surrounded by several layers of histiocytes and macrophages with ovoid or elongated vesicular nuclei (thin arrow). Some of the macrophages are multinucleated, containing a cluster of tightly packed basophilic nuclei in the cytoplasm (double arrow). The urate crystals are very small and the deposits appear amorphous. The crystals however have been shown to be birefringent in polarized light. Collagenous fibrous tissue surrounds the deposits of urate crystals, but there is no evidence of an acute inflammatory reaction in the vicinity of the tophus. HE ×150

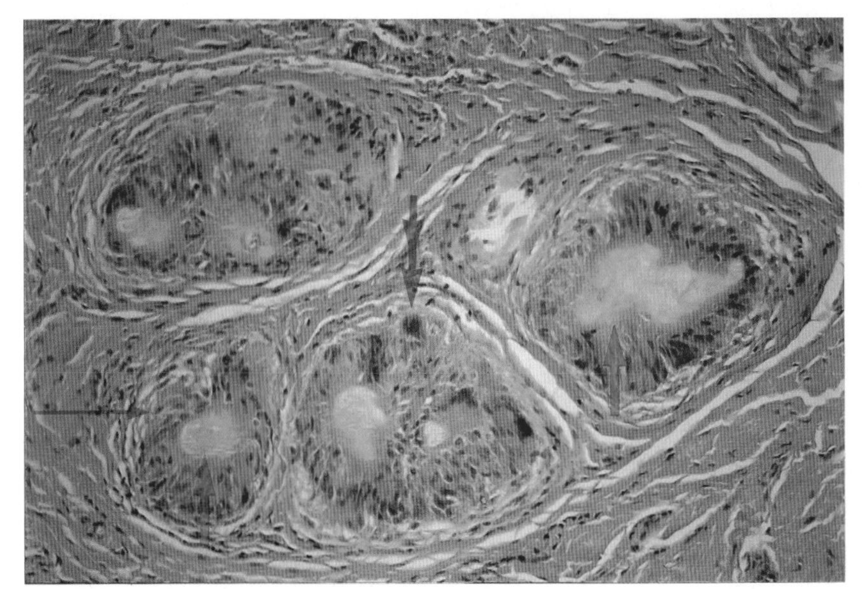

14.63 Lipoma ('hibernoma'): skin

Lipomas are common benign tumours of adipose tissue, which arise in any part of the body and are not infrequently multiple. Most of the patients are more than 40 years of age. Lipomas are usually composed of mature greatly swollen fat (adipose) cells with a very large clear (fat-containing) cytoplasmic vacuole, but this tumour is a rare variant, composed largely of 'brown fat'. Since brown fat is also abundant in hibernating animals, the name of the neoplasm is 'hibernoma'. Brown fat is found in the fetus but only in small amounts in later life, whereas a hibernoma is usually a well-defined lobulated brown mass in a young adult. In this lesion, the ordinary (clear) fat cells (thick arrow) are larger than the much more numerous closely apposed brown fat cells (thin arrows) and generally accompany them. The fat in the brown fat cells is distributed throughout the cytoplasm in multiple small vacuoles, and the cells are appropriately called 'mulberry cells'. In the centre of the cytoplasm in each brown fat cell there is a small round hyperchromatic nucleus. HE ×235

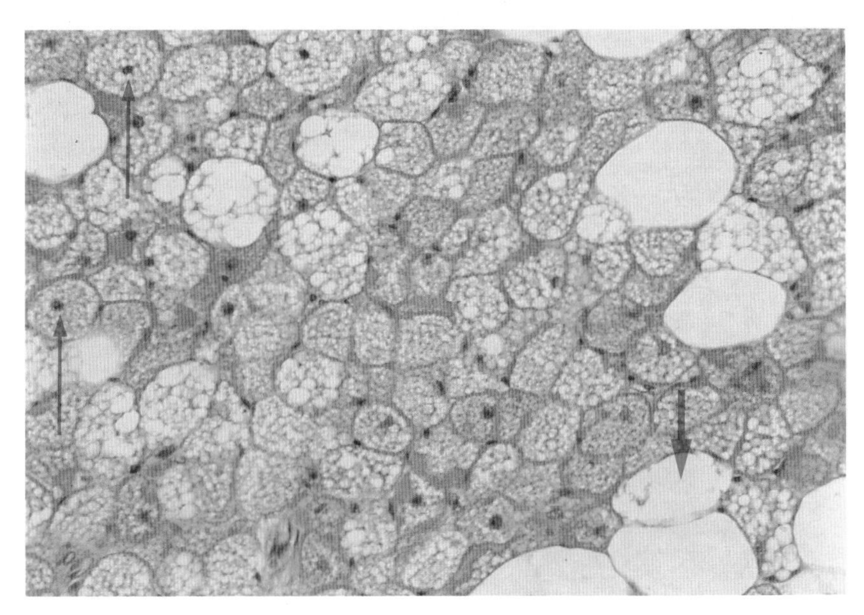

14.64 Xanthelasma: skin

When the levels of lipids and lipoproteins in the serum are raised (hyperlipidemia), lipid may be deposited in the tissues, where it is ingested by macrophages. This is the basis for the formation of xanthoma. The lipid-laden macrophages take a variety of forms and generally give rise to multiple lesions. In time, there is usually progressive fibrosis around each deposit. When a plane xanthoma develops on an eyelid, it is called a xanthelasma. However, the fat is neutral in the majority of xanthelasmas, the small yellow plaques that form in the eyelids of some individuals, and in only a minority of cases is there an association with hyperlipidemia. Xanthelasmas are noteworthy for their superficial location in the upper dermis, and this xanthelasma is situated in the subepithelial zone at the inner canthus. This part of the lesion consists of a sheet of closely packed large discrete lipid-laden foamy macrophages (thin arrow) , many of them multinucleated (thick arrow) with a large amount of well-defined very finely granular ('frosted--glass') cytoplasm. Xanthelasmas are also noted for the absence of fibrosis around the plaques. The structure on the right is a normal pilosebaceous follicle (double arrow). HE ×335

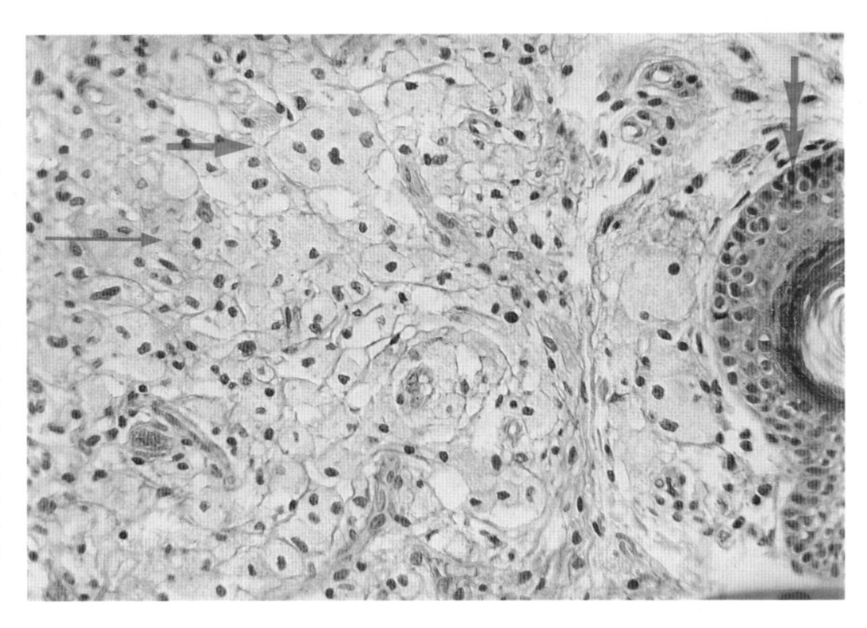

14.65 Tuberous xanthoma (xanthoma tuberosum): skin

Tuberous xanthomas develop in individuals with raised levels of beta-lipoproteins in the plasma. The lesions take the form of large nodules in the skin on extensor surfaces such as elbows, knees, ankles, fingers and the buttocks, and are often associated with trauma. The cut surface of a nodule is yellow or orange. Histologically, early lesions consist of aggregates of xanthoma cells (foamy macrophages), mixed with smaller numbers of histiocytes, lymphocytes and neutrophil polymorphs. As the lesions mature, fibroblasts appear in increasing numbers. This is a mature lesion. It consists of large macrophages, mostly elongated, with varying amounts of pale finely granular cytoplasm; and among them there are already elongated fibroblasts and collagenous fibrous tissue (thin arrow). Scattered throughout this tissue are very large multinucleated cells. These are Touton giant cells. Each cell contains large numbers of nuclei (double arrow), grouped around eosinophilic cytoplasm, and beyond (more peripheral than) the nuclei there is a large zone of finely granular (foamy) cytoplasm (thick arrows). HE ×360

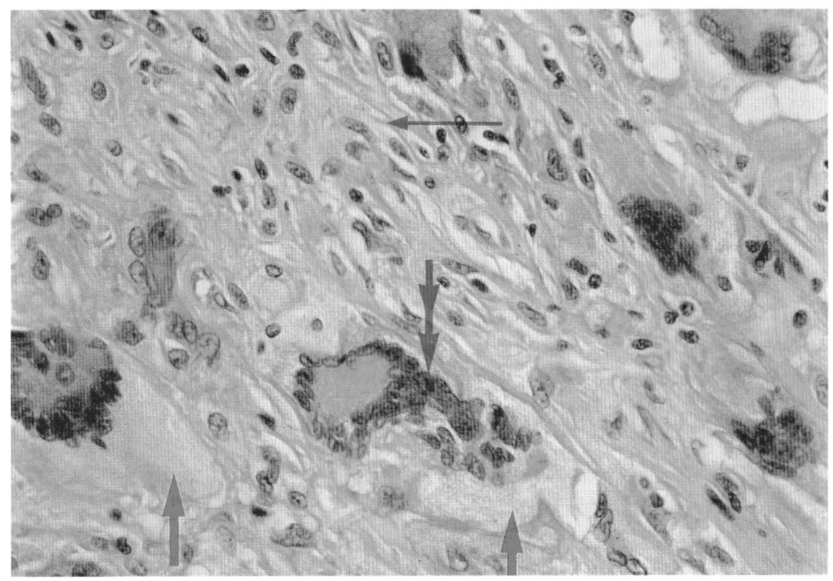

14.66 Tuberous xanthoma (xanthoma tuberosum): skin

Tuberous xanthomas contain higher concentrations of cholesterol esters than other types of xanthoma, and they are particularly common in people with hereditary hyperlipemia type IIA and less often in those with hyperlipemia types IIB or III or IV. Control of the hyperlipemia however does not cause tuberous xanthomas to regress. The lesions generally consist of macrophages filled with fat, along with a mixture of inflammatory cells in the early stages and an increasing amount of fibrous tissue in the late stages. This lesion consisted initially of macrophages with granular (foamy) cytoplasm, and it has now been largely replaced by a large collection of pale cholesterol-rich debris and a sheet of elongated fibroblasts and collagenous fibrous tissue. Between the bundles of collagenous fibres (thin arrows) there are many clefts (thick arrow), now empty but previously containing crystals of cholesterol (the cholesterol having dissolved in the tissue-processing reagents). Long spindle-shaped cells and large multinucleated (foreign body-type) cells lie alongside empty clefts which contained crystals. Fairly numerous lymphocytes are also present in the lesion. HE ×235

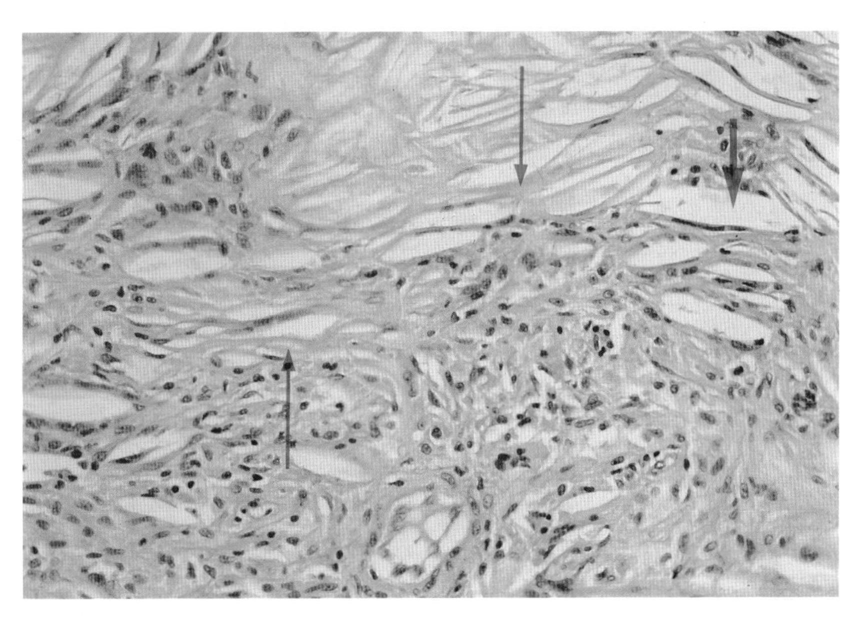

14.67 Dermatofibroma: skin

Dermatofibroma (termed nodular subepidermal fibrosis or cutaneous fibrous histiocytoma) is a common neoplasm in the 20-50 age range and affecting women more often than men. The tumour is often located on a limb, and minor trauma seems to play a role at the site. There is usually only one ovoid or round lesion in the skin (less than 0.5cm dia) but sometimes two or three. It is generally dome-shaped but may be depressed. Most dermatofibromas are brown but may be bluish, reddish or yellowish. The earliest lesion is a collection in the mid-dermis of mature histiocytes, many of which appear foamy. This was a large mushroom-shaped 'papilloma' on the knee of a woman of 52. In this frozen section, in which lipid is retained, the histiocytes contain numerous droplets of fat (stained orange-red) (arrow). The histiocytes lie between collagenous fibres, which are unstained. The cells with elongated nuclei and no lipid in their cytoplasm are fibroblasts and endothelial cells. Hemosiderin was also present. Sudan IV x150

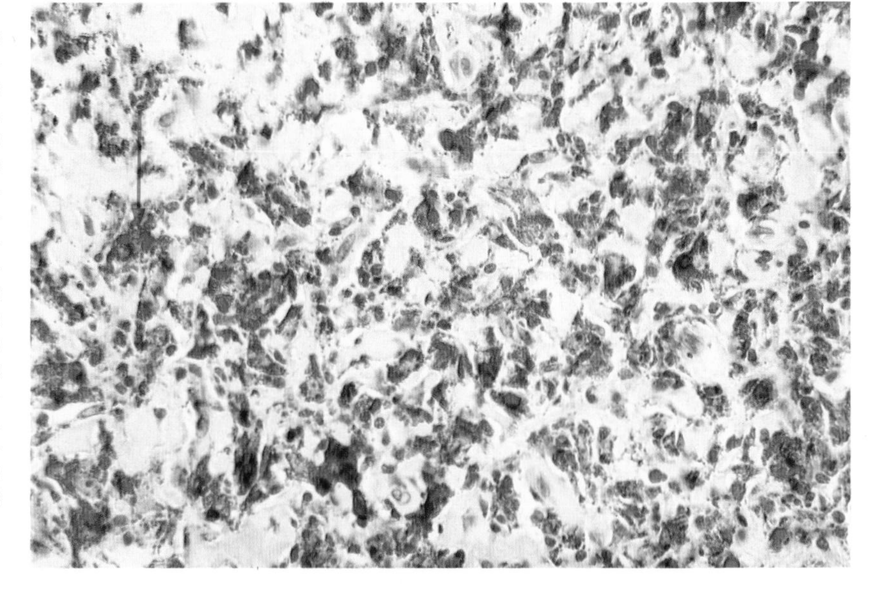

14.68 Dermatofibroma: skin

Some dermatofibromas, composed mainly very vascular connective tissue, tend to bleed. Most dermatofibromas however consist of interlacing bundles of spindle-shaped fibrocytes and collagenous fibrous tissue. Sometimes the collagen is dominant and the fibrocytes are small and inconspicuous. In other lesions, the fibrocytes are larger and more numerous, and the collagenous fibres between them are comparatively slender. This tissue is from a raised smooth cutaneous nodule (1.2cm dia) on the back of the thigh of a woman of 23, the cut surface of which looked characteristically brownish-yellow. The lesion consists of a network of strands of cellular eosinophilic connective tissue which enclose relatively large vascular channels. The channels are dilated (thin arrows) and lack a well-formed endothelial lining, and some of the blood is extravascular. Within the connective tissue there are many macrophages heavily laden with hemosiderin (thick arrow), and a frozen section would reveal large numbers of lipid-laden cells, the lipid presumably having the same origin as the hemosiderin. HE x215

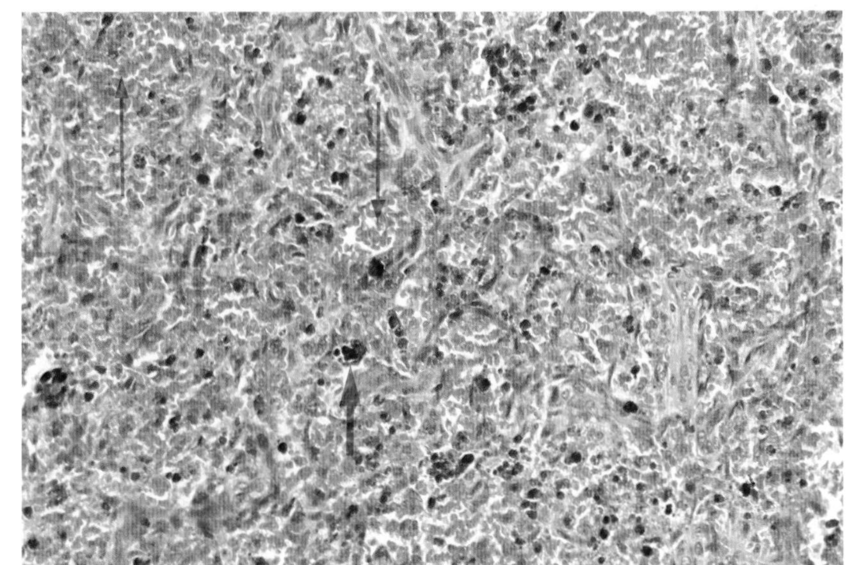

14.69 Dermatofibroma: skin

There is a storiform pattern in many dermatofibromas, and the fibrocytes exhibit little atypia. There is also minimal mitotic activity. However the neoplastic cells sometimes resemble ovoid macrophages with abundant well-defined cytoplasm and round or ovoid vesicular nuclei. In some of the macrophage-like cells there are droplets of fat or granules of hemosiderin. This firm nodule 1.5cm dia on the leg of a 43-year-old man represents the end-stage of nodular subepidermal fibrosis. The nodule is a dermatofibroma consisting of curved bundles of cells and fibrous tissue which form a well-developed storiform (basket-weave) pattern (see 14.71). The tissues are mainly interlacing strands of collagenous fibrous tissue (thick arrow) and, closely associated with them, a large population of curved or stellate fibroblasts (thin arrow). Many vacuolated cells are also present, and special stains would reveal histiocytes containing lipid and hemosiderin. The nodule looks well-demarcated to the naked eye but histologically it merges gradually into the dermis and subcutaneous fat. It is nevertheless benign. HE x235

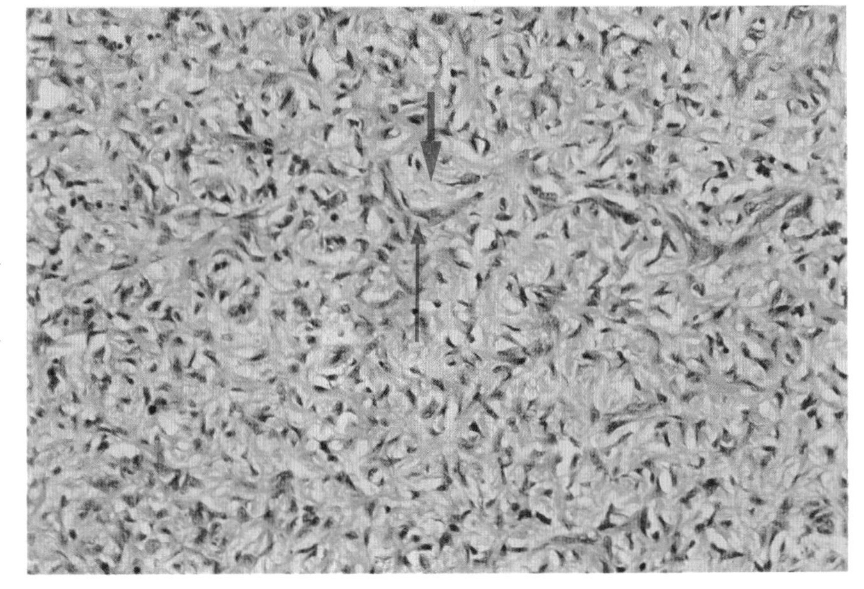

14.70 Dermatofibrosarcoma protuberans

Dermatofibrosarcoma is a slow-growing nodular lesion, peculiar to the dermis and usually on the trunk. It protrudes above the skin surface but also grows downwards, so that early lesions have an hour-glass shape. It may also reach a large size, and the skin over its surface may ulcerate. Although its malignancy is low-grade, it is not encapsulated and notoriously liable to recur, unless a wide margin of normal-looking skin around the tumour is resected. Metastases are very uncommon, but may recur after many years, especially after previous recurrent removals. This tumour also is a recurrent mass, in the skin of the back of a woman of 46. It is a firm white nodule 2 × 2 × 1.5cm. Histologically it is a well-differentiated fibrosarcoma, consisting of broad interlacing bands of collagenous fibrous tissue (arrow) in which there are numerous fibrocytes and proliferating fibroblastic cells with elongated spindle-shaped nuclei. Nuclear pleomorphism is slight, but occasional mitoses are present. The tumour has invaded the adjacent subcutaneous fat and probably also fascia and muscle. HE ×150

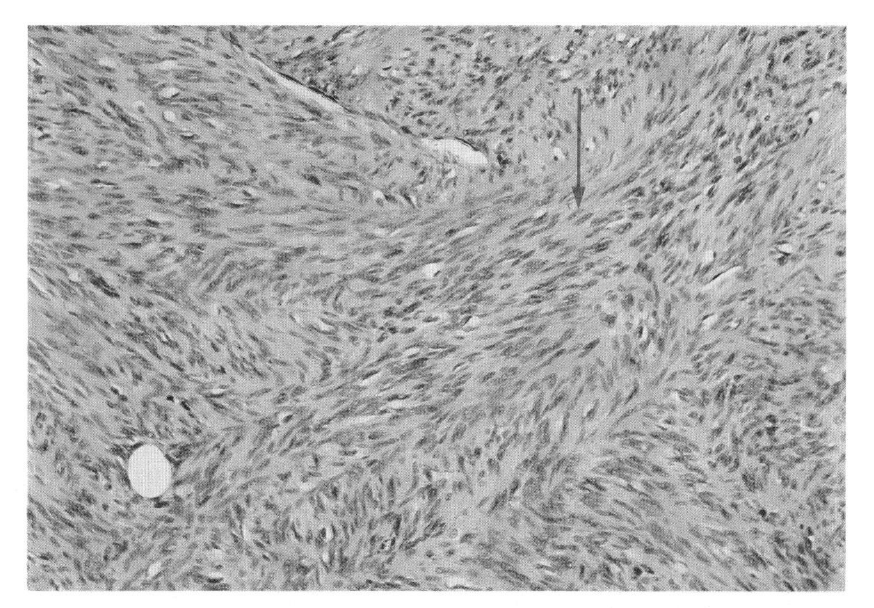

14.71 Dermatofibrosarcoma protuberans

Dermatofibrosarcoma protuberans invades slowly, but is persistent and tends to merge irregularly with the subcutaneous tissue or even more deeply. This tissue is from a raised nodule 1cm wide, on the right shoulder of a man of 26. It consists of relatively narrow interlacing bundles of apparently well-differentiated but mildly atypical elongated spindle-shaped cells and eosinophilic connective tissue. The spindle-shaped cells and connective tissue are arranged as tight whorls which form a very distinct storiform pattern (arrow), with nuclei tending to radiate out like spokes from the hub of a wheel (cart-wheel or basket-weave pattern) (see also 14.69). Special stains have revealed abundant reticulin but only a relatively small amount of collagen. The spindle-shaped cells show moderate mitotic activity. The tumour has invaded the subdermal tissues, but metastasis to regional lymph nodes and/or viscera is extremely unlikely. It has been suggested that dermatofibrosarcoma protuberans has a histiocytic origin and belongs to an increasing group of fibrous histiocytomas. This is uncertain, and demonstration of antigen CD34 (immunohistochemically) is diagnostically helpful. HE ×235

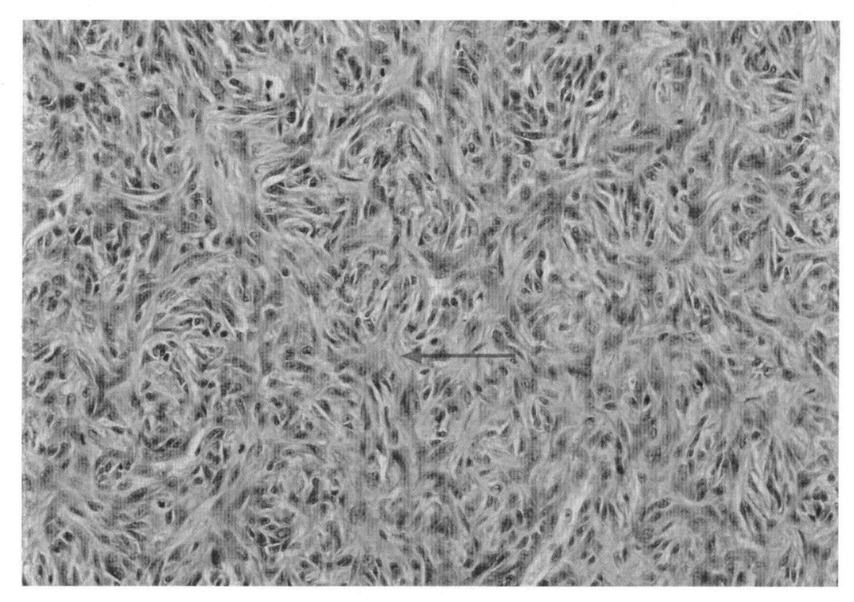

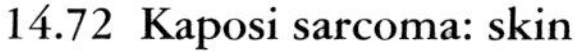

14.72 Kaposi sarcoma: skin

Kaposi sarcoma was a rare neoplasm in the USA and Europe until 1979, when it occurred in epidemic proportions in patients with AIDS, in whom a much more aggressive variant of Kaposi sarcoma, of uncertain histogenesis, was discovered. Macroscopically, the red or purplish lesions of the variant may or may not be confined to the skin but are widely distributed throughout the body, occurring particularly in lymph nodes, gastrointestinal tract and liver. Histologically, it is an infiltrative lesion, composed of spindle-shaped endothelial cells which form poorly developed vascular slits. Extravasation of red cells and deposition of hemosiderin often occurs. The appearance of this tumour is mainly angiosarcomatous. The cells are spindle-shaped (thin arrow) and resemble poorly-differentiated fibroblasts, smooth muscle cells or endothelial cells. They also readily form large numbers of narrow blood-filled channels. Mitotic figures are numerous among them (thick arrow). There is considerable hemorrhage throughout the tumour, and beneath the epidermis there is a thick compressed layer of red cells and deeply eosinophilic fibrin (double arrow). HE ×200

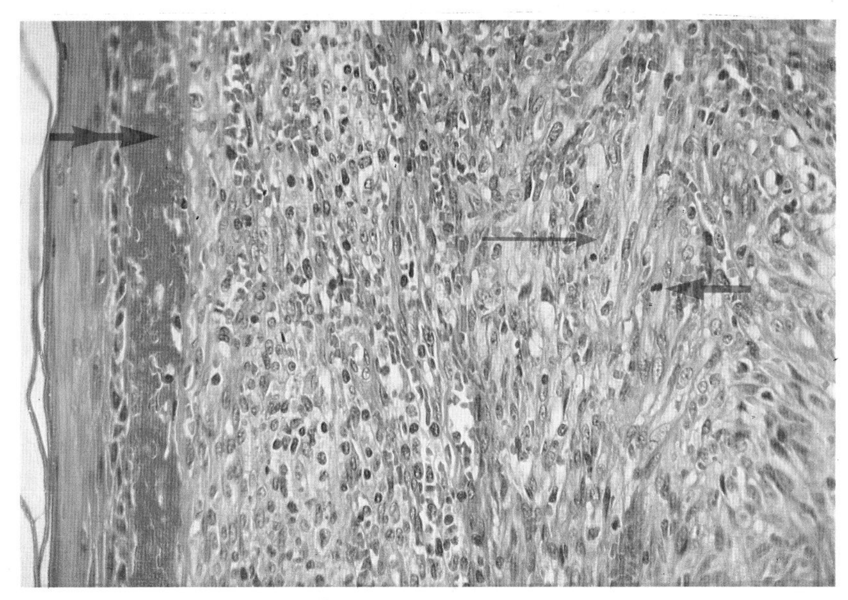

14.73 Neurofibroma: skin

Neurofibromas are slow-growing benign tumours that originate in the peripheral nerve sheaths of large nerve trunks or of very small nerves in peripheral tissues such as skin. They are generally well-circumscribed but not encapsulated, and (histologically) consist of a mixed (hamartomatous) population of spindle-shaped Schwann cells and fibroblasts. A neurofibroma may be a solitary neoplasm in the skin, usually in adult life, or it may be one of the many neurofibromas in neurofibromatosis (von Recklinghausen's syndrome), a condition usually manifest in childhood. Plexiform neuromas are typically large, pendulous and flabby, and generally multiple. They are composed of thickened tortuous nerves. This lesion is a plexiform neuroma in the upper lip of a woman of 22 but it is small. The epidermis (left) is stretched over a plexus of enormously thickened small nerves (double arrow) beneath the dermis. The sheaths (thin arrows) of the nerves are intact, but each nerve is greatly expanded by the presence within it of a considerable amount of pale-staining myxoid connective tissue, produced by the Schwann cells. There are numerous axons within the myxoid tissue but they are not visible in this type of illustration. A sebaceous gland (thick arrow) is present. HE ×70

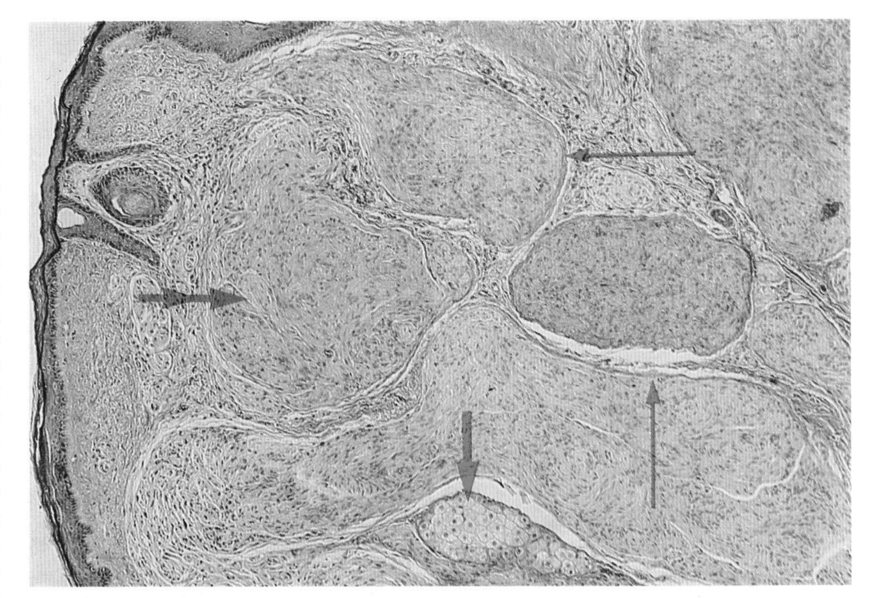

14.74 Neurofibroma: skin

Neurofibroma of skin is a non-encapsulated neoplasm, consisting of spindle-shaped cells and axons, in a myxoid stroma with variable amounts of collagen. The cells are a mixture of Schwann cells, perineural cells and fibroblasts. In this case, a neurofibroma of skin reacted with an antibody to the neural marker S100 protein, showing positive (brown) reactivity in the component cells. The presence of S100 protein is a reliable (immunohistochemical) method of confirming the identities of Schwannomas (neurilemmomas) and neurofibromas. The malignant potential of neurofibromas is very slight in solitary lesions, but malignant transformation is more common in the very numerous lesions of neurofibromatosis.

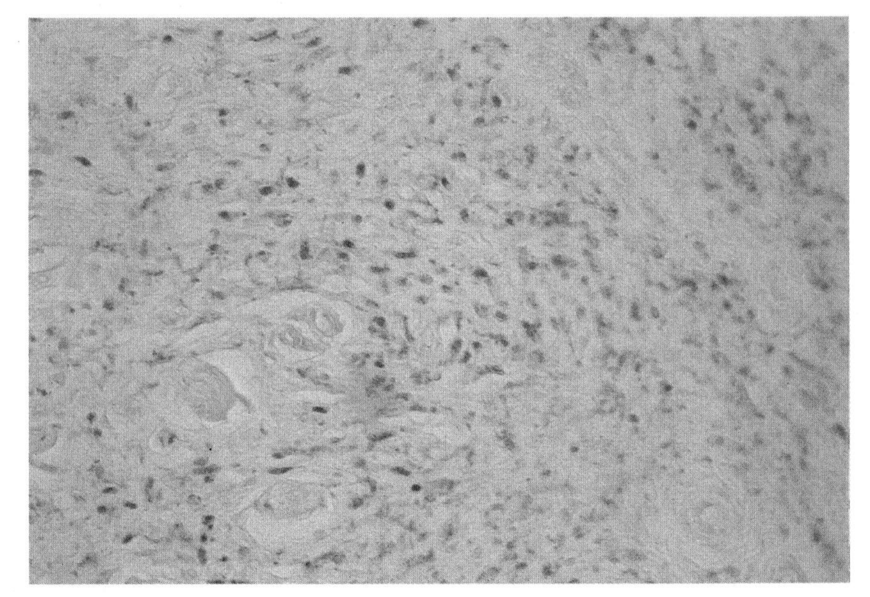

14.75 Neurofibroma: skin

Neurofibromas of large nerves are firm rubbery masses, the result of expansion of the affected nerve and removable only by sacrificing the nerve. Cellularity varies in neurofibromas, and the stroma often undergoes myxomatous change. The tumour is also liable to become cystic. The nuclei of the neoplastic cells are often atypical and pleomorphic, but their appearance does not predict malignancy. On the other hand, mitotic activity does generally indicate a significant trend towards malignancy. This lesion has the structure of the more common type of neurofibroma. The overlying epidermis is hyperkeratotic (thick arrow) and the papillary dermis is spared. In the deeper dermis, the tumour consists of elongated cells (thin arrow) with poorly defined cell margins and deeply basophilic ovoid or elongated nuclei of fairly uniform size and shape. There is no mitotic activity. The cells are distributed randomly throughout loosely-textured connective tissue. Special stains showed the presence of considerable amounts of delicate connective tissue (reticulin) but little collagen. There is no fibrous capsule. Nerve fibres are present in most neurofibromas but require special stains for their demonstration. Although malignant change rarely takes place in a neurofibroma in a person with neurofibromatosis, a small but significant number are the product of preexisting neurofibromas. HE ×150

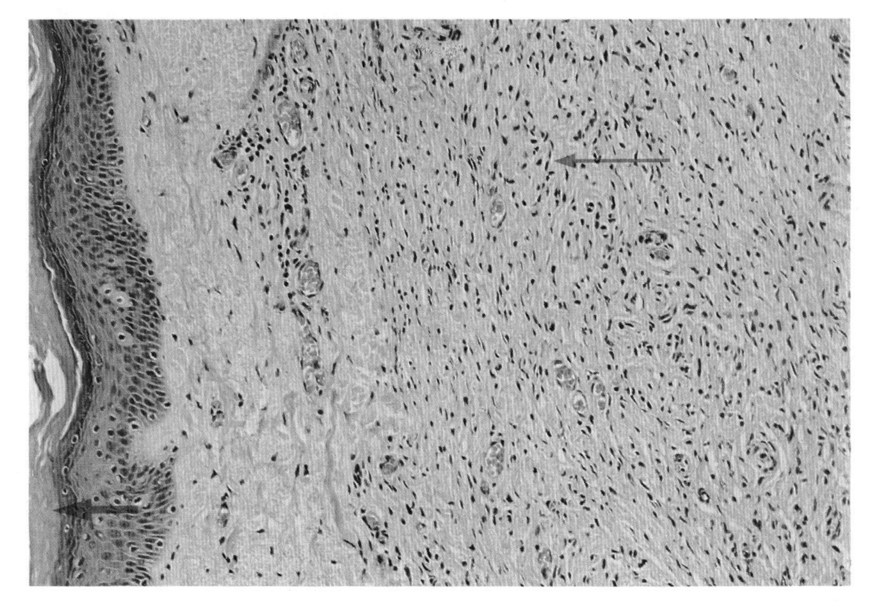

14.76 Neurofibroma: skin

There is a small but significant risk of neurofibromas becoming malignant, and more so in patients with von Recklinghausen's syndrome (neurofibromatosis). Neurofibromatosis is the most common hereditary neurocutaneous syndrome, with an estimated prevalence of one in three thousand in the USA. There are two types of syndrome, neurofibromatosis 1 (with an abnormal gene on chromosome 17) and neurofibromatosis 2 (with the gene on chromosome 22). This lesion is one of two subcutaneous nodules, each 1cm dia, in the subcutaneous tissues of the chest wall of a man of 34. Histologically they were identical, each consisting of irregular spindle-shaped cells with ill-defined cytoplasmic margins and ovoid or elongated moderately pleomorphic hyperchromatic nuclei (thin arrow). The neoplastic cells are surrounded by a considerable amount of loose (vacuolated) eosinophilic extracellular matrix and numerous delicate collagenous fibrils (thick arrow). There is no mitotic activity. Neither lesion is encapsulated and elsewhere some dermal appendages are caught up in both. HE ×235

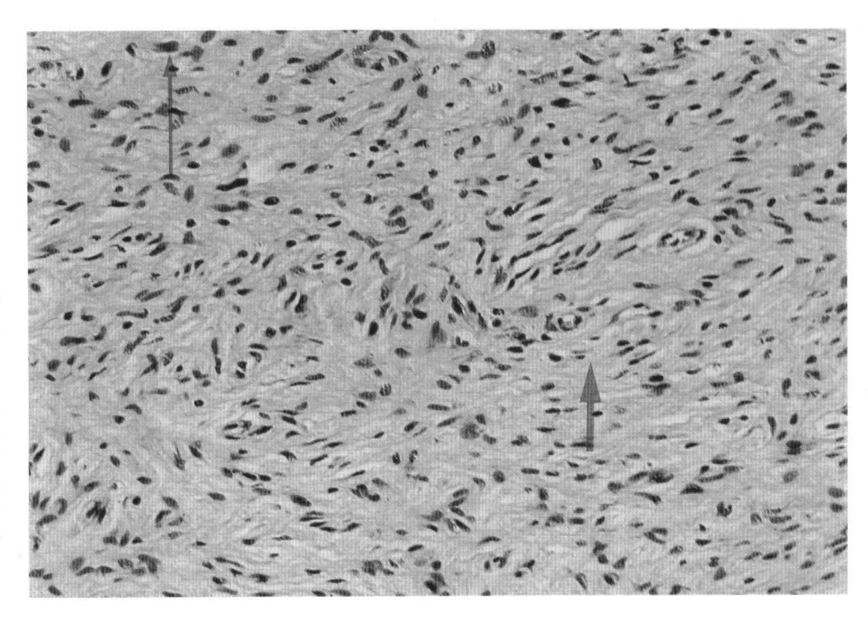

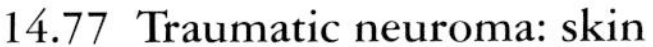

14.77 Traumatic neuroma: skin

When a segment of a peripheral nerve trunk is severely injured by trauma, the internal structure of the individual nerve bundles within the nerve trunk is considerably disorganized. The axons are disrupted and grow out from the cut ends of the nerve fibres. Their distal parts undergo Wallerian degeneration. Fibroblasts and Schwann cells proliferate, and if the cut ends of the nerve are not accurately apposed, the various elements continue to grow and form a disorderly mass of fibrous tissue and nerve fibres. Fibrous tissue forms within the damaged segment and acts as a barrier to the growing (proximal) axons. Schwann cells also grow out from the proximal part of the nerve, and along with the fibroblasts and axonal sprouts, create a fusiform swelling, termed a 'traumatic neuroma'. In this case, a firm white mass, 2cm in its long axis, was removed from the side of the neck from a woman of 55. It consists of bundles of nerve fibres (thin arrow) of various sizes and alignment, mingled with and separated by bands of loose connective tissue (thick arrow). The whole mass is enclosed in a collagenous fibrous capsule (double arrow). HE ×235

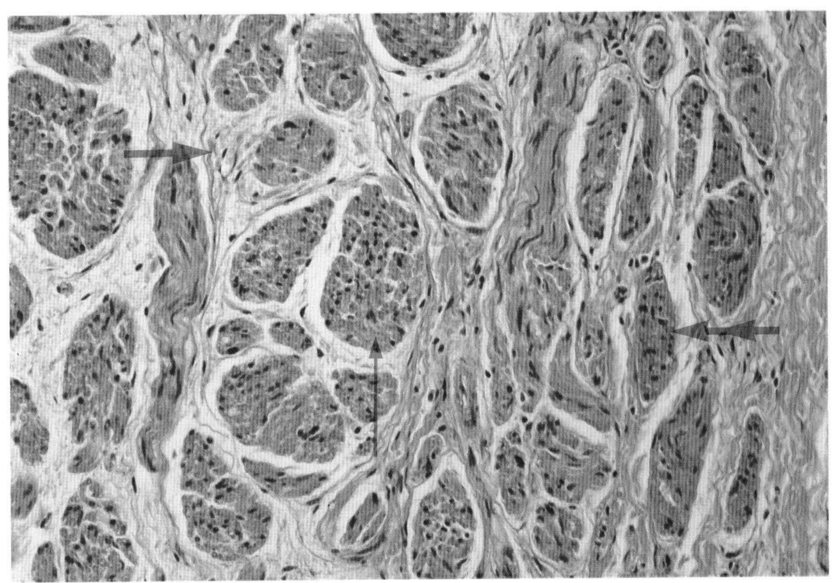

14.78 Hemangioma: skin

Hemangiomas are vascular hamartomas and take a variety of forms. Cavernous hemangiomas occur in the skin and also in the viscera. They are soft spongy lesions which grow slowly, up to 2-3cm dia. In the liver they are discovered incidentally and found to consist (histologically) of large endothelium-lined spaces filled with blood. Hemangiomas in deep subcutaneous tissues and muscle tend to be ill-defined and liable to recur unless widely excised. Capillary hemangiomas are usually small (less than 1cm dia) reddish-blue plaques or nodules which grow at the same rate as the individual, apart from 'strawberry' hemangiomas which grow rapidly in the first few months of life and then regress, often completely. This lesion, on the right cheek of a 6-year-old girl, is a capillary hemangioma. It consists of small thick-walled blood vessels, capillary-like but markedly distended, and lined by prominent endothelial cells (arrow). The blood vessels ramify throughout the subcutaneous fat of the cheek and have extended laterally for a considerable distance. Large 'feeding' blood vessels are present elsewhere in the lesion. HE ×150

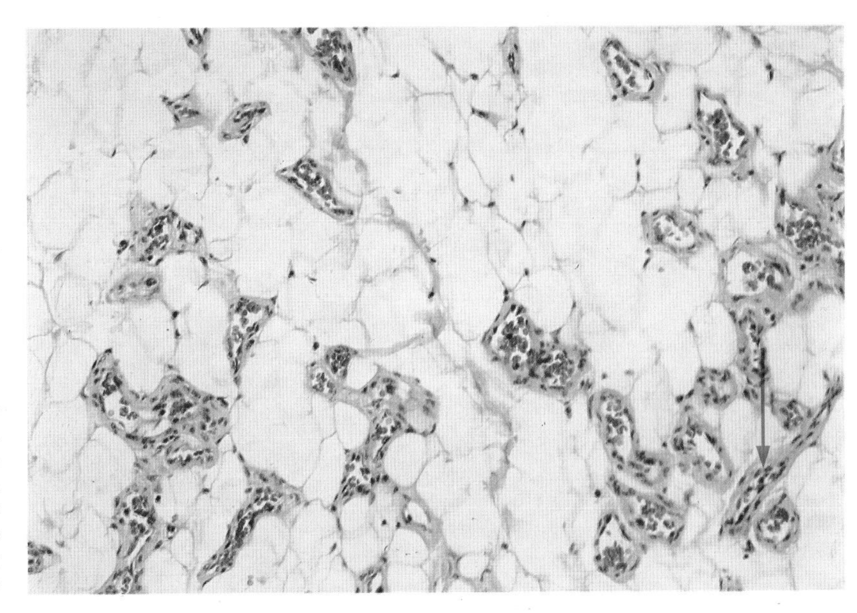

14.79 Glomus tumour (glomangioma) : skin

Glomus tumours (glomangiomas) arise from glomus bodies situated in small arterioles, in small arteriovenous anastomoses, which control blood flow and temperature. The tumour is usually a small firm purplish nodule, 1-10mm dia, encapsulated and benign, but sensitive to touch and liable to cause paroxysms of severe pain. Glomus tumours may be located anywhere in the skin, but most often under fingernails and toenails. Histologically they are composed of vascular spaces, separated by nests of small round cells with scant cytoplasm. Unusually however, this nodule, 2mm dia, in the subcutaneous tissue of the knee of a 33-year-old man, consists of dilated vascular channels, lined by a single layer of elongated very flat endothelium-like cells (thick arrows). The vessels are closely associated with slender cords and small groups of round or cuboidal glomus ('myoid') cells (thin arrow) with eosinophilic ill-defined cytoplasm and pale-staining uniformly round or ovoid nuclei which show no pleomorphism or mitotic activity. In some areas the glomus cells are surrounded by eosinophilic stroma. Special stains reveal large numbers of medullated and non-medullated nerve fibres in the tumour. HE x235

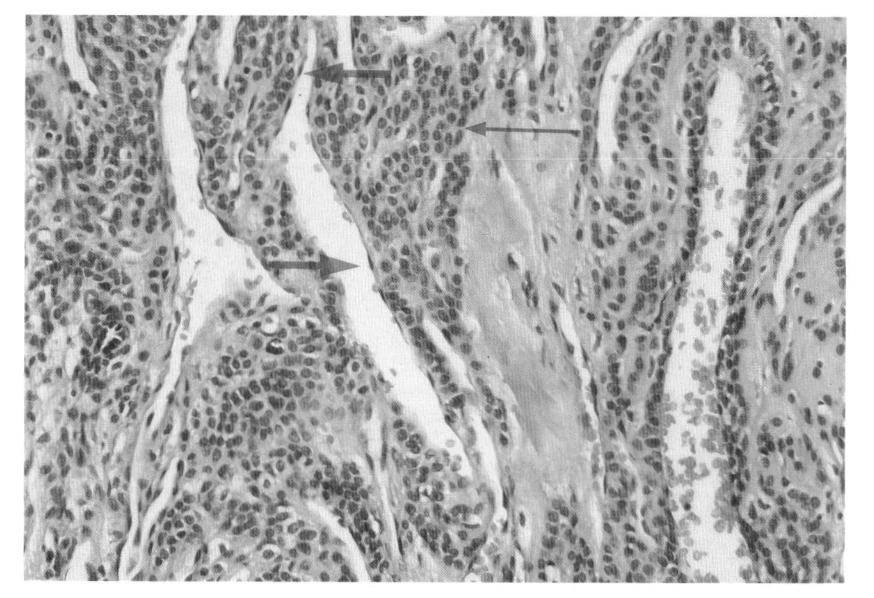

14.80 Metastatic renal carcinoma: skin

Renal carcinomas are usually large, with a variegated appearance, and probably originate in epithelial cells lining proximal renal tubules. They have a pseudocapsule and tend to invade a renal vein and form metastases. Uncommonly they occur in the skin, where they are usually multiple and a sign of widely disseminated malignancy. However, a solitary metastasis may form in the skin, and it may be sufficiently distinctive histologically to suggest the identity and source of the primary, namely renal carcinoma. In this case, the same sequence has occurred. A solitary deposit which appeared in the skin consists of clusters of large cells with a considerable amount of pale (almost unstained) finely granular or vacuolated (clear) cytoplasm (thin arrow). The cytoplasm is 'clear' from the presence of abundant glycogen, although lipid is also present. The groups of tumour cells are separated by strands, some broad, of highly vascular stroma which consists of fibrous connective tissue (thick arrow) and dilated thin-walled (sinusoidal) blood vessels (double arrow). Further clinical investigation confirmed the presence of a primary carcinoma of kidney. HE x235

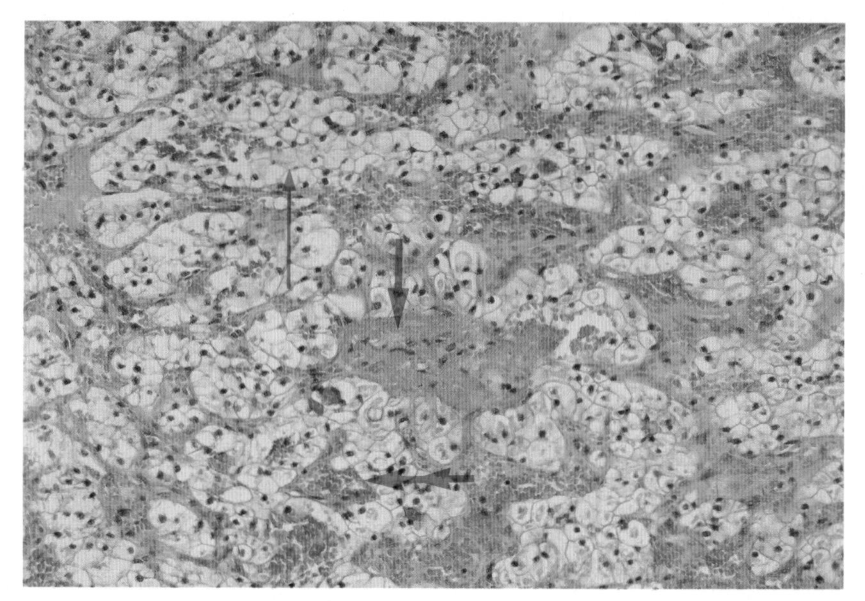

14.81 Extramammary Paget's disease: skin

In Paget's disease, there are adenocarcinomatous cells in the epidermis. In addition to adenocarcinoma of the breast, which gives rise to Paget's disease of the nipple, carcinomas in other sites and particularly neoplasms arising in apocrine or modified apocrine glands in the scrotum, perineum and labia majora may cause extramammary Paget's disease. This lesion was in the anal canal. The surface of the epidermis is out of the field on the left. In the rete ridges there are many large cells (arrows) with abundant pale finely granular or vacuolated cytoplasm. The cytoplasmic boundaries are well-defined, and the nuclei are large, round or ovoid and vesicular. The chromatin is also pale, apart from occasional small basophilic nucleolus-like clumps. The cells, singly or in small clusters, tend to lie close to the basal layers of the epidermis but they are also extending into the stratum spinosum. Mucin has been demonstrated in their cytoplasm. The prognosis of extramammary Paget's disease is poor if it is associated with an underlying invasive adenocarcinoma. In some cases the underlying carcinoma can not be detected.

HE x375

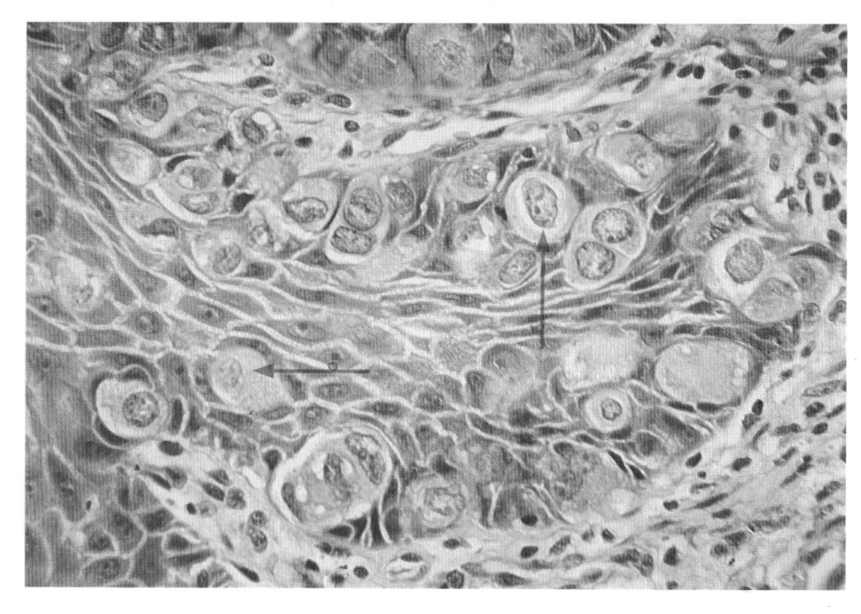

14.82 Chronic lymphocytic leukemia (CLL): vulva

Chronic lymphocytic leukemia (CLL) is characterized by the proliferation of small mature lymphocytes which resemble the resting small lymphocytes of the peripheral blood. The chromosomal abnormality is +12. Most (95%) of the lymphocytes are B cells and the remainder are T cells. Deposits of leukemic cells may form in any tissue, and CLL in lymph nodes are identical to small lymphocytic lymphoma (B or T type). Infiltrates of CLL in the skin and mucous membranes are also fairly common, usually taking the form of macules or papules. In this case a woman with long-standing chronic lymphocytic leukemia (CLL) developed lesions in the vulva. The epidermis (thin arrow) appears normal, apart from the presence of small numbers of lymphocytes in the basal layers, but in the deeper dermis there is a very dense infiltrate of small lymphocytes with round deeply basophilic nuclei. Remarkably however, in the papillary dermis the majority of cells are plasma cells (thick arrow), each with a relatively large amount of cytoplasm and an eccentric nucleus. Also present in the dermis are small blood vessels and scattered macrophages.
HE ×150

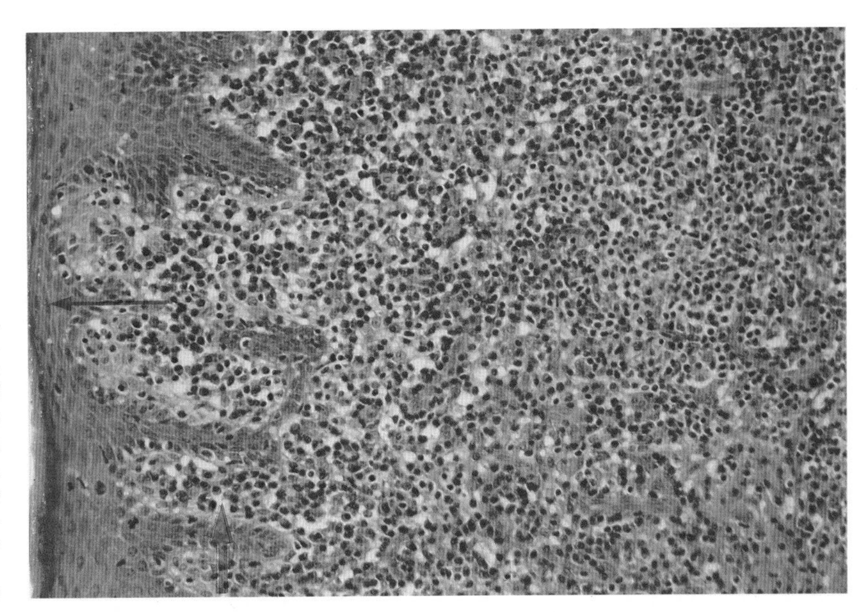

14.83 Mycosis fungoides (cutaneous T cell lymphoma): skin

Mycosis fungoides is a T cell lymphoma, characterized by large malignant T lymphocytes (mycosis cells) with irregularly lobed nuclei (cerebriform or brain-like) nuclei and a helper T cell phenotype. The condition is of a very chronic nature, and its course may last more than 20 years. The lesions are primarily in the skin, but later in the course of the disease they disseminate to lymph nodes and viscera. The condition may declare itself through non-specific eruptions in the skin, but eventually plaques form which slowly grow and become elevated, even to the extent of becoming mushroom-shaped - hence the name. Adjacent plaques may coalesce. In this case, a well-demarcated indurated erythematous plaque has developed on the left upper arm of a 57-year-old man. Histologically, the epidermis looks fairly normal, apart from a slightly thickened layer of eosinophilic keratin on its surface. Within the epidermis however there are several distinct groups of mycosis cells (Pautrier microabscesses) (thin arrow) and a dense infiltrate of closely packed polymorphous lymphocytes in the upper dermis and around the dermal appendages. The infiltrate in the upper dermis is band-like and well-demarcated from the subcutaneous tissues (thick arrow). HE ×150

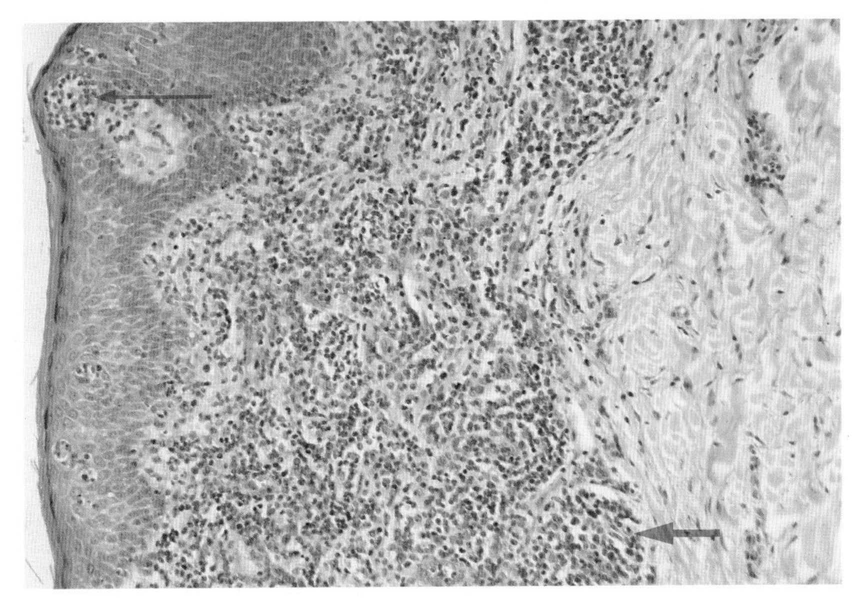

14.84 Mycosis fungoides (cutaneous T cell lymphoma): skin

An infiltrate of individual mycosis cells and groups of them (Pautrier microabsceses) in the epidermis is pathognomonic of mycosis fungoides. Subsequently the plaque stage of mycosis fungoides is superseded by the tumour stage, which is characterized by reddish-brown nodules that ulcerate. This is part of the same lesion as in **14.83**, at higher magnification. The majority of the cells infiltrating the upper dermis are mycosis cells, with compact ovoid or round dark nuclei and very little cytoplasm. They are accompanied by histiocytes, with larger vesicular nuclei. Small numbers of eosinophil leukocytes and plasma cells are also present. There are also fairly large compact groups of mycosis cells within the epidermis (Pautrier microabscesses) (thick arrows). This pleomorphic mixture of cell types in the upper dermis and epidermis is characteristic of mycosis fungoides. Sometimes a leukemic variant of mycosis fungoides develops. It is termed Sezary syndrome, and there are Sezary cells, indistinguishable from mycosis cells, in the peripheral blood. HE ×360

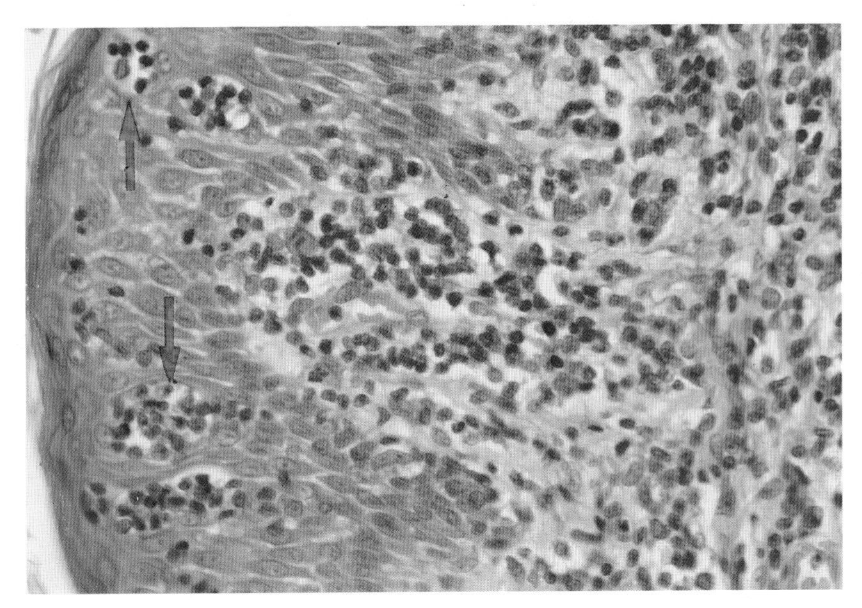